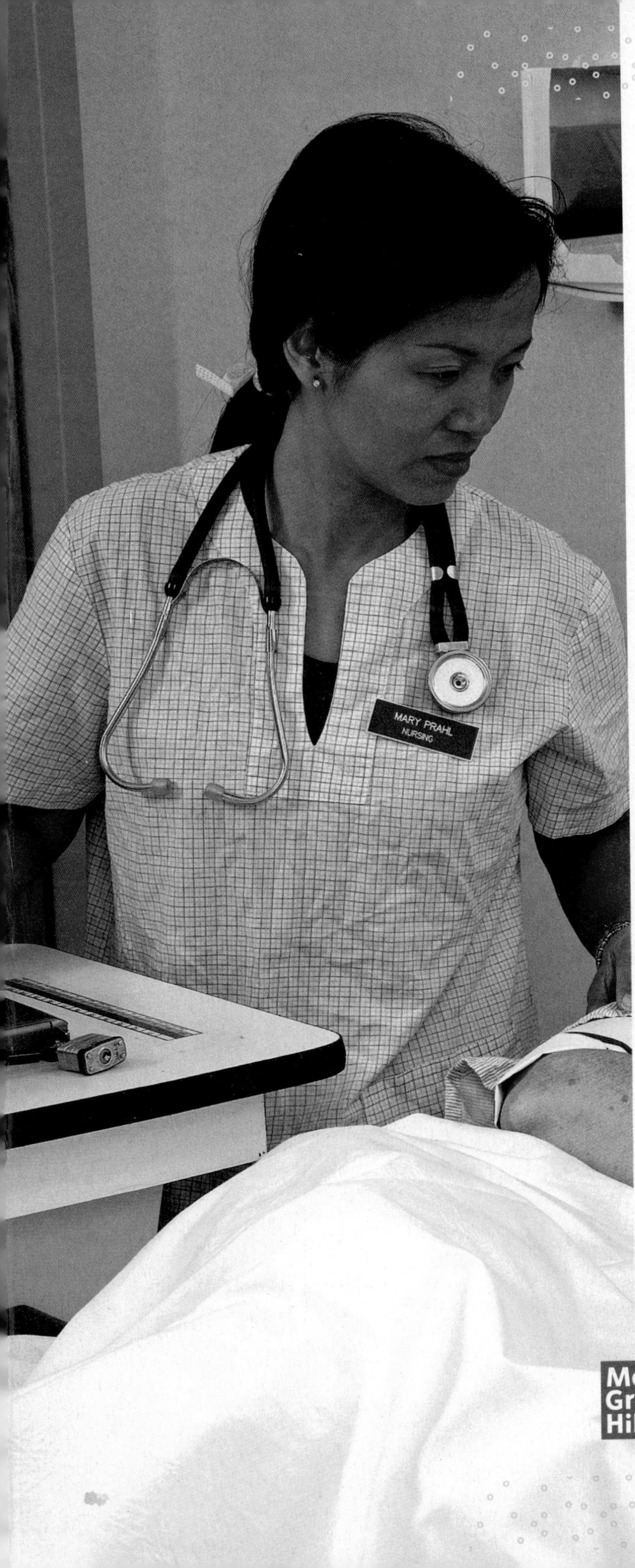

Essentials of Medical Language

Fourth Edition

David M. Allan, MA, MD

Rachel C. Basco, MHS, RRT

Mc Graw Hill

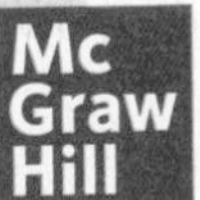

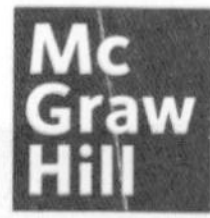

ESSENTIALS OF MEDICAL LANGUAGE, FOURTH EDITION

This book is printed on acid-free paper.

2 3 4 5 6 7 8 9 LMN 24 23 22 21 20

ISBN 978-1-259-90006-8 (bound edition)
MHID 1-259-90006-1 (bound edition)
ISBN 978-1-260-42672-4 (loose-leaf edition)
MHID 1-260-42672-6 (loose-leaf edition)

Portfolio Manager: *William Lawrensen*
Product Developer: *Christine Scheid*
Marketing Manager: *James Connely*
Content Project Managers: *Ann Courtney/Tammy Juran*
Buyer: *Susan K. Culbertson*
Designer: *David W. Hash*
Content Licensing Specialist: *Melissa Homer*
Cover Image: *©Ingram Publishing/SuperStock*
Compositor: *SPi Global*

Library of Congress Cataloging-in-Publication Data

Names: Allan, David, 1942- author. | Basco, Rachel C., author.
Title: Essentials of medical language / David M. Allan, MA, MD, Rachel C. Basco, MHS, RRT.
Description: Fourth edition. | New York, NY : McGraw-Hill Education, 2020. | Includes index.
Identifiers: LCCN 2019022187 | ISBN 9781259900068 (alk. paper)
Subjects: LCSH: Medicine–Terminology–Programmed instruction. | Medicine–Terminology–Problems, exercises, etc. | Communication in medicine–Programmed instruction. | Communication in medicine–Problems, exercises, etc.
Classification: LCC R123 .A44 2020 | DDC 610.1/4–dc23
LC record available at https://lccn.loc.gov/2019022187

mheducation.com/highered

Brief Contents

Appendices

Contents

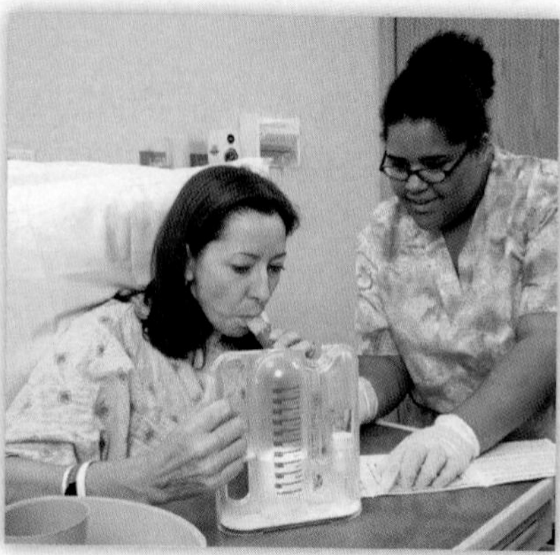
McGraw-Hill Education/Rick Brady

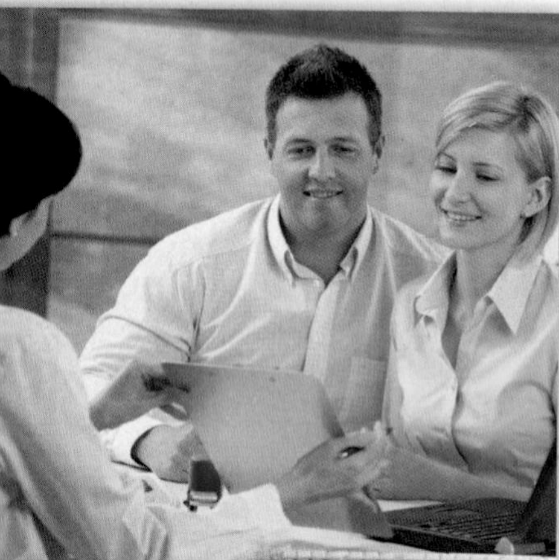
Classic Collection/Shotshop GmbH/Alamy Images

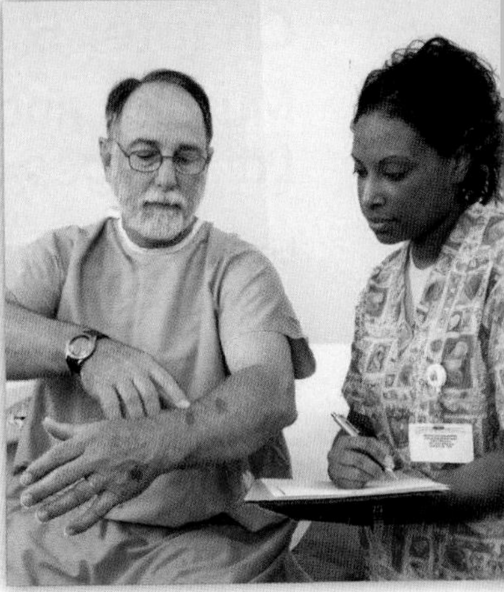
Rick Brady/McGraw-Hill Education

Chapter 3
The Integumentary System: *The Essentials of the Language of Dermatology* 35

Rick Brady/McGraw-Hill Education

Chapter 4
The Skeletal System: *The Essentials of the Language of Orthopedics* 63

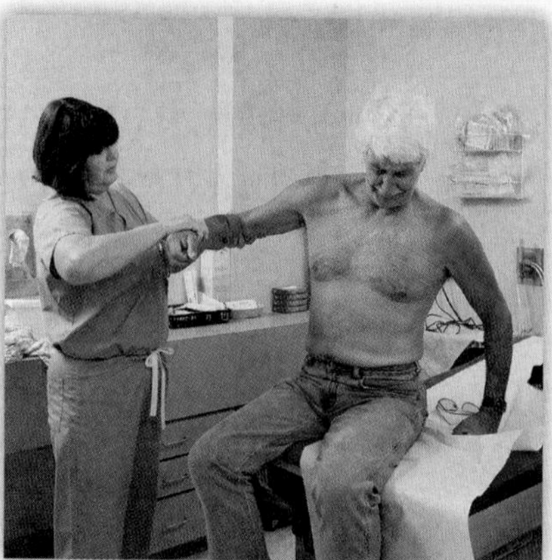
McGraw-Hill Education/Rick Brady

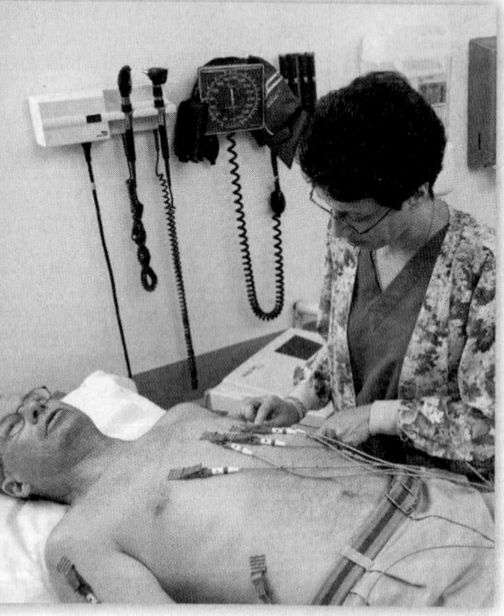
Rick Brady/McGraw-Hill Education

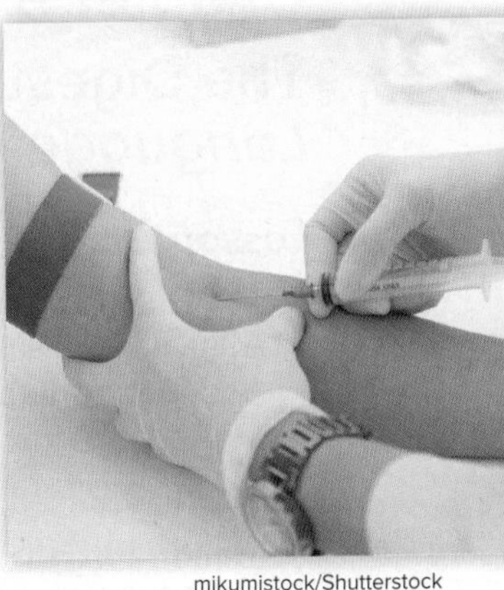
mikumistock/Shutterstock

Chapter 7
The Blood, Lymphatic, and Immune Systems: *The Essentials of the Languages of Hematology and Immunology* 147

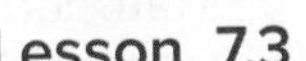

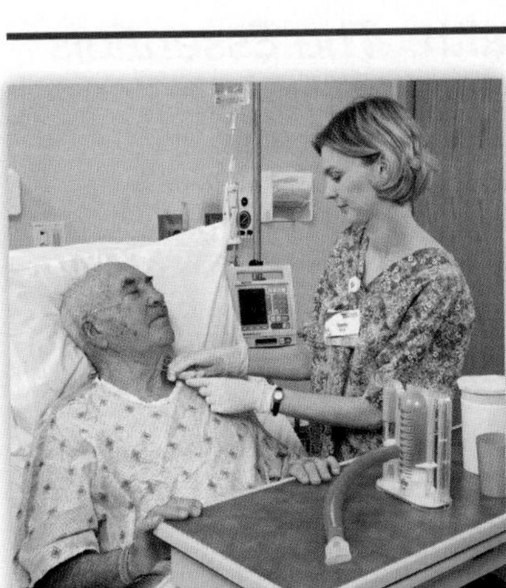
Rick Brady/McGraw-Hill Education

Chapter 8
The Respiratory System: *The Essentials of the Language of Pulmonology* 185

Chapter 9

The Digestive System: *The Essentials of the Language of Gastroenterology* 207

Rick Brady/McGraw-Hill Education

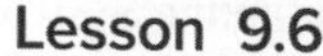

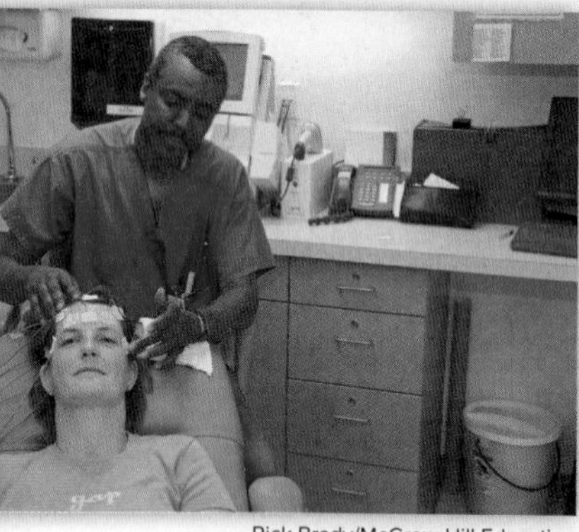

Rick Brady/McGraw-Hill Education

Chapter 10

The Nervous System and Mental Health: *The Essentials of the Languages of Neurology and Psychiatry* 243

Rick Brady/McGraw-Hill Education

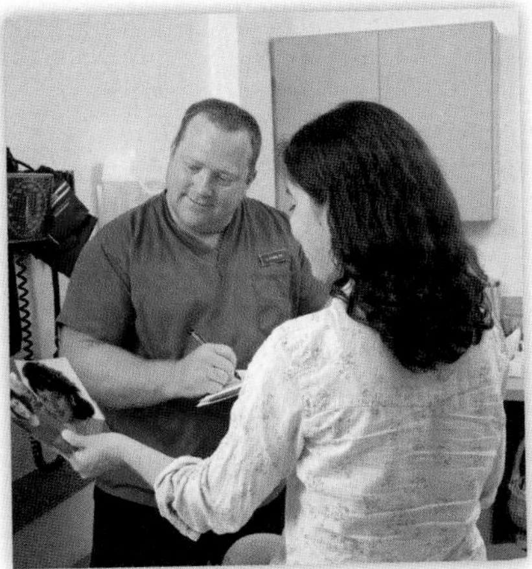

Rick Brady/McGraw-Hill Education

Chapter 13

The Urinary System: *The Essentials of the Language of Urology* 351

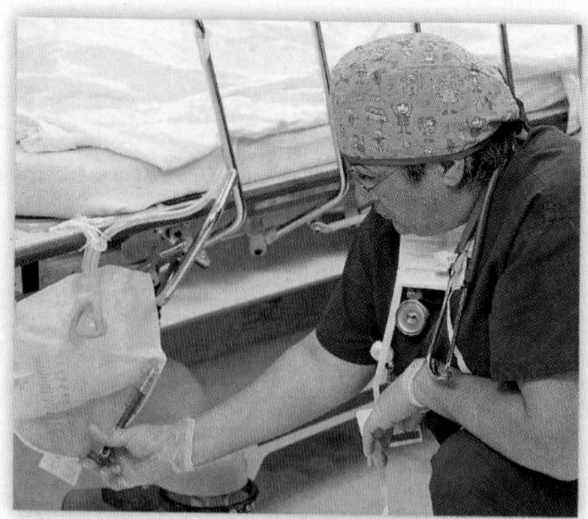

Rick Brady/McGraw-Hill Education

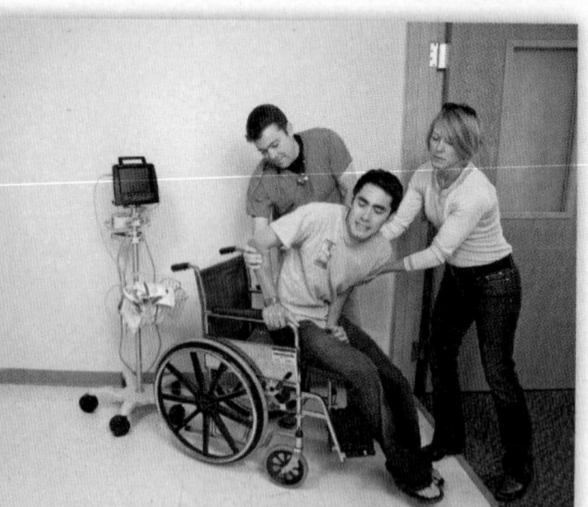

Rick Brady/McGraw-Hill Education

Chapter 14

The Male Reproductive System: *The Essentials of the Language of the Male Reproductive System* 371

Rick Brady/McGraw-Hill Education

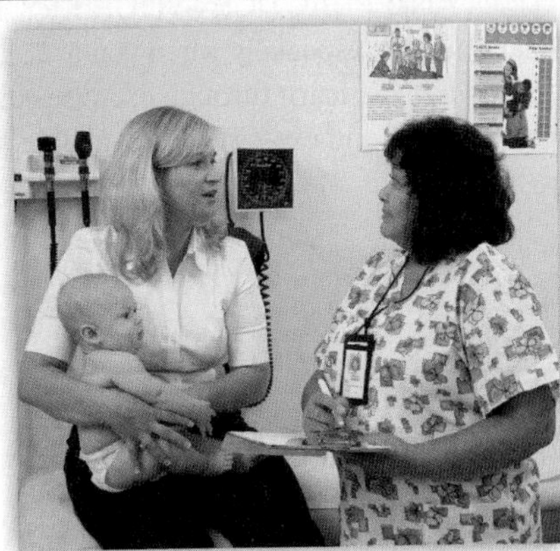

Rick Brady/McGraw-Hill Education

Preface

What Helps Students Learn Medical Terminology

This Textbook Incorporates Features Designed to Address These Four Factors:

Motivation to learn	→	In order for students to be motivated to learn, what they are learning must be meaningful and relevant. To ensure the chapters in *Essentials of Medical Language* fit these criteria, the student is asked to step into the role of an allied health professional in each chapter. Authentic patient cases are used to illustrate how medical language is used on the job.
Retention of the material	→	When students encounter new medical terms within the context of a patient case, they are able to remember it more effectively. In addition, each chapter presents medical terms from one body system or medical specialty, which further serves to "tie it all together" to help students retain the knowledge and skills.
Opportunities for application and practice	→	Practice makes perfect. This is especially true for learning medical terminology. This textbook provides many opportunities for students to apply what they are learning. Exercises are included in the lessons, and are available in Connect for practice. Chapter review questions are also included in Connect to reinforce students' mastery of the terminology in each chapter.
Readily available information	→	In this book, all the information needed for a specific topic is presented in self-contained two-page spreads. On the left-hand page, new medical terms are introduced. On the right-hand page, for each new term, the pronunciation, color-coded word elements, and definition are provided in a ***Word Analysis and Definition (WAD) Table.***

Essentials of Medical Language will help you learn the terminology and language of modern health care in a way that bridges the gap between the classroom and a clinical setting.

RELEVANT MATERIALS—YOUR MOTIVATION TO LEARN!

Essentials of Medical Language 4e provides you with terminology, exercises, images and examples you can apply to other courses and within your career. You will step into the role of a health professional in every chapter and experience medical language illustrated through authentic patient cases.

BODY SYSTEMS AND MEDICAL SPECIALTIES—REMEMBER AND APPLY THE MATERIAL!

Encountering new medical terms within the context of each patient case will help you remember them more effectively. Every chapter presents medical terms from one body system or medical specialty, which helps tie it all together!

APPLICATION AND PRACTICE—YOUR KEY TO MASTERING MEDICAL TERMINOLOGY!

Practice makes perfect, especially when you are learning medical terminology. You will have plenty of opportunity to apply what you learn through exercises during the lessons and at the end of every chapter. Additional practice opportunities and exercises are available through LearnSmart and Connect (see pages xviii and xv, respectively).

To The Instructor

McGraw-Hill Education knows how much effort it takes to prepare for a new course. Through focus groups, symposia, reviews, and conversations with instructors like you, we have gathered information about what materials you need in order to facilitate successful courses. We are committed to providing you with high-quality, accurate instructor support.

Meeting Your Needs

New to This Edition!

1. The Word Analysis and Definition (WAD) tables and review exercises have been updated, and new terms have been added.
2. End of section exercises have been updated providing clear questions requiring specific answers.
3. The Case Reports have been re-designed for further emphasis.
4. Updated material on Genetics, Genetic Therapy, Immunotherapy, Precision Medicine, Personal Medicine.
5. Continued inclusion and enhancement of the Diagnostic and Therapeutic Procedures and Pharmacology section.
6. Chapter 16: Infancy to Old Age: *The Languages of Pediatrics and Geriatrics* is now available with the print text.
7. **NEW!** Application-Based Activities (ABAs): a game-based learning experience, students dive into a micro-sim environment using their medical terminology knowledge to work through a real-life medical situation. More about the ABAs in the Connect section below.

When you use *Essentials of Medical Language,* you will be supported at every point in the program. Each chapter in the book is broken down into lessons, and the Instructor's Manual provides lesson plans and additional materials for each lesson. Following are features of the textbook designed to address student needs.

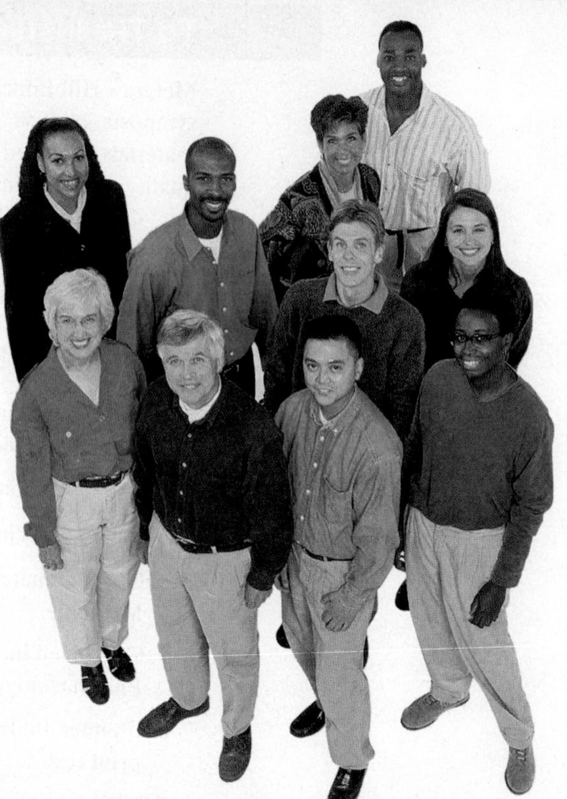

C Squared Studios/Getty Images

Lesson-Based Approach

Each chapter of *Essentials of Medical Language* is divided into lessons covering different aspects of the overall chapter subject. Lessons within a chapter break down into topics. Each topic is designed so your students will not have to flip back and forth when completing exercises or looking at figures, tables, and boxes. All main concepts and ideas presented in topics begin and end within a two-page "spread." These spreads help learning flow smoothly by ensuring that valuable class and reading time is not wasted on flipping pages.

You Are . . . Your Patient Is . . . Case Scenarios

Each chapter and most lessons begin by immediately placing your students in the role of an allied health professional faced with a situation in which medical communication is necessary. Many different professional allied health and LPN-level nursing roles are utilized so your students can "experience" various specialties and positions. The patient cases introduced at the beginning of the chapters and lessons are referenced throughout the lessons to further unify the students' experience.

Chapter Outcomes and Lesson Objectives

The major learning outcomes for each chapter are presented in the beginning so you and your students can focus on what they need to know and be able to do by the end of the chapter. Each lesson has outcome-based learning objectives. Accomplishing each lesson's objectives helps ensure students will be able to achieve the chapter outcomes and, ultimately, the goal of the textbook: to help them learn the essential terminology and language of modern health care.

Word Analysis and Definition (WAD) Tables

Each lesson contains tables listing important medical terms and their pronunciation, elements, and definition. Prefixes, suffixes, and combining forms are color-coded. These tables provide your students with an at-a-glance view of the terms covered. The tables are excellent for reference as well as for studying and reviewing.

Exercises

In addition to the exercises at the end of topic areas in the book, the chapter review exercises are included in the Test Bank in *Connect* **(http://connect.mheducation.com)**. All these exercises are graded in their difficulty according to Bloom's Taxonomy and are tied to Chapter Learning Outcomes.

Attention is given to developing skills in spelling, forming plurals, using accepted abbreviations, writing medical language, and pronunciation. The exercises take the learner beyond memorization and teach how to think critically about the realistic application of the medical language being learned.

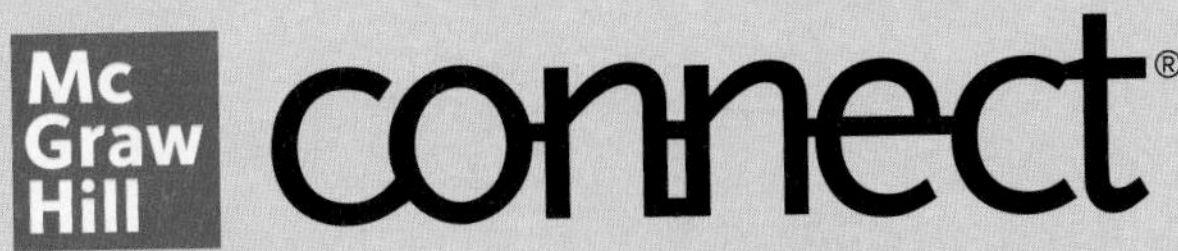

FOR INSTRUCTORS

You're in the driver's seat.

Want to build your own course? No problem. Prefer to use our turnkey, prebuilt course? Easy. Want to make changes throughout the semester? Sure. And you'll save time with Connect's auto-grading too.

65%
Less Time Grading

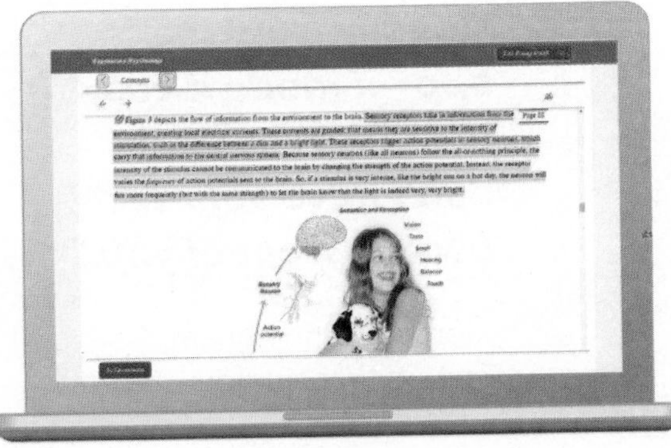

Laptop: McGraw-Hill; Woman/dog: George Doyle/Getty Images

They'll thank you for it.

Adaptive study resources like SmartBook® 2.0 help your students be better prepared in less time. You can transform your class time from dull definitions to dynamic debates. Find out more about the powerful personalized learning experience available in SmartBook 2.0 at **www.mheducation.com/highered/connect/smartbook**

Make it simple, make it affordable.

Connect makes it easy with seamless integration using any of the major Learning Management Systems—Blackboard®, Canvas, and D2L, among others—to let you organize your course in one convenient location. Give your students access to digital materials at a discount with our inclusive access program. Ask your McGraw-Hill representative for more information.

Padlock: Jobalou/Getty Images

Solutions for your challenges.

A product isn't a solution. Real solutions are affordable, reliable, and come with training and ongoing support when you need it and how you want it. Our Customer Experience Group can also help you troubleshoot tech problems—although Connect's 99% uptime means you might not need to call them. See for yourself at **status.mheducation.com**

Checkmark: Jobalou/Getty Images

FOR STUDENTS

Effective, efficient studying.

Connect helps you be more productive with your study time and get better grades using tools like SmartBook 2.0, which highlights key concepts and creates a personalized study plan. Connect sets you up for success, so you walk into class with confidence and walk out with better grades.

Study anytime, anywhere.

Download the free ReadAnywhere app and access your online eBook or SmartBook 2.0 assignments when it's convenient, even if you're offline. And since the app automatically syncs with your eBook and SmartBook 2.0 assignments in Connect, all of your work is available every time you open it. Find out more at **www.mheducation.com/readanywhere**

> ***"I really liked this app—it made it easy to study when you don't have your text-book in front of you."***
>
> \- Jordan Cunningham,
> Eastern Washington University

Calendar: owattaphotos/Getty Images

No surprises.

The Connect Calendar and Reports tools keep you on track with the work you need to get done and your assignment scores. Life gets busy; Connect tools help you keep learning through it all.

Learning for everyone.

McGraw-Hill works directly with Accessibility Services Departments and faculty to meet the learning needs of all students. Please contact your Accessibility Services office and ask them to email accessibility@mheducation.com, or visit **www.mheducation.com/about/accessibility** for more information.

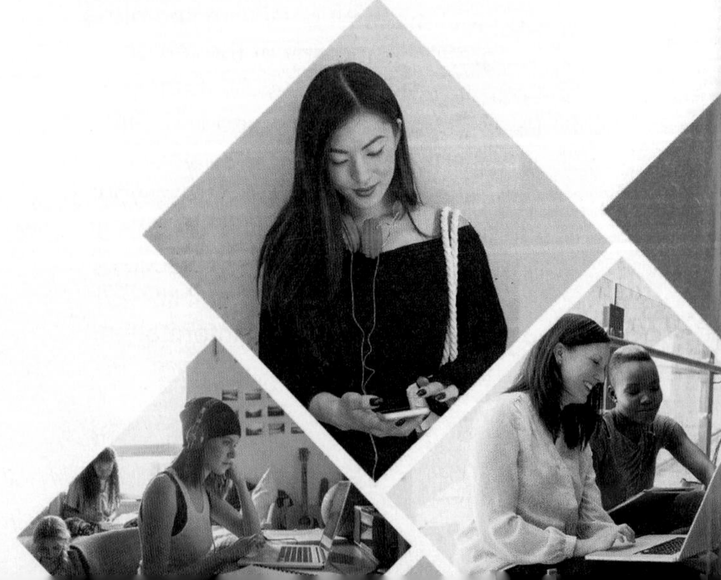

Top: Jenner Images/Getty Images, Left: Hero Images/Getty Images, Right: Hero Images/Getty Images

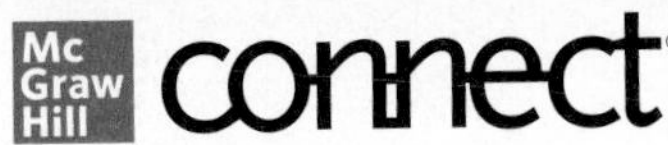

A One-Stop Spot to Present, Deliver, and Assess Digital Assets Available from McGraw-Hill: McGraw-Hill Essentials of Medical Terminology

McGraw-Hill Connect® Essentials of Medical Terminology provides online presentation, assignment, and assessment solutions. It connects your students with the tools and resources they'll need to achieve success. With Connect, you can deliver assignments, quizzes, and tests online. A robust set of questions and activities, including all of the lesson and end-of-chapter exercises, case studies, animation questions, and interactives, are presented and aligned with the textbook's learning outcomes. As an instructor, you can edit existing questions and author entirely new problems. Connect enables you to track individual student performance–by question, by assignment, or in relation to the class overall–with detailed grade reports. You can integrate grade reports easily with learning management systems (LMSs), such as Blackboard, Desire2Learn, and eCollege, plus much more.

NEW! **Application-Based Activities (ABAs) McGraw-Hill's** *new* ABAs are game-based learning activities that call upon decision making and application of medical terminology knowledge. They're not only an opportunity for students to practice skills and apply them in real-world scenarios, but also where they can see the *repercussions* of their choices or actions in a safe environment. With topics like Diagnostic Testing or Interpreting Reports, or even as the private practice psychologist in "A Shared Experience," students apply knowledge to define medical terms, disorders, treatments; choose appropriate diagnostic procedures; interpret medical documents; translate medical terms into everyday language; or even learn the meanings of medical abbreviations. Best of all, ABAs are found and assignable within Connect, and auto-gradable for the instructor.

Connect Essentials of Medical Terminology also provides students with 24/7 online access to an ebook. This media-rich version of the textbook is available through the McGraw-Hill Connect platform and allows seamless integration of text, media, and assessments. To learn more, visit **http://connect.mheducation.com.**
Connect Insight™ is the first and only analytics tool of its kind, which highlights a series of visual data displays–each framed by an intuitive question–to provide at-a-glance information regarding how your class is doing. As an instructor or administrator, you receive an instant, at-a-glance view of student performance matched with student activity. It puts real-time analytics in your hands so you can take action early and keep struggling students from falling behind. It also allows you to be empowered with a more valuable, transparent, and productive connection between you and your students. Available on demand wherever and whenever it's needed, Connect Insight travels from office to classroom!

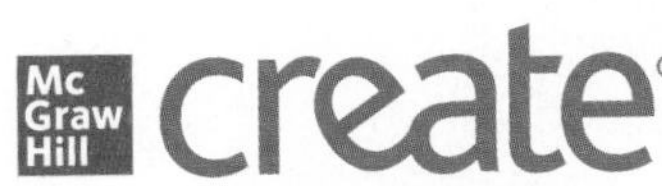

Create a Textbook Organized the Way You Teach: McGraw-Hill Create

With **McGraw-Hill Create®,** you can easily rearrange chapters, combine material from other content sources, and quickly upload content you have written, such as your course syllabus or teaching notes. Find the content you need in Create by searching through thousands of leading McGraw-Hill Education textbooks. Arrange your book to fit your teaching style. Create even allows you to personalize your book's appearance by selecting the cover and adding your name, school, and course information. Order a Create book and you'll receive a complimentary print review copy in three to five business days or a complimentary electronic review copy (eComp) via e-mail in minutes. Go to **www.mcgrawhillcreate.com** today and register to experience how McGraw-Hill Create empowers you to teach *your* students *your* way.

Tegrity: Lectures 24/7

Tegrity in Connect is a tool that makes class time available 24/7 by automatically capturing every lecture. With a simple one-click start-and-stop process, you capture all computer screens and corresponding audio in a format that is easy to search, frame by frame. Students can replay any part of any class with easy-to-use, browser-based viewing on a PC, Mac, iPod, or other mobile device.

Educators know that the more students can see, hear, and experience class resources, the better they learn. In fact, studies prove it. Tegrity's unique search feature helps students efficiently find what they need, when they need it, across an entire semester of class recordings. Help turn your students' study time into learning moments immediately supported by your lecture. With Tegrity, you also increase intent listening and class participation by easing students' concerns about note-taking. Using Tegrity in Connect will make it more likely you will see students' faces, not the tops of their heads.

LearnSmart® is one of the most effective and successful adaptive learning resources available on the market today and is again available for *Essentials of Medical Terminology.* More than 2 million students have answered more than 1.3 billion questions in LearnSmart since 2009, making it the most widely used and intelligent adaptive study tool. It has proven to strengthen memory recall, keep students in class, and boost grades. Students using LearnSmart are 13% more likely to pass their classes and 35% less likely to drop out. This revolutionary learning resource is available only from McGraw-Hill Education, so join the learning revolution, and start using LearnSmart today!

SmartBook® is the first and only adaptive reading experience currently available. SmartBook personalizes content for each student in a continuously adapting reading experience. Reading is no longer a passive and linear experience, but an engaging and dynamic one where students are more likely to master and retain important concepts, thus coming to class better prepared. Valuable reports provide instructors with insight into how students are progressing through textbook content, and are useful for shaping in-class time and assessments. As a result of the adaptive reading experience found in SmartBook, students are more likely to retain knowledge, stay in class, and get better grades. This revolutionary technology is available only from McGraw-Hill Education for hundreds of course areas as part of the LearnSmart Advantage series.

Instructors' Resources

The Instructor Online Learning Center is available through your Connect course. Your McGraw-Hill sales representative can provide you with the access you need to easily prepare for using *Essentials of Medical Language,* 4e. Our Online Learning Centers include:

- The Instructors' Manual, which contains valuable information that makes course prep a snap!
    - This manual includes information about student learning styles and instructor strategies; innovative learning activities; assessment techniques and strategies; classroom management tips; and answer keys.
    - **Lesson Planning Guide.** Our Lesson Planning Guide comes complete with a customizable lesson plan for each of the lessons in this text. Each plan contains a step-by-step 50-minute teaching plan and master copies of handouts. Use these lessons alone or combined to accommodate different class schedules–you can even revise them to reflect your preferred topic or sequence. Each lesson plan is designed to be used with a corresponding PowerPoint® presentation that is also available on the OLC.
- **PowerPoint® Lecture Outlines.** The PowerPoint lectures with speaking notes correlate to the Lesson Plans mentioned above and include the art and photos from the text. Covering the most important parts of every lesson, the slides are customizable to fit your course needs.
- **Test Builder in Connect,** making creating tests easy!

  Available within Connect, Test Builder is a cloud-based tool that enables instructors to format tests that can be printed or administered within a LMS. Test Builder offers a modern, streamlined interface for easy content configuration that matches course needs, without requiring a download.

  Test Builder allows you to:

    - access all test bank content from a particular title.
    - easily pinpoint the most relevant content through robust filtering options.
    - manipulate the order of questions or scramble questions and/or answers.
    - pin questions to a specific location within a test.
    - determine your preferred treatment of algorithmic questions.
    - choose the layout and spacing.
    - add instructions and configure default settings.

  Test Builder provides a secure interface for better protection of content and allows for just-in-time updates to flow directly into assessments.

Contextual Approach Promotes Active Learning

Chapters in the textbook are organized by body system in accordance with an overall anatomy and physiology (A & P) approach. Lessons introduce and define terminology through the context of A & P, pathology, and clinical and diagnostic procedures/tests. The organization of the body systems into chapters is based on an "outside to inside" sequence that reflects a physician's differential diagnosis method used during an examination.

To provide students with an authentic context, the medical specialty associated with each body area or system is introduced along with relevant anatomy and physiology. Students actually step into the role of an allied health professional associated with each specialty. Patient cases and documentation are used to illustrate the real-life application of medical terminology in modern health care: to care for and communicate with patients and to interact with other members of the health care team.

The A & P organizational approach, used in conjunction with an authentic medical setting and patient cases, encourages student motivation and facilitates active, engaged learning.

Innovative Pedagogical Aids Provide a Coherent Learning Program

Each chapter is structured around a consistent and unique framework of pedagogic devices. No matter what the subject matter of a chapter, the structure enables students to develop a consistent learning strategy, making *Essentials of Medical Language* a superior learning tool.

YOU ARE COMMUNICATING WITH . . .

Each chapter opens by placing the student in the role of an allied health professional related to the specialty and associated body systems/areas covered by the chapter. The student is also introduced to a patient and given information about the patient's case.

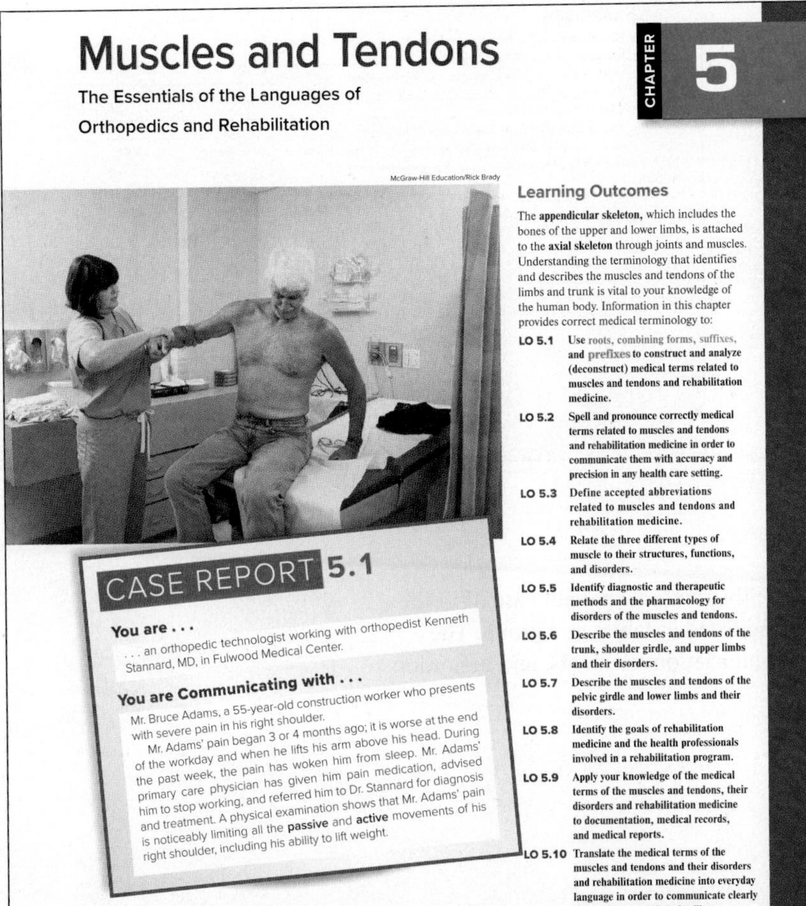

Muscles and Tendons

The Essentials of the Languages of Orthopedics and Rehabilitation

CHAPTER 5

McGraw-Hill Education/Rick Brady

CASE REPORT 5.1

You are . . .

. . . an orthopedic technologist working with orthopedist Kenneth Stannard, MD, in Fulwood Medical Center.

You are Communicating with . . .

Mr. Bruce Adams, a 55-year-old construction worker who presents with severe pain in his right shoulder.

Mr. Adams' pain began 3 or 4 months ago; it is worse at the end of the workday and when he lifts his arm above his head. During the past week, the pain has woken him from sleep. Mr. Adams' primary care physician has given him pain medication, advised him to stop working, and referred him to Dr. Stannard for diagnosis and treatment. A physical examination shows that Mr. Adams' pain is noticeably limiting all the **passive** and **active** movements of his right shoulder, including his ability to lift weight.

Learning Outcomes

The **appendicular skeleton,** which includes the bones of the upper and lower limbs, is attached to the **axial skeleton** through joints and muscles. Understanding the terminology that identifies and describes the muscles and tendons of the limbs and trunk is vital to your knowledge of the human body. Information in this chapter provides correct medical terminology to:

- **LO 5.1** Use roots, combining forms, suffixes, and prefixes to construct and analyze (deconstruct) medical terms related to muscles and tendons and rehabilitation medicine.
- **LO 5.2** Spell and pronounce correctly medical terms related to muscles and tendons and rehabilitation medicine in order to communicate them with accuracy and precision in any health care setting.
- **LO 5.3** Define accepted abbreviations related to muscles and tendons and rehabilitation medicine.
- **LO 5.4** Relate the three different types of muscle to their structures, functions, and disorders.
- **LO 5.5** Identify diagnostic and therapeutic methods and the pharmacology for disorders of the muscles and tendons.
- **LO 5.6** Describe the muscles and tendons of the trunk, shoulder girdle, and upper limbs and their disorders.
- **LO 5.7** Describe the muscles and tendons of the pelvic girdle and lower limbs and their disorders.
- **LO 5.8** Identify the goals of rehabilitation medicine and the health professionals involved in a rehabilitation program.
- **LO 5.9** Apply your knowledge of the medical terms of the muscles and tendons, their disorders and rehabilitation medicine to documentation, medical records, and medical reports.
- **LO 5.10** Translate the medical terms of the muscles and tendons and their disorders and rehabilitation medicine into everyday language in order to communicate clearly with patients and their families.

LEARNING OUTCOMES

At the same time, **Learning Outcomes** are presented to let students know what they will learn in the chapter. This technique immediately engages students, motivating them to read on to learn how this patient's case (and their role in the patient's care) relates to the medical terminology being introduced in the chapter.

Lesson-Based Organization

The chapter content is broken down into chunks, or lessons, to help students digest new information and relate it to previously learned information. Rather than containing many various topics within a chapter, these lessons group the chapter material into logical, streamlined learning units designed to help students achieve the chapter outcomes. Lessons within a chapter build on one another to form a cohesive, coherent experience for the learner.

Each lesson is based on specific **Lesson Objectives** designed to support the students' achievement of the overall chapter outcomes.

Each lesson in a chapter contains an Introduction, Lesson Objectives, Lesson Topics, Word Analysis and Definition Tables, and Lesson Exercises. Within each lesson, all topics and information are presented in **self-contained two-page spreads.** This means students will no longer have to flip back and forth to see figures on one page that are described on another.

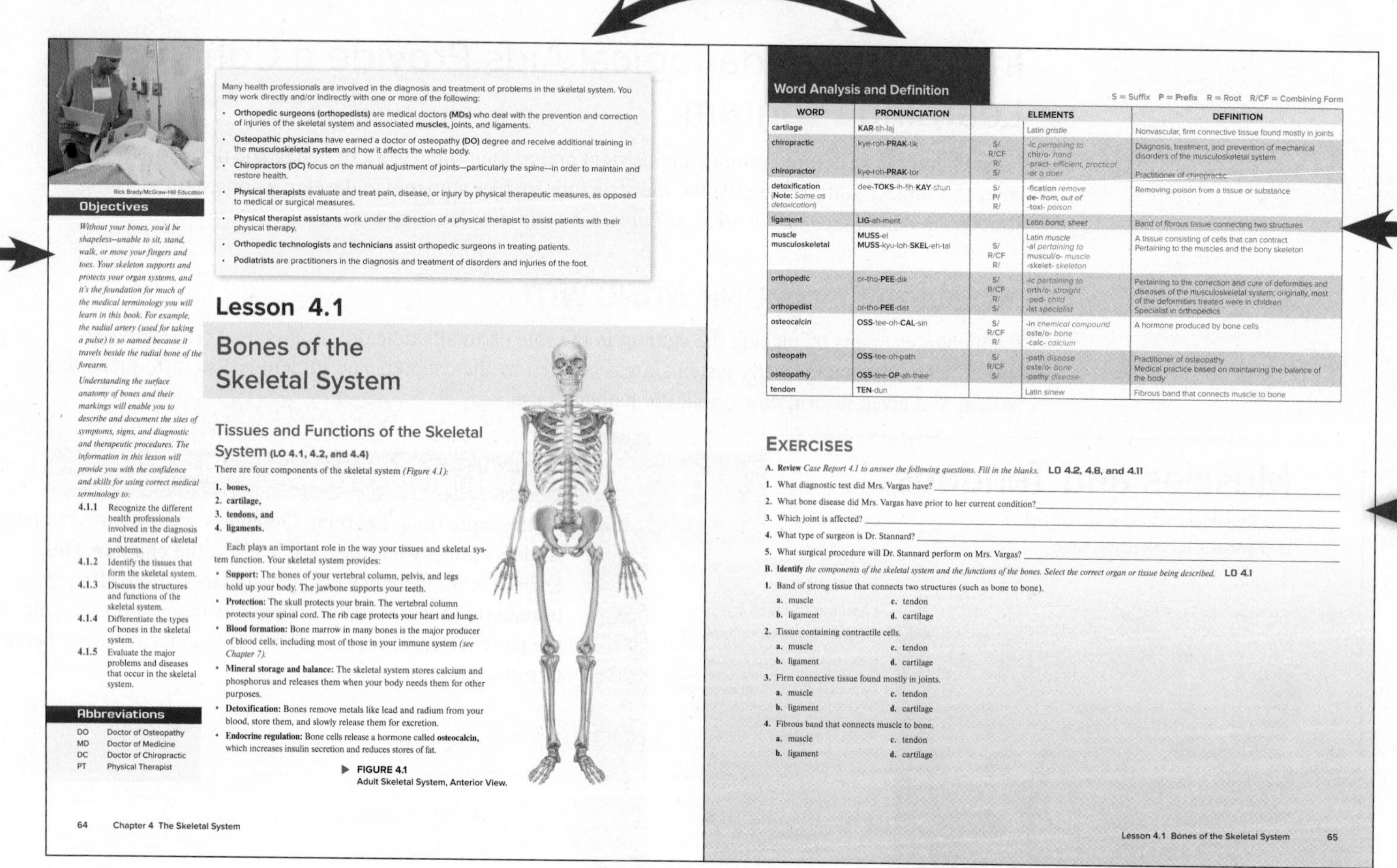

Rick Brady/McGraw-Hill Education

Objectives

Without your bones, you'd be shapeless–unable to sit, stand, walk, or move your fingers and toes. Your skeleton supports and protects your organ systems, and it's the foundation for much of the medical terminology you will learn in this book. For example, the radial artery (used for taking a pulse) is so named because it travels beside the radial bone of the forearm.

Understanding the surface anatomy of bones and their markings will enable you to describe and document the sites of symptoms, signs, and diagnostic and therapeutic procedures. The information in this lesson will provide you with the confidence and skills for using correct medical terminology to:

4.1.1 Recognize the different health professionals involved in the diagnosis and treatment of skeletal problems.
4.1.2 Identify the tissues that form the skeletal system.
4.1.3 Discuss the structures and functions of the skeletal system.
4.1.4 Differentiate the types of bones in the skeletal system.
4.1.5 Evaluate the major problems and diseases that occur in the skeletal system.

Abbreviations

DO Doctor of Osteopathy
MD Doctor of Medicine
DC Doctor of Chiropractic
PT Physical Therapist

Many health professionals are involved in the diagnosis and treatment of problems in the skeletal system. You may work directly and/or indirectly with one or more of the following:

- **Orthopedic surgeons (orthopedists)** are medical doctors **(MDs)** who deal with the prevention and correction of injuries of the skeletal system and associated **muscles,** joints, and ligaments.
- **Osteopathic physicians** have earned a doctor of osteopathy **(DO)** degree and receive additional training in the **musculoskeletal system** and how it affects the whole body.
- **Chiropractors (DC)** focus on the manual adjustment of joints—particularly the spine—in order to maintain and restore health.
- **Physical therapists** evaluate and treat pain, disease, or injury by physical therapeutic measures, as opposed to medical or surgical measures.
- **Physical therapist assistants** work under the direction of a physical therapist to assist patients with their physical therapy.
- **Orthopedic technologists** and **technicians** assist orthopedic surgeons in treating patients.
- **Podiatrists** are practitioners in the diagnosis and treatment of disorders and injuries of the foot.

Lesson 4.1

Bones of the Skeletal System

Tissues and Functions of the Skeletal System (LO 4.1, 4.2, and 4.4)

There are four components of the skeletal system *(Figure 4.1)*:

1. **bones,**
2. **cartilage,**
3. **tendons, and**
4. **ligaments.**

Each plays an important role in the way your tissues and skeletal system function. Your skeletal system provides:

- **Support:** The bones of your vertebral column, pelvis, and legs hold up your body. The jawbone supports your teeth.
- **Protection:** The skull protects your brain. The vertebral column protects your spinal cord. The rib cage protects your heart and lungs.
- **Blood formation:** Bone marrow in many bones is the major producer of blood cells, including most of those in your immune system *(see Chapter 7).*
- **Mineral storage and balance:** The skeletal system stores calcium and phosphorus and releases them when your body needs them for other purposes.
- **Detoxification:** Bones remove metals like lead and radium from your blood, store them, and slowly release them for excretion.
- **Endocrine regulation:** Bone cells release a hormone called **osteocalcin,** which increases insulin secretion and reduces stores of fat.

▶ **FIGURE 4.1**
Adult Skeletal System, Anterior View.

64 Chapter 4 The Skeletal System

Word Analysis and Definition

S = Suffix P = Prefix R = Root R/CF = Combining Form

WORD	PRONUNCIATION	ELEMENTS		DEFINITION
cartilage	**KAR**-tih-laj		Latin *gristle*	Nonvascular, firm connective tissue found mostly in joints
chiropractic chiropractor	kye-roh-**PRAK**-tik kye-roh-**PRAK**-tor	S/ R/CF R/ S/	-ic *pertaining to* chir/o- *hand* -pract- *efficient, practical* -or *a doer*	Diagnosis, treatment, and prevention of mechanical disorders of the musculoskeletal system Practitioner of chiropractic
detoxification (**Note:** *Same as detoxication*)	dee-**TOKS**-ih-fih-**KAY**-shun	S/ P/ R/	-fication *remove* de- *from, out of* -toxi- *poison*	Removing poison from a tissue or substance
ligament	**LIG**-ah-ment		Latin *band, sheet*	Band of fibrous tissue connecting two structures
muscle musculoskeletal	**MUSS**-el **MUSS**-kyu-loh-**SKEL**-eh-tal	S/ R/CF R/	Latin *muscle* -al *pertaining to* muscul/o- *muscle* -skelet- *skeleton*	A tissue consisting of cells that can contract Pertaining to the muscles and the bony skeleton
orthopedic orthopedist	or-tho-**PEE**-dik or-tho-**PEE**-dist	S/ R/CF R/ S/	-ic *pertaining to* orth/o- *straight* -ped- *child* -ist *specialist*	Pertaining to the correction and cure of deformities and diseases of the musculoskeletal system; originally, most of the deformities treated were in children Specialist in orthopedics
osteocalcin	**OSS**-tee-oh-**CAL**-sin	S/ R/CF R/	-in *chemical compound* oste/o- *bone* -calc- *calcium*	A hormone produced by bone cells
osteopath osteopathy	**OSS**-tee-oh-path **OSS**-tee-**OP**-ah-thee	S/ R/CF S/	-path *disease* oste/o- *bone* -pathy *disease*	Practitioner of osteopathy Medical practice based on maintaining the balance of the body
tendon	**TEN**-dun		Latin *sinew*	Fibrous band that connects muscle to bone

Exercises

A. Review *Case Report 4.1 to answer the following questions. Fill in the blanks.* **LO 4.2, 4.8, and 4.11**

1. What diagnostic test did Mrs. Vargas have? ____________
2. What bone disease did Mrs. Vargas have prior to her current condition? ____________
3. Which joint is affected? ____________
4. What type of surgeon is Dr. Stannard? ____________
5. What surgical procedure will Dr. Stannard perform on Mrs. Vargas? ____________

B. Identify *the components of the skeletal system and the functions of the bones. Select the correct organ or tissue being described.* **LO 4.1**

1. Band of strong tissue that connects two structures (such as bone to bone).
   a. muscle c. tendon
   b. ligament d. cartilage
2. Tissue containing contractile cells.
   a. muscle c. tendon
   b. ligament d. cartilage
3. Firm connective tissue found mostly in joints.
   a. muscle c. tendon
   b. ligament d. cartilage
4. Fibrous band that connects muscle to bone.
   a. muscle c. tendon
   b. ligament d. cartilage

Lesson 4.1 Bones of the Skeletal System 65

Word Analysis and Definition Tables

The medical terms covered in each lesson are introduced in context, either within a patient case or in the lesson topics. To facilitate easy reference and review, the terms are also listed in tables as a group. The **Word Analysis and Definition (WAD) Tables** list each term and its pronunciation, elements, and definition in a concise, color-coded, at-a-glance format.

Lesson and Chapter Exercises

Topics within a chapter end with exercises designed to allow students to check their basic understanding of the terms they just learned. These "checkpoints" can be used by instructors as assignments or for self-evaluation by students.

In *Connect* you will find additional review exercises that ask students to apply what they learned in all lessons of a chapter. These exercises reinforce learning and help students go beyond mere memorization to think critically about the medical language they use. In addition to reviewing and recalling the definitions of terms learned in the chapter, students are asked to use medical terms in new and different ways to ensure a thorough understanding.

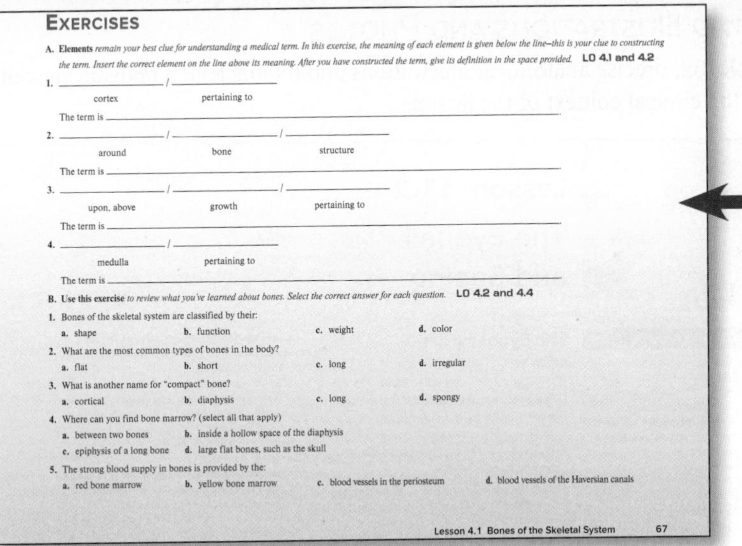

Exercises

A. **Elements** *remain your best clue for understanding a medical term. In this exercise, the meaning of each element is given below the line–this is your clue to constructing the term. Insert the correct element on the line above its meaning. After you have constructed the term, give its definition in the space provided.* LO 4.1 and 4.2

1. ________ / ________
   cortex / pertaining to
   The term is ________
2. ________ / ________ / ________
   around / bone / structure
   The term is ________
3. ________ / ________ / ________
   upon, above / growth / pertaining to
   The term is ________
4. ________ / ________
   medulla / pertaining to
   The term is ________

B. **Use this exercise** *to review what you've learned about bones. Select the correct answer for each question.* LO 4.2 and 4.4

1. Bones of the skeletal system are classified by their:
   a. shape b. function c. weight d. color
2. What are the most common types of bones in the body?
   a. flat b. short c. long d. irregular
3. What is another name for "compact" bone?
   a. cortical b. diaphysis c. long d. spongy
4. Where can you find bone marrow? (select all that apply)
   a. between two bones b. inside a hollow space of the diaphysis
   c. epiphysis of a long bone d. large flat bones, such as the skull
5. The strong blood supply in bones is provided by the:
   a. red bone marrow b. yellow bone marrow c. blood vessels in the periosteum d. blood vessels of the Haversian canals

Lesson 4.1 Bones of the Skeletal System 67

Chapter Review in Connect

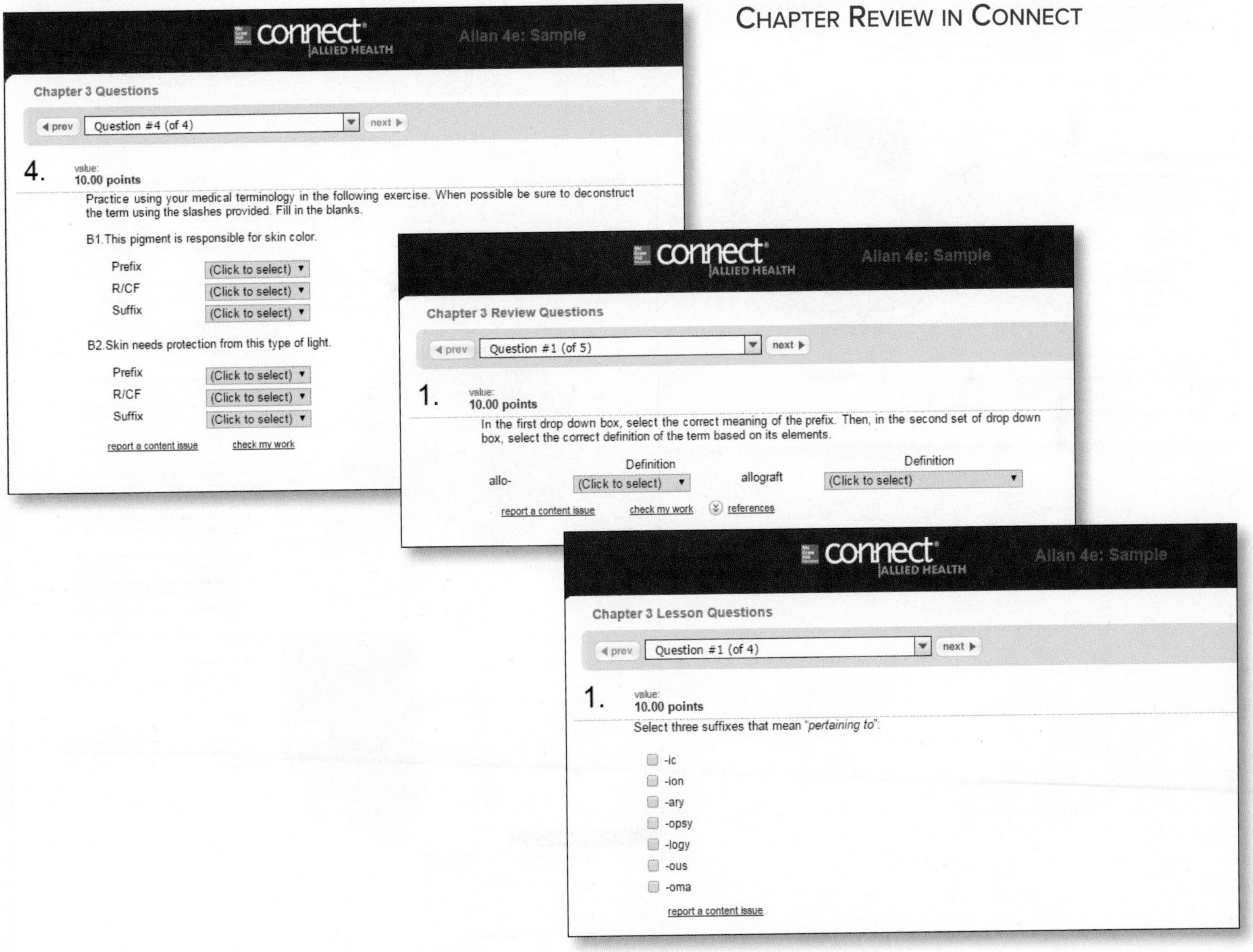

connect ALLIED HEALTH Allan 4e: Sample

Chapter 3 Questions

prev Question #4 (of 4) next

4. value: 10.00 points

Practice using your medical terminology in the following exercise. When possible be sure to deconstruct the term using the slashes provided. Fill in the blanks.

B1. This pigment is responsible for skin color.

Prefix (Click to select)
R/CF (Click to select)
Suffix (Click to select)

B2. Skin needs protection from this type of light.

Prefix (Click to select)
R/CF (Click to select)
Suffix (Click to select)

report a content issue check my work

connect ALLIED HEALTH Allan 4e: Sample

Chapter 3 Review Questions

prev Question #1 (of 5) next

1. value: 10.00 points

In the first drop down box, select the correct meaning of the prefix. Then, in the second set of drop down box, select the correct definition of the term based on its elements.

allo- Definition (Click to select) allograft Definition (Click to select)

report a content issue check my work references

connect ALLIED HEALTH Allan 4e: Sample

Chapter 3 Lesson Questions

prev Question #1 (of 4) next

1. value: 10.00 points

Select three suffixes that mean "*pertaining to*":

- -ic
- -ion
- -ary
- -opsy
- -logy
- -ous
- -oma

report a content issue

VIVID ILLUSTRATIONS AND PHOTOS

Colorful, precise anatomical illustrations and photos lend a realistic view of body structures and correlate to the clinical context of the lessons.

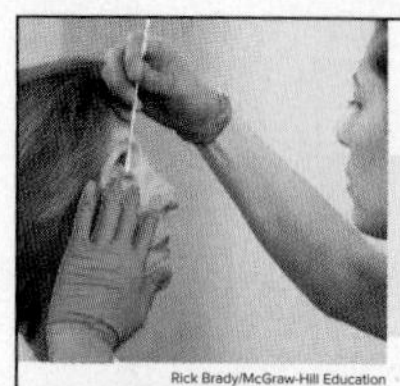

Rick Brady/McGraw-Hill Education

Lesson 11.2

The Eyeball and Seeing

Objectives

Although your eyeball may appear to be solid, it's actually a hollow sphere that measures around 1 inch in diameter. Knowledge of its terminology, structure, and function allows you to understand how we see and what major problems and disorders can arise with the eye. In this lesson, the information will enable you to use correct medical terminology to:

11.2.1 Identify the principal structures of the eyeball and their functions.
11.2.2 Explain the role of the cornea and the problems that can occur in that structure.
11.2.3 Describe the structures and functions of the lens and its associated structures.
11.2.4 Link the different components of the retina to their functions.
11.2.5 Discuss disorders of the eyeball.

Keynotes

- The cornea protects the eye and, by changing shape, provides about 60% of the eye's focusing power.
- The iris controls the amount of light entering the eye.
- The lens changes its shape to focus rays of light on the retina.
- Medical shorthand for a quick, normal eye examination can be PERRLA: Pupils Equal, Round, Reactive to Light and Accommodation.

The Eyeball (Globe)

(LO 11.5)

The functions of the eyeball are to continuously:

1. **Adjust** the amount of light it lets in to reach the retina;
2. **Focus** on near and distant objects; and
3. **Produce** images of those objects and instantly transmit them to the brain.

As shown earlier in this chapter, the front of the eyeball is covered by the conjunctiva. This thin layer of tissue lines the inside of the eyelids and curves over the eyeball to meet the **sclera** *(Figure 11.9)*, the tough, white outer layer of the eye.

At the center of the front of the eye is the **cornea,** a transparent, dome-shaped membrane. The cornea has no blood supply and obtains its nutrients from tears and from fluid in the anterior chamber behind it.

When light rays strike the eye, they pass through the cornea. Because of its dome curvature, those rays striking the edge of the cornea are bent toward its center.

The light rays then go through the **pupil,** the black opening in the center of the colored area (the **iris**) in the front of the eye.

The iris controls the amount of light entering the eye. For example, when you're in the dark outside at night the iris opens **(dilates)** to allow more light into the eye. When you're in bright sunlight or in a well-lit room, the iris closes **(constricts)** to allow less light into the eye.

After traveling through the pupil, the light rays pass through the transparent **lens.** This lens can become thicker and thinner, enabling it to bend light rays and focus them on the **retina** at the back of the eye. Accommodation is the process of changing focus, and **refraction** is the process of bending light rays.

The lens does not contain blood vessels **(avascular)** or nerves, and with increasing age, it loses its elasticity. Because of this reduced elasticity, when you reach your forties, your eyes may have difficulty focusing on near objects, a condition called **presbyopia.**

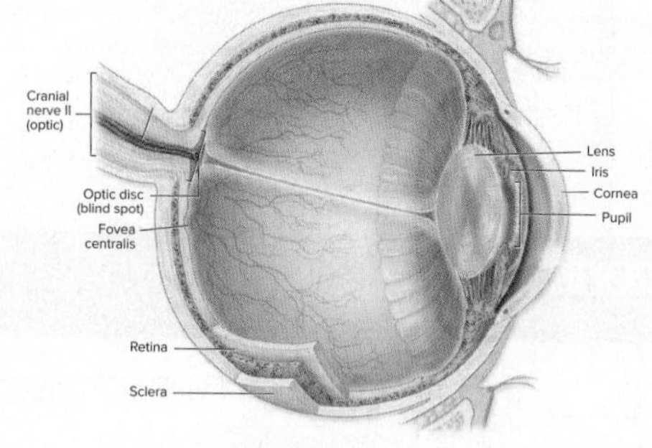

▲ FIGURE 11.9
Anatomy of the Eyeball.

290 Chapter 11 Special Senses of the Eye and Ear

tory tests for it. The only treatment options are pain management, physiotherapy, and stress reduction.

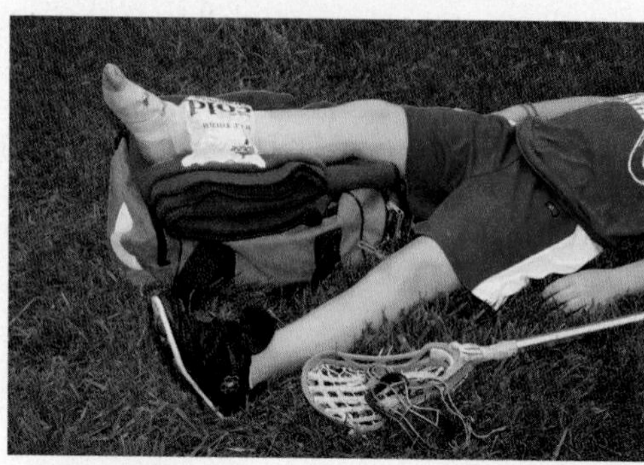

▲ **FIGURE 5.3**
RICE Treatment.

Rick Brady/McGraw-Hill Education

Lesson 4.2 (cont'd)

Skull and Face (LO 4.2 and 4.6)

The Skull (LO 4.2 and 4.6)

When you glance at your face in the mirror, chances are you're not thinking about what's behind your brown eyes or your slightly crooked smile. You see one image—not its layers, pieces, or parts. However, the human skull *(Figure 4.9)* is made up of 22 separate bones. Your **cranium,** the upper part of the skull that encloses the **cranial** cavity and protects the brain, contains 8 of these 22 bones; your facial skeleton contains the rest.

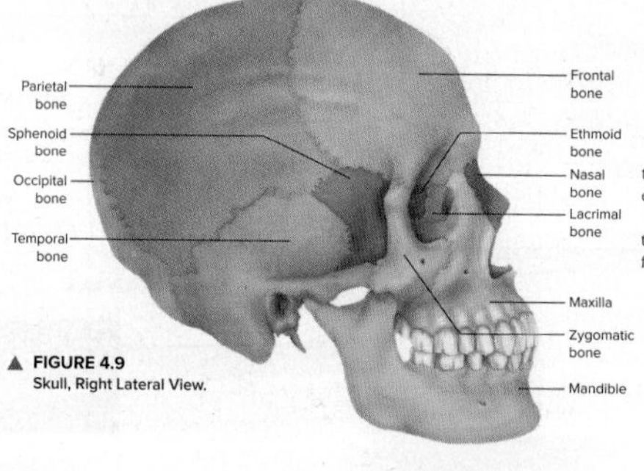

▲ FIGURE 4.9
Skull, Right Lateral View.

The bones of the cranium are joined together by sutures (joints that appear as seams), which are covered on the inside and outside by a thin layer of connective tissue. These bones have the following functions:

1. The **frontal** bone forms the forehead, roofs of the (eye) orbits, and part of the floor of the cranium and contains a pair of right and left frontal sinuses above the orbits.
2. **Parietal** bones form the bulging sides and roof of the cranium.
3. The **occipital** bone forms the back of and part of the base of the cranium.
4. **Temporal** bones form the sides of and part of the base of the cranium.
5. The **sphenoid** bone forms part of the base of the cranium and the orbits.
6. The **ethmoid** bone is hollow and forms part of the nose, the orbits, and the ethmoid sinuses.

These bones of the skull provide protection for the brain and the organs of vision, taste, hearing, equilibrium, and smell.

The lower part of the skull houses the bones of the facial skeleton *(Figure 4.10)*. These bones do the following:

1. **Maxillary** bones form the upper jaw **(maxilla),** hold the upper teeth, and are hollow, forming the maxillary sinuses.
2. **Palatine** bones are located behind the maxilla and cannot be seen on a lateral view of the skull.
3. **Zygomatic** bones are the prominences of the cheeks (cheekbones) below the eyes.
4. **Lacrimal** bones form the medial wall of each eye orbit.
5. **Nasal** bones form the sides and bridge of the nose.
6. **The mandible** is the lower jawbone, which holds the lower teeth. The mandible articulates (joins) with the temporal bone to form the **temporomandibular joint (TMJ).**

The bones of the facial skeleton provide a frame on which the muscles and other tissues of the face facilitate eating, facial expressions, breathing, and speech.

The third component of the axial skeleton, the rib cage, is discussed in Chapter 8, "Respiratory System."

Nasal bone
Palatine bone
Maxilla
Mandible

Abbreviation

TMJ temporomandibular joint

▲ FIGURE 4.10
Facial Bones.

74 Chapter 4 The Skeletal System

TABLES

Meaningful tables aid in summarizing concepts and lesson topics.

Lesson 4.1 (cont'd) Bone Fractures (FXs) (LO 4.2 and 4.5)

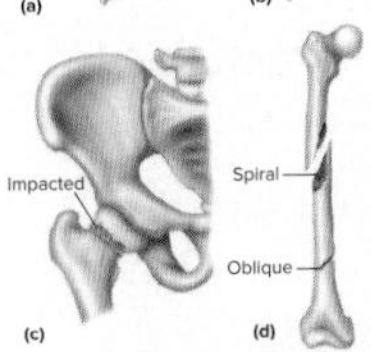

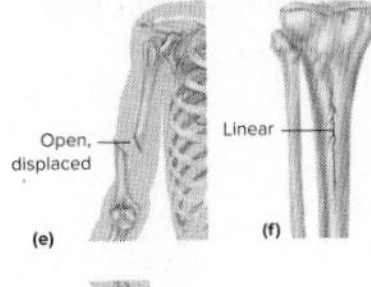

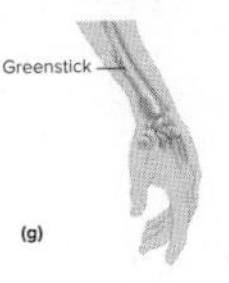

▲ FIGURE 4.6 Bone Fractures.

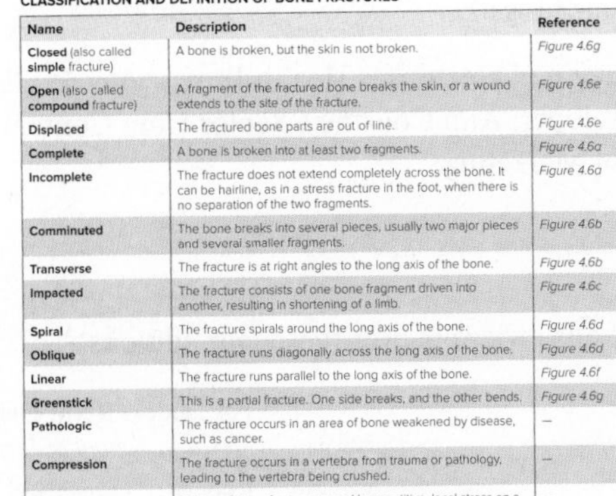

▼ TABLE 4.1

CLASSIFICATION AND DEFINITION OF BONE FRACTURES

Name	Description	Reference
Closed (also called **simple** fracture)	A bone is broken, but the skin is not broken.	*Figure 4.6g*
Open (also called **compound** fracture)	A fragment of the fractured bone breaks the skin, or a wound extends to the site of the fracture.	*Figure 4.6e*
Displaced	The fractured bone parts are out of line.	*Figure 4.6e*
Complete	A bone is broken into at least two fragments.	*Figure 4.6a*
Incomplete	The fracture does not extend completely across the bone. It can be hairline, as in a stress fracture in the foot, when there is no separation of the two fragments.	*Figure 4.6a*
Comminuted	The bone breaks into several pieces, usually two major pieces and several smaller fragments.	*Figure 4.6b*
Transverse	The fracture is at right angles to the long axis of the bone.	*Figure 4.6b*
Impacted	The fracture consists of one bone fragment driven into another, resulting in shortening of a limb.	*Figure 4.6c*
Spiral	The fracture spirals around the long axis of the bone.	*Figure 4.6d*
Oblique	The fracture runs diagonally across the long axis of the bone.	*Figure 4.6d*
Linear	The fracture runs parallel to the long axis of the bone.	*Figure 4.6f*
Greenstick	This is a partial fracture. One side breaks, and the other bends.	*Figure 4.6g*
Pathologic	The fracture occurs in an area of bone weakened by disease, such as cancer.	—
Compression	The fracture occurs in a vertebra from trauma or pathology, leading to the vertebra being crushed.	—
Stress	This is a fatigue fracture caused by repetitive, local stress on a bone, as occurs in marching or running.	—

Healing of Fractures (LO 4.2 and 4.5)

When a bone is fractured, blood vessels bleed into the fracture site, forming a hematoma *(Figure 4.7a)*. After a few days, bone-forming cells called **osteoblasts** move in and start to produce new bone cells (osteocytes), which form a **callus** *(Figure 4.7b)*. Osteblasts continue to produce bone cells, which form **cancellous** (spongy) bone to replace the callus *(Figure 4.7c)*. As more bone cells form, the spongy bone structure is replaced by compact bone, which fuses together the bone segments *(Figure 4.7d)*. Uncomplicated fractures take 8 to 12 weeks to heal. (Surgical procedures to help fractures heal are shown in Lesson 4.4.)

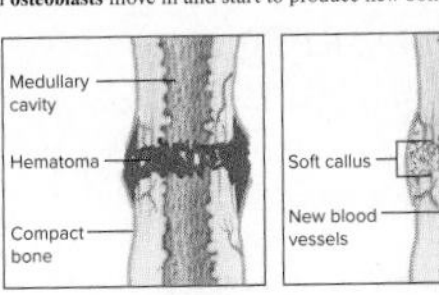

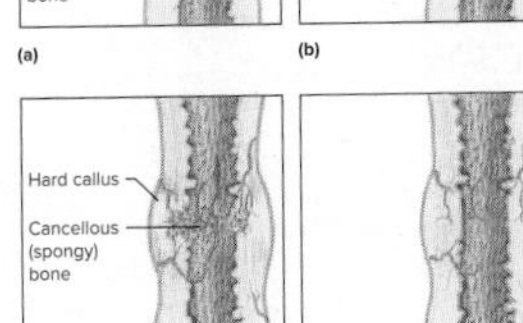

▶ FIGURE 4.7 Healing of Bone Fracture.

Abbreviation

Fx fracture

70 Chapter 4 The Skeletal System

KEYNOTES AND ABBREVIATIONS

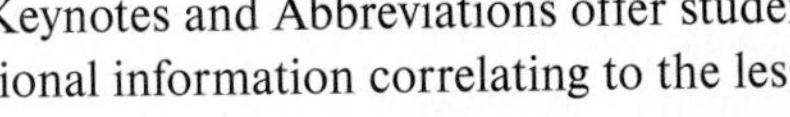

Keynotes and Abbreviations offer students additional information correlating to the lesson.

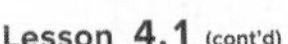

Lesson 4.1 (cont'd)

Keynote

- **Osteomalacia occurs in some developing nations and occasionally in this country when children drink soft drinks instead of milk fortified with vitamin D.**

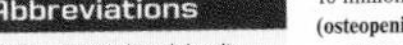

Abbreviations

BMD bone mineral density
DEXA dual energy X-ray absorptiometry
FDA Food and Drug Administration
IU international unit(s)
mg milligram

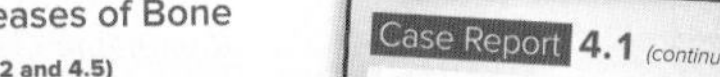

Diseases of Bone (LO 4.2 and 4.5)

Case Report 4.1 *(continued)*

On questioning, Amy Vargas demonstrated many of the risk factors for osteoporosis, including family history, lack of exercise, cigarette smoking, inadequate diet, post-menopause, and increasing age.

One of the major bone diseases is **osteoporosis,** which results from a loss of bone density *(Figure 4.4)*. More common in women than in men, the incidence of osteoporosis increases with age. In the United States alone, 10 million people are living with osteoporosis and 18 million more have low bone density **(osteopenia).** Osteopenia puts people at risk for developing osteoporosis.

In women, production of the hormone estrogen decreases after menopause, weakening the body's protection against bone loss and potentially resulting in fragile, brittle bones. In men, lower levels of testosterone have a similar but less noticeable effect.

Women at risk for osteoporosis should have a bone mineral density **(BMD)** screening using a **DEXA** scan, which is a measuring device that uses low-energy radiation beams. Men and women over 50 are often advised to follow a daily regimen of 1,200 milligrams **(mg)** of calcium, 400 to 600 international units **(IU)** of vitamin D, and 15 minutes of real sun exposure. In addition, there are several **FDA**-approved medications available for treating osteoporosis.

Other bone diseases that may not be as prevalent or publicized as osteoporosis are the following:

Osteomyelitis: an inflammation of bone and bone marrow caused by a bacterial infection, such as staphylococcus.

Osteomalacia: a disease (known as **rickets** in children) caused by vitamin D deficiency where the calcium-lacking bones become soft and flexible, lose their ability to bear weight, and become bowed.

Achondroplasia: a very rare condition where the long bones stop growing in childhood, but the axial skeleton bones are not affected *(Figure 4.5)*. People with this condition are short in stature, with the average adult measuring about 4 feet tall. Although intelligence and life span are normal, the disease is caused by a spontaneous gene mutation that then becomes a dominant gene for succeeding generations.

Osteogenesis imperfecta (OI): a rare genetic disorder producing very brittle bones that are easily fractured or broken, often **in utero** (while inside the uterus).

Primary bone cancer is found in three forms:

1. **Osteogenic sarcoma** occurs most often in bone cells around the knee in adolescents.
2. **Ewing sarcoma** occurs most often in children and adolescents.
3. **Chondrosarcoma** arises in cartilage cells, often in the pelvises of older people.

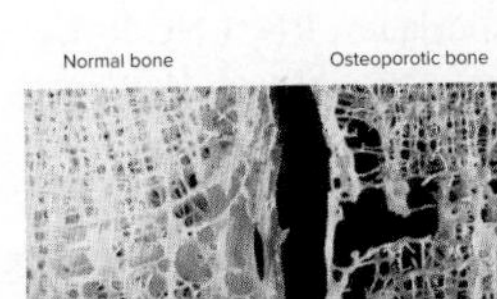

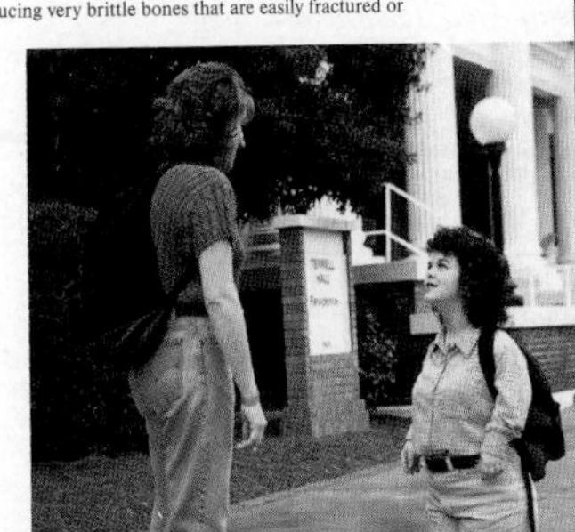

Acknowledgments

I wish to thank the talented efforts of a group of dedicated individuals at McGraw-Hill Education who have made this book and its digital ancillary products come together:

Thomas Timp, Managing Director for Health Professions; William Lawrensen, Executive Portfolio Manager; Christine "Chipper" Scheid, Senior Product Developer; Ann Courtney, Senior Core Content Project Manager; Yvonne Lloyd, Business Product Manager; and James Connely, Director of Marketing.

David Allan, MD
Author

Our thanks to all of our reviewers over these four editions:

Kathryn G. Aguirre, MA
UEI College-El Monte Campus

Theresa Allyn, BS, MEd
Edmonds Community College

Vanessa Austin, RMA, CAHI
Clarian Health Ed Sciences

Dr. Joseph H. Balabat, MD, RMA, RPT
Sanford-Brown Institute, New York

Dr. Seth Balogh, BS, MS, PhD
Brookline College

Rachel Basco, BS, MHS
Bossier Parish Community College

Michael Battaglia, MS
Greenville Technical College

Carole Berube, MA, BSN, MSN
Bristol Community College

Sue Biedermann, MSHP, RHIA, FAHIMA
Texas State University-San Marcos

Amy Bolinger Snow, MS
Greenville Technical College

Bonnie Bonner, RDA, LVN
Franklin Career College

Quiana Bost, RMA
Bohecker College-Cincinnati

Dorisann Brandt, MSPT
Greenville Technical College

Bill Burke, BA
Madison Area Technical College; Blackhawk Technical College

Jennifer Campbell, BS, M.Ed
Tulsa Community College

Kim Carlson, M.Ed
Delta College of Arts and Technology

Marie Cissell, MN, RN, C
South Dakota State University

Ursula Cole, M.Ed, CMA, AAMA
Harrison College

Rosalind Collazo, CMA
ASA Institute of Business and Technology

Dr. Brian Conroy, MD
Lehigh Valley College

Kimberly Corsi, LRCP, CCS
Davenport University

Carlos Cuervo, MD
Florida National University

Debra Mishoe Downs, LPN, AAS, RAM (AMT)
Okefenokee Technical College

Pat Dudek, RNM CHI, RMA
McCann School of Business and Technology

Robert E. Fanger, BS HCM, MSEd
Del Mar College

Tim Feltmeyer, MS
Erie Business Center

Jean Fennema, BA
Pima Medical Institute

Lance Followell, BS
Fremont College

Kenneth D. Franks
Bossier Parish Community College

Joanne Habenicht, MPA, RT, BS, ARRT
Manhattan College

Gregory Hartnett, BS, CPC
Sanford-Brown, Iselin, New Jersey

Diana Hollwedel, LPN
Career Institute of Florida

Mary W. Hood MS ARR(R)(CT)
William Rainey Harper College

Harold N. Horn MA
Lincoln Land Community College

Susan Horn, AAS, CMA
Indiana Business College-Lafayette

William J. Horton, RHIA
Hutchinson Community College

Janet Hunter, MS, MBA
Northland Pioneer College

Judy Johnson, RN
Nashville State Community College

Tim Jones, BA, MA
Oklahoma City Community College; University of Oklahoma

Angela C. Jording, CMA
Fortis College

Judith Karls, RN, BSN, M.Ed
Madison Area Technical College

Heather Kies, MHA, CMA (AAMA)
Goodwin College

Amy Kuehnl, BS
Central Ohio Technical College

Shelli Lampi, PhD, RDH, NREMT
Dunwoody College of Technology

Sandra Lehrke, RN, LNC, RMA
Anoka Technical College

James Lynch, MD
Florida Southern College

Nelly Mangarova, MD
Heald College

David McBride, MA, RT(R) (CT) (MR)
Westmoreland County Community College

Pam McConnell, MA, AS
High Tech Institute

Jacqueline McNair, MA, RHIT
Baltimore City Community College

Cari McPherson, LP, N.II, AHI
Ross Medical Education Center

Susan Meeks, CPC-A
Milan Institute

Roxanna Montoya, M.Ed
Pima Medical Institute

Steve Moon, MS CMI, FAMI
The Ohio State University

Steve Moon, MS, CMI, FAMI
Ohio State University, College of Medicine

Cathleen Murphy, DC
Katherine Gibbs School

Sheila Newberry, M.Ed, RHIT
Remington College

Evie O'Nan, RMA
National College

Professor Eva Oltman, MEd, CPC, CPC-I
Jefferson Community and Technical College

Jennifer S. Painter,
Ohio Business College

Mirella G Pardee, MSN, MA, RN
The University of Toledo

Fred Pearson, PhD
Brigham Young University–Idaho

Christina Rauberts Conklin, AA, RMA
Keiser University

Adrienne Reeves, BS, M.Ed
Westwood College

Becky Rodenbaugh, MBA, CMA
Baker College of Cadillac

Irma Rodriguez
South Texas College

Janette Rodriguez, RN, LNC RMA
Woot Tobe Coburn School, Manhattan, New York

Dr. Beth Roraback
Greenville Technical College, Spartanburg Community College

Shawn Marie Russell, BA, CPC
University of Alaska-Fairbanks

Rebecca Schultz, PhD
University of Sioux Falls

Gene Simon, RHIA, RMD
Florida Career College

Donna Slovensky, PhD, RHIA, FAHIMA
University of Alabama-Birmingham

Brian S. Spence
Tarrant County College

Alice L. Spencer, BS, MT, MS, CQA (ASQ)
National College-Florence, Kentucky

Susan Stockmaster, CMA (AAMA), MHS
Trident Technical College

Charlotte Susie Myers, MA
Kansas City Kansas Community College

Catherine A. Teel, AST, Health Care Technology, RMA
McCann School of Business and Technology

Lenette Thompson, CST
Piedmont Technical College

Jonathan Thorsen, BS, RRT
Long Beach Community College

Margaret A. Tiemann, RN, BS
St. Charles Community College

Lori A. Warren, MA, RN, CPC, CPC-I, CCP, CLNC
Spencerian College-Louisville, KY

Kathryn Whitley, MSN, FNP
Patrick Henry Community College

Stacy Wilson, MT/PBT, CMA, MHA Program Chair
Cabarrus College of Health Sciences

Dr. Barbara Worley, DPM, BS, RMA, Program Manager, Medical Assisting
King's College

Carole A. Zeglin, MS, BS, RMA
Westmoreland County Community College

Daphne Zito, M.Ed, LPN
Katharine Gibbs School

Susan Zolvinski, BS, MBA
Brown Mackie College

Digital and Instructor Resource Content Development

Special thanks to the instructors who assisted with the development of Connect and SmartBook materials.

Rachel Basco, BS, MHS
Bossier Parish Community College

Tammy Burnette, PhD.
Tyler Junior College

Vicky Navaroli, PhD
Goodwin University

Shauna Phillips, RMA, CCMA, CPT, AHI
Pima Medical Institute

Patricia Saccone, MA, RHIA, CCS-P, CDIP, CPB
Waubonsee Community College

About the Authors

David M. Allan

David Allan received his medical training at Cambridge University and Guy's Hospital in England. He was Chief Resident in Pediatrics at Bellevue Hospital in New York City before moving to San Diego, California.

Dr. Allan has worked as a family physician in England, a pediatrician in San Diego, and Associate Dean at the University of California, San Diego School of Medicine. He has designed, written, and produced more than 100 award-winning multimedia programs with virtual reality as their conceptual base. Dr. Allan resides happily in San Diego.

Rachel Curran Basco

Rachel Basco earned her BS in Cardiopulmonary Science and MS in Health Sciences from Louisiana State University Health Sciences Center, School of Allied Health Professions (SAHP). She worked as a registered respiratory therapist for ten years and then began her career in college instruction in respiratory therapy at LSU-SAHP in Shreveport, LA. She then found her interest to be in nonclinical education and began instructing biology courses at Bossier Parish Community College (BPCC) in Bossier City, LA. Ms. Basco is employed as an Assistant Professor of biology, instructing courses in medical terminology along with human anatomy I and II.

Ms. Basco resides in Shreveport with her husband. While very busy with her family, work, and studies, Rachel always finds time to visit her relatives in her home state of Wisconsin.

Essentials of Medical Language

Learning the Essentials of Medical Language

Welcome

Rick Brady/McGraw-Hill Education

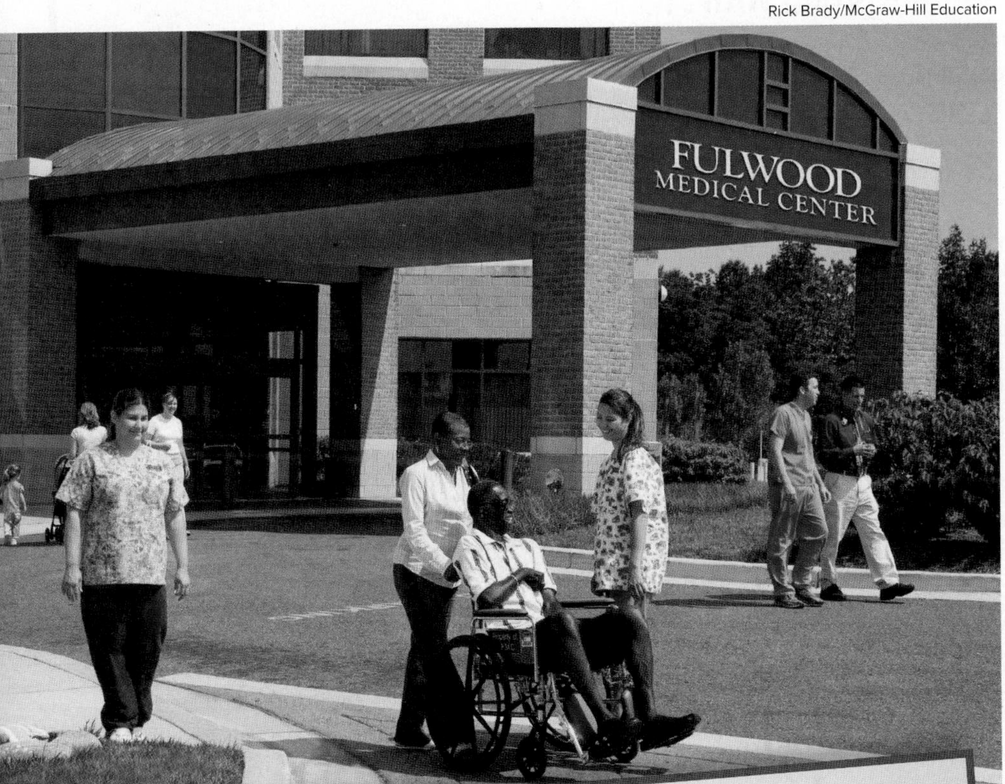

Learning Outcomes

In order to get the most out of your learning experiences and this textbook, you need to:

LO W.1 **Establish a commitment to learn medical terminology.**

LO W.2 **Recognize the knowledge and skills you will need to be an active learner.**

LO W.3 **Understand how the contextual approach of this book promotes active learning.**

LO W.4 **Utilize the pedagogical devices used in each chapter and lesson.**

LO W.5 **Use the vivid illustrations, photos, and tables in the book to enhance understanding of the concepts being taught.**

LO W.6 **Solve the exercises in each lesson and at the end of each chapter to demonstrate understanding of the material.**

LO W.7 **Implement the effective organizational strategies and study habits described in this chapter of the book.**

LO W.8 **Understand how a commitment to lifelong learning will enhance your professionalism.**

LO W.9 **Differentiate the roles of the various members of a health care team in different medical specialties and settings.**

CASE REPORT W.1

You are . . .

. . . a student preparing for a career as a health professional and allied health care worker.

You are communicating with . . .

. . . many different health professionals in health care teams as you go through an externship at Fulwood Medical Center. The center comprises a medical office building with physicians in a wide range of primary care, medical specialties, and complementary medicine therapies; a 300-bed hospital with a busy Emergency Room and operating rooms; a laboratory, pharmacy, X-Ray Department, Physiotherapy Department, and Patient Education Unit that serve both the hospital and the medical offices.

Between attending classes, doing your externship, working part-time, and bringing up two children, you have a full schedule. The knowledge and skills you are learning in the classroom and at Fulwood Medical Center will prepare you for a successful future.

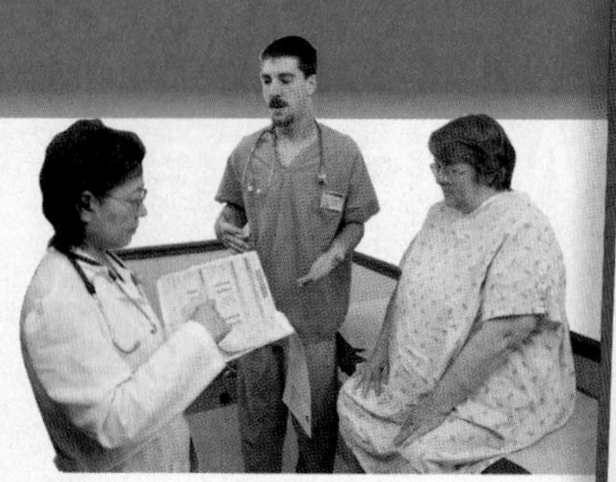

▲ **FIGURE W.1**
Direct Communication with Doctor and Patient.

McGraw-Hill Education/Rick Brady

CASE REPORT W.2

You are . . .

. . . Luis Guitterez, a certified medical assistant (CMA) working with Susan Lee, MD, a primary care physician at Fulwood Medical Center.

You are communicating with . . .

. . . Dr. Lee and Mrs. Martha Jones, a patient.

Luiz Guitterez, CMA: Dr. Lee, this is Mrs. Martha Jones, who is a type **2 diabetic** with **retinopathy** and **neuropathy.** She had a routine appointment with us today. Her temperature is 97.8, pulse 120, respirations 24, blood pressure 100/50.

Mrs. Martha Jones: Dr. Lee, I've had a cough and cold for the past few days, and today I'm feeling drowsy and nauseous and my chest hurts.

Dr. Lee: Did you give yourself your morning insulin?

Mrs. Jones: I can't remember.

Dr. Lee: Luis, she's confused, has **tachycardia** and **tachypnea,** and is **hypotensive.** I'm concerned she is going into diabetic **ketoacidosis.** Get the glucometer and test her blood glucose while I examine her. She may have **pneumonia.**

(Note: The pronunciations and meanings of the medical terms used in this Case Report are on page W-9.)

Keynote

As a **health professional,** you are part of a team of medical and other professionals who provide health care services designed to improve the health and well-being of their patients.

The Health Care Team (LO W.9)

Fulwood Medical Center is a realistic health care setting that allows you to experience the use of medical language. Each chapter in this book focuses on the medical terminology used in a specific medical specialty and the body systems related to that specialty. A variety of health professionals make up the teams caring for patients in each medical specialty.

The team leader is a medical doctor, or physician, who can be an **MD** (doctor of medicine) or a **DO** (doctor of osteopathy). Most **managed care systems** require the patient to have a **primary care physician.** This physician can be a **family practitioner, internist,** or **pediatrician** (for children) and is responsible for the continuing overall care of the patient. In managed care, the primary care physician acts as the "gatekeeper" for the patient to enter the system, supervising all care the patient receives.

If needed medical care is beyond the expertise of the primary care physician, the patient is referred to a medical specialist whose expertise is based on a specific body system or even a part of a body system. For example, a **cardiologist** has expertise in diseases of the heart and vascular system, whereas a **dermatologist** specializes in diseases of the skin and an **orthopedist** in problems with the musculoskeletal system. A **gastroenterologist** is an expert in diseases of the whole digestive system, whereas a **colorectal surgeon** specializes only in diseases of the lower gastrointestinal tract.

Other health professionals work under the supervision of the physician and provide direct care *(Figure W.1)* to the patient. These can include a **physician assistant, nurse practitioner, medical assistant,** and, in specialty areas, different therapists, technologists, and technicians with expertise in the use of specific therapeutic and diagnostic tools.

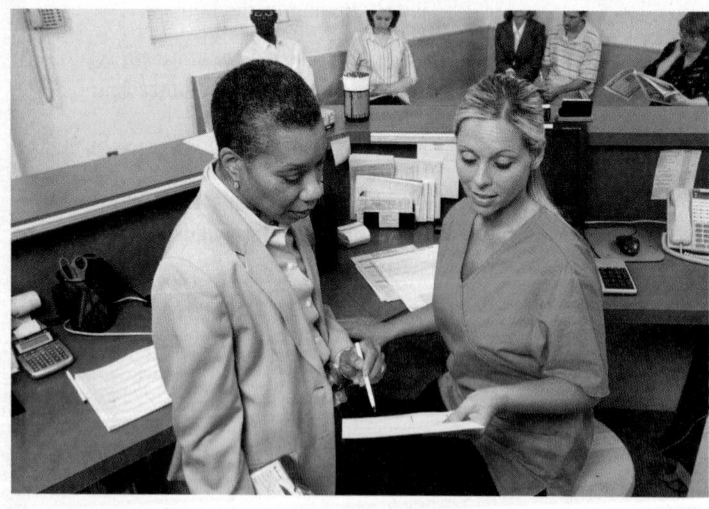

▲ **FIGURE W.2**
Administrative medical assistants are among the health professionals who provide indirect care to patients.

McGraw-Hill Education/Rick Brady

Still other health professionals on the team provide indirect patient care *(Figure W.2)*. These include **administrative medical assistants, transcriptionists, health information technicians, medical insurance billers,** and **coders,** all of whom are essential to providing high-quality patient care.

As you study the language of each medical specialty at Fulwood Medical Center, you will also meet the members of each specialty's health care team and learn more about their roles in caring for the patient.

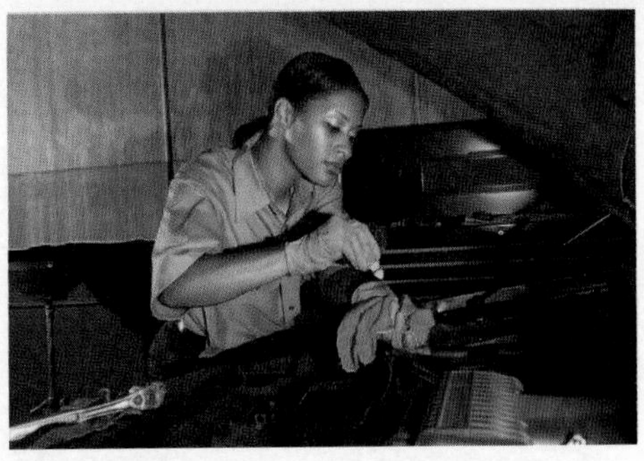

▲ **FIGURE W.3**
Every Profession Has Its Own Language
You may have difficulty understanding your auto mechanic when she tells you that the expansion valve, evaporator core, and orifice tubes in your air-conditioning system need to be replaced.
Jupiterimages/Comstock Images/Getty Images

"Why Do I Need to Learn Medical Terminology?"

Communication Needs

Throughout your career as a health professional, you will need to communicate with other health professionals. This need is present whether you are providing direct patient care–for example, as a CMA like Luis Guitterez–or whether you are providing indirect patient care–for example, as a medical transcriptionist, biller, or coder. In this book, you will find all the medical terms necessary to equip yourself with the essential medical vocabulary needed for work and further study in any of the allied health professional careers.

As you can see in Case Report W.2, health professionals use specific terms and a different language to describe to each other situations they encounter each day. You need to be able to understand, spell, and pronounce the terms they use.

Modern medical terminology is an artificial language constructed over centuries using words and elements from Greek and Latin origins (where healing professions began). Some 15,000 or more words are formed from 1,200 Greek and Latin roots. New words are being added continually as new medical discoveries are made. Medical terminology enables health professionals from different fields, different specialties, and different countries to communicate clearly and precisely with each other. Every profession has its own language *(Figure W.3)*.

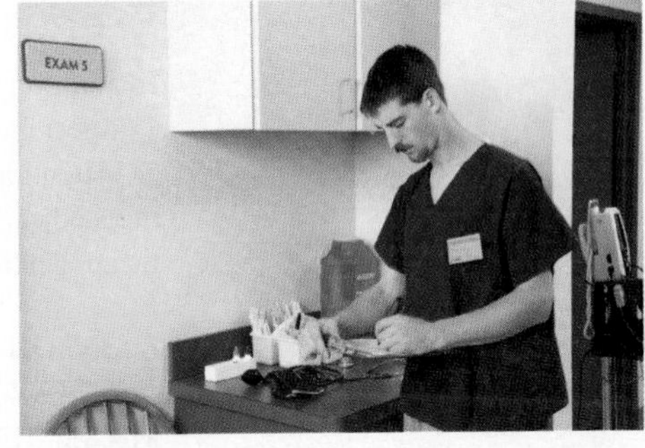

▲ **FIGURE W.4**
Accurate Documentation of Care Is Critical.
McGraw-Hill Education/Rick Brady

Listening, Speaking, Reading, Writing, and Critical Thinking

Daily in your practice as a health professional you will:

Listen to information from physicians about patient care, and carry out their instructions.

Listen to patients describing their symptoms, and translate their descriptions into medical terms.

Speak to physicians and other health professionals to report information and ask questions.

Speak to patients to translate and clarify information given to them by physicians and other health professionals.

Read physicians' comments and treatment plans in patient medical records and insurance reports.

Read the results of physical examinations, procedures, and laboratory and diagnostic tests.

Write to document actions taken by yourself and other members of the health care team *(Figure W.4)*.

Write to precisely record verbal orders, test results given over the phone, and other phone messages.

Think critically to evaluate medical documentation for accuracy.

Think critically to analyze and discover the meaning of unfamiliar medical terms using the strategies outlined in *Chapter 1* of this book.

IF YOU CANNOT SPEAK AND UNDERSTAND THE LANGUAGE, YOU CANNOT JOIN THE CLUB.

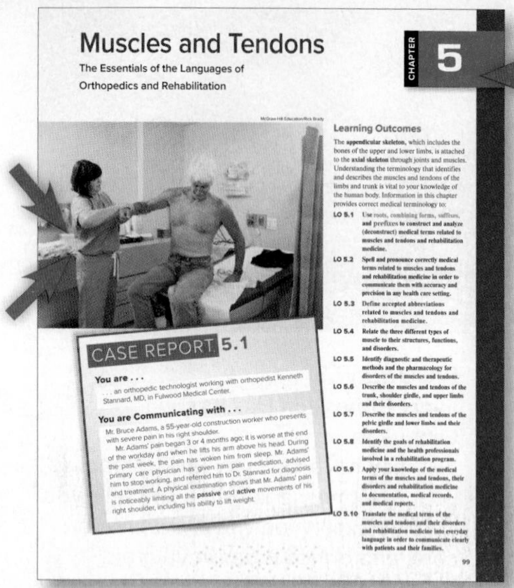

Muscles and Tendons

The Essentials of the Languages of Orthopedics and Rehabilitation

CHAPTER 5

McGraw-Hill Education/Rick Brady

CASE REPORT 5.1

You are . . .

. . . an orthopedic technologist working with orthopedist Kenneth Stannard, MD, in Fulwood Medical Center.

You are Communicating with . . .

Mr. Bruce Adams, a 55-year-old construction worker who presents with severe pain in his right shoulder.

Mr. Adams' pain began 3 or 4 months ago; it is worse at the end of the workday and when he lifts his arm above his head. During the past week, the pain has woken him from sleep. Mr. Adams' primary care physician has given him pain medication, advised him to stop working, and referred him to Dr. Stannard for diagnosis and treatment. A physical examination shows that Mr. Adams' pain is noticeably limiting all the **passive** and **active** movements of his right shoulder, including his ability to lift weight.

Learning Outcomes

The **appendicular skeleton,** which includes the bones of the upper and lower limbs, is attached to the **axial skeleton** through joints and muscles. Understanding the terminology that identifies and describes the muscles and tendons of the limbs and trunk is vital to your knowledge of the human body. Information in this chapter provides correct medical terminology to:

LO 5.1 Use roots, combining forms, suffixes, and prefixes to construct and analyze (deconstruct) medical terms related to muscles and tendons and rehabilitation medicine.

LO 5.2 Spell and pronounce correctly medical terms related to muscles and tendons and rehabilitation medicine in order to communicate them with accuracy and precision in any health care setting.

LO 5.3 Define accepted abbreviations related to muscles and tendons and rehabilitation medicine.

LO 5.4 Relate the three different types of muscle to their structures, functions, and disorders.

LO 5.5 Identify diagnostic and therapeutic methods and the pharmacology for disorders of the muscles and tendons.

LO 5.6 Describe the muscles and tendons of the trunk, shoulder girdle, and upper limbs and their disorders.

LO 5.7 Describe the muscles and tendons of the pelvic girdle and lower limbs and their disorders.

LO 5.8 Identify the goals of rehabilitation medicine and the health professionals involved in a rehabilitation program.

LO 5.9 Apply your knowledge of the medical terms of the muscles and tendons, their disorders and rehabilitation medicine to documentation, medical records, and medical reports.

LO 5.10 Translate the medical terms of the muscles and tendons and their disorders and rehabilitation medicine into everyday language in order to communicate clearly with patients and their families.

99

"What's Unique About This Book?"

Although the chapters in this book are organized by body system, as in many other textbooks on medical terminology, this book has many unique features that enhance learning, create interest, and provide a consistent learning strategy for you.

Each chapter is broken down into lessons; each lesson is broken down into self-contained topic areas so that there are smaller "chunks" of information to master.

You Are . . . You Are Communicating With . . .

At the beginning of each chapter and lesson, you are placed in the role of a health professional in a field related to the body system and medical specialty covered in the material. At the same time, learning objectives (**LOs**) are presented for each chapter and lesson. These techniques immediately engage your attention, motivate you to read on to discover how this patient's diagnosis and care progress, and illustrate the medical terminology being introduced in the lessons.

Word Analysis And Definition

All the information needed for a topic area is presented in self-contained two-page spreads.

On the left-hand page, the new medical terms are introduced. On the right-hand page, for each new medical term the pronunciation, color-coded word elements, and definition are provided in a **Word Analysis and Definition (WAD)** box. For example, in Case Report W.2 earlier in this chapter, the medical terms diabetic, retinopathy, neuropathy, tachycardia, tachypnea, hypotensive, ketoacidosis, glucometer, and pneumonia were used. On the right-hand page here, you can see an example of how these terms are analyzed. All these terms will appear again in the appropriate body-system chapter.

Also, below each WAD are exercises that test your understanding of key components of the terminology analyzed in the WAD.

Keynotes

- **Study Hints** provide ways to help retain knowledge.
- **Abbreviation Boxes** show commonly accepted abbreviations.
- **Illustrations and photos** are vivid and clear and correlate precisely to the appropriate terms in the text.

Exercises

In addition to the exercises at the end of each topic area, there are chapter review questions exercises included in Connect (see below).

Attention is given to developing skills in pronunciation, spelling, forming plurals, using abbreviations, and writing medical language. The exercises take you beyond memorization and teach you to think critically about the realistic application of the medical language you are learning.

Mc Graw Hill connect

A ONE-STOP SPOT TO PRESENT, DELIVER, AND ASSESS DIGITAL ASSETS AVAILABLE WITH ESSENTIALS OF MEDICAL LANGUAGE:

McGraw-Hill Connect® Essentials of Medical Language provides online presentation, assignment, and assessment solutions. It connects students with the tools and resources they'll need to achieve success. With *Connect,* students can complete assignments, quizzes, and tests online. A robust set of questions and activities, including all of the lesson exercises and end-of-chapter questions, additional case studies, and interactives, are presented and aligned with the textbook's learning outcomes.

Connect Essentials of Medical Language also provides students with 24/7 online access to an ebook. This media-rich version of the textbook is available through the McGraw-Hill Education Connect platform and allows seamless integration of text, media, and assessments. To learn more, visit **http://connect.mheducation.com.**

MCGRAW-HILL EDUCATION'S ADAPTIVE SUITE

New from McGraw-Hill Education, LearnSmart Advantage is a series of adaptive learning products, which include LearnSmart, Smartbook, LearnSmart Prep, LearnSmart Achieve, and Learnsmart Labs. Since 2009, LearnSmart has been the most widely used and intelligent adaptive learning resource proven to improve learning. Developed to deliver demonstrable results in boosting grades, increasing course retention, and strengthening memory recall, the LearnSmart Advantage series spans the entire learning process from course preparation to providing the first adaptive reading experience, and it's found only in SmartBook. Distinguishing what students know from what they don't, and honing in on concepts they are most likely to forget, each product in the series helps students study smarter and retain more knowledge. A smarter learning experience for students coupled with valuable reporting tools for instructors, and available in hundreds of course areas, LearnSmart Advantage is advancing learning like no other products in higher education today. **Go to www.LearnSmartAdvantage.com** for more information.

Word Analysis and Definition

S = Suffix P = Prefix R = Root R/CF = Combining Form

WORD	PRONUNCIATION	ELEMENTS		DEFINITION
diabetes mellitus	dye-ah-**BEE**-teez **MEL**-ih-tus		diabetes, Greek *a siphon* mellitus, Latin *sweetened with honey*	Metabolic syndrome caused by absolute or relative insulin deficiency and/or insulin ineffectiveness
diabetic (adj)	dye-ah-**BET**-ik	S/ R/	-ic *pertaining to* diabet- *diabetes*	Pertaining to or suffering from diabetes
hypotension	**HIGH**-poh-**TEN**-shun	S/ P/ R/	-ion *action, condition* hypo- *below* -tens- *pressure*	Persistent low arterial blood pressure
hypotensive (adj)	**HIGH**-poh-**TEN**-siv	S/	-ive *pertaining to, quality of*	Pertaining to or suffering from hypotension
ketoacidosis	**KEY**-toe-ass-ih-**DOE**-sis	S/ R/CF R/CF	-sis *abnormal condition* ket/o- *ketone* -acid/o- *acid*	Excessive production of ketones, making the blood acidic
neuropathy	nyu-**ROP**-ah-thee	S/ R/CF	-pathy *disease* neur/o- *nerve*	Any disorder affecting the nervous system
pneumonia (**Note:** *The initial "p" is silent.*)	new-**MOH**-nee-ah	S/ R/	-ia *condition* pneumon- *air, lung*	Inflammation of the lung parenchyma
retinopathy	ret-ih-**NOP**-ah-thee	S/ R/CF	-pathy *disease* retin/o- *retina*	Any disease of the retina
tachycardia	tack-ih-**KAR**-dee-ah	S/ P/ R/	-ia *condition* tachy- *rapid* -card- *heart*	Rapid heart rate, above 100 beats per minute
tachypnea	tack-ip-**NEE**-ah	P/ R/	tachy- *rapid* -pnea *breathe*	Rapid breathing

The elements of a term are discussed in Chapter 1.

SmartBook is the first and only adaptive reading experience currently available. SmartBook personalizes content for each student in a continuously adapting reading experience. Reading is no longer a passive and linear experience, but an engaging and dynamic one where students are more likely to master and retain important concepts, thus coming to class better prepared. Valuable reports provide instructors with insight into how students are progressing through textbook content, and are useful for shaping in-class time and assessments. As a result of the adaptive reading experience found in SmartBook, students are more likely to retain knowledge, stay in class, and get better grades. This revolutionary technology is available only from McGraw-Hill Education for hundreds of course areas as part of the LearnSmart Advantage series.

Exercises

Elements *are your best tool for understanding medical terms. In the chart below, the elements are listed in column 1. Identify the meaning of each element in column 2, and give an example of a term containing that element in column 3. Some terms will apply to more than one element. The first one is done for you.*

Element	Meaning of Element	Medical Term Containing This Element
hypo	**below**	**hypotension**
tens		
ion		
neuro		
retino		
pathy		
ia		
pneumon		
pnea		
tachy		

1. Choose any term from column 3, and use it in a sentence of your choice:

___

___

___

"What Is Lifelong, Active Learning?"

Lifelong Learning

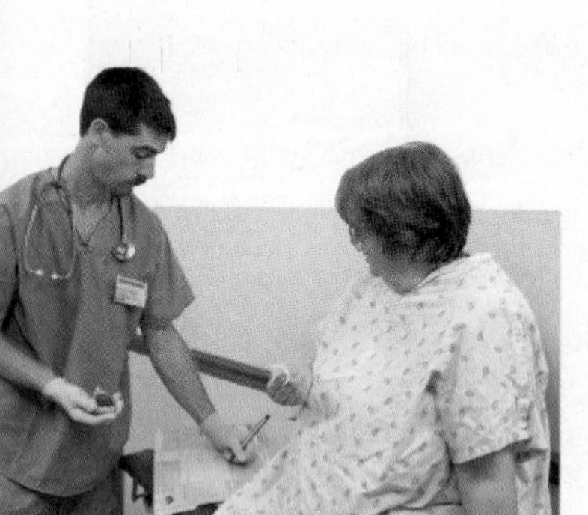

▲ **FIGURE W.5**
Every Patient Interaction Is an Opportunity for Learning.

McGraw-Hill Education/Rick Brady

Your current training in medical terminology is necessary for you to be able to continue your education in your health care profession. But it is important to recognize that school is only one of the many places where you acquire knowledge.

You also acquire knowledge:

- Each time you ask a question about a patient or a report and receive an answer.
- Each time you analyze an unfamiliar medical term and discover its meaning.
- Each time you interact with a patient and see how that patient is coping with his or her problems *(Figure W.5)*.

All these are opportunities for learning to discover ***your own*** answers to ***your own*** problems or lack of knowledge.

This type of knowledge–discovered through your own experience and driven by your own needs and goals–is genuine, real, and trustworthy for you. It is not like what you learn in school, which is determined by some distant authority.

The authentic knowledge you gain from solving your own problems, whether by yourself or with the help of other people or resources, motivates you to acquire still more knowledge and helps you grow as a person and as a professional.

Throughout your working life, additional classroom training will be needed to keep your skills and professional knowledge up to date with new developments in medicine. You will also continue to learn through your own experience. Everything you do in life can result in learning.

Your own experience and judgment become your most valuable resources for making your life vibrant, strong, creative, and what ***you*** want ***it*** to be.

Your own experience and judgment maximize your professional and personal success.

Your own learning never ends.

Keynote

Novelist Lillian Smith said, "When you stop learning, stop listening, stop looking, and stop asking new questions, then it is time to die."

Actively Experiencing Medical Language

Medical terms were created to provide health care professionals a way to communicate with each other and document the care they provide. To provide effective patient care, all health care professionals must be fluent in medical language. One misused or misspelled medical term on a patient record can cause errors that can result in injury or death to patients, incorrect coding or billing of medical claims, and possible fraud charges.

When medical terms are separated from their intended context, as they are in other medical terminology textbooks, it is easy to lose sight of how important it is to use them accurately and precisely. Learning medical terminology in the context of the medical setting reinforces the importance of correct usage and precision in communication.

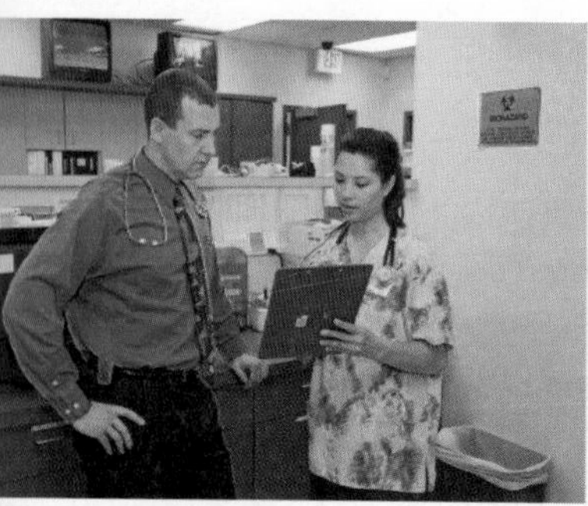

▲ **FIGURE W.6**
Medical assistant interacts with a physician.

McGraw-Hill Education/Rick Brady

During your externship at Fulwood Medical Center, you will *experience* medical language. Just as in a real medical center, you will encounter and apply medical terminology in a variety of ways. Actively experiencing medical language will help ensure that you are truly learning, and not simply memorizing, the medical terms in each chapter. Memorizing a term allows you to use it in the same situation (e.g., repeating a definition) but doesn't help you apply it in new situations. Whether you are reading chart notes in a patient's medical record ***(Figure W.6)*** or a description of the treatment prescribed by a physician, you will see medical terms being used for the purpose they were intended.

Active Learning

It's no good sitting back and expecting someone else to pour knowledge into your head. You have to **actively work at learning** *(Figure W.7)*.

Get the Most Out of Lectures

- ***Prepare*** for your classroom experiences. Preview the book chapter before class ***(Figure W.7)***, and the material will be much easier to understand.
- ***Listen actively.*** You cannot do this if you are looking at your cell phone, daydreaming, or worrying about what you have to get for dinner.
- ***Ask*** a question if you do not comprehend something the instructor is saying.
- ***Write*** good notes. Focus on the main points, and capture key ideas; review and edit your notes within 24 hours of the class.

Get the Most Out of Reading

- ***Concentrate*** on what you are reading. Review the titles, objectives, headings, and visuals for each lesson to identify what the lesson is all about.
- ***Read*** actively using the SQ3R method (see the Study Hint) to help you.
- ***Write*** down any questions you have.

Study with a Partner or Group

- ***Find*** a study partner. Schedule study dates, compare notes, talk through concepts and questions, and quiz each other.
- ***Establish*** a small study group, including your study partner. Again, compare notes and quiz each other.

Perform Well on Tests

- ***Read*** the directions carefully, and scan the entire test so that you know how long it is and what types of activities it contains.
- ***Answer*** the easy questions or sections first so that you finish as much as possible before doing the difficult questions, which might slow you down.
- ***Use*** any extra time, after you have finished the test, to check that you have answered all the questions and then to confirm your answers.

Know and Motivate Yourself

- What type of learner are you? **Visual**–who responds best by **seeing** information. **Auditory**–who works best by listening. **Tactile**–who prefers hands-on applications. Recognize your type and motivate yourself by emphasizing your best method of learning to help achieve your goals.

A few months of committed study now is a small price to pay for a lifetime of professionalism.

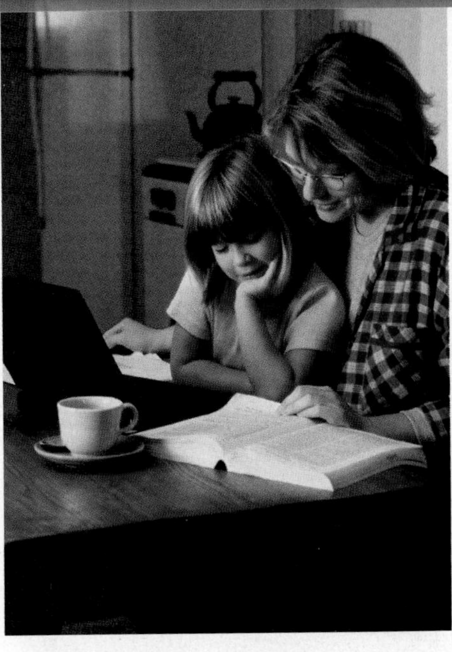

▲ **FIGURE W.7**
Identify your own personal preferences for learning, and seek out the resources that will best help you with your studies. Recognize your weaknesses, and try to compensate for or work to improve them.

Scott T. Baxter/Getty Images

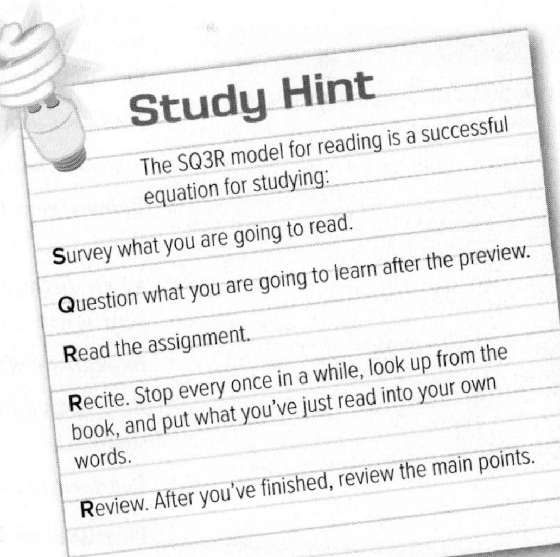

Study Hint

The SQ3R model for reading is a successful equation for studying:

Survey what you are going to read.

Question what you are going to learn after the preview.

Read the assignment.

Recite. Stop every once in a while, look up from the book, and put what you've just read into your own words.

Review. After you've finished, review the main points.

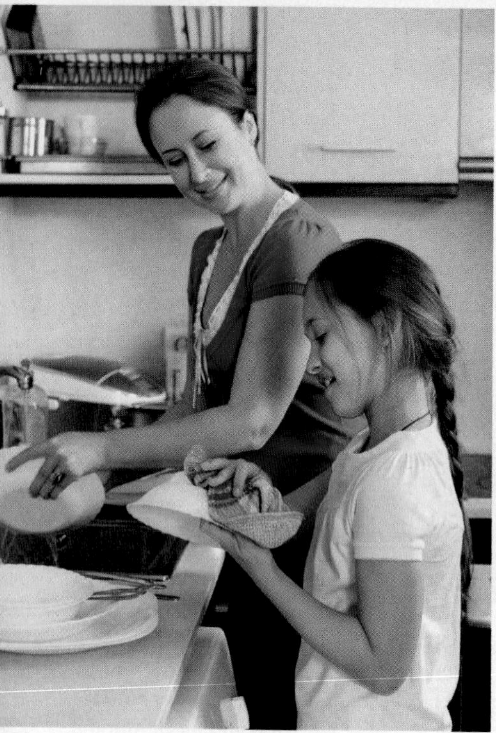

▲ **FIGURE W.8**
An Evening at Home.

Iakov Filimonov/123RF.com

CASE REPORT W.3

Your first day of externship at Fulwood Medical Center went well. You enjoyed being in the Primary Care Clinic with Dr. Lee and Luis Guitterez, CMA. You wonder if this could be a career choice for you. Now it's 6:15 p.m. at home, and you have yet to feed the kids, get them to bed, pay some bills, pick up around the house, and review a whole chapter in your medical terminology text to prepare for a test in class tomorrow. How are you going to do all this?

"How Can I Help Myself Learn Better?"

You have a lot of time and money invested in your education. To succeed, you need to be able to focus and manage your time and your studies. To manage the difficulties described in Case Report W.3 *(Figure W.8),* you need to:

- ***Recognize*** the stresses in your life at different times.
- ***Prioritize*** mentally, and handle each task in the order of importance. In this case, eat a healthy meal with your kids, enjoy putting them to bed, pay the bills, and then relax (or meditate) for 10 minutes. When you are relaxed, settle down to review the text, and go to bed at a reasonable hour. Picking up around the house will have to wait because study and sleep are a higher priority. Sounds too easy? What other choices do you have to be able to study in an effective way?
- ***Actively develop a support group.*** Enlist the support of your spouse, parents, siblings, friends–any people you can trust and rely on. If you have a test every Thursday, get one of them to come over Wednesday night and put the kids to bed while you go over to his or her house or the library to study.
- ***Find your own space.*** Create a place where you keep everything for your courses at your fingertips, clutter-free.
- ***Study when you are most productive.*** Are you a night owl or an early bird? Set a daily study time for yourself.
- ***Balance your life.*** While studying should be a main focus, plan time for family, friends, leisure, exercise, and sleep.
- ***Resist distractions.*** Avoid the temptation to surf the Web, send instant messages, and make phone calls. Stick to your schedule.
- ***Be realistic*** when planning–know your limits and priorities.
- ***Be prepared*** for the unexpected (child's illness, your illness, inclement weather) that can turn your schedule into shambles.
- ***Reprioritize*** daily on the basis of schedule disruptions and other conflicts.
- ***Identify*** clear goals for what you need to get done today, this week, this month, before the end of the semester, and so on.

Keynote

Life, living, and learning are constant choices of priority.

EXERCISES

Write out *all of your activities for a typical week. On average, how many hours each week do you spend sleeping, grooming, eating, working, running errands, studying, attending your children's activities, and watching TV? Add all the hours up. There are 168 hours in the week. How many hours do you have left for studying? A sample time budget is shown below.*

Activity	Number of Hours per Day	Number of Days per Week	Number of Hours per Week
Sleeping	8	7	56
Grooming	1	7	7
Meals: preparation, eating, cleanup	1	7	7
Cleaning, laundry	1	3	3
Commuting to and from school	1	5	5
In class	4	5	20
Doing errands	1	3	3
Family time	3	7	21
Church, workout, hobbies			5
Job			30
Friends, going out, TV, entertainment			6
TOTAL			163
TOTAL HOURS IN A WEEK			168
Hours remaining for study			5

- ARE 5 HOURS ENOUGH FOR STUDY?
- WHEN ARE THEY AVAILABLE?
- WHAT CAN YOU DO TO INCREASE THEM?

STUDY HOURS SHOULD BE SPENT IN A SETTING THAT ALLOWS YOU TO CONCENTRATE ON YOUR WORK AND NOT BE DISTRACTED. TURN OFF YOUR CELL PHONE AND TV. THE BIGGEST QUESTION TO ASK YOURSELF IS, "AM I INVESTING MY TIME WISELY?" IF NOT, HOW CAN YOU BUDGET YOUR TIME DIFFERENTLY SO THAT MORE TIME IS SPENT ON HIGHER-PRIORITY ACTIVITIES?

The Anatomy of Medical Terms

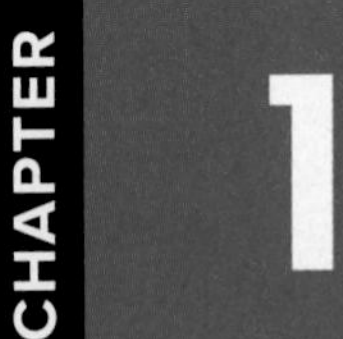

The Essential Elements of the Language of Medicine

McGraw-Hill Education/Rick Brady

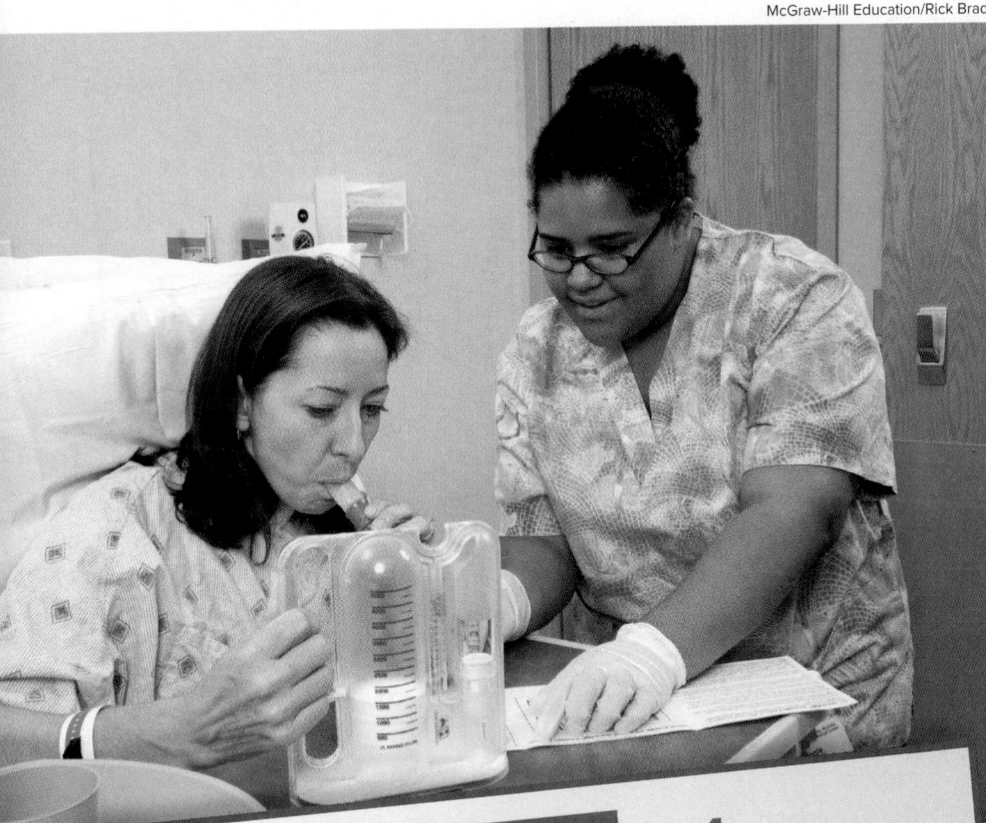

CASE REPORT 1.1

You are . . .

. . . a **respiratory therapist** working with Tavis Senko, MD, a pulmonologist at Fulwood Medical Center.

You are communicating with . . .

. . . Mrs. Sandra Schwartz, a 43-year-old woman referred to Dr. Senko by her primary care physician, Dr. Andrew McDonald, an **internist.** Mrs. Schwartz has a persistent abnormality on her chest **X-ray**. You have been asked to determine her **pulmonary** function prior to a scheduled **bronchoscopy.**

This summary of a Case Report illustrates for you the use of some simple medical terms. Modern health care and medicine have their own language. The medical terms all have precise meanings, which enable you, as a health professional, to communicate clearly and accurately with other health professionals involved in the care of a patient. This communication is critical for patient safety and the delivery of high-quality patient care.

Learning Outcomes

The technical language of medicine has been developed logically from Latin and Greek roots. In fact, it was in Latin and Greek cultures that the concept of treating patients began. Medical terms are built from their individual parts, or **elements,** which form the **anatomy** of the word. The information in this chapter will enable you to:

LO 1.1 **Select the roots, combining vowels, and combining forms of medical terms.**

LO 1.2 **Demonstrate the importance of suffixes and prefixes in forming medical terms.**

LO 1.3 **Construct (build) medical terms from separate elements.**

LO 1.4 **Deconstruct (break down) medical terms into their elements.**

LO 1.5 **Use correctly the plurals of medical terms.**

LO 1.6 **Articulate the correct pronunciations of medical terms.**

LO 1.7 **Demonstrate precision and accuracy in documentation and other written and verbal communication of medical terms.**

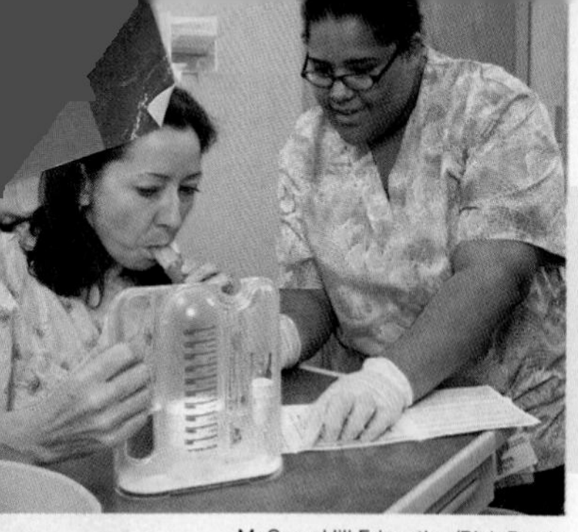

McGraw-Hill Education/Rick Brady

Lesson 1.1

The Construction of Medical Words

Objectives

Your confidence in using and understanding the medical terms in this book will increase as you become familiar with the logic of how these terms are constructed. The information in this lesson will enable you to:

1.1.1 Build and construct medical terms using their elements.

1.1.2 Select and identify the meaning of essential medical term **roots**.

1.1.3 Define the elements **combining vowel** and **combining form**.

1.1.4 Identify the **combining vowel** and **combining form** of essential medical terms.

1.1.5 Define the elements **suffix** and **prefix**.

1.1.6 Select and identify the meaning of the **suffixes** and **prefixes** of essential medical terms.

Roots

- A **root** is the constant foundation and core of a medical term.
- **Roots** are usually of Greek or Latin origin.
- All medical terms have *one* or *more* **roots**.
- A **root** can appear anywhere in the term.
- More than one **root** can have the same meaning.
- A **root** plus a **combining vowel** creates a **combining form**.

Abbreviations

CXR chest X-ray
RUL right upper lobe

Roots (LO 1.1)

Every medical term has a **root**—the element that provides the core meaning of the word. For example, in Case Report 1.1:

- The word *pneumonia* has the **root** ***pneumon-***, taken from the Greek word meaning *lung* or *air.* The Greek **root** ***pneum-*** also means *lung* or *air. Pneumonia* is an infection of the lung tissue.
- Dr. Tavis Senko is a *pulmonologist.* The **root** ***pulmon-*** is taken from the Latin word meaning *lung.* A *pulmonologist* is a specialist who treats lung diseases.

Case Report 1.1 *(continued)*

From her medical records, you can see that 2 months ago Mrs. Schwartz developed a right upper lobe (**RUL**) **pneumonia.** After treatment with an **antibiotic,** a follow-up chest **X-ray (CXR)** showed some residual collapse in the right upper lobe and a small right **pneumothorax.** Mrs. Schwartz has smoked a pack a day since she was a teenager. Dr. Senko is concerned that she has lung cancer and has scheduled her for a **bronchoscopy.**

Combining Forms (LO 1.1)

Roots are often joined to other elements in a medical term by adding a **combining vowel**, such as the letter "o," to the end of the **root**, like ***pneum-***, to form **pneum/o-**.

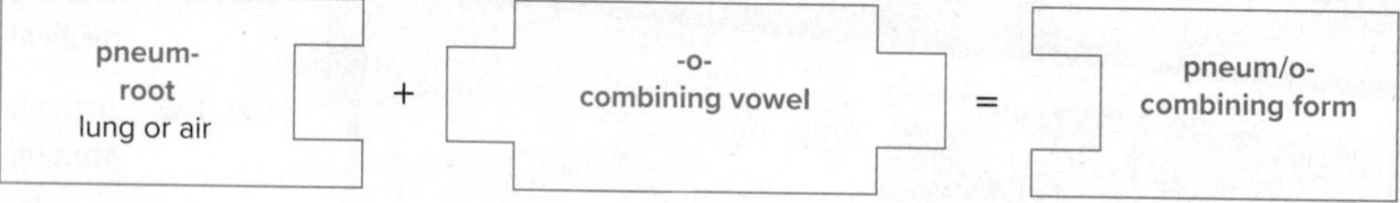

Throughout this book, whenever a term is presented, a **slash** (/) will be used to separate the combining vowel from the **root.** Other examples of this approach are as follows:

- Adding the **combining vowel** "o" to the Latin **root** ***pulmon-*** makes the **combining form** ***pulmon/o-.***

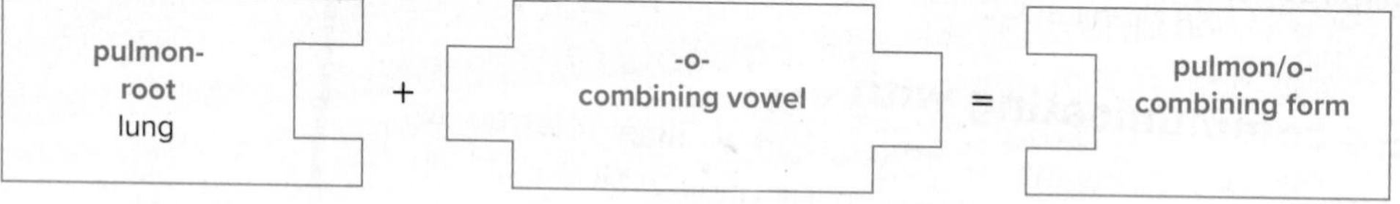

Any vowel, "a," "e," "i," "o," or "u," can be used as a **combining vowel.**

- The **root** ***respir-*** means *to breathe.* Adding the **combining vowel** "a" makes the **combining form** ***respir/a-.***

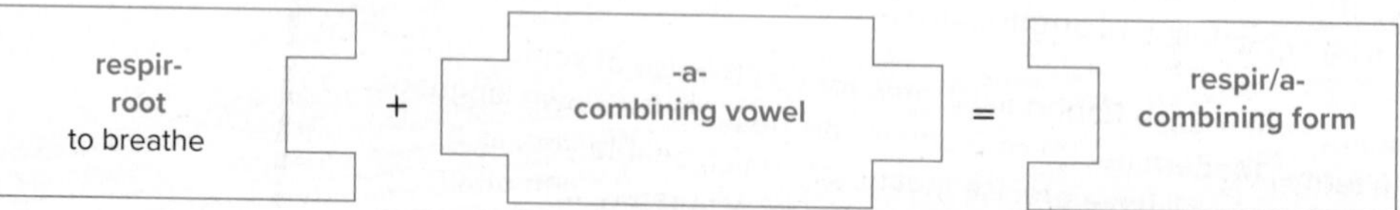

- The **root** *bronch-* is derived from the Greek word for *windpipe* and is one of the two subdivisions of the trachea that carry air to and from the lungs. Adding the **combining vowel "o"** to the **root** *bronch-* makes the **combining form** *bronch/o-*.

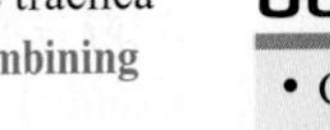

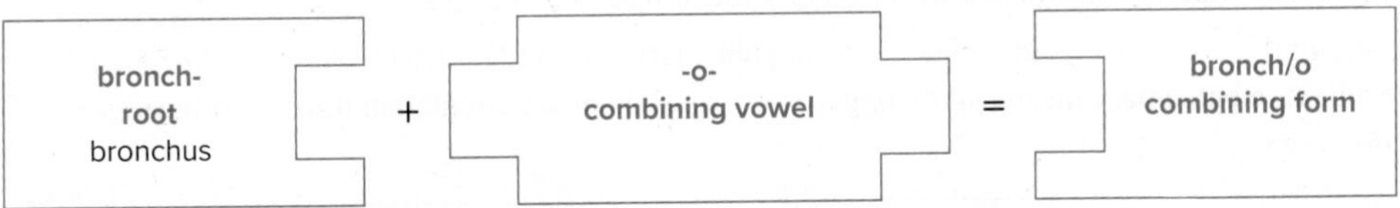

Combining Forms

- Combine a **root** and a **combining vowel.**
- Can be attached to another **root** or **combining form.**
- Can precede another word element called a **suffix.**
- Can follow a **prefix.**

Many medical terms contain more than one **root**; when two roots occur together, they are always joined by a **combining vowel,** as in the following example:

- The word **hemopneumothorax** has the **root** *hem-,* from the Greek word meaning *blood,* and the **root** *pneum-,* from the Greek word meaning *air* or *lung,* and the **suffix** *-thorax,* from the Greek word meaning *chest.* The **combining vowel "o"** joins these two roots together to make the **combining form,** *pneum/o-.* A **hemopneumothorax** is the presence of air and blood in the space that surrounds the lungs in the chest. As blood and air fill the pleural cavity, the lungs cannot expand and respiration is not possible, thus forcing the affected lung to collapse.

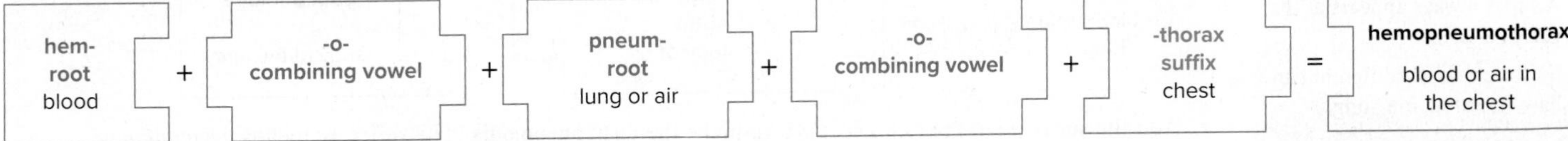

Keynotes

- Throughout this book, look for the following patterns:

  Roots, combining forms, and combining vowels will be colored red.

  Prefixes will be colored green.

  Suffixes will be colored blue.

- Different roots can have the same meaning. *Pulmon-* and *pneumon-* both mean *lung, air.*

EXERCISES

A. Review *what you have just learned about roots and combining forms. Select the correct answer to the statement.* **LO 1.1**

root | combining form | combining vowel | suffix | prefix

1. Roots and combining forms can go before a ____________________
2. This element does not have a meaning; it serves to make the word easier to pronounce: ____________________
3. A ____________ can go before a root, but never after.
4. The ____________ is the root plus a combining vowel.

B. Identify *the word parts of a medical term. Use the provided medical term to correctly answer the questions.* **LO 1.1**

1. In the word **pneumonia,** the root is:

   a. pneum- **c.** -ia

   b. pneumon- **d.** -nia

2. In the medical term **pulmonologist,** the root is:

   a. pulm- **c.** -logist

   b. pulmon- **d.** -gist

3. The combining vowel in the medical term **respiratory** is:

   a. -a- **c.** -i-

   b. -o- **d.** -e-

Suffixes

- A suffix is a group of letters attached to the end of a root or combining form.
- A suffix changes the meaning of the word.
- If the suffix begins with a consonant, it must follow a combining vowel.
- If the suffix begins with a vowel, no combining vowel is needed.
- A few medical terms can have two suffixes.
- A suffix always appears at the end of a term.
- Suffixes that are different can have the same meaning.

Keynote

Adjectival suffixes meaning *pertaining to:*

-ac, -al, -ale, -alis, -ar, -aris, -ary, atic, -ative, -eal, -ent, -etic, -ial, -ic, -ica, -ical, -ine, -ior, -iosum, -ious, -istic, -ius, -nic, -ous, -tic, -tiz, -tous, -us.

Suffixes (LO 1.2)

A suffix is an element added to the end of a root or combining form to give it a new meaning. You can add different suffixes to the same root to build new words, all with different meanings. For example:

- Add the suffix *-ary* to the root *pulmon-* to create the term **pulmonary.** The suffix *-ary* means *pertaining to* or *relating to.* The adjective **pulmonary** means *pertaining to the lung.* **Pulmonary circulation** means the *passage of blood through the lungs.*

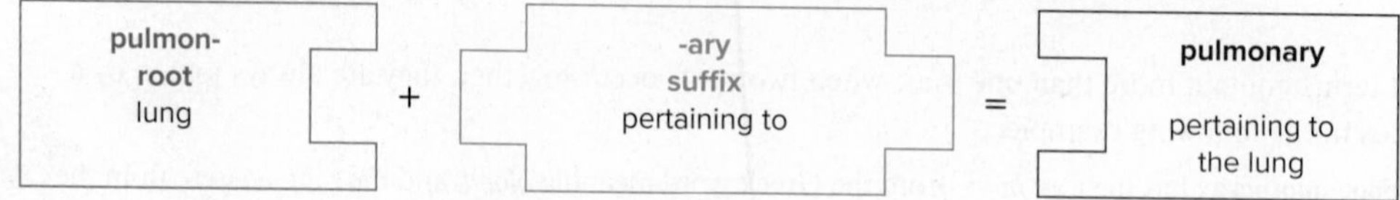

- Add the suffix *-logy* to the combining form *pulmon/o-* to make the term **pulmonology.** The suffix *-logy* means *study of.* **Pulmonology** is the study of the structure, functions, and diseases of the lungs.

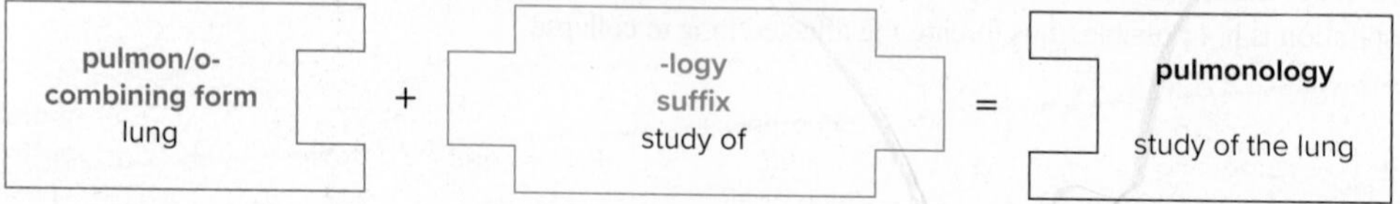

- Add the suffix *-ia* to the root *pneumon-* to make the term **pneumonia.** The suffix *-ia* means *a condition of.* **Pneumonia** is a condition of the lungs that involves an infection of the lung tissue.

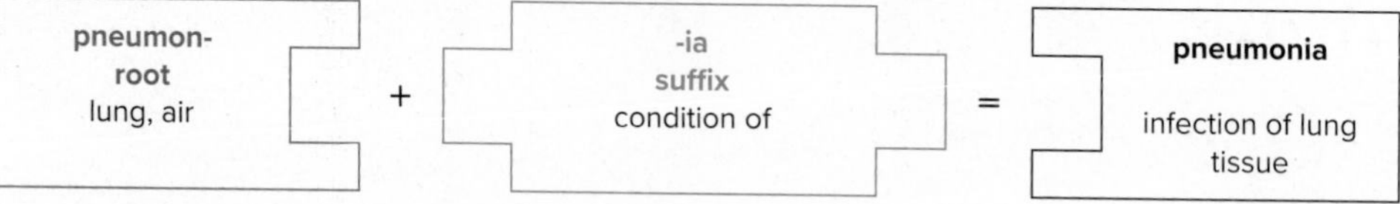

- Add the suffix *-ation* to the root *respir-* to make the term **respiration.** The suffix *-ation* means *a process.* **Respiration** is the process of breathing in and out.

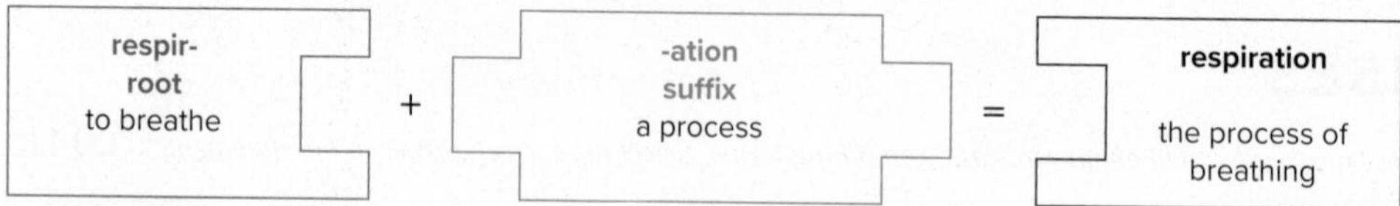

- Add the suffix *-itis* to the root *bronch-* to make the term **bronchitis.** The suffix *-itis* means *inflammation.* **Bronchitis** is an inflammation of the bronchial tubes.

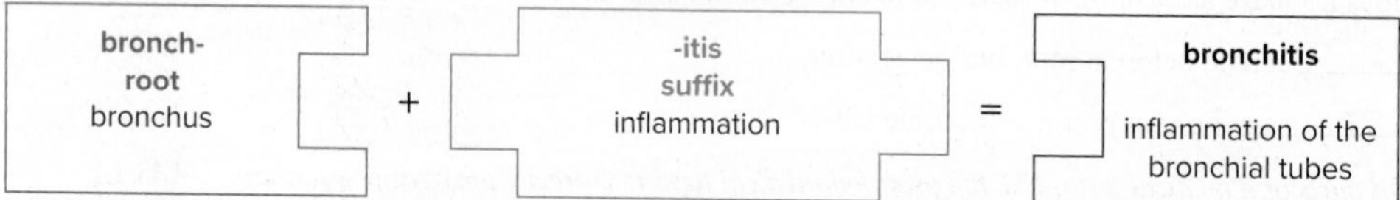

Although most roots are specific to body systems and medical specialties, suffixes are universal and can be applied to all body systems and specialties.

One user-friendly design concept of this book is that all the information you will need for any given topic is presented on the left-hand page of the two-page spread open in front of you. As part of this, you will find a Word Analysis and Definition (WAD) box on the right-hand side of each two-page spread. This section provides the elements, definition, and pronunciation of every new and repeated significant medical term that appears in the two-page spread.

Review all the terms in the WAD before you start any exercise.

Word Analysis and Definition

S = Suffix P = Prefix R = Root R/CF = Combining Form

WORD	PRONUNCIATION	ELEMENTS		DEFINITION
bronchitis	brong-**KI**-tis	S/ R/	-itis *inflammation* bronch- *bronchus*	Inflammation of the bronchi
pneumonia pneumonitis (same as *pneumonia*)	new-**MOH**-nee-ah new-moh-**NI**-tis	S/ R/ S/	-ia *condition* pneumon- *lung, air* -itis *inflammation*	Inflammation of the lung parenchyma (tissue)
pulmonary pulmonology pulmonologist	**PULL**-moh-**NAR**-ee **PULL**-moh-**NOL**-oh-jee **PULL**-moh-**NOL**-oh-jist	S/ R/ S/ R/CF S/	-ary *pertaining to* pulmon- *lung* -logy *study of* pulmon/o- *lung* -logist *one who studies, specialist*	Pertaining to the lungs Study of the lungs, or the medical specialty of disorders of the lungs Specialist in treating disorders of the lungs
respiration respiratory (adj)	**RES**-pih-**RAY**-shun **RES**-pih-rah-tor-ee	S/ R/ S/	-ation *process* respir- *to breathe* -atory *pertaining to*	Process of breathing; fundamental process of life used to exchange oxygen and carbon dioxide Pertaining to respiration

EXERCISES

Elements: *It is important for you to recognize the identity of an element. Is it a root, combining form, or suffix? This will help you to determine its place in the term when you are building terms.*

A. Build the appropriate medical term *to match the definitions given. The placement of the elements is noted for you under the line; each different element is separated on the line. Insert the correct elements on the line. The first one is done for you.* **LO 1.1 and 1.2**

1. Study of the lungs: ______ pulmon/o ______ / ______ logy ______
   R/CF S
2. Pertaining to the lung: ______ / ______
   R/CF S
3. The process of breathing: ______ / ______
   R/CF S
4. Condition of the lung: ______ / ______
   R/CF S

B. Suffixes *can provide clues to the meanings of terms. Answer the following questions using terms related to the respiratory system. Fill in the blanks.* **LO 1.1 and 1.2**

1. What is another term with the same meaning as pneumonia? ______
2. Which term is a body process? ______
3. Which suffix can be applied to a specialist? ______

Lesson 1.1 (cont'd)

Prefixes

- A prefix always appears at the beginning of a term.
- A prefix precedes a root to change its meaning.
- Prefixes can have more than one meaning.
- Prefixes never require a combining vowel.
- An occasional medical term can have two prefixes.
- Not every term has a prefix.

Practical Points

- A root can start a term and does not become a prefix.
- A root can end a term and does not become a suffix.

Prefixes (LO 1.2)

A **prefix** is an element added to the beginning of a **root** or **combining form** to further expand the meaning of a medical term. **Prefixes** usually indicate time, number, size, or location.

Examples of **prefixes** defining time are as follows:

- The term **mature** can refer to an infant born after a normal length of pregnancy, between 37 and 42 weeks.
- An infant born before 37 weeks is called **premature.** The **prefix** *pre-* means *before.* **Premature** means that the infant was born *before 37 weeks.*
- An infant born after 42 weeks is called **postmature.** The **prefix** *post-* means *after.* **Postmature** means that the *infant was born after 42 weeks.*

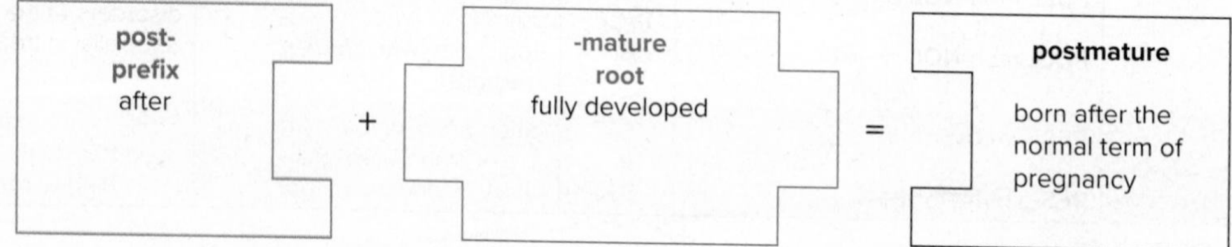

- The term **natal** contains the **root** *nat- (birth* or *born)* and the **suffix** *-al (pertaining to);* it means *pertaining to birth.*
- Add the **prefix** *pre- (before)* to form **prenatal,** which means *the time before birth.*
- Add the **prefix** *post- (after)* to form **postnatal,** which means *the time after birth.*
- Add the **prefix** *peri- (around)* to form **perinatal,** which means *around the time of birth.* This includes the time immediately *before, during,* and *directly after birth.*

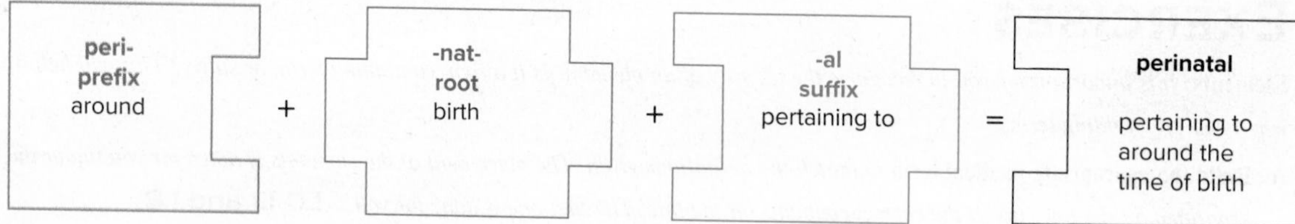

Examples of **prefixes** indicating number are as follows:

- The term **lateral** contains the **root** *later- (side)* and the **suffix** *-al (pertaining to).* **Lateral** means *pertaining to a side of the body.*
- Add the **prefix** *uni- (one)* to form **unilateral,** which means *pertaining to one side of the body only.*
- Add the **prefix** *bi- (two)* to form **bilateral,** which means *pertaining to both sides of the body.*

Examples of prefixes indicating location are as follows:

- The term **gastric** contains the **root** *gastr- (stomach)* and the **suffix** *-ic (pertaining to).* **Gastric** means *pertaining to the stomach.*
- Add the **prefix** *epi- (above)* to form **epigastric,** which means *pertaining to above the stomach.*
- Add the **prefix** *hypo- (below)* to form **hypogastric,** which means *pertaining to below the stomach.*

Examples of **prefixes** indicating size are as follows:

- The **root** *-cyte* means *cell.*
- Add the **prefix** *macro- (large)* to form **macrocyte,** which means *a large cell.*
- Add the **prefix** *micro- (small)* to form **microcyte,** which means *a small cell.*

Word Analysis and Definition

S = Suffix P = Prefix R = Root R/CF = Combining Form

WORD	PRONUNCIATION	ELEMENTS		DEFINITION
gastric	**GAS**-trik	S/	-ic *pertaining to*	Pertaining to the stomach
		R/	**gastr-** *stomach*	
epigastric	ep-ih-**GAS**-trik	P/	**epi-** *above*	Abdominal region above the stomach
hypogastric	high-poh-**GAS**-trik	P/	**hypo-** *below*	Abdominal region below the stomach
lateral	**LAT**-er-al	S/	-al *pertaining to*	Pertaining to one side of the body
		R/	later- *side*	
bilateral	by-**LAT**-er-al	P/	**bi-** *two*	Pertaining to both sides of the body
unilateral	you-nih-**LAT**-er-al	P/	**uni-** *one*	Pertaining to one side of the body only
macrocyte	**MACK**-roh-site	P/	**macro-** *large*	Large cell
		R/	**-cyte** *cell*	
macrocytic (adj) (**Note:** *The "e" in cyte is deleted to allow the word to flow.*)	mack-roh-**SIT**-ik	S/	-ic *pertaining to*	Pertaining to a macrocyte
mature	mah-**TYUR**		Latin *ready*	Fully developed
postmature	post-mah-**TYUR**	P/	**post-** *after*	Infant born after 42 weeks of gestation
		R/	**-mature** *fully developed*	
premature	pree-mah-**TYUR**	P/	**pre-** *before*	Occurring before the expected time; e.g., an infant born before 37 weeks of gestation.
microcyte	**MY**-kroh-site	P/	**micro-** *small*	Small cell
		R/	**-cyte** *cell*	
microcytic (adj) (**Note:** *The "e" in cyte is deleted to allow the word to flow.*)	my-kroh-**SIT**-ik	S/	-ic *pertaining to*	Pertaining to a small cell
natal	**NAY**-tal	S/	-al *pertaining to*	Pertaining to birth
		R/	nat- *birth, born*	
perinatal	per-ih-**NAY**-tal	P/	**peri-** *around*	Around the time of birth
postnatal	post-**NAY**-tal	P/	**post-** *after*	After the birth
prenatal	pree-**NAY**-tal	P/	**pre-** *before*	Before the birth
pneumothorax	new-moh-**THOR**-ax	R/CF	**pneum/o-** *air, lung*	Air in the pleural cavity
		S/	-thorax *chest*	

EXERCISES

Prefixes: *Solid knowledge of prefixes will quickly help increase your medical vocabulary.*

A. Answer the first question, *and then build the correct term on the line next to the definitions in 2 through 4.* **LO 1.1, 1.2, and 1.4**

natal **prenatal** **postnatal** **perinatal**

1. The term *natal* means ______________________________

2. Pertaining to around the time of birth: __________ / __________ / __________
P R/CF S

3. Pertaining to after the birth: __________ / __________ / __________
P R/CF S

4. Pertaining to before the birth: __________ / __________ / __________
P R/CF S

B. Prefixes usually indicate time, number, size, or location. *Given the prefix, select the correct category of meaning.* **LO 1.2**

1. hypo

a. time **b.** number **c.** size **d.** location

2. uni

a. time **b.** number **c.** size **d.** location

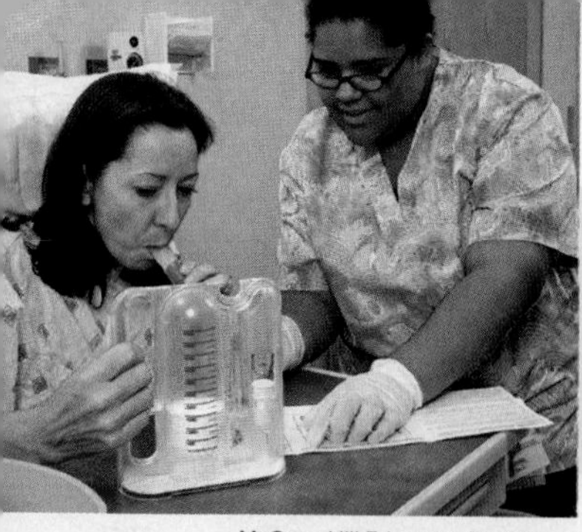
McGraw-Hill Education/Rick Brady

Lesson 1.2

Word Deconstruction, Plurals, Pronunciation, and Precision

Objectives

When you see an unfamiliar medical term, you can learn its meaning by ***deconstructing*** *it–reducing it to its basic elements. In this lesson you will learn to:*

1.2.1 Break down or deconstruct a medical term into its elements.

1.2.2 Use word analysis to help ensure the precise use of medical terms.

1.2.3 Use the word elements to analyze and determine the meaning of the term.

1.2.4 Apply the correct pronunciation to medical terms.

CASE REPORT 1.2

You are . . .

. . . a medical assistant working in the office of Lokesh Bannerjee, MD, a cardiologist in Fulwood Medical Center.

You are communicating with . . .

. . . the 70-year-old wife and the 45-year-old son of James Donovan, a 75-year-old man who will be admitted to the hospital's acute care **cardiology** unit.

Dr. Bannerjee has **diagnosed** Mr. Donovan with an acute myocardial infarction **(AMI),** confirmed by changes in his **electrocardiogram (ECG/EKG).** One of your tasks is to explain Mr. Donovan's **diagnosis** and reasons for admission to the hospital to Mrs. Donovan and her son. While Mr. Donovan is waiting to be admitted, he is receiving oxygen through nasal prongs. He is **hypotensive**, and an intravenous **(IV)** infusion of normal saline has been started. His medical record indicates that he is being seen in the neurology clinic for early dementia.

The bold terms in the Case Report are used as examples in the text and/or are deconstructed in the Word Analysis and Definition box (opposite page).

Keynotes

- Always begin deconstructing a medical term by identifying its suffix.
- Abbreviations are listed in Abbreviations Boxes throughout the book.

Abbreviations

AMI	acute myocardial infarction
CXR	chest X-ray
ECG/EKG	electrocardiogram
IV	intravenous

Word Deconstruction (LO 1.1, 1.2, and 1.4)

When you see an unfamiliar medical term, first identify the suffix. Take the term **cardiologist.** Here, the suffix at the end of the word is *-logist,* which means *one who studies and is a specialist in.* This leaves the element *cardi/o-,* which is the combining form for *heart.* The term **cardiologist** means *a specialist in the heart and its diseases.* It has a combining form and a suffix.

In the term **myocardial,** the suffix at the end of the word is -al, which means *pertaining to,* as you learned earlier in this chapter. The combining form *my/o-,* which means *muscle,* is at the beginning of the word. The root *-cardi-,* which means *heart,* is in the middle of the word. So, the term **myocardial** means *pertaining to the heart muscle.* It has a combining form, a root, and a suffix.

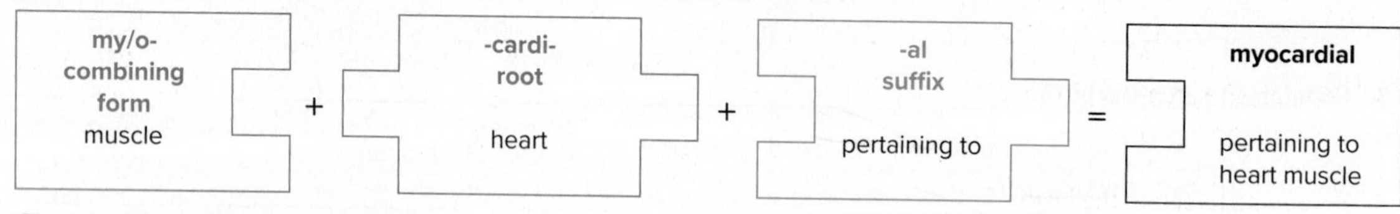

Changing the suffix to *-um,* meaning *a structure,* results in the term **myocardium,** *the structure called the heart muscle.*

The term **cardiomyopathy** contains the suffix -pathy, meaning *a disease,* the combining form *cardi/o-,* meaning the *heart,* and the combining form *my/o-,* meaning *muscle.* When you put this all together, the term **cardiomyopathy** means *a disease of the heart muscle.*

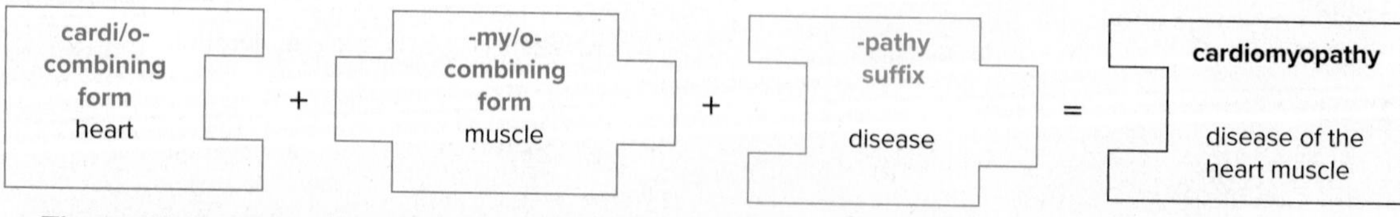

The term **ischemia** has the suffix *-emia,* which means *a blood condition.* The root *isch-* means *to block.* **Ischemia** means *a blockage of blood flow.* The term **myocardial ischemia** means *a blockage of blood flow to the heart muscle*–better known as a heart attack.

Word Analysis and Definition

S = Suffix P = Prefix R = Root R/CF = Combining Form

WORD	PRONUNCIATION	ELEMENTS		DEFINITION
cardiologist	kar-dee-**OL**-oh-jist	S/ R/CF	-logist *one who studies and is a specialist in* cardi/o- *heart*	A medical specialist in the diagnosis and treatment of disorders of the heart
cardiology	kar-dee-**OL**-oh-jee	S/	-logy *study of*	Medical specialty of diseases of the heart
cardiomyopathy	KAR-dee-oh-my-**OP**-ah-thee	S/ R/CF R/CF	-pathy *disease* cardi/o- *heart* -my/o- *muscle*	Disease of the heart muscle, the myocardium
diagnosis (noun)	die-ag-**NO**-sis	P/ R/	**dia-** *complete* **-gnosis** *knowledge of an abnormal condition*	The determination of the cause of a disease
diagnoses (pl) **diagnostic (adj)** (**Note:** *The "is" in -gnosis is deleted to allow the word to flow.*)	die-ag-**NO**-seez die-ag-**NOS**-tik	S/	-tic *pertaining to*	Pertaining to or establishing a diagnosis
diagnose (verb)	die-ag-**NOSE**	R/	-gnose *recognize an abnormal condition*	To make a diagnosis
electrocardiogram	ee-lek-troh-**KAR**-dee-oh-gram	S/ R/CF R/CF	-gram *record* electr/o- *electricity* -cardi/o- *heart*	Record of the heart's electrical signals
hypotensive (adj)	**HIGH**-po-**TEN**-siv	S/ P/ R/	-ive *pertaining to* hypo- *low* -tens- *pressure*	Pertaining to or suffering from low blood pressure
infarct	in-**FARKT**	P/ R/	in- *in* -farct *area of dead tissue*	An area of cell death resulting from blockage of its blood supply
infarction	in-**FARK**-shun	S/	-ion *action, condition*	Sudden blockage of an artery
ischemia	is-**KEY**-me-ah	S/ R/	-emia *a blood condition* isch- *to block*	Lack of blood supply to tissue
ischemic (adj)	is-**KEY**-mik	S/	-emic *pertaining to a condition of the blood*	Pertaining to the lack of blood supply to tissue
myocardial (adj)	MY-oh-**KAR**-dee-al	S/ R/CF R/	-al *pertaining to* my/o- *muscle* -cardi- *heart*	Pertaining to heart muscle
myocardium	MY-oh-**KAR**-dee-um	S/	-um *structure*	All the heart muscle
prognosis (noun)	prog-**NO**-sis	P/ R/	**pro-** *before, project forward* **-gnosis** *knowledge of an abnormal condition*	A forecast of the probable course and outcome of a disease

Changing the suffix *-emia* to *-emic,* which means *pertaining to a condition of the blood,* creates a new term, **ischemic,** that is an adjective. It means *pertaining to a blockage of blood flow.* It has a root and a suffix.

EXERCISES

Precision in communication: *In addition to using the precise medical terms and speaking and spelling them correctly, you must use the appropriate form of the term as well.*

A. There are several forms for the term diagnosis. *Note that there are singular and plural forms of the term, as well as the noun, adjective, and verb forms. Insert the correct form of the term in the documentation below.* **LO 1.1, 1.2, and 1.7**

Note: A noun is a person, place, or thing. Singular: One
A verb denotes action. Plural: More than one
An adjective usually describes something.

1. The primary ___________ for this patient is myocardial ischemia.
2. Dr. Bannerjee is unable to ____________ this patient until he receives the lab results.
3. The ___________ tests have been ordered for this patient first thing in the morning.
4. It is possible for this patient to have multiple _________ if there is more than one condition present.

B. Identify the form of the term diagnosis. *Fill in the blanks.* **LO 1.4 and 1.7**

1. The verb form: ______________________________
2. Plural form: ______________________________
3. Singular noun: ______________________________
4. Adjective form: ______________________________

Lesson 1.2 (cont'd)

Communication

Some medical terms are pronounced the same but spelled differently. For example:

- Both *ilium* and *ileum* are pronounced **ILL**-ee-um. *Ilium* is a bone in the pelvis; *ileum* is a segment of the small intestine.
- Both *mucus* and *mucous* are pronounced **MYU**-kus. *Mucus* is a noun and is the name of a fluid secreted by *mucous* (adjective) membranes that line body cavities.

A medical term may relate to more than one anatomical structure.

- The term *cervical* means relating to a neck in any sense.
- It can pertain to the neck that joins the head to the trunk with the cervical vertebrae.
- It can also pertain to the cervix of the uterus, with its cervical canal.

Some words, when incorrectly pronounced, sound the same. For example:

- The term *prostate,* pronounced **PROS**-tate, refers to the gland at the base of the male bladder. The term *prostrate* means to be physically weak or exhausted, or to lie flat on the ground.
- Train your ear to hear the differences—*reflex* is not *reflux.*

Many medical terms form a verb, a noun, a plural, and an adjective, and you have to know them all, as in diagnose, diagnosis, diagnoses, and diagnostic (see the WAD on the previous spread).

Plurals (LO 1.5)

Many words in the English language allow you to change them from singular to plural by adding an "s." For medical terms, this rarely happens, as these plurals are formed in ways that were once logical to Greeks and Romans but now have to be learned by memory in English. Examples of medical terms with Greek and Latin plurals are shown in *Table 1.1*.

Throughout this book, the Greek and Latin plurals of medical terms appear in the Word Analysis and Definition box with the singular medical term, as with the term **diagnosis** in the previous spread.

▼ TABLE 1.1

SINGULAR AND PLURAL FORMS

Singular Ending	Plural Ending	Examples
-a		axilla
	-ae	axillae
-ax		thorax
	-aces	thoraces
-en		lumen
	-ina	lumina
-ex		cortex
	-ices	cortices
-is		diagnosis
	-es	diagnoses
-is		epididymis
	-ides	epididymides
-ix		appendix
	-ices	appendices
-ma		carcinoma
	-mata	carcinomata
-on		ganglion
	-a	ganglia
-um		septum
	-a	septa
-us		viscus
	-era	viscera
-us		villus
	-i	villi
-us		corpus
	-ora	corpora
-x		phalanx
	-ges	phalanges
-y		ovary
	-ies	ovaries
-yx		calyx
	-ices	calices

Pronunciation (LO 1.6)

Being able to pronounce words correctly is essential to effective communication. In the medical world, this concept is especially important. As a health professional, you will routinely use medical terms and your colleagues must be able to understand what you are saying. Correct pronunciation is crucial to patient safety and your ability to provide high-quality patient care.

Throughout this book, the pronunciation of medical terms is spelled out phonetically using modern English forms to show you exactly how the terms are pronounced. The word part to be emphasized is shown in bold, uppercase letters.

For example, **pulmonary** is phonetically written **PUL**-moh-nar-ee, and **pulmonology** is written **PUL**-moh-**NOL**-oh-jee. This illustrates that words derived from the same root can have their emphasis placed on different parts of the word and that the emphasized part can be from different elements. The emphasized syllable **NOL** comes partly from the **combining form** *pulmon/o-* and partly from the suffix *-logy.* You can hear glossary terms pronounced correctly by visiting the audio glossary in Connect® (connect.mheducation.com).

Word Analysis and Definition

S = Suffix P = Prefix R = Root R/CF = Combining Form

WORD	PRONUNCIATION	ELEMENTS		DEFINITION
axilla **axillae (pl)** **axillary (adj)**	**AK**-sill-ah **AK**-sill-ee **AK**-sill-air-ee	 S/ R/	Latin *armpit* -ary *pertaining to* axill- *armpit*	Medical term for the armpit Pertaining to the armpit
dementia	dee-**MEN**-she-ah	S/ P/ R/	-ia *condition* de- *without* -ment- *mind*	Chronic, progressive, irreversible loss of intellectual and mental functions
ganglion **ganglia (pl)**	**GANG**-lee-on **GANG**-lee-ah		Greek *a swelling* or *knot*	A fluid-filled cyst or a collection of nerve cells outside the brain and spinal cord
ileum **ilium** **ilia (pl)**	**ILL**-ee-um **ILL**-ee-um **ILL**-ee-ah		Latin *to twist* or *roll up* Latin *groin*	Third portion of the small intestine. Large wing-shaped bone at the upper and posterior part of the pelvis
mucus (noun) **mucous (adj)** **mucosa**	**MYU**-kus **MYU**-kus myu-**KOH**-sah	 S/ R/ S/	Greek *slime* -ous *pertaining to* muc- *mucus* -osa *full of; like*	Sticky secretion of cells in mucous membranes Pertaining to mucus or the mucosa Lining of a tubular structure that secretes mucus
prostate **prostrate** **prostration (noun)**	**PROS**-tate pros-**TRAYT** pros-**TRAY**-shun		Greek *one who stands before* Latin *to stretch out*	Organ surrounding the urethra at the base of the male urinary bladder To lay flat or to be overcome by physical weakness and exhaustion
reflex **reflux**	**REE**-fleks **REE**-fluks		Latin *bend back* Latin *backward flow*	An involuntary response to a stimulus Backward flow
septum **septa (pl)**	**SEP**-tum **SEP**-tah		Latin *a partition*	A thin wall separating two cavities or two tissue masses

EXERCISES

A. Medical language: *Many terms in medicine sound and/or look very similar. The difference of only one letter can make a new term. Train your eye and ear to know the difference. Select the correct choice of terms in the following documentation.* **LO 1.6 and 1.7**

1. The patient's nasal (mucus/mucous) membrane is severely infected.
2. Schedule this patient for a (prostrate/prostate) exam at his next annual physical.
3. The doctor checked the (reflex/reflux) in the patient's knee.
4. The patient's (ilium/ileum) was severely fractured in the motor vehicle accident.

B. Plurals: *Select the correct form of the plural in the following sentences.* **LO 1.5**

1. Because of additional medical problems needing treatment, this patient's insurance claim form will have multiple (diagnoses/diagnosis).
2. Check both (axilla/axillae) for any evidence of enlarged lymph nodes.
3. Several (septa/septum) exist in the body—e.g., in the heart and in the nose.
4. A cluster of (ganglia/ganglion) has formed on her left wrist.

C. Terminology challenge: *Use your knowledge of the new medical terms you have learned in this chapter and choose the correct answer.* **LO 1.7**

1. The term *cervical* can apply to two different places in the body. Where are they?
   a. neck of the body and neck of the femur
   b. neck of the uterus and neck of the humerus
   c. neck of the femur and neck of the humerus
   d. neck of the body and neck of the uterus
2. The terms *ileum* and *ilium* are pronounced the same but are in two different body systems. Where are they?
   a. muscular and nervous systems
   b. digestive and skeletal systems
   c. circulatory and integumentary systems
   d. endocrine and respiratory systems

Precision in Communication (LO 1.7)

Keynotes

- Many words, when they are written or pronounced, have an element that if misspelled or mispronounced gives the intended word an entirely different meaning. A treatment response to the different meaning could cause a medical error or even the death of a patient.
- Precision in written and verbal communication is essential to prevent errors in patient care.
- The medical record in which you document a patient's care and your actions is a legal document. It can be used in court as evidence in professional medical liability cases.

It's important for you to note that being accurate and precise in both your written and verbal communication with your health care team can save someone's life. Each year in the United States, more than 400,000 people die because of drug reactions and medical errors, many of which are the result of poor communication. On the next page, you will find some specific examples of how certain medical terms could be seriously miscommunicated and misinterpreted.

Case Report 1.2 *(continued)*

Mr. Donovan is waiting to be admitted to the hospital and is receiving oxygen through nasal prongs. He is **hypotensive,** and an **intravenous (IV) infusion** of normal saline has been started. According to his medical record, he is being seen in the **neurology** clinic for early dementia.

In the above Case Report involving Mr. Donovan, if **hypotensive** (suffering from **low** blood pressure) were confused with **hypertensive** (suffering from **high** blood pressure), incorrect and dangerous treatments could be prescribed.

- In the word **hypotensive,** the suffix-*ive* means *pertaining to.* The prefix *hypo-* means *below or less than normal.* The root-*tens-* means *pressure.* The term **hypotensive** means *pertaining to or suffering from a below normal or low blood pressure.*
- In the word **hypertensive,** the prefix *hyper-* means *above or higher than normal.* The term **hypertensive** means *pertaining to or suffering from an above normal or high blood pressure.*

Abbreviation

IV intravenous

To deconstruct the term **hypotensive,** start with the suffix-*ive,* which means *pertaining to* or *suffering from.* Next, the prefix *hypo-* means *below or less than normal.* Then the root-*tens-* means *pressure.* Now, place the pieces together to form a word meaning *suffering from a below-normal pressure* or *low blood pressure.*

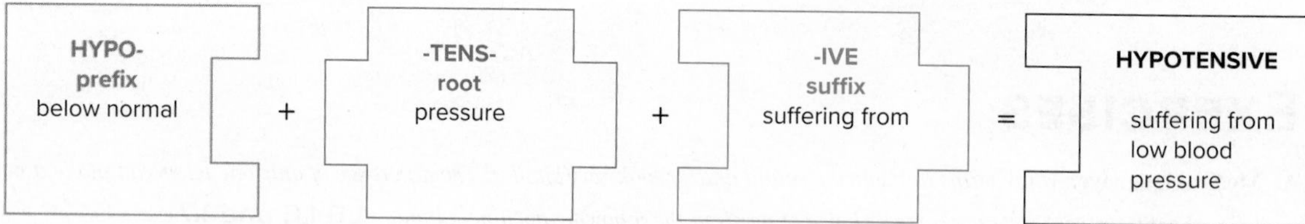

Keynotes

- Communicate verbally and in writing with attention to detail, accuracy, and precision.
- When you understand the individual word elements that make up a medical term, you are better able to understand clearly the medical terms you are using.

Also in the above Case Report, the term **neurology,** the specialty of the nervous system *(see Chapter 10),* can sound very similar to **urology,** the study of the urinary system *(see Chapter 13).* In the urinary system, if a patient's **ureter** (the tube from the kidney to the bladder) were confused with the **urethra** (the tube from the bladder to the outside), the consequences could be serious.

As you can see from the above examples, your ability to correctly identify, spell, and pronounce different medical terms is essential. Being a health professional requires the utmost attention to detail, as a patient's life could be in your hands. Incorrect spelling and poor pronunciation not only reflect badly on you and your health team—it could also be a matter of life and death.

Word Analysis and Definition

S = Suffix P = Prefix R = Root R/CF = Combining Form

WORD	PRONUNCIATION	ELEMENTS		DEFINITION
cervical (adj) cervix	**SER**-vih-kal **SER**-viks	S/ R/	**-al** *pertaining to* **cervic-** *neck* Latin *neck*	Pertaining to the cervix or to the neck region Lower part of the uterus
hypertension hypertensive (adj) hypotension hypotensive (adj)	**HIGH**-per-**TEN**-shun **HIGH**-per-**TEN**-siv **HIGH**-poh-**TEN**-shun **HIGH**-poh-**TEN**-siv	S/ P/ R/ S/ P/	**-ion** *condition, action* **hyper-** *above normal* **-tens-** *pressure* **-ive** *pertaining to* **hypo-** *below normal*	Persistent high arterial blood pressure Pertaining to or suffering from high blood pressure Persistent low arterial blood pressure Pertaining to or suffering from low blood pressure
infusion transfusion	in-**FYU**-zhun trans-**FYU**-zhun	P/ R/ P/	**in-** *in* **-fusion** *to pour* **trans-** *across, through*	Introduction of a substance other than blood intravenously Transfer of blood or a blood component from a donor to a recipient
intravenous	**IN**-trah-**VEE**-nus	S/ P/ R/	**-ous** *pertaining to* **intra-** *within, inside* **-ven-** *vein*	Inside a vein
neurology neurologist	nyu-**ROL**-oh-jee nyu-**ROL**-oh-jist	S/ R/CF S/	**-logy** *study of* **neur/o-** *nerve* **-logist** *one who studies and is a specialist in*	Medical specialty of disorders of the nervous system Medical specialist in disorders of the nervous system
protocol	**PRO**-toe-kol		Latin *contents page of a book*	Detailed plan; in this case, for a regimen of therapy
ureter urethra urology	you-**REE**-ter you-**REE**-thrah you-**ROL**-oh-jee	S/ R/CF	Greek *urinary canal* Greek *passage for urine* **-logy** *study of* **ur/o-** *urine*	Tube that connects a kidney to the urinary bladder Canal leading from the bladder to the outside Medical specialty of disorders of the urinary system
uterus	**YOU**-ter-us		Latin *womb*	Organ in which an egg develops into a fetus
vertebra vertebrae (pl)	**VER**-teh-brah **VER**-teh-brae		Latin *bone in the spine*	One of the bones of the spinal column

EXERCISES

A. Patient documentation: *Read the following excerpts from patient charts and insert the medical term that correctly completes each sentence.* **LO 1.7**

1. This patient has several badly fractured ________________ in his spinal column.
2. This patient has nerve damage. Refer him to the department of ________________.
3. Schedule this patient for an ________________ of chemotherapy drugs today.
4. This patient has low blood pressure–he is ________________ and anemic.
5. I am ordering an immediate ________________ of 2 units of whole blood for this patient.
6. Send this patient for ________________ X-rays of his neck immediately.

B. Brain teaser: *Challenge yourself to analyze the question and insert the correct answers.* **LO 1.1, 1.2, and 1.7**

1. If a medical specialist in the study of disorders of the nervous system is a neurologist, what is a medical specialist in the study of disorders of the urinary system called?
   (Hint: Use your knowledge of suffixes and roots to help you.)
2. What element is the difference between high blood pressure and low blood pressure? ________________
3. What is the tube that connects a kidney to the bladder? ________________
4. What substance goes through a transfusion but not through an infusion? ________________

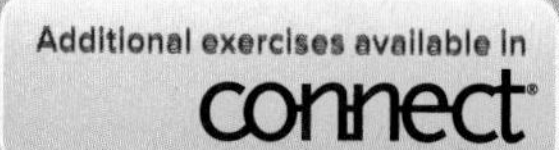

Chapter Review exercises, along with additional practice items, are available in Connect!

The Body as a Whole, Cells, and Genes

CHAPTER 2

The Essentials of the Languages of Anatomy and Genetics

Classic Collection/Shotshop GmbH/Alamy Images

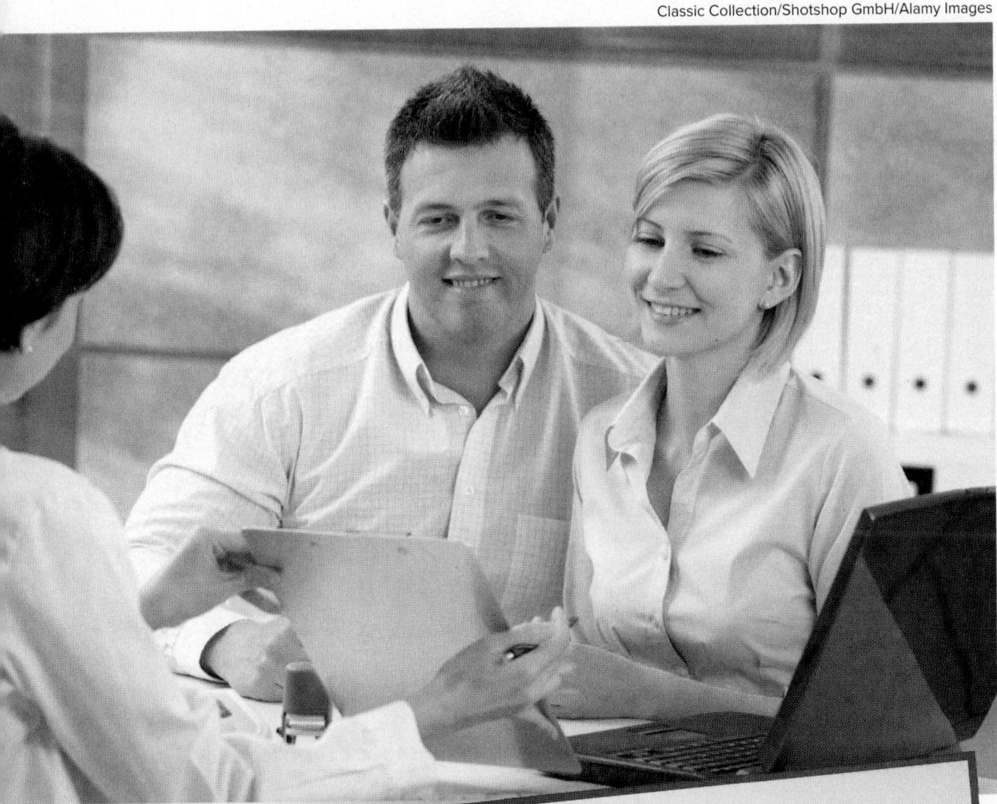

CASE REPORT 2.1

You are . . .

. . . a certified medical assistant (**CMA**) employed as an in vitro fertilization coordinator in the Assisted Reproduction Clinic at Fulwood Medical Center.

You are communicating with . . .

. . . Mrs. Mary Arnold, a 35-year-old woman who has been unable to **conceive. In vitro fertilization (IVF)** was recommended. After **hormone** therapy, several healthy and mature eggs were recovered from her **ovary.** The eggs were combined with her husband's **sperm** in a laboratory dish where **fertilization** occurred to form a single cell, called a **zygote.** The cells were allowed to divide for five days to become **blastocysts,** and then four blastocysts were implanted in her uterus.

Your role is to guide, counsel, and support Mrs. Arnold and her husband through the implementation and follow-up for the IVF process.

Learning Outcomes

Effective medical treatment recognizes that each organ, tissue, and cell in your body, no matter where it's located, is connected to and functions in harmony with every other organ, tissue, and cell. To understand these concepts, you need to be able to:

- **LO 2.1** **Use roots, combining forms, suffixes, and prefixes to construct and analyze (deconstruct) medical terms related to the anatomy and physiology of the body as a whole.**
- **LO 2.2** **Spell and pronounce correctly medical terms related to the body as a whole in order to communicate with accuracy and precision in any health care setting.**
- **LO 2.3** **Discuss the medical terms associated with cells and tissues.**
- **LO 2.4** **Explain the terms genes, genetics, and gene therapy.**
- **LO 2.5** **Describe the primary tissue groups and their functions.**
- **LO 2.6** **Relate individual organs and organ systems to the organization and function of the body as a whole.**
- **LO 2.7** **Integrate the medical terms of the different anatomic positions, planes, and directions of the body into everyday medical language.**
- **LO 2.8** **Describe the nine regions of the abdomen.**
- **LO 2.9** **Map the body cavities.**
- **LO 2.10** **Apply your knowledge of the medical terms of the body as a whole to documentation, medical records, and medical reports.**
- **LO 2.11** **Translate the medical terms of the body as a whole into everyday language in order to communicate clearly with patients and their families.**

Abbreviations

CMA	certified medical assistant
IVF	in vitro fertilization

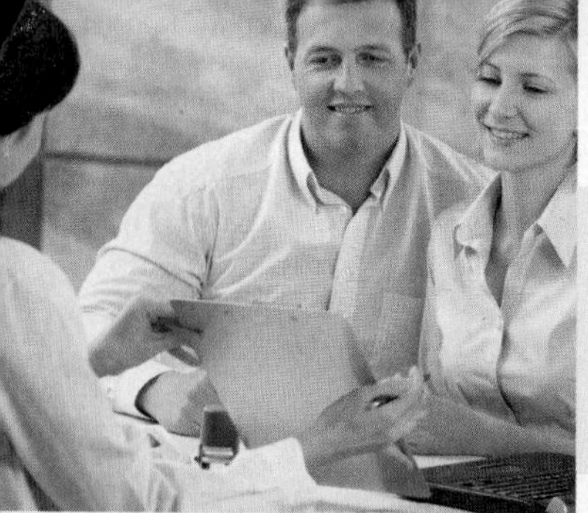

Classic Collection/Shotshop GmbH/Alamy Images

Lesson 2.1

Composition of Body and Cells

Objectives

All the different elements of your body interact with each other to support constant change as your body reacts to your environment and to the nourishment you give it. To understand the structure and function of the elements of your body, you need to be able to:

2.1.1 Name the medical terms associated with cells, tissues, and organs.

2.1.2 Discuss the medical terminology for the major structures and functions of a cell.

Composition of the Body (LO 2.1 and 2.2)

- The whole body or organism is composed of **organ systems** *(Figure 2.1).*
    - Organ systems are composed of **organs.**
        - Organs are composed of **tissues.**
            - Tissues are composed of **cells.**
                - Cells are composed in part of **organelles.**
                    - Organelles are composed of **molecules.**
                        - Molecules are composed of **atoms.**

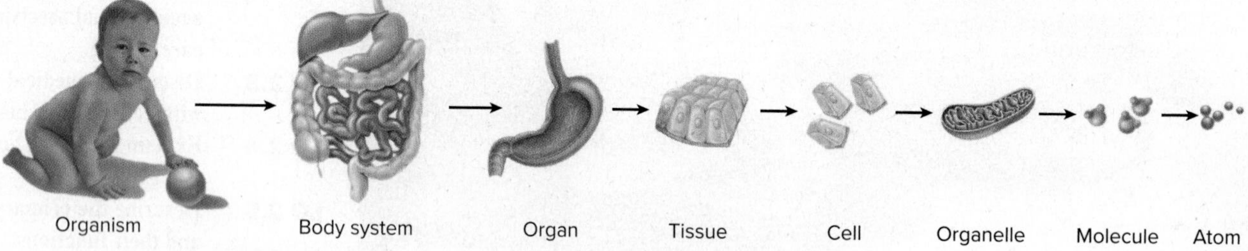

▲ **FIGURE 2.1**
Composition of the Body.

The Cell (LO 2.3)

The result of the **fertilization** of an egg by a sperm is a single fertilized cell called a **zygote** *(Figure 2.2).* This process is also called **conception.** This zygote is the origin of every cell in your body. It divides and multiplies into trillions of cells, which become the basic unit of every tissue and organ. These cells are responsible for the structure and all the functions of your tissues and organs.

Cytology is the study of cell structure and function, and this forms the basis of the knowledge of the anatomy and physiology of every tissue and organ.

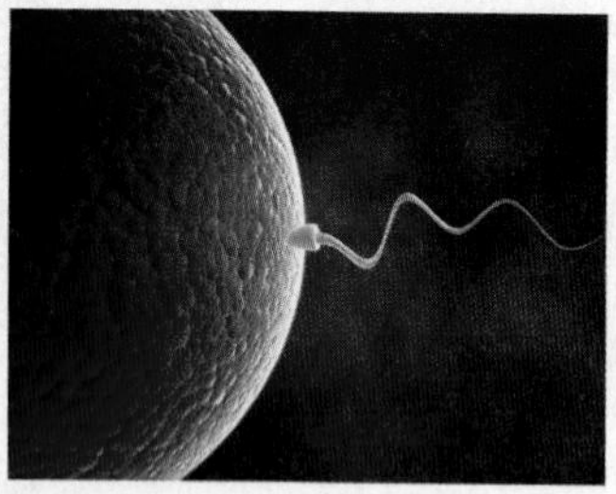

▲ **FIGURE 2.2**
Fertilization of Egg by Single Sperm.

Jezper/Shutterstock

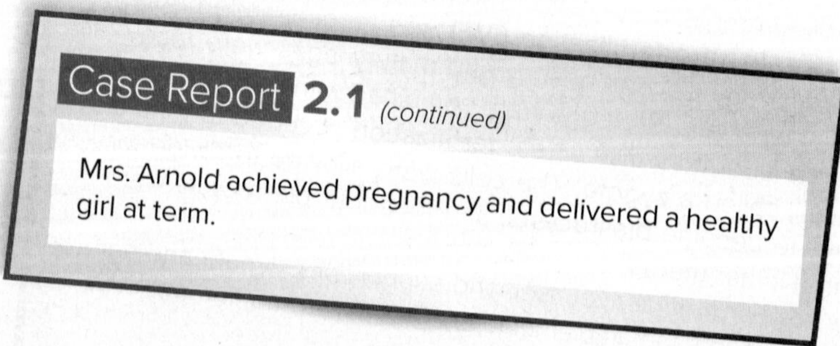

Case Report 2.1 *(continued)*

Mrs. Arnold achieved pregnancy and delivered a healthy girl at term.

Word Analysis and Definition

S = Suffix P = Prefix R = Root R/CF = Combining Form

WORD	PRONUNCIATION	ELEMENTS		DEFINITION
cell	**SELL**		Latin a *storeroom*	The smallest unit of the body capable of independent existence
conception	kon-**SEP**-shun		Latin *something received*	Fertilization of the egg by sperm to form a zygote
cytology	**SIGH**-tol-oh-jee	S/ R/CF	**-logy** *study of* **cyt/o-** *cell*	Study of the cell
cytologist	**SIGH**-tol-oh-jist	S/	**-logist** *one who studies, a specialist*	Specialist in the structure, chemistry, and pathology of the cell
fertilization (noun)	**FER**-til-eye-**ZAY**-shun	S/ R/	**-ation** *process* **fertiliz-** *to make fruitful*	Union of a male sperm and a female egg
fertilize (verb)	**FER**-til-ize		Greek *to bear*	Penetration of the egg by sperm
in vitro	en-**VEE**-troh		Latin *glass*	In vitro fertilization is the process of combining sperm and eggs in a laboratory dish and placing resulting embryos inside a uterus
organ	**OR**-gan		Latin *instrument, tool*	Structure with specific functions in a body system
organelle	**OR**-gah-nell	S/ R/	**-elle** *small* **organ-** *organ*	Part of a cell having specialized function(s)
organism	**OR**-gan-izm	S/	**-ism** *condition, process*	Any whole living, individual plant or animal
tissue	**TISH**-you		Latin *to weave*	Collection of similar cells
zygote	**ZYE**-goat		Greek *yolk*	Cell resulting from the union of sperm and egg

EXERCISES

A. Review *the terms related to the composition of the body and the cell. Pay careful attention to word elements and meanings. Fill in the blanks.* **LO 2.1 and 2.3**

1. Put the following terms in ascending order of their size:

organism **cells** **molecules** **organs**

organ systems **organelles** **atoms** **tissues**

a. ______________________________

b. ______________________________

c. ______________________________

d. ______________________________

e. ______________________________

f. ______________________________

g. ______________________________

h. ______________________________

B. Use the terms *and their elements related to the cell to answer the questions.* **LO 2.1 and 2.2**

1. The suffix ______________ means *study of.* The suffix that means *specialist (in the study of)* is ______________________________.

2. What part of *cyt/o* makes it a combining form rather than a root? ______________________________

3. What is the medical term for *union of a male sperm and a female egg?* ______________________________

4. What suffix related to the composition of the body and the cell describes the size of something? ______________________________

5. What does a cytologist study? ______________________________

Keynote

- The cytoplasm is a clear, gelatinous substance crowded with different organelles.

Abbreviations

DNA deoxyribonucleic acid
RNA ribonucleic acid

Structure and Function of Cells (LO 2.3)

As the zygote divides, every cell it creates becomes a complex little factory that carries out these basic life functions:

- **Manufacture** of **proteins** and **lipids;**
- **Production** and use of energy;
- **Communication** with other cells;
- **Replication** of **deoxyribonucleic acid (DNA);** and
- **Reproduction** of itself.

All cells contain a fluid called **cytoplasm** (intracellular fluid) surrounded by a cell **membrane** *(Figure 2.3).* Your cell membrane–made of **proteins** and **lipids**–allows water, oxygen, glucose, **electrolytes, steroids,** and alcohol to pass through it. On the outside of the cell membrane, you have receptors that bind to chemical messengers like **hormones** sent by other cells. These are the chemical signals by which your cells communicate with each other.

Organelles (LO 2.2)

Organelles are small structures in the cytoplasm of the cell that carry out special **metabolic** tasks (the chemical processes that occur in the cell).

The **nucleus** is the largest organelle *(Figure 2.3).* It is surrounded by its own membrane and directs all the cell's activities. The 46 molecules of DNA in the nucleus form 46 **chromosomes.**

A **nucleolus** is a small, dense body composed of **ribonucleic acid (RNA)** and protein found in the nucleus. It is involved in the manufacture of proteins from simple materials–a process called **anabolism.**

Mitochondria are the cell's powerhouses. They produce energy by breaking down compounds like glucose and fat in a process called **catabolism.**

- **Metabolism** is the sum of the constructive processes of anabolism and the destructive processes of catabolism within a cell **(intracellular).**

The **endoplasmic reticulum** manufactures steroids, cholesterol and other lipids, and proteins. It also detoxifies alcohol and other drugs.

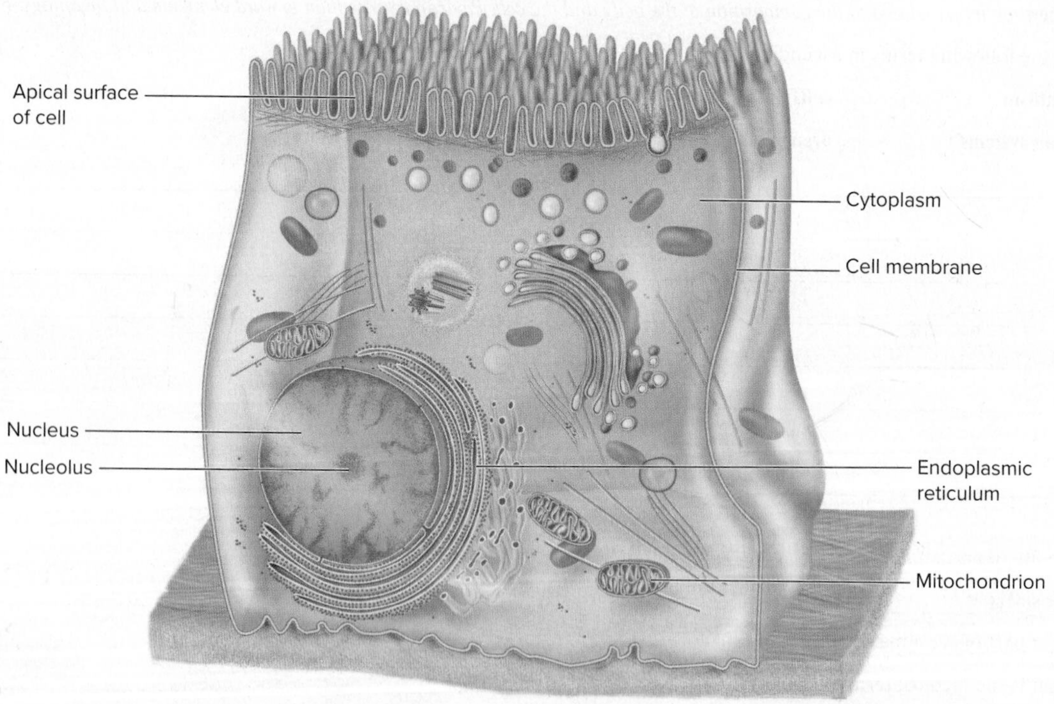

▲ **FIGURE 2.3**
Structure of a Representative Cell.

Word Analysis and Definition

S = Suffix P = Prefix R = Root R/CF = Combining Form

WORD	PRONUNCIATION		ELEMENTS	DEFINITION
anabolism	an-**AB**-oh-lizm	S/ R/	-ism *process, condition* anabol- *build up*	The buildup of complex substances in the cell from simpler ones as a part of metabolism
catabolism	kah-**TAB**-oh-lizm	S/ R/	-ism *process, condition* catabol- *break down*	The breakdown of complex substances into simpler ones as a part of metabolism
chromosome	**KROH**-moh-sohm	S/ R/CF	-some *body* chrom/o- *color*	Body in the nucleus that contains DNA and genes
cytoplasm	**SIGH**-toh-plazm	S/ R/CF	-plasm *something formed* cyt/o- *cell*	Clear, gelatinous substance that forms the substance of a cell, except for the nucleus
deoxyribonucleic acid (DNA)	dee-**OCK**-see-rye-boh-nyu-**KLEE**-ik **ASS**-id		deoxyribose *a sugar* nucleic acid *a protein*	Source of hereditary characteristics found in chromosomes
electrolyte	ee-**LEK**-troh-lite	S/ R/CF	-lyte *soluble* electr/o- *electricity*	Substance that, when dissolved in a suitable medium, forms electrically charged particles
hormone hormonal (adj)	**HOR**-mohn hor-**MOHN**-al	S/ R/	Greek *set in motion* -al *pertaining to* hormon- *hormone*	Chemical formed in one tissue or organ and carried by the blood to stimulate or inhibit a function of another tissue or organ Pertaining to a hormone
intracellular	in-trah-**SELL**-you-lar	S/ P/ R/	-ar *pertaining to* intra- *within* -cellul- *small cell*	Within the cell
lipid	**LIP**-id		Greek *fat*	General term for all types of fatty compounds; for example, cholesterol, triglycerides, and fatty acids
membrane membranous (adj)	**MEM**-brain **MEM**-brah-nus	S/ R/	Latin *parchment* -ous *pertaining to* membran- *cover, skin*	Thin layer of tissue covering a structure or cavity Pertaining to a membrane
metabolism metabolic (adj)	meh-**TAB**-oh-lizm met-ah-**BOL**-ik	S/ R/ S/	-ism *condition, process* metabol- *change* -ic *pertaining to*	The constantly changing physical and chemical processes occurring in the cell that are the sum of anabolism and catabolism Pertaining to metabolism
mitochondria (pl) mitochondrion (singular)	my-toe-**KON**-dree-ah my-toe-**KON**-dree-on	S/ R/CF R/ S/	-ia *condition* mit/o- *thread* -chondr- *granule* -ion *condition*	Organelles that generate, store, and release energy for cell activities
nucleolus	nyu-**KLEE**-oh-lus	S/ R/CF	-lus *small* nucle/o- *nucleus*	Small mass within the nucleus
nucleus nuclear (adj)	**NYU**-klee-us **NYU**-klee-ar	S/ R/	Latin *command center* -ar *pertaining to* nucle- *nucleus*	Functional center of a cell or structure Pertaining to a nucleus
protein	**PRO**-teen		Greek *protein*	Class of food substances based on amino acids
ribonucleic acid (RNA)	RYE-boh-nyu-**KLEE**-ik **ASS**-id	S/ P/ R/	-ic *pertaining to* ribo- *from ribose, a sugar* -nucle- *nucleus*	The information carrier from DNA in the nucleus to an organelle to produce protein molecules
steroid	**STAIR**-oyd	S/ R/	-oid *resembling* ster- *solid*	Large family of chemical substances found in many drugs, hormones, and body components

EXERCISE

A. Knowledge *of elements is your best clue to determining the meaning of medical terminology. Deconstruct the elements in these questions to find your answers. Select the BEST ANSWER to the question.* **LO 2.3**

1. Which term relates to electrically charged particles?

a. protein **b.** hormonal **c.** electrolyte

2. Which term relates to change?

a. steroid **b.** metabolic **c.** lipid

3. Which term has an element meaning "condition"?

a. metabolism **b.** cytoplasm **c.** hormone

4. What is a thin layer of tissue that covers a structure or cavity?

a. lipid **b.** membrane **c.** hormone

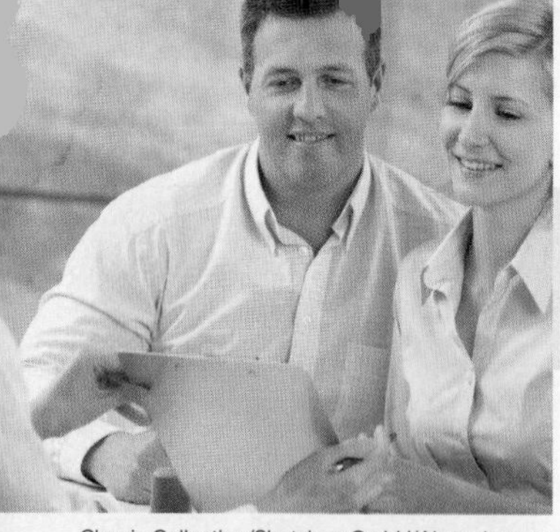

Classic Collection/Shotshop GmbH/Alamy Images

Lesson 2.2

Genes and Genetics

Objectives

- **2.2.1** Describe the structure and functions of deoxyribonucleic acid (DNA).
- **2.2.2** Discuss the roles of genes in heredity.
- **2.2.3** Define mitosis.
- **2.2.4** Discuss mutations and epigenetic changes.

DNA and Genes (LO 2.4)

Inside the cell nucleus are packed 46 molecules of **deoxyribonucleic acid (DNA)** as thin strands called **chromatin**. When cells divide, the chromatin condenses with **histone** proteins to form 23 pairs (46 total) of densely coiled bodies called **chromosomes**. Twenty-two of these pairs look the same in both males and females. In the 23rd pair, females have two copies of the X chromosome; males have one X and one Y. The picture of the human chromosomes lined up in pairs is called a **karyotype** *(Figure 2.4)*.

The information in DNA is stored as a code of four chemical bases: adenine (A), guanine (G), cytosine (C), and thymine (T). The total human DNA contains about 3 billion bases, and more than 99% of those bases are the same in all people. The sequence of these bases determines the building and maintaining of the organism's cells, similar to the way in which letters of the alphabet appear in order to form words and sentences.

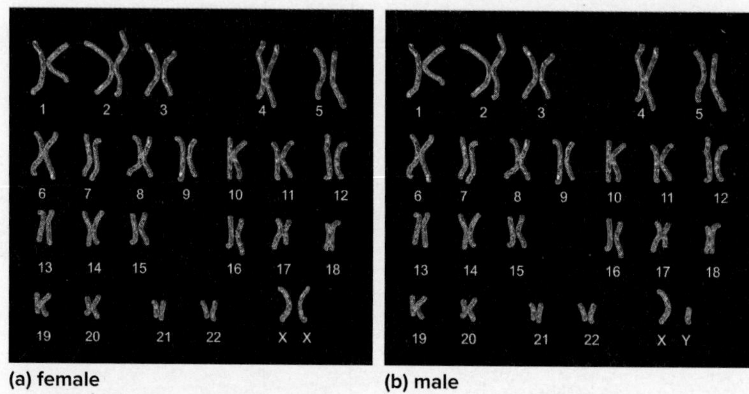

(a) female (b) male

FIGURE 2.4 Human Karyotype.

(a, b) Kateryna Kon/Shutterstock

The **chromosomal** DNA bases pair with each other–A with T and C with G–and are attached to a sugar molecule and a phosphate molecule. A base, sugar, and phosphate form a **nucleotide**. Nucleotides are arranged in two long strands to form a spiral called a double **helix**.

The nuclear DNA in the chromosomes is the **hereditary** material, each unit of which is called a **gene**. The genes act as instructions to make molecules of different proteins. Each person has two copies of each gene, one inherited from each parent. Most genes are the same in all people; only less than one percent is slightly different between people. These small differences contribute to each person's unique physical features. Humans are thought to have between 20,000 and 25,000 genes. This total is called the **genome**.

Abbreviations

A	adenosine
C	cytosine
DNA	deoxyribonucleic acid
G	guanine
T	thymine

Mitosis

The critical property of DNA is that it can **replicate**, make copies of itself, so that when cells divide, each new cell has an exact copy of the DNA present in the old cell. This cell division is called **mitosis**, in which a cell duplicates all of its contents, including its chromosomes, to form two identical daughter cells. When mitosis is not performed correctly, abnormal cells, such as cancer cells, can result.

Mutations and Epigenetic Changes

A permanent alteration of the nucleotide sequence of the genome of an organism is called a **mutation**. Mutations may or may not produce visible changes in the observable characteristics (**phenotype**) of an organism. Mutations play a part in both normal and abnormal biological processes including evolution, cancer, and the development of the immune system.

Chemical compounds that become added to single genes can regulate their activity to produce modifications known as **epigenetic** changes. These changes can remain as cells divide and can be inherited through generations. Environmental influences from pollution, drugs, pharmaceuticals, aging, and diets can also produce epigenetic modifications, such as cancers, mental disorders, and degenerative and metabolic disorders.

Keynotes

- Deoxyribonucleic acid (DNA) is the hereditary material in humans.
- DNA molecules are packaged into chromosomes.
- Genes are the basic functional and physical unit of **heredity** and are made up of DNA.
- Genes regulate the division and replication of cells.
- Cancer can result when cell division and replication are abnormal.
- Chemical compounds can be added to a gene and can lead to abnormal **genetic** (epigenetic) activity producing cancers and degenerative and metabolic diseases.

Word Analysis and Definition

S = Suffix P = Prefix R = Root R/CF = Combining Form

WORD	PRONUNCIATION	ELEMENTS		DEFINITION
chromatin	**KROH**-ma-tin	S/ R/CF	-tin *pertaining to* **chrom/a-** *color*	DNA that forms chromosomes during cell division
chromosome **chromosomal (adj)**	**KROH**-moh-sohm **KROH**-moh-**SO**-mal	R/CF R/ S/	**chrom/o-** *color* -some *body* -al *pertaining to*	The body in the cell nucleus that carries the genes Pertaining to a chromosome
deoxyribonucleic acid (DNA)	dee-**OCK**-see-**RYE**-boh-noo-**KLEE**-ik **ASS**-id	S/ P/ P/ R/ R/ R/	-ic *pertaining to* **de-** *without* **-oxy-** *oxygen* -ribo- *ribose* -nucle- *nucleus* acid *acid, low pH*	The chemical repository of hereditary characteristics
epigenetics	**EP**-ih-jeh-**NET**-iks	S/ P/ R/	-etics *pertaining to* **epi-** *above, over* -gen- *to create*	The study of disorders produced by the effects of chemical compounds (e.g., pollutants) or environmental influences (such as diet) on genes
gene **genetic (adj)** **genome**	JEEN jeh-**NET**-ik **JEE**-nome	S/ R/ R/	Greek *birth* -etic *pertaining to* **gen-** *to create* -ome *body*	The functional unit of heredity on a chromosome Pertaining to genetics A complete set of chromosomes
helix	**HEE**-liks		Greek *a coil*	A spiral of nucleotides in the structure of DNA
heredity **hereditary**	heh-**RED**-ih-tee heh-**RED**-ih-ter-ee	S/ R/	Latin *an heir* -ary *pertaining to* **heredit-** *inherited through genes*	The transmission of characteristics from parent to offspring Transmissible from parent to offspring
histone	**HIS**-tone	S/ R/	-one *chemical* **hist-** *tissue*	A simple protein found in the cell nucleus
karyotype	**KAIR**-ee-oh-type	S/ R/CF	-type *model* **kary/o-** *nucleus*	The chromosome characteristics of an individual cell
mitosis	my-**TOE**-sis		Greek *thread*	Cell division to create two identical cells, each with 46 chromosomes
mutation	myu-**TAY**-shun		Latin *to change*	A permanent alteration in the nucleotide sequence of the genome
nucleotide	**NYU**-klee-oh-tide	R/CF R/	**nucle/o-** *nucleus* -tide *time*	Combination of a DNA base, a sugar molecule, and a phosphate molecule
phenotype	**FEE**-noh-type	S/ R/CF	-type *model* **phen/o-** *appearance*	Manifestation of a genome
replicate	**REP**-lih-kate		Latin *a reply*	To produce an exact copy

EXERCISE

A. Use your knowledge of medical terminology related to genetics. Insert the correct term in the appropriate statement. **LO 2.4**

gene genome mitosis chromosomes chromatin

1. When the cell is maintaining normal function, DNA and proteins are contained within thin strands of ______________________.
2. When the cell is dividing, DNA wraps around the proteins and is contained within densely coiled bodies called ______________________.
3. The unit of nuclear DNA in the chromosomes is called a ______________________.
4. A ______________________ is a complete set of chromosomes.
5. The process of ______________________ occurs when a cell creates an exact copy of itself and divides into two identical cells.

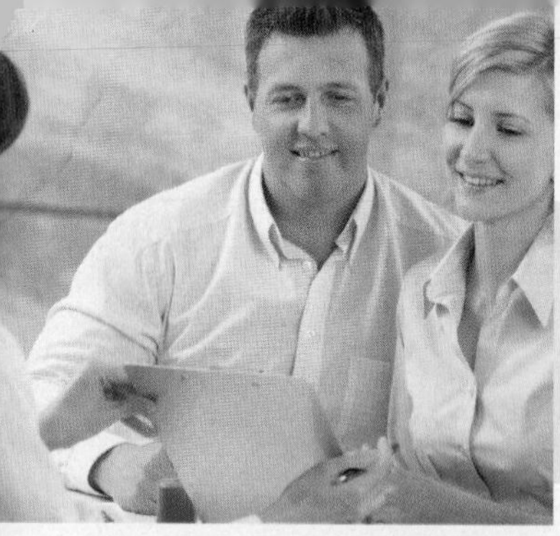

Classic Collection/Shotshop GmbH/Alamy Images

Lesson 2.3

Genetic Medicine

CASE REPORT 2.2

You are

. . . a physician's assistant (**PA**) in the Genetic Counseling Clinic at Fulwood Medical Center.

Your patient is

. . . Mrs. Patricia Bennet, a 52-year-old office manager with two daughters, aged 30 and 25. Mrs. Bennett's sister, aged 55, recently had a mastectomy for breast cancer and is now receiving chemotherapy. Their mother died of ovarian cancer in her late fifties. Mrs. Bennet wants to know her risk for breast or ovarian cancer, what she can do to prevent it, and what her daughters' risks are.

Objectives

- **2.3.1** Discuss the applications of medical genetics.
- **2.3.2** Define the concept of personalized medicine and its advantages.
- **2.3.3** Describe gene therapy.
- **2.3.4** Explain the values of predictive medicine.

Abbreviations

ADHD	attention deficit hyperactivity disorder
BRCA	breast cancer
PA	physician's assistant

Genetic Medicine (LO 2.4)

Medical genetics is the application of genetics to medical care. Genetic medicine is the newer term for medical genetics and incorporates areas such as gene therapy, personalized (precise) medicine, and predictive medicine.

Every person has a unique variation of the human genome and an individual's health stems from this genetic variation interacting with behaviors (drinking, smoking, etc.) and influences from the environment (chemical pollution in some form). Knowing the genetic makeup will enable more accurate diagnoses to be made, the source of the disease to be understood, and earlier, more accurate treatments or the prevention of progression of the disease provided. This concept is called *personalized medicine.*

One way that the biological variant is seen is responsiveness to drugs. Attention deficit hyperactivity disorder (ADHD) medications only work for one out of ten preschoolers, cancer drugs are effective for only one out of four patients, and depression drugs work for six out of ten patients. The drug Tamoxifen used to be prescribed to women with a form of breast cancer (BRCA), but 65% developed resistance to it. These women were found to have a mutation in their CYP2D6 gene that made Tamoxifen an ineffective treatment.

Personalized medicine can assist with preventive care. Women, such as Patricia Bennet in Case Report 2.2, are already being genotyped for mutations in the BRCA1 and BRCA2 genes if they have a family history of breast or ovarian cancer. In Mrs. Bennet's case, she is positive for both mutations and is now considering surgical measures that can then be taken to prevent the disease from developing. Her daughters have appointments to receive genetic testing in their own health plans.

Cytogenetics is the study of chromosome abnormalities to determine a cause for developmental delay, mental retardation, birth defects, and **dysmorphic** features, and chromosomal abnormalities are often detected in cancer cells.

Gene therapy is an experimental technique to replace a mutated gene that causes disease with a healthy copy, inactivate a mutated gene that is functioning improperly, or introduce a new gene into the body to prevent or help cure a disease. The **therapeutic** genes are introduced into body cells, and some 600 clinical trials utilizing this form of therapy are underway in the United States.

Predictive medicine looks at the probability of a disease and allows preventive measures to be taken. Examples are newborn screening to identify genetic disorders that can be treated early in life, and **prenatal** testing to look for diseases and conditions in an **embryo** or **fetus** whose parents have an increased risk of having a baby with a genetic or chromosomal disorder.

Word Analysis and Definition

S = Suffix P = Prefix R = Root R/CF = Combining Form

WORD	PRONUNCIATION	ELEMENTS		DEFINITION
cytogenetics	**SIGH**-toh-jeh-**NET**-iks	S/ R/CF R/	-etics *pertaining to* cyto- *cell* -gen- *create*	Study of chromosomal abnormalities in a cell
dysmorphology **dysmorphic**	dis-mor-**FOLL**-oh-jee dis-**MOR**-fik	S/ P/ R/CF S/	-logy *study of* **dys-** *difficult, bad* -morph/o- *form* -ic *pertaining to*	The study of developmental structural defects Possessing a developmental structural defect
embryo	**EM**-bree-oh		Greek *a young one*	Developing organism from conception until the end of the eighth week
fetus	**FEE**-tus		Latin *offspring*	Human organism from the end of the eighth week to birth
predictive	pree-**DIK**-tiv	S/ P/ R/	-ive *quality of* **pre-** *before* -dict- *consent*	The likelihood of a disease or disorder being present or occurring in the future
prenatal	pree-**NAY**-tal	S/ P/ R/	-al *pertaining to* **pre-** *before* -nat- *born*	Before birth
therapy **therapeutic**	**THAIR**-ah-pee **THAIR**-ah-**PYU**-tik		Greek *medical treatment* Greek *curing of a disorder or disease*	Systematic treatment of a disease, dysfunction, or disorder Curing or capable of curing a disorder or disease

EXERCISES

A. Discuss *the applications of medical genetics. Choose the correct answer to complete the following statements.* **LO 2.4**

1. The replacement of a mutated gene with a healthy copy is termed:

a. predictive medicine

b. cytogenetics

c. gene therapy

d. personalized medicine

2. The study of chromosome abnormalities in a cell is:

a. cytogenetics

b. dysmorphology

c. prenatal therapy

d. precise medicine

3. ________________ medicine uses genetics to determine accurate treatments for an existing condition.

a. Personalized

b. Preventative

c. Cytogenetic

d. Predictive

B. Not all terms can be deconstructed. *It is sometimes necessary to memorize the medical terms of Greek and Latin origin. Given the definition, provide the term that is being described. Fill in the blanks.* **LO 2.4**

1. Systematic treatment of a disease, dysfunction, or disorder. ________________________________

2. Human organism from conception to the end of the eighth week. ________________________________

3. Human organism from the end of the eighth week to birth. ________________________________

4. Curing or capable of curing a disorder or disease. ________________________________

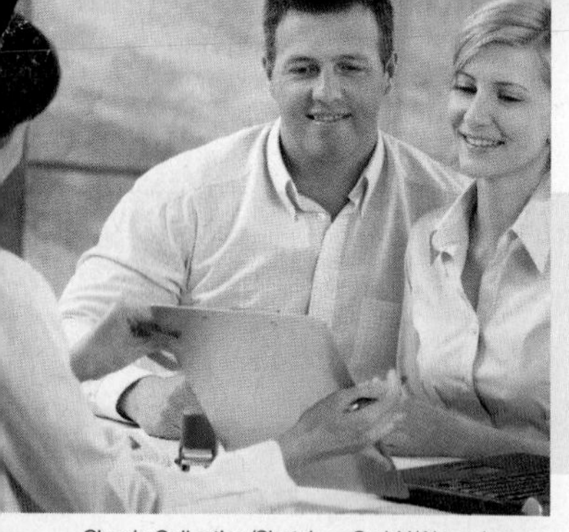

Classic Collection/Shotshop GmbH/Alamy Images

Lesson 2.4

Tissues, Organs, and Organ Systems

Objectives

Your tissues, organs, and organ systems must continually adapt and adjust in order to work in sync with each other. The information in this lesson will enable you to:

2.4.1 Define the four primary tissue groups.

2.4.2 Discuss the medical terminology for the structure and functions of each tissue group.

2.4.3 Name the organ systems.

2.4.4 Describe the medical terminology for the strucure and functions of each organ system.

Tissues (LO 2.5)

Tissues hold your body together. Each tissue is different but made of similar cells with unique materials around them manufactured by the cells. The many tissues of your body have different structures that enable them to perform specialized functions. **Histology** is the study of the structure and function of tissues. The four primary tissue groups are outlined in *Table 2.1.*

CASE REPORT 2.3

You are . . .

. . . a physical therapy assistant employed in the Rehabilitation Unit in Fulwood Medical Center.

You are communicating with . . .

. . . Mr. Richard Josen, a 22-year-old man who injured tissues in his left knee while playing football (Figure 2.5). Using **arthroscopy,** the orthopedic surgeon removed his torn **anterior cruciate ligament (ACL)** and replaced it with a **graft** from his **patellar tendon**. The torn medial collateral ligament was **sutured** together. The tear in his medial **meniscus** was repaired. Rehabilitation is focused on strengthening the **muscles** around his knee joint and regaining joint mobility and stability.

▼ **TABLE 2.1**

THE FOUR PRIMARY TISSUE GROUPS (LO 2.5)

Type	Function	Location
Connective	Bind, support, protect, fill spaces, store fat	Widely distributed throughout the body, e.g., in blood, bone, cartilage, and fat
Epithelial	Protect, secrete, absorb, excrete	Cover body surface, cover and line internal organs, compose glands
Muscle	Movement	Attached to bones; found in the walls of hollow tubes, organs, and the heart
Nervous	Transmit impulses for coordination, sensory reception, motor actions	Brain, spinal cord, nerves

Adapted from David Shier, Jackie L. Butler, and Ricki Lewis, *Hole's Human Anatomy and Physiology,* 10th ed. Copyright © 2004 The McGraw-Hill Companies, Inc. Adapted with permission.

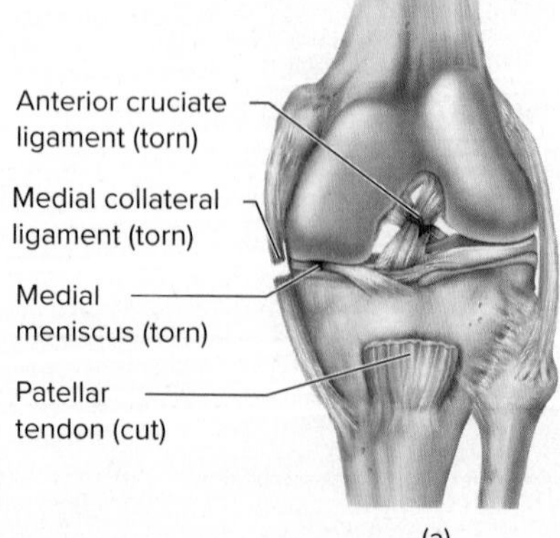

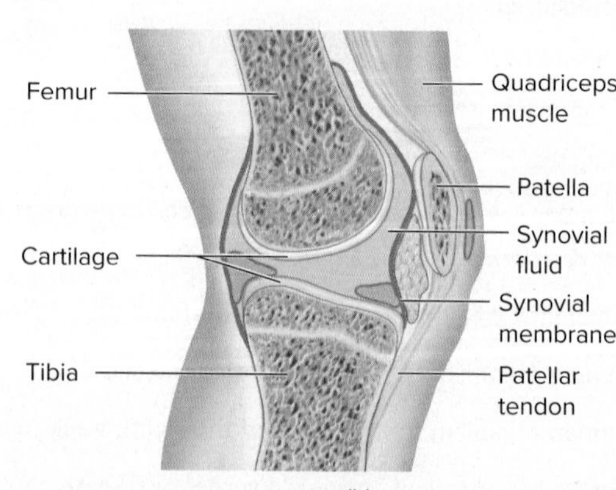

▶ **FIGURE 2.5**
Knee Anatomy.
(a) Injury to left knee.
(b) Normal knee.

Abbreviation

ACL anterior cruciate ligament

Word Analysis and Definition

S = Suffix P = Prefix R = Root R/CF = Combining Form

WORD	PRONUNCIATION	ELEMENTS		DEFINITION
arthroscopy	ar-**THROS**-koh-pee	S/ R/CF	**-scopy** *to examine, to view* **arthr/o-** *joint*	Visual examination of the interior of a joint
connective tissue	koh-**NECK**-tiv **TISH**-you	S/ R/	-ive *pertaining to* **connect-** *join together* tissue Latin *to weave*	The supporting tissue of the body
cruciate	**KRU**-she-ate		Latin *cross*	Shaped like a cross
graft	**GRAFT**		French *transplant*	Transplantation of living tissue
histology	his-**TOL**-oh-jee	S/ R/CF	**-logy** *study of* **hist/o-** *tissue*	Study of the structure and function of cells, tissues, and organs
histologist	his-**TOL**-oh-jist	S/	**-logist** *one who studies, specialist*	Specialist in histology
ligament	**LIG**-ah-ment		Latin *band*	Band of fibrous tissue connecting two structures
meniscus	meh-**NISS**-kuss		Greek *crescent*	Disc of cartilage between the bones of a joint
muscle	**MUSS**-el		Latin *muscle*	A tissue consisting of contractile cells
patella (singular) patellae (pl)	pah-**TELL**-ah pah-**TELL**-ee		Latin *small plate*	Thin, circular bone embedded in the patellar tendon in front of the knee joint; also called the kneecap
patellar (adj)	pah-**TELL**-ar	S/ R/	-ar *pertaining to* **patell-** *patella*	Pertaining to the patella
therapy	**THAIR**-ah-pee		Greek *medical treatment*	Systematic treatment of a disease, dysfunction, or disorder
therapeutic	**THAIR**-ah-**PYU**-tik	S/ R/	-ic *pertaining to* **therapeut-** *treatment*	Relating to the treatment of a disease or disorder
therapist	**THAIR**-ah-pist	S/ R/	-ist *specialist* **therap-** *treatment*	Professional trained in the practice of a particular therapy

EXERCISES

A. Review *Case Report 2.3. Then answer the following questions. Fill in the blanks.* **LO 2.2, 2.5, and 2.10**

1. Which therapeutic procedure was performed on Mr. Josen? ____________________
2. Which tendon contributed a graft to repair the ACL? ____________________
3. What type of surgeon performed the procedures? ____________________
4. Which of the structures repaired is a type of cartilage? ____________________
5. Which structure was repaired by suturing? ____________________

B. Dictionary exercise: *When you are working in the medical field, you will be exposed to medical terms you may not recognize. Learn to use the glossary or a good medical dictionary, or practice going online to find the definitions you need. Case Report 2.3 contains some terms that are not defined within the reading. Insert the correct term in the appropriate statement.* **LO 2.2 and 2.10**

orthopedic **collateral** **sutured**

1. Placing stitches to bind the wound edges together to close an incision or laceration of a body part. ____________________
2. Accessory or secondary ____________________
3. Medical specialty that diagnosis and treats diseases and conditions of bones ____________________

Lesson 2.4 (cont'd)

Keynotes

- Different tissues are made of specialized cells that manufacture unique fluids. The epithelial layer of the connective tissue synovial membrane is an example, as it produces the lubricant synovial fluid.
- Each connective tissue has distinct functions that enable a structure or organ to function correctly.
- There are four major ligaments of the knee joint:
  1. anterior cruciate ligament (ACL)
  2. posterior cruciate ligament (PCL)
  3. medial collateral ligament (MCL)
  4. lateral collateral ligament (LCL)

Connective Tissues (LO 2.5)

The relation of structure to function in your body tissues is key. To help you understand this important connection, this lesson uses the knee joint to illustrate the structures and functions of the different tissues found in this joint.

Connective Tissues in the Knee Joint (LO 2.5)

The connective tissues in your knee joint make it possible for you to enjoy your daily life–from standing, sitting, walking, bending, and running. These tissues and their roles are listed below:

- The **bones** of the knee joint are the **femur, tibia,** and **patella** *(see Chapter 4)*. Bone is the hardest connective tissue in your body because it contains calcium mineral salts (mainly calcium phosphate). Bones have a good blood supply so they can heal well after a fracture. Bones in general are covered with a thick fibrous tissue called the **periosteum.**
- **Cartilage** has a flexible, rubbery **matrix** (in the knee as a **meniscus)** that allows it to function as a shock absorber and a gliding surface where two bones meet to form a joint. Cartilage has very few blood vessels and heals poorly–sometimes not at all. When it is injured or torn, surgery is often needed. Cartilage also forms the shape of your ear, the tip of your nose, and your larynx.
- **Ligaments** hold the knee joint together. Two ligaments outside the joint cavity on each side of the joint are the **medial collateral ligament (MCL)** and the **lateral collateral ligament (LCL)** *(Figure 2.6)*. Two other ligaments located inside the joint cavity are called the **anterior collateral ligament (ACL)** and the **posterior collateral ligament**); they cross over each other to form an "X". *(Figure 2.6)*.
- **Ligaments** are strips or bands of fibrous connective tissue made of **collagen** fibers. The knee joint has four major ligaments that hold it together. The blood supply to these ligaments is poor, so they do not heal well without surgery *(Figure 2.6)*.
- **Tendons** are thick, strong ligaments that attach muscles to bone.
- The **joint capsule** of the knee joint encloses the joint cavity. It's made of thin, fibrous connective tissue and strengthened by fibers that extend over it from the surrounding ligaments and muscles. These features are common to most joints.
- The **synovial membrane** lines many joint capsules and secretes **synovial fluid**–a slippery lubricant stored in the joint cavity. This fluid makes joint movement almost friction-free. It distributes **nutrients** to the cartilage on the joint surfaces of bone.
- **Muscle tissue** stabilizes the joint. Extensions of the large muscle tendons in the front and the rear of the thigh are major stabilizers of the knee joint. The muscles alone extend and flex the knee joint *(see Chapter 4)*.
- **Nervous tissue** carries messages between the brain and the knee structures. All the knee structures are packed with nerves, which is why a knee injury is excruciatingly painful.

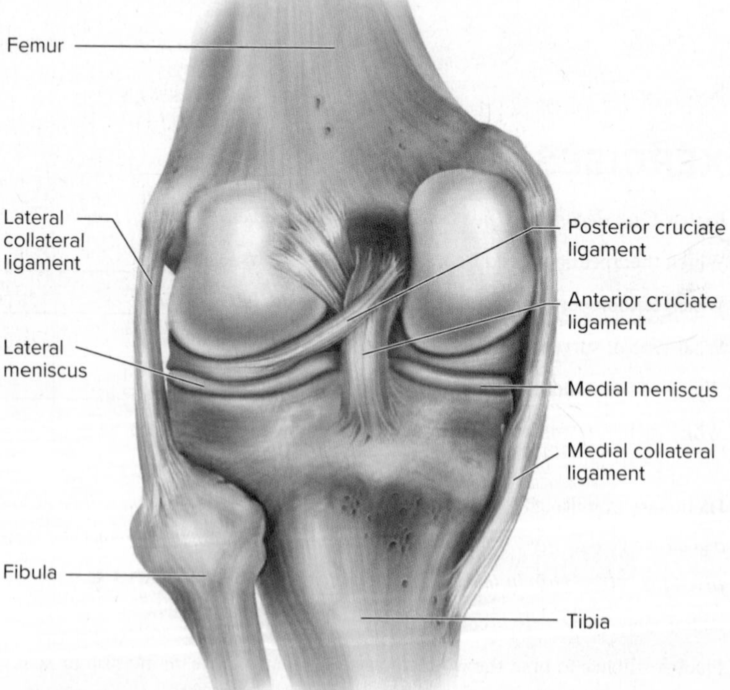

FIGURE 2.6
Ligaments of Knee Joint, with the Patellar Tendon Removed.

Word Analysis and Definition

S = Suffix P = Prefix R = Root R/CF = Combining Form

WORD	PRONUNCIATION	ELEMENTS		DEFINITION
capsule	**KAP**-syul		Latin *little box*	Fibrous tissue layer surrounding a joint or other structure
capsular (adj)	**KAP**-syu-lar	S/ R/	-ar *pertaining to* capsul- *box*	Pertaining to a capsule
cartilage	**KAR**-tih-lage		Latin *gristle*	Nonvascular, firm connective tissue found mostly in joints
collagen	**KOLL**-ah-jen	S/ R/CF	-gen *produce, form* coll/a- *glue*	Major protein of connective tissue, cartilage, and bone
matrix	**MAY**-triks		Latin mater *mother*	Substance that surrounds and protects cells, is manufactured by the cells, and holds them together
nutrient	**NYU**-tree-ent	S/ R/	-ent *end result* nutri- *nourish*	A substance in food required for normal physiologic function
periosteum	**PER**-ee-**OSS**-tee-um	S/ P/ R/	-um *tissue* peri- *around* -oste- *bone*	Fibrous membrane covering a bone
synovial	si-**NOH**-vee-al	S/ P/ R/CF	-al *pertaining to* syn- *together* -ov/i- *egg*	Pertaining to the synovial membrane or fluid
tendon	**TEN**-dun		Latin *sinew*	Fibrous band that connects muscle to bone

EXERCISES

A. Construct the appropriate medical term *to match the definitions given. The placement of the elements is noted for you under the line; each different element is separated on the line. Write the correct elements on the line. If a term does not have a particular element, leave it blank.* **LO 2.5**

1. Fibrous membrane covering a bone: ________ / ________ / ________
   P R/CF S

2. Major protein of connective tissue: ________ / ________ / ________
   P R/CF S

3. Pertaining to the synovial membrane ________ / ________ / ________
   P R/CF S

4. Substance in food that nourishes ________ / ________ / ________
   P R/CF S

B. Match *each connective tissue term to its correct description.* **LO 2.5**

1. Term that contains a word element meaning bone
2. Term that contains a word element that means glue
3. Term that contains a word element meaning egg
4. Term that is Latin and means gristle
5. Term that is Latin and means sinew

a. cartilage
b. tendon
c. periosteum
d. synovial
e. collagen

Keynote

- Homeostasis is the coordinated response of all the organs to maintain the internal physiologic stability of an organism.

Organs and Organ Systems (LO 2.6)

An **organ** is a structure composed of several tissues that work together to carry out specific functions. For example, your skin is an organ that has different tissues in it, such as epithelial cells, hair, nails, and glands *(see Chapter 3).*

An **organ system** is a group of organs with a specific collective function, like digestion, circulation, or respiration. For example, your nose, pharynx, larynx, trachea, bronchi, and lungs all work together to achieve the total function of respiration *(see Chapter 8).*

The different organs in an organ system are usually interconnected. For example, in the **urinary** organ system *(Figure 2.7),* the organs are the kidneys, ureters, bladder, and urethra, and they are all connected *(see Chapter 13).*

All your organ systems work together to ensure that your body's internal environment remains relatively constant. This process is called **homeostasis.** It ensures that cells receive adequate nutrients and oxygen. It also ensures that cell waste products are removed so your cells can function normally. Disease affecting an organ or organ system disrupts the homeostasis game plan.

Your body has 11 organ systems, as shown in *Table 2.2.* Muscular and **skeletal** are considered one organ system called the musculoskeletal system *(see Chapters 4 and 5).* Each body system has a chapter in this book where the terms associated with it are defined.

▼ **TABLE 2.2**

ORGAN SYSTEMS (LO 2.6)

Organ System	Major Organs	Major Functions
Integumentary	Skin, hair, nails, sweat glands, sebaceous glands	Protect tissues, regulate body temperature, support sensory receptors
Skeletal	Bones, ligaments, cartilage	Provide framework, protect soft tissues, provide attachments for muscles, produce blood cells, store inorganic salts
Muscular	Muscles	Cause movements, maintain posture, produce body heat
Nervous	Brain, spinal cord, nerves, sense organs	Receive and interpret sensory information and, in response, stimulate muscles, glands, and other organ systems
Endocrine	Glands that secrete hormones: pituitary, thyroid, parathyroid, adrenal, pancreas, ovaries, testes, pineal, thymus	Control metabolic activities of organs
Cardiovascular	Heart, blood vessels	Move blood and transport substances throughout body
Lymphatic	Lymph vessels and nodes, thymus, spleen	Defend body against infection, return tissue fluid to blood, carry certain absorbed food molecules
Digestive	Mouth, tongue, teeth, salivary glands, pharynx, esophagus, stomach, liver, gallbladder, pancreas, small and large intestines	Receive, break down, and absorb food; eliminate unabsorbed material
Respiratory	Nasal cavity, pharynx, larynx, trachea, bronchi, lungs	Intake and output air, exchange gases between air and blood
Urinary	Kidneys, ureters, urinary bladder, urethra	Remove wastes from blood, maintain water and electrolyte balance, store and transport urine
Reproductive	Male: scrotum, testes, epididymides, vasa deferentia, seminal vesicles, prostate, bulbourethral glands, urethra, penis	Produce and maintain sperm cells, transfer sperm cells into female reproductive tract
	Female: ovaries, fallopian tubes, uterus, vagina, vulva	Produce and maintain egg cells, receive sperm cells, support development of an embryo, function in birth process

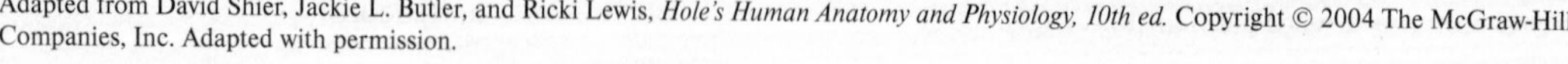
Adapted from David Shier, Jackie L. Butler, and Ricki Lewis, *Hole's Human Anatomy and Physiology, 10th ed.* Copyright © 2004 The McGraw-Hill Companies, Inc. Adapted with permission.

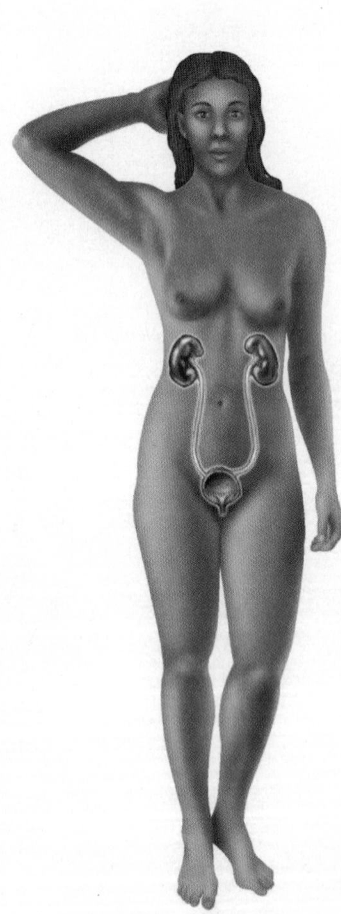

▲ **FIGURE 2.7**
The Urinary System.

Word Analysis and Definition

S = Suffix P = Prefix R = Root R/CF = Combining Form

WORD	PRONUNCIATION	ELEMENTS		DEFINITION
cardiovascular	**KAR**-dee-oh-**VAS**-kyu-lar	S/ R/CF R/	-ar *pertaining to* **cardi/o-** *heart* **-vascul-** *blood vessel*	Pertaining to the heart and blood vessels
digestion **digestive (adj)**	die-**JEST**-shun die-**JEST**-iv	S/ R/ S/	-ion *action* **digest-** *break down food* -ive *pertaining to*	Breakdown of food into elements suitable for cell metabolism Pertaining to digestion
endocrine	**EN**-doh-krin	P/ R/	**endo-** *within* -crine *to secrete*	A gland that produces an internal or hormonal substance
homeostasis (**Note:** *Hemostasis is the arrest of bleeding.*)	hoh-mee-oh-**STAY**-sis	S/ R/CF	-stasis *standstill, control* **home/o-** *the same*	Maintaining the stability of a system or the body's internal environment
integument **integumentary (adj)**	in-**TEG**-you-ment in-**TEG**-you-**MENT**-ah-ree	 S/ R/	Latin *a covering* -ary *pertaining to* **integument-** *covering of the body*	Organ system that covers the body, the skin being the main organ within the system Pertaining to the covering of the body
lymph **lymphatic (adj)**	**LIMF** lim-**FAT**-ic	 S/ R/	Latin *clear spring water* -atic *pertaining to* **lymph-** *lymph, lymphatic system*	Clear fluid collected from body tissues and transported by lymph vessels to the venous circulation Pertaining to lymph or the lymphatic system
nervous **nervous system**	**NER**-vus **NER**-vus **SIS**-tem	S/ R/	-ous *pertaining to* **nerv-** *nerve* **system** Greek *an organized whole*	Pertaining to a nerve or the nervous system; or easily excited or agitated The whole, integrated nerve apparatus
respiration **respiratory (adj)**	**RES**-pih-**RAY**-shun **RES**-pih-rah-tor-ee	S/ R/ S/	-ation *process* **respir-** *to breathe* -atory *pertaining to*	Process of breathing; fundamental process of life used to exchange oxygen and carbon dioxide Pertaining to respiration
skeleton **skeletal (adj)**	**SKEL**-eh-ton **SKEL**-eh-tal	 S/ R/	Greek *skeleton or mummy* -al *pertaining to* **skelet-** *skeleton*	The bony framework of the body Pertaining to the skeleton
urinary (adj)	**YUR**-in-ary	S/ R/	-ary *pertaining to* **urin-** *urine*	Pertaining to urine

Exercises

A. Construct *the correct medical terms by working with the literal meaning of the elements a. Enter the correct elements on each line to complete the term.* **LO 2.6**

1. ______________ / ______________
lymph — pertaining to

2. ______________ / ______________
heart and blood vessels — pertaining to

3. ______________ / ______________
skeleton — pertaining to

4. ______________ / ______________
covering of the body — pertaining to

5. ______________ / ______________
break down food — pertaining to

B. Continue *working with the medical terms related to the organs and organ systems.* **LO 2.6** Remember

1. When referring to a body system, add a suffix that means: ______________
2. Which element type is different between the terms *homeostasis* and *hemostasis?* ______________
3. What is the main organ in the integumentary system? ______________
4. What is the bony framework of the body called? ______________
5. What term refers to clear fluid? ______________

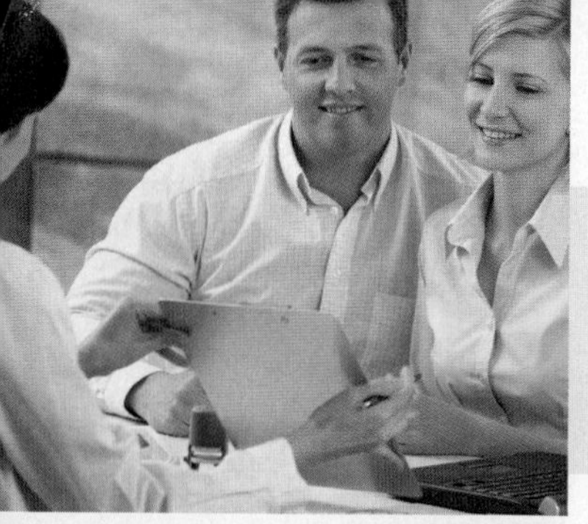

Classic Collection/Shotshop GmbH/Alamy Images

Lesson 2.5

Anatomical Positions, Planes, and Directions

Objectives

Medical terms have been developed over the past several thousand years to help you describe clearly the location of different anatomical structures and lesions and their relation to each other in the human body. To do this, you need to be able to:

2.5.1 Define the fundamental anatomical position on which all descriptions of anatomical locations are based.

2.5.2 Describe the medical terminology of the different anatomical planes and directions.

2.5.3 Relate these terms to physical sites on the body.

2.5.4 Locate the body cavities.

2.5.5 Identify the medical terminology of the four abdominal quadrants and the nine main regions.

Keynote

- The transverse plane is the only horizontal body plane.

Fundamental Anatomical Position (LO 2.7)

When all anatomical descriptions are used, it's assumed that the body is in the "anatomical position" *(Figure 2.8).* Here is how this position looks if you're standing in front of a full-length mirror: your body is standing erect, your feet are flat on the floor, your face and eyes are facing forward, and your arms are at your sides with your palms facing forward.

When you lie down flat on your back with your palms upward, you are **supine.** When you lie down flat on your belly with your palms facing the floor, you are **prone.**

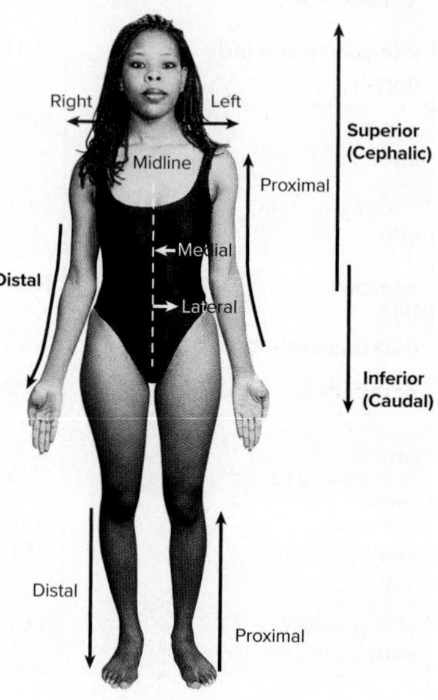

▼ **FIGURE 2.8** Anatomical Position, with Directional Terms.

Joe DeGrandis/McGraw-Hill Education

Anatomical Directional Terms (LO 2.7)

Directional terms describe the position of one body structure or part relative to another body structure or part. These directional terms are shown in *Figures 2.8* and *2.9.*

Anatomical Planes (LO 2.7)

Different views of your body are based on imaginary "slices," which produce flat surfaces called **planes** that pass through your body *(Figure 2.10).* The **three major anatomical planes** are the following:

▼ **FIGURE 2.9** Other Directional Terms.

Aaron Roeth Photography

- **Transverse or horizontal:** a plane passing across the body parallel to the floor and perpendicular to the body's long axis. It divides the body into an upper/superior portion and a lower/inferior portion.
- **Sagittal:** a vertical plane that divides the body into right and left portions.
- **Frontal (coronal):** a vertical plane that divides the body into front **(anterior)** and back **(posterior)** portions.

▼ **FIGURE 2.10** Anatomical Planes.

Joe DeGrandis/McGraw-Hill Education

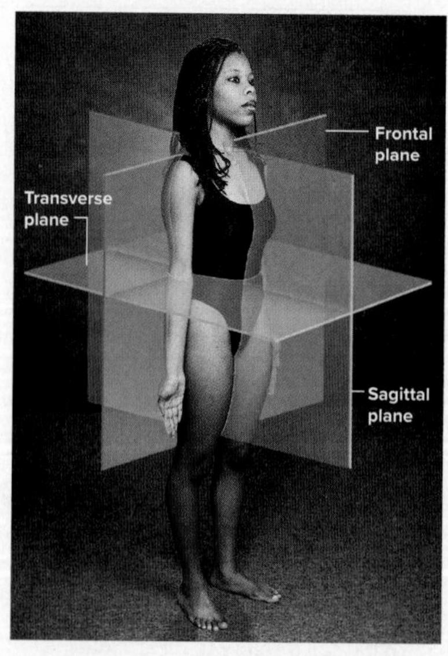

Word Analysis and Definition

S = Suffix P = Prefix R = Root R/CF = Combining Form

WORD	PRONUNCIATION	ELEMENTS		DEFINITION
anatomy anatomical (adj)	ah-**NAT**-oh-mee an-ah-**TOM**-ik-al	S/ R/ S/	-tomy *process of separating* ana- *apart from* -ical *pertaining to*	Study of the structures of the human body Pertaining to anatomy
anterior *(opposite of posterior)*	an-**TEER**-ee-or	S/ R/	-ior *pertaining to* anter- *before, front part*	The front surface of the body; situated in front
caudal *(opposite of cephalic, same as inferior)*	**KAW**-dal	S/ R/	-al *pertaining to* caud- *tail*	Pertaining to or nearer to the tailbone
cephalic *(opposite of caudal, same as superior)*	seh-**FAL**-ik	S/ R/	-ic *pertaining to* cephal- *head*	Pertaining to or nearer to the head
coronal *(same as frontal)*	**KOR**-oh-nal	S/ R/	-al *pertaining to* coron- *crown*	Pertaining to the vertical plane dividing the body into anterior and posterior portions
distal *(opposite of proximal)*	**DISS**-tal	S/ R/	-al *pertaining to* dist- *away from the center*	Situated away from the center of the body
dorsal *(same as posterior)*	**DOOR**-sal	S/ R/	-al *pertaining to* dors- *back*	Pertaining to the back or situated behind
inferior *(opposite of superior)*	in-**FEER**-ee-or	S/ R/	-ior *pertaining to* infer- *below*	Situated below
lateral *(opposite of medial)*	**LAT**-er-al	S/ R/	-al *pertaining to* later- *side*	Situated at the side of a structure
medial *(opposite of lateral)*	**ME**-dee-al	S/ R/	-al *pertaining to* medi- *middle*	Nearer to the middle of the body
posterior *(opposite of anterior)*	pohs-**TEER**-ee-or	S/ R/	-ior *pertaining to* poster- *back part*	Pertaining to the back surface of the body; situated behind
prone *(opposite of supine)*	**PROHN**		Latin *bending forward*	Lying face down, flat on your belly
proximal *(opposite of distal)*	**PROK**-sih-mal	S/ R/	-al *pertaining to* proxim- *nearest to the center*	Situated nearest to the center of the body
sagittal	**SAJ**-ih-tal	S/ R/	-al *pertaining to* sagitt- *arrow*	Vertical plane through the body dividing it into right and left portions
superior *(opposite of inferior)*	soo-**PEER**-ee-or	S/ R/	-ior *pertaining to* super- *above*	Situated above
supine *(opposite of prone)*	soo-**PINE**		Latin *lying on the back*	Lying face up, flat on your spine
transverse	trans-**VERS**		Latin *crosswise*	Horizontal plane dividing the body into upper and lower portions
ventral *(same as anterior)*	**VEN**-tral	S/ R/	-al *pertaining to* ventr- *belly*	Pertaining to the belly or situated nearer the surface of the belly

Study Hint

Help your memory with little tricks of association for medical terms. Example: The medical term *supine* has the word up in it. The meaning of *supine* is *lying with the face and the anterior part of the body UP*. Associate UP with sUPine and you will have no trouble remembering its definition. Then associate the opposite term and you will know the meaning of *prone* as well.

EXERCISES

A. *Review Case Report 2.1. Use directional terms to correctly answer each question. Fill in the blanks.* **LO 2.2 and 2.7**

1. To examine Mrs. Arnold's abdomen, in which position would you place her? ____________
2. To examine Mrs. Arnold's spine, in which position would you place her? ____________
3. Mrs. Arnold's spine is ____________ to her abdomen.

B. Identify *the following pairs of terms as either opposites or synonyms.* **LO 2.7**

1. anterior/posterior ____________
2. ventral/anterior ____________
3. prone/supine ____________
4. coronal/frontal ____________
5. cephalic/caudal ____________
6. cephalic/superior ____________

Lesson 2.5 (cont'd)

Abbreviations

LLQ	left lower quadrant
LUQ	left upper quadrant
RLQ	right lower quadrant
RUQ	right upper quadrant

Abdominal Quadrants (LO 2.8)

To simplify your job of locating and identifying abdominal structures and sites of abdominal pain and other abnormalities, you can mentally divide the abdomen into **quadrants,** as shown in *Figure 2.11a.* This approach allows you to separate these locations into manageable parts. So, here you have the right upper quadrant **(RUQ),** left upper quadrant **(LUQ),** right lower quadrant **(RLQ),** and left lower quadrant **(LLQ).**

In addition, there are three main regions of your abdomen–the epigastric, umbilical, and hypogastric regions, as shown in *Figure 2.11b.*

Body Cavities (LO 2.9)

Your body contains many **cavities** or hollow spaces. Some, like the nasal cavity, open to the outside of your body. Five cavities that do not open to the outside are shown in *Figure 2.12* and listed below.

1. The **cranial cavity** contains the brain within the skull.
2. The **thoracic cavity** contains the heart, lungs, thymus gland, trachea and esophagus, and numerous blood vessels and nerves.
3. The **abdominal cavity,** separated from the thoracic cavity by the **diaphragm,** contains the stomach, intestines, liver, spleen, pancreas, and kidneys. There are nine regions in the abdomen, as shown in *Figure 2.11b.*
4. The **pelvic cavity,** surrounded by the pelvic bones, contains the urinary bladder, part of the large intestine, the rectum and anus, and the internal reproductive organs.
5. The **spinal cavity** contains the spinal cord.

The abdominal cavity and pelvic cavity can be combined as the **abdominopelvic cavity.**

FIGURE 2.11 Regional Anatomy.

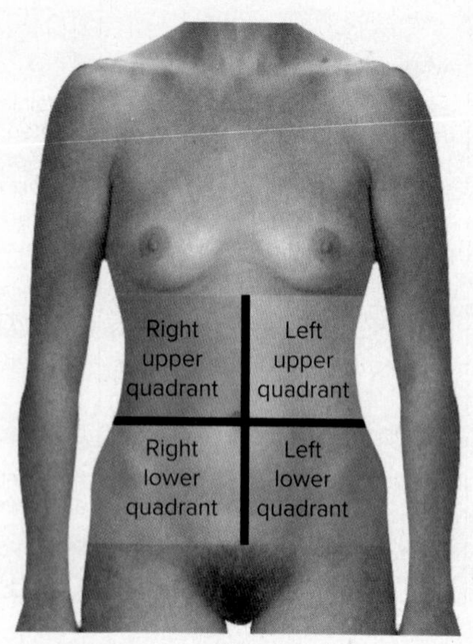

(a) Abdominal quadrants

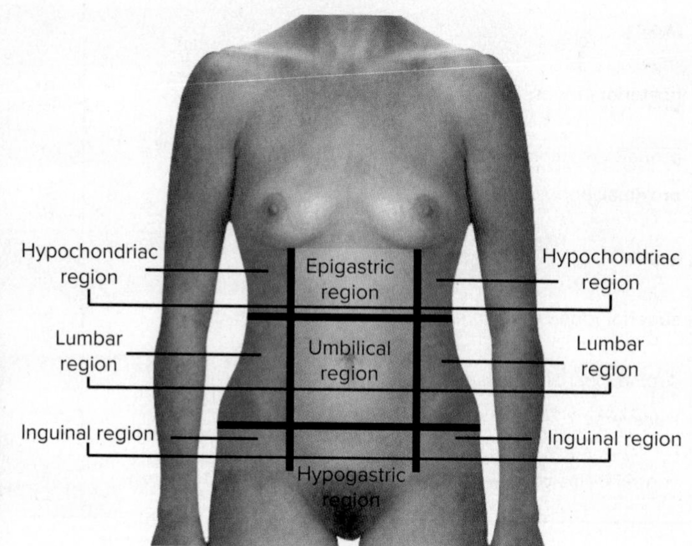

(b) Abdominal regions

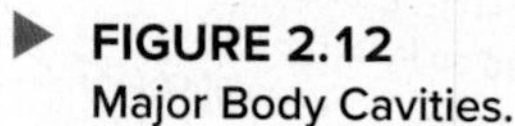

FIGURE 2.12 Major Body Cavities.

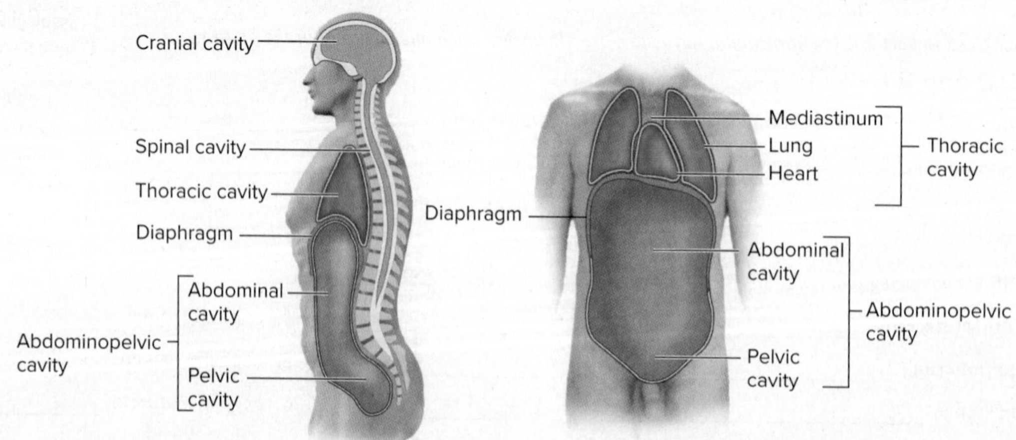

Word Analysis and Definition

S = Suffix P = Prefix R = Root R/CF = Combining Form

WORD	PRONUNCIATION		ELEMENTS	DEFINITION
abdomen	**AB**-doh-men		Latin *abdomen*	Part of the trunk between the thorax and the pelvis
abdominal (adj)	ab-**DOM**-in-al	S/ R/	-al *pertaining to* abdomin- *abdomen*	Pertaining to the abdomen
abdominopelvic	ab-**DOM**-ih-no-**PEL**-vik	S/ R/CF R/	-ic *pertaining to* abdomin/o- *abdomen* -pelv- *pelvis*	Pertaining to the abdomen and pelvis
cavity cavities (pl)	**KAV**-ih-tee **KAV**-ih-teez	S/ R/	-ity *state, condition* cav- *hollow space*	A hollow space or body compartment
cranial (adj)	**KRAY**-nee-al	S/ R/	-al *pertaining to* crani- *skull*	Pertaining to the cranium
cranium	**KRAY**-nee-um	S/	-um *structure*	The skull
diaphragm	**DIE**-ah-fram		Greek *diaphragm, fence*	Muscular sheet separating the abdominal and thoracic cavities
diaphragmatic (adj)	**DIE**-ah-frag-**MAT**-ik	S/ R/	-ic *pertaining to* diaphragmat- *diaphragm*	Pertaining to the diaphragm
quadrant	**KWAD**-rant		Latin *one quarter*	One quarter of a circle; one of four regions of the surface of the abdomen
spine	**SPYN**		Latin *spine*	The vertebral column or a short bony projection
spinal (adj)	**SPY**-nal	S/ R/	-al *pertaining to* spin- *spine*	Pertaining to the spine
thoracic (adj)	**THOR**-ass-ik	S/ R/	-ic *pertaining to* thorac- *chest*	Pertaining to the chest (thorax)
thorax	**THOR**-acks		Greek *chest*	The part of the trunk between the abdomen and the neck
umbilical (adj)	um-**BILL**-ih-kal	S/ R/	-al *pertaining to* umbilic- *navel (belly button)*	Pertaining to the umbilicus or the center of the abdomen
umbilicus	um-**BILL**-ih-kuss		Latin *navel (belly button)*	Pit in the abdomen where the umbilical cord entered the fetus

EXERCISES

A. Deconstruct the following terms *into their basic elements. Note that not every type of element will appear in every term. The only element every term needs is a root or a combining form. Fill in the blanks.* **LO 2.1 and 2.9**

1. diaphragmatic ______________ / ______________
   R/CF S
2. abdominopelvic ______________ / ______________ / ______________
   R/CF R/CF S
3. umbilical ______________ / ______________
   R/CF S
4. cranial ______________ / ______________
   R/CF S
5. thoracic ______________ / ______________
   R/CF S
6. cavity ______________ / ______________
   R/CF S

B. Select *the correct answer to answer each question or complete the statement.* **LO 2.8 and 2.9**

1. Which term contains a root and a combining form?
   - **a.** abdominopelvic
   - **b.** diaphragmatic
   - **c.** thoracic
   - **d.** spinal
2. Which term is a muscle that separates body cavities?
   - **a.** abdominopelvic
   - **b.** diaphragm
   - **c.** thoracic
   - **d.** spinal
3. The term "quadrant" represents what number?
   - **a.** two
   - **b.** four
   - **c.** six
   - **d.** eight
4. The term "spine" also refers to
   - **a.** diaphragm
   - **b.** skull
   - **c.** chest
   - **d.** vertebral column
5. Which of the following terms is a dentist likely to use?
   - **a.** cavity
   - **b.** abdomen
   - **c.** spinal
   - **d.** thoracic

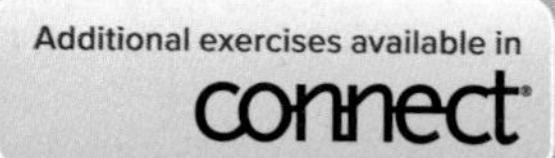

Chapter Review exercises, along with additional practice items, are available in Connect!

The Integumentary System

The Essentials of the Language of Dermatology

Rick Brady/McGraw-Hill Education

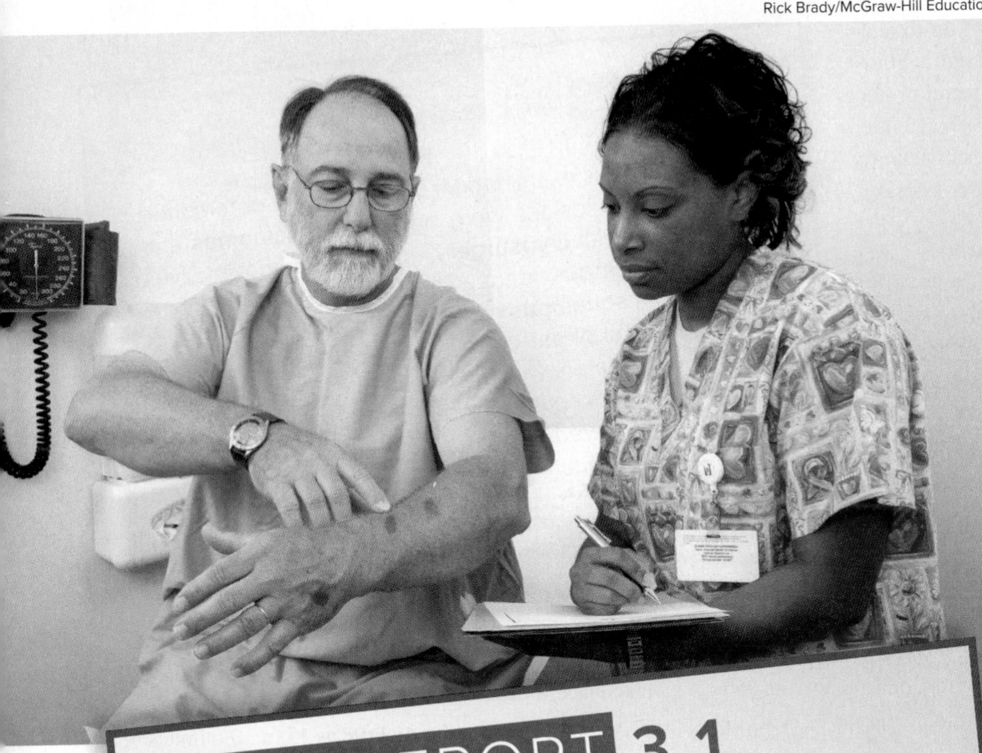

CASE REPORT 3.1

You are . . .

. . . a **dermatology technologist** working with **dermatologist** Laura Echols, MD, a member of the Fulwood Medical Group.

You are communicating with . . .

. . . Mr. Rod Andrews, a 60-year-old man, who shows you three skin lesions—two on his left forearm and one on the back of his left hand. You learn that he has been living in Arizona for the past 10 years but has recently returned to this area in order to live near his daughter and young grandchildren. You find no other skin lesions on his body.

The health professionals involved in the diagnosis and treatment of problems with the integumentary system include the following:

- **Dermatologists** are medical doctors who are specialists in skin disorders.
- **Dermatology technologists** are medical assistants who have an additional year of training in dermatology.

Learning Outcomes

In addition to anticipating Dr. Echols' needs for equipment to **biopsy,** diagnose, and treat the lesions, you also have to be able to communicate clearly with her in medical terms and understand her language as she communicates with you and the patient about the **etiology** (cause) and structure of the lesions. You will then need to document the medical history and treatment and communicate clearly with Mr. Andrews about the treatment of his lesions and their **prognosis.**

To perform these tasks, you must be able to:

LO 3.1 **Use roots, combining forms, suffixes, and prefixes to construct and analyze medical terms related to the integumentary system.**

LO 3.2 **Spell and pronounce correctly medical terms and their plurals related to the integumentary system to communicate them with accuracy and precision in any health care setting.**

LO 3.3 **Define accepted abbreviations related to the integumentary system.**

LO 3.4 **Relate the anatomical structures of the integumentary system and their locations to their functions.**

LO 3.5 **Describe common disorders of and injuries to the skin and its accessory glands.**

LO 3.6 **Identify diagnostic and therapeutic procedures and pharmacology used to treat disorders of the integumentary system.**

LO 3.7 **Apply your knowledge of medical terms relating to the integumentary system to documentation, medical records, and medical reports.**

LO 3.8 **Translate the medical terms relating to the integumentary system into everyday language in order to communicate clearly with patients and their families.**

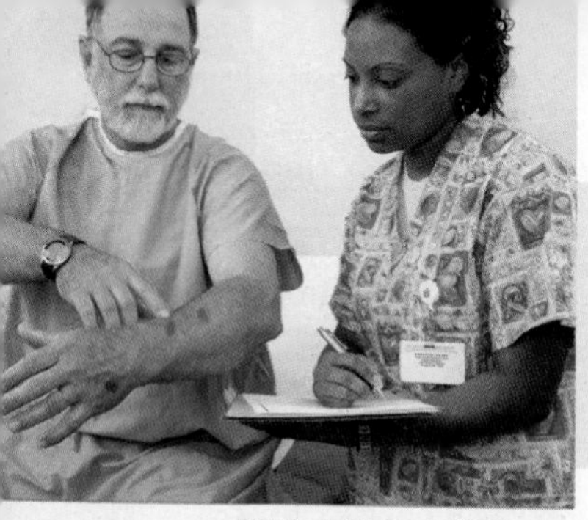

Rick Brady/McGraw-Hill Education

Lesson 3.1

Functions and Structure of the Skin

Objectives

Your skin is your largest organ—it covers your entire body. The three lesions on Mr. Andrews' arm and hand developed in the outer layer of the skin, the ***epidermis.*** *This lesson looks at the structure and function of the skin so that you will be able to use correct medical terminology to:*

3.1.1 Describe the functions of the skin.

3.1.2 Name the tissues in the different layers of the skin.

3.1.3 Specify the functions of the different layers of the skin.

Your skin's nerves allow you to feel heat, cold, pain, and comfort. Your skin wards off infections and protects your body from harmful environmental elements. Your skin is constantly shedding old cells in order to make room for new skin growth.

The **integumentary system** consists of your skin and its associated organs. **Dermatology** is the study and treatment of the integumentary system. A **dermatologist** is a medical specialist in the disorders of the skin.

Case Report 3.1 *(continued)*

When Dr. Echols examined Mr. Andrews, she determined that two of his lesions were basal cell **carcinomas** and treated them with **cryosurgery,** an approach that involves freezing cancerous tissue. She believed that the third lesion was a **squamous cell** carcinoma and performed a biopsy removal of the **cutaneous** (skin) lesion. You sent this to the laboratory with a request for a pathologic diagnosis and determination of whether the lesion had been completely removed.

Functions of the Skin (LO 3.1, 3.2, and 3.4)

Your skin functions in several ways to keep you healthy and safe. These important functions include the following:

- **Protection:** Your skin is a physical barrier against injury, chemicals, ultraviolet rays, microbes, and toxins and is not easily breached *(Figure 3.1).* Bacteria and other pathogens, called normal **flora,** populate your skin's surface.
- **Water resistance:** You don't swell up every time you take a bath because your skin is water resistant. It also prevents water from leaking out of body tissues.
- **Temperature regulation:** A network of capillaries in your skin opens up or dilates **(vasodilation)** when your body is too hot. When your body is cold, this capillary network narrows **(vasoconstriction),** blood flow decreases, and your body retains heat.

The structure of the skin to enable these functions to take place is detailed in the next section.

- **Vitamin D synthesis:** As little as 15 to 30 minutes of sunlight each day allow your skin cells to initiate the metabolism of vitamin D, which is essential for bone growth and maintenance.
- **Sensation:** Nerve endings that detect touch, pressure, heat, cold, pain, vibration, and tissue injury are particularly numerous in the skin of your face, fingers, palms, soles, nipples, and genitals.
- **Excretion and secretion:** Water and small amounts of waste products from cell metabolism are lost through your skin by **excretion** and **secretion** from your sweat glands.
- **Social functions:** The skin reflects your emotions: it blushes when you are self-conscious, goes pale when you are frightened, and wrinkles when you register disgust.

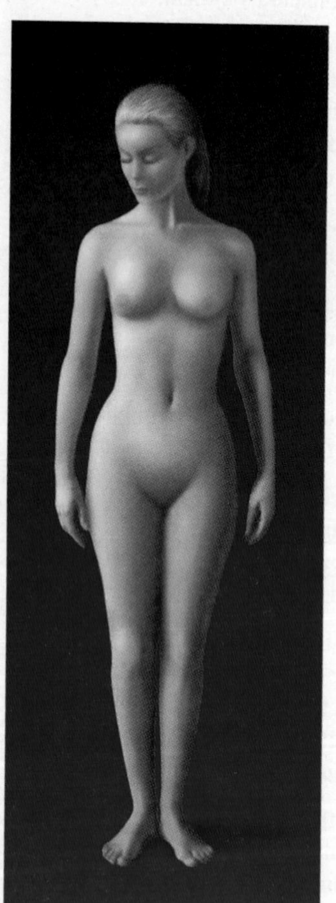

FIGURE 3.1
Integumentary System.
The skin provides protection, contains sensory organs, and helps control body temperature.

Word Analysis and Definition

S = Suffix P = Prefix R = Root R/CF = Combining Form

WORD	PRONUNCIATION	ELEMENTS		DEFINITION
biopsy	BI-op-see	S/ R/	-opsy *to view* bi- *life*	Removing tissue from a living person for laboratory examination
carcinoma	kar-sih-**NOH**-mah	S/ R/	-oma *tumor, mass* carcin- *cancer*	A malignant and invasive epithelial tumor
cryosurgery	cry-oh-**SUR**-jer-ee	S/ R/CF R/	-ery *process of* cry/o- *icy cold* -surg- *operate*	Use of liquid nitrogen or argon gas in a probe to freeze and kill abnormal tissue
cutaneous	kyu-**TAY**-nee-us	S/ R/CF	-ous *pertaining to* cutan/e- *skin*	Pertaining to the skin
dermatology	der-mah-**TOL**-oh-jee	S/ R/CF	-logy *study of* dermat/o- *skin*	Medical specialty concerned with disorders of the skin
dermatologist	der-mah-**TOL**-oh-jist	S/	-logist *one who studies, specialist*	Medical specialist in diseases of the skin
dermatologic (adj)	der-mah-toh-**LOJ**-ik	S/	-ic *pertaining to*	Pertaining to the skin and dermatology
etiology	ee-tee-**OL**-oh-jee	S/ R/CF	-logy *study of* eti/o- *cause*	The study of the causes of a disease
excrete (verb)	eks-**KREET**	P/ R	ex- *out of, away from* -crete *separate*	To pass waste products of metabolism out of the body
excretion (noun)	eks-**KREE**-shun	S/	-ion *action*	Removal of waste products of metabolism out of the body
flora	**FLO**-rah		Latin *flower*	The population of microorganisms covering the exterior and interior surfaces of healthy animals
integument	in-**TEG**-you-ment		Latin *a covering*	Organ system that covers the body, the skin being the main organ within the system
integumentary (adj)	in-**TEG**-you-**MENT**-ah-ree	S/ R/	-ary *pertaining to* integument- *covering of the body*	Pertaining to the covering of the body
prognosis	prog-**NO**-sis	P/ R/	pro- *projecting forward* -gnosis *knowledge*	Forecast of the probable future course and outcome of a disease
secrete (verb)	seh-**KREET**	R/	secret- *produce*	To produce a chemical substance in a cell and release it from the cell
secretion (noun)	seh-**KREE**-shun	S/	-ion *action*	Production by a cell(s) of a physiologically active substance and its movement out of the cell.
squamous cell	**SKWAY**-mus **SELL**		squamous Latin *scaly*	Flat, scale-like epithelial cell
synthesis	**SIN**-the-sis	P/ R/	syn- *together* -thesis *to organize, arrange*	The process of building a compound from different elements
synthetic (adj)	sin-**THET**-ik	S/ R/	-ic *pertaining to* -thet- *arrange, organize*	Built up or put together from simpler compounds
vasoconstriction	**VAY**-soh-con-**STRIK**-shun	S/ R/CF R/	-ion *action* vas/o- *blood vessel* -constrict- *narrow*	Reduction in diameter of a blood vessel
vasodilation	**VAY**-soh-die-**LAY**-shun	R/	-dilat- *widen, open up*	Increase in diameter of a blood vessel

EXERCISE

A. Review *Case Report 3.1 to select the correct answer the following questions.* **LO 3.2 and 3.8**

1. Which two types of skin lesions did Dr. Echols remove from Mr. Andrews?

a. squamous cell carcinoma and cryosurgery
b. basal cell carcinoma and squamous cell carcinoma
c. cutaneous and integumentary
d. cryosurgery and excisional biopsy

2. What different types of treatment did Dr. Echols use to remove these lesions?

a. squamous cell carcinoma and cryosurgery
b. basal cell carcinoma and squamous cell carcinoma
c. cutaneous and integumentary
d. cryosurgery and excisional biopsy

3. What two questions did Dr. Echols need the pathologist to answer?

a. What kind of cancer is present and has the lesion been completely removed?
b. What are the results of the biopsy and what type of flora is present?
c. What is Mr. Andrews' prognosis and has the lesion been completely removed?
d. What is Mr. Andrews' prognosis and should he see a dermatologist?

4. What treatment approach involves freezing cancerous tissue?

a. excretion **b.** vasoconstriction **c.** excisional biopsy **d.** cryosurgery

5. Cutaneous means:

a. pertaining to the skin **b.** action of the skin **c.** pertaining to icy cold **d.** process of covering the body

Structure of the Skin (LO 3.1, 3.2, and 3.4)

Epidermis (LO 3.1, 3.2, 3.3, and 3.4)

Mr. Andrews' three lesions were present in his **epidermis,** the most superficial layer of his skin.

The outer layer of your epidermis *(Figure 3.2)* is a keratin-packed cover of compact, dead cells that you continually shed. **Keratin**–a tough, scaly protein that is also the basis for your hair and nails–shields your body from harmful elements like chemicals and bacteria. **Dandruff** is essentially clumps of these dead keratin cells stuck together with **sebum** (oil) from **sebaceous glands.**

In the lower layers of your epidermis, cells are filled with a protein that becomes keratin. Other cells produce a brown/black pigment called **melanin,** which determines the color of your skin and protects it from **ultraviolet (UV)** light damage.

Dermis (LO 3.1, 3.2, and 3.4)

Figure 3.3 shows that the **dermis** is a much thicker connective tissue layer than the epidermis. Your dermis is the middle layer of your skin between your epidermis and **hypodermis.** It consists mostly of collagen fibers. Your dermis is well supplied with blood vessels and nerves. It contains your other skin organs: sweat glands, sebaceous glands, hair **follicles,** and nail roots.

Abbreviations

IM	intramuscular
SC	subcutaneous
TB	tuberculosis
UV	ultraviolet

▼ **FIGURE 3.2**
Epidermis.

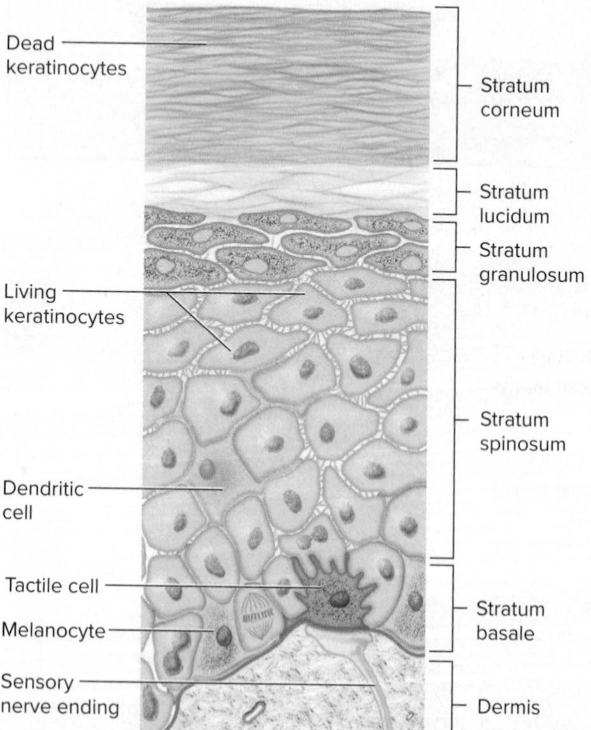

Hypodermis or Subcutaneous Tissue Layer (LO 3.1, 3.2, and 3.4)

This layer beneath your dermis is the site of **subcutaneous** fat (**adipose** tissue), nerves, and blood vessels. Also called the subcutaneous tissue layer, it regulates your body's temperature and helps protect your vital organs. When this layer becomes thinner or deteriorates, as with the aging process, your skin begins to sag.

Clinical Applications (LO 3.1, 3.2, 3.3, and 3.4)

Injections are given into the three areas of the skin using the following approaches:

- **Intradermal,** in which a short, thin needle is introduced into the epidermis, raising a small **wheal** on the skin. This site is used for allergy testing or a tuberculosis **(TB)** test.
- **Subcutaneous (SC),** in which a longer needle pierces the epidermis and dermis to reach the hypodermis (subcutaneous) layer. This site is used for insulin injections and immunizations.
- **Intramuscular (IM),** in which a long needle penetrates the epidermis, dermis, and hypodermis to reach into the muscles underneath. Some antibiotics and immunizations are given this way.

In addition, there are **transdermal** applications. Here, medications are administered through the skin by an adhesive transdermal patch applied to the skin. The medication diffuses across the epidermis and enters the blood vessels in the dermis. Contraceptive hormones, **analgesics,** and antinausea/antiseasickness medications are examples of transdermal applications.

▼ **FIGURE 3.3**
Dermis and Its Organs.

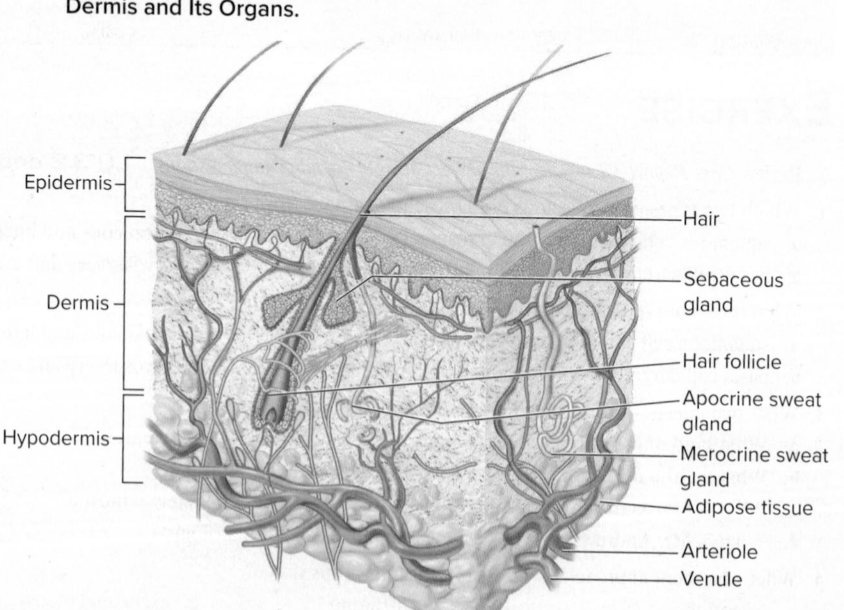

Word Analysis and Definition

S = Suffix P = Prefix R = Root R/CF = Combining Form

WORD	PRONUNCIATION	ELEMENTS		DEFINITION
adipose	**ADD**-ih-pose	S/ R/	-ose *full of* adip- *fat*	Containing fat
analgesic (adj) analgesia	an-al-**JEE**-sic an-al-**JEE**-zee-ah	S/ P/ R/ S/	-ic *pertaining to* an- *without* -alges- *sensation of pain* -ia *condition*	Substance that reduces or relieves the response to pain without producing loss of consciousness State in which pain is reduced or relieved
dandruff	**DAN**-druff		Source unknown	Scales in hair from shedding of the epidermis
dermis dermal	**DER**-miss **DER**-mal	S/ R/	Greek *skin* -al *pertaining to* derm- *skin*	Connective tissue layer of the skin beneath the epidermis Pertaining to the skin
epidermis epidermal (adj)	ep-ih-**DER**-miss ep-ih-**DER**-mal	P/ R/ S/ R/	epi- *above, upon* -dermis *skin* -al *pertaining to* -derm- *skin*	Top layer of the skin Pertaining to the epidermis
follicle	**FOLL**-ih-kull		Latin *small sac*	Spherical mass of cells containing a cavity or a small cul-de-sac, such as a hair follicle
hypodermis hypodermic (adj) *(same as subcutaneous)*	high-poh-**DER**-miss high-poh-**DER**-mik	P/ R/ S/ R/	hypo- *below* -dermis *skin* -ic *pertaining to* -derm- *skin*	Loose connective tissue layer of skin below the dermis Pertaining to the hypodermis
intradermal	in-trah-**DER**-mal	S/ P/ R/	-al *pertaining to* intra- *within* -derm- *skin*	Within the epidermis
intramuscular	in-trah-**MUSS**-kew-lar	S/ P/ R/	-ar *pertaining to* intra- *within* -muscul- *muscle*	Within the muscle
keratin	**KER**-ah-tin	S/ R/	-in *substance* kerat- *hard protein*	Protein present in skin, hair, and nails
melanin	**MEL**-ah-nin	S/ R/	-in *substance* melan- *black pigment*	Black pigment found in skin, hair, and the retina
sebaceous glands sebum	seh-**BAY**-shus **GLANZ** **SEE**-bum	S/ R/CF	-ous *pertaining to* sebac/e- *wax* Latin *tallow*	Glands in the dermis that open into hair follicles and secrete a waxy fluid called sebum Waxy secretion of the sebaceous glands
subcutaneous *(same as hypodermic)*	sub-kew-**TAY**-nee-us	S/ P/ R/CF	-ous *pertaining to* sub- *below* -cutan/e- *skin*	Below the skin
transdermal	trans-**DER**-mal	S/ P/ R/	-al *pertaining to* trans- *across, through* -derm- *skin*	Going across or through the skin
ultraviolet	ul-trah-**VIE**-oh-let	P/ R/	ultra- *beyond* -violet *violet, bluish purple*	Light rays at a higher frequency than the violet end of the spectrum
wheal *(same as hives)*	**WHEEL**		Old English *wheal*	Small, itchy swelling of the skin (wheals raised by an injection do not itch)

Exercises

A. Review *Case Report 3.1 to answer the following questions.* **LO 3.5**

1. What type of physician is Dr. Echols? ______
2. What treatments were given for Mr. Andrews' skin cancer? ______
3. What future precautions should Mr. Andrews take? ______

B. Practice *using your medical terminology in the following exercise. When possible, be sure to deconstruct the term using the slashes provided. Fill in the blanks.* **LO 3.1, 3.4, and 3.5**

1. This pigment is responsible for skin color: ______ / ______
   R/CF S
2. Skin needs protection from this type of light: ______ / ______
   P R/CF

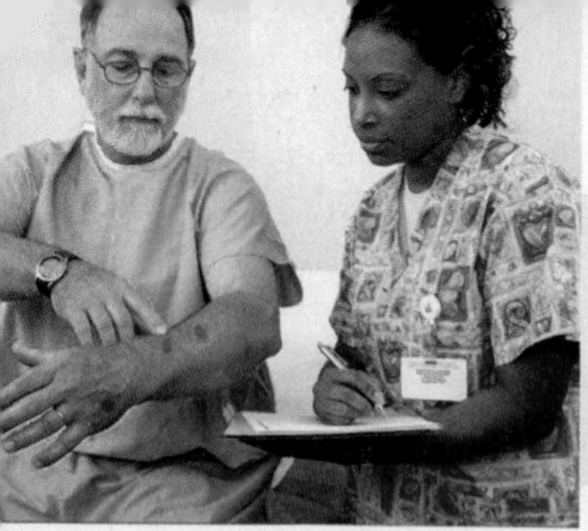

Rick Brady/McGraw-Hill Education

Lesson 3.2

Disorders of the Skin

Objectives

Your skin provides your body's first line of defense against injury, disease, ***allergens,*** *and pollutants. Because your skin is continually exposed to the elements, it's susceptible to various problems and disorders. The skin shows the same types of disease as most organs–infections, tumors, cancers–but because of its protective covering, it's the first responder to many irritant and* ***allergenic*** *agents. The information in this lesson will enable you to use correct medical terminology to:*

3.2.1 Name common disorders of the skin.

3.2.2 Describe the effects of these disorders on health.

CASE REPORT 3.2

You are . . .

. . . a medical assistant working with dermatologist Dr. Lenore Echols in Fulwood Medical Center.

You are communicating with . . .

. . . Ms. Cheryl Fox, a 37-year-old nursing assistant working in a surgical unit in Fulwood Medical Center.

Recently, Ms. Fox's fingers have become red and itchy, with occasional **vesicles.** She has also noticed irritation and swelling of her earlobes and **pruritus.** Over the weekends, both the itching and the **rash** on her hands worsen. A patch test by Dr. Echols showed that Ms. Fox is **allergic** to nickel, which is present in the rings she wears on both hands and in her earrings. She only wears this jewelry on the weekends, not during her workdays.

Dermatitis (LO 3.5)

Dermatitis is an inflammation that produces swollen, red, itchy skin. Ms. Fox has a dermatitis *(Figure 3.4)* resulting from direct exposure to an irritating agent.

The different types of dermatitis and their related causes are as follows:

- **Contact dermatitis** results from direct contact with irritants or allergens, including soaps, detergents, cleaning products, and solvents.
- **Atopic** or **allergic dermatitis** is due to allergens that include nickel in jewelry (as with Ms. Fox), perfume, cosmetics, poison ivy, and latex.
- **Eczema** is a general term used for inflamed and itchy skin conditions. When the itchy skin is scratched, it becomes **excoriated** and produces the dry, red, scaly patches characteristic of eczema. The atopic dermatitis that Ms. Fox developed is a common form of eczema.
- **Seborrheic dermatitis** produces a red rash overlaid with a yellow, oily scale and is common in people with oily skin or hair.
- **Stasis dermatitis** occurs in the lower leg when varicose veins slow the return of blood and the accumulation of fluid interferes with the nourishment of the skin.

Case Report 3.2 *(continued)*

For Ms. Fox, the **allergy** is not just a local reaction to an irritant. Her form of **atopic** or allergic **dermatitis** develops when the whole body becomes sensitive to an allergen. This whole-body involvement is shown by her systemic symptoms of **pruritus** distant from the local irritant site. Ms. Fox has stopped wearing rings and earrings that contain nickel. Her dermatitis was treated with topical steroids *(see Lesson 3.4).*

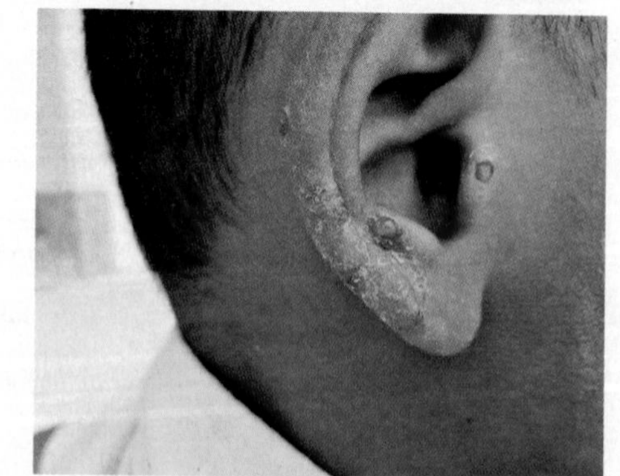

▲ **FIGURE 3.4**
Dermatitis of the Ear.

Paosun Rt/Shutterstock

Word Analysis and Definition

S = Suffix P = Prefix R = Root R/CF = Combining Form

WORD	PRONUNCIATION		ELEMENTS	DEFINITION
allergen *(The duplicate "g" is deleted.)*	**AL**-er-jen	S/ R/ R/ S/	-gen- *produce* **all-** *strange, other* **-erg-** *work, activity* -ic *pertaining to*	Substance producing a hypersensitivity (allergic) reaction
allergenic (adj)	al-er-**JEN**-ik			Pertaining to the capacity to produce an allergic reaction
allergy allergic (adj)	**AL**-er-jee ah-**LER**-jik			Hypersensitivity to an allergen Pertaining to being hypersensitive
atopy atopic (adj)	**AT**-oh-pee ay-**TOP**-ik		Greek *strangeness*	State of hypersensitivity to an allergen—allergic
dermatitis	der-mah-**TYE**-tis	S/ R/	-itis *inflammation* **dermat-** *skin*	Inflammation of the skin
eczema	**EK**-zeh-mah		Greek *to boil* or *ferment*	Inflammatory skin disease, often with a serous discharge
eczematous (adj)	ek-**ZEM**-ah-tus	S/ R/CF	-tous *pertaining to* **eczem/a-** *eczema*	Pertaining to or marked by eczema
excoriate (verb)	eks-**KOR**-ee-ate	S/ P/ R/	-ate *pertaining to* **ex-** *away from* **-cori-** *skin*	To scratch
excoriation (noun)	eks-**KOR**-ee-**AY**-shun	S/	-ation *process*	Scratch mark
pruritus pruritic (adj)	proo-**RYE**-tus proo-**RIT**-ik	S/ R/	Latin *to itch* -ic *pertaining to* **prurit-** *itch*	Itching Itchy
antipruritic	**AN**-tee-proo-**RIT**-ik	P/	**anti-** *against*	Medication against itching
rash	**RASH**		French *skin eruption*	Skin eruption
seborrhea	seb-oh-**REE**-ah	S/ R/CF	-rrhea *flow* **seb/o-** *sebum*	Excessive amount of sebum
seborrheic (adj) *(The "a" is deleted to enable the word to flow.)*	seb-oh-**REE**-ik	S/	-ic *pertaining to*	Pertaining to seborrhea
stasis	**STAY**-sis		Greek *staying in one place*	Stagnation in the flow of any body fluid
vesicle	**VES**-ih-kull		Latin *blister*	Small sac containing liquid; e.g., a blister

EXERCISES

A. Review *Case Report 3.2 to answer the following questions.* **LO 3.4 and 3.5**

1. Which two parts of Ms. Fox's body were exhibiting symptoms? __________
2. Does Ms. Fox experience itching on her earlobes? __________
3. What test did Dr. Echols use to determine the cause of the symptoms? __________
4. What is Ms. Fox allergic to? __________
5. Which of the symptoms means blisters? __________

B. Medical documentation *should always be neat, legible, and spelled correctly for patient safety. Also remember that the patient record is a legal document. After you finish this exercise, you can hear terms pronounced correctly by visiting the audio glossary contained in your Connect® course (http://connect.mheducation.com) and practice them yourself. Below, insert the correct spelling of the term on the line.* **LO 3.5, 3.6, and 3.7**

1. Medication has been prescribed for this patient's case of __________ dermatitis.

   seborheic **seborrheic**

2. The __________ rash on the patient's face is slowly clearing after she tried the new medication.

   eczematous **exzematous**

3. Ms. Fox's __________ is an allergic reaction to her jewelry, which contains nickel.

   purritis **pruritus**

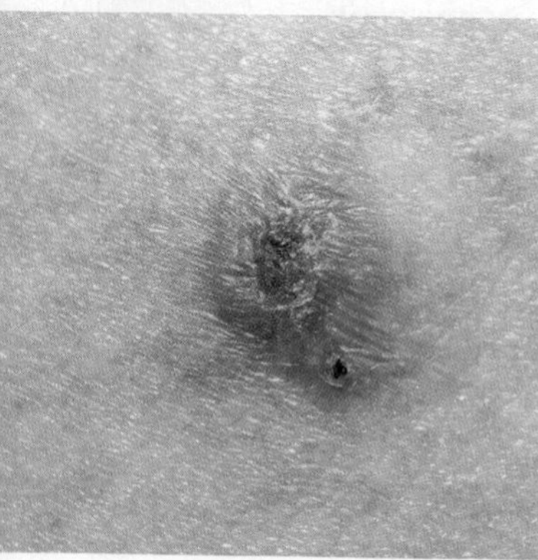

▲ FIGURE 3.5
Basal Cell Carcinoma.

jax10289/Shutterstock

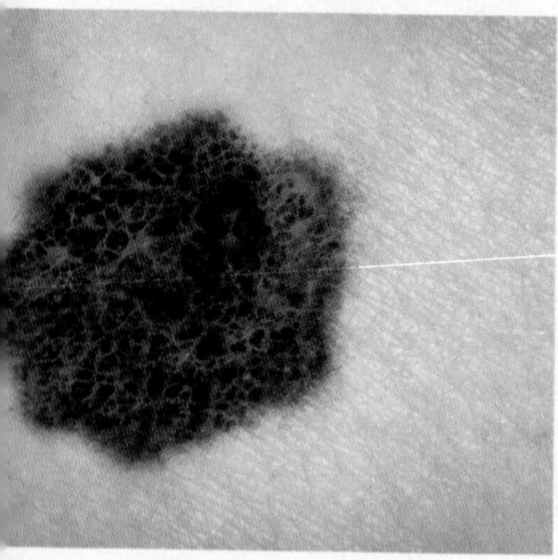

▲ FIGURE 3.6
Malignant Melanoma.

Australis Photography/Shutterstock

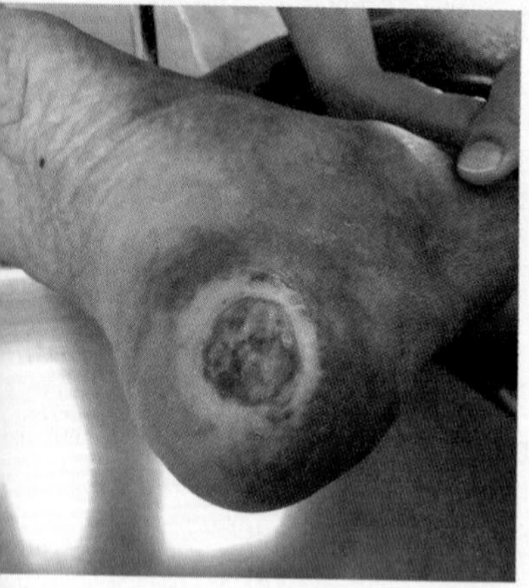

▲ FIGURE 3.7
Decubitus (Pressure) Ulcer on the Heel.

Duangnapa Kanchanasakun/Shutterstock

Skin Cancers (LO 3.5)

The two basal cell carcinomas *(Figure 3.5)* on Mr. Andrews' arm arose from the basal (bottom) layer of his epidermis. This is the most common and the least dangerous form of skin cancer because it does not **metastasize** (spread to elsewhere in the body).

The squamous cell carcinoma on Mr. Andrews' hand arose from cells in the middle layers of the epidermis. This skin cancer responds well to surgical removal but can metastasize to lymph glands if neglected.

Malignant melanoma *(Figure 3.6)* is the least common but most dangerous skin cancer. It arises in melanin-producing cells in the basal layer of the epidermis and metastasizes quickly. If neglected, this cancer is fatal.

Excess **sunlight** can also be an irritant to the skin. Too much sun can burn the skin and may lead to cancer, as it did for Mr. Andrews.

Pressure Ulcers (LO 3.5)

When a patient lies in one position for a long period, the pressure between the bed and the body's bony projections, such as the lower spine or heel, cuts off the blood supply to the skin. Under these circumstances, **pressure** or **decubitus ulcers** can appear *(Figure 3.7)*. When this happens, the skin's protective function is compromised, making it easy for germs to enter the body. The elderly are often at risk for pressure ulcers because their skin is usually thin and dry. In addition, poor nutritional status can deplete the fatty protective layer in the hypodermis under the skin, making the body more susceptible to pressure ulcers.

Congenital Lesions (LO 3.5)

A birthmark caused by abnormal pigmentation or proliferation of blood vessels is called a nevus. Vascular nevi produce the port-wine stain or stork bite on the back of the neck and face; they resolve spontaneously in the first few years of life. The blue-gray, benign, flat Mongolian spot on the lower back of blacks, Native Americans, and Latin Americans usually fades by two years of age.

Infections of the Skin (LO 3.5)

The skin can be susceptible to many different types of infections, including viral, fungal, parasitic, and bacterial infections.

Viral Infections (LO 3.5)

Warts (verrucas) are skin growths caused by the human **papillomavirus** invading the epidermis *(Figure 3.8)*.

Varicella-zoster virus causes chickenpox in unvaccinated people. Here, **macules** (small, flat spots different in color from the surrounding skin), **papules** (small, solid elevations), and **vesicles** (small sacs containing fluid) form. The virus can then remain dormant in the peripheral nerves (near the skin's surface) for decades before erupting as the painful vesicles of **herpes zoster,** also called **shingles** *(Figure 3.9)*.

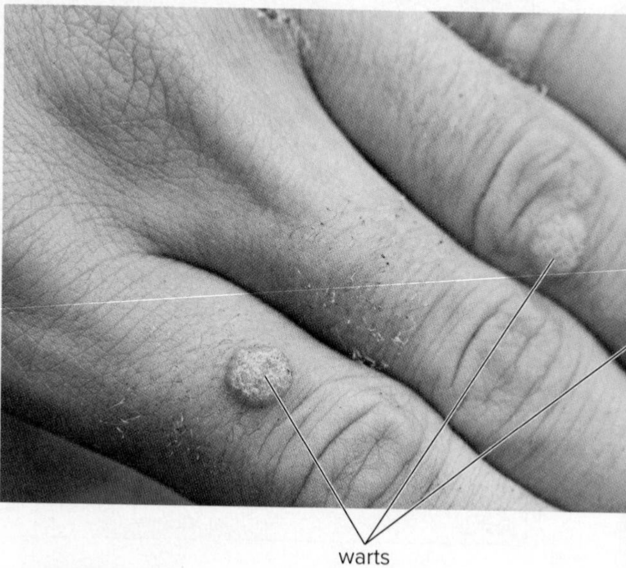

▲ FIGURE 3.8
Warts on Hands.

Marcel Jancovic/Shutterstock

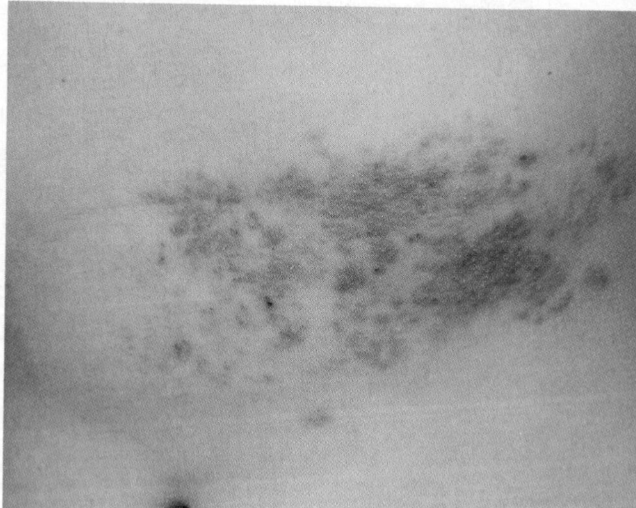

▲ FIGURE 3.9
Shingles.

Franciscodiazpagador/Getty Images

Word Analysis and Definition

S = Suffix P = Prefix R = Root R/CF = Combining Form

WORD	PRONUNCIATION	ELEMENTS		DEFINITION
congenital	con-**JEN**-ih-tal	S/ P/ R/	-al *pertaining to* **con-** *with* -genit- *bring forth*	Present at birth
decubitus ulcer (pressure ulcer)	deh-**KYU**-bit-us **UL**-ser	P/ R/ R/	de- *from* -cubitus *lying down* ulcer *sore*	Sore caused by lying down for long periods of time
herpes zoster (shingles)	**HER**-peez **ZOS**-ter		herpes Greek *to creep or spread* zoster Greek *belt, girdle*	Painful eruption of vesicles that follows a nerve root on one side of the body
macule	**MACK**-yul		Latin *spot*	Small, flat spot or patch on the skin
malignant	mah-**LIG**-nant	S/ R/	-ant *forming, pertaining to* **malign-** *harmful, bad*	Tumor that invades surrounding tissues and metastasizes to distant organs
malignancy	mah-**LIG**-nan-see	S/	-ancy *state of*	State of being malignant
melanin melanoma	**MEL**-ah-nin mel-ah-**NO**-mah	 S/ R/	Greek *black* **-oma** *tumor, mass* **melan-** *black pigment*	Black pigment found in skin, hair, and retina Malignant neoplasm formed from cells that produce melanin
metastasis (noun) metastasize (verb) metastatic (adj)	meh-**TAS**-tah-sis meh-**TAS**-tah-size meh-tah-**STAT**-ik	P/ R/ S/ R/ S/	**meta-** *beyond, subsequent to* **-stasis** *stagnate, stay in one place* **-ize** *affect in a specific way* **-stat-** *stationary* **-ic** *pertaining to*	Spread of a disease from one part of the body to another To spread to distant parts Pertaining to the character of cells that can metastasize
nevus nevi (pl)	**NEE**-vus **NEE**-veye		Latin *mole, birthmark*	Congenital lesion of the skin
papillomavirus	pap-ih-**LOH**-mah-vi-rus	S/ R/CF	**-oma** *mass, tumor* **papill/o-** *papilla, pimple* **virus** Latin *poison*	Virus that causes warts and is associated with cancer
papule	**PAP**-yul		Latin **pimple**	Small, circumscribed elevation on the skin
verruca	ver-**ROO**-cah		Latin **wart**	Wart caused by a virus

Exercises

A. Identify *the italicized element* in the first column of the chart, define it, and use it to determine the meaning of the medical term. **LO 3.1 and 3.5**

Medical Term	Identity of Element (P, S, R, or CF)	Meaning of Element	Meaning of Medical Term
meta*stasis*	1.	2.	3.
*malign*ant	4.	5.	6.
melan*oma*	7.	8.	9.
*de*cubitus	10.	11.	12.

B. Demonstrate *that you are able to spell medical terms related to disorders of the skin. Fill in the blank with the correct term from the list below. Not all terms will be used.* **LO 3.5**

congenital **herpes zoster** **macule** **nevi** **nevus** **papillomavirus**

1. The medical term that means the same as *mole* is ____________________
2. Shingles is caused by the ____________________ virus.
3. The plural form of the term *nevus* is ____________________.
4. A birthmark is a ____________________ accumulation of pigment in the skin.

Fungal Infections (LO 3.5)

Tinea is a general term for a group of related skin infections caused by different species of **fungi.**

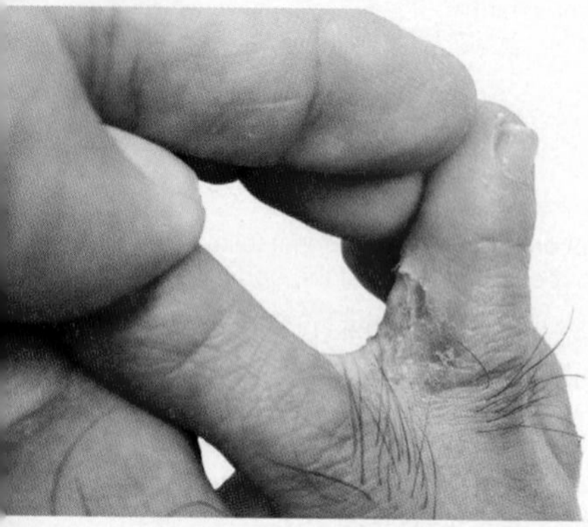

▲ **FIGURE 3.10**
Tinea Pedis between the Toes.
Thiti Sukapan/Shutterstock

Tinea pedis, or athlete's foot, causes itching, redness, and peeling of the skin of the foot, particularly between the toes *(Figure 3.10).* **Tinea capitis** describes an infection of the scalp (ringworm). **Tinea corporis** refers to ringworm infections of the body's skin and hands. **Tinea cruris,** or jock itch, is the name for infections of the groin. The fungus spreads from animals, from the soil, and by direct contact with infected individuals.

A yeast-like fungus, ***Candida albicans,*** can produce recurrent infections of the skin, nails, and mucous membranes. The first sign can be a frequent diaper rash or oral **thrush** in infants. Older children can show repeated or persistent lesions on the scalp. In adults, chronic **mucocutaneous candidiasis** can affect the mouth (thrush) *(Figure 3.11),* vagina, and skin. It can also occur with diseases of the immune system *(see Chapter 7),* as those with a compromised immune system are more susceptible to chronic infections, including fungal infections.

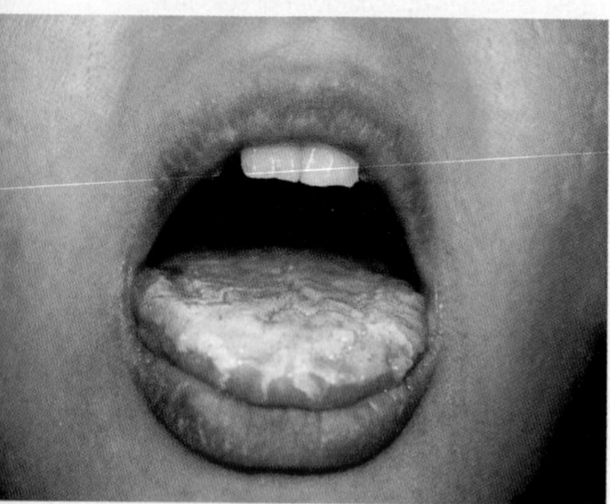

▲ **FIGURE 3.11**
Thrush.
Timonina/Shutterstock

Parasitic Infestations (LO 3.5)

A **parasite** is an organism that lives in contact with and feeds off another organism or host. This process is called an **infestation** and is different from an **infection.**

Lice *(Figure 3.12)* are small, wingless, blood-sucking parasites that produce the disease **pediculosis** by attaching their nits (eggs) to hair and clothing.

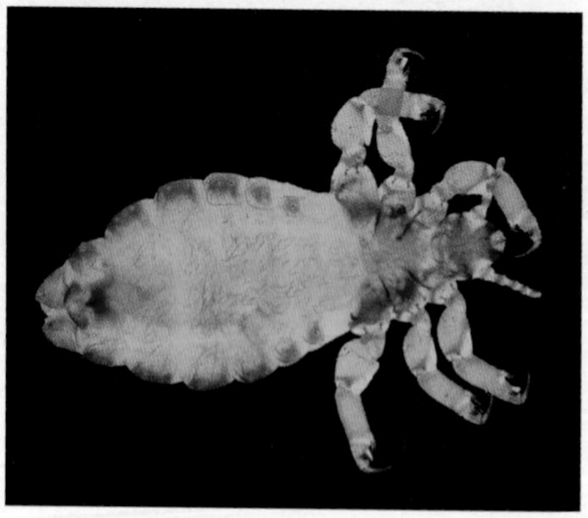

▲ **FIGURE 3.12**
Body Louse.
STEVE GSCHMEISSNER/Getty Images

Itch mites *(Figure 3.13)* produce an intense, itching rash called **scabies,** which generally occurs in the genital area or near the waist, breasts, and armpits. These mites lay eggs under the skin.

Bacterial Infections (LO 3.5)

Staphylococcus aureus (commonly called "staph") is the most common bacterium to invade the skin. Staph causes pimples, boils, **carbuncles,** and **impetigo** *(Figure 3.14).* It can also produce a **cellulitis** of the epidermis and dermis. *Group A Streptococcus* (strep) can also cause cellulitis.

Occasionally, some strains of both staph and strep can be extremely **toxic,** especially when their enzymes digest the connective tissues and spread into the muscle layers. This condition is called **necrotizing fasciitis** and requires highly aggressive surgical and antibiotic treatment.

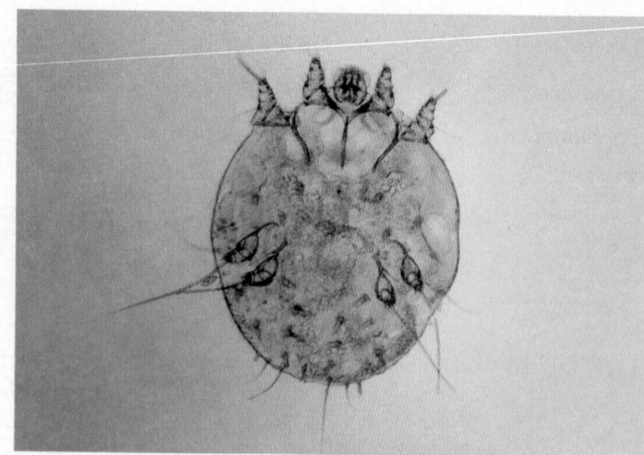

▲ **FIGURE 3.13**
The Itch Mite of Scabies.
Aliaksei Marozau/Shutterstock

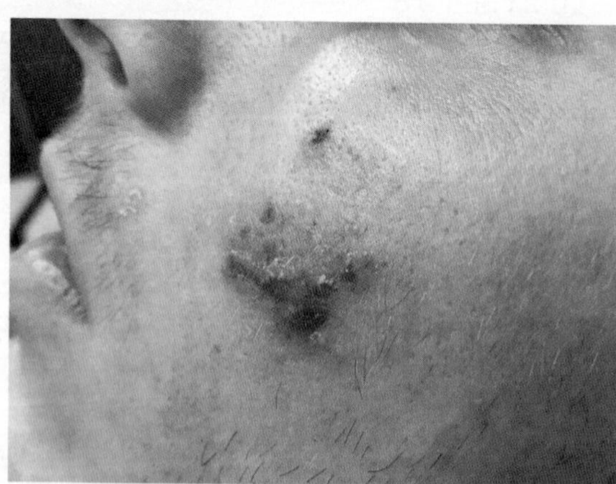

▲ **FIGURE 3.14**
Impetigo.
TisforThan/Shutterstock

Word Analysis and Definition

S = Suffix P = Prefix R = Root R/CF = Combining Form

WORD	PRONUNCIATION	ELEMENTS		DEFINITION
Candida candidiasis *Candida albicans* thrush	**KAN**-did-ah kan-dih-**DIE**-ah-sis **KAN**-did-ah **AL**-bih-kanz **THRUSH**	S/ R/	Latin *dazzling white* -iasis *state of, condition* candid- *Candida* albicans *Latin white*	A yeastlike fungus Infection with the yeastlike fungus The most common form of *Candida* Another name for infection with *Candida*
carbuncle	**KAR**-bunk-ul		Latin *carbuncle*	Infection of many hair follicles in a small area, often on the back of the neck
cellulitis	sell-you-**LIE**-tis	S/ R/	-itis *inflammation* cellul- *cell*	Infection of subcutaneous connective tissue
contagious	kon-**TAY**-jus		Latin *touch closely*	Can be transmitted from person to person or from a person to a surface to a person
fungus fungi (pl)	**FUN**-gus **FUN**-jee or **FUN**-gee		Latin *mushroom*	General term used to describe yeasts and molds
impetigo	im-peh-**TIE**-go		Latin *scabby eruption*	Infection of the skin producing thick, yellow crusts
infection infectious (adj)	in-**FECK**-shun in-**FECK**-shus	S/ R/ S/	-ion *action* infect- *internal invasion, infection* -ious *pertaining to*	Invasion of the body by disease-producing microorganisms Capable of being transmitted, or a disease caused by the action of a microorganism
infestation	in-fes-**TAY**-shun	S/ R/	-ation *process* infest- *invade*	Act of being invaded on the skin by a troublesome other species, such as a parasite
louse lice (pl)	**LOWSE** **LISE**		Old English *louse*	Parasitic insect
mucocutaneous	**MYU**-koh-kyu-**TAY**-nee-us	S/ R/CF R/CF	-ous *pertaining to* muc/o- *mucous membrane* -cutan/e- *skin*	Junction of skin and mucous membrane; e.g., the lips
necrotizing fasciitis *(Note the spelling.)*	**NEH**-kroh-**TIZE**-ing fash-eh-**EYE**-tis	S/ S/ R/CF S/ R/CF	-ing *quality of* -tiz- *pertaining to* necr/o- *death* -itis *inflammation* fasc/i *fascia*	Inflammation of fascia producing death of the tissue
parasite parasitic (adj)	**PAR**-ah-site par-ah-**SIT**-ik	S/ R/	Greek *guest* -ic *pertaining to* parasit- *parasite*	An organism that attaches itself to, lives on or in, and derives its nutrition from another species Pertaining to a parasite
pediculosis	peh-dick-you-**LOH**-sis	S/ R/	-osis *condition* pedicul- *louse*	An infestation with lice
scabies	**SKAY**-beez		Latin *to scratch*	Skin disease produced by mites
tinea	**TIN**-ee-ah		Latin *worm*	General term for a group of related skin infections caused by different species of fungi
toxin toxic (adj) toxicity *(Contains two suffixes)*	**TOK**-sin **TOK**-sick tok-**SIS**-ih-tee	S/ R/ S/	Greek *poison* -ic *pertaining to* tox- *poison* -ity *state, condition*	Poisonous substance formed by a cell or organism Pertaining to a toxin The state of being poisonous

EXERCISE

A. Demonstrate *that you are able to spell medical terms related to disorders of the skin. Fill in the blanks.* **LO 3.2 and 3.5**

1. A condition caused by lice infestation: ______________________________
2. Inflammation of subcutaneous connective tissue: ______________________________
3. What are lice eggs called? ______________________________
4. A skin disease caused by mites: ______________________________
5. An infection of the fascia that results in the death of the tissue: ______________________________

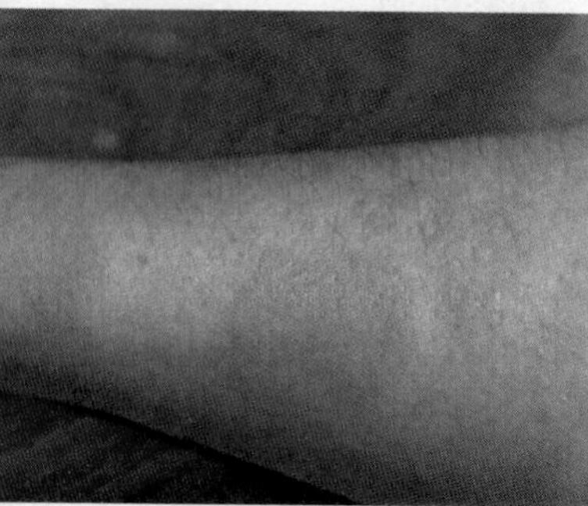

▲ **FIGURE 3.15**
Systemic Lupus Erythematosus.

korn ratchaneekorn/Shutterstock

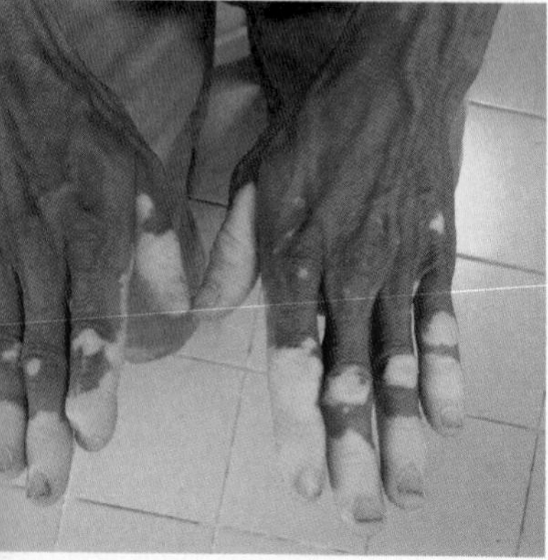

▲ **FIGURE 3.16**
Scleroderma.

Numstocker/Shutterstock

Abbreviations

HIV	human immunodeficiency virus
SLE	systemic lupus erythematosus

Collagen Diseases (LO 3.5)

Collagen, a fibrous protein, comprises 30% of your total body protein. Because your body contains so much of this protein, collagen diseases can have a dramatic effect throughout the body and in the skin.

Systemic lupus erythematosus (SLE) is an **autoimmune** disease that occurs most commonly in women. It produces characteristic skin lesions like a butterfly-shaped, red rash on both cheeks that is joined across the bridge of the nose *(Figure 3.15).* This disease also affects multiple organs, including the kidneys, brain, heart, and joints.

Rosacea produces a similar facial rash to that of SLE, but there are no systemic complications.

Scleroderma is a chronic, persistent autoimmune disease that also occurs more often in women. It's characterized by a hardening and shrinking of the skin that makes it feel leathery *(Figure 3.16).* Joints show swelling, pain, and stiffness. Internal organs, including the heart, lungs, kidneys, and digestive tract, are involved in a similar process. The etiology is unknown, and there is no effective treatment.

Breast cancer can often occur in a patient with scleroderma.

Other Skin Diseases (LO 3.5)

Psoriasis *(Figure 3.17)* is marked by itchy, flaky, red patches of skin of various sizes covered with white or silvery scales. It appears most commonly on the scalp, elbows, and knees, and its cause is unknown.

Skin Manifestations of Internal Disease (LO 3.1, 3.2, 3.3 and 3.5)

The presence of cancer inside the body is often shown by skin lesions visible on the body's surface, even before the cancer or other disease has produced **symptoms** or been diagnosed. **Dermatomyositis** *(Figure 3.18)* is often associated with ovarian cancer, which can appear within 4 to 5 years after the skin disease is diagnosed. This skin disease presents with a reddish-purple rash around the eyes. Muscle weakness commonly follows weeks or months after the appearance of the rash.

Kaposi sarcoma mostly develops in association with **HIV** infection. Raised red or brown blotches or bumps in tissues occur below the skin's surface and eventually spread throughout the body.

Herpes zoster, referred to earlier in this chapter, is common in immunocompromised patients, including the elderly, individuals with HIV, and patients on chemotherapy *(see Chapter 7).*

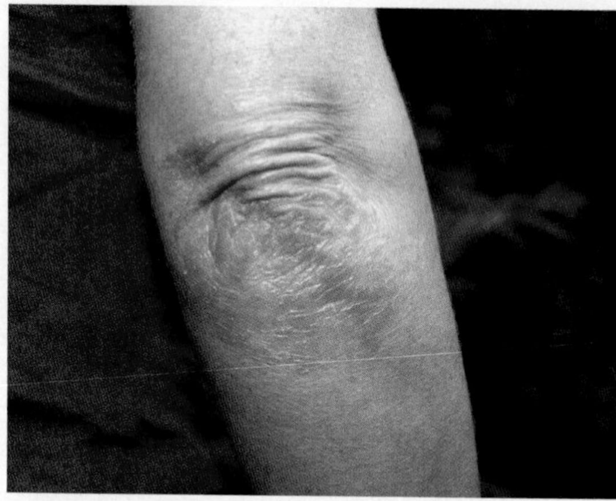

▲ **FIGURE 3.17**
Psoriasis Patch on the Elbow.

Dave Bolton/Getty Images

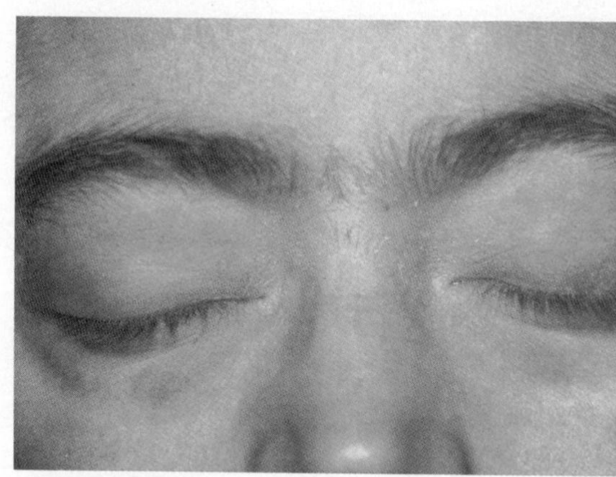

▲ **FIGURE 3.18**
Periorbital Rash of Dermatomyositis.

Mediscan/Alamy Images

Word Analysis and Definition

S = Suffix P = Prefix R = Root R/CF = Combining Form

WORD	PRONUNCIATION	ELEMENTS		DEFINITION
autoimmune	awe-toe-im-**YUNE**	P/ R/	auto- *self* -immune *protected from*	Diseases in which the body makes antibodies directed against its own tissues
dermatomyositis	**DER**-mah-toe-**MY**-oh-site-is	S/ R/CF R/	-itis *inflammation* dermat/o- *skin* -myos- *muscle*	Inflammation of the skin and muscles
Kaposi sarcoma	kah-**POH**-see sar-**KOH**-mah		Moritz Kaposi, Hungarian dermatologist, 1837–1902	A form of skin cancer seen in AIDS patients
psoriasis	so-**RYE**-ah-sis		Greek *the itch*	Rash characterized by reddish, silver-scaled patches
rosacea	roh-**ZAY**-she-ah		Latin *rosy*	Persistent erythematous rash of the central face
scleroderma	sklair-oh-**DERM**-ah	S/ R/CF	-derma *skin* scler/o- *hard*	Thickening and hardening of the skin due to new collagen formation
symptom *(subjective)* symptomatic (adj) sign *(objective)*	**SIMP**-tum simp-toe-**MAT**-ik SINE	 S/ R/	Greek *event or feeling that has happened to someone* -atic *pertaining to* symptom *symptoms* Latin *mark*	Departure from normal health experienced by the patient Pertaining to the symptoms of a disease Physical evidence of a disease process
systemic lupus erythematosus	sis-**TEM**-ik **LOO**-pus er-ih-**THEE**-mah-**TOE**-sus	S/ R/ S/ R/	-ic *pertaining to* system- *the body as a whole* lupus Latin *wolf* -osus *condition* erythemat- *redness*	Inflammatory connective tissue disease affecting the whole body

EXERCISES

A. Document *using the language of dermatology by inserting the correct term in the space provided. Fill in the blanks.* **LO 3.2, 3.5, and 3.7**

1. According to the patient's symptoms, the physician diagnosed a/an (body attacks its own tissues) ______________________ disease.
2. What we thought was originally a localized problem has now spread, and the patient's final diagnosis is (inflammatory connective tissue disease affecting the whole body) ______________________.
3. Because of this patient's past history of HIV, his new skin lesions have been diagnosed by the pathologist as (a form of skin cancer seen in AIDS patients) ______________________.
4. Patients with (rash with reddish, silver-scaled patches) ______________________ often wear long sleeves to hide their elbows.

B. Building medical terms and taking them apart *force you to focus on the elements they contain. Understanding elements is the key to increasing your medical vocabulary. Deconstruct the following terms to increase your knowledge of their elements.* **LO 3.1 and 3.5**

1. In the term **erythematosus,** the root means:
   a. condition of **b.** blemish **c.** red **d.** inflammation
2. In the term **symptomatic,** the suffix means:
   a. pertaining to **b.** inflammation **c.** painful **d.** condition of
3. In the term **dermatomyositis,** the word element that means skin is a:
   a. root/combining form **b.** prefix **c.** suffix
4. In the term **autoimmune,** the word element that means self is a:
   a. root/combining form **b.** prefix **c.** suffix

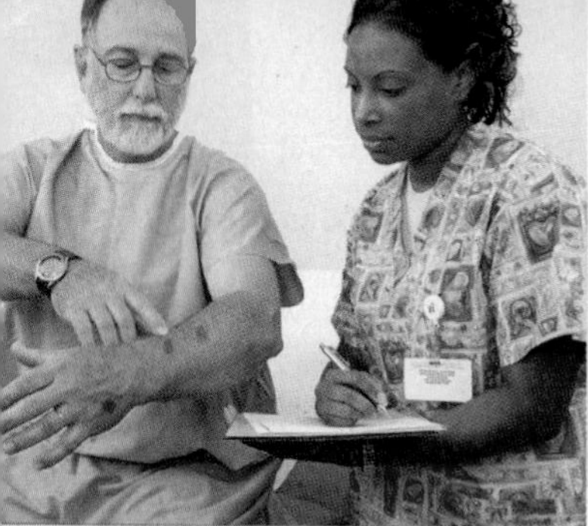
Rick Brady/McGraw-Hill Education

Lesson 3.3
Accessory Skin Organs

Objectives

***Hair follicles, sebaceous glands, sweat glands,** and **nails** are **accessory organs** located in your skin. Each of these skin organs has specific anatomical and physiological characteristics. This lesson will enable you to use correct medical terminology to:*

3.3.1 Distinguish the different accessory skin organs.

3.3.2 Identify the structure and functions of the accessory skin organs.

3.3.3 Describe certain disorders affecting the accessory skin organs.

CASE REPORT 3.3

You are . . .

. . . a pharmacist working in the pharmacy at Fulwood Medical Center.

You are communicating with . . .

. . . Mr. Wayne Winter, an 18-year-old man who will be starting college in a few months.

Mr. Winter has had acne since the age of 15. He has tried several over-the-counter products, all of which have been unsuccessful in treating his acne. He's even tried retinoic acid. He has numerous **comedones,** papules, **pustules,** and **scars** on his face and forehead and has severe **cystic** lesions and scars on his back. His social life is nonexistent, and his peers frequently tease him. He wishes to change all this before he gets to college.

Your role is to explain to him how to use the medications Dr. Echols, a dermatologist, has prescribed, what their effects will be, and what possible complications may occur.

Hair Follicles and Sebaceous Glands (LO 3.4 and 3.5)

Each hair follicle on your face has a sebaceous gland opening into it *(Figure 3.19).* This gland secretes into the follicle oily, acidic sebum, which mixes with broken-down keratin cells from the base of the follicle.

Around puberty, **androgens,** male sex hormones, are thought to trigger an excessive production of sebum from the sebaceous glands. Sebum brings with it excessive numbers of broken-down keratin cells. This blocks the hair follicle, forming a **comedo** (whitehead or blackhead). Comedones can stay closed, leading to papules, or can rupture, allowing bacteria to get in and produce **pustules.** These are the classic signs of **acne.** Acne affects about 85% of people between the ages of 12 and 25 years *(Figure 3.20).*

Another skin problem involving the sebaceous glands is seborrheic dermatitis. Here, the glands are thought to be inflamed and to produce a different sebum. The skin around the face and scalp is reddened and covered with yellow, greasy scales. In infants, this condition is called "cradle cap." Seborrheic dermatitis of the scalp produces dandruff.

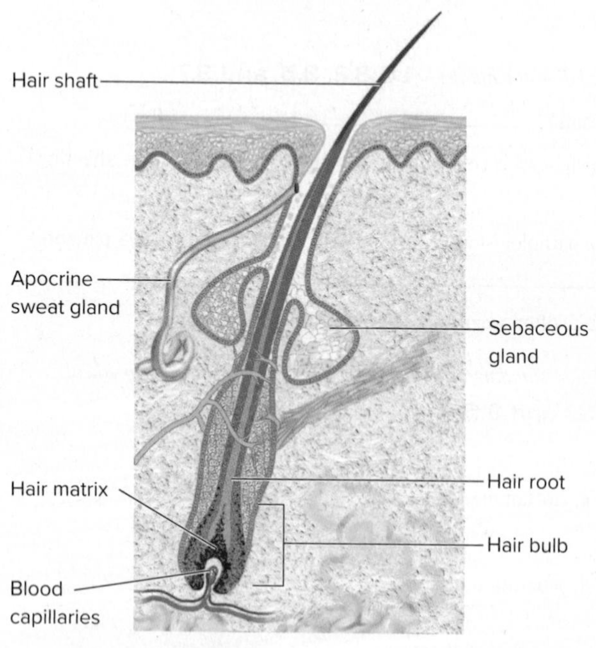

▲ **FIGURE 3.19**
Hair Follicle and Sebaceous Gland.

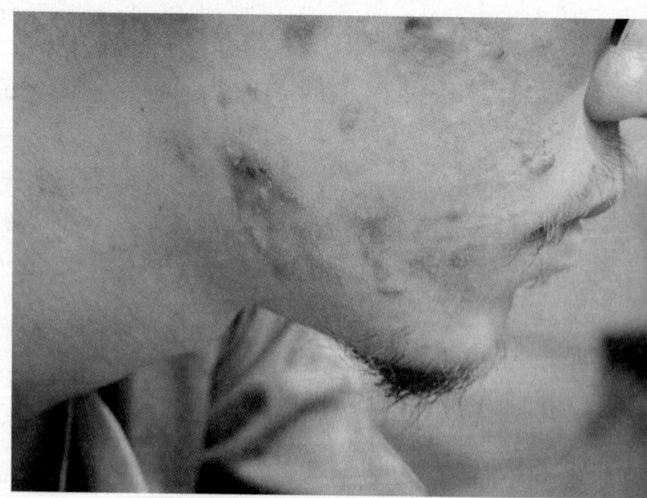

▲ **FIGURE 3.20**
Acne –showing pustules and papules.
NikomMaelao Production/Shutterstock

Word Analysis and Definition

S = Suffix P = Prefix R = Root R/CF = Combining Form

WORD	PRONUNCIATION	ELEMENTS		DEFINITION
acne	**AK**-nee		Greek *point*	Inflammatory disease of sebaceous glands and hair follicles
androgen	**AN**-droh-jen	S/ R/CF	-gen *to produce, create* andr/o- *male*	Hormone that promotes masculine characteristics
comedo *(whitehead or blackhead)* comedones (pl)	**KOM**-ee-doh kom-ee-**DOH**-nz		Latin *eat up*	Too much sebum and too many keratin cells block the hair follicle to produce the comedo
cyst	**SIST**		Greek *sac, bladder*	Abnormal fluid-filled sac surrounded by a membrane
cystic (adj)	**SIS**-tik	S/	-ic *pertaining to*	Pertaining to a cyst
pustule	**PUS**-tyul		Latin *pustule*	Small protuberance on the skin containing pus
scar	**SKAR**		Greek *scab*	Fibrotic seam that forms when a wound heals

Exercises

A. Review *Case Report 3.3 to answer the following questions. Fill in the blanks.* **LO 3.4, 3.5, and 3.6**

1. Does an over the counter medication require a prescription? ______
2. Does Mr. Winter have blackheads, whiteheads, or both? ______
3. Which hormone is likely triggering Mr. Winter's acne? ______
4. Evidence of previous pustules and cystic lesions are noted as: ______
5. What type of specialist did Mr. Winter consult? ______

B. Indicate if the statement is true or false. **LO 3.4**

1. A pustule is filled with pus. True False
2. Acne is a degenerative disease of the skin. True False
3. A cystic lesion is filled with hard, packed cells. True False
4. A comedo can be either a whitehead or a blackhead. True False

C. List *the plural term of the following:* **LO 3.2**

1. scar ______
2. cyst ______
3. comedo ______

Accessory Skin Organs (LO 3.4 and 3.5)

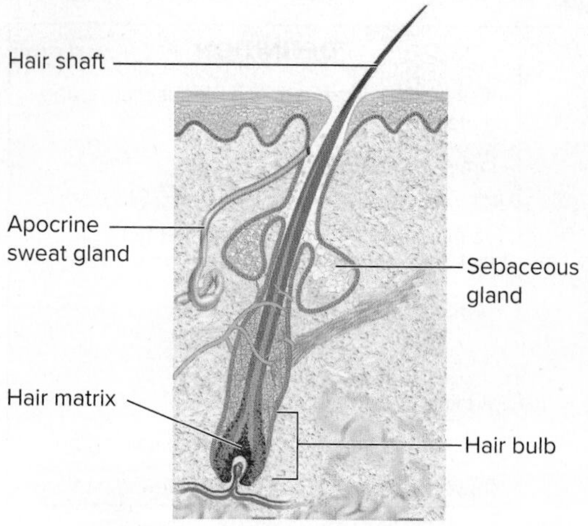

▲ **FIGURE 3.21**
Hair Follicle.

Hair (LO 3.4 and 3.5)

Every hair on your body or scalp originates from epidermal cells at the base (**matrix**) of a hair follicle. As these cells divide and grow, they push older cells upward, away from the source of nutrition in the hair papilla *(Figure 3.21)*. The older cells become keratinized and die.

In most people, aging causes **alopecia,** thinning of the hair, and baldness as the follicles shrink and produce thin, wispy hairs.

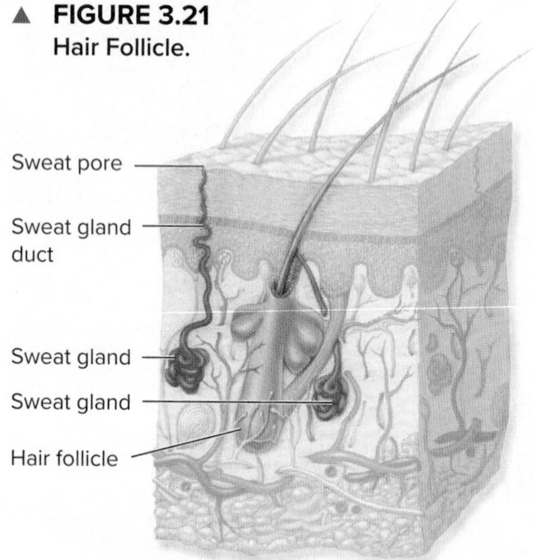

▲ **FIGURE 3.22**
Sweat Glands.

Sweat Glands (LO 3.4 and 3.5)

You have 3 million to 4 million sweat glands scattered all over your skin, with clusters on your palms, soles, and forehead *(Figure 3.22)*. Their main function is to produce the watery perspiration (sweat) that cools your body. Some sweat glands open directly onto the surface of your skin. Others open into your hair follicles *(Figure 3.22)*.

In the dermis, the sweat gland is a coiled tube lined with epithelial, sweat-secreting cells. In your armpits (axillae), around your nipples, in your groin, and around your anus, different sweat glands produce a thick, cloudy secretion. This interacts with your normal skin bacteria to produce a distinct, noticeable smell. The ducts of these glands lead directly into your hair follicles *(see Figure 3.21)*.

Nails (LO 3.4 and 3.5)

Your nails consist of closely packed, thin, dead skin cells that are filled with parallel fibers of hard keratin. On the average, your fingernails grow about 1 millimeter (mm) per week. New cells are added by cell division in the nail matrix, which is protected by the nail fold of skin and the **cuticle** at the base of your nail *(Figure 3.23)*.

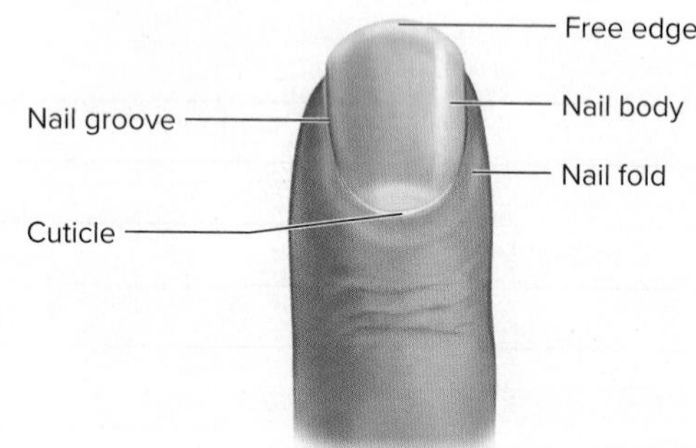

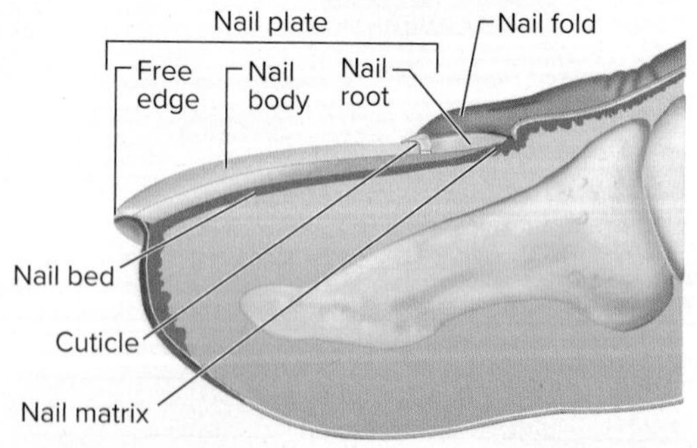

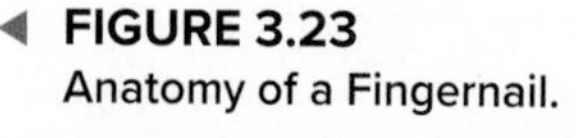

◀ **FIGURE 3.23**
Anatomy of a Fingernail.

Diseases of Nails (LO 3.4 and 3.5)

Fifty percent of all nail disorders are caused by fungal infections and are called **onychomycosis** *(Figure 3.24)*. With these infections, the fungus grows under the nail and leads to yellow, brittle, cracked nails that separate from the underlying nail bed.

Paronychia *(Figure 3.25)* is a bacterial infection, usually staphylococcal, of the nail base. The nail fold and cuticle become swollen, red, and painful, and pus forms under the nail.

With an **ingrown toenail,** the nail grows into the skin at the side of the nail, particularly if pressured by tight, narrow shoes. An infection can then grow underneath this ingrown toenail.

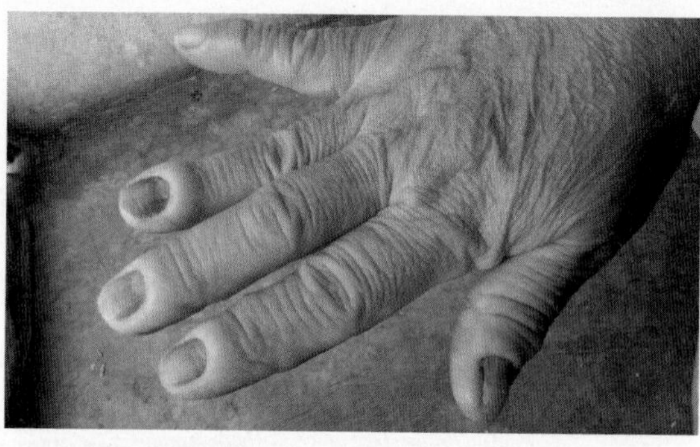

▲ **FIGURE 3.24**
Onychomycosis (Fungal Infection).

jeeraphon/Shutterstock

Pus

▲ **FIGURE 3.25**
Paronychia.

Robert Kirk/Getty Images

Word Analysis and Definition

S = Suffix P = Prefix R = Root R/CF = Combining Form

WORD	PRONUNCIATION	ELEMENTS		DEFINITION
alopecia	al-oh-**PEE**-shah		Greek *mange*	Partial or complete loss of hair, naturally or from medication
cuticle	**KEW**-tih-cul		Diminutive of cutis *skin*	Nonliving epidermis at base of fingernails and toenails
matrix	**MAY**-tricks		Latin *mother*	The formative portion of a hair, nail, or tooth
onychomycosis	oh-nih-koh-my-**KOH**-sis	S/ R/CF R/	-osis *condition* onych/o- *nail* -myc- *fungus*	Condition of a fungus infection in a nail
paronychia (**Note:** *The vowel "a" at the end of para is dropped to make the composite word flow more easily.*)	par-oh-**NICK**-ee-ah	S/ P/ R/	-ia *condition* para- *alongside* -onych- *nail*	Infection alongside the nail

EXERCISES

A. Elements *are clues to the meaning of a medical term. Identify each given element in the following chart and list its meaning.* **LO 3.1**

Element	Identity of Element (P, R, CF, or S)	Meaning of Element
para	1.	2.
ia	3.	4.
myc	5.	6.
onycho	7.	8.
osis	9.	10.
onych	11.	12.

B. Answer the following questions regarding the diseases of the nail. Select the correct answer that completes each statement. **LO 3.4 and 3.5**

1. The structure that protects the nail matrix:

a. nail root

b. free edge

c. cuticle

d. dermis

2. Fungal infection of the nail:

a. paronychia

b. alopecia

c. ingrown toenail

d. onychomycosis

3. Sweat glands open:

a. into hair follicles only

b. onto the surface of the skin only

c. into the hair follicles and onto the surface of the skin

4. Alopecia is defined as a(n):

a. infection of a hair follicle

b. partial or complete hair loss

c. infection alongside the nail

d. fluid- filled sac

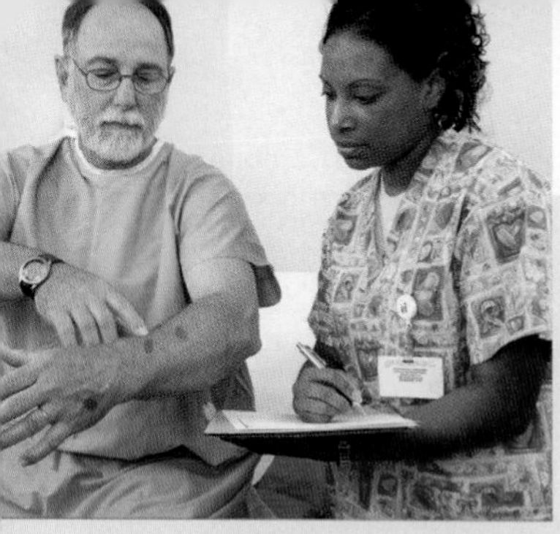
Rick Brady/McGraw-Hill Education

Lesson 3.4

Diagnostic and Therapeutic Procedures and Pharmacology for Skin Disorders (LO 3.6)

Objectives

This lesson will enable you to use correct medical terminology to:

3.4.1 Describe common diagnostic procedures used in dermatology.

3.4.2 Identify common therapeutic procedures used in dermatology.

3.4.3 Define the types of pharmacological agents used in the treatment of skin disorders.

Diagnostic Procedures (LO 3.6)

The most important procedures in making a diagnosis of a skin lesion are a careful history of the etiology and progression of the lesion and a careful visual examination to define the clinical appearance of the lesion.

Diascopy, in which a finger or a microscope slide is pressed against a lesion to see if it blanches, helps define a vascular (inflammatory) lesion, which blanches, from a hemorrhagic lesion (petechia or purpura) which does not blanch.

Microscopic examination of skin scrapings helps diagnose fungal infections and scabies. Tzanck testing by scraping the base of vesicles and staining them with a Giemsa stain shows multinucleated giant cells of herpes simplex or zoster under microscopy.

Cultures using swabs taken from lesions and implanted in the appropriate growth medium are utilized to diagnose some viruses (e.g., herpes simplex) and certain bacteria.

Biopsy (Bx) of a skin lesion using a punch biopsy, excision of a whole lesion, or shaving of the lesion for microscopic examination is valuable in diagnosing malignancies, fungal diseases, and immune diseases.

Wood's light (black light) is used to define the borders of pigmented lesions before excision, show the presence of *Pseudomonas* infection (**fluoresces** green), and distinguish the **hypopigmentation** of vitiligo, which fluoresces a deep ivory white.

Therapeutic Procedures (LO 3.6)

Photodynamic therapy (PDT) in a series of sessions exposes the skin in acne to a high-intensity blue light and creates a toxic environment in which bacteria in the sebaceous glands cannot live. In addition to treating acne, PDT can be used to treat precancerous lesions called **actinic keratoses**, which have the potential to develop into squamous cell carcinomas.

Laser therapy is used for the management of birthmarks, vascular lesions, warts, and skin disorders like vitiligo.

Chemical peels are performed on the face, neck, or hands. An acid solution such as glycolic acid, salicylic acid, or carbolic acid (phenol) is applied to small areas of skin to reduce fine facial lines and wrinkles, treat sun damage, and reduce age spots and dark patches (**melasma**).

Cryotherapy is used frequently to treat acne, scars, sebaceous plaques, and some skin cancers. Liquid nitrogen is sprayed onto the affected area of skin to cause peeling or scabbing.

Used purely for **cosmetic** procedures, Botox is a prescription medicine that blocks signals from nerves to muscles. When injected into superficial muscles, the injected muscle can no longer contract, causing facial wrinkles and lines to temporarily relax and soften.

Dermal fillers such as Restylane and Juvederm help to diminish facial lines and wrinkles by restoring subcutaneous volume and fullness to the face as subcutaneous fat is lost in the natural aging process.

Abbreviations

Bx	biopsy
PDT	Photodynamic therapy

Word Analysis and Definition

S = Suffix P = Prefix R = Root R/CF = Combining Form

WORD	PRONUNCIATION	ELEMENTS		DEFINITION
actinic	ak-**TIN**-ik	S/ R/	-ic *pertaining to* **actin-** *ray*	Pertaining to the sun
cosmetic	koz-**MET**-ik		Greek *an adornment*	A concern for appearance
cryotherapy	**CRY**-oh-**THAIR**-ah pee	P/ R/	**cryo-** *cold* **-therapy** *medical treatment*	The use of cold in the treatment of disease
culture	**KUL**-chur		Latin *tillage*	The growth of microorganisms on or in media
diascopy	di-**AS**-koh-pee	P/ R/	**dia-** *through* **scopy** *to examine, to view*	Examination of superficial skin lesions with pressure
fluoresce	flor-**ESS**		Greek *bright color*	Emit a bright-colored light when irradiated with ultraviolet or violet-blue rays
keratosis keratoses (pl)	ker-ah-**TOH**-sis ker-ah-**TOH**-seez	S/ R/	-osis *condition* **kerat-** *horny*	Epidermal lesion of circumscribed overgrowth of the horny layer
melasma	meh-**LAZ**-mah		Greek *black spot*	Patchy pigmentation of the skin
pigment hypopigmentation	**PIG**-ment **HIGH**-poh-pig-men-**TAY**-shun	S/ P/ R/	Latin *paint* -ation *process* **hypo-** *below normal* **-pigment-** *color*	A coloring matter or stain Below normal melanin relative to the surrounding skin

Exercises

A. Identify *the proper diagnostic procedure or treatment for each condition. Use the words from the provided word bank to complete the sentences. Fill in the blanks.* **LO 3.6**

diascopy **Juvederm** **cryotherapy** **Botox** **fluoresce**

1. Injecting ______________ into the skin will fill areas to reduce the appearance of aging.
2. Acne can be treated with _________ to freeze the cells of the affected area.
3. Pigmented or hypopigmented areas can be better seen when they _________ with Wood's light.
4. Pressing on an area of skin to see if it blanches is termed ________________.
5. The injection of _____ can reduce the appearance of wrinkles by paralyzing the affected muscles.

B. Defining the meaning of word elements can help you to quickly decipher the meaning of medical terms. *Choose the correct answer to each question.* **LO 3.1**

1. The word element that means *cold:*

   a. *dia-* **b.** *-therapy* **c.** *cry/o-* **d.** *hypo-*

2. The word element *dia-* means:

   a. to view **b.** through **c.** light **d.** two

3. The word element *-scopy* means:

   a. to view **b.** scrape **c.** suture **d.** inject

4. The suffix that means *condition of* is:

   a. *-osis* **b.** *-ic* **c.** *-itis* **d.** *-al*

Dermatologic Pharmacology (LO 3.6)

A wide range of **topical pharmacologic** agents of different types can be used in the treatment of skin lesions either to relieve symptoms or to cure the disease.

- **Anesthetics**: topical agents that relieve pain or itching on the skin's surface. Benzocaine is used for this purpose as a numbing **cream.** It is used prior to injections, for oral ulcers, for hemorrhoids, and for infant teething.
- **Antibacterials:** topical agents that eliminate bacteria that cause skin lesions. Neomycin **ointment** is commonly used.
- **Antifungals:** topical agents that eliminate or inhibit the growth of fungi. Nystatin (*Mycostatin, Nilstat*) is used as a cream or ointment. Terbinafine (*Lamisil*) is used as a cream or ointment. Clotrimazole (*Canesten, Clomazol*) and ketaconazole (*Ketopine, Daktagold*) are *imadazoles* available in creams, sprays, **lotions,** and **shampoos.** Amphotericin B (*Fungizone*) is used locally to treat oral candidiasis (thrush), and in IV therapy for systemic fungal infections.
- **Antipruritics**: topical lotions, ointments, creams, or sprays that relieve itching. **Corticosteroids** such as hydrocortisone are most frequently used.
- **Keratolytics:** topical agents that peel away the skin's stratum corneum from the other epidermal layers. Salicylic acid is used for this purpose in the treatment of acne, psoriasis, ichthyoses, and dandruff. It is available in the form of wipes, creams, **lotions, gels,** ointments, and **shampoos** in strengths varying from 3% to 20%.
- **Parasiticides:** topical agents that kill parasites living on the skin. Hexachlorocyclohexane (*Lindane 1%*) is used in lotion or shampoo form to kill lice if other methods have failed.
- **Retinoids**: derivatives of retinoic acid (vitamin A) used under the strict supervision of a physician in the treatment of acne, sun spots, and psoriasis. Tretinoin (*Retin-A*) is used topically for acne; isoretinoin (*Accutane*) is taken orally for severe acne; etretinate (*Tegison*) is taken orally to treat severe psoriasis; and adapalene (*Differin*) is used topically for psoriasis.

Classes of Topical Medications
Solutions are usually a powder dissolved in water or alcohol.
Lotions are usually a powder mixed with oil and water to be thicker than a solution.
Gels are a semisolid **emulsion** in an alcohol base.
Creams are an emulsion of oil and water that is thicker than a lotion and holds its shape when removed from its container. They penetrate the outer stratum corneum layer of skin.
Ointments are a homogenous semisolid preparation, 80% a thick oil and 20% water, that lies on the skin. They can also be used on the mucous membranes of the eye, vulva, anus, and nose, and are emulsifiable with the mucous membrane secretions.
Transdermal patches are a very precise time-released method to deliver a drug. Release of the drug can be controlled by **diffusion** through the adhesive that covers the whole patch or through a membrane with adhesive only on the patch rim.

Word Analysis and Definition

S = Suffix P = Prefix R = Root R/CF = Combining Form

WORD	PRONUNCIATION	ELEMENTS		DEFINITION
anesthetic	an-es-**THET**-ik	S/ P/ R/	-ic *pertaining to* an- *without* -esthet- *sensation, perception*	Substance that takes away feeling and pain.
antibacterial	**AN**-tee-bak-**TEER**-ee-al	S/ P/ R/CF	-al *pertaining to* anti- *against* -bacter/i-	Destroying or preventing the growth of bacteria
antifungal	**AN**-tee-**FUN**-gul	R/	fung- *fungus*	Destroying or preventing the growth of a fungus
antipruritic	**AN**-tee-pru-**RIT**-ik	S/ P/ R/	-ic *pertaining to* anti- *against* -prurit- *itch*	Medication against itching
cream	KREEM		Latin *thick juice*	A semisolid emulsion
diffusion	dih-**FYU**-zhun	S/ R/	-ion *process* diffus- *movement*	The process by which small particles move between tissues
emulsion	ee-**MUL**-shun	S/ R/	-ion *process* emuls- *suspension in a liquid*	Very small particles suspended in a solution
keratolytic	**KER**-ah-toh-**LIT**-ik	S/ R/CF R/	-ic *pertaining to* kerat/o- *horn* -lyt- *loosening*	Causing separation or loosening of the horny layer (stratum corneum) of the skin
parasiticide	par-ah-**SIT**-ih-side	S/ R/CF	-cide *to kill* parasit/i *parasite*	Agent that destroys parasites
retinoid	**RET**-ih-noyd		Derived from retinoic acid	A cream that is a derivative of vitamin A used to treat acne and wrinkles
topical	**TOP**-ih-kal	S/ R/	-al *pertaining to* topic- *local*	Medication applied to the skin to obtain a local effect

EXERCISES

A. Practice *your language of pharmacology by correctly filling in the blanks of each sentence.* **LO 3.6 and 3.7**

Mrs. Robison brought in her 8-year-old daughter to the doctor because the child had a red ring-like rash on her abdomen. Dr. Palmer examined the child and diagnosed her with tinea corporis. She prescribed terbenafine cream to be applied to the site twice daily for 6 weeks.

1. Dr. Palmer prescribed an ________________ cream to cure the patient's tinea corporis.

2. She prefers to provide ___________________ application of the medication because it stays local to the site of the infection.

B. Define *the classes of topical medications. Topical medications come in a variety of forms to best deliver medication to the skin. Match the description of the form of the medication to its term.* **LO 3.7**

	Term	Meaning
_____	**1.** gel	**a.** adhesive membrane attached to the surface of the skin
_____	**2.** lotion	**b.** semisolid emulsion in an alcohol base
_____	**3.** ointment	**c.** powder dissolved in alcohol or water
_____	**4.** transdermal patch	**d.** powder mixed with oil and water; thicker than a solution
_____	**5.** solution	**e.** semisolid preparation of oil and water

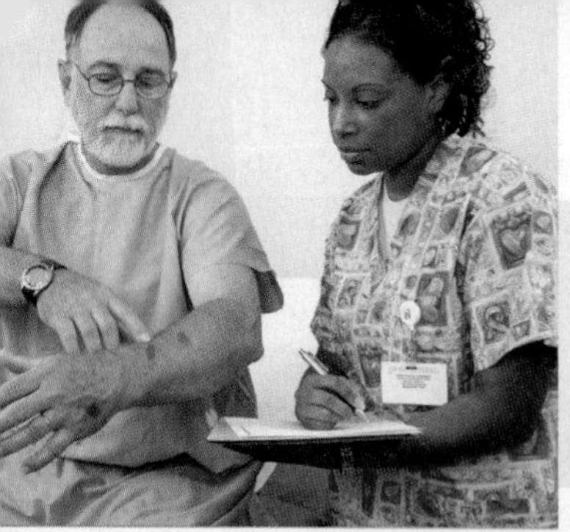

Rick Brady/McGraw-Hill Education

Lesson 3.5

Burns and Injuries to the Skin

Objectives

Your role is to participate in patient care as a member of the Burn Unit team. You will be communicating with family members about the extent of the patient's injuries, the necessary and available treatment options, and the patient's prognosis. You need to be able to use correct medical terminology to:

3.5.1 Distinguish the four classes of burns.

3.5.2 Describe the **inflammatory** and repair process of the skin when it is injured.

3.5.3 Identify local and systemic complications of burns.

CASE REPORT 3.5

You are . . .

. . . a burn technologist employed in the Burn Unit at Fulwood Medical Center.

You are communicating with . . .

. . . the son and daughter of Mr. Steven Hapgood, a 52-year-old man.

Mr. Hapgood has been admitted to the Fulwood Burn Unit with severe burns over his face, chest, and abdomen. After an evening of drinking, he began smoking in bed and fell asleep. His next-door neighbors smelled smoke and called 911. In the Burn Unit, his initial treatment included large volumes of intravenous fluids to prevent shock.

Keynotes

- Sunburn causes a first-degree burn.
- **Scalds** can cause second-degree burns.
- House fires with prolonged flame contact can cause third-degree burns.
- High-voltage electrical injury can cause fourth-degree burns.

Burns (LO 3.4 and 3.5)

In burns, the immediate threats to life are from fluid loss, infection, and the systemic effects of burned dead tissue. Burn injury to the lungs through damage from heat or smoke inhalation is responsible for 60% or more of burn-related fatalities.

Burns are classified according to the depth of burnt tissue involved *(Figure 3.26):*

First-degree (superficial) burns involve only the epidermis and produce superficial **inflammation,** with redness, pain, and slight edema. Healing takes 3 to 5 days without scarring.

Second-degree (partial-thickness) burns involve the epidermis and dermis but leave some of the dermis intact. They produce redness, blisters, and more severe pain. Healing takes 2 to 3 weeks, with minimal scarring.

Third-degree (full-thickness) burns involve the epidermis, dermis, and subcutaneous tissues, which are often completely destroyed. Healing takes a long time and involves skin **grafts.**

Fourth-degree burns destroy all layers of the skin and involve underlying tendons, muscles, and, sometimes, bones.

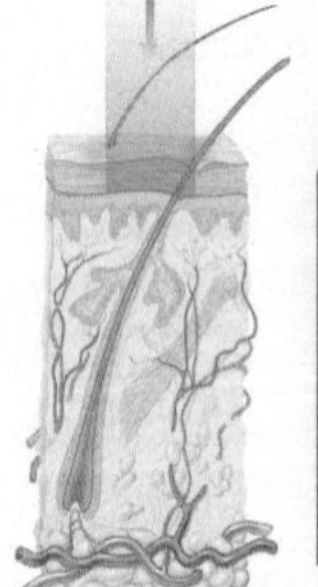
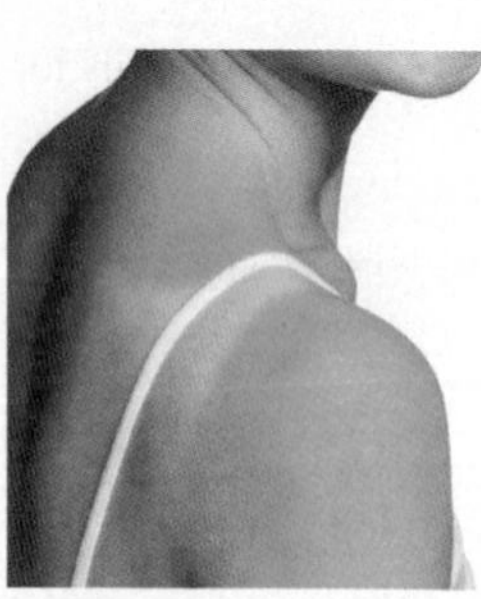

(a)

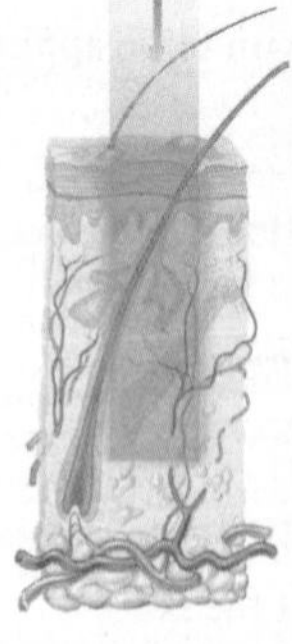
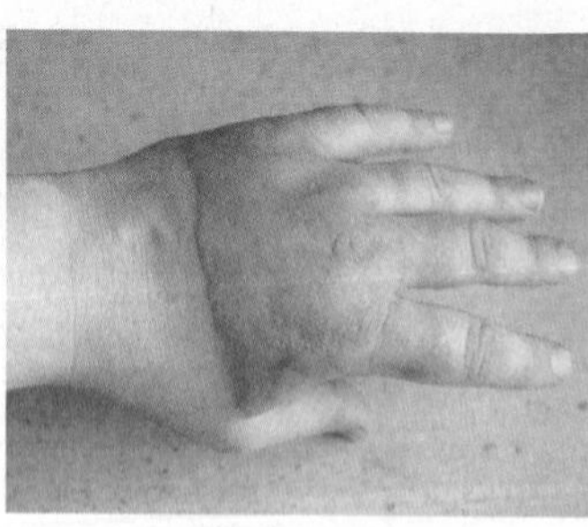

(b)

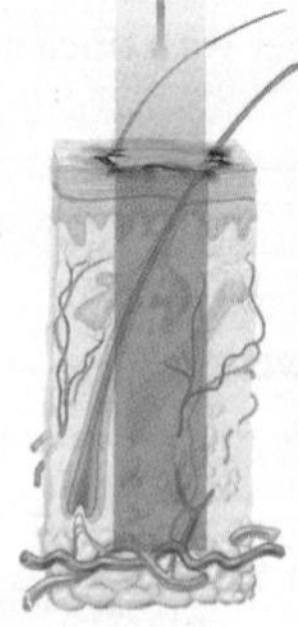
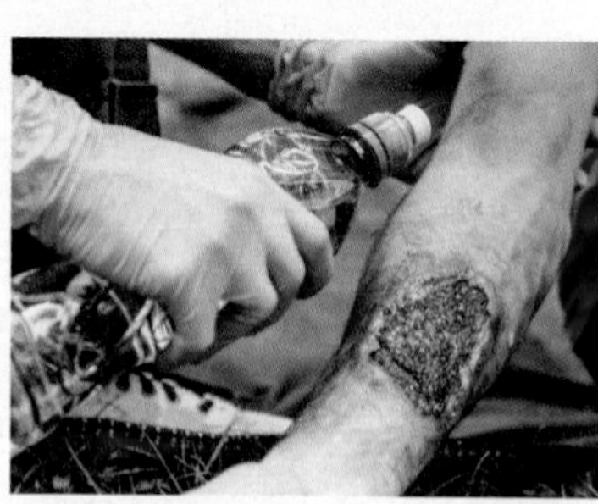

(c)

▲ **FIGURE 3.26**
Partial- and Full-Thickness Burns.
(a) First degree (superficial thickness). (b) Second degree (partial thickness). (c) Third degree (full thickness).

Dmitrii Kotin/Alamy Stock Photo Oksana_Slepko/Shutterstock Microgen/Shutterstock

Word Analysis and Definition

S = Suffix P = Prefix R = Root R/CF = Combining Form

WORD	PRONUNCIATION	ELEMENTS		DEFINITION
inflammation	in-flah-**MAY**-shun	S/ P/ R/	-ion *action, condition* in- *in* -flammat- *flame*	A complex of cell and chemical reactions occurring in response to an injury or chemical or biologic agent
inflammatory (adj)	in-**FLAM**-ah-tor-ee	S/	-ory *having the function of*	Causing or affected by inflammation
scald	SKAWLD		Latin *wash in hot water*	Burn from contact with hot liquid or steam
shock	SHOCK		German *to clash*	Sudden physical or mental collapse or circulatory collapse

EXERCISES

A. Review *Case Report 3.5 to answer the following.* **LO 3.5 and 3.7**

1. What areas of his body have the most severe burns? ______________________
2. How did Mr. Hapgood sustain these burns? ______________________
3. How do intravenous fluids get into the body? ______________________
4. What is the fluid treatment designed to prevent in Mr. Hapgood's case? ______________________

B. Lesson objectives: *Meet the lesson objectives with this exercise on burns. Employ your knowledge of medical terms from the integumentary system. Fill in the blanks.* **LO 3.2, 3.5, and 3.7**

1. High-voltage electrocution typically causes:

   Degree of burn: ______________________

   ____

   Layers of skin involved: ______________________

2. Scalding typically causes:

   Degree of burn: ______________________

   ____

   Layers of skin involved: ______________________

3. Prolonged flame contact in a house fire typically causes:

   Degree of burn: ______________________

   ____

   Layers of skin involved: ______________________

   What specific surgical procedure is used to promote healing for this type of burn? ______________________

4. Sunburn typically causes:

   Degree of burn: ______________ Signs: ______________________

   ____

   Layers of skin involved: ______________________

Burns (continued) (LO 3.4 and 3.5)

Keynote

- In third- and fourth-degree burns, there is no dermal tissue left for regeneration, and skin grafts are necessary.

In full-thickness burns, because there is no dermal tissue left for **regeneration,** skin grafts are necessary. The ideal graft is an **autograft,** taken from another location on the patient's body, because it is not rejected by the immune system. Mr. Hapgood had autografts taken from his unburned legs and back.

If the patient's burns are too extensive, **allografts**–grafts from another person–are used. **Homograft** is another name for allograft. These grafts are provided by skin banks, which acquire them from deceased people **(cadavers).** A **xenograft** or **heterograft** is a graft from another species, such as a pig for heart valves.

In addition, artificial skin is being developed commercially and can stimulate the growth of new connective tissues from the patient's underlying tissue.

Case Report 3.5 (continued)

Mr. Hapgood's burns were mostly third-degree. The burned, dead tissue formed an eschar that can have toxic effects on the digestive, respiratory, and cardiovascular systems. The **eschar** was surgically removed by debridement.

Anterior head and neck 4½%
4½%
Anterior trunk 18%
Anterior upper extremities 9%
4½%
4½%
Genitalia 1%
9%
9%
Anterior lower extremities 18%

Rule of Nines (LO 3.4 and 3.5)

The treatment and prognosis for a burn patient also depend on how much of the body surface is affected. This is estimated by subdividing the skin's surface into regions, each one of which is a fraction of or multiple of 9% of the total surface area *(Figure 3.27).* To give you a clearer idea of how these numbers come into play, the body's surface areas are assigned the following percentages:

- Head and neck = 9% (4½% anterior and 4½% posterior).
- Each arm = 9% (4½% anterior and 4½% posterior).
- Each leg = 18% (9% anterior and 9% posterior).
- The anterior trunk = 18%.
- The posterior trunk = 18%.
- Genitalia = 1%.

Aging of the Skin (LO 3.4 and 3.5)

With aging, the epidermis thins and the number of melanocytes decreases, but the remaining melanocytes increase in size. Aging skin, therefore, appears thinner, paler, and more translucent, and large pigmented spots **(lentigos)** appear in sun-exposed areas. The blood vessels of the dermis become fragile, leading to bruising and bleeding under the skin. Sebaceous glands produce less oil, leading to dryness and itching. Sweat glands produce less sweat, making it harder to keep cool. The subcutaneous fat layer thins, connective tissue becomes less elastic, and the skin wrinkles and tears easily. Aging skin repairs slowly and wound healing takes up to 4 times longer. Most of these skin changes are hastened and increased by sun exposure.

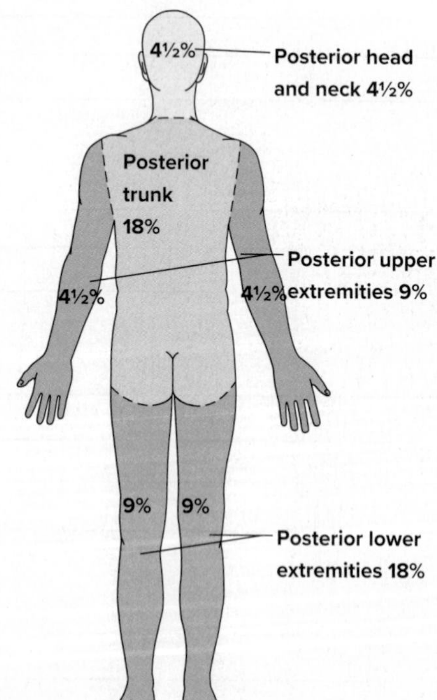

FIGURE 3.27
Rule of Nines.

Word Analysis and Definition

S = Suffix P = Prefix R = Root R/CF = Combining Form

WORD	PRONUNCIATION	ELEMENTS		DEFINITION
allograft	**AL**-oh-graft	P/ R/	**allo-** *other* -graft *transplant*	Skin graft from another person or a cadaver
autograft	**AWE**-toe-graft	P/ R/	auto- *self, same* -graft *transplant*	A graft removed from the patient's own skin
cadaver	kah-**DAV**-er		Latin *dead body*	A dead body or corpse
debridement	day-**BREED**-mon (French pronunciation of -ment)	S/ P/ R/	-ment *resulting state* de- *take away* -bride- *rubbish*	The removal of injured or necrotic tissue
eschar	**ESS**-kar		Greek *scab of a burn*	The burnt, dead tissue lying on top of third-degree burns
heterograft *(same as xenograft)*	**HET**-er-oh-graft	P/ R/	hetero- *different* -graft *transplant*	A graft from another species (not human)
homograft *(same as allograft)*	**HOH**-moh-graft	P/ R/	homo- *same, alike* -graft *transplant*	Skin graft from another person or a cadaver
lentigo	len-**TIH**-go		Greek *lentil*	Age spot; small, flat, brown-black spot in the skin of older people
regenerate (verb) **regeneration (noun)**	ree-**JEN**-eh-rate ree-**JEN**-eh-**RAY**-shun	S/ P/ R/ S/	-ate *composed of* re- *again* -gener- *produce* -ation *process*	Reconstitution of a lost part The process of reconstitution
xenograft *(same as heterograft)*	**ZEN**-oh-graft	P/ R/	xeno- *foreign* -graft *transplant*	A graft from another species (not human)

EXERCISES

A. Review *Case Report 3.5 to answer the following questions.* **LO 3.2, 3.5, and 3.7**

1. What degree of burns did Mr. Hapgood suffer? ______________________________
2. The burned, dead tissue is referred to as: ______________________________
3. What is the surgical procedure called that removes burned, dead tissue? ______________________________

B. Compare and contrast *the meanings of word elements that describe the types of skin grafts. Fill in each blank with the correct term that completes each sentence.* **LO 3.4 and 3.5**

1. A graft from another species is a **xenograft** and a __________.
2. A graft from another person is an **allograft** and a __________.
3. A graft taken from one part of a person's body and placed elsewhere on the same body: ______.

C. Remembering *the meaning of the word element can help you easily identify the type of skin grafts. Match the prefix to its meaning.* **LO 3.4 and 3.5**

1. hetero-	**a.** other
2. allo-	**b.** same, alike
3. xeno-	**c.** self
4. homo-	**d.** different
5. auto-	**e.** foreign

Wounds and Tissue Repair (LO 3.5 and 3.6)

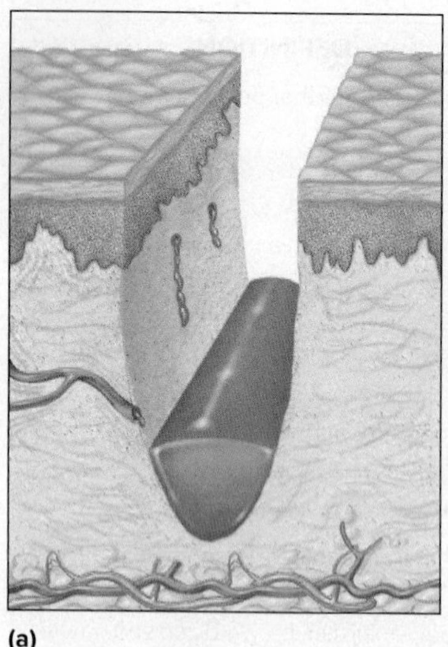

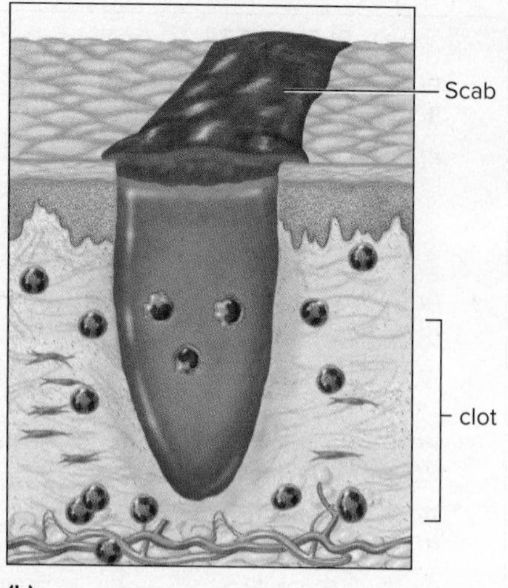

(a) (b)

▲ **FIGURE 3.28**
Wound Healing.
(a) Bleeding into the wound. (b) Scab formation.

If you cut yourself when shaving and produce a superficial **laceration** in the epidermis, the epithelial (surface tissue) cells along the laceration's edges will split rapidly and fill in the gap to heal it.

If you cut yourself more deeply, creating a **wound** in the dermis or hypodermis, blood vessels in the dermis break and blood escapes into the wound *(Figure 3.28a).* The same happens when a surgeon makes an **incision.** On the other hand, a surgeon would perform an **excision** if he or she removed a lesion from the skin or any other tissue.

Escaped blood from a wound or surgical procedure forms a **clot** in the wound. The clot consists of the protein fibrin together with platelets, blood cells, and dried tissue fluids trapped in the fibers. Cells that digest and clean up the tissue debris enter the wound *(see Chapter 7).* The surface of the clot dries and hardens in the air to form a **scab.** The scab seals and protects the wound from becoming infected *(Figure 3.28b).*

New capillaries from the surrounding dermis then invade the clot. Three or four days after the injury, other cells migrate into the wound. These cells form new collagen fibers that pull the wound together. This soft tissue in the wound is called **granulation** tissue *(Figure 3.29),* which is later replaced by a scar *(Figure 3.30).*

Suturing brings together the edges of the wound to enhance tissue healing.

In some patients, there is excessive fibrosis and scar tissue, producing raised, irregular, lumpy, shiny scars called **keloids** *(Figure 3.31).* Keloids, most commonly found on the upper body and earlobes, can extend beyond the edges of the original wound and often return if they are surgically removed.

A superficial scraping of the skin, a mucous membrane, or the cornea *(Chapter 11)* is called an **abrasion.**

Surgery on the skin is now being performed using focused light beams called lasers. These lasers remove lesions like birthmarks and tattoos and create a fresh surface over which skin can grow.

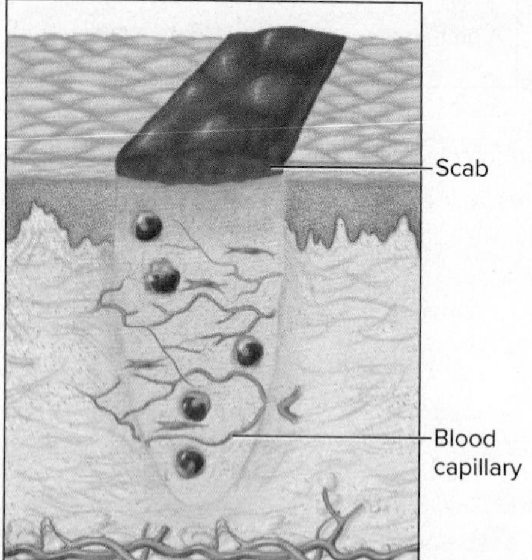

▲ **FIGURE 3.29**
Formation of Granulation Tissue.

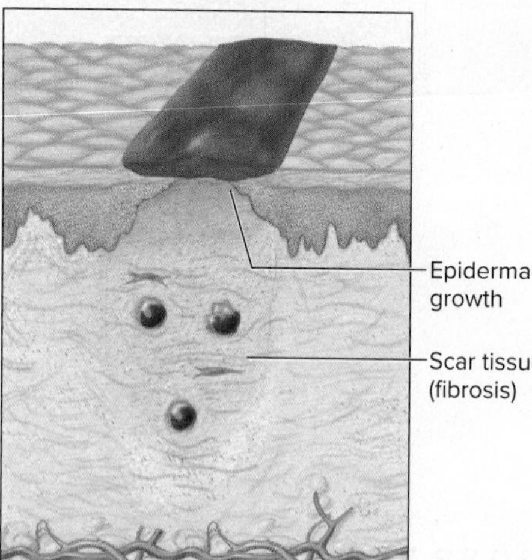

▲ **FIGURE 3.30**
Scar Formation.

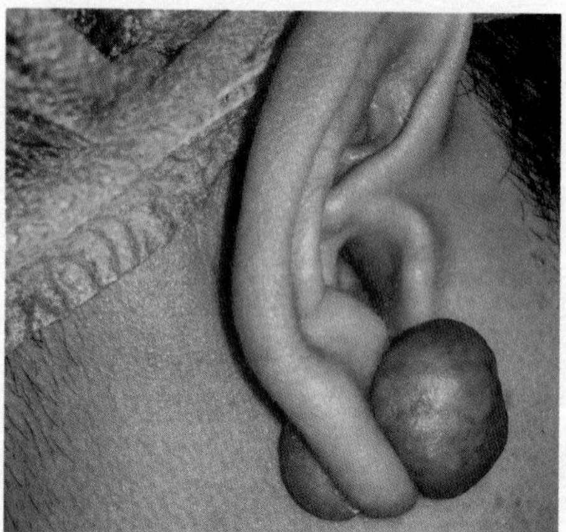

▲ **FIGURE 3.31**
Keloid of the Earlobe—resulting from piercing of the earlobe.

Karan Bunjean/Shutterstock

Cosmetic Procedures (LO 3.1, 3.2, 3.5, 3.6, and 3.8)

Surgical procedures that cosmetically alter or improve the appearance of your face or body are becoming more and more common. These cosmetic procedures include:

Abdominoplasty: a "tummy tuck."

Blepharoplasty: the correction of defects in the eyelids.

Dermabrasion: the removal of upper layers of skin using a high-powered rotating brush.

Lipectomy: the surgical removal of fatty tissue by excision.

Liposuction: the surgical removal of fatty tissue using suction.

Mammoplasty: the surgical procedure to alter the size or shape of the breasts.

Rhinoplasty: the surgical procedure to alter the size or shape of the nose.

Word Analysis and Definition

S = Suffix P = Prefix R = Root R/CF = Combining Form

WORD	PRONUNCIATION	ELEMENTS		DEFINITION
abdominoplasty (tummy tuck)	ab-**DOM**-ih-noh-plas-tee	S/ R/CF	-plasty *surgical repair* abdomin/o- *abdomen*	Surgical removal of excess subcutaneous fat from abdominal wall
abrasion	ah-**BRAY**-zhun		Latin *to scrape*	Area of skin or mucous membrane that has been scraped off
blepharoplasty	**BLEF**-ah-roh-plas-tee	S/ R/CF	-plasty *surgical repair* blephar/o- *eyelid*	Surgical repair of an eyelid
clot	**KLOT**		German *to block*	The mass of fibrin and cells that is produced in a wound
dermabrasion	der-mah-**BRAY**-zhun	S/ R/ R/	-ion *action* derm- *skin* -abras- *scrape off*	Removal of upper layers of skin by rotary brush
granulation	gran-you-**LAY**-shun	S/ R/	-ation *process* granul- *small grain*	New fibrous tissue formed during wound healing
incision excision	in-**SIZH**-un ek-**SIZH**-un	S/ R/ R/	-ion *action, condition* incis- *cut into* excis- *cut out*	A cut or surgical wound Surgical removal of part or all of a structure
keloid	**KEY**-loyd		Greek *stain*	Raised, irregular, lumpy scar due to excess collagen fiber production during healing of a wound
laceration	lass-eh-**RAY**-shun	S/ R/	-ation *process* lacer- *to tear*	A tear or jagged wound of the skin caused by blunt trauma; not a cut
lipectomy liposuction	lip-**ECK**-toe-me **LIP**-oh-suck-shun	S/ R/ S/ R/CF R/	-ectomy *surgical excision* lip- *lipid, fat* -ion *action* lip/o- *fat* -suct- *suck*	Surgical removal of adipose tissue Surgical removal of adipose tissue using suction
mammoplasty	**MAM**-oh-plas-tee	S/ R/CF	-plasty *surgical repair* mamm/o- *breast*	Surgical procedure to change the size or shape of the breast
rhinoplasty	**RYE**-no-plas-tee	S/ R/CF	-plasty *surgical repair* rhin/o- *nose*	Surgical procedure to change the size or shape of the nose
scab	**SKAB**		Old English *crust*	Crust that forms over a wound or sore during healing
suture (noun) suture (verb)	**SOO**-chur		Latin *seam*	Stitch to hold the edges of a wound together To stitch the edges of a wound together
wound	**WOOND**		Old English *wound*	Any injury that interrupts the continuity of skin or a mucous membrane

EXERCISES

A. Wounds: *Use your knowledge of the meaning of the following medical terms to put them in the correct order of their appearance and give a brief description of each term. Fill in the chart.* **LO 3.2, 3.5, and 3.7**

keloid **scab** **clot** **laceration** **wound** **granulation**

Medical Term	Brief Description
1.	**2.**
3.	**4.**
5.	**6.**
7.	**8.**
9.	**10.**
11.	**12.**

B. Construct *medical terms related to therapeutic procedures of the skin.* **LO 3.1**

1. Surgical repair of the nose: ________________/________________
   R/CF S

2. Surgical removal of adipose tissue: ________________/________________
   R/CF S

3. Surgical repair of an eyelid: ________________/________________
   R/CF S

4. Surgical repair of the breast: ________________/________________
   R/CF S

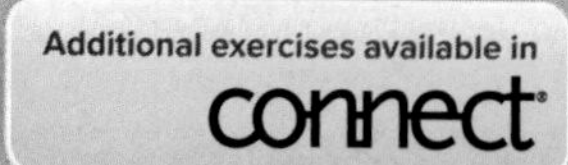

Chapter Review exercises, along with additional practice items, are available in Connect!

The Skeletal System

The Essentials of the Language of Orthopedics

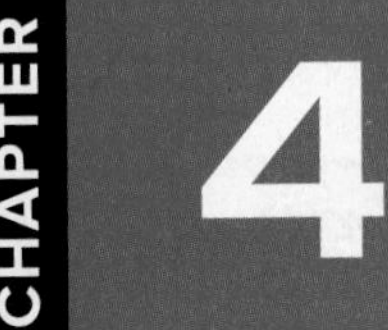

Rick Brady/McGraw-Hill Education

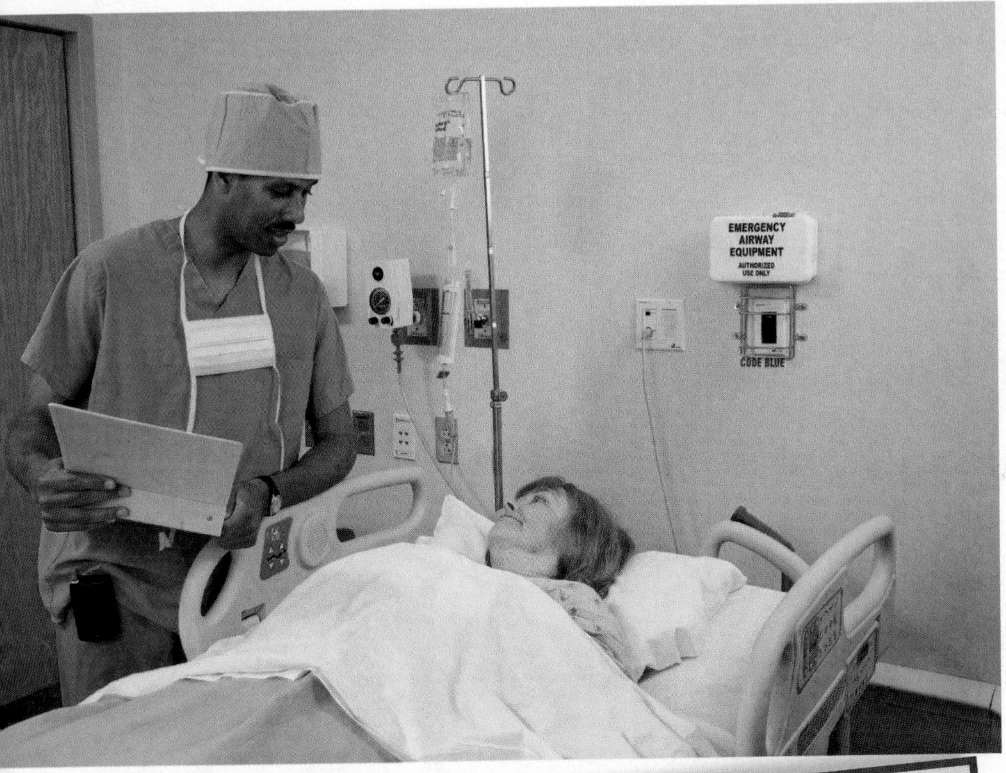

CASE REPORT 4.1

You are . . .

. . . an **orthopedic** technologist working for Kenneth Stannard, MD, an **orthopedist** in the Fulwood Medical Group.

You are communicating with . . .

. . . Mrs. Amy Vargas, a 70-year-old housewife, who tripped while walking down the front steps of her house. She has severe pain in her right hip and is unable to stand. An X-ray shows a hip fracture and marked **osteoporosis**. Dr. Stannard examined her in the Emergency Department, and Mrs. Vargas is being admitted for a hip replacement.

Learning Outcomes

In order for you to work with Dr. Stannard to give optimal care to Mrs. Vargas, and to help her and her family understand the significance of her bone disorder and injury, you will need to be able to use correct medical terminology to:

LO 4.1 Use roots, combining forms, suffixes, and prefixes to construct and analyze (deconstruct) medical terms related to the skeletal system.

LO 4.2 Spell and pronounce correctly medical terms related to the skeletal system to communicate them with accuracy and precision in any health care setting.

LO 4.3 Define accepted abbreviations related to the skeletal system.

LO 4.4 Relate the different types of bones and their structure to their functions.

LO 4.5 Describe the causes, appearances, methods of diagnosis, and treatment of bone and joint disorders and bone fractures, and their methods of healing.

LO 4.6 Identify the structures of the axial skeleton and their disorders and treatments.

LO 4.7 Describe the bones and joints of the shoulder girdle and upper limb and their disorders and treatments.

LO 4.8 Relate the structure of the pelvic girdle, hip joint, and thigh bone to their functions and disorders and treatments.

LO 4.9 Relate the structures of the knee joint, ankle, and foot to their functions and disorders and treatments.

LO 4.10 Specify the diagnostic and therapeutic procedures and the pharmacology for treating disorders of bones.

LO 4.11 Apply your knowledge of the medical terms of the skeletal system to documentation, medical records, and medical reports.

LO 4.12 Translate the medical terms of the skeletal system into everyday language in order to communicate clearly with patients and their families.

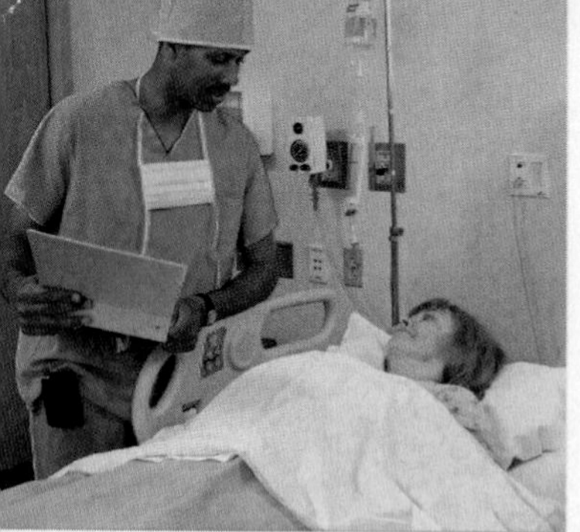

Rick Brady/McGraw-Hill Education

Many health professionals are involved in the diagnosis and treatment of problems in the skeletal system. You may work directly and/or indirectly with one or more of the following:

- **Orthopedic surgeons (orthopedists)** are medical doctors **(MDs)** who deal with the prevention and correction of injuries of the skeletal system and associated **muscles,** joints, and ligaments.
- **Osteopathic physicians** have earned a doctor of osteopathy **(DO)** degree and receive additional training in the **musculoskeletal system** and how it affects the whole body.
- **Chiropractors (DC)** focus on the manual adjustment of joints—particularly the spine—in order to maintain and restore health.
- **Physical therapists** evaluate and treat pain, disease, or injury by physical therapeutic measures, as opposed to medical or surgical measures.
- **Physical therapist assistants** work under the direction of a physical therapist to assist patients with their physical therapy.
- **Orthopedic technologists** and **technicians** assist orthopedic surgeons in treating patients.
- **Podiatrists** are practitioners in the diagnosis and treatment of disorders and injuries of the foot.

Objectives

Without your bones, you'd be shapeless–unable to sit, stand, walk, or move your fingers and toes. Your skeleton supports and protects your organ systems, and it's the foundation for much of the medical terminology you will learn in this book. For example, the radial artery (used for taking a pulse) is so named because it travels beside the radial bone of the forearm.

Understanding the surface anatomy of bones and their markings will enable you to describe and document the sites of symptoms, signs, and diagnostic and therapeutic procedures. The information in this lesson will provide you with the confidence and skills for using correct medical terminology to:

4.1.1 Recognize the different health professionals involved in the diagnosis and treatment of skeletal problems.

4.1.2 Identify the tissues that form the skeletal system.

4.1.3 Discuss the structures and functions of the skeletal system.

4.1.4 Differentiate the types of bones in the skeletal system.

4.1.5 Evaluate the major problems and diseases that occur in the skeletal system.

Abbreviations

DO	Doctor of Osteopathy
MD	Doctor of Medicine
DC	Doctor of Chiropractic
PT	Physical Therapist

Lesson 4.1

Bones of the Skeletal System

Tissues and Functions of the Skeletal System (LO 4.1, 4.2, and 4.4)

There are four components of the skeletal system *(Figure 4.1)*:

1. **bones,**
2. **cartilage,**
3. **tendons, and**
4. **ligaments.**

Each plays an important role in the way your tissues and skeletal system function. Your skeletal system provides:

- **Support:** The bones of your vertebral column, pelvis, and legs hold up your body. The jawbone supports your teeth.
- **Protection:** The skull protects your brain. The vertebral column protects your spinal cord. The rib cage protects your heart and lungs.
- **Blood formation:** Bone marrow in many bones is the major producer of blood cells, including most of those in your immune system *(see Chapter 7).*
- **Mineral storage and balance:** The skeletal system stores calcium and phosphorus and releases them when your body needs them for other purposes.
- **Detoxification:** Bones remove metals like lead and radium from your blood, store them, and slowly release them for excretion.
- **Endocrine regulation:** Bone cells release a hormone called **osteocalcin,** which increases insulin secretion and reduces stores of fat.

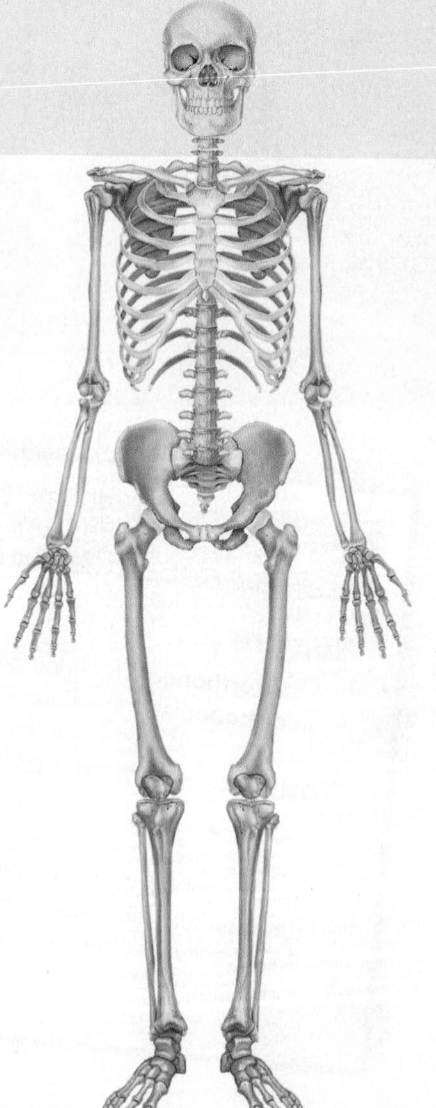

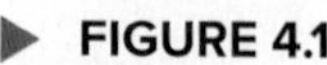

FIGURE 4.1
Adult Skeletal System, Anterior View.

Word Analysis and Definition

S = Suffix P = Prefix R = Root R/CF = Combining Form

WORD	PRONUNCIATION		ELEMENTS	DEFINITION
cartilage	**KAR**-tih-laj		Latin *gristle*	Nonvascular, firm connective tissue found mostly in joints
chiropractic chiropractor	kye-roh-**PRAK**-tik kye-roh-**PRAK**-tor	S/ R/CF R/ S/	-ic *pertaining to* chir/o- *hand* -pract- *efficient, practical* -or *a doer*	Diagnosis, treatment, and prevention of mechanical disorders of the musculoskeletal system Practitioner of chiropractic
detoxification (**Note:** *Same as detoxication*)	dee-**TOKS**-ih-fih-**KAY**-shun	S/ P/ R/	-fication *remove* de- *from, out of* -toxi- *poison*	Removing poison from a tissue or substance
ligament	**LIG**-ah-ment		Latin *band, sheet*	Band of fibrous tissue connecting two structures
muscle musculoskeletal	**MUSS**-el **MUSS**-kyu-loh-**SKEL**-eh-tal	 S/ R/CF R/	Latin *muscle* -al *pertaining to* muscul/o- *muscle* -skelet- *skeleton*	A tissue consisting of cells that can contract Pertaining to the muscles and the bony skeleton
orthopedic orthopedist	or-tho-**PEE**-dik or-tho-**PEE**-dist	S/ R/CF R/ S/	-ic *pertaining to* orth/o- *straight* -ped- *child* -ist *specialist*	Pertaining to the correction and cure of deformities and diseases of the musculoskeletal system; originally, most of the deformities treated were in children Specialist in orthopedics
osteocalcin	**OSS**-tee-oh-**CAL**-sin	S/ R/CF R/	-in *chemical compound* oste/o- *bone* -calc- *calcium*	A hormone produced by bone cells
osteopath osteopathy	**OSS**-tee-oh-path **OSS**-tee-**OP**-ah-thee	S/ R/CF S/	-path *disease* oste/o- *bone* -pathy *disease*	Practitioner of osteopathy Medical practice based on maintaining the balance of the body
tendon	**TEN**-dun		Latin *sinew*	Fibrous band that connects muscle to bone

Exercises

A. Review *Case Report 4.1 to answer the following questions. Fill in the blanks.* **LO 4.2, 4.8, and 4.11**

1. What diagnostic test did Mrs. Vargas have? ____________________
2. What bone disease did Mrs. Vargas have prior to her current condition?____________________
3. Which joint is affected? ____________________
4. What type of surgeon is Dr. Stannard? ____________________
5. What surgical procedure will Dr. Stannard perform on Mrs. Vargas? ____________________

B. Identify *the components of the skeletal system and the functions of the bones. Select the correct organ or tissue being described.* **LO 4.1**

1. Band of strong tissue that connects two structures (such as bone to bone).
   a. muscle **c.** tendon
   b. ligament **d.** cartilage
2. Tissue containing contractile cells.
   a. muscle **c.** tendon
   b. ligament **d.** cartilage
3. Firm connective tissue found mostly in joints.
   a. muscle **c.** tendon
   b. ligament **d.** cartilage
4. Fibrous band that connects muscle to bone.
   a. muscle **c.** tendon
   b. ligament **d.** cartilage

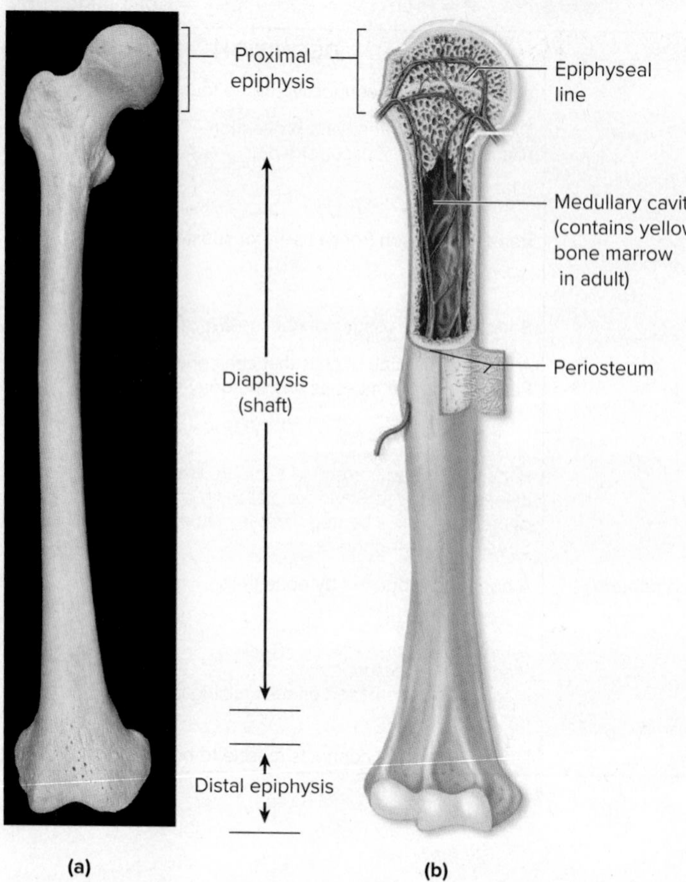

▲ **FIGURE 4.2**
Femur: Long Bone of the Thigh.
(a) Anterior view. (b) Interior view.

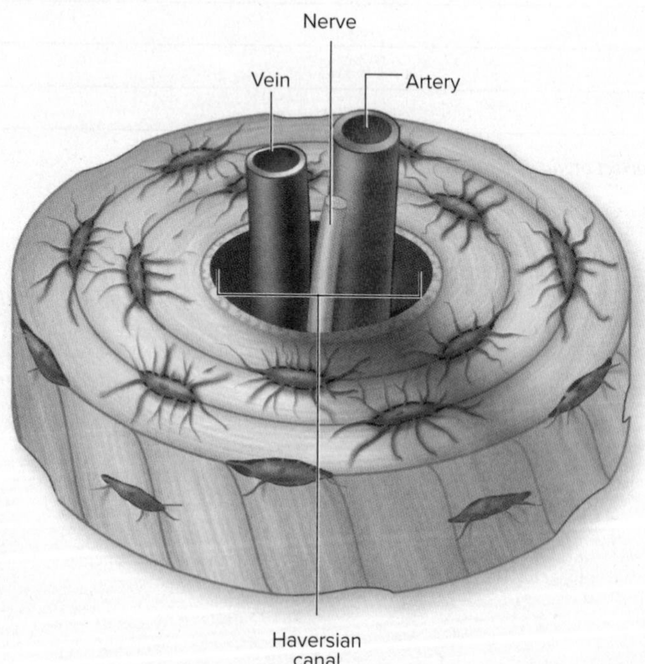

▲ **FIGURE 4.3**
Blood Supply to Bone.

Classification of Bones (LO 4.2 and 4.4)

The bones of your skeletal system are classified by their shape. Each falls into one of the following four shape categories:

- **Long** (considerably longer than they are wide), like the main bones of the limbs, palms, soles, fingers, and toes;
- **Short** (nearly as long as they are wide), like the patella (kneecap) and the bones of the wrists and ankles;
- **Flat,** like the bones of the skull and the ribs; or
- **Irregular,** like the vertebrae.

Structure of Bones (LO 4.2 and 4.4)

Think about how long your arms and legs are, and then consider how few bones make up all that length. In that context, it's likely no surprise that **long bones** are the most common bones in your body *(Figure 4.2)*. The shaft **(diaphysis)** of a long bone contains compact bone (also called **cortical** bone), while each end of the bone (the **epiphysis)** is composed of spongy bone. Sandwiched between the diaphysis and epiphysis are thin layers of cartilage cells in the **epiphysial plate** or **line** that allow your bones to grow longer.

A tough, connective tissue sheath called **periosteum** covers the outer surface of all bones; it protects the bone and anchors blood vessels and nerves to the bone's surface. Strong collagen fibers attach the periosteum to the cortical bone.

Inside the diaphysis is a hollow cylinder called the **medulla** *(Figure 4.2b),* which contains bone **marrow,** a fatty tissue in adults. Red bone marrow with blood cells in varying stages of development can be found in the epiphyseal ends of the bone and in the flat bones of the skull, the sternum, and the hip bones. Because red bone marrow is normally concentrated here, the medulla of the sternum and hip bone is the ideal source for bone marrow aspiration, a procedure where a needle is inserted into the bone to withdraw a sample of bone marrow fluid and cells to be checked for abnormalities.

Most bones have a strong blood supply *(Figure 4.3)* because of the blood vessels that travel through them in a system of small **Haversian canals.** The good supply of blood through your bones promotes healing.

Word Analysis and Definition

S = Suffix   P = Prefix   R = Root   R/CF = Combining Form

WORD	PRONUNCIATION		ELEMENTS	DEFINITION
cortex cortical (adj)	**KOR**-teks **KOR**-tih-cal	 S/ R/	Latin *bark* -al *pertaining to* cortic- *cortex*	Outer portion of an organ, such as bone Pertaining to a cortex
diaphysis	die-**AF**-ih-sis		Greek *growing between*	The shaft of a long bone
epiphysis	ep-ih-**FI**-sis	P/ R/	**epi-** *upon, above* **-physis** *growth*	Expanded area at the proximal and distal ends of a long bone to provide increased surface area for attachment of ligaments and tendons
epiphysial (adj) (**Note:** *The part "is" is deleted to enable the word to flow.*)	ep-ih-**FIZ**-ee-al	S/	**-ial** *pertaining to*	Pertaining to an epiphysis
Haversian canals	hah-**VER**-shan ka-NALS		Clopton Havers, English physician, 1655–1702	Vascular canals in bone
marrow	**MAH**-roe		Old English *marrow*	Fatty, blood-forming tissue in the cavities of long bones
medulla medullary (adj)	meh-**DULL**-ah meh-**DULL**-ah-ree	 S/ R/	Latin *marrow* **-ary** *pertaining to* **medulla-** *medulla*	Central portion of a structure surrounded by cortex Pertaining to a medulla
periosteum	**PER**-ee-**OSS**-tee-um	S/ P/ R/	**-um** *structure* **peri-** *around* **-oste-** *bone*	Strong membrane surrounding a bone
periosteal (adj)	**PER**-ee-**OSS**-tee-al	S/	**-al** *pertaining to*	Pertaining to the periosteum

EXERCISES

A. Elements *remain your best clue for understanding a medical term. In this exercise, the meaning of each element is given below the line–this is your clue to constructing the term. Insert the correct element on the line above its meaning. After you have constructed the term, give its definition in the space provided.* **LO 4.1 and 4.2**

1. _______________ / _______________
cortex — pertaining to

The term is ____

2. _______________ / _______________ / _______________
around — bone — structure

The term is ____

3. _______________ / _______________ / _______________
upon, above — growth — pertaining to

The term is ____

4. _______________ / _______________
medulla — pertaining to

The term is ____

B. Use this exercise *to review what you've learned about bones. Select the correct answer for each question.* **LO 4.4**

1. Bones of the skeletal system are classified by their:

a. shape   **b.** function   **c.** weight   **d.** color

2. What are the most common types of bones in the body?

a. flat   **b.** short   **c.** long   **d.** irregular

3. What is another name for "compact" bone?

a. cortical   **b.** diaphysis   **c.** long   **d.** spongy

4. Where can you find bone marrow? (select all that apply)

a. between two bones   **b.** inside a hollow space of the diaphysis

c. epiphysis of a long bone   **d.** large flat bones, such as the skull

5. The strong blood supply in bones is provided by the:

a. red bone marrow   **b.** yellow bone marrow   **c.** blood vessels in the periosteum   **d.** blood vessels of the Haversian canals

Diseases of Bone

(LO 4.2 and 4.5)

Keynote

- **Osteomalacia occurs in some developing nations and occasionally in this country when children drink soft drinks instead of milk fortified with vitamin D.**

Abbreviations

BMD	bone mineral density
DEXA	dual energy X-ray absorptiometry
FDA	Food and Drug Administration
IU	international unit(s)
mg	milligram

Case Report 4.1 *(continued)*

On questioning, Amy Vargas demonstrated many of the risk factors for **osteoporosis**, including family history, lack of exercise, cigarette smoking, inadequate diet, post-menopause, and increasing age.

One of the major bone diseases is **osteoporosis,** which results from a loss of bone density *(Figure 4.4)*. More common in women than in men, the incidence of osteoporosis increases with age. In the United States alone, 10 million people are living with osteoporosis and 18 million more have low bone density **(osteopenia).** Osteopenia puts people at risk for developing osteoporosis.

In women, production of the hormone estrogen decreases after menopause, weakening the body's protection against bone loss and potentially resulting in fragile, brittle bones. In men, lower levels of testosterone have a similar but less noticeable effect.

Women at risk for osteoporosis should have a bone mineral density **(BMD)** screening using a **DEXA** scan, which is a measuring device that uses low-energy radiation beams. Men and women over 50 are often advised to follow a daily regimen of 1,200 milligrams **(mg)** of calcium, 400 to 600 international units **(IU)** of vitamin D, and 15 minutes of real sun exposure. In addition, there are several **FDA**-approved medications available for treating osteoporosis.

Other bone diseases that may not be as prevalent or publicized as osteoporosis are the following:

Osteomyelitis: an inflammation of bone and bone marrow caused by a bacterial infection, such as staphylococcus.

Osteomalacia: a disease (known as **rickets** in children) caused by vitamin D deficiency where the calcium-lacking bones become soft and flexible, lose their ability to bear weight, and become bowed.

Achondroplasia: a very rare condition where the long bones stop growing in childhood, but the axial skeleton bones are not affected *(Figure 4.5)*. People with this condition are short in stature, with the average adult measuring about 4 feet tall. Although intelligence and life span are normal, the disease is caused by a spontaneous gene mutation that then becomes a dominant gene for succeeding generations.

Osteogenesis imperfecta (OI): a rare genetic disorder producing very brittle bones that are easily fractured or broken, often **in utero** (while inside the uterus).

Primary bone cancer is found in three forms:

1. **Osteogenic sarcoma** occurs most often in bone cells around the knee in adolescents.
2. **Ewing sarcoma** occurs most often in children and adolescents.
3. **Chondrosarcoma** arises in cartilage cells, often in the pelvises of older people.

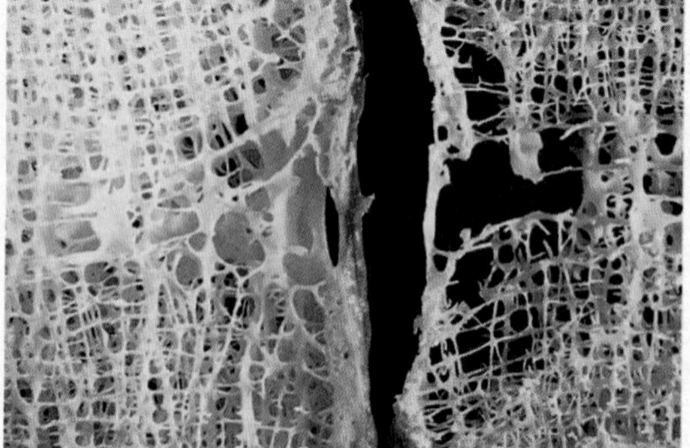

▲ **FIGURE 4.4** Normal Bone and Osteoporotic Bone.

Michael Klein/Photolibrary/Getty Images

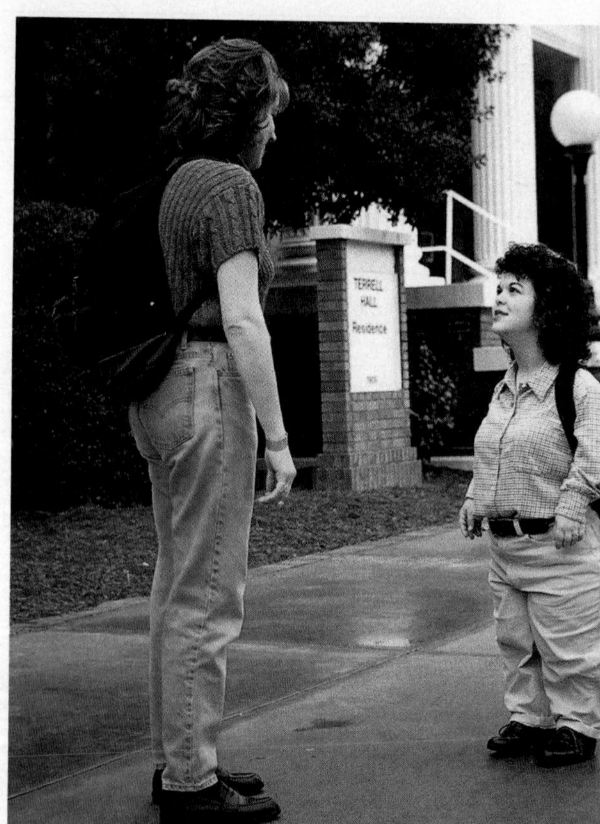

▶ **FIGURE 4.5** Achondroplastic Dwarf with College Roommate.

Joe DeGrandis/McGraw-Hill Education

Word Analysis and Definition

S = Suffix P = Prefix R = Root R/CF = Combining Form

WORD	PRONUNCIATION	ELEMENTS		DEFINITION
achondroplasia	a-kon-droh-**PLAY**-zee-ah	S/ P/ R/CF	-plasia *formation* a- *without* -chondr/o- *cartilage*	Condition with abnormal, early conversion of cartilage into bone, leading to dwarfism
osteogenesis imperfecta	**OSS**-tee-oh-**JEN**-eh-sis im-per-**FEK**-tah	S/ R/CF	-genesis *creation, formation* oste/o- *bone* imperfecta, Latin *unfinished*	Inherited condition in which bone formation is incomplete, leading to fragile, easily broken bones
osteomalacia	**OSS**-tee-oh-mah-**LAY**-she-ah	S/ R/CF	-malacia *abnormal softness* oste/o- *bone*	Soft, flexible bones lacking in calcium (rickets)
osteomyelitis	**OSS**-tee-oh-my-eh-**LIE**-tis	S/ R/CF R/	-itis *inflammation* oste/o- *bone* -myel- *bone marrow*	Inflammation of bone and bone marrow
osteopenia	**OSS**-tee-oh-**PEE**-nee-ah	S/ R/CF	-penia *deficient* oste/o- *bone*	Decreased calcification of bone
osteoporosis	**OSS**-tee-oh-poh-**ROE**-sis	S/ R/CF R/CF	-sis *condition* oste/o- *bone* -por/o- *opening*	Condition in which the bones become more porous, brittle, and fragile and more likely to fracture
rickets	**RICK**-ets		Old English *to twist*	Disease due to vitamin D deficiency, producing soft, flexible bones
sarcoma	sar-**KOH**-mah	S/ R/	-oma *tumor, mass* sarc- *flesh*	Malignant tumor originating in connective tissue
chondrosarcoma	**CHON**-droh-sar-**KOH**-mah	R/CF	chondr/o *cartilage*	Malignant tumor originating in cartilage cells
osteogenic sarcoma	**OSS**-tee-oh-**JEN**-ik sar-**KOH**-mah	S/ R/CF R/	-ic *pertaining to* oste/o- *bone* -gen- *creation*	Malignant tumor originating in bone-producing cells

Exercises

A. Review *Case Report 4.1 (continued) to answer the following questions. Select the correct answer to each question.* **LO 4.5**

1. What is a risk factor?

a. an inherited condition

b. a characteristic, condition, or behavior that decreases the possibility of disease

c. a characteristic, condition, or behavior that increases the possibility of disease

d. a behavior that promotes wellness

2. Which of the following risk factors is one that is out of a person's control?

a. lack of exercise **c.** cigarette smoking

b. inadequate diet **d.** increasing age

3. Which bone disease contributed to causing her hip fracture?

a. osteomyelitis **c.** achrondroplasia

b. osteoporosis **d.** sarcoma

4. What does it mean if this diagnosis is in her family history?

a. people in her family are in poor health

b. no one in her family has had the same problem

c. other people in her family have had the same problem

B. Suffixes: *The combining form* oste/o *means bone, and it is the main element in each of the following terms. You choose the correct suffix to complete the term. Fill in the blanks.* **LO 4.1 and 4.5**

genesis **genic** **sarcoma** **penia** **malacia** **porosis** **myelitis**

1. Disease caused by vitamin D deficiency osteo/ ______________________

2. Low bone density osteo/ ______________________

3. Porous, brittle, fragile bones osteo/ ______________________

4. Most common malignant bone tumor osteo/ ______________________

5. Rare genetic disorder producing easily fractured bones, often in utero osteo/ ______________________

6. Inflammation of bone and bone marrow osteo/ ______________________

Note: *The meaning of the combining form never changes. The addition of six different suffixes has helped you learn six new terms in orthopedic vocabulary!*

Bone Fractures (FXs) (LO 4.2 and 4.5)

Incomplete
Complete
(a)
Comminuted
Transverse
(b)

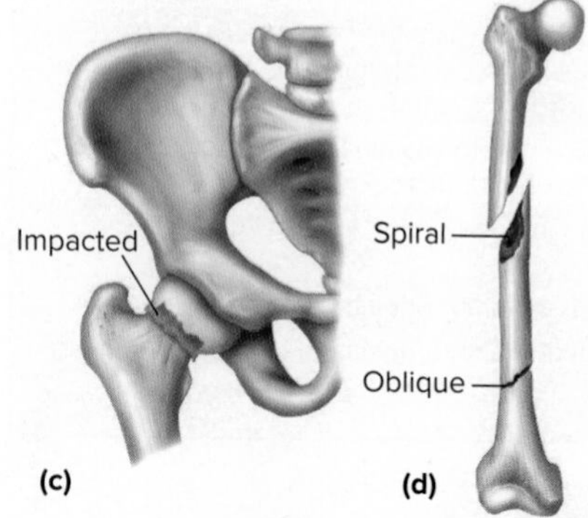

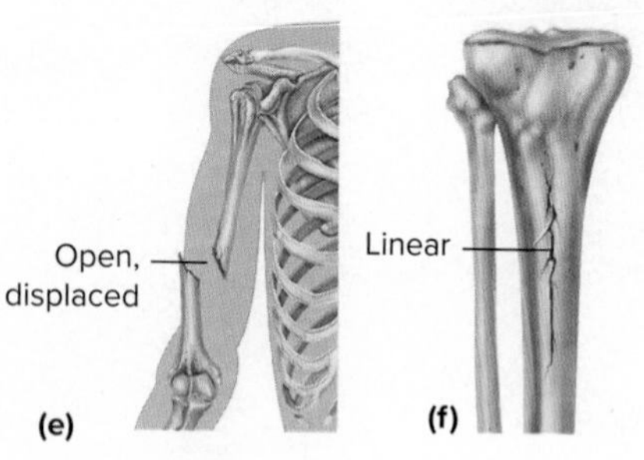

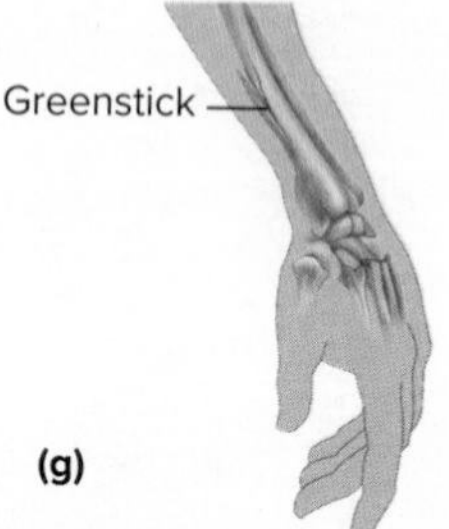

▲ **FIGURE 4.6**
Bone Fractures.

▼ **TABLE 4.1**

CLASSIFICATION AND DEFINITION OF BONE FRACTURES

Name	Description	Reference
Closed (also called **simple** fracture)	A bone is broken, but the skin is not broken.	*Figure 4.6g*
Open (also called **compound** fracture)	A fragment of the fractured bone breaks the skin, or a wound extends to the site of the fracture.	*Figure 4.6e*
Displaced	The fractured bone parts are out of line.	*Figure 4.6e*
Complete	A bone is broken into at least two fragments.	*Figure 4.6a*
Incomplete	The fracture does not extend completely across the bone. It can be hairline, as in a stress fracture in the foot, when there is no separation of the two fragments.	*Figure 4.6a*
Comminuted	The bone breaks into several pieces, usually two major pieces and several smaller fragments.	*Figure 4.6b*
Transverse	The fracture is at right angles to the long axis of the bone.	*Figure 4.6b*
Impacted	The fracture consists of one bone fragment driven into another, resulting in shortening of a limb.	*Figure 4.6c*
Spiral	The fracture spirals around the long axis of the bone.	*Figure 4.6d*
Oblique	The fracture runs diagonally across the long axis of the bone.	*Figure 4.6d*
Linear	The fracture runs parallel to the long axis of the bone.	*Figure 4.6f*
Greenstick	This is a partial fracture. One side breaks, and the other bends.	*Figure 4.6g*
Pathologic	The fracture occurs in an area of bone weakened by disease, such as cancer.	—
Compression	The fracture occurs in a vertebra from trauma or pathology, leading to the vertebra being crushed.	—
Stress	This is a fatigue fracture caused by repetitive, local stress on a bone, as occurs in marching or running.	—

Healing of Fractures (LO 4.2 and 4.5)

When a bone is fractured, blood vessels bleed into the fracture site, forming a hematoma *(Figure 4.7a)*. After a few days, bone-forming cells called **osteoblasts** move in and start to produce new bone cells (osteocytes), which form a **callus** *(Figure 4.7b)*. Osteblasts continue to produce bone cells, which form **cancellous** (spongy) bone to replace the callus *(Figure 4.7c)*. As more bone cells form, the spongy bone structure is replaced by compact bone, which fuses together the bone segments *(Figure 4.7d)*. Uncomplicated fractures take 8 to 12 weeks to heal. (Surgical procedures to help fractures heal are shown in Lesson 4.4.)

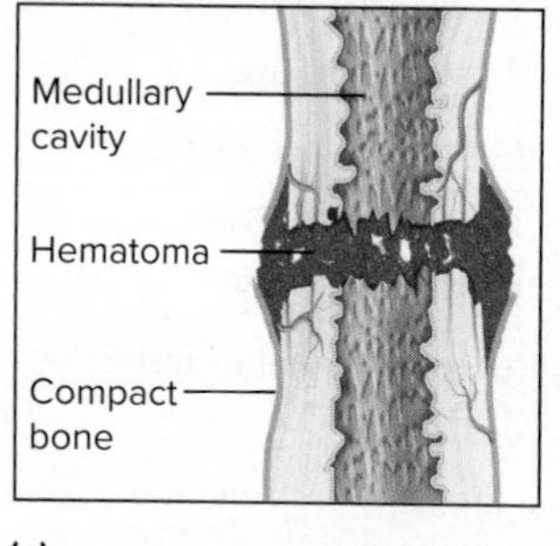

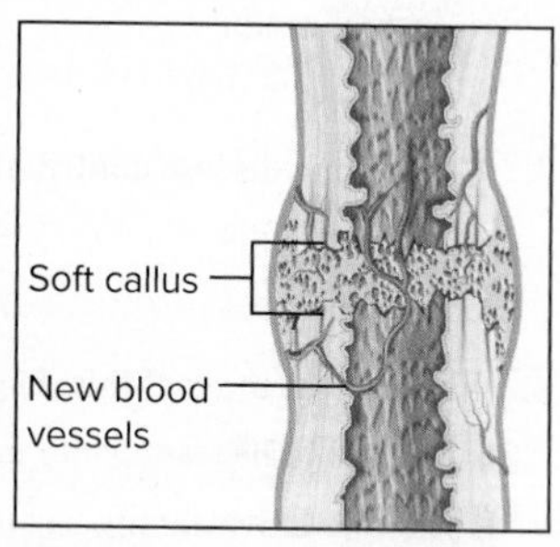

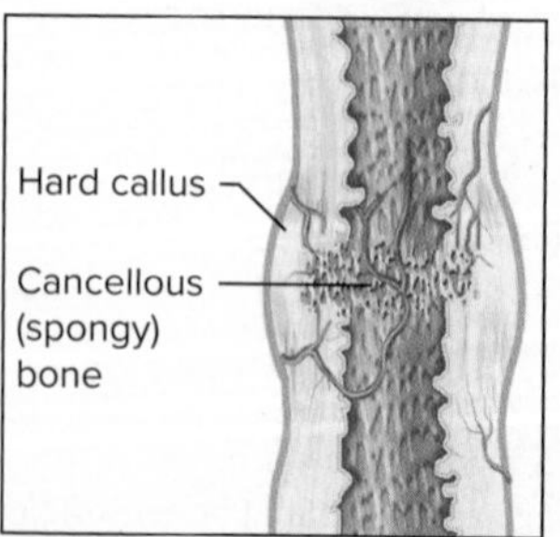

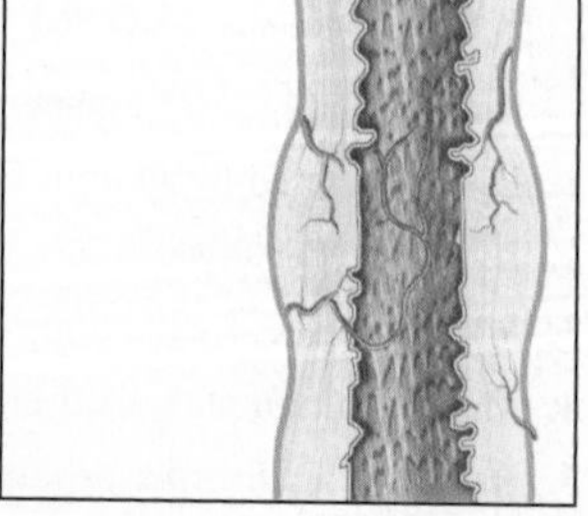

▶ **FIGURE 4.7**
Healing of Bone Fracture.

Abbreviation

Fx	fracture

Word Analysis and Definition

S = Suffix P = Prefix R = Root R/CF = Combining Form

WORD	PRONUNCIATION	ELEMENTS		DEFINITION
callus	**KAL**-us		Latin *hard skin*	Bony tissue that forms at a fracture site early in healing
cancellous	**KAN**-sell-us		Latin *lattice*	Bone that has a spongy or lattice-like structure
comminuted	**KOM**-ih-nyu-ted	S/ R/	**-ed** *pertaining to* **comminut-** *break into pieces*	A fracture in which the bone is broken into pieces
hematoma	he-mah-**TOH**-mah	S/ R/	**-oma** *tumor, mass* **hemat-** *blood*	Collection of blood that has escaped from blood vessels into tissue
osteoblast osteocyte	**OSS**-tee-oh-blast **OSS**-tee-oh-site	S/ R/CF R/	**-blast** *immature cell* **oste/o-** *bone* **-cyte** *cell*	A bone-forming cell A bone-maintaining cell
pathologic fracture	path-oh-**LOJ**-ik **FRAK**-chur	S/ R/CF R/ S/ R/	**-ic** *pertaining to* **path/o-** *disease* **-log-** *to study* **-ure** *result of* **fract-** *to break*	Fracture occurring at a site already weakened by a disease process, such as cancer

EXERCISES

A. Place in order *the steps the body takes to heal a bone fracture. The first event will be "1," and the last event will be "4."* **LO 4.2 and 4.5**

________ spongy bone

________ callus

________ compact bone

________ hematoma

B. Match the description of the fracture *in the first column with the fracture it is describing in the second column. Refer to Table 4.1.* **LO 4.2 and 4.5**

	Fracture Seen on the Film	Type of Fracture
______	**1.** Fracture at a right angle to the long axis of the radius	**a.** open fracture
______	**2.** Femur broken into two clean pieces	**b.** oblique fracture
______	**3.** Cancer patient with vertebral fracture	**c.** closed fracture
______	**4.** Broken ankle but no broken skin	**d.** transverse fracture
______	**5.** Diagonal fracture across the long axis of the femur	**e.** pathologic fracture
______	**6.** Fractured hand with bone fragments sticking out	**f.** displaced fracture

C. Deconstruct *the following medical terms into their basic elements. Then provide a brief definition for each term. Fill in the chart.* **LO 4.1 and 4.2**

Medical Term	Prefix	Root/CF	Suffix	Definition of Medical Term
pathologic	**1.**	**2.**	**3.**	**4.**
osteoblast	**5.**	**6.**	**7.**	**8.**
comminuted	**9.**	**10.**	**11.**	**12.**

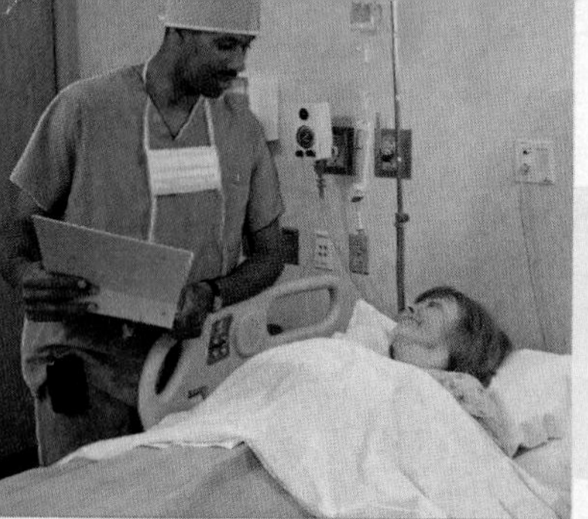

Rick Brady/McGraw-Hill Education

Lesson 4.2

Axial Skeleton

Objectives

In order to best evaluate, treat, and educate patients, understanding the medical terminology for the structures and functions of the vertebral column, its joints, and its ligaments is a must. The vertebral column is part of the axial skeleton, and in this lesson, information about the axial skeleton will enable you to use correct medical terminology to:

4.2.1 Identify the regions and bones of the vertebral column.

4.2.2 Describe the joints and ligaments of the vertebral column.

4.2.3 Distinguish the different bones of the skull.

4.2.4 Differentiate the major problems and diseases that affect the vertebral column and skull.

CASE REPORT 4.2

You are . . .

. . . an orthopedic technologist working in the orthopedic department of Fulwood Medical Center with Dr. Kenneth Stannard.

You are communicating with . . .

. . . Ms. Nancy Cardenas, a 27-year-old jeweler whose car was rear-ended by another car at a traffic light 3 days ago. Ms. Cardenas suffers from severe neck pain radiating down her left arm, as well as dizziness and headaches. She is unable to go to work. Dr. Stannard has examined her and diagnosed her condition as a **whiplash** injury. An MRI shows herniation (rupture) of intervertebral discs between C5-C6 and C6-C7. Your role is to assist Dr. Stannard and document the care Ms. Cardenas receives to relieve her symptoms. Ms. Cardenas' whiplash injury caused protrusion of two cervical intervertebral discs. The centers of the discs bulge into the vertebral canal and pinch the nerves in such a way that the pain radiates to her left arm.

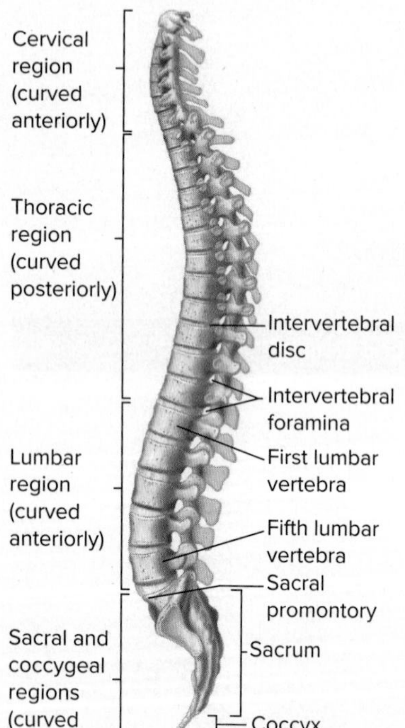

FIGURE 4.8
Vertebral Column, Lateral View.

Structure of the Axial Skeleton (LO 4.2 and 4.6)

Your axial skeleton, the upright axis of your body, includes the:

1. **vertebral column,**
2. **skull, and**
3. **rib cage.**

The axial skeleton protects the brain, **spinal cord,** heart, and lungs–most of the major centers of human physiology.

Within the vertebral column, there are 26 bones divided into the following five regions *(Figure 4.8)*:

- **Cervical** region, with 7 **vertebrae,** labeled C1 to C7 and curved anteriorly;
- **Thoracic** region, with 12 vertebrae, labeled T1 to T12 and curved posteriorly;
- **Lumbar** region, with 5 vertebrae, labeled L1 to L5 and curved anteriorly;
- **Sacral** region, with 5 bones that in early childhood fuse into 1 bone curved posteriorly; and
- **Coccyx** (tailbone), with 4 small bones fused together into 1 bone curved posteriorly.

The spinal cord lies protected in the vertebral canal of the vertebral column. Spinal nerves travel from the spinal cord to other parts of the body through the intervertebral **foramina.**

Intervertebral discs consisting of fibrocartilage (a form of cartilage) are also found in the axial skeleton. These discs inhabit the intervertebral space between the bodies of adjacent vertebrae and provide extra support and cushioning (acting as shock absorbers) for the vertebral column.

The vertebral column, like any other body part, is susceptible to injury and disease. One common disorder of the vertebral column is **scoliosis,** an abnormal lateral curvature of the **spine** that occurs in both children and adults. Abnormal curvature of the spine is more common in older people, particularly those with osteoporosis; in this case, the normal anteriorly concave curvature in the thoracic region **(kyphosis)** is exaggerated.

Abbreviations

C5	the fifth cervical vertebra
C5-C6	the intervertebral space between the fifth and sixth cervical vertebrae
C6	the sixth cervical vertebra
MRI	magnetic resonance imaging (diagnostic technique that produces focused slices of images of structures)

Word Analysis and Definition

S = Suffix P = Prefix R = Root R/CF = Combining Form

WORD	PRONUNCIATION	ELEMENTS		DEFINITION
cervical	**SER**-vih-kal	S/ R/	**-al** *pertaining to* **cervic-** *neck*	Pertaining to the neck region
coccyx	**KOK**-sicks		Greek *coccyx*	Small tailbone at the lowest end of the vertebral column
foramen	foh-**RAY**-men		Latin *an opening*	An opening through a structure
foramina (pl)	foh-**RAM**-in-ah			
kyphosis **kyphotic (adj)**	ki-**FOH**-sis ki-**FOT**-ik	S/ R/ S/ R/CF	**-osis** *condition* **kyph-** *bent, humpback* **-tic** *pertaining to* **kyph/o-** *bent, humpback*	A normal posterior curve of the spine that can be exaggerated in disease Pertaining to or suffering from kyphosis
lumbar	**LUM**-bar		Latin *loin*	The region of the back and sides between the ribs and pelvis
sacrum **sacral (adj)**	**SAY**-crum **SAY**-kral	 S/ R/	Latin *sacred* **-al** *pertaining to* **sacr-** *sacrum*	Segment of the vertebral column that forms part of the pelvis Pertaining to or in the region of the sacrum
scoliosis **scoliotic (adj)**	skoh-lee-**OH**-sis **SKOH**-lee-**OT**-ik	S/ R/ S/ R/CF	**-osis** *condition* **scoli-** *crooked* **-tic** *pertaining to* **scoli/o-** *crooked*	An abnormal lateral curvature of the vertebral column Pertaining to or suffering from scoliosis
spine **spinal (adj)**	**SPINE** **SPY**-nal	 S/ R/	Latin *spine* **-al** *pertaining to* **spin-** *spine*	Vertebral column or a short projection from a bone Pertaining to the spine
vertebra **vertebrae (pl)** **vertebral (adj)**	**VER**-teh-brah **VER**-teh-brae **VER**-teh-bral	 S/ R/	Latin *spinal joint* **-al** *pertaining to* **vertebr-** *vertebra*	One of the bones of the spinal column Pertaining to a vertebra
whiplash	**WHIP**-lash	R/ R/	**whip-** *to swing* **-lash** *end of whip*	Symptoms caused by sudden, uncontrolled extension, and flexion of the neck, often in an automobile accident

EXERCISES

A. Review *Case Report 4.2 to select the correct answer to the following questions.* **LO 4.2, 4.3, and 4.6**

1. The abbreviation MRI stands for:

a. multiple reading interpretations
b. magnetic radiographic imaging
c. maximal recording indices
d. magnetic resonance imaging

2. Describe herniation of a disc:

a. lateral displacement of cartilage in the knee
b. rupture of a disc into surrounding tissue
c. displacement of a vertebra into the spinal canal
d. fracture of a bone of the spine

3. The term *intervertebral* means:

a. condition around the spine
b. pertaining to within the backbones
c. pertaining to between the backbones
d. condition between the spine

4. The "C" in "C5-C6" means:

a. cavity
b. cervical
c. central
d. cartilage

B. Apply *the correct form of the bolded similar terms appropriately in the following documentation, and you will meet a chapter objective! Fill in the blanks.* **LO 4.2, 4.3, and 4.6**

vertebra **vertebral** **vertebrae**

1. The patient's C5 ______________________ was fractured in the accident.

2. A part of the axial skeleton is the ______________________ column.

3. The patient's C5 and C6 ______________________ were fractured in the accident.

Now supply the missing terms to complete the following sentence.

4. The designations C5-C6 and C6-C7 are for locations of ______________________.

Skull and Face (LO 4.2 and 4.6)

The Skull (LO 4.2 and 4.6)

When you glance at your face in the mirror, chances are you're not thinking about what's behind your brown eyes or your slightly crooked smile. You see one image—not its layers, pieces, or parts. However, the human skull *(Figure 4.9)* is made up of 22 separate bones. Your **cranium,** the upper part of the skull that encloses the **cranial** cavity and protects the brain, contains 8 of these 22 bones; your facial skeleton contains the rest.

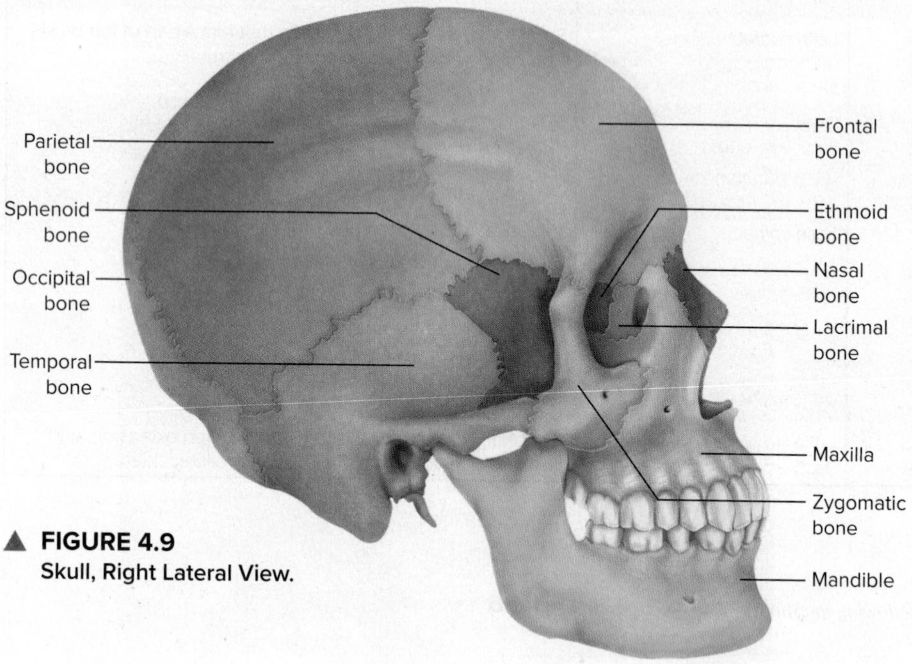

▲ **FIGURE 4.9**
Skull, Right Lateral View.

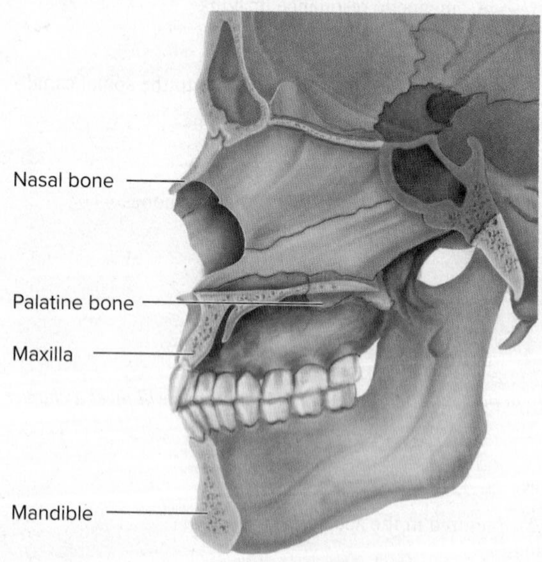

▲ **FIGURE 4.10**
Facial Bones.

The bones of the cranium are joined together by sutures (joints that appear as seams), which are covered on the inside and outside by a thin layer of connective tissue. These bones have the following functions:

1. The **frontal** bone forms the forehead, roofs of the (eye) orbits, and part of the floor of the cranium and contains a pair of right and left frontal sinuses above the orbits.
2. **Parietal** bones form the bulging sides and roof of the cranium.
3. The **occipital** bone forms the back of and part of the base of the cranium.
4. **Temporal** bones form the sides of and part of the base of the cranium.
5. The **sphenoid** bone forms part of the base of the cranium and the orbits.
6. The **ethmoid** bone is hollow and forms part of the nose, the orbits, and the ethmoid sinuses.

These bones of the skull provide protection for the brain and the organs of vision, taste, hearing, equilibrium, and smell.

The lower part of the skull houses the bones of the facial skeleton *(Figure 4.10)*. These bones do the following:

1. **Maxillary** bones form the upper jaw **(maxilla),** hold the upper teeth, and are hollow, forming the maxillary sinuses.
2. **Palatine** bones are located behind the maxilla and cannot be seen on a lateral view of the skull.
3. **Zygomatic** bones are the prominences of the cheeks (cheekbones) below the eyes.
4. **Lacrimal** bones form the medial wall of each eye orbit.
5. **Nasal** bones form the sides and bridge of the nose.
6. **The mandible** is the lower jawbone, which holds the lower teeth. The mandible articulates (joins) with the temporal bone to form the **temporomandibular joint (TMJ).**

The bones of the facial skeleton provide a frame on which the muscles and other tissues of the face facilitate eating, facial expressions, breathing, and speech.

The third component of the axial skeleton, the rib cage, is discussed in Chapter 8, "Respiratory System."

Abbreviation

TMJ	temporomandibular joint

Word Analysis and Definition

S = Suffix P = Prefix R = Root R/CF = Combining Form

WORD	PRONUNCIATION		ELEMENTS	DEFINITION
cranium	**KRAY**-nee-um		Greek *skull*	The upper part of the skull that encloses and protects the brain
cranial (adj)	**KRAY**-nee-al	S/ R/	-al *pertaining to* crani- *skull*	Pertaining to the skull
ethmoid	**ETH**-moyd	S/ R/	-oid *resembling* ethm- *sieve*	Bone that forms the back of the nose and encloses numerous air cells
lacrimal	**LAK**-rim-al	S/ R/	-al *pertaining to* lacrim- *tears*	Lacrimal bone forms part of the medial wall of the orbit, *or* pertaining to tears
mandible mandibular (adj)	**MAN**-di-bel man-**DIB**-you-lar	S/ R/	Latin *jaw* -ar *pertaining to* mandibul- *mandible*	Lower jaw bone Pertaining to the mandible
maxilla	mak-**SILL**-ah		Latin *jawbone*	Upper jawbone, containing right and left maxillary sinuses
maxillary (adj)	mak-**SILL**-ah-ree	S/ R/	-ary *pertaining to* maxilla- *maxilla*	Pertaining to the maxilla
occipital	ock-**SIP**-it-al	S/ R/	-al *pertaining to* occipit- *back of the head*	The back of the skull
palatine	**PAL**-ah-tine	S/ R/	-ine *pertaining to* palat- *palate*	Bone that forms the hard palate and parts of the nose and orbits
parietal	pah-**RYE**-eh-tal	S/ R/	-al *pertaining to* pariet- *wall*	The two bones forming the sidewalls and roof of the cranium
sphenoid	**SFEE**-noyd	S/ R/	-oid *resemble* sphen- *wedge*	Wedge-shaped bone at the base of the skull
temporal	**TEM**-pore-al	S/ R/	-al *pertaining to* tempor- *time, temple*	Bone that forms part of the base and sides of the skull
temporomandibular joint (TMJ)	**TEM**-pore-oh-man-**DIB**-you-lar **JOYNT**	S/ R/CF R/	-ar *pertaining to* tempor/o- *temple* -mandibul- *mandible*	The joint between the temporal bone and the mandible
zygoma zygomatic (adj)	zye-**GO**-mah zye-go-**MAT**-ik	S/ R/	French *yoke* -ic *pertaining to* zygomat- *cheekbone*	Bone that forms the prominence of the cheek Pertaining to the cheekbone

EXERCISES

A. Construct medical terms related to the bones of the skull. *Given the definition, complete the medical term with the correct word element. Fill in the blanks.* **LO 4.1 and 4.6**

1. Wedge-shaped bone at the base of the skull: ____________ /oid
2. Bone that forms part of the base and sides of the skull: ____________ /al
3. Bone that forms the back of the nose and encloses numerous air cells: ____________ /oid
4. The two bones forming the sidewalls and roof of the cranium: ____________ /al

B. Apply *the language of orthopedics and select the correct answer.* **LO 4.6**

1. The mandible is the:
   a. lower jawbone **b.** base of the cranium **c.** upper jawbone
2. Which of these bones is a bone of the cranium?
   a. lacrimal **b.** frontal **c.** patella
3. How many bones are in the cranium?
   a. 8 **b.** 14 **c.** 22
4. What does *articulate* mean?
   a. stretches **b.** fractures **c.** joins
5. What is a *suture*?
   a. seam **b.** bend **c.** sharp point

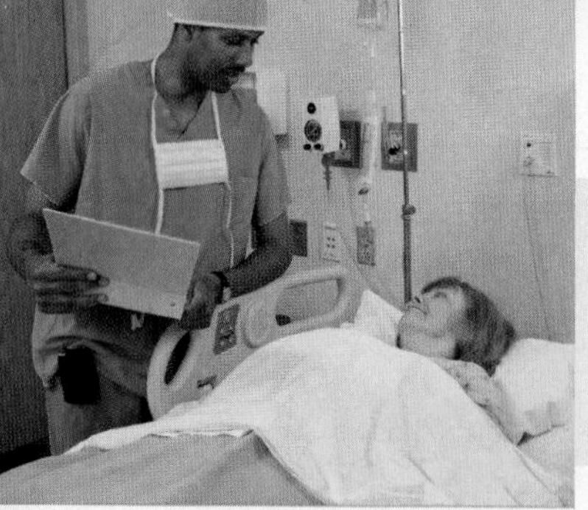
Rick Brady/McGraw-Hill Education

Lesson 4.3

Bones and Joints of the Shoulder Girdle and Upper Limb

Objectives

Your shoulders, arms, hands, and fingers are used nearly every time you move your body, no matter where you are—at work, at home, at the gym, in the car, or relaxing on the beach. Because these bones and joints get so much use, it's necessary to understand how they work and how to care for them. The information in this lesson will enable you to use correct medical terminology to:

- **4.3.1** Recognize the structures and functions of the bones and joints of the shoulder girdle.
- **4.3.2** Explain common disorders of the bones and joints of the shoulder girdle.
- **4.3.3** Identify the structures and functions of the bones and joints of the arm, elbow, and wrist.
- **4.3.4** Describe common disorders of the bones and joints of the arm, elbow, and wrist.
- **4.3.5** Specify the structures and functions of the bones and joints of the hand.
- **4.3.6** Define common disorders of the bones and joints of the hand.

Abbreviation

AC acromioclavicular

CASE REPORT 4.3

You are . . .

. . . an orthopedic technologist working with Kenneth Stannard, MD, at Fulwood Medical Center.

You are communicating with . . .

. . . James Fox, a 17-year-old male who complains of severe pain in his right wrist. While playing soccer a few hours earlier, he fell. James pushed his hand out to break his fall and heard his wrist snap. The wrist is now swollen and deformed.

T 98.2, P 92, R 15, BP 110/76. On examination, his right wrist is swollen and tender and has a dinner-fork **deformity.** An IV has been started, and he has been given 3 mg of morphine IV. An X-ray of the wrist has been ordered.

Shoulder Girdle

(LO 4.2 and 4.7)

The bones and joints of your shoulder girdle connect your axial skeleton to your upper limbs.

The bones of the shoulder girdle are the **scapulae** (shoulder blades) and **clavicles** (collarbones). The scapula extends over the top of the shoulder joint to form a roof called the **acromion,** which is attached to the clavicle at the **acromioclavicular (AC)** joint. Several ligaments hold together the **articulating** surfaces of the humerus and scapula.

The shoulder joint between the scapula and the **humerus** bone of the upper arm *(Figure 4.11)* is a ball-and-socket joint, allowing the head of the humerus greater range of motion than any other joint in the body. This broad range of motion does have one drawback; because the shoulder joint is very unstable, it's prone to **dislocation.**

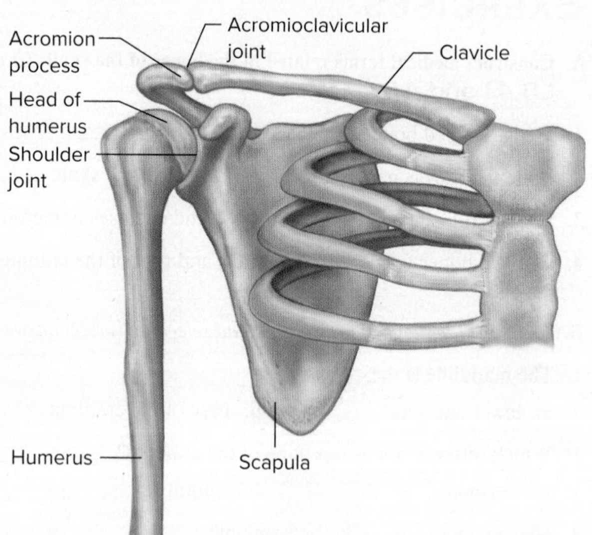

FIGURE 4.11
Pectoral Girdle and Humerus.

Disorders of the Shoulder Girdle (LO 4.2 and 4.7)

Shoulder separation is a dislocation of the acromioclavicular joint, often caused by a fall onto the point of the shoulder.

Shoulder dislocation occurs when the ball of the humerus slips out of the scapula's socket, usually anteriorly.

Shoulder subluxation occurs when the ball of the humerus slips partially out of position in the socket, and then moves back in.

Word Analysis and Definition

S = Suffix P = Prefix R = Root R/CF = Combining Form

WORD	PRONUNCIATION		ELEMENTS	DEFINITION
acromion	ah-**CROW**-mee-on		Greek *tip of the shoulder*	Lateral end of the scapula, extending over the shoulder joint
acromioclavicular	ah-**CROW**-mee-oh-klah-**VICK**-you-lar	S/ R/CF R/	-ar *pertaining to* acromi/o- *acromion* -clavicul- *clavicle*	The joint between the acromion and the clavicle
articulate articulation	ar-**TIK**-you-late ar-tik-you-**LAY**-shun	S/ R/ S/	-ate *composed of* articul-*joint* -ation *process*	Two separate bones have formed a joint A joint
clavicle clavicular (adj)	**KLAV**-ih-kul klah-**VICK**-you-lar	 S/ R/	Latin *collarbone* -ar *pertaining to* clavicul- *clavicle*	Curved bone that forms the anterior part of the pectoral girdle Pertaining to the clavicle
deformity	dee-**FOR**-mih-tee	S/ P/ R/	-ity *condition* de- *change of* -form- *appearance, form*	A permanent structural deviation from the normal
dislocation	dis-low-**KAY**-shun	S/ P/ R/	-ion *action, condition* dis- *apart, away from* -locat- *place*	Completely out of joint
humerus	**HYU**-mer-us		Latin *shoulder*	Single bone of the upper arm
pectoral pectoral girdle	**PEK**-tor-al **PEK**-tor-al **GIR**-del	S/ R/	-al *pertaining to* pector- *chest* girdle, Old English *encircle*	Pertaining to the chest Incomplete bony ring that attaches the upper limb to the axial skeleton
scapula scapulae (pl) scapular (adj)	**SKAP**-you-lah **SKAP**-you-lee **SKAP**-you-lar	 S/ R/	Latin *shoulder blade* -ar *pertaining to* scapul- *scapula*	Shoulder blade Pertaining to the shoulder blade
subluxation	sub-luck-**SAY**-shun	S/ P/ R/	-ion *action, condition* sub- *under, below, slightly* -luxat- *dislocate*	An incomplete dislocation when some contact between the joint surfaces remains

EXERCISES

A. Review *Case Report 4.3 and then select the correct answer for the question or that completes the statement.* **LO 4.2, 4.7, and 4.11**

1. Which of the following are Mr. Fox's complaints?

a. wrist snapped **b.** fever **c.** shortness of breath **d.** severe pain

2. What is discovered on Mr. Fox's physical examination?

a. high blood pressure **b.** swollen deformed wrist **c.** fever **d.** hematoma of fingers

3. IV is the abbreviation for the medical term:

a. intravertebral **b.** intervertebral **c.** intravenous **d.** intervenous

4. Morphine is given to treat Mr. Fox's:

a. low blood pressure **b.** pain **c.** swelling **d.** fever

B. Build medical terms *using the language of orthopedics to complete this exercise. Each term is defined and partially complete. Add the rest of the elements to complete the term. The first one is done for you. Fill in the blanks.* **LO 4.1, 4.2, 4.7, and 4.11**

1. incomplete dislocation ____sub____ / ____luxat____ / ____ion____
P R S

2. joint between acromion and clavicle ________ / ________ / ____ar____
R/CF R S

3. a joint ________ / ________ / ____ation____
P R S

4. pertaining to the shoulder blade ________ / ________ / ____ar____
P R S

Upper Arm and Elbow Joint

(LO 4.2 and 4.7)

Your upper arm extends from your shoulder to your elbow and contains only one bone, the **humerus** *(Figure 4.12).* The smooth surface of the hemispherical head that articulates with the socket of the scapula is covered with articular cartilage. At the lower end of the humerus, the **trochlea** articulates with the **ulna** bone of the forearm and the **capitulum** articulates with the **radius** *(Figure 4.13).*

Elbow Joint (LO 4.2 and 4.7)

The elbow joint has two articulations:

1. A hinge joint between the humerus and the ulna bone of the forearm, which allows flexion and extension of the elbow; and
2. A gliding joint between the humerus and the radius bone of the forearm, which allows **pronation** and **supination** of the forearm and hand.

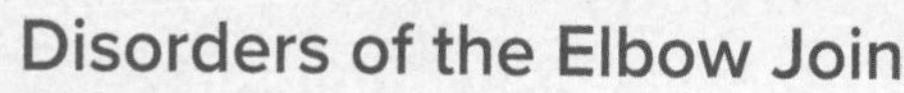

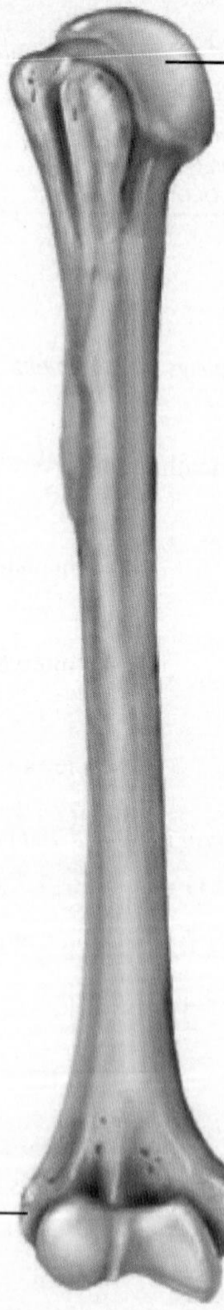

Disorders of the Elbow Joint

(LO 4.2 and 4.7)

When you bend your elbow, you can easily feel the bony prominence (the **olecranon** *Figure 4.13*) that extends from the ulna. The olecranon can be easily fractured by a direct blow to the elbow or by a fall on a bent elbow.

The olecranon **bursa** is a thin, slippery sac between the skin and the prominence of the olecranon bone. It contains a small amount of fluid to enable the skin to move freely over the bone. If the bursa becomes irritated or inflamed, fluid accumulates and **bursitis** occurs. Treatment is **aspiration** and an antibiotic if indicated by laboratory investigation of the aspirated fluid.

Tennis elbow is caused by overuse of the elbow joint or poor form when playing tennis or golf. The pain occurs when ligaments and muscle tendons around the joint tear. Treatment is rest, ice, pain medication, massage, and stretching exercises.

When a child falls on an outstretched arm, the force of hitting the ground can be transmitted up the arm to cause a fracture of the elbow joint. This accounts for about 10% of all fractures in children.

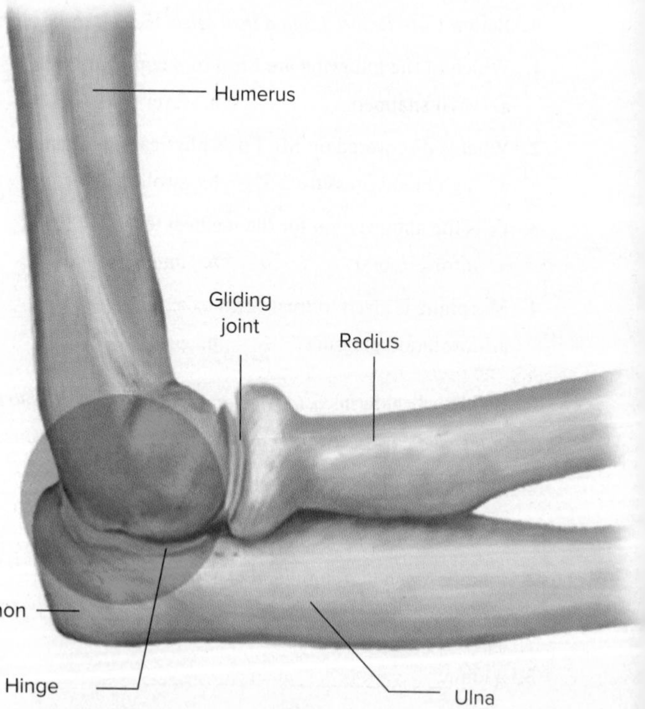

Anterior surface

Head

Lateral epicondyle

Medial epicondyle

▶ **FIGURE 4.12**
Humerus.

Humerus

Gliding joint

Radius

Olecranon

Hinge

Ulna

▲ **FIGURE 4.13**
Elbow Joint.

Word Analysis and Definition

S = Suffix P = Prefix R = Root R/CF = Combining Form

WORD	PRONUNCIATION	ELEMENTS		DEFINITION
aspiration aspirate (verb)	as-pih-**RAY**-shun **AS**-pih-rate	S/ R/	**-ion** *process* **aspirat-** *to breathe on*	Removal by suction of fluid or gas from a body cavity
bursa bursae (pl)	**BURR**-sah **BURR**-see		Latin *purse*	A closed sac containing synovial fluid
bursitis	burr-**SIGH**-tis	S/ R/	**-itis** *inflammation* **burs-** *bursa*	Inflammation of a bursa
capitulum	kah-**PIT**-you-lum	S/ R/CF	**-lum** *small structure* **capit/u** *small head*	A small head or rounded extremity of a bone
olecranon	oh-**LECK**-rah-non		Greek *point of elbow*	Prominent, proximal extremity of ulna
pronation pronate (verb) prone	pro-**NAY**-shun **PRO**-nate **PRONE**	S/ R/	**-ion** *action, condition* **pronat-** *bend down* Latin, *lying down*	Process of lying face down or of turning a hand or foot with the volar (palm or sole) surface down Lying face down, flat on your belly
radius radial (adj)	**RAY**-dee-us **RAY**-dee-al	 S/ R/	Latin *spoke of a wheel* **-al** *pertaining to* **radi-** *radius*	The forearm bone on the thumb side Pertaining to the radius or to any of the structures (artery, vein, nerve) named after it
supination supine	soo-pih-**NAY**-shun soo-**PINE**	S/ R/	**-ion** *action, condition* **supinat-** *bend backward* Latin *bend backward*	Process of lying face upward or of turning a hand or foot so that the palm or sole is facing up Lying face up, flat on your spine
trochlea trochlear	**TROHK**-lee-ah **TROHK**-lee-ar	 S/ R/	Latin *pulley* **-ar** *pertaining to* **trochle-** *pulley*	Smooth articular surface of bone on which another glides Pertaining to a trochlea
ulna ulnar (adj)	**UL**-nah **UL**-nar	 S/ R/	Latin *elbow, arm* **-ar** *pertaining to* **uln-** *ulna*	The medial and larger bone of the forearm Pertaining to the ulna or to any of the structures (artery, vein, nerve) named after it

EXERCISES

A. Meet lesson *and chapter objectives by answering these questions using the language of orthopedics. Select the correct answer to complete each statement.* **LO 4.2, 4.7, and 4.11**

1. The two types of joints fond in the elbow are:

a. hinge and cruciate **b.** ball-and-socket and gliding **c.** hinge and gliding **d.** gliding and pivot

2. The upper arm consists of the bone(s):

a. humerus **b.** humerus and scapula **c.** radius **d.** radius and ulna

3. The lower arms consists of the bone(s):

a. humerus **b.** humerus and scapula **c.** radius **d.** radius and ulna

4. The bony projection that means *pulley*:

a. capitulum **b.** ulna **c.** trochlea **d.** olecranon

5. A bursa can be found:

a. between a bone and skin **b.** between a bone and a bone **c.** under the periosteum **d.** connecting muscle to bone

B. The statement *is either true or false. Select T if the statement is true. Select F if the statement is false.* **LO 4.7**

1. The opposite of pronation is supination. T F

2. The capitulum articulates with the scapula. T F

3. A sports-related injury is very common in the elbow. T F

4. The radius is on the thumb side of the hand. T F

5. A hinge joint allows pronation of the hand and forearm. T F

Forearm, Wrist, and Hand (LO 4.2 and 4.7)

The Wrist (LO 4.2 and 4.7)

In your forearm, the radius bone on the thumb side and the larger ulna bone on the little-finger side articulate at your wrist joint with the small **carpal** bones *(Figure 4.14)*.

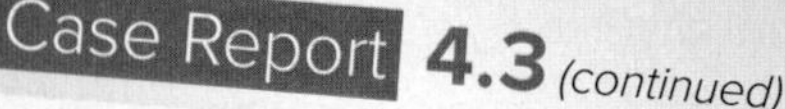

Case Report 4.3 *(continued)*

The X-ray of James Fox's wrist showed a **Colles fracture** of the radius, 1 inch above the end of the bone. Dr. Stannard applied a cast with the **distal** fragment of the fracture in palmar flexion and ulnar deviation. Mr. Fox was sent home with Vicodin 500 mg **po, prn,** for pain, and an appointment to return to the clinic in a week.

Keynote

- **Colles fracture is an eponym. An eponym is a procedure or a diagnosis with a name derived from the name of the person who discovered it (if it is a disease or condition) or originated it (if it is a procedure). This text contains several examples of eponyms—be on the lookout for them.**

Abbreviations

po	by mouth
prn	when necessary

Disorders of the Wrist (LO 4.2 and 4.7)

A **Colles fracture** is a common fracture of the radius just above the wrist joint *(Figure 4.15)* that occurs when a person tries to break a fall with an outstretched hand.

Fracture of the scaphoid bone *(Figure 4.14)*—the most common fracture of a carpal bone—also results from breaking a fall with an outstretched hand, but poor blood supply here makes healing slow and difficult.

Carpal tunnel syndrome is inflammation of the tendon synovial sheaths on the back of the wrist arising from repetitive movements such as computer keyboard operation.

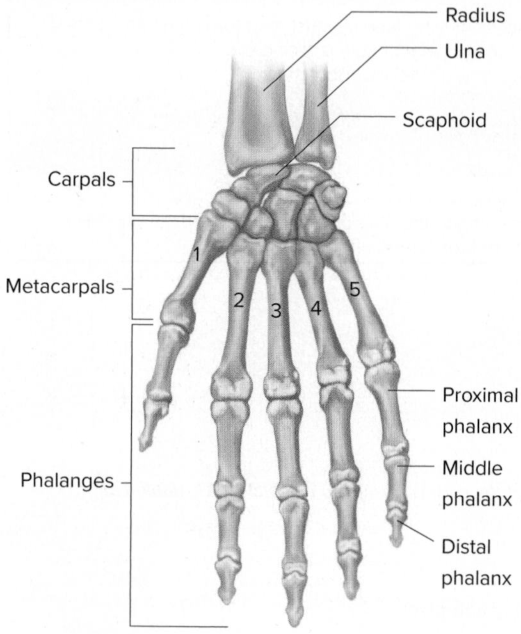

▲ **FIGURE 4.14**
Bones of the Wrist and Hand.

The Hand (LO 4.2 and 4.7)

The five fingers of your single hand have 14 bones called **phalanges.** The thumb has two phalanges, and each of the remaining four fingers has three *(Figure 4.14)*. In your palm, the five bones closest to the fingers are **metacarpals;** these connect to the phalanges at the **metacarpophalangeal** joints. The metacarpals connect at the wrist to eight small carpal bones, which then connect the hand to the bones of the forearm. All of these bones require numerous joints with ligaments to connect and stabilize them.

Disorders of the Hand (LO 4.2 and 4.7)

Osteoarthritis (OA) in the hand joints occurs from wear and tear leading to deterioration of joint cartilage. Small bony spurs called **Heberden nodes** form over the joint *(Figure 4.16)*.

Rheumatoid arthritis (RA), with destruction of joint surfaces, joint capsules, and ligaments, leads to noticeable deformity and joint instability *(Figure 4.17)*. RA occurs mostly in women, between ages 40 and 60, and affects the synovial membrane lining the joints and tendons. Lumps known as **rheumatic** nodules form over the small joints of the hand and wrist.

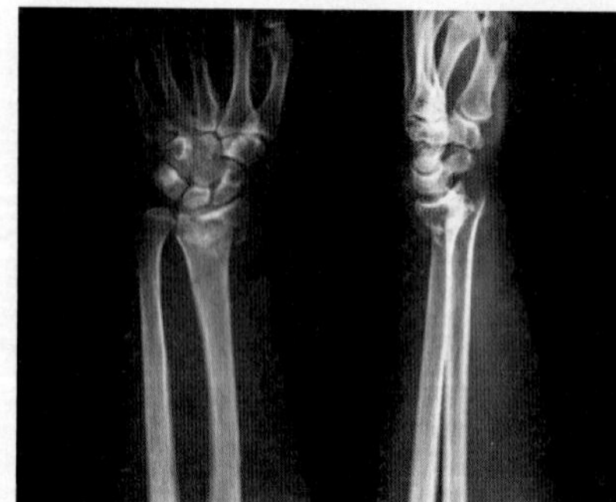

▲ **FIGURE 4.15**
X-Ray of Colles Fracture.

Puwadol Jaturawutthichai/Shutterstock

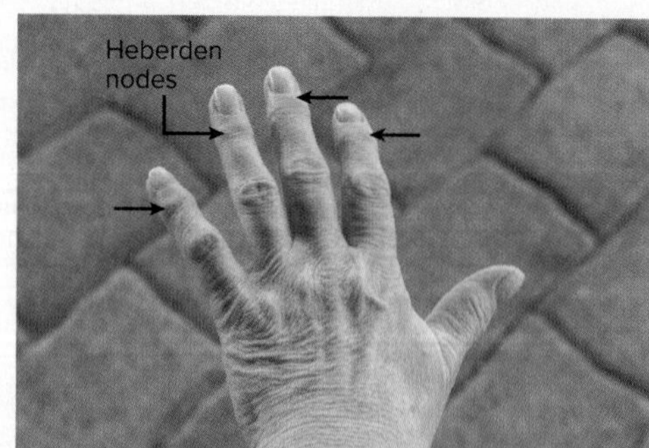

▲ **FIGURE 4.16**
Hand with Osteoarthritis.

Vincent Scherer/Alamy Images

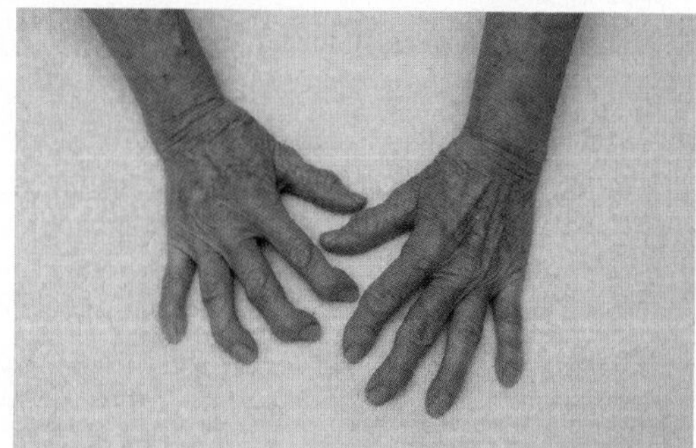

▲ **FIGURE 4.17**
Hands with Rheumatoid Arthritis.

Aaron Roeth

Word Analysis and Definition

S = Suffix P = Prefix R = Root R/CF = Combining Form

WORD	PRONUNCIATION	ELEMENTS		DEFINITION
arthritis	ar-**THRI**-tis	S/ R/	-itis *inflammation* arthr- *joint*	Inflammation of a joint or joints
carpus carpal (adj) metacarpal	**KAR**-pus **KAR**-pal **MET**-ah-**KAR**-pal	 S/ R/ P/	Greek *wrist* -al *pertaining to* carp- *wrist bones* meta- *after, subsequent to*	The eight carpal bones of the wrist Pertaining to the wrist The five bones between the carpus and the fingers
Colles fracture	**KOL**-ez **FRAK**-chur		Abraham Colles, Irish surgeon, 1773–1843	Fracture of the distal radius at the wrist
eponym	**EH**-po-nim		Greek *epōnymos, meaning eponymous*	A procedure or a diagnosis with a name derived from the name of the person who discovered it (if it is a disease or condition) or originated it (if it is a procedure)
Heberden node	**HEH**-ber-den **NOHD**		William Heberden, English physician, 1710–1801	Bony lump on the terminal phalanx of the fingers in osteoarthritis
metacarpophalangeal	**MET**-ah-**KAR**-poh-fay-**LAN**-jee-al	S/ P/ R/CF R/CF	-al *pertaining to* meta- *after, subsequent to* -carp/o- *bones of the wrist* -phalang/e- *phalanx, finger or toe*	The joints between the metacarpal bones and the phalanges
osteoarthritis	**OSS**-tee-oh-ar-**THRI**-tis	S/ R/CF R/	-itis *inflammation* oste/o- *bone* arthr- *joint*	Chronic inflammatory disease of joints
phalanx phalanges (pl)	**FAY**-lanks fay-**LAN**-jeez		Latin *bone of finger* or *toe*	One of the bones of the digits (fingers or toes)
rheumatism rheumatic (adj) rheumatoid arthritis	**RU**-ma-tizm ru-**MA**-tik **RU**-mah-toyd ar-**THRI**-tis	S/ R/ S/ S/	-ism *condition* rheumat- *a flow* -ic *pertaining to* -oid *resembling*	Pain in various parts of the musculoskeletal system Pertaining to or characterized by rheumatism Systemic disease affecting many joints

EXERCISES

A. Deconstruct *the following terms by filling in the blanks:* **LO 4.1, 4.7, and 4.11**

1. Metacarpophalangeal: ________ / ________ / ________ / ________
   P — R, R/CF — R, R/CF — S

2. Osteoarthritis: ________ / ________ / ________
   R, R/CF — R, R/CF — S

B. Review *Case Report 4.3 (continued) to select the correct answer to complete each statement.* **LO 4.7 and 4.11**

1. The specific type of fracture Mr. Fox has is a ____ fracture.
   a. comminuted **b.** Colles **c.** open **d.** greenstick
2. The presence of a fracture was confirmed by a(n):
   a. Vicodin **b.** X-ray **c.** cast **d.** pronation
3. The treatment for the fracture was a(n):
   a. Vicodin **b.** X-ray **c.** cast **d.** pronation

C. Review *Figure 4.14 to formulate your answers to the following questions. Fill in the blanks.* **LO 4.2, 4.7, and 4.11**

1. The bones of the hand are called: ________
2. The bones of the wrist are called: ________
3. The tip of each finger is made up of a ________ phalanx.

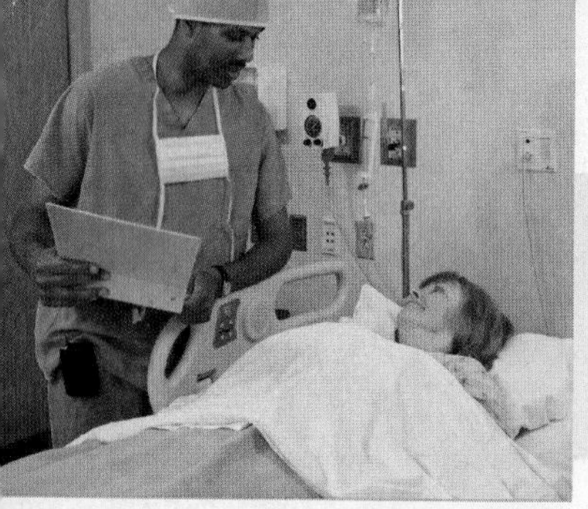

Rick Brady/McGraw-Hill Education

Lesson 4.4

Pelvic Girdle and Lower Limb

Objectives

You use your legs and feet constantly, every day of your life, whether you are standing, walking, or changing positions. The information in this lesson will enable you to use correct medical terminology to:

4.4.1 Identify the structures and functions of the bones and joints of the pelvic girdle.

4.4.2 Describe common disorders of the bones and joints of the pelvic girdle.

4.4.3 Identify the structures and functions of the bones and joints of the leg, knee, and ankle.

4.4.4 Recognize common disorders of the hip joint, knee, and ankle.

4.4.5 Identify the structures and functions of the bones and joints of the foot.

4.4.6 Name common disorders of the bones and joints of the foot.

The Pelvic Girdle (LO 4.2 and 4.8)

Your pelvic girdle consists of your two hip bones that articulate anteriorly with each other at the **symphysis pubis** and posteriorly with the **sacrum** (a triangular-shaped bone in your lower back). This forms the bowl-shaped **pelvis.** The two joints between your hip bones and the sacrum are called **sacroiliac joints.**

The pelvic girdle has these functions:

1. Supports the axial skeleton;
2. Transmits the upper body's weight to the lower limbs;
3. Provides attachments for the lower limbs; and
4. Protects the internal reproductive organs, urinary bladder, and distal segment of the large intestine.

Each of your hip bones is actually a fusion of three bones: the **ilium, ischium,** and **pubis** *(Figure 4.18a).* This fusion occurs in the region of the **acetabulum,** a cup-shaped cavity on the lateral surface of the hip bone that receives the head of the **femur,** or thigh bone *(Figure 4.18b).*

The lower part of the pelvis is formed by the lower ilium, ischium, and pubic bones that surround a short canal-like pelvic cavity, through which the rectum, vagina, and urethra pass. In females, the infant passes down this canal during childbirth.

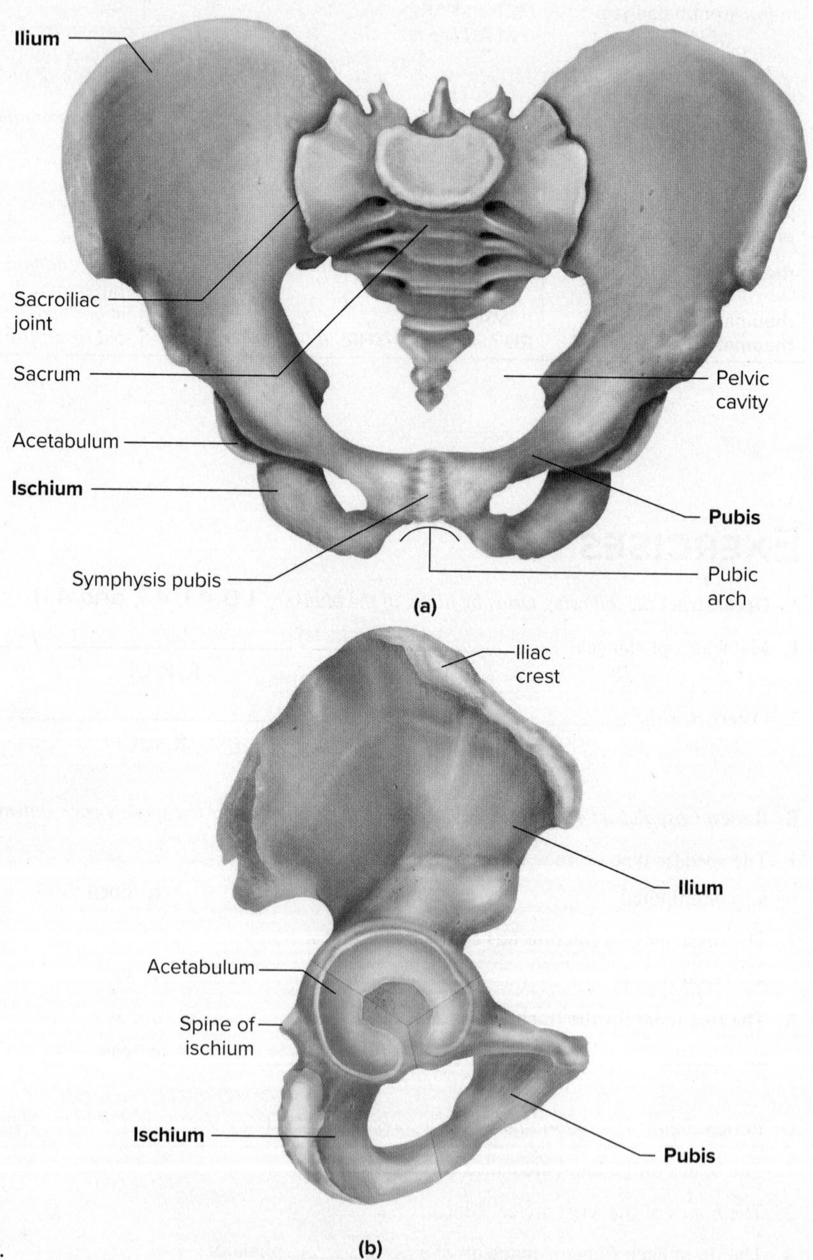

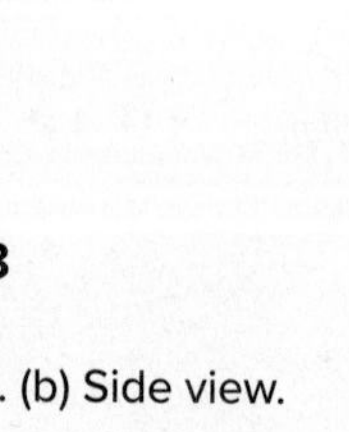

FIGURE 4.18
Pelvic Girdle.
(a) Front view. (b) Side view.

Word Analysis and Definition

S = Suffix P = Prefix R = Root R/CF = Combining Form

WORD	PRONUNCIATION		ELEMENTS	DEFINITION
acetabulum	ass-eh-**TAB**-you-lum		Latin *vinegar cup*	The cup-shaped cavity of the hip bone that receives the head of the femur to form the hip joint
femur	**FEE**-mur		Latin *thigh*	The thigh bone
femoral (adj)	**FEM**-oh-ral	S/ R/	**-al** *pertaining to* **femor-** *femur*	Pertaining to the femur
ilium	**ILL**-ee-um		Latin *groin*	Large wing-shaped bone at the upper and posterior part of the pelvis
ischium **ischia (pl)** **ischial (adj)**	**IS**-kee-um **IS**-kee-ah **IS**-kee-al	S/ R/	Greek *hip* **-al** *pertaining to* **ischi-** *ischium, hip bone*	Lower and posterior part of the hip bone Pertaining to the ischium
pelvis	**PEL**-viss		Latin *basin*	Basin-shaped ring of bones, ligaments, and muscles at the base of the spine. Also, any basin-shaped cavity, like the pelvis of the kidney
pelvic (adj)	**PEL**-vik	S/ R/	**-ic** *pertaining to* **pelv-** *pelvis*	Pertaining to the pelvis
pubis **pubic (adj)**	**PYU**-bis **PYU**-bik	S/ R/	Latin *pubis* **-ic** *pertaining to* **pub-** *pubis*	Alternative name for the pubic bone Pertaining to the pubic bone
sacroiliac joint	say-kroh-**ILL**-ih-ak **JOINT**	S/ R/CF R	**-ac** *pertaining to* **sacr/o-** *sacrum* **-ili-** *ilium*	The joint between the sacrum and the ilium
symphysis **symphyses (pl)**	**SIM**-feh-sis **SIM**-feh-seez		Greek *grow together*	Two bones joined by fibrocartilage; in this case, the two pubic bones

EXERCISES

A. Demonstrate your knowledge *of the precise medical term to answer the following questions. Fill in the blanks with the term that is:* **LO 4.2, 4.8, and 4.11**

1. another name for the thigh bone ______________________
2. a basin-shaped ring of bones ______________________
3. the joint between the sacrum and the ilium ______________________
4. the lower posterior part of the hip bone ______________________
5. the wing-shaped bone in the pelvis ______________________

B. Meet lesson objectives *and select the correct medical term based on the statement.* **LO 4.8**

1. The hip bone is a fusion of three bones: the ilium, the ischium, and the
   a. femur **b.** pubis **c.** acetabulum
2. The pelvis is shaped like a
   a. bowl **b.** box **c.** basket
3. One function of the pelvic girdle is to:
   a. support the cranium **b.** attach lower limbs **c.** transport waste products
4. What organs does the pelvic girdle protect?
   a. lungs **b.** pancreas and gallbladder **c.** bladder, intestines, reproductive
5. A triangular-shaped bone in the lower back is the
   a. scapula **b.** sacrum **c.** symphysis

Disorders of the Pelvic Girdle (LO 4.1, 4.2, and 4.8)

Keynote

- **The sciatic nerve lies directly behind the lower third of the SI joint. Many patients with SI joint strain will have pain radiating down the back of the leg.**

CASE REPORT 4.4

You are . . .

. . . a physical therapist assistant working in the physical therapy department of Fulwood Medical Center.

You are communicating with . . .

. . . Sandra Halpin, a 38-year-old female who is complaining of persistent low back pain on her left side. The pain began about two years previously, when she and her husband were moving and she was lifting heavy boxes. Her family physician has prescribed rest, back exercises, muscle relaxants, and painkillers, but she has had no relief.

On examination, she exhibits tenderness over the left sacroiliac joint, and when she presses her left knee to her chest, she experiences considerable pain over the **SI** joint. X-rays of the pelvis and hips, and an angle study of the SI joints, showed narrowing of the left SI joint space. A diagnosis of left sacroiliac joint strain has been made.

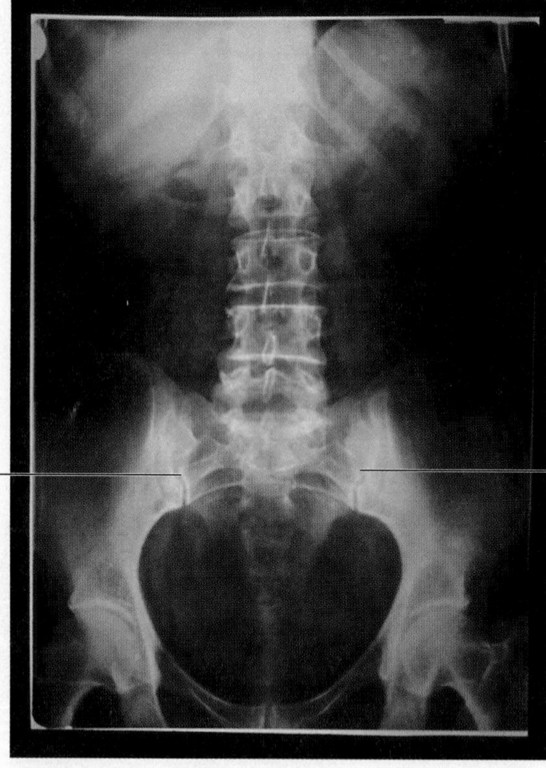

▲ **FIGURE 4.19**
X-ray of the Sacroiliac (SI) Joints—showing narrowing of the joint space in the left SI joint.

Andre Thijssen/Getty Images

Sacroiliac (SI) joint strain is a common cause of lower back pain. Unlike most joints, the SI joint *(Figure 4.19)* is designed to move only 1/4 of an inch during weight-bearing and forward-bending movements. Its main function is to provide shock absorption for the spine.

Because stretching in the SI joint ligaments makes this joint overly mobile, it's susceptible to wear and tear, including painful arthritis. Another cause of pain in the SI joint is trauma, when tearing of the joint ligaments allows too much motion.

A clinical examination, joint X-ray **(radiology),** and CT scan may be used to diagnose the presence of sacroiliac strain. For temporary pain relief, a local anesthetic can be injected into the joint. Standard treatment involves **stabilizing** the joint with a **brace** and strengthening the lower back muscles with physical therapy. Occasionally, **arthrodesis** of the joint is necessary.

Diastasis symphysis pubis sometimes occurs during pregnancy. It is caused by excessive stretching of pelvic ligaments, which widens the joint between the two pubic bones. This leads to pain and difficulty in walking, climbing stairs, and turning over in bed. During pregnancy, however, hormones generally enable connective tissue in the SI joint area to relax so the pelvis can expand enough to allow birth without causing SI joint strain.

Abbreviation

SI	sacroiliac

Word Analysis and Definition

S = Suffix P = Prefix R = Root R/CF = Combining Form

WORD	PRONUNCIATION		ELEMENTS	DEFINITION
arthrodesis	ar-**THROW**-dee-sis	S/ R/CF	-desis *to fuse together* arthr/o- *joint*	Fixation or stiffening of a joint by surgery
brace	BRACE		Old English *to fasten*	Appliance to support a part of the body in its correct position
diastasis	die-**ASS**-tah-sis		Greek *separation*	Separation of normally joined parts
radiology	ray-dee-**OL**-oh-jee	S/ R/CF	-logy *study of* radi/o- *radiation, X-rays*	The study of medical imaging
radiologist	ray-dee-**OL**-oh-jist	S/	-logist *one who studies, specialist*	Medical specialist in the use of X-rays and other imaging techniques
stable	**STAY**-bell		Latin *steady*	Steady, not varying
stabilize	**STAY**-bill-ize	S/ R/	-ize *action* stabil- *steady, fixed*	To make or hold firm and steady

Exercises

A. Review *Case Report 4.4 to select the correct answer the following questions.* **LO 4.8 and 4.11**

1. What is Sandra Halpin's chief complaint?
   - **a.** prescription pain killers are not strong enough
   - **b.** narrowing of the left SI joint space
   - **c.** persistent low back pain on her left side
   - **d.** left knee pain on standing
2. How did Ms. Halpin injure herself?
   - **a.** lifting and moving heavy boxes
   - **b.** pressing her left knee to her chest
   - **c.** tripping on the stairs in front of her house
   - **d.** overuse injury while exercising
3. Which of the following is a therapy prescribed by her physician to help Ms. Halpin's pain?
   - **a.** acupuncture
   - **b.** chiropractic manipulation
   - **c.** deep tissue massage
   - **d.** rest
4. What is Ms. Halpin's final diagnosis?
   - **a.** subluxation of the left sacroiliac joint
   - **b.** right sacroiliac joint strain
   - **c.** left sacroiliac joint strain
   - **d.** subluxation of the right sacroiliac joint

B. Construct medical terms related to the bones of the pelvic girdle. *Given the definition, complete the medical term with the correct word element. The first one has been done for you. Fill in the blanks.* **LO 4.1 and 4.8**

1. The joint that is made up of the sacrum and ilium bones: **sacro** (S) / **ili** (P) / **ac** (R)
2. Study of medical imaging: ______________ / ______________
3. Surgical fixation of a joint: ______________ / ______________

C. Read *the answer choices for each question and immediately discard the ones you know are not correct. Select the correct answer in the remaining possibilities.* **LO 4.8 and 4.11**

1. What can the physician do to provide temporary pain relief from SI joint strain?
   - **a.** stretching
   - **b.** a brace
   - **c.** PT
   - **d.** heat application
   - **e.** local anesthetic injected into the joint
2. The expertise of a radiologist is in:
   - **a.** skin diseases
   - **b.** tissue study
   - **c.** disorders of the brain
   - **d.** interpreting X-rays
   - **e.** lung conditions
3. Fixation or stiffening of a joint by surgery is called
   - **a.** arthroscopy
   - **b.** arthroplasty
   - **c.** arthrodesis
   - **d.** arthrotomy
   - **e.** none of these
4. What substance allows the SI joint to relax enough for delivery of a baby?
   - **a.** lymph
   - **b.** blood
   - **c.** enzymes
   - **d.** synovial fluid
   - **e.** hormones

Bones and Joints of the Hip and Thigh (LO 4.2 and 4.8)

Your **hip joint** is a ball-and-socket mechanism formed by the head of your femur (thigh bone) and the acetabulum (cup-shaped hip socket) of your hip bone *(Figure 4.20)*. The **labrum** is the articular cartilage that forms a rim around the hip joint socket, cushioning the joint and helping to keep your femoral head in place in the socket. Finally, the hip joint is secured by a thick joint capsule reinforced by strong ligaments that connect the neck of the femur to the rim of the hip socket.

Disorders and Injuries of the Hip Joint (LO 4.2 and 4.8)

Hip pointer, often a football-related injury, is a blow to the rim of the pelvis that leads to bruising of the bone and surrounding tissues.

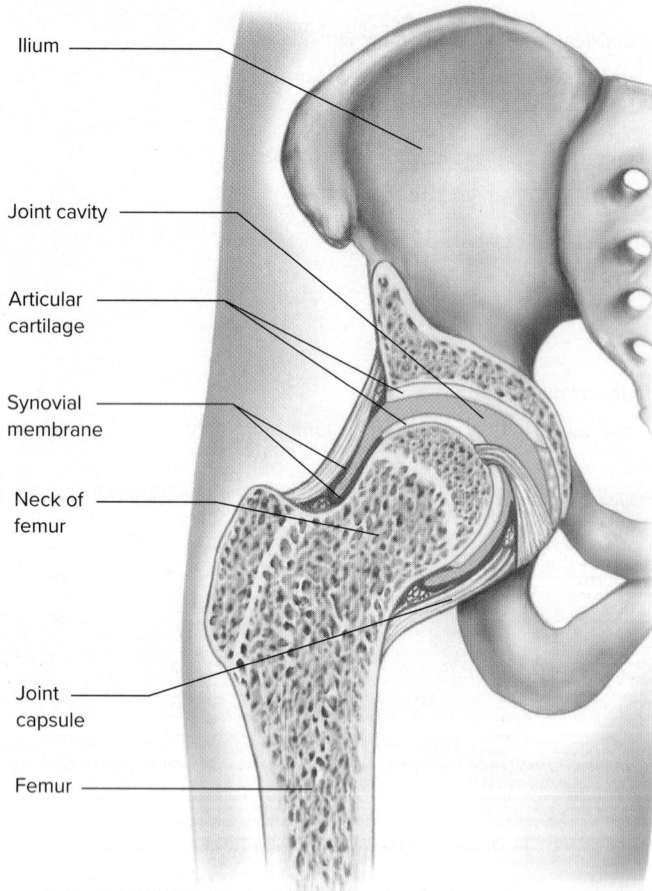

▲ **FIGURE 4.20**
Hip Joint.
Right frontal view of a section of the hip joint.

Osteoarthritis is common in the hip as a result of aging, weight bearing, and repetitive use of the joint. The cartilage on both the acetabulum and the head of the femur deteriorates, causing friction between the bones of the femoral head and the acetabulum that leads to pain and loss of mobility.

Rheumatoid arthritis can also affect the hip, beginning in the synovial membrane and progressing to destroy cartilage and bone.

Avascular necrosis of the femoral head is the death (necrosis) of bone tissue when the blood supply is cut off (avascular), usually as a result of trauma.

Fractures of the neck of the femur occur as a result of a fall, most commonly in elderly women with osteoporosis.

Surgical Procedures of the Hip Joint (LO 4.2 and 4.8)

There are two standard surgical procedures for replacing or repairing the hip joint. **Arthroplasty,** a total replacement of the hip joint with a metal **prosthesis,** is the most common hip surgery today. Here, the diseased parts of the joint are removed and replaced with artificial parts made of titanium and other metals, ceramics, and plastics *(Figure 4.21)*.

Arthrodesis is a surgical procedure that fixates or stiffens a joint.

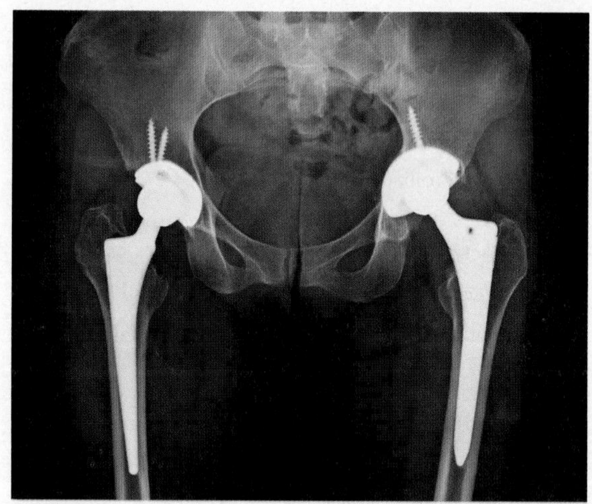

▲ **FIGURE 4.21**
Total Hip Replacement.
Colored X-ray of prosthetic hip.

Tridsanu Thopet/Shutterstock

Word Analysis and Definition

S = Suffix P = Prefix R = Root R/CF = Combining Form

WORD	PRONUNCIATION	ELEMENTS		DEFINITION
arthrodesis	ar-**THROW**-dee-sis	S/ R/CF	**-desis** *to fuse together* **arthr/o-** *joint*	Fixation or stiffening of a joint by surgery
arthroplasty	**AR**-throw-plas-tee	S/ R/CF	**-plasty** *reshaping by surgery* **arthr/o-** *joint*	Surgery to repair, as far as possible, the function of a joint
avascular	a-**VAS**-cue-lar	S/ P/ R/	**-ar** *pertaining to* **a-** *without* **-vascul-** *blood vessel*	Without a blood supply
labrum	**LAY**-brum		Latin *lip-shaped*	Cartilage that forms a rim around the socket of the hip joint
necrosis necrotic (adj)	neh-**KROH**-sis neh-**KROT**-ik	 S/ R/CF	Greek *death* **-tic** *pertaining to* **necr/o-** *death*	Pathologic death of cells or tissue Pertaining to or affected by necrosis
prosthesis prosthetic (adj)	**PROS**-thee-sis pros-**THET**-ik	 S/ R/CF	Greek *addition* **-ic** *pertaining to* **prosthet-** *prosthesis*	An artificial part to remedy a defect in the body Pertaining to a prosthesis

EXERCISES

A. Match *the correct medical term in column one with its meaning in column two.* **LO 4.2 and 4.5**

1. ________ synovial — **a.** artificial body part
2. ________ arthroplasty — **b.** bloodless
3. ________ prosthesis — **c.** death of cells
4. ________ avascular — **d.** lubricating
5. ________ necrosis — **e.** joint repair

B. Select *the best choice after you have discounted the answers you know are not correct.* **LO 4.2 and 4.5**

1. What is the purpose of synovial fluid?
   - **a.** balance
   - **b.** alignment
   - **c.** lubrication
   - **d.** weight bearing
   - **e.** mobility
2. What is the purpose of a prosthesis?
   - **a.** restore well being
   - **b.** remedy a defect in the body
   - **c.** maintain balance
   - **d.** support the skeleton
   - **e.** repair a joint
3. The head of the femur fits into the _____________ of the pelvis.
   - **a.** sacrum
   - **b.** acetabulum
   - **c.** labrum
   - **d.** foramen
4. Inflammation of the bone and joints:
   - **a.** arthritis
   - **b.** osteoarthritis
   - **c.** necrosis
   - **d.** avascular
5. Hip pointer injury results from a blow to the:
   - **a.** femur
   - **b.** sacrum
   - **c.** pelvis
   - **d.** pubic symphysis
6. The cartilage that forms a ring around the hip joint:
   - **a.** labrum
   - **b.** pubis
   - **c.** acetabulum
   - **d.** symphysis

Abbreviations

ACL anterior cruciate ligament
PCL posterior cruciate ligament

The Knee Joint

(LO 4.2 and 4.9)

Your knees do plenty of bending, whether you're climbing the stairs, exercising, sitting cross-legged, or squatting down to collect something from the floor. Each of your knees is a hinged joint formed with these four bones:

1. **The lower end of the femur,** shaped like a horseshoe;
2. **The flat upper end of the tibia;**
3. **The flat triangular patella** (kneecap), embedded in the **patellar** tendon and articulating with the femur *(Figure 4.22a)*; and
4. **The fibula,** which forms a separate joint—the **tibiofibular joint** *(Figure 4.22b)*—by articulating with the tibia.

CASE REPORT 4.5

You are . . .

. . . an Emergency Technician working in the Emergency Department of Fulwood Medical Center.

You are communicating with . . .

. . . Gail Griffith, a 17-year-old high school student and her mother, Mrs. Cindy Griffith. Gail landed awkwardly after jumping for a ball during a basketball game.

Gail: "My knee kinda popped as I landed."

Gail had to be assisted off the court. In the Emergency Department, the knee was swollen and unstable. An MRI showed a partial tear of the medial **collateral** ligament, a complete **rupture** of the anterior **cruciate** ligament, and a partial tear of the medial **meniscus.** Gail decided to have surgery, even though full recovery would take 6 months to 1 year of rehabilitation.

Mechanically, the patella's role is to provide a 30% strength increase in the extension of the knee joint.

Within the knee joint, two crescent-shaped pads of cartilage—the **medial** and **lateral menisci**—lie on top of the tibia and articulate with the femur. This cartilage helps to distribute weight more evenly across the joint surface to minimize wear and tear.

The knee joint has a fibrous capsule, lined with synovial membrane that secretes synovial fluid to lubricate the joint. Four ligaments hold the knee joint together: the **medial** and **lateral collateral ligaments** located outside the joint and the **anterior cruciate ligament (ACL)** and **posterior cruciate ligament (PCL)** located inside the joint cavity, crossing over each other to form an "X" *(Figure 4.22b)*.

The thigh muscles which move the knee joint are described in Lesson 5.3 of the next chapter.

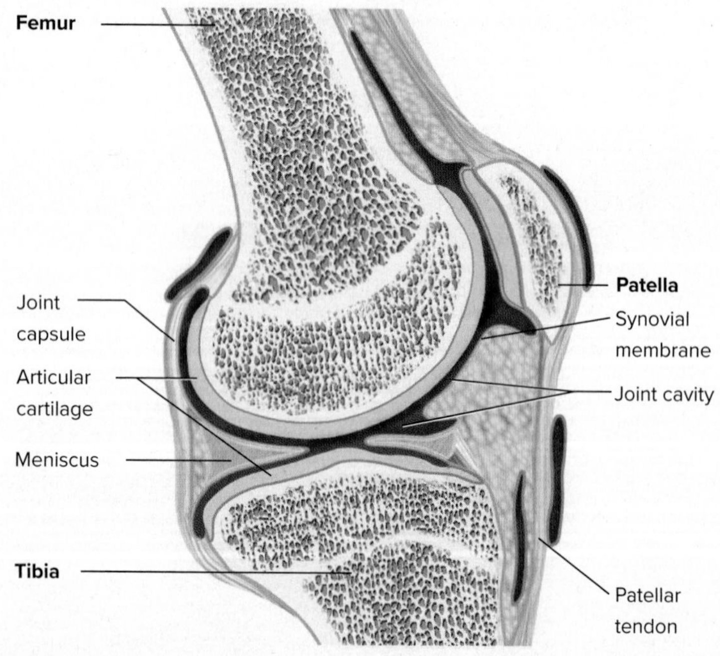

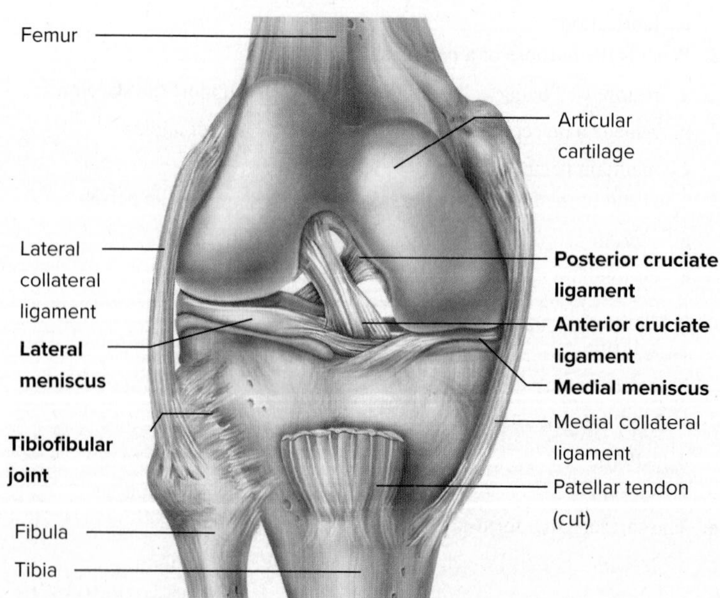

▼ FIGURE 4.22
Knee Joint.
(a) Section of knee joint.
(b) Right knee joint, anterior view.

Word Analysis and Definition

S = Suffix P = Prefix R = Root R/CF = Combining Form

WORD	PRONUNCIATION	ELEMENTS		DEFINITION
collateral (**Note:** *An extra "l" has been inserted.*)	koh-**LAT**-er-al	S/ P/ R/	-al *pertaining to* co- *together* -later- *side*	Situated at the side, often to bypass an obstruction
cruciate	**KRU**-she-ate		Latin *cross*	Shaped like a cross. In this case, the two internal ligaments of the knee joint cross over each other to form an "X"
fibula fibular (adj)	**FIB**-you-lah **FIB**-you-lar	 S/ R/	Latin *clasp* or *buckle* -ar *pertaining to* fibul- *fibula*	The smaller of the two bones of the lower leg Pertaining to the fibula
meniscus menisci (pl)	meh-**NISS**-kuss meh-**NISS**-key		Greek *crescent*	Disc of cartilage between the bones of a joint, in this case, the knee joint
patella (kneecap) patellae (pl) patellar (adj)	pah-**TELL**-ah pah-**TELL**-ee pah-**TELL**-ar	 S/ R/	Latin *small plate* -ar *pertaining to* patell- *patella*	Thin, circular bone in front of the knee joint, embedded in the patellar tendon Pertaining to the patella bone or the tendon
rupture	**RUP**-tyur		Latin *break*	Break or tear of any body part
tibia tibial (adj)	**TIB**-ee-ah **TIB**-ee-al	 S/ R/	Latin *large shinbone* -al *pertaining to* tibi- *tibia*	The larger bone of the lower leg Pertaining to the tibia

EXERCISES

A. Review *the Case Report 4.5 to select the correct answer for each question.* **LO 4.2, 4.9, and 4.11**

1. What are Gail's symptoms when she presents to the ER?
   - **a.** dislocated hip
   - **b.** swollen and dislocated knee
   - **c.** swollen and painful foot
   - **d.** painful and dislocated ankle
2. What does MRI mean?
   - **a.** multiple recurring images
   - **b.** maximal reasonable intensity
   - **c.** minimal recorded interference
   - **d.** magnetic resonance imaging
3. As a diagnostic test, what did the MRI show? (choose all that apply)
   - **a.** partial tear of the medial meniscus
   - **b.** complete rupture of the anterior cruciate ligament
   - **c.** complete rupture of the lateral collateral ligament
   - **d.** partial tear of the medial collateral ligament
4. The meaning of collateral means situated:
   - **a.** beneath
   - **b.** in front of
   - **c.** at the side
   - **d.** behind
5. In her treatment plan, what will Gail be doing after surgery?
   - **a.** limiting basketball practice for six months
   - **b.** limiting all after-school activities
   - **c.** six months to one year of rehabilitation
   - **d.** two to six months of rehabilitation
6. What is the most severe of the injuries to Gail's knees?
   - **a.** complete rupture of the lateral collateral ligament
   - **b.** complete rupture of the anterior cruciate ligament
   - **c.** partial tear of the medical meniscus
   - **d.** partial tear of the medial collateral ligament

B. Spelling *medical terms is a skill that is necessary for communicating in written documentation. Given the definition, correctly spell the medical term it is defining. Fill in the blanks.* **LO 4.2, 4.9, and 4.11**

1. The lateral bone of the lower leg: ____________________
2. The medical term for the kneecap: ____________________
3. Situated to the side: ____________________
4. Disc of cartilage between the bones of a joint: ____________________
5. Shaped like a cross: ____________________

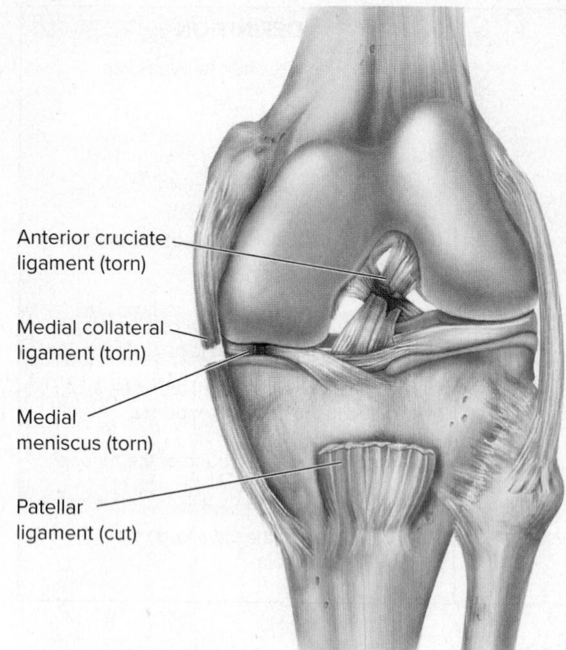

▲ **FIGURE 4.23**
Gail Griffith's Knee Injuries.

Operative Report: Fulwood Medical Center

Patient: Gail Griffith, aged 17.
Preoperative Diagnosis: Traumatic **ACL** tear, medial collateral ligament tear, and tear of medial meniscus, right knee.

Case Report 4.5 *(continued)*

Postoperative Diagnosis: Same.
Procedure Performed: Arthroscopy, repair of medial collateral ligament, **ACL** reconstruction, repair of torn medial meniscus, right knee.
Operative Findings: An avulsed anterior cruciate ligament **(ACL)** of the femur with a tear of the posterior horn of the medial meniscus and tear of medial collateral ligament.

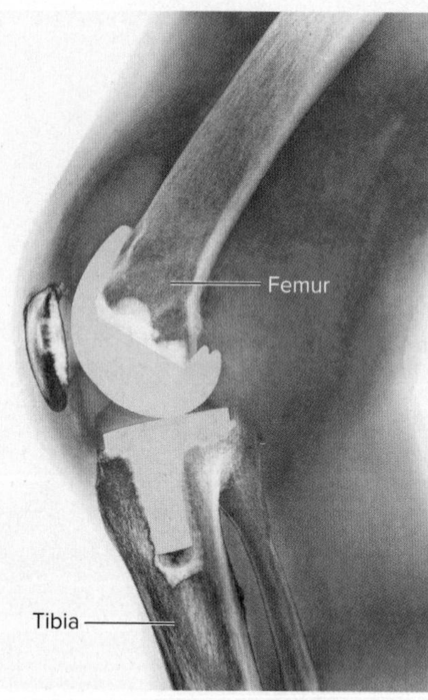

▲ **FIGURE 4.24**
Colored X-ray of Total Knee Replacement.

Dr. P. Marazzi/Science Photo Library/Getty Images

The Knee Joint (continued) (LO 4.2 and 4.9)

Injuries to the Knee Joint (LO 4.2 and 4.9)

The **anterior cruciate ligament (ACL)** is the most commonly injured ligament in the knee *(Figure 4.23),* particularly in football players and female athletes. The injury is often caused by a sudden **hyperflexion** of the knee joint when landing awkwardly on flat ground, as in Gail Griffith's case. Because of its poor vascular (blood) supply, the torn ligament does not heal and has to be surgically mended.

Other commonly injured major ligaments are the medial and lateral collateral ligaments and the posterior cruciate ligament.

Meniscus injuries result from a twist to the knee that tears the meniscus. The torn meniscus flips in and out of the joint as it moves, locking the knee and creating pain. Losing a meniscus leads to arthritic changes, so repair of the meniscus, as in Ms. Griffith's case, instead of removal (a **meniscectomy**) is preferred.

Patellar subluxation or dislocation produces an unstable, painful kneecap.

Prepatellar bursitis ("housemaid's knee") produces painful swelling over the **bursa** at the front of the knee and is seen in people who kneel for extended periods of time, like carpet layers.

Tendinitis of the patellar tendon results from overuse during activities like cycling, running, or dancing. Pain is felt where the tendon is inserted into the tibia, and this is treated with R.I.C.E (rest, ice, compression, elevation).

Surgical Procedures of the Knee Joint (LO 4.2 and 4.9)

There are several procedures and surgery options for those who sustain knee injuries. **Arthrocentesis** is the aspiration of knee joint fluid, which is examined to establish a diagnosis. Infected fluid may be drained off or medication, such as local corticosteroids, may be inserted.

Arthrography is an X-ray of a joint after injection of a contrast medium (harmless dye) into the joint to make the inside details of the joint visible.

Diagnostic arthroscopy is an exploratory procedure performed using an arthroscope to examine the internal compartments of the knee joint.

Surgical arthroscopy is performed through an arthroscope. This can be a **debridement** or removal of torn tissue like a meniscus or a ligament. It can also be a repair of a torn ligament by suturing, or tendon autograft, or repair of a torn meniscus.

Arthroplasty involves a total replacement of the knee joint *(Figure 4.24),* usually because of osteoarthritis. The damaged cartilage and bone from the knee joint's surface are removed and replaced with metal and plastic.

Word Analysis and Definition

S = Suffix P = Prefix R = Root R/CF = Combining Form

WORD	PRONUNCIATION	ELEMENTS		DEFINITION
arthrocentesis	**AR**-throw-sen-**TEE**-sis	S/ R/CF	**-centesis** *puncture* **arthr/o-** *joint*	Aspiration of fluid from a joint
arthrography	ar-**THROG**-rah-fee	S/ R/CF	**-graphy** *process of recording* **arthr/o-** *joint*	X-ray of a joint taken after the injection of a contrast medium into the joint
arthroscopy	ar-**THROS**-koh-pee	S/ R/CF	**-scopy** *the process of using an instrument to examine visually* **arthr/o-** *joint*	Visual examination of the interior of a joint
arthroscope	**AR**-thro-skope	S/	**-scope** *instrument to examine visually*	Endoscope used to examine the interior of a joint
bursa bursitis	**BURR**-sah burr-**SIGH**-tis	 S/ R/	Latin *purse* **-itis** *inflammation* **burs-** *bursa*	A closed sac containing synovial fluid Inflammation of a bursa
debridement	day-**BREED**-mon ("Mon" is the French pronunciation of *ment.*)	S/ P/ R/	**-ment** *action* **de-** *removal, out of* **-bride-** *rubble, rubbish*	The removal of injured or necrotic tissue
hyperflexion	high-per-**FLEK**-shun	S/ P/ R/	**-ion** *action, condition* **hyper-** *excessive* **-flex-** *bend*	Flexion of a limb or part beyond the normal limits
meniscectomy	men-ih-**SEK**-toh-me	S/ R/	**-ectomy** *surgical excision* **menisc-** *crescent, meniscus*	Excision (cutting out) of all or part of a meniscus
prepatellar	pree-pah-**TELL**-ar	S/ P/ R/	**-ar** *pertaining to* **pre-** *before, in front of* **-patell-** *patella*	In front of the patella
tendinitis *(also spelled tendonitis)*	ten-dih-**NYE**-tis	S/ R/	**-itis** *inflammation* **tendin-** *tendon*	Inflammation of a tendon

EXERCISES

A. Review *Case Report 4.5 (continued) to select the correct answer(s) in the following questions.* **LO 4.2, 4.9, and 4.11**

1. Select all the structures that were torn in Gail's knee. (choose all that apply)

a. medial meniscus
b. posterior cruciate ligament
c. medial collateral ligament
d. lateral collateral ligament
e. anterior cruciate ligament

2. In the abbreviation ACL, the "C" stands for

a. cross **b.** collateral **c.** cruciate **d.** combined

3. Define the procedure performed.

a. CT scan is taken of the knee to determine the ligament damage.
b. Laser is aimed at the knee joint and the ligaments are fused.
c. Incision is made into the knee joint and ligaments are sutured.
d. Arthroscope is inserted into the joint and repairs are made through the scope.

4. Select all of the directional terms that are used in Case Report 4.5 (continued). (choose all that apply)

a. medial
b. collateral
c. anterior
d. posterior
e. cruciate

B. Elements: *Recognition of word elements will help you understand a medical term. For each of the following terms, identify the type of element shown in bold italics, and then define that element. Fill in the chart, and answer the questions below it.* **LO 4.1, 4.2, and 4.9**

Remember: An element that begins a term is not necessarily a prefix!

Medical Term	Type of Element (P, R/CF, or S)	Meaning of Element	Meaning of Term
tendin*itis*	1.	2.	3.
***pre*patellar**	4.	5.	6.
de*brid*ement	7.	8.	9.
***burs*itis**	10.	11.	12.
arthro*centesis*	13.	14.	15.

Lesson 4.4 (cont'd) Bones and Joints of the Lower Leg, Ankle, and Foot

(LO 4.2 and 4.9)

Your lower leg has two differently sized bones: the large medial tibia and the thin lateral fibula. The lower end of your tibia on its medial border forms a prominent process called the medial malleolus. The lower end of your fibula forms the lateral malleolus *(Figure 4.25).* You can palpate (feel) both these prominences at your own ankle, which has two joints:

- One between the lateral malleolus of the fibula and the talus; and
- One between the medial malleolus of the tibia and the talus.

The **talus** is the most superior of the seven **tarsal** bones of the ankle *(Figure 4.25),* and its upper surface articulates with the tibia. The heel bone is called the **calcaneus.** The tarsal bones help the ankle bear the body's weight. Strong ligaments on both sides of the ankle joint hold the joint together.

Attached to the tarsal bones are the five parallel **metatarsal** bones *(Figure 4.26).* These bones form the instep and the ball of the foot, where they bear weight. Each toe has three phalanges, except for the big toe, which has only two. This configuration is identical to the thumb and its relation to the hand.

Disorders and Injuries of the Ankle and Foot (LO 4.2 and 4.9)

Podiatry is a health care specialty concerned with the diagnosis and treatment of disorders and injuries of the foot and toenails. A **podiatrist** is not an MD but is a doctor of podiatric medicine (DPM).

Bunions, deformities that appear as swollen bones, often occur at the base of the big toe. A bunion is also called a **hallux valgus,** and it causes the metatarsophalangeal joint to misalign and stick out.

Pott fracture is a fracture of the fibula near the ankle, often accompanied by a fracture of the medial malleolus of the tibia.

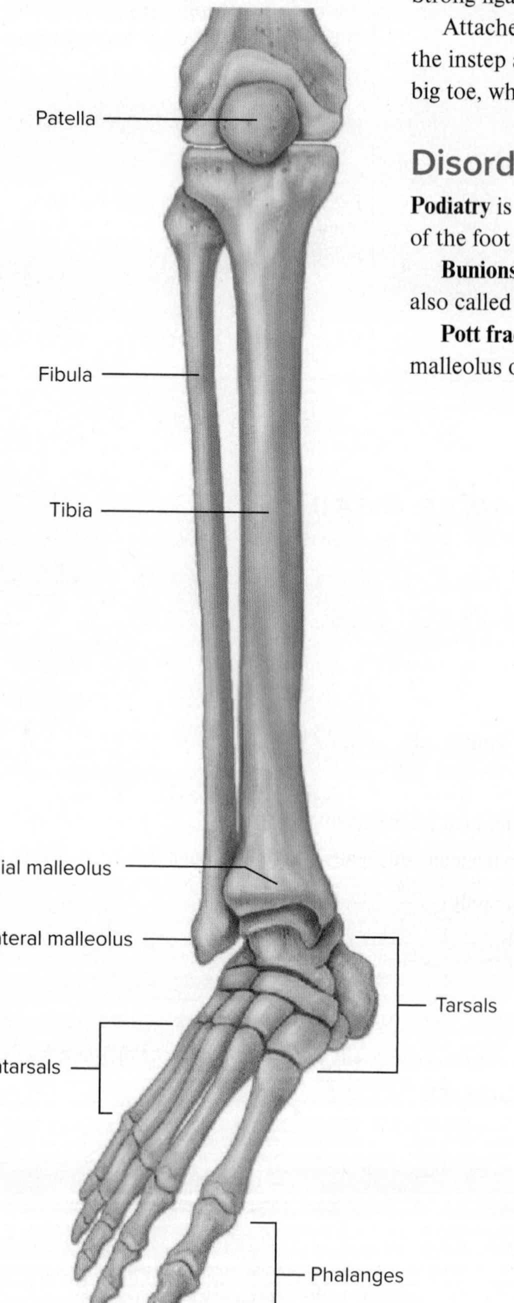

▲ **FIGURE 4.25**
Bones of the Lower Leg and Foot.

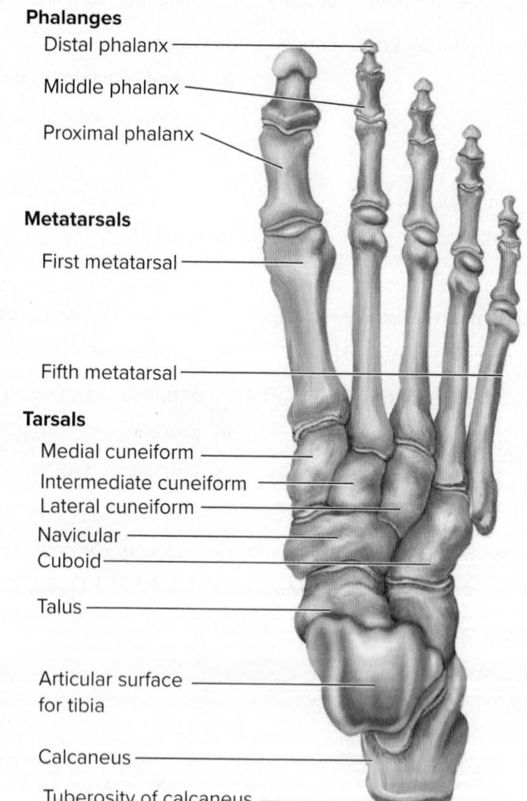

▲ **FIGURE 4.26**
Twenty-Six Bones and 33 Joints of Right Foot.

Word Analysis and Definition

S = Suffix P = Prefix R = Root R/CF = Combining Form

WORD	PRONUNCIATION	ELEMENTS		DEFINITION
bunion	**BUN**-yun		French *bump*	A swelling at the base of the big toe
calcaneus calcaneal (adj)	kal-**KAY**-knee-us kal-**KAY**-knee-al	S/ R/	Latin *heel* -eal *pertaining to* calcan- *calcaneus*	Bone of the tarsus that forms the heel Pertaining to the calcaneus
hallux valgus	**HAL**-uks **VAL**-gus	R/ R/	hallux *big toe* valgus *turn out*	Deviation of the big toe toward the medial side of the foot
metatarsus metatarsal (adj)	**MET**-ah-**TAR**-sus **MET**-ah-**TAR**-sal	S/ P/ R/ S/	-us *pertaining to* meta- *after, subsequent to* -tars- *ankle* -al *pertaining to*	The five parallel bones of the foot between the tarsus and the phalanges Pertaining to the metatarsus
podiatry podiatrist	poh-**DIE**-ah-tree poh-**DIE**-ah-trist	S/ R/ S/	-iatry *treatment* pod- *foot* -iatrist *practitioner*	The diagnosis and treatment of disorders and injuries of the foot Practitioner of podiatry
Pott fracture	**POT FRAK**-shur		Percival Pott, London surgeon, 1714–1788	Fracture of the lower end of the fibula, often with fracture of the tibial malleolus
talus	**TAY**-luss		Latin *heel bone*	The tarsal bone that articulates with the tibia to form the ankle joint
tarsus tarsal (adj)	**TAR**-sus **TAR**-sal	S/ R/	Latin *ankle* -al *pertaining to* tars- *ankle*	The collection of seven bones in the foot that form the ankle and instep Pertaining to the tarsus

EXERCISES

A. Challenge your knowledge *of the language of orthopedics. Fill in the blanks with the correct medical terms.* **LO 4.2, 4.9, and 4.11**

1. On which bone does a Pott fracture occur? ____________________
2. Metacarpal bones appear in the hand; what are the similar bones called in the foot? ____________________
3. Another name for a bunion is ____________________.
4. What is another name for the heel bone? ____________________
5. The big toe is similar in construction to the ____________________ of the hand.
6. What is the prominent process called at the lower end of the tibia on its medial border? ____________________.
7. A medical specialist that treats disorders of the foot: ____________________
8. How many bones form the instep? ____________ Are these bones classified as tarsals, metatarsals, or phalanges? ____________

B. Demonstrate *your knowledge of elements that construct medical terms. Select the correct answer that completes each statement.* **LO 4.2 and 4.9**

1. The suffix in the term *podiatry* means:
   - **a.** pertaining to
   - **b.** specialist
   - **c.** structure
   - **d.** treatment
2. The prefix in the term *metatarsus* means:
   - **a.** ankle
   - **b.** after
   - **c.** foot
   - **d.** bone
3. The root in the term *tarsal* means:
   - **a.** ankle
   - **b.** foot
   - **c.** bump
   - **d.** big toe

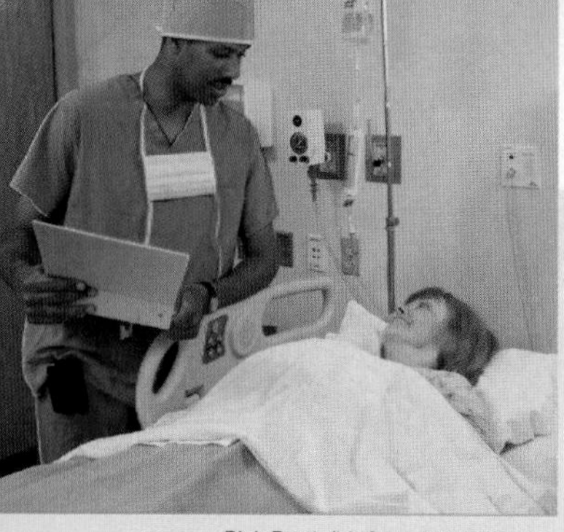
Rick Brady/McGraw-Hill Education

Lesson 4.5

Diagnostic and Therapeutic Procedures and Pharmacology for Bone Disorders (LO 4.5, 4.6, 4.7, 4.8, and 4.9)

Objectives

The procedures and methods, other than clinical examination, that are used to assess, diagnose, and treat bone disorders, particularly bone cancer, can be complicated and expensive and have to be used with discretion. The treatments can also cause unpleasant side effects. In order to understand and relate to this arena, you need to be able to:

4.5.1 Discuss the types of procedures used in diagnosing metabolic bone disorders.

4.5.2 Describe the types of procedures used to diagnose primary and metastatic bone cancer.

4.5.3 Define the types of chemicals used to treat metabolic bone disorders.

4.5.4 Identify the types of treatments used for primary and metastatic bone cancer.

Keynotes

- **Malignant tumors that begin in bone tissue are called primary bone cancer.**
- **Cancer that spreads to the bones from other organs and sites of the body, such as the lung, breast, or prostate, is called metastatic cancer.**
- **Primary bone cancer is uncommon.**

Abbreviations

BMD	bone mineral density
CAT (CT)	computed tomography scan
DEXA (DXA)	dual-energy X-ray absorptiometry
ERT	estrogen replacement therapy
MRI	magnetic resonance imaging
PET	positron emission tomography
SERM	selective estrogen receptor modulator

Diagnostic Procedures for Metabolic Bone Disorders (LO 4.5, 4.6, 4.7, 4.8, 4.9, and 4.10)

- **Bone mineral density (BMD)** screening using dual-energy X-ray absorptiometry (**DEXA or DXA scan**) is used to diagnose and follow osteoporosis.
- **Nuclear bone scan** involves a radioactive substance injected into the bloodstream. From there, it travels into the bones and is detected by a special camera. It can show a bone infection, a fracture not clearly seen on X-ray, arthritis, and primary or metastatic cancer.
- **Blood tests** examine serum calcium, serum alkaline phosphate, and serum phosphate, which can be abnormal in metabolic bone disorders.
- **Bone biopsy** is the ultimate way to establish a diagnosis of osteomalacia.

Diagnostic Procedures for Bone Cancer (LO 4.5, 4.6, 4.7, 4.8, 4.9, and 4.10)

- **X-ray** shows the location, shape, and size of a bone tumor.
- **Nuclear bone scan** (described above).
- **Computed tomography (CAT or CT) scan** provides a series of detailed pictures of parts of the body, taken from different angles, that are created by an X-ray machine linked to a computer.
- **Magnetic resonance imaging (MRI)** uses a magnet linked to a computer to create detailed pictures of body parts without using X-rays.
- **Positron emission tomography (PET) scan** uses radioactive **glucose** that is injected into the bloodstream and a scanner that makes a computerized picture of body parts where the glucose is being used. Cancer cells can use more glucose than normal cells and can be detected by the scan.
- **Biopsy** can be a **needle** or **incisional** biopsy.

Therapeutic Procedures for Bone Disorders (LO 4.5, 4.6, 4.7, 4.8, 4.9, and 4.10)

- **Surgery** is a common treatment for many bone disorders. In bone cancer, the surgeon removes the entire tumor with margins that are negative for cancer cells. Modern surgical techniques have reduced the need for **amputation** in limb bone cancer. Surgical techniques used for specific bones, joints, and their disorders have been discussed previously in this chapter.
- **Chemotherapy** is the use of anticancer drugs, often in combinations, to kill cancer cells. Numerous drugs are available.
- **Radiotherapy** uses high-energy X-rays to kill cancer cells and is often used with surgery.
- **Cryosurgery** uses liquid nitrogen to freeze and kill cancer cells.
- **Drug therapy** for metabolic bone disorders includes, for osteoporosis, **estrogen replacement therapy (ERT),** anti-estrogens **(SERMs),** or bone-preserving medications such as calcitonin. A class of drugs called **bisphosphonates** prevents the loss of bone mass and is used in the treatment of osteoporosis, Paget disease, osteogenesis imperfecta, and any condition that features bone fragility.

Word Analysis and Definition

S = Suffix P = Prefix R = Root R/CF = Combining Form

WORD	PRONUNCIATION	ELEMENTS		DEFINITION
amputation (noun)	am-pyu-**TAY**-shun	S/ R/	-ation *a process* amput- *to prune, top off*	Process of removing a limb, part of a limb, a breast, or other projecting part
biopsy *(one of the "o"s is not pronounced)*	**BI**-op-see	S/ R/	-opsy *to view* bi/o- *life*	Process of removing tissue from a living person for laboratory examination
biphosphonate	bi-**PHOS**-fon-ate	S/ P/ R/ R/	-ate *composed of* bi- *two* -phos- *phosphate* -phon- *sound*	A class of drugs used to prevent and treat fragile bones
chemotherapy	**KEY**-moh-**THAIR**-ah-pee	R/ R/CF	-therapy *medical treatment* chem/o- *chemical*	Treatment using chemical agents
cryosurgery	cry-oh-**SUR**-jer-ee	S/ R/CF R/	-ery *process of* cry/o- *icy cold* -surg- *operate*	Use of liquid nitrogen or argon gas in surgery to freeze and kill abnormal tissue
estrogen	**ESS**-troh-jen	S/ R/CF	-gen *produce, create* estr/o- *woman*	Generic term for hormones that stimulate female secondary sex characteristics
glucose	**GLUE**-kose	S/ R/	-ose *full of* gluc- *sugar, glucose*	The final product of carbohydrate digestion and the main sugar in blood
incision incisional (adj)	in-**SIZH**-un in-**SIZH**-un-al	S/ R/ S/	-ion *action, condition* incis- *cut into* -al *pertaining to*	A cut or surgical wound Pertaining to an incision
radiotherapy	**RAY**-dee-oh-**THAIR**-ah-pee	R/CF R/	radi/o- *X-ray, radiation* -therapy *medical treatment*	Treatment using radiation

EXERCISES

A. Match *the abbreviation in the first column with its correct application in the diagnosis and treatment of bone disorders described in the second column.* **LO 4.3 and 4.12**

_____ 1 MRI — **a.** provide detailed images of organs without the use of radiation

_____ 2. CT scan — **b.** determines the presence of osteoporosis

_____ 3. BMD — **c.** used to determine the presence of cancer

_____ 4. PET — **d.** used to treat osteoporosis

_____ 5. ERT — **e.** provide detailed images at different angles using X-rays

B. Identify *the diagnostic procedures to determine the presence of bone disorders including cancer.* **LO 4.5**

1. The physician wishes to definitively determine if a patient has a bone infection.

   a. X-ray **b.** DEXA scan **c.** nuclear bone scan **d.** CT scan

2. The gynecologist suspects that his patient has osteoporosis. He will order a:

   a. BMD **b.** bone biopsy **c.** MRI **d.** PET scan

3. It is necessary to decisively determine if the patient has osteomalacia. The physician should order a:

   a. BMD **b.** bone biopsy **c.** MRI **d.** PET scan

C. Construct *medical terms that are treatments used to treat bone disorders.* **LO 4.1 and 4.5**

1. Treatment using chemical agents: ____________ / ____________
   R/CF R

2. Treatment using radiation: ____________ / ____________
   R/CF R

3. Treatment that freezes and kills abnormal tissue: ____________ / ____________ / ____________
   R/CF R S

4. Process of removing a limb: ____________ / ____________
   R S

Pharmacology (LO 4.10)

Abbreviations

DMARD	disease modifying anti-rheumatic drug
FDA	Food and Drug Administration
NSAID	nonsteroidal anti-inflammatory drug
OTC	over the counter
RA	rheumatoid arthritis
TNF	tumor necrosis factor

For osteoporosis, calcium (1200 mg daily) and vitamin D (800 IU daily) are both the accepted baseline prevention and treatment.

For patients at risk of fractures, several medications approved by the U.S. **Food and Drug Administration (FDA)** are available for the treatment of osteoporosis. Most inhibit osteoclast activity to reduce the rate of loss of bone **(resorption),** but some produce a direct increase in bone mass. As the turnover of bone is very slow, the time needed for assessing the effects of medications takes several years. Drugs that reduce the rate of bone resorption include estrogen, bisphosphonates, and calcitonin. **Bisphosphonates** (*Alendronate, Risedronate,* and others) are poorly absorbed from the gastrointestinal tract and can be given intravenously. **Calcitonin** also decreases osteoclast activity and is available as a subcutaneous injection or nasal spray. Several other drugs are available in other countries and/or are undergoing clinical trials in the United States.

Medications for osteoarthritis are numerous. **Acetaminophen** reduces mild pain but does not affect inflammation or swelling. It is used in combination with aspirin and/or caffeine *(Excedrin)* as an **OTC** medicine, and with codeine, propoxyphene (*Darvon*), or the narcotics hydrocodone *(Vicodin)* or oxycodone *(Percocet)* as prescription medications. Nonsteroidal anti-inflammatory drugs **(NSAIDs)** such as ibubrofen *(Advil)* and naproxen *(Aleve)* work well for pain but cause gastrointestinal problems and an increased risk of heart attacks and strokes.

Corticosteroids such as cortisone, prednisone, triamcinalone, and betamethsone, are used to reduce the pain and inflammation of severe osteoarthritis and are given orally or injected directly into the joint **(intra-articular).** Corticosteroids are also used to reduce inflammation in rheumatoid arthritis (**RA**) but do not slow the progression of the disease. **Disease modifying anti-rheumatic drugs (DMARDs)** such as methotrexate *(Trexall)* are effective in reducing the signs and symptoms of RA, and other DMARDs such as hydrochloroquine *(Plaquenil)* and sulfasalazine *(Azulfidine)* can be added to methotrexate to enhance its effects. **Tumor necrosis factor (TNF)** is produced in RA joints by synovial macrophages and lymphocytes to attack the joint tissues and TNF **inhibitors** such as abatacept *(Orencia)* and rituximab *(Rituxan)* slow or halt the destruction.

Word Analysis and Definition

S = Suffix P = Prefix R = Root R/CF = Combining Form

WORD	PRONUNCIATION	ELEMENTS		DEFINITION
acetaminophen	ah-seat-ah-**MIN**-oh-fen		Generic drug name	Medication that modifies or relieves pain
bisphosphonate	bis-**FOSS**-foh-nate	S/ P/ R/ R/	-ate *composed of* **bi-** *two* -phos- *light* -phon- *sound*	Drug that delays the rate of bone resporption
calcitonin	kal-sih-**TONE**-in	S/ R/CF R/	-in *chemical compound* calci- *calcium* -ton- *tension, pressure*	Hormone that moves calcium from blood to bones
corticosteroid	**KOR**-tih-koh-**STEHR**-oyd	S/ R/CF R/	-oid *resembling* cortic/o- *cortisone* -ster- *steroid*	A hormone produced by the adrenal cortex
inhibit (verb) **inhibitor** (noun)	in-**HIB**-it in-**HIB**-it-or		Latin *to keep back*	To curb or restrain Agent that curbs or restrains
intra-articular	**IN**-trah-ar-**TIK**-you-lar	S/ P/ R/	-ar *pertaining to* **intra-** *inside* -articul- *joint*	Pertaining to the inside of a joint

EXERCISES

A. Use terms related to pharmacology. *Using the terms provided, correctly complete the paragraph. Not all terms will be used. Fill in the blanks.* **LO 4.10 and 4.11**

DMARD **podiatrist** **RA** **OTC** **chiropractor** **acetaminophen** **calcitonin** **corticosteroid**

Ms. Walker made an appointment with a ____________________ for pain in her shoulder. She participates in high-intensity weightlifting and fitness training. She has been taking ____________________ medication to treat the pain; specifically, the medication ____________________. She denies a personal or family history of ____________________.

B. Construct medical terms related to the pharmacology of the skeletal system. *Insert the correct word element that completes each term. Fill in the blanks.* **LO 4.1 and 4.10**

1. Hormone that moves calcium from the blood to the bone: calci/______________/in
2. Hormone produced by the adrenal cortex: ______________/ster/oid
3. Pertaining to the inside of a joint: intra-______________/ar

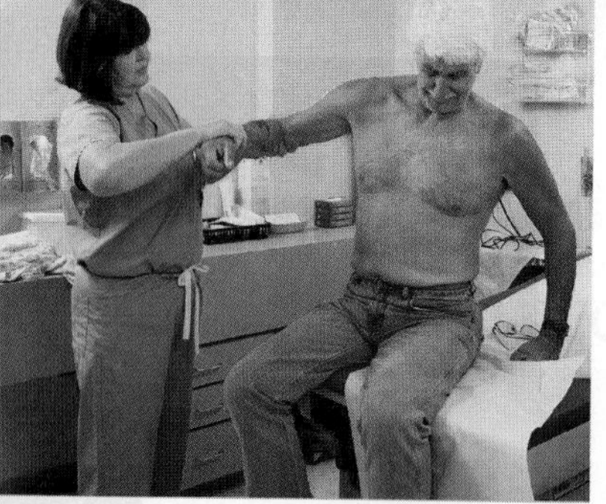
McGraw-Hill Education/Rick Brady

Rehabilitation programs involve a **multidisciplinary** team approach where each team member manages different rehabilitation activities. The members of a rehabilitation team include the following health professionals and their respective roles (see the WADs in this chapter for these terms):

- A **physiatrist,** often the team leader, is a physician specializing in physical medicine and rehabilitation.
- **Medical specialists** manage acute or chronic illnesses and pain.
- **Occupational therapists** practice occupational therapy **(OT)** to help improve a patient's activities of daily living **(ADLs)** and adapt to visual and other perceptual deficits.
- **Occupational therapy assistants (OTAs)** assist occupational therapists.
- **Physical therapists** practice **physical therapy (PT)** to help patients improve their strength, **range of motion (ROM),** balance, and endurance. Physical therapists are assisted by **restorative aids** and teach patients how to use these devices.
- **Physical therapy assistants (PTAs)** assist physical therapists.
- **Rehabilitation psychologists** and counselors are specialists who help patients undergoing rehabilitation and those with resulting disabilities to reclaim their sense of belonging, contributing to, and participating in the world around them.
- **Social workers** provide support and assistance with social issues, such as health insurance, care facilities, and employment.
- **Speech therapists** evaluate and treat communication, speech, and swallowing disorders.
- **Orthotists** make and fit orthopedic appliances **(orthotics).**
- **Nutritionists** evaluate and improve a patient's nutritional status.

Objectives

In Chapter 4, you learned how the bones of your skeleton support your body and how your joints provide mobility throughout your body. However, neither of these functions can occur without your **muscles,** *which provide posture and movement. Information in this lesson will enable you to use correct medical terminology to:*

5.1.1 Identify the functions of skeletal muscle and tendons.

5.1.2 Describe the structure of skeletal muscle and tendons.

5.1.3 Demonstrate an understanding of the major problems and diseases that occur in muscles and tendons.

5.1.4 Discuss diagnostic and therapeutic methods used to diagnose muscle disorders.

Abbreviations

ADL	activities of daily living
DC	Doctor of Chiropractic
DO	Doctor of Osteopathy
OT	occupational therapy
PT	physical therapy
ROM	range of motion
MD	Doctor of Medicine

Lesson 5.1 Muscles and Tendons

Types, Functions and Structure of Muscle

Types of Muscle (LO 5.4)

There are three types of **muscle: skeletal, cardiac,** and **smooth.** Skeletal muscles contract on demand to provide posture and locomotion. Cardiac and smooth muscle contract without conscious thought, cardiac muscle to power the heart contractions and smooth muscle to power the movement of food through the digestive system via **peristalsis.**

Functions and Structure of Skeletal Muscle (LO 5.4)

Functions of Skeletal Muscle (LO 5.4)

Skeletal muscles, which are attached to one or more bones, are also called **voluntary** muscles. This means that you have conscious control of your muscles, which perform your movements. Each muscle consists of bundles of muscle cells (often called **fibers** because of their length), blood vessels, and nerves. Connective tissue sheets hold your muscle fibers together and connect the muscles to your bones.

Your skeletal muscle has the following functions:

1. **Movement.** All skeletal muscles are attached to bones so when a muscle **contracts,** your bones move, too *(Figure 5.1).* This allows you to walk, run, and work with your hands.
2. **Posture.** The **tone** of your skeletal muscles holds you straight when sitting, standing, or moving.
3. **Body heat.** When skeletal muscles contract, they produce the heat needed to maintain your body temperature.
4. **Respiration.** Skeletal muscles move the chest wall as you breathe.
5. **Communication.** Skeletal muscles enable you to speak, write, type, gesture, and smile.

Word Analysis and Definition

S = Suffix P = Prefix R = Root R/CF = Combining Form

WORD	PRONUNCIATION		ELEMENTS	DEFINITION
active activity	**ACK**-tiv ack-**TIV**-ih-tee	 S/ R/	Latin *movement* **-ity** *condition, state* **activ-** *movement*	Causing action or change The state of being active
contract	kon-**TRAKT**	P/ R/	**con-** *with, together* **-tract** *draw*	Draw together or shorten
fiber	**FIE**-ber		Latin *fiber*	A strand or filament
multidisciplinary	mul-tee-**DIS**-ih-plih-**NAR**-ee	S/ P/ R/	**-ary** *pertaining to* **multi-** *many* **-disciplin-** *instruction*	Involving health care providers from more than one profession
muscle	**MUSS**-el		Latin *muscle*	A tissue consisting of cells that can contract
passive	**PASS**-iv		Latin *to endure*	Not active
peristalsis	pear-ih-**STAL**-sis	P/ R/	**peri-** *around* **-stalsis** *constrict*	Waves of alternate constriction and relaxation in a tube
skeletal (adj)	**SKEL**-eh-tal	S/ R/	**-al** *pertaining to* **skelet-** *skeleton*	Pertaining to the skeleton
tone	**TONE**		Greek *tone*	Tension present in resting muscles
voluntary muscle	**VOL**-un-tare-ee **MUSS**-el	S/ R/	**-ary** *pertaining to* **volunt-** *free will*	Muscle that is under the control of the will

EXERCISES

A. Review *Case Report 5.1 to answer the following questions.*

1. What type of physician is Dr. Stannard?________________
2. Did Mr. Adams see another physician before seeing Dr. Stannard?________________
3. What is Mr. Adams's chief complaint?________________
4. The one word that describes "movement in which in which Dr. Stannard moves the arm while Mr. Adams does not contract his muscle" is termed: ______

B. Deconstruct *the following medical terms into their basic elements. Fill in the chart.* **LO 5.1**

Medical Term	Prefix	Root(s)/CF	Suffix
contract	**1.**	**2.**	**3.**
voluntary	**4.**	**5.**	**6.**
skeletal	**7.**	**8.**	**9.**

C. Meet lesson and chapter objectives *and use the correct medical terminology to answer the questions. Fill in the blanks.* **LO 5.2 and 5.4**

1. Muscle cells are also referred to as muscle ____________.
2. Skeletal muscle attaches to one or more ____________.
3. Skeletal muscle is under conscious control; therefore, it is considered a _________ muscle.
4. Peristalsis is a function of _________ muscle.

Functions of Skeletal Muscle (continued) (LO 5.4)

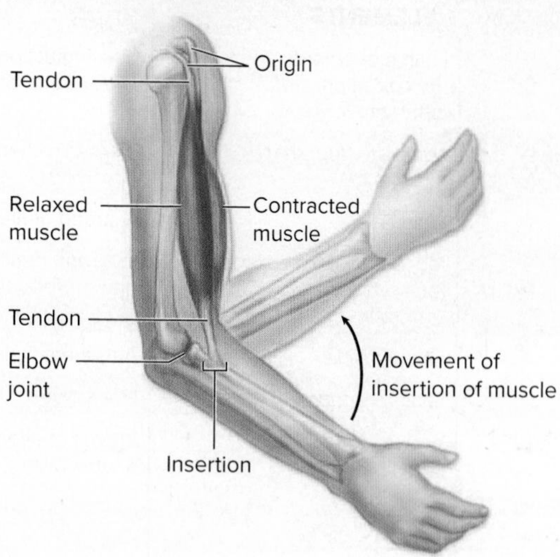

▶ **FIGURE 5.1**
Muscle Contraction to Flex the Elbow Joint.

Abbreviations

NSAID	nonsteroidal anti-inflammatory drug
RICE	rest, ice, compression, and elevation

Structure of Skeletal Muscle (LO 5.4)

Your skeletal muscle fibers are narrow and measure up to 1½ inches long. Bundles of these fibers create separate muscles, which are held in place by **fascia** *(Figure 5.2),* a thick layer of connective tissue. Fascia extends beyond the muscle to form a **tendon,** which attaches to a bone's periosteum at the origin and insertion of the muscle.

Because skeletal muscle fibers contain **striations** (alternating dark and light bands of protein filaments responsible for muscle contraction), skeletal muscle can also be called **striated muscle.**

You have the same number of muscle fibers as an adult that you had in late childhood. Exercise and/or weightlifting will enlarge **(hypertrophy)** your muscles, increasing the thickness of your muscle fibers. If you neglect these muscles, they will shrink **(atrophy).**

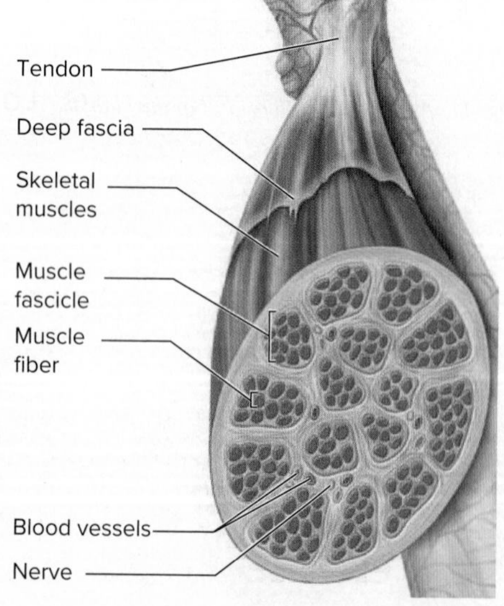

▶ **FIGURE 5.2**
Structure of Skeletal Muscle.

Disorders of Skeletal Muscles (LO 5.4)

Because you use so many different muscles for various activities, the likelihood of experiencing some form of skeletal muscle disorder in your lifetime is almost certain. **Muscle soreness** can result from vigorous exercise, particularly if your muscles are not used to it. Exercise increases the lactic acid in your muscle fibers, causing inflammation, and produces soreness in the muscles and nearby connective tissue.

Muscle cramps are sudden, short, painful contractions of a muscle or group of muscles. The cause of these cramps is unknown. A poor diet that leads to low blood potassium, calcium, and magnesium levels; caffeine and tobacco use; and reduced blood supply may contribute to muscle cramps. There are no effective medications available.

Muscle strains range from a simple stretch to a partial or complete tear in the muscle, tendon, or muscle-tendon combination. Most strains heal with RICE *(Figure 5.3),* followed by basic exercises to relieve pain and restore mobility. A complete tear may require surgery.

A **sprain** is a stretch or tear of a ligament, often in the ankle, knee, or wrist, and is also treated by RICE.

Anabolic steroids are related to testosterone but altered to make skeletal muscle hypertrophy. Used illegally in many sports to boost muscle strength, steroids have noticeable, often irreversible side effects. These include stunted growth in adolescents, shrinking testes and reduced sperm counts, masculinization of women's bodies and voices, delusions, and paranoid jealousy. Long-term effects may be increased risk of heart attack and stroke, kidney failure, and liver tumors.

Fibromyalgia affects muscles and tendons all over the body, causing chronic pain, fatigue, and depression. Its cause is unknown and there are currently no laboratory tests for it. The only treatment options are pain management, physiotherapy, and stress reduction.

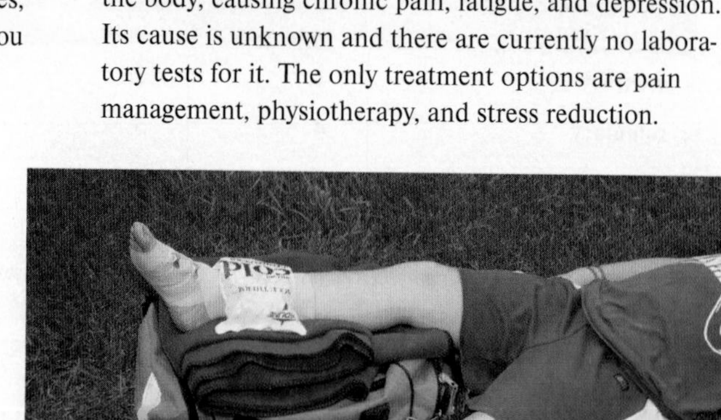

▲ **FIGURE 5.3**
RICE Treatment.

Word Analysis and Definition

S = Suffix P = Prefix R = Root R/CF = Combining Form

WORD	PRONUNCIATION	ELEMENTS		DEFINITION
atrophy	**A**-troh-fee	P/ R/	a- *without* **-trophy** *nourishment*	The wasting away or diminished volume of tissue, an organ, or a body part
hypertrophy	high-**PER**-troh-fee	P/ R/	**hyper-** *above, excessive* **-trophy** *nourishment*	Increase in size, but not in number, of an individual tissue element
fascia	**FASH**-ee-ah		Latin *a band*	Sheet of fibrous connective tissue
fibromyalgia	fie-broh-my-**AL**-jee-ah	S/ R/CF R/	-algia *pain* **fibr/o-** *fiber* **-my-** *muscle*	Pain in the muscle fibers
sprain	**SPRAIN**		root unknown	A wrench or tear in a ligament
strain	**STRAIN**		Latin *to bind*	Overstretch or tear in a muscle or tendon
tendon	**TEN**-dun		Latin *sinew*	Fibrous band that connects muscle to bone
tendinitis (*also spelled* tendonitis)	ten-dih-**NYE**-tis	S/ R/	-itis *inflammation* **tendin-** *tendon*	Inflammation of a tendon

Exercises

A. Remembering *the meanings of word elements makes short work of defining medical terms. Select the correct answer.* **LO 5.1**

1. The suffix *-itis* means: **a.** condition **b.** disease **c.** inflammation
2. Hyper- is a: **a.** suffix **b.** prefix **c.** root
3. The root *trophy-* means: **a.** condition **b.** procedure **c.** nourishment
4. *Fibro* is a: **a.** combining form **b.** root **c.** suffix
5. The root *my-* means: **a.** tendon **b.** ligament **c.** muscle
6. The suffix *-algia* means: **a.** inflammation **b.** pain **c.** swelling

B. Select *the answer that correctly completes each statement.* **LO 5.4**

1. Muscle that has decreased in size is said to have the condition of:
   a. edema **b.** hypertrophy **c.** atrophy **d.** paralysis
2. Lifting heavy objects over a long period of time can result in muscle:
   a. polymyalgia **b.** tenosynovitis **c.** atrophy **d.** hypertrophy
3. An overstretch or tear in a muscle is termed a:
   a. strain **b.** fasciotomy **c.** sprain **d.** tenosynovitis
4. Use of anabolic steroids can result in muscle:
   a. polymyalgia **b.** strain **c.** atrophy **d.** hypertrophy
5. The symptoms of fibromyalgia include: (choose all that apply)
   a. pain in muscles **b.** depression **c.** pain in tendons **d.** fatigue

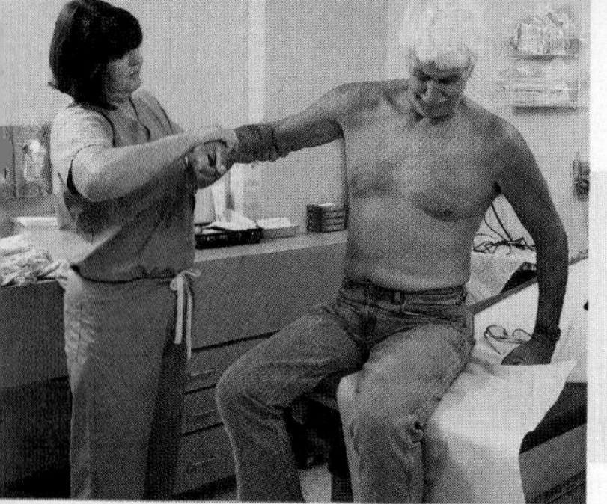

McGraw-Hill Education/Rick Brady

Lesson 5.2

Muscles and Tendons of the Shoulder Girdle, Trunk, and Upper Limb

Objectives

The muscles and tendons of your shoulders, arms, and hands are nearly always in motion. You shake hands, point your finger, turn doorknobs, and lift various objects throughout the course of any given day. The information in this lesson will enable you to use correct medical terminology to:

5.2.1 Describe the structures and functions of the muscles and tendons of the shoulder girdle.

5.2.2 Identify common disorders of the muscles and tendons of the shoulder girdle.

5.2.3 Specify the major muscles that join the arm to the trunk.

5.2.4 Explain the structures and functions of the muscles of the arm, elbow, forearm, and wrist.

5.2.5 Name common disorders of the joints, muscles, and tendons of the elbow.

5.2.6 Define common disorders of the joints and muscles of the hand.

Shoulder Girdle (LO 5.6)

Your **pectoral** (shoulder) **girdle** connects your axial skeleton to your upper limbs and helps you to move these limbs. Without your shoulder girdle, you wouldn't be able to throw a ball, drive a car, or reach that top shelf of your closet or kitchen cabinet. In fact, you wouldn't be able to move your upper limbs.

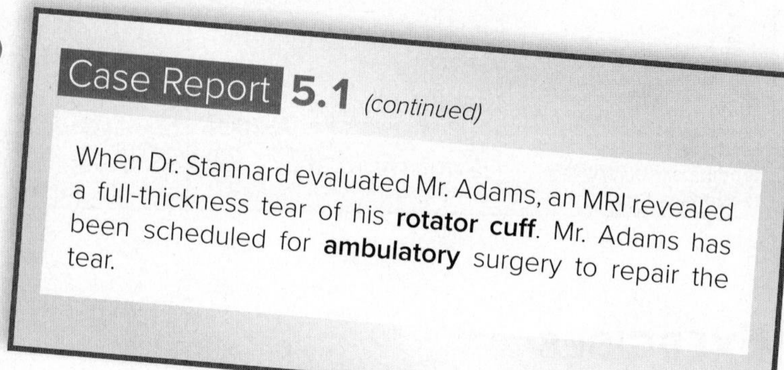

Case Report 5.1 *(continued)*

When Dr. Stannard evaluated Mr. Adams, an MRI revealed a full-thickness tear of his **rotator cuff**. Mr. Adams has been scheduled for **ambulatory** surgery to repair the tear.

The muscles and tendons in your shoulder girdle get plenty of use. Four muscles that **originate** on your scapula wrap around the shoulder joint and fuse together. This fusion forms one large tendon (the **rotator cuff**), which is **inserted** into the humerus *(Figure 5.4).* Your rotator cuff keeps the ball of the humerus tightly in the scapula's socket and provides the kind of strength needed by baseball pitchers.

Common Disorders of the Shoulder Girdle (LO 5.6)

Rotator cuff tears (a frequent injury to the shoulder girdle) are caused by wear and tear from overuse in work situations or in certain sports, such as baseball, football, and golf. These tears can be partial or complete.

Tendonitis of the shoulder joint is caused when the rotator cuff and/or biceps tendon becomes inflamed from overuse.

Bursitis, inflammation of the lubricating sac of the rotator cuff, can also be produced by overuse.

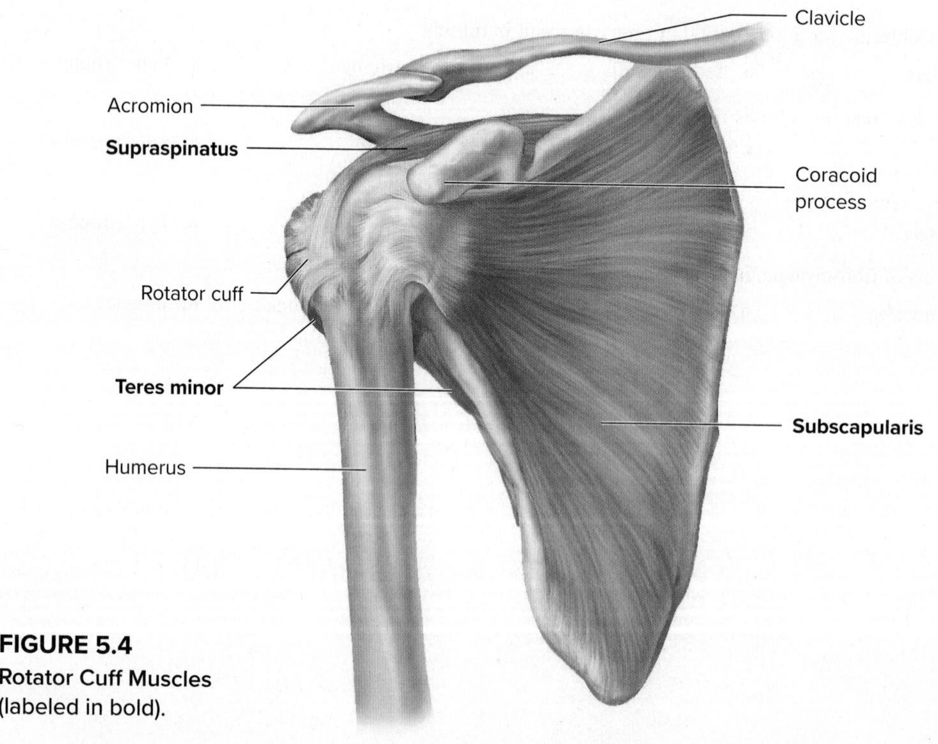

FIGURE 5.4
Rotator Cuff Muscles (labeled in bold).

Word Analysis and Definition

S = Suffix P = Prefix R = Root R/CF = Combining Form

WORD	PRONUNCIATION	ELEMENTS		DEFINITION
ambulatory	AM-byu-LAY-tor-ee	S/ R/	-ory *having the function of* ambulat- *walking*	Surgery or any other care provided without an overnight stay in a medical facility
insertion insert (verb)	in-SIR-shun in-SIRT	S/ R/	-ion *action, condition* insert- *put together*	The insertion of a muscle is the attachment of a muscle to a more movable part of the skeleton, as distinct from the origin
origin	OR-ih-gin		Latin *source of*	Fixed source of a muscle at its attachment to bone
pectoral pectoral girdle	PEK-tor-al PEK-tor-al GIR-del	S/ R/	-al *pertaining to* pector- *chest* girdle, Old English *encircle*	Pertaining to the chest Incomplete bony ring that attaches the upper limb to the axial skeleton
rotator cuff	roh-TAY-tor CUFF	S/ R/	-or *one who does* rotat- *rotate* cuff, Old English *band*	Part of the capsule of the shoulder joint

EXERCISES

A. Review *Case Report 5.1 (continued) to correctly answer the following questions. Fill in the blanks.* **LO 5.2, 5.5, and 5.6**

1. What type of diagnostic test did Mr. Adams have? ________________

2. What muscular structure was injured? ________________

3. Mr. Adams experiences pain when he moves his arm because the muscles ________________ (*insert or originate*) on the humerus.

4. Is Mr. Adams scheduled to spend the night in the hospital? ________________

B. Construct *medical terms related to the muscles of the upper limb. Fill in the blanks.* **LO 5.1, 5.2, and 5.6**

1. Pertaining to the chest: ____________/al

2. Function of walking: ____________/ory

3. Part of the capsule of the shoulder joint: ____________/or cuff

4. Point of attachment of a muscle to the more moveable part of the skeleton: ____________/tion

5. Inflammation of the lubricating sac near a joint: ____________/itis

6. Inflammation of the connective tissue that connects muscle to bone: ____________/itis

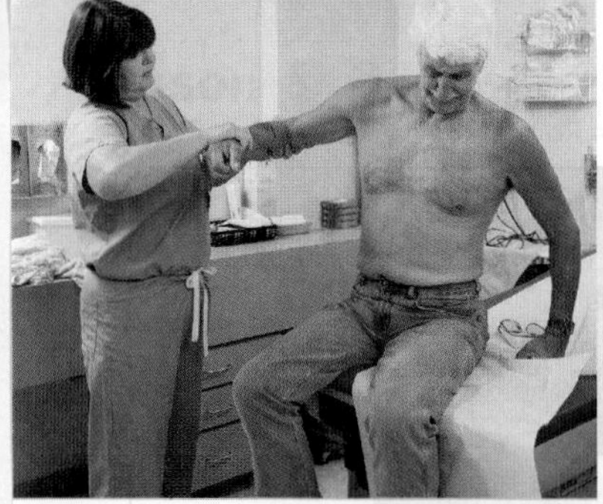

McGraw-Hill Education/Rick Brady

Lesson 5.3

Pelvic Girdle, Thigh, Leg, and Foot

Objectives

You use the muscles and tendons of your legs and feet so routinely that sometimes you might forget that these "separate pieces" exist until one of them begins to ache or is injured. The information in this lesson will enable you to use correct medical terminology to:

5.3.1 Discuss the muscles of the hip and thigh.

5.3.2 Describe the muscles and tendons of the lower leg, ankle, and foot.

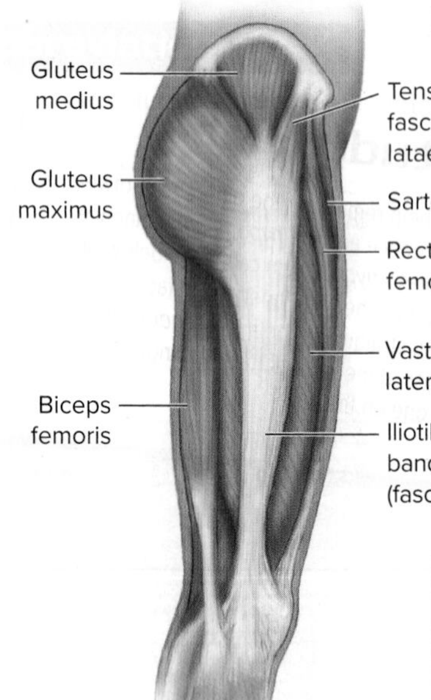

▼ **FIGURE 5.7**
Hip Joint.
Muscles of the hip and thigh, lateral view.

Muscles of the Hip and Thigh

(LO 5.4 and 5.7)

Some of your body's most powerful muscles support your hip joint and move your thigh. These muscles originate on the pelvic girdle and are inserted into the femur. Among these prominent muscles are your three **gluteus** muscles—**maximus, medius,** and **minimus** *(Figure 5.7)*—and the **adductor** muscles that run down your inner thigh.

Thigh Muscles (LO 5.4 and 5.7)

Your thigh muscles move your knee joint and lower leg. Your anterior thigh (the front of your thigh) contains your large **quadriceps femoris** muscle. This muscle has four heads: the rectus femoris, vastus lateralis, vastus medialis, and the vastus intermedius (which lies beneath the rectus femoris). These four muscle heads join into the **quadriceps tendon** (which contains the patella) and continue as the patellar tendon to be inserted into the tibia *(Figure 5.8)*. The quadriceps muscle **extends** (straightens) the knee joint and, because of the lower leg's weight, it has to be a very strong muscle.

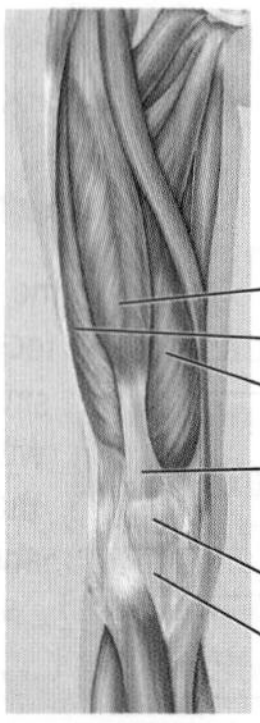

◀ **FIGURE 5.8**
Anterior Muscles of the Thigh.

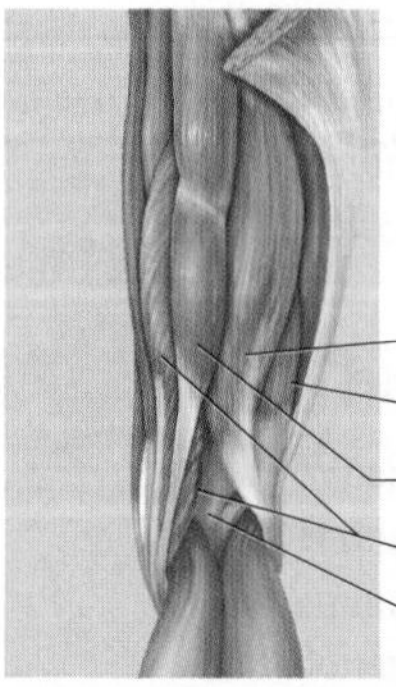

◀ **FIGURE 5.9**
Posterior Thigh Muscles.

Your posterior (rear) thigh is composed mostly of your three **hamstring muscles**—the **biceps femoris, semimembranosus,** and **semitendinosus** *(Figure 5.9)*. These muscles flex (bend) your knee joint and rotate your leg. The hollow area at the back of your knee between your hamstring tendons is the **popliteal fossa.**

Muscles and Tendons of the Lower Leg, Ankle, and Foot

(LO 5.4 and 5.7)

The muscles of your lower leg move your ankle, foot, and toes. Your front leg muscles bend your foot backward at the ankle and extend your toes. The side or lateral leg muscles turn your foot outward or evert it. Your back leg muscles plantar-flex your foot at the ankle, flex your toes, and turn in or invert your foot. The **gastrocnemius** muscle *(Figure 5.10(b))*, located at the back of your leg, forms a large part of your calf. The distal end of this muscle joins the tendon of the smaller calf (soleus) muscle to create the **Achilles (calcaneal) tendon,** which is attached to the heel bone **(calcaneus)** *(Figure 5.10(b))*. Together, your gastrocnemius muscle and Achilles tendon make it possible for you to "push off" when jumping or running. For more detailed foot movement descriptions, you may review the terms in Chapter 2.

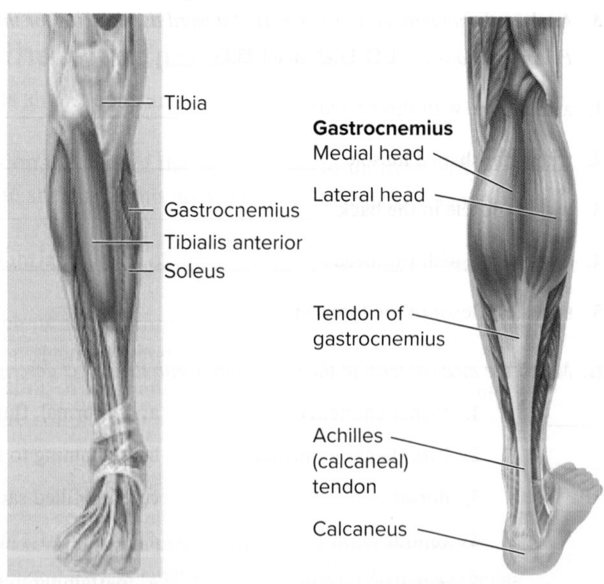

▲ **FIGURE 5.10**
Muscles of Lower Leg and Foot.
(a) Muscles of the front of the right leg.
(b) Muscles of the back of the right leg.

Word Analysis and Definition

S = Suffix P = Prefix R = Root R/CF = Combining Form

WORD	PRONUNCIATION	ELEMENTS		DEFINITION
abduction **abduct (verb)**	ab-**DUCK**-shun ab-**DUKT**	S/ P/ R/	-ion *process, action* **ab-** *away from* **-duct-** *lead*	Action of moving away from the midline To move away from the midline
adductor	ah-**DUCK**-tor	S/ P/ R/	-or *that which does something* **ad-** *toward* **-duct-** *lead*	Muscle that moves the thigh toward the midline
adduction	ah-**DUCK**-shun	S/	-ion *action, condition*	Action of moving toward the midline
calcaneus	cal-**KAY**-knee-us		Latin *the heel*	The heel bone
calcaneal tendon (*same as* **Achilles tendon**) **Achilles**	kal-**KAY**-knee-al ah-**KILL**-eeze	S/ R/	-eal *pertaining to* **calcan-** *calcaneus* mythical Greek warrior	The tendon of the heel formed from gastrocnemius and soleus muscles and inserted into the calcaneus
gastrocnemius	gas-trok-**KNEE**-me-us	S/ R/	-ius *pertaining to* **gastrocnem-** *calf of leg*	Major muscle in back of the lower leg (the calf)
gluteus **gluteal (adj)**	**GLUE**-tee-us **GLUE**-tee-al	 S/ R/	Greek *buttocks* -eal *pertaining to* **glut-** *buttocks*	Refers to one of three muscles in the buttocks Pertaining to the buttocks
maximus	**MAKS**-ih-mus		Latin *the biggest* or *the greatest*	The gluteus maximus muscle is the largest muscle in the body, covering a large part of each buttock
medius	**MEE**-dee-us		Latin *middle*	The gluteus medius muscle is partly covered by the gluteus maximus
minimus	**MIN**-ih-mus		Latin *smallest*	The gluteus minimus is the smallest of the gluteal muscles and lies under the gluteus medius
popliteal fossa	pop-**LIT**-ee-al **FOSS**-ah	S/ R/CF	-al *pertaining to* **poplit/e-** *ham, back of knee* fossa, Latin *trench, ditch*	The hollow at the back of the knee
quadriceps femoris	**KWAD**-rih-seps **FEM**-or-is	P/ R/ S/ R/	**quadri-** *four* **-ceps** *head* -is *belonging to, pertaining to* **femor-** *femur*	An anterior thigh muscle with four heads (origins)

EXERCISES

A. Defining *the word element provides a clue to its meaning. Select the correct answer for each statement.* **LO 5.1**

1. The prefix that means *four*:

a. ad- **b.** quadri- **c.** ab-

2. The root that means *lead*:

a. calcan- **b.** femor- **c.** glut- **d.** duct-

3. The suffix that means *that which does something*:

a. -is **b.** -ion **c.** -al **d.** -or

4. The suffix *-ceps* means:

a. trench, ditch **b.** muscle **c.** head **d.** belong to

B. Identify medical terms that come from Latin. *Given the Latin meaning, insert the medical term that it is defining. Fill in the blanks.* **LO 5.2**

1. buttocks: ____________________

2. smallest: ____________________

3. the heel: ____________________

4. middle: ____________________

5. biggest: ____________________

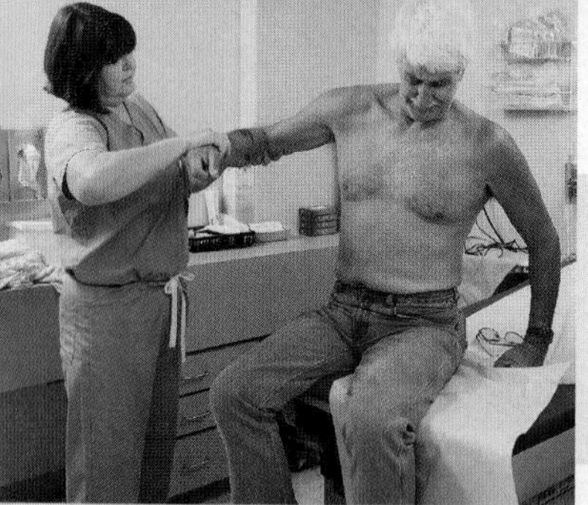
McGraw-Hill Education/Rick Brady

Lesson 5.4

Physical Medicine and Rehabilitation (PM&R)

Objectives

As a health professional, you may be directly involved in helping a patient through the rehabilitation and recovery process after an illness, surgery, or medical procedure. The information in this lesson will enable you to use correct medical terminology to:

5.4.1 Identify the members of the rehabilitation team.

5.4.2 Discuss the purposes of rehabilitation medicine.

5.4.3 Define the goals for a restorative rehabilitation program for specific common problems.

5.4.4 Define the different types of rehabilitation.

5.4.5 Use the activities of daily living as a measure to assess therapy needs and effectiveness.

CASE REPORT 5.2

You are . . .

. . . a **certified occupational therapist assistant** working in the Rehabilitation Unit at Fulwood Medical Center.

You are communicating with . . .

. . . Mr. Hank Johnson, a 65-year-old print shop owner.

One year ago, Mr. Johnson had an elective left total-hip replacement for osteoarthritis. Four months later, he had a myocardial infarction. Two weeks ago, while on his exercise bike, he had a stroke. His right arm and leg were paralyzed, he lost his speech, and he had difficulty swallowing. He arrived in the Emergency Department within 3 hours of the stroke and received **thrombolytic therapy** *(see Chapter 6).* Mr. Johnson is now receiving **physical therapy, occupational therapy,** and speech therapy in the inpatient Rehabilitation Unit. He is able to say some simple words and has begun to have voluntary movements in the arm and leg. Your roles are to help him regain function in his arm and leg and to monitor and record his progress.

Physical Medicine and Rehabilitation (PM&R)

(LO 5.5 and 5.8)

PM&R health professionals are listed and defined at the beginning of this chapter.

Physical medicine and rehabilitation is also called **physiatry.** Its goal is to develop a comprehensive program to put together the different pieces of a person's life—medical, social, emotional, and **vocational**—after injury or disease. PM&R programs cover a wide spectrum, from prevention of injury in athletes to treating sports-related injuries in sports medicine to coping with complicated multiple trauma.

Mr. Hank Johnson *(see Case Report 5.2)* will need a program designed specifically to get him back on his feet literally and in so many other ways.

Stroke Rehabilitation

(LO 5.5 and 5.8)

The goals of Mr. Johnson's **rehabilitation** program are to enable him to:

- Walk safely using an **assistive device.**
- Use his hands with accuracy.
- Restore his speech abilities.
- Prevent a second stroke.

Because he received thrombolytic therapy *(see Chapter 6)* within 3 hours of his stroke's onset, he has a 50% chance of being left with little or no residual difficulty, compared to a 35% chance had he not received the therapy.

Social workers are helping Mr. Johnson's wife to make their home safe for his return, including obtaining **adaptive equipment.** Raised toilet seats, handrails in the bath and shower, eating devices, and other adaptive equipment will help Mr. Johnson perform activities of daily living during his recovery. Social workers will also help Mrs. Johnson to work with Medicare to obtain the maximum allowable benefits. Anyone who has had one stroke is at high risk for having a second stroke. Therefore, during this rehabilitative period, Mr. Johnson will be evaluated for such risk factors as narrowing of the carotid arteries with plaque, thrombosis *(see Chapter 6),* and the presence of atrial fibrillation *(see Chapter 6).*

Abbreviation

PM&R	physical medicine and rehabilitation

Word Analysis and Definition

S = Suffix P = Prefix R = Root R/CF = Combining Form

WORD	PRONUNCIATION	ELEMENTS		DEFINITION
assistive device	ah-**SIS**-tiv de-**VICE**	S/ R/ R/	**-ive** *nature of* **assist-** *aid, help* **device** *an appliance*	Tool, software, or hardware to assist in performing daily activities
occupational therapy	**OCK**-you-**PAY**-shun-al **THAIR**-ah-pee	S/ R/ R/	**-al** *pertaining to* **occupation-** *work* **therapy** *treatment*	Use of work and recreational activities to increase independent function
orthotic orthotist	or-**THOT**-ik or-**THOT**-ist	S/ R/ S/	**-ic** *pertaining to* **orthot-** *correct* **-ist** *specialist*	Orthopedic appliance to correct an abnormality Specialist who makes and fits orthopedic appliances
physiatry physiatrist physical medicine	fih-**ZIE**-ah-tree fih-**ZIE**-ah-trist **FIZ**-ih-cal **MED**-ih-sin	 S/ R/ R/ S/ R/	Greek *science of nature* **-ist** *specialist* **phys-** *nature* **-iatr-** *treatment* **-al** *pertaining to* **physic-** *body*	Physical medicine Specialist in physical medicine Diagnosis and treatment by means of remedial agents, such as exercises, manipulation, heat, etc.
physical therapy *(also known as physiotherapy)* physiotherapy (syn)	**FIZ**-ih-cal **THAIR**-ah-pee **FIZ**-ee-oh-**THAIR**-ah-pee	S/ R/ R/ R/CF	**-al** *pertaining to* **physic-** *body* **therapy** *treatment* **physi/o-** *body*	Use of remedial processes to overcome a physical defect Another term for physical therapy
rehabilitation	**REE**-hah-bill-ih-**TAY**-shun	S/ P/ R/	**-ion** *action, condition* **re-** *again* **-habilitat-** *restore*	Therapeutic restoration of an ability to function as before
therapy therapeutic (adj) therapist	**THAIR**-ah-pee **THAIR**-ah-**PYU**-tik **THAIR**-ah-pist	 S/ R/ S/ R/	Greek *medical treatment* **-ic** *pertaining to* **therapeut-** *treatment* **-ist** *specialist* **therap-** *treatment*	Systematic treatment of a disease, dysfunction, or disorder Relating to the treatment of a disease or disorder Professional trained in the practice of a particular therapy

EXERCISES

A. Review *Case Report 5.2. Apply your knowledge of medical language to select the correct answer(s) for each question.* **LO 5.5 and 5.9**

1. Mr. Johnson needed a hip replacement due to:

a. myocardial infarction **b.** osteoarthritis **c.** stroke **d.** hemiplegia

2. What two major medical events did Mr. Johnson suffer recently? (choose two)

a. stroke **b.** muscle strain **c.** rotator cuff tear **d.** myocardial infarction

3. Which of the following are the goals of Mr. Johnson's rehabilitation? (choose all that apply)

a. walk safely using an assistive device **c.** restore his speech abilities
b. prevent congestive heart failure **d.** prevent a second stroke

4. Of his goals for rehabilitation, which one are you tasked with you helping him meet?

a. walk safely using an assistive device **c.** restore his speech abilities
b. prevent congestive heart failure **d.** prevent a second stroke

B. Deconstruct *the following medical terms into their word elements. Some terms will not have every element present. Fill in the chart.* **LO 5.1, 5.2, and 5.8**

Medical Term	Prefix	Root/CF	Suffix
therapeutic	1.	2.	3.
rehabilitation	4.	5.	6.
orthotic	7.	8.	9.
multidisciplinary	10.	11.	12.
orthotist	13.	14.	15.
assistive	16.	17.	18.

Rehabilitation Definitions (LO 5.2, 5.3, and 5.8)

Definitions (LO 5.2, 5.3, and 5.8)

The following definitions of terms or phrases specific to rehabilitation will help you to understand more precisely the different kinds of rehabilitation in which you may be involved as a health professional.

Rehabilitation medicine focuses on function. Being able to function is essential to an individual's independence and ability to have a good quality of life.

Restorative rehabilitation restores a function that has been lost, such as after a hip fracture, hip replacement, or stroke. This process can be intense, but it's also usually short term.

Maintenance rehabilitation strengthens and maintains a function that is gradually being lost. It is less intense than restorative rehabilitation but often long term. Problems of senescence (old age), like difficulty with balance or flexibility, require this long-term approach.

Rehabilitation medicine is also involved with the **prevention** of function loss and the prevention of injury. In sports medicine, an example is the prevention of shoulder and elbow injuries often experienced by baseball pitchers.

Activities of daily living (ADLs) are the routine activities of personal care. The six basic ADLs are eating, bathing, dressing, grooming, toileting, and transferring. Assistive devices are designed to make ADLs easier to perform and help maintain the patient's independence. Examples of these devices include reachers and grabbers, easy-pull sock aids, long shoehorns, jar openers, and eating aids *(Figure 5.11)*. ADLs are also a measurement to assess therapy needs and monitor its effectiveness.

Instrumental activities of daily living (IADLs) relate to independent living. These activities include managing money, using a telephone, cooking, driving, shopping for groceries and personal items, and doing housework.

Keynote

- **Coordinated multidisciplinary evaluation, management, and therapy add significantly to the chances of a good recovery.**

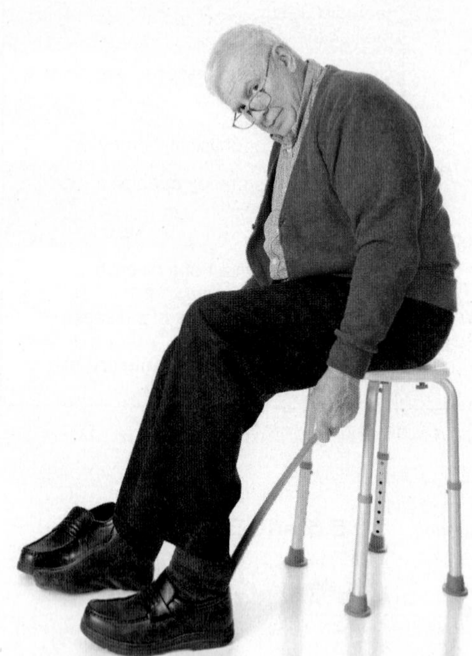

▲ **FIGURE 5.11** Assistive Device for Dressing.

glenda/Shutterstock

Abbreviations

ADLs	activities of daily living
BKA	below-the-knee amputation
COTA	certified occupational therapist assistant
IADLs	instrumental activities of daily living
PVD	peripheral vascular disease

Amputations (LO 5.2, 5.3, and 5.8)

Seventy-five percent of all amputations are performed on people over 65 years of age with **peripheral vascular disease (PVD)**. This includes complications from arteriosclerosis and diabetes. Most of these cases involve **below-the-knee amputations (BKAs)**. On the other hand, the wars in Iraq and Afghanistan led to soldiers losing their arms and legs from have the detonation of explosive devices. In some of these cases, amputations are also required, depending on the level of damage an explosion has caused to the soldier's body.

Rehabilitation after amputation is an increasingly important component in rehabilitation programs. Immediately after surgery, the objectives of the rehabilitation team are to:

- Promote healing of the stump;
- Strengthen the muscles above the site of the amputation;
- Strengthen arm muscles to assist in ambulation or help with walking using a cane, crutches, or other assistive devices;
- Prevent **contractures** or **tightening** of the joints above the amputation (knee and hip for BKAs);
- Shrink the post-amputation stump with elastic cuffs or bandages to fit the socket of a temporary **prosthesis** *(Figure 5.12)*; and
- Provide emotional, psychological, and family support.

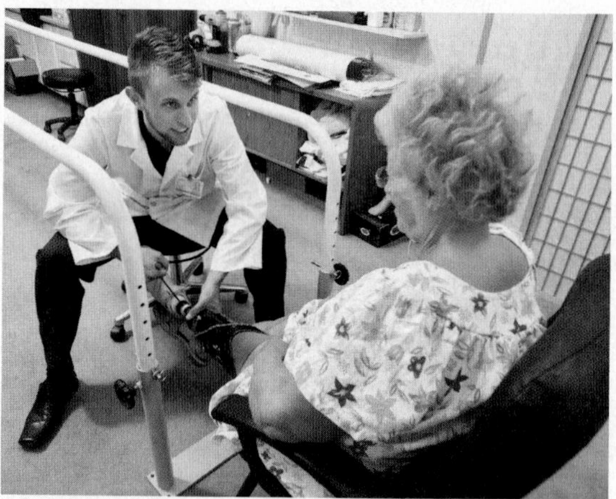

▲ **FIGURE 5.12** A physical therapist explains to a patient how to use her prosthesis.

Mood Board/Shutterstock

Word Analysis and Definition

S = Suffix P = Prefix R = Root R/CF = Combining Form

WORD	PRONUNCIATION	ELEMENTS		DEFINITION
amputation	am-pyu-**TAY**-shun	S/ R/	-ation *a process* amput- *prune*	Removal of a limb, part of a limb, or other projecting body part
contracture	kon-**TRAK**-chur	S/ R/	-ure *result of* contract- *pull together*	Muscle shortening due to spasm or fibrosis
prevention	pree-**VEN**-shun	S/ R/	-ion *action, condition* prevent- *prevent*	Process to prevent occurrence of a disease or health problem
prosthesis	**PROS**-thee-sis		Greek *an addition*	An artificial part to remedy a defect in the body
restorative rehabilitation	ree-**STOR**-ah-tiv **REE**-hah-bill-ih-**TAY**-shun	S/ R/	-ative *quality of* restor- *renew*	Therapy that promotes renewal of health and strength

Exercises

A. Deconstruct *the following terms:* **LO 5.1, 5.2, and 5.8**

1. Prevention: ______________ / ______________
R, R/CF S

2. Contracture: ______________ / ______________
R, R/CF S

3. Restorative: ______________ / ______________
R, R/CF S

B. Identify *abbreviations that describe medical terms. Match the abbreviation in the first column to its correct description in the second column.* **LO 5.3**

_____ **1.** COTA **a.** removal of the lower leg and foot

_____ **2.** ADL **b.** a professional that assists people in improving their activities of daily living

_____ **3.** IADL **c.** examples include toileting, brushing one's hair, brushing one's teeth

_____ **4.** PVD **d.** example include reachers, grabbers, and long shoehorns

_____ **5.** BKA **e.** condition that is responsible for a large percentage of below the knee amputations

C. Utilize *the correct language of rehabilitation in the following paragraph. The word bank contains more terms than you need to use–some terms you may use more than once. When you have finished the exercise, proofread it again to see if it makes sense. Fill in the blanks.* **LO 5.2, 5.8, and 5.9**

adapt	**contracture**	**amputation(s)**	**prosthesis**
amputee	**assistive devices**	**elective**	**amputate**
residual	**PVD**	**assistive**	**protocol**

Seventy-five percent of all (1) ______________ are performed on patients over 65 years of age with (2) ______________ complicating arteriosclerosis and diabetes. Loss of blood flow to a limb area produces necrotic tissue, which in time can become infected or gangrenous and makes the need for this procedure urgent, rather than (3) ______________ ______________. The decision to (4) ______________ is a serious one and must be undertaken by a qualified surgeon.

The (5) ______________ will require a physical therapist to help the patient learn to (6) ______________ to the use of a (7) ______________. Hopefully, there will be no muscle (8) ______________ or (9) ______________ pain after the surgery.

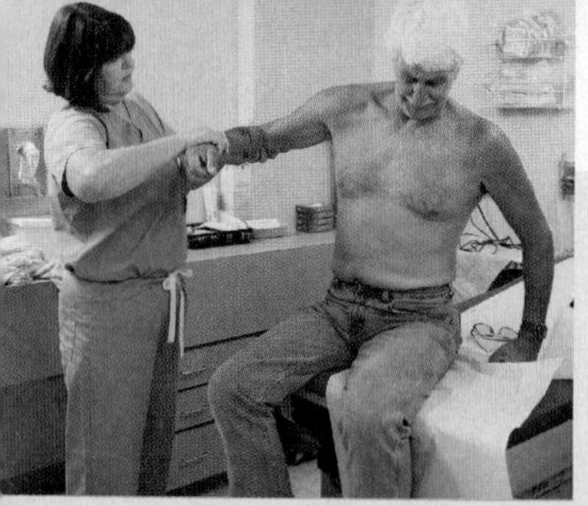

McGraw-Hill Education/Rick Brady

Lesson 5.5

Diagnostic and Therapeutic Procedures and Pharmacology for Disorders of the Muscles and Tendons

Objectives

Many different health professionals are involved in the diagnosis and treatment of disorders of muscles and tendons in their acute phase, primary care and rehabilitation. It is essential to have a common language and understanding to ensure a high quality of patient care. The information in this lesson will enable you to:

5.5.1 Explain the diagnostic procedures used for disorders of muscles and tendons.

5.5.2 Discuss the treatment procedures used for disorders of the wrist.

5.5.3 Describe the medications used for disorders of muscles and tendons.

Abbreviations

Bx	biopsy
CK	creatine kinase
CT	computed tomography
EMG	electromyography
ESR	erythrocyte sedimentation rate
MRI	magnetic resonance imaging
MSA	myositis specific antibodies

Diagnostic Procedures for Disorders of Muscles and Tendons (LO 5.5)

A medical history and physical examination are essential components of a diagnostic examination. Additional diagnostic tests include:

- **Blood tests.** Damaged muscles release **enzymes** such as **creatine kinase** (CK) and aldolase into the blood, and their levels can be measured. An **erythrocyte sedimentation rate (ESR)** is not specific for any disease process, but it indicates the presence of **inflammation,** and serial readings can be used to measure changes in an inflammatory process.
- **Electromyography** (EMG), in which an **electrode** needle is inserted into the muscle to be tested to measure and record the electrical activity in that muscle as the muscle is contracted and relaxed.
- **Nerve conduction studies** are used to measure the speed at which motor or sensory nerves conduct impulses and also can show problems at the neuromuscular junction; for example, in myasthenia gravis.
- **Magnetic resonance imaging** (MRI) and **computed tomography scan (CT scan)** show detailed images of damage or disease in muscles.
- **Ultrasonography** can identify tears and inflammation of tendons and involves no exposure to radiation, unlike MRI and CT scan.
- **Muscle biopsy** (Bx) is performed by removing a small piece of the abnormal muscle through a hollow needle or a small incision to be sent to the laboratory for examination and analysis.
- **Genetic testing** of blood or tissues can show the mutations in some of the genes that cause the different types of muscular dystrophy.
- **Myositis specific antibodies** (MSA) can confirm a diagnosis of **dermatomyositis** or polymyositis. Dozens of these antibodies have been identified and research is ongoing to define their significance.

Therapeutic Methods for Disorders of Muscles and Tendons (LO 5.3 and 5.5)

RICE (rest, ice, compression, and elevation) is used in the acute phase for muscle and tendon strains and sprains.

- **Physical therapy (PT)** and **exercise** are important in the treatment of muscle diseases and involve **range of motion** exercises to prevent **contracture** of joints and exercises and resistance training to restore muscle mass and strength.
- **Medications** are used frequently in muscle diseases. Acetaminophen (paracetamol) and hydrocodone can be used for pain in the acute stages following injury. For the inflammatory myopathies, **oral corticosteroids** are often the first line of treatment, sometimes with the **anti-metabolite** drugs methotrexate or azathioprine. For patients who do not respond to standard treatments, **immunosuppressive** drugs can be used.
- **Surgical** treatments include **tendon reconstruction,** in which the two ends of a ruptured or torn tendon are **sutured** back together. In ligament injuries of the elbow joint in high-level, overhead-throwing athletes, such as baseball pitchers, reconstruction techniques and tendon grafting are often used with success.
- **Orthopedic appliances** such as braces and walkers are used during recovery from muscle and tendon injury.

Musculoskeletal Drugs (LO 5.5)

NSAIDs inhibit the two cyclooxygenase (**COX**) enzymes that are involved in producing the inflammatory process. They have **analgesic** and **antipyretic** effects and are used for treatment of tissue injury, pyrexia, rheumatoid arthritis, osteoarthritis, gout, and nonspecific joint and tissue pains. The three major NSAIDs, each of which is available OTC, are:

1. **Acetylsalicylic acid** (aspirin), which, in addition to the above effects and uses, also has an antiplatelet effect due to its inhibition of one of the COX enzymes; thus, it is often used in the prevention of heart attacks.
2. **Ibuprofen** (*Advil, Motrin,* and several other trade names), which acts by inhibiting both the COX enzymes, essential elements in the enzyme pathways involved in pain, inflammation, and fever. It is taken orally, but in 2009 an injectable form of ibuprofen (*Caldolor*) was approved for use. In some studies, ibuprofen has been associated with the prevention of Alzheimer and Parkinson diseases, but further studies are needed.
3. **Naproxen** (*Aleve* and many other trade names), which is taken orally once a day and also inhibits both the COX enzymes.

Indomethacin, an NSAID that inhibits both COX enzymes, is a potent drug with many serious side effects. It is not used as an analgesic for minor aches and pains or for fever.

Paracetamol (acetaminophen), an active **metabolite** of phenacetin (not an NSAID), is a widely used OTC analgesic and antipyretic. It is used for the relief of minor aches and pains and is an **ingredient** in many cold and flu remedies.

Skeletal muscle relaxants are FDA-approved for spasticity (baclofen, dantrolene, tizanidine) or for muscular conditions like multiple sclerosis (carisoprodol, chlorzoxazone, cyclobenzaprine, metaxalone, methocarbamol, orphenadrine). The only drug with available evidence of efficacy in spasticity is tizanidine (*Zanaflex, Sirdalud*), but cyclobenzaprine (*Amrix*) appears to be somewhat effective.

Anabolic steroids are related to testosterone but have been altered so that their main effect is to cause skeletal muscle to hypertrophy. They are used illegally in many sports to increase muscle strength. They have marked, often irreversible, side effects, including stunting the height of growing adolescents, shrinking testes and sperm counts, masculinizing women, and causing delusions and paranoid jealousy. In the long term, there are increased risks of heart attacks and strokes, kidney failure, and liver tumors.

Keynote

Spasticity is a state of increased muscular tone with exaggeration of the tendon reflexes.

Abbreviations

COX	cyclooxygenase enzymes
NSAID	nonsteroidal anti-inflammatory drug

Word Analysis and Definition

S = Suffix P = Prefix R = Root R/CF = Combining Form

WORD	PRONUNCIATION	ELEMENTS		DEFINITION
antibody	**AN**-tih-body	P/ R/	anti- *against* -body *substance*	Protein produced in response to an antigen
biopsy	**BY**-op-see	S/ R/	-opsy *to view* bi- *life*	Removal of a tissue from a living person for laboratory examination
electromyography	ee-**LEK**-troh-my-**OG**-rah-fee	S/ R/CF R/CF	-graphy *process of recording* electr/o- *electricity* -my/o- *muscle*	Recording of electrical activity in a muscle
enzyme	**EN**-zime	P/ R	en- *in* -zyme *fermenting*	Protein that induces change in other substances
inflammation	in-flah-**MAY**-shun	S/ P/ R/	-ation *process* in- *in* -flamm- *flame*	A basic complex of reactions in blood vessels and adjacent tissues in response to injury or abnormal stimulation
ultrasonography	**UL**-trah-soh-**NOG**-rah-fee	S/ P/ R/CF	-graphy *process of recording* ultra- *beyond* -son/o- *sound*	Delineation of deep structures using sound waves
antimetabolite	**AN**-teh-meh-**TAB**-oh-lite	S/ P/ R/	-ite *pertaining to* anti- *against* metabol- *change*	A substance that replaces or inhibits a specific part of a cell's normal metabolism
corticosteroid	**KOR**-tih-koh-**STEHR**-oyd	S/ R/	-steroid *steroid* cortic/o *from the cortex*	A hormone produced by the adrenal cortex
immunosuppressive	**IM**-you-noh-suh-**PRESS**-iv	S/ R/CF R/	-ive *nature of* immune/o *immune response* -suppress- *press under*	Substance that causes failure of the immune system

Exercises

A. Determine the appropriate diagnostic test. *Read each scenario and determine which diagnostic test is indicated to support the diagnosis. Fill in the blanks. Not all answers will be used.* LO 5.3 and 5.9

ESR **EMG** **CK** **Bx** **MSA**

1. The physician ordered a(n) ______________ to determine the strength of muscular contraction in the patient with polio.
2. In order to support the diagnosis of myositis, a(n) ______________ of the muscle tissue was ordered.
3. Dr. Novak sent a blood sample to the lab to have the medical technologist measure the ______________ to determine if the patient had rhabdomyolysis.
4. The patient's blood was sent to the lab with an order for the medical technologist to measure the ______________ in order to determine if the patient had a chronic inflammatory condition.

Word Analysis and Definition

S = Suffix P = Prefix R = Root R/CF = Combining Form

WORD	PRONUNCIATION	ELEMENTS		DEFINITION
anabolic steroid	an-ah-**BOL**-ik **STER**-oyd	S/ R/ S/ R/	-ic *pertaining to* **anabol-** *to raise up* -oid *resembling* **ster-** *solid*	Prescription drug used by some athletes to increase muscle mass
analgesia **analgesic**	an-al-**JEE**-zee-ah	S/ P/ R/ S/	-ia *condition* **an-** *without* **-alges-** *sensation of pain* -ic *pertaining to*	State in which pain is reduced Agent that produces analgesia
antimetabolite	**AN**-teh-meh-**TAB**-oh-lite	S/ P/ R/	-ite *pertaining to* **anti-** *against* **-metabol-** *change*	A substance that replaces or inhibits a specific part of a cell's normal metabolism
antipyretic	**AN**-tee-pie-**RET**-ik	S/ P/ R/	-ic *pertaining to* **anti-** *against* **-pyret-** *fever*	Agent that reduces fever
contracture	kon-**TRAK**-chur	S/ R/	-ure *result of* **contract-** *pull together*	Muscle shortening due to spasm or fibrosis
corticosteroid	**KOR**-tih-koh-**STEHR**-oyd	S/ R/CF	**-steroid** *steroid* **cortic/o** *from the cortex*	A hormone produced by the adrenal cortex
Duchenne muscular dystrophy	**DOO**-shen **MUSS**-kyu-lar **DISS**-troh-fee	 P/ R/	Guillaume Benjamin Duchenne, French neurologist, 1806–1875 **dys-** *bad, difficult* **-trophy** *nourishment*	A condition with symmetrical weakness and wasting of pelvic, shoulder, and proximal limb muscles
immunosuppressive	**IM**-you-noh-suh-**PRESS**-iv	S/ R/CF R/	-ive *nature of* **immune/o** *immune response* **-suppress-** *press under*	Substance that causes failure of the immune system
ingredient	in-**GREE**-dee-ent	S/ P/ R/	-ent *end result, pertaining to* **in-** *in, into* **-gredi-** *to go*	An element in a mixture
metabolism **metabolite**	meh-**TAB**-oh-lizm meh-**TAB**-oh-lite	S/ R/ S/	-ism *condition* **metabol-** *change* -ite *associated with*	The constantly changing physical and chemical processes in the cell Any product of metabolism
myoglobin	**MY**-oh-**GLOW**-bin	S/ R/CF R/	-in *substance* **my/o-** *muscle* **-glob-** *globe*	Protein of muscle that stores and transports oxygen
myopathy **myositis**	my-**OP**-ah-thee my-oh-**SI**-tis	S/ R/CF S/	-pathy *disease* **my/o-** *muscle* -sitis *inflammation*	Any disease of muscle Inflammation of muscle tissue
rhabdomyolysis	**RAB**-doh-my-oh-**LIE**-sis	S/ R/CF R/CF	-lysis *destruction* **rhabd/o-** *rod-shaped* **-my/o-** *muscle*	Destruction of muscle to produce myoglobin
statin	**STAH**-tin		Greek *stationary*	A class of drug used to lower blood cholesterol levels
tenosynovitis	**TEN**-oh-sine-oh-**VIE**-tis	S/ R/CF R/	-itis *inflammation* **ten/o-** *tendon* **- synov-** *synovial membrane*	Inflammation of a tendon and its surrounding synovial sheath
thymectomy	thigh-**MEK**-toe-me	S/ R/	-ectomy *surgical excision* **thym-** *thymus gland*	Surgical removal of the thymus gland

EXERCISES

A. The following statement is *written in the medical record. Explain its meaning of the term in bold to your patient.* **LO 5.5 and 5.10**

1. In order to diagnose the cause of Mrs. Patricia Keene's muscle weakness, an **EMG** will be performed.

a. test to measure the electrical activity of a muscle

b. X-ray that views organs in different slices

c. test to measure the presence of inflammatory substances in your blood

d. examination of the genetic make up of one's body

EXERCISES

B. Select the correct medical term to complete the following questions. *Choose the correct answer.* **LO 5.5**

1. NSAIDS inhibit enzymes that are involved in the ____________________ process.

a. respiratory

b. digestive

c. urinary

d. pulmonary

e. inflammatory

2. The class of medication that treats muscle spasticity:

a. COX inhibitor

b. analgesic

c. muscle relaxant

d. antipyretic

3. The analgesic listed that is NOT an NSAID:

a. naproxen

b. ibuprofen

c. aspirin

d. paracetamol

4. An NSAID that is described as a potent pain reliever but is not used for minor aches and pains due to its serious side effects:

a. orphenadrine

b. naproxen

c. indomethacin

d. cyclobenzaprine

5. A medication that lowers a fever is termed a(n):

a. metabolite

b. antipyretic

c. ingredient

d. anti-inflammatory

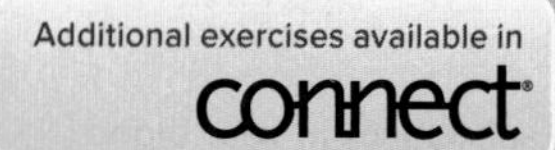

Chapter Review exercises, along with additional practice items, are available in Connect!

The Cardiovascular and Circulatory Systems

CHAPTER

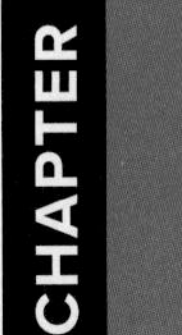

The Essentials of the Language of Cardiology

Rick Brady/McGraw-Hill Education

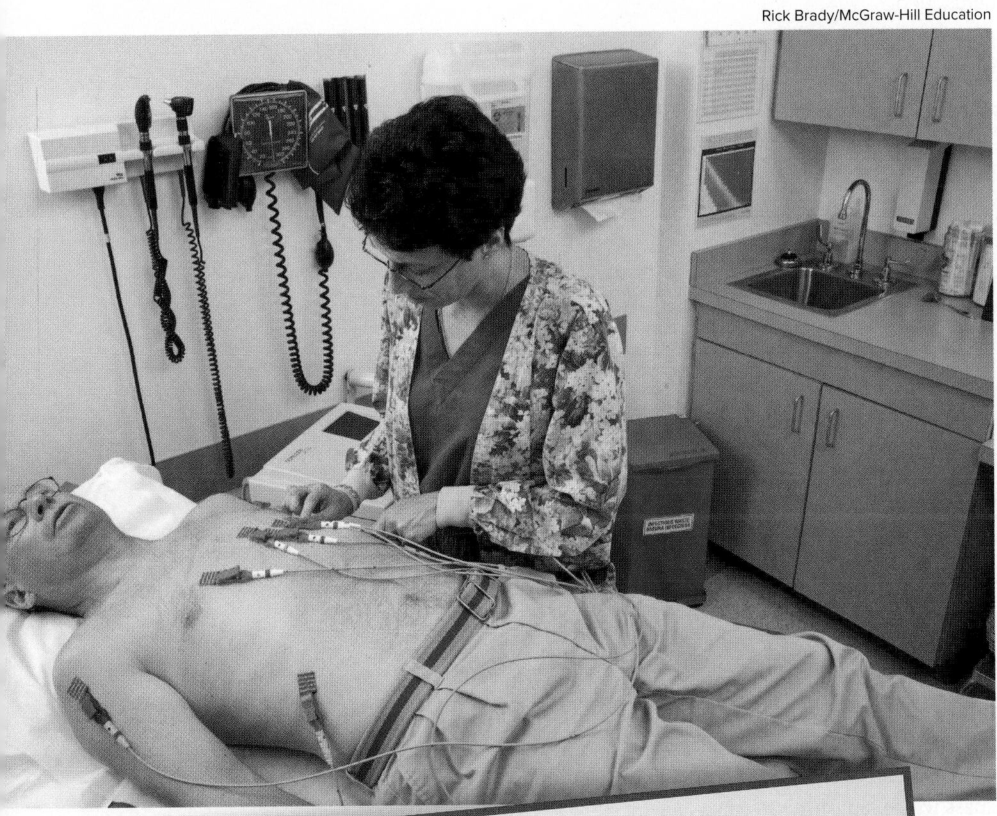

CASE REPORT 6.1

You are . . .

. . . a cardiovascular technologist (CVT) employed by the **Cardiology** Department at Fulwood Medical Center. You have been called to the Emergency Department (ED) to perform an **electrocardiogram (ECG** or **EKG)**, STAT.

You are communicating with . . .

. . . Mr. Hank Johnson, a 64-year-old owner of a printing company. Eight months ago, he had a left total hip replacement. In the past 3 months, Mr. Johnson has returned to his daily workouts. This morning, while riding his exercise bike, he felt a tightness in his chest, but continued cycling. He developed pain in the center of his chest, radiating down his left arm and up into his jaw, and became **diaphoretic.** His personal trainer called 911. You perform the ECG and the automatic report describes abnormalities in the chest leads. As you remove the **electrodes,** Mr. Johnson complains that he is feeling faint and having difficulty breathing (DOB). You are the only person in the room.

Learning Outcomes

The health of a patient's heart—in fact, the entire cardiovascular system—will always be a factor in the diagnosis and treatment of any condition, no matter what discipline or setting you find yourself working in as a health professional. From routine blood pressure checks to ultrasounds to surgical procedures, the condition of a patient's cardiovascular system must be carefully monitored. In order to best understand, communicate, and document conditions affecting the heart, blood vessels, and blood, you need to be able to:

LO 6.1 **Use roots, combining forms, suffixes, and prefixes to construct and analyze (deconstruct) medical terms related to the cardiovascular and circulatory systems.**

LO 6.2 **Spell and pronounce correctly medical terms and their plurals related to the cardiovascular and circulatory systems to communicate them with accuracy and precision in any health care setting.**

LO 6.3 **Define accepted abbreviations related to the cardiovascular and circulatory systems.**

LO 6.4 **Relate the anatomical structure of the heart to its functions, the blood flow through it, and disorders of its wall and valves.**

LO 6.5 **Describe the blood supply to the heart, and the electrical properties of the heart.**

LO 6.6 **Identify the different circulatory systems and the disorders of arteries and veins.**

LO 6.7 **Discuss the diagnostic and therapeutic procedures and pharmacologic agents used for cardiovascular and circulatory disorders.**

LO 6.8 **Apply your knowledge of the medical terms of the cardiovascular and circulatory systems to documentation, medical records, and medical reports.**

LO 6.9 **Translate the medical terms of the cardiovascular and circulatory systems into everyday language in order to communicate clearly with patients and their families.**

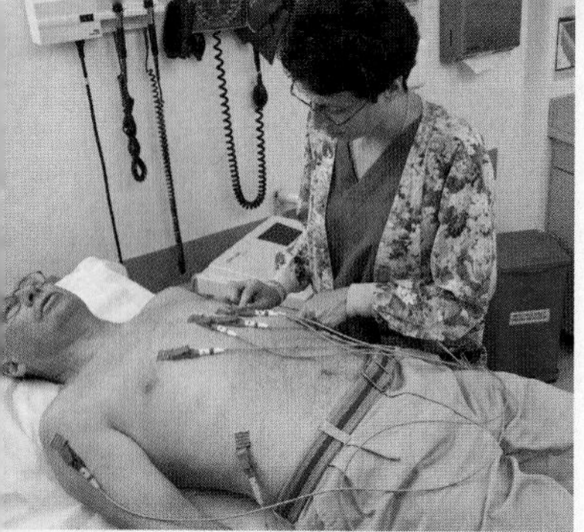

Rick Brady/McGraw-Hill Education

The health professionals involved in the diagnosis and treatment of problems with the cardiovascular system include the following:

- **Cardiologists** are medical doctors who specialize in disorders of the cardiovascular system.
- **Cardiovascular surgeons** are surgeons who specialize in surgery of the heart and the peripheral blood vessels.
- **Cardiovascular technologists** and technicians assist physicians in the diagnosis and treatment of cardiovascular disorders.
- **Vascular technologists** are practitioners who assist physicians by performing diagnostic and monitoring procedures using ultrasound.
- **Cardiac sonographers** or echocardiographers are technologists who use ultrasound to observe the heart chambers, valves, and blood vessels.
- **Phlebotomists** or phlebotomy technicians assist physicians by drawing patient blood samples for laboratory testing.
- **Perfusionists** are highly trained health care professionals who use the heart-lung machine during cardiac and other surgeries that require cardiopulmonary bypass.

Objectives

Your heart is roughly the size of your fist, weighs approximately 8 to 10 ounces, and pumps around 2,000 gallons of blood each day. Your heart is always working. When your heart fails to work, your blood stops circulating, your tissues stop receiving oxygen and nutrients, your metabolic wastes accumulate, and your cells die. The information in this lesson will enable you to use correct medical terminology to:

6.1.1 Describe the location of the heart.
6.1.2 Relate the structure of the heart to its functions.
6.1.3 Discuss the blood flow through the heart.
6.1.4 Explain the heart cycle.
6.1.5 Identify the blood supply to the heart.
6.1.6 Detail the electrical properties of the heart.

Lesson 6.1

The Heart

Location of the Heart (LO 6.4)

It is important to know precisely where the heart is located so that you can perform effective **cardiopulmonary resuscitation (CPR).** The heart is located in the **thoracic cavity** between the lungs, in an area called the **mediastinum** *(Figure 6.1a).* The heart is shaped like a blunt cone, pointing down and to the left. It rests at an angle with the majority of its mass to the left of the **sternum** *(Figure 6.1b).*

Abbreviations

CPR	cardiopulmonary resuscitation
CVT	cardiovascular technologist
ECG	electrocardiogram
ED	emergency department
EKG	electrocardiogram
DOB	difficulty of breathing
STAT	immediately

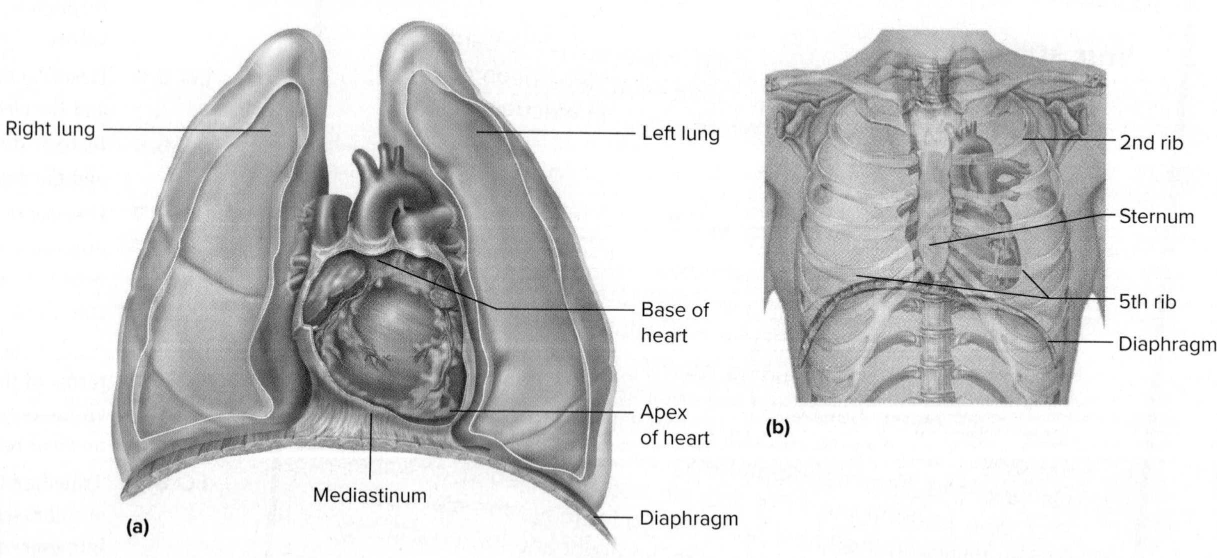

FIGURE 6.1
Position of Heart in Thoracic Cavity.
(a) Position of heart in mediastinum.
(b) Relationship of heart to sternum.

Word Analysis and Definition

S = Suffix P = Prefix R = Root R/CF = Combining Form

WORD	PRONUNCIATION	ELEMENTS		DEFINITION
cardiac	**KAR**-dee-ak	S/ R/	-ac *pertaining to* cardi- *heart*	Pertaining to the heart
cardiologist	kar-dee-**OL**-oh-jist	S/ R/CF	-logist *one who studies, specialist* cardi/o- *heart*	A medical specialist in the diagnosis and treatment of the heart (cardiology)
cardiology	kar-dee-**OL**-oh-jee	S/	-logy *study of*	Medical specialty of diseases of the heart
cardiopulmonary resuscitation (CPR)	**KAR**-dee-oh-**PUL**-mo-nar-ee ree-sus-ih-**TAY**-shun	S/ R/CF R/ S/ R/-	-ary *pertaining to* cardi/o- *heart* -pulmon- *lung* -ation *a process* resuscit- *revive from apparent death*	The attempt to restore cardiac and pulmonary function
cardiovascular	**KAR**-dee-oh-**VAS**-kyu-lar	S/ R/CF R/	-ar *pertaining to* cardi/o- *heart* -vascul- *blood vessel*	Pertaining to the heart and blood vessels
diaphoresis (noun)	**DIE**-ah-foh-**REE**-sis	S/ R/	-esis *condition* diaphor- *sweat*	Sweat, perspiration, or sweaty
diaphoretic (adj)	**DIE**-ah-foh-**RET**-ic	S/	-etic *pertaining to*	Pertaining to sweat or perspiration
electrocardiogram (ECG, EKG)	ee-lek-troh-**KAR**-dee-oh-gram	S/ R/CF R/CF	-gram *a record* electr/o- *electricity* -cardi/o- *heart*	Record of the electrical signals of the heart
electrocardiograph	ee-lek-troh-**KAR**-dee-oh-graf	S/	-graph *to record*	Machine that produces the electrocardiogram
electrocardiography	ee-**LEK**-troh-kar-dee-**OG**-rah-fee	S/	-graphy *process of recording*	The method of recording and the interpretation of electrocardiograms
electrode	ee-**LEK**-trode	S/ R/	-ode *way, road* electr- *electricity*	A device for conducting electricity
mediastinum	**ME**-dee-ass-**TIE**-num	S/ P/ R/	-um *structure* media- *middle* -stin- *partition*	Area between the lungs containing the heart, aorta, venae cavae, esophagus, and trachea
perfusion	per-**FYU**-zhun	S/ R/	-ion *action* perfus- *to pour*	The act of forcing blood to flow through a lumen or a vascular bed
phlebotomist	fleh-**BOT**-oh-mist	S/ R/CF R/	-ist *specialist in* phleb/o- *vein* -tom- *incise, cut*	Person skilled in taking blood from veins
phlebotomy	fleh-**BOT**-oh-me	S/	-tomy *surgical incision*	Withdrawing blood from a vein through a needle or catheter
sternum	**STIR**-num		Latin *the chest*	Long, flat bone forming the center of the anterior wall of the chest
thoracic cavity	**THOR**-ass-ik **KAV**-ih-tee	S/ R/	-ic *pertaining to* thorac- *chest* cavity, Latin *hollow*	Space within the chest containing the lungs, heart, esophagus, trachea, aorta, venae cavae, and pulmonary vessels

Exercises

A. Review *Case Report 6.1 and correctly answer the following questions. Fill in the blanks.* **LO 6.2, 6.3, 6.7, and 6.8**

1. The following abbreviations all appear in the Case Report. Demonstrate your understanding of the abbreviations by providing the terms they represent.

a. EKG ______________________

b. ED ______________________

c. CVT ______________________

d. DOB ______________________

e. ECG ______________________

B. Apply the language *of cardiology in the following documentation. Be sure to use the correct form (noun, adjective) of the term. There is only one best answer for each blank.* **LO 6.2 and 6.8**

cardiologist **cardiovascular** **cardiology** **cardiopulmonary**

1. The ____________ Department sent a specialist to examine the patient in the Emergency Room because of his symptoms. The ____________ ordered an angioplasty, which found that the patient had three obstructed arteries in his heart, so the ____________ surgeon prepared to operate immediately. Before surgery could begin, the patient suffered a heart attack and ____________ resuscitation was needed.

Functions and Structure of the Heart (LO 6.4)

Functions of the Heart (LO 6.4)

In order to keep your body alive, your heart must work all the time, without stopping. Its three most important functions are to:

1. **Pump blood.** As your heart contracts, it generates pressure that moves your blood through your blood vessels.
2. **Route blood.** Your heart essentially has two pumps: one on the right side that sends blood through the **pulmonary** circulation of your lungs and back to the second pump on your left side, which sends blood through the **systemic** circulation of your body. Your heart valves make this one-way flow of blood possible.
3. **Regulate blood supply.** The changing metabolic needs of your tissues and organs–for example, when you exercise–are met by changes in the rate and force of your heart's contractions.

Case Report 6.1 *(continued)*

A **myocardial infarction** (heart attack) is what was happening to Mr. Johnson at the beginning of this chapter. The changes on the ECG showed this event. A doctor should be called.

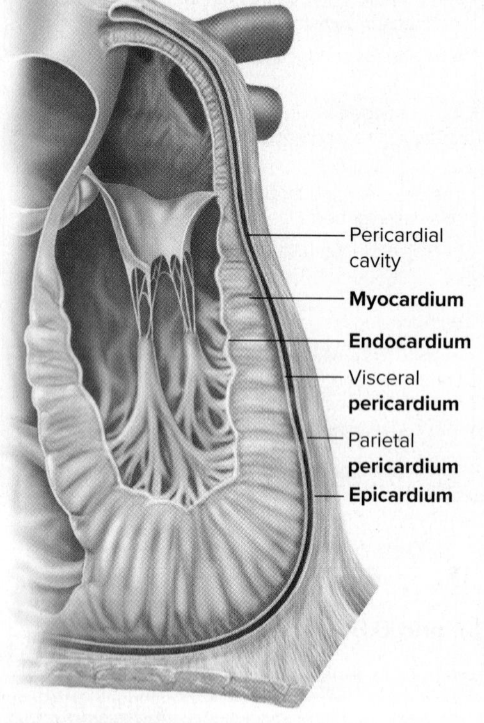

▲ **FIGURE 6.2**
Heart Wall.

Structure of the Heart (LO 6.4)

The heart wall consists of three layers *(Figure 6.2)*:

1. **Endocardium:** Connective tissue lining the inside of your heart.
2. **Myocardium:** Cardiac muscle cells that contract to enable your heart to pump blood.
3. **Epicardium:** An outer single layer of cells overlying a thin layer of connective tissue.

The **pericardium** is a double-layered connective tissue sac that surrounds and protects your heart.

Blood Supply to Heart Muscle (LO 6.5)

Because your heart beats continually and forcefully, it requires an abundant supply of oxygen and nutrients. To meet this need, your cardiac muscle has its own blood circulation called the **coronary circulation** *(Figure 6.3)*. This system of arteries arises directly from the **aorta.**

If any of your coronary arteries become blocked, the blood supply to a part of your cardiac muscle is cut off **(ischemia)** and the cells supplied by that artery die **(necrosis)** within minutes. This is a **myocardial infarction (MI)** or a "heart attack."

Aortic arch
Pulmonary trunk
Left coronary artery
Circumflex artery
Right coronary artery
Right ventricle
Left ventricle

▲ **FIGURE 6.3**
Coronary Arterial Circulation.

Abbreviation

MI	myocardial infarction

Word Analysis and Definition

S = Suffix P = Prefix R = Root R/CF = Combining Form

WORD	PRONUNCIATION	ELEMENTS		DEFINITION
aorta aortic (adj)	a-**OR**-tuh a-**OR**-tik	 S/ R/	Greek *lift up* -ic *pertaining to* aort- *aorta*	Main trunk of the systemic arterial system Pertaining to the aorta
coronary circulation	**KOR**-oh-nair-ee **SER**-kyu-**LAY**-shun	S/ R/ S/ R/	-ary *pertaining to* coron- *crown, coronary* -ion *action, condition* circulat- *circular route*	Blood vessels supplying the heart muscle
endocardium endocardial (adj)	**EN**-doh-**KAR**-dee-um **EN**-doh-**KAR**-dee-al	S/ P/ R/ S/	-um *structure* endo- *inside* -cardi- *heart* -al *pertaining to*	The inside lining of the heart Pertaining to the endocardium
epicardium epicardial (adj)	**EP**-ih-**KAR**-dee-um **EP**-ih-**KAR**-dee-al	S/ P/ R/ S/	-um *structure* epi- *upon, above* -cardi- *heart* -al *pertaining to*	The outer layer of the heart wall Pertaining to the epicardium
infarct infarction	in-**FARKT** in-**FARKT**-shun	P/ R/ S/	in- *in* -farct- *area of dead tissue* -ion *action, condition*	Area of cell death resulting from an infarction Sudden blockage of an artery
ischemia ischemic (adj)	is-**KEY**-me-ah is-**KEY**-mik	S/ R/ S/	-emia *a blood condition* isch- *to keep back* -emic *a condition of the blood*	Lack of blood supply to a tissue Pertaining to or affected by the lack of blood supply to a tissue
myocardium myocardial (adj)	**MY**-oh-**KAR**-dee-um my-oh-**KAR**-dee-al	S/ R/CF R/ S/	-um *structure* my/o- *muscle* -cardi- *heart* -al *pertaining to*	Muscular layer of the heart Pertaining to heart muscle
necrosis necrotic (adj)	neh-**KROH**-sis neh-**KROT**-ik	S/ R/ S/ R/CF	-osis *condition* necr- *death* -tic *pertaining to* necr/o- *death*	Pathologic death of cells or tissue Pertaining to or affected by necrosis (death)
pericardium (noun) pericardial (adj)	per-ih-**KAR**-dee-um per-ih-**KAR**-dee-al	S/ P/ R/ S/	-um *structure* peri- *around* -cardi- *heart* -al *pertaining to*	A double layer of membranes surrounding the heart Pertaining to the pericardium
pulmonary	**PULL**-moh-**NAR**-ee	S/ R/	-ary *pertaining to* pulmon- *lung*	Pertaining to the lungs and their blood supply

EXERCISES

A. Review *Case Report 6.1 (continued) and correctly answer the following questions. Fill in the blanks.* **LO 6.1, 6.2, 6.3, and 6.5**

1. Based on the patient's ECG, what was his final diagnosis? _______
2. What is the abbreviation for this condition? ____________________
3. **Deconstruct** *Mr. Johnson's diagnosis. If the term does not have a particular element, insert N/A. Fill in the blanks.*

________/________/________
R/CF R/CF S

________/________/________
P R/CF S

B. Construct medical terms. *Provide the correct word to the term to correctly complete each sentence.* **LO 6.1 and 6.4**

1. The **inside** heart is termed the _______/cardium.
2. The **muscular** part of the heart is termed the _____/cardium.
3. The **outer** layer of the heart is termed the _____/cardium.
4. An area of tissue that is not getting an adequate amount of blood flow is termed______/mic.
5. Over time, the lack of blood flow to the tissue can lead to an in/_________/ion.
6. Dead tissue is described as being ______/tic.

Lesson 6.1 (cont'd)

Keynote

- **The pulmonary circulation is the only place in the body where deoxygenated blood is carried in arteries and oxygenated blood is carried in veins.**

Abbreviations

CO_2	carbon dioxide
O_2	oxygen

Blood Flow through the Heart (LO 6.4)

Your heart *(Figures 6.4 and 6.6)* has four chambers through which your blood flows. These chambers are the:

1. Right **atrium**
2. Right **ventricle**
3. Left atrium
4. Left ventricle

Your right and left atria are separated by a thin muscle wall called the **interatrial septum.** Your right and left ventricles are divided by a thicker muscle wall called the **interventricular septum.**

Your left ventricle pumps blood to all the parts of your body (except the lungs) through the **systemic circulation.** Oxygen **(O_2)** and nutrients are delivered to your body's cells, and carbon dioxide **(CO_2)** and metabolic waste products are removed from the cells. This **deoxygenated** blood, via the veins, returns to the heart where the right ventricle pumps blood into the **pulmonary circulation** to the lungs. In the lungs, the carbon dioxide waste material is exchanged for oxygen from inhaled air *(Figure 6.5)*. This oxygenated blood then travels through the pulmonary veins back to the left side of the heart.

You have four valves that work together to ensure the correct flow of blood through your heart; on the right side are the **tricuspid** and **pulmonary** valves, and on the left side are the **mitral (bicuspid)** and **aortic** valves *(Figure 6.4)*.

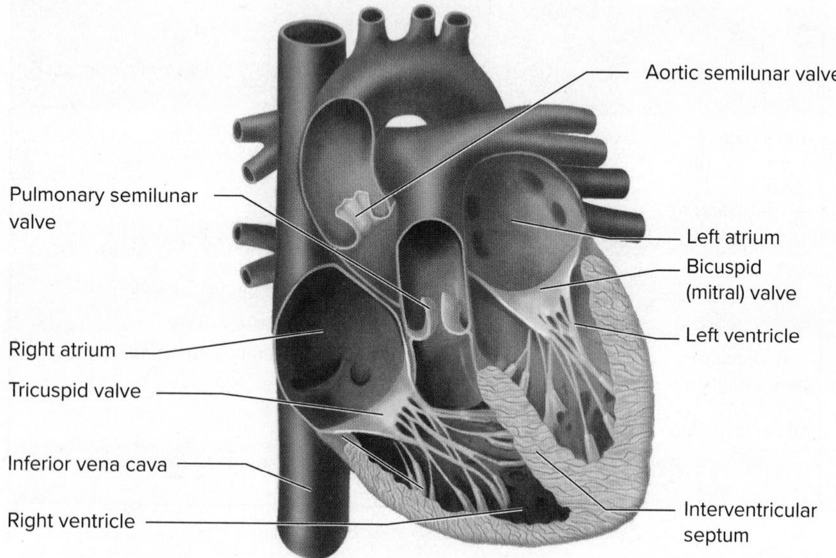

▲ **FIGURE 6.4**
Anatomy of the Heart.

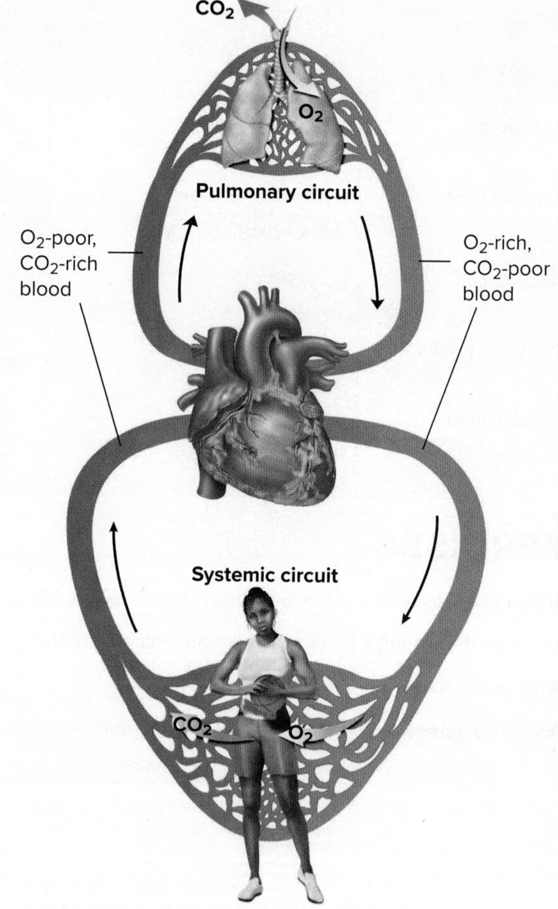

▲ **FIGURE 6.5**
Schematic of Cardiovascular System.

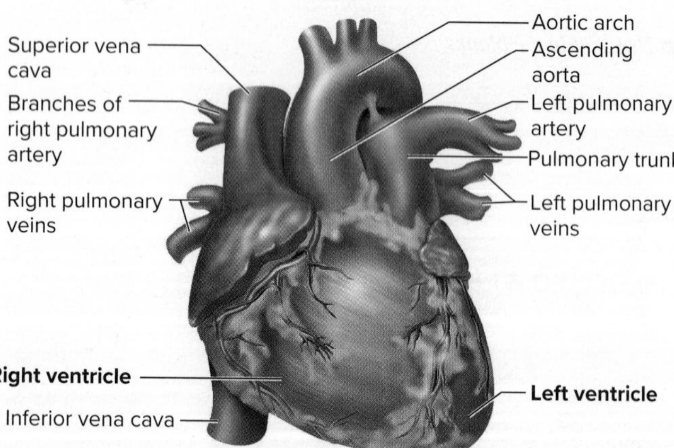

▲ **FIGURE 6.6**
External Anatomy of the Heart: Frontal View.

Word Analysis and Definition

S = Suffix P = Prefix R = Root R/CF = Combining Form

WORD	PRONUNCIATION	ELEMENTS		DEFINITION
atrium atria (pl) atrial (adj)	A-tree-um A-tree-ah A-tree-al	S/ R/ S/	-um *structure* atri- *entrance, atrium* -al *pertaining to*	Chamber where blood enters the heart on both the right and left sides Pertaining to the atrium
bicuspid	by-**KUSS**-pid	S/ P/ R/	-id *having a particular quality* bi- *two* -cusp- *point*	Having two points; a bicuspid heart valve has two flaps
interatrial	**IN**-ter-**AY**-tree-al	S/ P/ R/	-al *pertaining to* inter- *between* -atri- *atrium*	Between the atria of the heart
interventricular (IV)	**IN**-ter-ven-**TRIK**-you-lar	S/ P/ R/	-ar *pertaining to* inter- *between* -ventricul- *ventricle*	Between the ventricles of the heart
mitral	**MY**-tral		Latin *turban*	Shaped like the headdress of a Catholic bishop
septum septa (pl)	**SEP**-tum **SEP**-tah		Latin *partition*	A thin wall dividing two cavities
tricuspid	try-**KUSS**-pid	S/ P/ R/	-id *having a particular quality* tri- *three* -cusp- *point*	Having three points; a tricuspid heart valve has three flaps
ventricle	**VEN**-trih-kel		Latin *small belly*	Chamber of the heart (pumps blood) or a cavity in the brain (produces cerebrospinal fluid)

Study Hint

Try to relate these same prefixes to common English words. It will help you remember the meaning of the prefix in the medical terms.

Exercises

A. Define *the words in bold using the correct medical term. Use the terms related to the function and structure of the heart to correctly complete each statement.* **LO 6.2 and 6.4**

The right side of the heart pumps blood through arteries to the **lungs** to pick up oxygen. The left side of the heart pumps blood through arteries to deliver oxygenated blood to the organs of each body **system**.

1. The right side of the heart pumps blood to the ______ circulation.
2. The left side of the heart pumps blood to the ______ circulation.

When learning how to ride a bike, children might first learn to ride a **three**-wheeled cycle, and then learn to ride a **two**-wheeled cycle.

When learning blood flow through the heart, students usually start with the right side of the heart and trace flow to the left side of the heart.

3. Blood returns from the systemic circulation and passes through the ______/cuspid valve.
4. Blood returns from the pulmonary circulation and passes through the ______/cuspid valve.

B. Plurals of medical terms *follow established rules. Apply these rules and change the singular form of each terms to its plural form.* **LO 6.2**

1. Singular: **atrium** Plural: ________________
2. Singular: **septum** Plural: ________________
3. Singular: **vena cava** Plural: ________________
4. Singular: **ventricle** Plural: ________________

C. Meet lesson objectives *and use the language of cardiology to answer the following questions.* **LO 6.2, 6.4, and 6.6**

1. Name the four chambers in the heart. ________________
2. List the four valves in the heart. ________________
3. What is the function of a valve? ________________
4. What is the purpose of the systemic circulation? ________________

Keynotes

- **Vital signs (VS) measure temperature (T), pulse (P), respiration (R), and blood pressure (BP) to assess cardiorespiratory function.**
- **A heart rate slower than 60 is called bradycardia. *(Figure 6.9)* A heart rate faster than 100 is called tachycardia *(Figure 6.10)*.**

Abbreviations

AV	atrioventricular
BP	blood pressure
P	pulse
R	respiration
SA	sinoatrial
T	temperature
VS	vital signs

The Heartbeat (LO 6.4 and 6.5)

The actions of the four heart chambers are coordinated. When the atria contract (atrial **systole**), the ventricles relax (ventricular **diastole**). When the atria relax (atrial diastole), the ventricles contract (ventricular systole). Then the atria and ventricles all relax briefly. This series of events is a complete cardiac cycle, or heartbeat.

The "lub-dub, lub-dub" sounds heard through the stethoscope are made by the heart valves snapping as they close. If there is an abnormality in valve closure, it will produce an extra, abnormal sound called a **murmur.**

Electrical Properties of the Heart (LO 6.4 and 6.5)

As your heart muscles contract, they generate a small electrical current that sustains your heartbeat rhythm through a conduction system *(Figure 6.7)*. Here is how this conduction system works:

1. A small region of specialized muscle cells in the right atrium's **sinoatrial (SA) node** initiates your heartbeat. The SA node is the **pacemaker** of your heart's rhythm.
2. Electrical signals from the SA node spread out through the atria and rejoin at the **atrioventricular (AV) node.** The AV is the electrical gateway to the ventricles.
3. Electrical signals leave the AV node and travel to the ventricular myocardium where they stimulate the ventricular myocardium to contract, creating your heartbeat.

Sinus rhythm is the term used to describe a normal heartbeat, where normal electrical conduction leads to a ventricular rate of about 60 to 80 beats per minute. An abnormal cardiac rhythm is called an **arrhythmia** or a **dysrhythmia.**

An **electrocardiograph** is a device that picks up the heart muscle's electrical changes and amplifies them to record an electrocardiogram in the form of waves *(Figure 6.8)*.

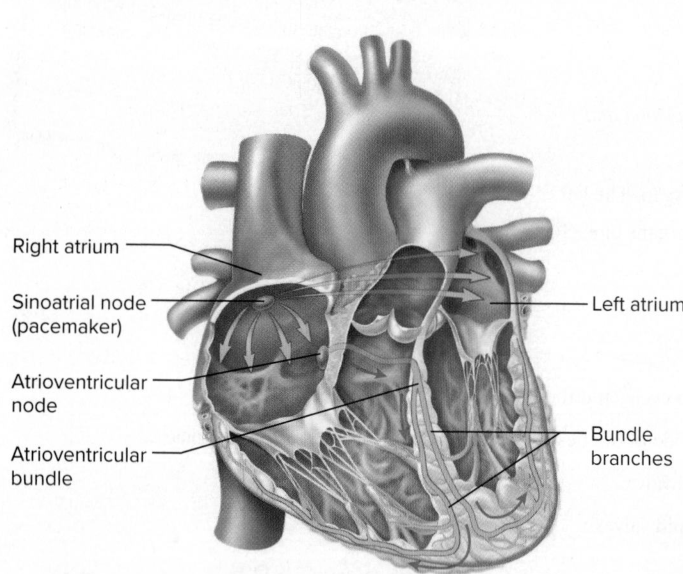

▲ **FIGURE 6.7**
Cardiac Conduction System.

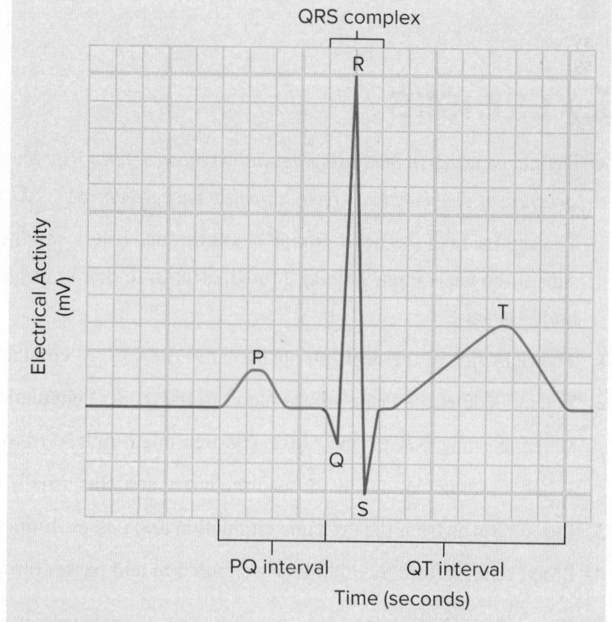

▲ **FIGURE 6.8**
Normal Electrocardiogram.

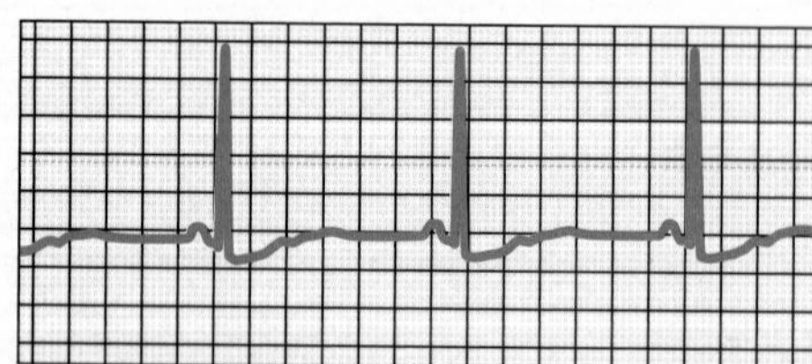

▲ **FIGURE 6.9**
Bradycardia.

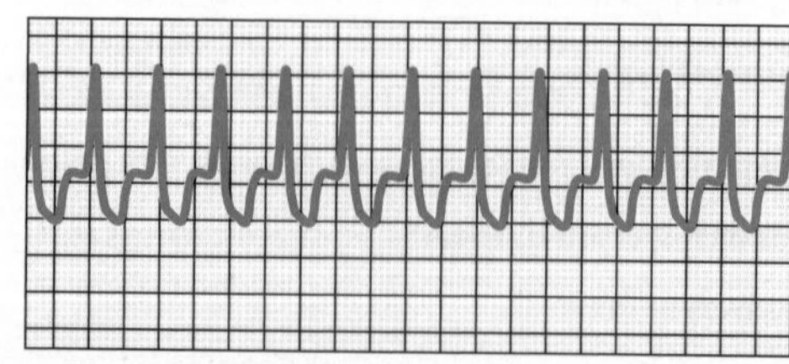

▲ **FIGURE 6.10**
Tachycardia.

Word Analysis and Definition

S = Suffix P = Prefix R = Root R/CF = Combining Form

WORD	PRONUNCIATION	ELEMENTS		DEFINITION
arrhythmia **(Note:** *double "rr"*)	a-**RITH**-me-ah	S/ P/ R/	-ia *condition* a- *without* -rrhythm- *rhythm*	Condition when the heart rhythm is abnormal
atrioventricular (AV)	A-tree-oh-ven-**TRICK**-you-lar	S/ R/CF R/	-ar *pertaining to* atri/o- *entrance, atrium* -ventricul- *ventricle*	Pertaining to both the atrium and the ventricle
bradycardia	**BRAY**-dih-kard-ia	S/ R/ P/	-ia condition -card- *heart* brady- *slow*	Condition of slow heart beat
diastole (noun) **diastolic (adj)**	die-**AS**-toe-lee die-as-**TOL**-ik	 S/ R/	Greek *dilation* -ic *pertaining to* diastol- *diastole*	Dilation of heart cavities, during which they fill with blood Pertaining to diastole
dysrhythmia **(Note:** *single "r"*)	dis-**RITH**-me-ah	S/ P/ R/	-ia condition dys- *bad, difficult* -rhythm- *rhythm*	An abnormal heart rhythm
murmur	**MUR**-mur		Latin *low voice*	Abnormal heart sound heard with a stethoscope when a valve closes or opens abnormally
sinoatrial (SA) node	sigh-noh-**AY**-tree-al NODE	S/ R/CF R/	-al *pertaining to* sin/o- *sinus* -atri- *atrium*	The center of modified cardiac muscle fibers in the wall of the right atrium that acts as the pacemaker for the heart rhythm
sinus rhythm	**SIGH**-nus **RITH**-um		sinus Latin *channel, cavity* rhythm Greek *to flow*	The normal (optimal) heart rhythm arising from the sinoatrial node
systole (noun) **systolic (adj)**	**SIS**-toe-lee sis-**TOL**-ik	 S/ R/	Greek *contraction* -ic *pertaining to* systol- *systole, contraction*	Contraction of the heart muscle Pertaining to systole
tachycardia	**TAK**-ih-kard-ia	S/ R/ P/	-ia *condition* -card- *heart* tachy- *rapid*	Condition of rapid heart beat
vital signs (VS)	**VI**-tal SIGNS		vital Latin *life* signs Latin *mark*	A procedure during a physical examination in which temperature (T), pulse (P), respirations (R), and blood pressure (BP) are measured to assess general health and cardiorespiratory function

EXERCISES

A. Match *the correct element to its meaning.* **LO 6.1**

_____ **1.** atrio	**a.** without
_____ **2.** ar	**b.** contraction
_____ **3.** ia	**c.** bad, difficult
_____ **4.** systol	**d.** entrance
_____ **5.** dys	**e.** condition
_____ **6.** a	**f.** pertaining to

B. Spelling: *The following terms commonly occur in the cardiology department. Select the correct choice for the documentation.* **LO 6.4 and 6.5**

1. An (arhythmia/arrhythmia) has been confirmed with the EKG.

2. Her (sysstolic/systolic) blood pressure is dangerously high.

3. The (murrmur/murmur) was detected during ventricular (dyastole/diastole).

4. Cardiac (dysrrhythmia/dysrhythmia) can be a symptom of a serious underlying condition.

5. The (sinoatrial/synoatrial) node is the pacemaker for the heart rhythm.

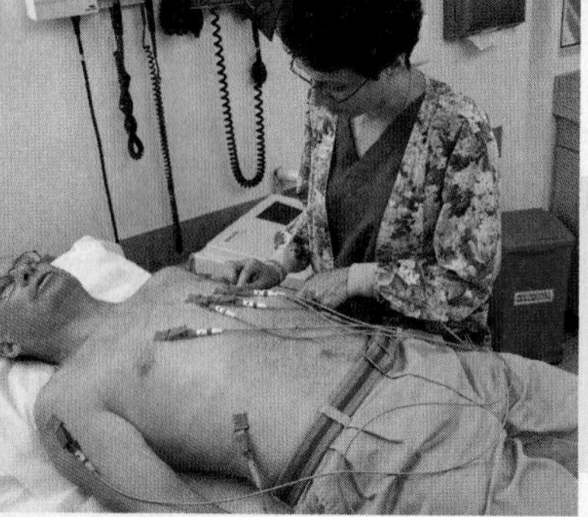

Rick Brady/McGraw-Hill Education

Lesson 6.2

Disorders of the Heart

Objectives

Any loss of consciousness precipitated by exertion can be due to a cardiac arrhythmia or a ***cardiomyopathy.*** *In this lesson, the information will enable you to:*

6.2.1 Name common cardiac arrhythmias.

6.2.2 Discuss common disorders of the heart and heart valves.

6.2.3 Describe coronary heart disease.

6.2.4 Explain hypertensive heart disease.

6.2.5 Define the term *cardiomyopathy.*

CASE REPORT 6.2

You are . . .

. . . an EMT-P called to the gymnasium of Fulwood University.

You are communicating with . . .

. . . Danny Gitlin, a 21-year-old guard on the university basketball team. Danny lost consciousness during a strenuous practice. He had no pulse but was revived by the coach, who used an automatic external **defibrillator (AED).** Danny has never lost consciousness before, but he has noticed episodes of rapid **palpitations** after games. On examination, he is fully conscious and appears to be fit. His pulse is 70 but irregular in rate and force. His blood pressure is 110/65 mmHg. He has no known family history of heart disease.

Abbreviations

AED	automatic external defibrillator
A-fib	atrial fibrillation
EMT-P	Emergency Medical Technician–Paramedic
ICD	implantable cardioverter/defibrillator
PVC	premature ventricular contraction
V-fib	ventricular fibrillation
V-tach	ventricular tachycardia

Disorders of the Heart

(LO 6.4 and 6.5)

Abnormal Heart Rhythms (LO 6.5)

Arrhythmias are abnormal or irregular heartbeats, and six types are commonly seen:

1. **Premature beats** occur most often in elderly people and are usually associated with caffeine and stress.
2. **Atrial fibrillation (A-fib)** occurs when the two atria quiver rather than contract correctly to pump blood. This causes blood to pool in the atria and sometimes clot.
3. **Ventricular tachycardia (V-tach)** is a rapid heartbeat occurring in the ventricles.
4. **Ventricular arrhythmias** include:
   a. **Premature ventricular contractions (PVCs),** which result when extra impulses arise from a ventricle; and
   b. **Ventricular fibrillation (V-fib),** which occurs when the ventricles lose control, quivering instead of pumping.
5. **Heart block** occurs when interference in cardiac electrical conduction prevents the atria's contractions from coordinating with the ventricles' contractions.
6. **Palpitations** are brief but unpleasant sensations of a rapid or irregular heartbeat. They can be brought on by exercise, anxiety, and stimulants like caffeine.

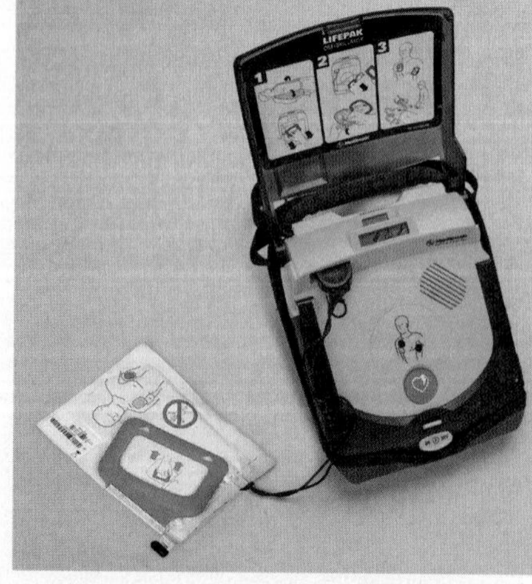

▶ **FIGURE 6.11** Automatic External Defibrillator.

Rick Brady/McGraw-Hill Education

Arrhythmias can be treated with medications, but some patients require mechanical **pacemakers.** Pacemakers consist of a battery, electronic circuits, and computer memory to generate electronic signals. These signals are carried along thin, insulated wires to the heart muscle. Pacemakers are ideal for patients with a very slow heart rate (bradycardia).

In emergency situations, external **defibrillation** is performed through **automatic external defibrillators,** or **AEDs** *(Figure 6.11).* AEDs send an electric shock to the heart in order to stop the heart temporarily so that a normal contraction rhythm can resume. This procedure was used for Danny Gitlin.

People with life-threatening arrhythmias may need an **implantable defibrillator (ICD),** which senses abnormal rhythms. An ICD gives the heart a small electric shock to return its rhythm to normal.

Defibrillation is the nonsynchronized delivery of energy to the heart during any phase of the cardiac cycle used in emergency situations. **Cardioversion** is the delivery of lower levels of energy synchronized to the large R waves of the QRS complex and is mostly used for A-fib or flutter and V-tach.

Word Analysis and Definition

S = Suffix P = Prefix R = Root R/CF = Combining Form

WORD	PRONUNCIATION	ELEMENTS		DEFINITION
cardioversion	**KAR**-dee-oh-**VER**-zhun	S/ R/CF	-version *change* cardi/o- *heart*	Restoration of a normal heart rhythm by electric shock or medications
defibrillation defibrillator	dee-fib-rih-**LAY**-shun dee-**FIB**-rih-lay-tor	S/ P/ R/ S/	-ation *process* de- *from, out of* -fibrill- *small fiber* -ator *instrument*	Restoration of normal cardiac activity in life-threatening cardiac arrhythmias Instrument for defibrillation
fibrillation	fi-brih-**LAY**-shun	S/ R/	-ation *a process* fibrill- *small fiber*	Uncontrolled quivering or twitching of the heart muscle
implantable	im-**PLAN**-tah-bul	S/ P/ R/	-able *capable* im- *in* -plant- *insert*	A device that can be inserted into tissues
pacemaker	**PACE**-may-ker	S/ R/	-maker *one who makes* pace- *step*	Device that regulates cardiac electrical activity
palpitation	pal-pih-**TAY**-shun	S/ R/	-ation *a process* palpit- *throb*	Forcible, rapid beat of the heart felt by the patient

EXERCISES

A. Review *Case Report 6.2 and correctly answer the following questions. Select the correct answer to complete the statement or answer the question.* **LO 6.3, 6.7, and 6.8**

1. When a person *loses consciousness,* they:
   - **a.** are not aware of their surroundings and cannot be aroused.
   - **b.** appear to be asleep and are easily aroused.
   - **c.** have no pulse.
   - **d.** have a have a rapid heartbeat.
2. What seems to be the trigger for causing his symptoms?
   - **a.** high temperature
   - **b.** increased physical activity
   - **c.** dehydration
   - **d.** lack of exercise
3. How might Danny describe his *palpitations?*
   - **a.** "I have times that I black out and forget what has happened."
   - **b.** "I feel like my heart quits beating for a moment."
   - **c.**"I have a dizzy feeling that makes me feel like I will faint."
   - **d.**"My heart beats hard and feels like it is beating out of my chest."
4. Which of the following describes an AED?
   - **a.** blood pressure is measured by a machine
   - **b.** the heart rate is counted by a computer
   - **c.** machine displays the electrical activity of the heart
   - **d.** machine determines when to deliver an electrical shock to the heart

B. Construct *the correct medical terms to match the definitions given. If a term does not have a particular element, insert N/A on that blank. Fill in the blanks.* **LO 6.1, 6.4, and 6.5**

1. Forceful, rapid beat of the heart

   ______________ / ______________ / ______________
   P R/CF S

2. Uncontrolled heart muscle twitching

   ______________ / ______________ / ______________
   P R/CF S

3. Device that restores uncontrolled twitching of cardiac muscle to normal rhythm

   ______________ / ______________ / ______________
   P R/CF S

4. Implanted device that regulates cardiac electrical activity

   ______________ / ______________ / ______________
   P R/CF S

Lesson 6.2 (cont'd)

Keynotes

- **Cor pulmonale is failure of the right ventricle to pump properly. Almost any chronic lung disease causing low blood oxygen (hypoxia) can cause this disorder.**
- **Malfunctions of the valves on the right side of the heart are much less common than those on the left side.**

Disorders of the Heart (continued)

Disorders of Heart Valves (LO 6.4)

The heart valves can malfunction in two basic ways. Malfunctions most often occur in the heart's left side.

1. **Stenosis:** The valve cannot open fully, and its opening is narrowed (constricted). Because blood cannot flow freely through the valve, it accumulates in the chamber behind the valve.
2. **Incompetence** or **insufficiency** is a condition where the heart valve cannot close fully, allowing blood to leak or **regurgitate** (flow back) through the valve to the heart chamber from which it came.

Mitral valve stenosis can occur following rheumatic fever. Because the blood cannot flow freely through the valve, the left atrium becomes dilated (enlarged). Eventually, chronic heart failure results.

Mitral valve prolapse (MVP) occurs when the cusps of the valve bulge back into the left atrium when the left ventricle contracts. This allows blood to flow back into the atrium.

Aortic valve stenosis is common in the elderly when the valves become calcified due to atherosclerosis. Blood flow into the systemic circulation is diminished, leading to dizziness and fainting. The left ventricle dilates, **hypertrophies,** ceases to beat strongly, and ultimately fails.

Aortic valve incompetence initially produces few symptoms other than a murmur. Eventually the left ventricle is unable to cope with the excess volume of blood and fails. *(Figure 6.12* enables you to review the locations of the valves and chambers.)

When a valve replacement is necessary, there are two types of artificial valves available:

1. Mechanical or **prosthetic** valves, which are made from metal alloys and plastics; or
2. **Tissue** valves, which can come from a pig or cow, a human cadaver (dead person), or a patient's own pericardium.

Disorders of the Heart Wall (LO 6.4)

Endocarditis is an inflammation of the heart's lining, which is usually secondary to an infection elsewhere. Intravenous drug users and people with damaged heart valves are at high risk for endocarditis.

Case Report 6.2 *(continued)*

The physical findings on Danny Gitlin suggested a **cardiomyopathy**, which was confirmed by echocardiography. Exercise testing (a cardiac stress test), with close medical supervision, produced a ventricular arrhythmia that returned to normal on cessation of the test. Danny was treated with beta blockers and restricted to nonstrenuous sports.

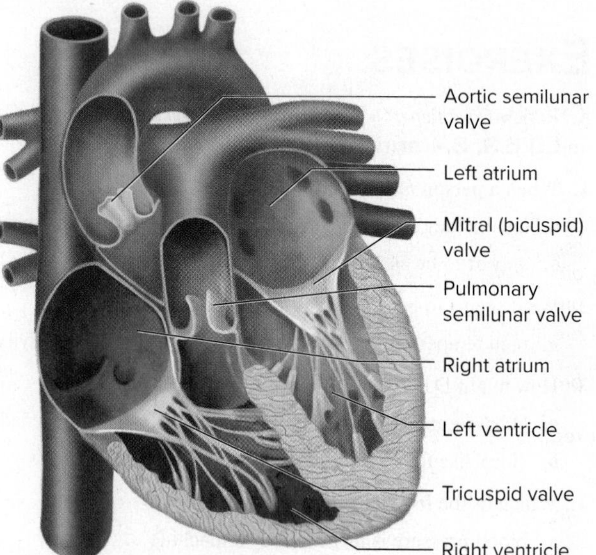

▲ **FIGURE 6.12**
Heart Valves.

Myocarditis is an inflammation of the heart muscle. It can be bacterial, viral, or fungal in origin, or can arise as a complication of other diseases like influenza.

Pericarditis is inflammation of the covering of the heart. The inflammation causes an **exudate** (pericardial effusion) to be released into the pericardial space between the two layers of the pericardium. This interferes with the heart's ability to contract and expand normally, which reduces cardiac output **(CO)** and leads to a life-threatening condition called **cardiac tamponade.**

Cardiomyopathy is a weakening of the heart muscle that makes it pump inadequately. This causes the heart to enlarge **(cardiomegaly)** and leads to heart failure.

Abbreviations

CO	cardiac output
MVP	mitral valve prolapse

Word Analysis and Definition

S = Suffix P = Prefix R = Root R/CF = Combining Form

WORD	PRONUNCIATION	ELEMENTS		DEFINITION
cardiomegaly	**KAR**-dee-oh-**MEG**-ah-lee	S/ R/CF	**-megaly** *enlargement* **cardi/o-** *heart*	Enlargement of the heart
cardiomyopathy	**KAR**-dee-oh-my-**OP**-ah-thee	S/ R/CF R/CF	**-pathy** *disease* **cardi/o** *-heart* **-my/o-** *muscle*	Disease of the heart muscle, the myocardium
cor pulmonale	**KOR** pul-moh-**NAH**-lee	 S/ R/	**cor** Latin *heart* **-ale** *pertaining to* **pulmon-** *lung*	Right-sided heart failure arising from chronic lung disease
endocarditis (**Note:** The extra "i" from the root *cardi* is dropped when joined to the suffix *-itis.)*	**EN**-doh-kar-**DIE**-tis	S/ P/ R/	**-itis** *inflammation* **endo-** *within* **-cardi-** *heart*	Inflammation of the lining of the heart
exudate	**EKS**-you-date	S/ P/ R/	**-ate** *pertaining to* **ex-** *out of* **-sud-** *sweat*	Fluid that has passed out of a tissue or capillaries as a result of inflammation or injury
hypertrophy (can be a noun or a verb)	high-**PER**-troh-fee	P/ R/	**hyper-** *above, excessive* **-trophy** *development*	Increase in size, but not in number, of an individual tissue element
incompetence	in-**KOM**-peh-tense	S/ P/ R/	**-ence** *quality of* **in-** *not* **-compet-** *strive together*	Failure of a valve to close completely
insufficiency	in-suh-**FISH**-en-see	S/ P/ R/CF	**-ency** *quality of* **in-** *not* **–suffic/i-** *enough*	Lack of completeness of function; e.g., a heart valve that fails to close properly
myocarditis (**Note:** The extra "i" from the root *cardi* is dropped when joined to the suffix *-itis.)*	**MY**-oh-kar-**DIE**-tis	S/ R/CF R/	**-itis** *inflammation* **my/o-** *muscle* **-cardi-** *heart*	Inflammation of the heart muscle
pericarditis (**Note:** The extra "i" from the root *cardi* is dropped when joined to the suffix *-itis.)*	**PER**-ih-kar-**DIE**-tis	S/ P/ R/	**-itis** *inflammation* **peri-** *around* **-cardi-** *heart*	Inflammation of the pericardium, the covering of the heart
prolapse	pro-**LAPS**		Latin *a falling*	An organ slips out of its normal position
prosthesis (noun) prosthetic (adj)	pros-**THEE**-sis pros-**THET**-ik	 S/ R/	Greek *an addition* **-ic** *pertaining to* **prosthet-** *artificial part*	A manufactured substitute for a missing or diseased part of the body Pertaining to a prosthesis
regurgitate	ree-**GUR**-jih-tate	S/ P/ R/	**-ate** *pertaining to* **re-** *back* **-gurgit-** *flood*	To flow backward; e.g., blood through a heart valve
stenosis	ste-**NOH**-sis	S/ R/CF	**-sis** *abnormal condition* **sten/o-** *narrow*	Narrowing of a canal or passage, e.g., of a heart valve
tamponade	tam-poh-**NAID**	S/ R/	**-ade** *a process* **tampon-** *plug*	Pathologic compression of an organ, such as the heart

Exercises

A. Use your knowledge *of the language of cardiology to match the description in the left column with the correct medical term in the right column. Match the term to its correct meaning.* **LO 6.4**

______	**1.** Weakening of heart muscle	**a.** prolapse
______	**2.** Inflammation that causes exudates	**b.** cardiomegaly
______	**3.** Cusps of valve bulge back into atrium	**c.** cor pulmonale
______	**4.** Constricted valve opening	**d.** pericarditis
______	**5.** Failure of right ventricle to pump properly	**e.** stenosis
______	**6.** Cardiomyopathy can be the cause	**f.** cardiomyopathy

B. Spell *the term that correctly completes each statement.* **LO 6.2 and 6.4**

1. The MVP caused the blood to ______ into the left atrium.

2. In heart disease, the left ventricle can ______ in an effort to increase CO.

3. Right heart failure is termed _______.

4. Inflammation of the tissue lining the inside of the heart is termed ________.

Keynotes

- **Risk factors for CAD include:**
  - **Heredity**
  - **Age**
  - **Obesity**
  - **Lack of exercise**
  - **Tobacco**
  - **Diabetes mellitus**
  - **Stress**
  - **High blood pressure**
  - **Elevated serum cholesterol**
- **All these risk factors—except heredity and age—can be reduced by lifestyle changes.**

Coronary Artery Disease (CAD) (LO 6.5)

Coronary artery disease occurs when the coronary arteries supplying blood to the myocardium are constricted by **atherosclerotic plaques** called **atheroma** (compare *Figure 6.13(a)* to *6.13(b)*). This reduces the blood supply to the cardiac muscle. Platelet clumping can occur on the plaque and form a blood clot **(coronary thrombosis). Atherosclerosis** is the most common form of **arteriosclerosis** (hardening of the arteries), and it can lead to **arteriosclerotic** heart disease **(ASHD).**

Case Report 6.1 (continued)

For Mr. Johnson in the Emergency Department, the ECG (EKG) indicated that he was having an MI affecting the anterior wall of his left ventricle. The cardiovascular technician, who did not want to leave the patient alone, used the call system to obtain nursing and medical help.

Angina pectoris (pain in the chest on exertion) is often the first symptom of a reduced oxygen supply to the myocardium. **Myocardial infarction (MI)** is the death of myocardial cells, caused by the lack of blood supply **(ischemia)** when an artery eventually becomes blocked **(occluded).** If the ischemia is not reversed within 4 to 6 hours, the myocardial cells die **(necrosis).**

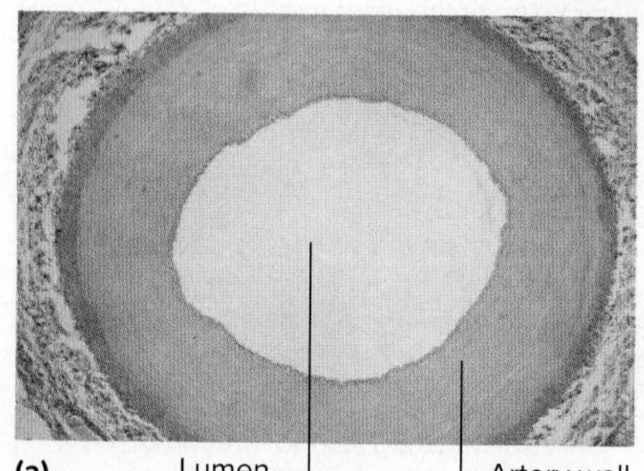

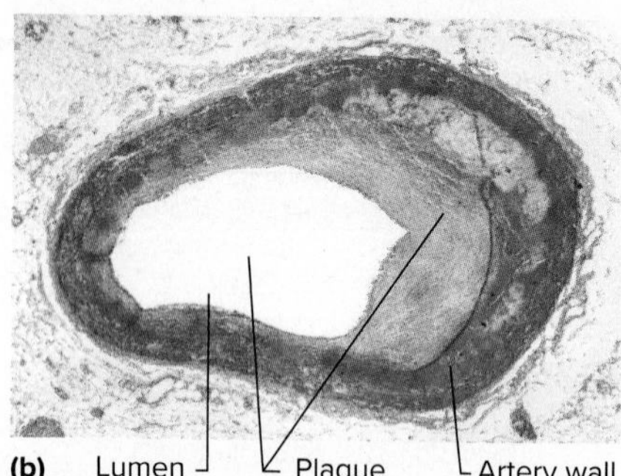

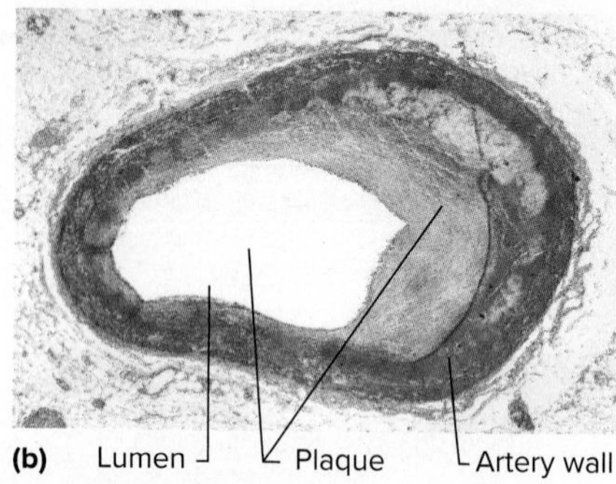

▲ **FIGURE 6.13**
Arterial Structure.
(a) Normal coronary artery.
(b) Advanced atherosclerosis.

Shock is a life-threatening condition that occurs when the body is not getting sufficient blood flow; this can damage multiple organs. A classification of shock includes:

- **Cardiogenic shock** occurs when the heart fails to pump blood effectively through the body's organs and tissues.
- **Hypovolemic shock** occurs from a loss of blood volume, often due to excessive bleeding (hemorrhage) or dehydration.
- **Anaphylactic shock** is caused by a severe allergic reaction.
- **Septic shock** is caused by a severe infection.
- **Neurogenic shock** is associated with damage to the nervous system.

Cardiac arrest is the sudden cessation of cardiac activity that results from **anoxia** (lack of oxygen in the body tissues). Most patients show **asystole** (no heartbeat) on the cardiac monitor *(Figure 6.14).* A person in cardiac arrest has no pulse, is not breathing, and can be referred to as a **pulseless nonbreather (PNB).**

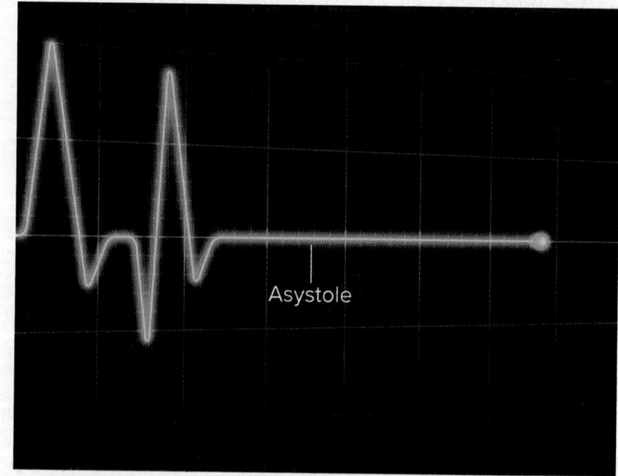

▶ **FIGURE 6.14**
Electrocardiogram (ECG) Showing Asystole.
angelhell/Getty Images

Abbreviations

ASHD	arteriosclerotic heart disease
CAD	coronary artery disease
MI	myocardial infarction
PNB	pulseless nonbreather

Word Analysis and Definition

S = Suffix P = Prefix R = Root R/CF = Combining Form

WORD	PRONUNCIATION	ELEMENTS		DEFINITION
anoxia (noun) **anoxic (adj)**	an-**OCK**-see-ah an-**OCK**-sik	S/ P/ R/ S/	-ia *condition* an- *without* -ox- *oxygen* -ic *pertaining to*	Without oxygen Pertaining to or suffering from lack of oxygen
arteriosclerosis **arteriosclerotic (adj)**	ar-**TIER**-ee-oh-skler-**OH**-sis ar-**TIER**-ee-oh-skler-**OT**-ik	S/ R/CF R/CF S/	-sis *abnormal condition* arteri/o- *artery* -scler/o- *hardness* -tic *pertaining to*	Hardening of the arteries Pertaining to or affected by arteriosclerosis
asystole	a-**SIS**-toe-lee	P/ R/CF	a- *without* -systol/e *contraction*	Absence of contractions of the heart
atheroma (plaque) **atherectomy** **atherosclerosis**	ath-er-**ROE**-mah ath-er-**EK**-toe-me **ATH**-er-oh-skler-**OH**-sis	S/ R/ S/ S/ R/CF R/CF	-oma *tumor, mass* ather- *porridge, gruel* -ectomy *surgical excision* -sis *abnormal condition* ather/o- *porridge, gruel* -scler/o- *hardness*	Fatty deposit in the lining of an artery Surgical removal of the atheroma Hardening of the arteries due to atheroma (plaque)
cardiogenic	**KAR**-dee-oh-**JEN**-ik	S/ R/CF R/	-ic *pertaining to* cardi/o- *heart* -gen- *produce*	Of cardiac origin
hypovolemia **hypovolemic**	**HIGH**-poh-vo-**LEE**-me-ah **HIGH**-poh-vo-**LEE**-mik	S/ S/ P/ R/ S/	-emia *a blood condition* -emic *a condition in the blood* hypo- *below* -vol- *volume* -ic *pertaining to*	Decreased blood volume in the body Pertaining to a decreased blood volume in the body
occlude (verb) **occlusion (noun)**	oh-**KLUDE** oh-**KLU**-zhun		Latin *to close*	To close, plug, or completely obstruct A complete obstruction
substernal	sub-**STER**-nal	S/ P/ R/	-al *pertaining to* sub- *under* -stern- *chest*	Under (behind) the sternum or breastbone

Exercises

A. Review *Case Report 6.1 (continued) and answer the following questions. Select the correct answer.* **LO 6.3, 6.4, 6.7, and 6.8**

1. What specific place in Mr. Johnson's heart was affected by his MI?

a. posterior wall of his left ventricle
b. anterior wall of his left ventricle
c. anterior wall of his right ventricle
d. posterior wall of his left ventricle

2. What does an MI do to the living tissue in Mr. Johnson's heart?

a. increases oxygen delivery to myocardial cells
b. causes death to myocardial cells
c. produces myocardial hypertrophy
d. results in valve insufficiency

3. The device that indicated that Mr. Johnson was having an MI is the:

a. echocardiograph
b. automatic electronic defibrillator
c. electrocardiogram
d. patient call system

B. Precision *in communication and documention is required for patient safety in health care. Match the term in the first column with its correct definition in the second column.* **LO 6.6**

_____ **1.** arteriosclerosis — **a.** fatty deposit in an artery
_____ **2.** atherosclerosis — **b.** hardening of an artery due to a fatty deposit
_____ **3.** atheroma — **c.** hardening of an artery

Keynotes

- Hypertension is the major cause of heart failure, stroke, and kidney failure.
- The risk factors for hypertension are:
  - Overweight
  - Alcohol
  - Lack of exercise
  - Tobacco
  - Stress
- All these risk factors can be reduced by lifestyle changes.

Disorders of the Heart (continued)

Hypertensive Heart Disease (LO 6.4 and 6.5)

Hypertension (HTN), the most common cardiovascular disorder in this country, affects more than 20% of the adult population. It results from a prolonged elevated blood pressure in the vascular system, which forces the ventricles to work harder to pump blood.

High blood pressure is indicated by a blood pressure reading of 140/90 mmHg (millimeters of mercury) or higher. A normal blood pressure is below 120/80 mmHg. The first number, or **systolic** reading, reflects the blood pressure when the heart is contracting. The second number, or **diastolic** reading, reflects the blood pressure when the heart is relaxed between contractions.

Primary or **essential hypertension** is the most common type of hypertension. Its etiology is **idiopathic** (unknown).

Secondary hypertension results from other diseases like kidney disease, atherosclerosis, and hyperthyroidism.

Malignant hypertension is a rare, severe, life-threatening form of hypertension that involves a blood pressure reading of greater than 200/120 mmHg. Aggressive intervention is mandatory to reduce the blood pressure.

Congestive Heart Failure (CHF) (LO 6.4 and 6.5)

CHF occurs when the heart is unable to supply enough cardiac output to meet the body's metabolic needs, and the blood backs up to congest the lungs. The most common conditions leading to CHF are:

- Cardiac ischemia
- Severe hypertension
- Valvular regurgitation
- Aortic stenosis
- Cardiomyopathy

Congenital Heart Disease (CHD) (LO 6.4)

CHD is the result of an abnormal development of the heart in the fetus. Common **congenital** defects or abnormalities can usually be surgically repaired, and can include the following:

1. **Atrial septal defect (ASD)** is a hole in the interatrial septum *(Figure 6.15).*
2. **Ventricular septal defect (VSD)** is a gap in the interventricular septum *(Figure 6.15).*
3. **Patent ductus arteriosus (PDA)** arises from a failure of the ductus arteriosus (a normal blood vessel in the fetus) to close within 24 hours of birth.
4. **Coarctation of the aorta** is a narrowing of the aorta anywhere along its length. This causes **hypertension** in the arms behind the narrowing and **hypotension** in the lower limbs and organs (like the kidney) below the narrowing.
5. **Tetralogy of Fallot** (**TOF**) is a **syndrome** in which four congenital heart defects prevent enough blood from reaching the lungs. TOF occurs in about 5 out of every 10,000 newborns. Babies and children with TOF have episodes of cyanosis and are often called "blue babies." Treatment is with open heart surgery soon after birth or in infancy.

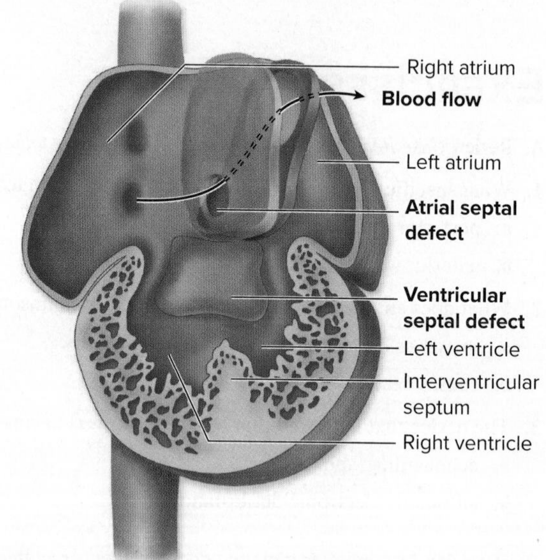

▲ **FIGURE 6.15**
Atrial and Ventricular Septal Defects.

Abbreviations

ASD	atrial septal defect
CHD	congenital heart disease
CHF	congestive heart failure
HTN	hypertension
PDA	patent ductus arteriosus
TOF	tetralogy of Fallot
VSD	ventricular septal defect

Word Analysis and Definition

S = Suffix P = Prefix R = Root R/CF = Combining Form

WORD	PRONUNCIATION	ELEMENTS		DEFINITION
coarctation	koh-ark-**TAY**-shun	S/ R/	-ation *process* coarct- *press together, narrow*	Constriction, stenosis, particularly of the aorta
congenital	kon-**JEN**-ih-tal	S/ P/ R/	-al *pertaining to* con- *together, with* -genit- *bring forth*	Present at birth, either inherited or due to an event during gestation up to the moment of birth
cyanosis	sigh-ah-**NO**-sis	S/ R/	-osis *condition* cyan- dark blue	Blue discoloration of the skin, lips, and nail beds due to low blood oxygen
hypertension hypotension	**HIGH**-per-**TEN**-shun **HIGH**-poh-**TEN**-shun	S/ P/ R/ P/	-ion *condition, action* hyper- *excessive* -tens- *pressure* hypo- *low*	Persistent high arterial blood pressure Persistent low arterial blood pressure
idiopathic	**ID**-ih-oh-**PATH**-ik	S/ R/CF R/	-ic *pertaining to* idi/o- *unknown* -path- *disease*	Pertaining to a disease of unknown etiology
patent ductus arteriosus (PDA) (**Note:** *This term is composed only of roots.*)	**PAY**-tent **DUK**-tus ar-ter-ee-**OH**-sus		patent Latin *lie open* ductus Latin *leading* arteriosus Latin *artery*	An open, direct channel between the aorta and the pulmonary artery in the newborn
syndrome	**SIN**-drohm	P/ R/	syn- *together* -drome *running*	Combination of signs and symptoms associated with a particular disease process
tetralogy of Fallot (TOF)	te-**TRA**-loh-jee of fah-**LOW**	P/ R/	tetra- *four* -logy *study of* Etienne-Louis Fallot, French physician, 1850–1911	Set of four congenital heart defects occurring together

EXERCISES

A. Abbreviations *need to be used carefully so that you communicate exactly what is necessary. Match the abbreviation to the correct condition it describes.* **LO 6.3, 6.4, and 6.5**

_____ **1.** ASD **a.** force of blood pushing on the vessel walls

_____ **2.** TOF **b.** artery remains open instead of normally closing after birth

_____ **3.** VSD **c.** chronic elevated blood pressure

_____ **4.** PDA **d.** congenital heart defect that is made up of four congenital abnormalities

_____ **5.** CHF **e.** abnormal opening between the atria

_____ **6.** BP **f.** abnormal opening between the ventricles

_____ **7.** HTN **g.** heart is unable to pump enough blood to meet the body's needs

Lesson 6.2 (cont'd)

Keynotes

- **A Holter monitor *(Figure 6.16)* is a continuous ECG recorded on a tape-recorder cassette as you work, play, and rest for at least 24 hours.**
- **An ambulatory blood pressure monitor provides a record of your blood pressure over a 24-hour period as you go about your daily activities.**

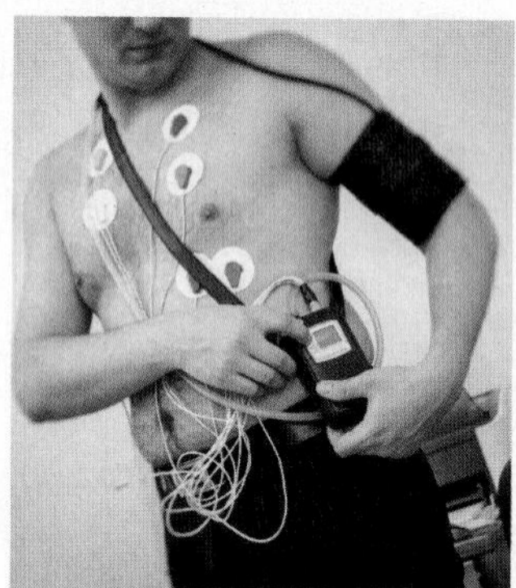

▲ FIGURE 6.16
Holter Monitor.

Lena Ivanova/Shutterstock

Abbreviations

CABG	coronary artery bypass graft
ECG or EKG	electrocardiogram
HDL	high-density lipoprotein
LDL	low-density lipoprotein
MI	myocardial infarction
MRI	magnetic resonance imaging
PTCA	percutaneous transluminal coronary angioplasty

Diagnostic and Therapeutic Procedures and Pharmacology (LO 6.3 and 6.7)

Blood Tests (LO 6.2, 6.3, and 6.7)

A **lipid profile** helps determine the risk of CAD and comprises:

- Total cholesterol;
- High-density **lipoprotein (HDL)** ("good cholesterol");
- Low-density lipoprotein **(LDL)** ("bad cholesterol"); and
- **Triglycerides.**

Troponin I and **T** are part of a protein complex in muscle that is released into the blood during a muscle injury. Troponin I is found in heart muscle but not in skeletal muscle, which makes it a highly-sensitive indicator of a recent MI.

Diagnostic Tests (LO 6.3 and 6.7)

Several diagnostic tests are used to measure heart health.

An **electrocardiogram (ECG** or **EKG)** is a paper record of the electrical signals of your heart.

Cardiac stress testing is an exercise tolerance test that raises your heart rate through exercise (like jogging on a treadmill) and monitors its effect on cardiac function. **Nuclear imaging** of the heart, which involves the injection of a radioactive substance, can be used with the stress test.

Echocardiography uses ultrasound waves to study cardiac function.

Magnetic resonance imaging (MRI) can produce detailed images of the heart and identify sections of cardiac muscle that are not receiving an adequate blood supply.

Cardiac catheterization detects pressure and blood flow patterns in the heart. A thin tube is inserted into a vein or artery and is then threaded into the heart under X-ray guidance.

A **coronary angiogram** uses a contrast dye injected during cardiac catheterization to identify coronary artery blockages.

Treatment Procedures (LO 6.3 and 6.7)

The most immediate need in the treatment of MI is to get blood and oxygen to the affected myocardium. This can be attempted in several ways:

1. **Injection of clot-busting (thrombolytic) drugs:** These drugs are injected within 3½ hours of the MI to dissolve the **thrombus.**
2. **Artery-cleaning angioplasty (percutaneous transluminal coronary angioplasty, or PTCA):** A balloon-tipped **catheter** is guided to the blockage site and inflated. The inflated balloon expands the artery from the inside by compressing the plaque against the artery's walls.
3. **Stent placement:** To reduce the likelihood that the artery will close up again (occlude), a wire-mesh tube, or **stent,** is placed inside the vessel. **Drug-eluting** stents are covered with a special medication to help keep the artery open.
4. **Cardioversion** and **defibrillation** have been discussed earlier.
5. **Radiofrequency ablation** uses a catheter with an electrode in its tip that is guided into the heart to destroy cells from which abnormal cardiac rhythms are originating.
6. **Coronary artery bypass graft (CABG):** Healthy blood vessels harvested from the leg, chest, or arm are used to bypass (detour) the blood around blocked coronary arteries.
7. **Heart transplant:** The heart of a recently deceased person (donor) is transplanted into the recipient after the recipient's diseased heart has been removed.

Word Analysis and Definition

S = Suffix P = Prefix R = Root R/CF = Combining Form

WORD	PRONUNCIATION	ELEMENTS		DEFINITION
ablation	ab-**LAY**-shun	S/ R/	-ion *process* **ablat-** *take away*	Removal of a tissue to destroy its function
angiogram angiography	**AN**-jee-oh-gram **AN**-jee-**OG**-rah-fee	S/ R/CF S/	-gram *a record* **angi/o-** *blood vessel* -graphy *process of recording*	Radiograph obtained after injection of radiopaque contrast material into blood vessels Radiography of blood vessels after injection of contrast material
angioplasty	**AN**-jee-oh-**PLAS**-tee	S/ R/CF	-plasty *surgical repair* **angi/o-** *blood vessel*	Repair or unblocking of a blood vessel through surgery
catheter catheterize (verb) catheterization (noun)	**KATH**-eh-ter **KATH**-eh-teh-**RIZE** **KATH**-eh-ter-ih-**ZAY**-shun	 S/ R/ S/	Greek *to send down* -ize *action* **catheter-** *catheter* -ization *process of inserting*	Hollow tube to allow passage of fluid into or out of a body cavity, organ, or vessel To introduce a catheter Introduction of a catheter
echocardiography	**EK**-oh-kar-dee-**OG**-rah-fee	S/ R/CF R/CF	-graphy *process of recording* **ech/o-** *sound wave* **-cardi/o-** *heart*	Ultrasound recording of heart function
lipoprotein	**LIE**-poh-pro-teen	R/CF R/	**lip/o-** *fat* **-protein** *protein*	Bonding of molecules of fat and protein
percutaneous	**PER**-kyu-**TAY**-nee-us	S/ P/ R/	-ous *pertaining to* per- *through* **-cutane-** *skin*	Passage through the skin, in this case, by needle puncture
stent	STENT		Charles Stent, English dentist, 19th century	Wire-mesh tube used to keep arteries open
thrombus thrombi (pl) thrombolytic (adj) thrombolysis	**THROM**-bus **THROM**-bee throm-boh-**LIT**-ik throm-**BOH**-lih-sis	 S/ R/CF R/	Latin *clot* -lytic *pertaining to destruction* **thromb/o-** *blood clot* -lysis *dissolve*	A clot attached to a diseased blood vessel or heart lining Able to dissolve or break up a blood clot Dissolving of a thrombus (clot)
triglyceride	try-**GLISS**-eh-ride	S/ P/ R/	-ide *having a particular quality* tri- *three* **-glycer-** *sweet, glycerol*	Lipid containing three fatty acids

Exercises

A. Use the correct abbreviation *from the provided list to complete each statement. Not all choices will be used. Fill in the blanks.* **LO 6.3, 6.6, and 6.9**

CABG ECG HDL LDL MRI PTCA

1. The blood tests revealed that Ms. Nugrak's good cholesterol, her ___ , was high.
2. Mr. Tervo will undergo a ____ to open the occluded coronary artery.
3. The ____ showed that Mr. Welch's heart has normal electrical activity.
4. The ____ was high, which may place a person at risk of developing coronary artery disease.

B. Determine the type of condition *that is treated with a particular procedure.* **LO 6.3 and 6.7**

1. Coronary artery bypass grafting
   a. arrhythmia **b.** occluded coronary artery
2. Radiofrequency ablation
   a. arrhythmia **b.** occluded coronary artery
3. Cardioversion
   a. arrhythmia **b.** occluded coronary artery
4. Percutaneous transluminal coronary angioplasty
   a. arrhythmia **b.** occluded coronary artery

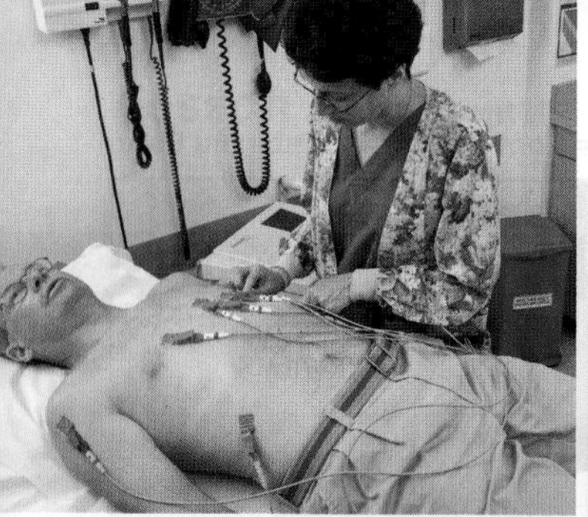
Rick Brady/McGraw-Hill Education

Lesson 6.3

Circulatory Systems

Objectives

In order to understand the **etiologies** *and effects of Mrs. Jones' problems (see Case Report 6.3), and to clearly communicate with her and Dr. Bannerjee, you first need to have the medical terminology and knowledge to be able to:*

6.3.1 Specify the functions of the systemic and pulmonary circulations.

6.3.2 Identify the major **arteries** and **veins** in the body.

6.3.3 Explain the **hemodynamics** and control of blood flow.

6.3.4 Describe common disorders of the circulatory system.

Abbreviations

BP	blood pressure
CMA	certified medical assistant
H/O	history of
NKA	no known allergies
OA	osteoarthritis
P	pulse rate

CASE REPORT 6.3

You are . . .

. . . a certified medical assistant **(CMA)** working for Dr. Lokesh Bannerjee, a cardiologist in Fulwood Medical Center.

You are communicating with . . .

. . . Mrs. Martha Jones. You are documenting her medical record after Dr. Bannerjee interviewed and examined her.

Fulwood Medical Center
Consultation Request and Report Form

Patient's Name: Jones, MARTHA Age: 52
To: Dr. LOKESH BANNERJEE Department: cardiology
From: Dr. Susan Lee Department: Primary Care
Patient's Location: FULWOOD MEDICAL CENTER
Type of Consultation Desired:
☐ Consultation Only
☐ Consulation and follow Jointly
☒ Accept in Transfer

Referring Diagnoses: CLAUDICATION, POSSIBLE DVT
Reason for Consultation: Severe pain in both legs on walking

Signature: [signature] Date: 2/21/09 Time 1105 hrs

Consultation Report: by Lokesh Bannerjee

Chief complaint: Pt. c/o severe pain in both legs on walking about 100 yards or climbing a flight of stairs. Pain is so severe she must stop and wait 5 mins. before she can go on. For the past two weeks she has noticed soreness and hardness along a vein in her left calf.

Past medical history: Known type 2 diabetic with hypertension, CAD, diabetic retinopathy, and OA of her hips and knees. Several episodes of ketoacidosis and one of pulmonary edema. Bariatric surgery performed 8 months prior at 275 lbs.

Medications: metformin, verapamil, propanolol, Mevacor

Allergies: NKA

Physical examination: Ht: 5'2" Wt: 190 lbs. BP: 170/100 sitting. P: 80, regular. Both feet show slight pitting edema and skin is pale, cold, and dry. Small ulcer on lateral margin of each big toe. Varicosities, both legs. Tender cord in superficial vein of left calf. Flexion of left foot produces pain in left calf. Chest clear. Heart sounds unremarkable. No loss of sensation in legs or feet.

Impression:
1. varicose veins, both legs.
2. severe claudication, both legs.
3. probable deep vein thrombosis, left leg
4. possible peripheral neuropathy
5. H/O diabetes type 2, CAD, hypertension, retinopathy, OA

Plan: Admit patient to cardiology unit stat for IV heparin and conversion to oral anticoagulant therapy with Coumadin. Doppler studies, venogram, and angiogram have been ordered.

Signature: [signature] Date 2/21/09 Time 1250 hrs

Word Analysis and Definition

S = Suffix P = Prefix R = Root R/CF = Combining Form

WORD	PRONUNCIATION		ELEMENTS	DEFINITION
artery	**AR**-ter-ee		Greek *artery*	Thick-walled blood vessel carrying oxygenated blood away from the heart
claudication	klaw-dih-**KAY**-shun	S/ R/	-ation *a process* claudic- *limping*	Intermittent leg pain and limping
Doppler	**DOP**-ler		Johann Doppler, Austrian mathematician and physician, 1803–1853	Diagnostic instrument that sends an ultrasonic beam into the body
hemodynamics	**HE**-mo-die-**NAM**-iks	S/ R/CF R/	-ics *knowledge* hem/o- *blood* -dynam- *power*	The science of the blood flow through the circulation
varix varices (pl) varicose (adj)	**VAIR**-iks **VAIR**-ih-seez **VAIR**-ih-kose	 S/ R/	Latin *dilated vein* -ose *full of* varic- *varicosity; dilated, tortuous vein*	Dilated, tortuous vein Characterized by or affected with varices
vein	**VANE**		Latin *vein*	Blood vessel carrying blood toward the heart
venous (adj)	**VEE**-nuss	S/ R/	-ous *pertaining to* ven- *vein*	Pertaining to a vein
venogram	**VEE**-noh-gram	S/ R/CF	-gram *recording* ven/o- *vein*	Radiograph of veins after injection of radiopaque contrast material

EXERCISES

A. Review *Case Report 6.3 and answer the following questions. Select the correct answer.* **LO 6.6 and 6.8**

1. Which of the following are Mrs. Jones's symptoms? (choose all that apply)

a. severe pain in legs while sitting
b. severe pain in legs when walking 100 yards
c. severe pain in legs when climbing stairs
d. pain in her left calf
e. chest pain on exertion

2. Which of the following are diseases and conditions that Mrs. Jones is suffering from? (choose all that apply)

a. hypertension **b.** pulmonary embolism **c.** osteoarthritis **d.** type 1 diabetes mellitus **e.** gout

3. Why did Mrs. Jones have bariatric surgery?

a. diabetic retinopathy **b.** osteoarthritis **c.** obesity **d.** hypertension

4. What is the purpose of anticoagulant therapy?

a. to prevent the formation of blood clots
b. to make the heart beat slower
c. treat the diabetes mellitus
d. lower the blood pressure

5. Of the studies ordered, which one uses ultrasound?

a. angiogram **b.** venogram **c.** Doppler studies **d.** IV anticoagulant therapy

6. What is pitting edema?

a. a finger that is pressed into a swollen area leaves an indentation in the tissue
b. swelling that moves toward the feet when a person is standing upright
c. swelling around a wound that indents into the surrounding tissue
d. small pockets of swelling that are distributed throughout body

B. Singulars and plurals, *nouns and adjectives: Terms from the WAD can all be correctly inserted into the following paragraph of radiology documentation. Fill in the blanks.* **LO 6.2, 6.6, and 6.7**

veins **varicosities** **varix** **vein** **varicose** **varices** **venogram** **venous**

1. A ____________________ performed on this patient's left saphenous and popliteal ____________________.

Abnormalities: One slightly engorged and dilated ____________________ at the midpoint of the saphenous ____________________ and several ____________________ at the terminal end of the popliteal vein where ____________________ blood is pooling.

Diagnosis: ________________ veins. These ________________ need immediate attention by a vascular surgeon.

Keynotes

- **All arteries of the systemic circulation arise either directly or indirectly from the aorta.**
- **Blood flows from arteries to veins through capillary beds.**

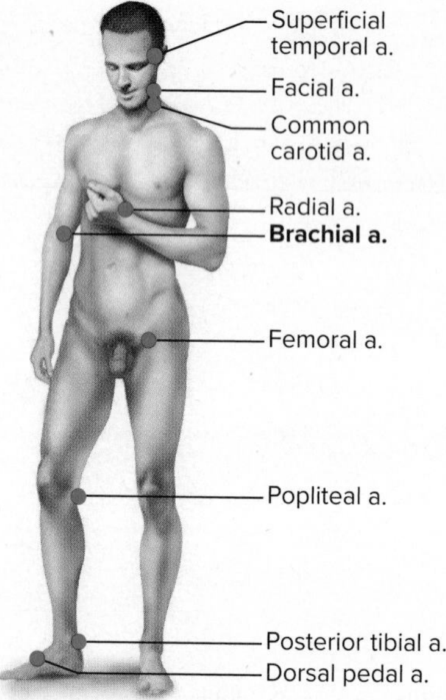

▲ **FIGURE 6.17**
Arterial Pulses—9 locations. (a. = artery)

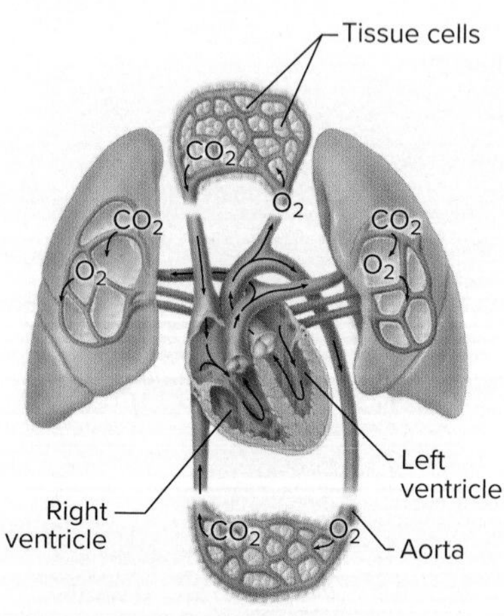

▲ **FIGURE 6.18**
Systemic and Pulmonary Circulations.

Circulatory System (LO 6.6)

The term **circulatory system** refers to your heart and blood vessels. It has two major divisions *(see Figure 6.18)*:

1. The **pulmonary circulation,** which carries deoxygenated blood from the heart to the lungs, and returns oxygenated blood to the heart; and
2. The **systemic circulation,** which supplies oxygenated blood to every organ except the lungs, and then returns deoxygenated blood to the heart, which pumps it into the pulmonary circulation.

Functions of the Circulatory System (LO 6.6)

The circulatory system has the following three functions:

- **Transportation.** It carries oxygen, nutrients, hormones, and enzymes that **diffuse** from the blood into the cells. Waste products and carbon dioxide diffuse back from the cells into the system and are carried to the lungs, liver, and kidney for excretion.
- **Homeostasis maintenance.** The systemic circulation directs blood flow to the tissues to enable them to meet their metabolic needs.
- **Blood pressure regulation.** In the systemic circulation, the arteries' ability to expand and contract in coordination with the systole and diastole of the heartbeat maintains a steady flow of blood and blood pressure to the tissues.

Arterial Pulses (LO 6.6)

The pulse is always part of a clinical examination because it can provide information about heart rate, heart rhythm, and the state of the arterial wall by **palpation** *(Figure 6.17)*. The most easily accessible artery is the radial artery at the wrist, where the pulse is usually taken.

Blood Pressure (BP) (LO 6.6)

Blood pressure is the force the blood exerts on arterial walls as it is pumped around the circulatory system by the left ventricle. The pressure is measured using a **sphygmomanometer** and a **stethoscope,** usually at the **brachial** artery *(Figure 6.17).*

Arterioles, Capillaries, and Venules (LO 6.6)

As the arteries branch farther away from the heart and distribute blood to specific organs, they become smaller, muscular vessels called **arterioles.** By contracting and relaxing, these arterioles are the primary controllers that help the body direct the amount of blood that the organs and structures receive.

From the arterioles, the blood flows into **capillaries** and **capillary beds** *(Figure 6.19)*. Red blood cells flow in single file through the small capillaries.

From the capillaries, tiny **venules** accept the blood and merge to form veins. The veins form reservoirs for blood. At any moment, 60% to 70% of the total blood volume is contained in the venules and veins.

Systemic Venous Circulation (LO 6.6)

There are three major types of veins:

1. **Superficial,** such as those you can see under the skin of your arms and hands;
2. **Deep,** which run parallel to arteries and drain the same tissues that the arteries supply; and
3. **Venous sinuses,** which are in the head and heart and have specific functions.

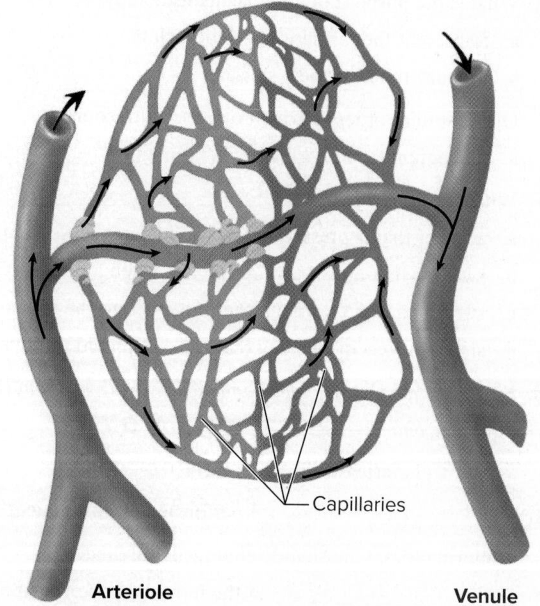

▲ **FIGURE 6.19**
Capillary Bed.

Word Analysis and Definition

S = Suffix P = Prefix R = Root R/CF = Combining Form

WORD	PRONUNCIATION	ELEMENTS		DEFINITION
arteriole	ar-**TER**-ee-ole	S/ R/	-ole *small* arteri- *artery*	Small terminal artery leading into the capillary network
brachial	**BRAY**-kee-al	S/ R/	-al *pertaining to* brachi- *arm*	Pertaining to the arm
capillary capillaries	**KAP**-ih-lair-ee **KAP**-ih-lair-eez	S/ R/	-ary *pertaining to* capill- *hairlike structure*	Minute blood vessel between the arterial and venous systems
diffuse	di-**FUZE**		Latin *to pull in different directions*	To disseminate or spread out
homeostasis	hoh-mee-oh-**STAY**-sis	S/ R/CF	-stasis *stand still* home/o- *the same*	Maintaining the stability, or equilibrium, of a system or the body's internal environment
palpate (verb) palpation (noun)	**PAL**-pate pal-**PAY**-shun	 S/ R/	Latin *touch, stroke* -ion *action, condition* palpat- *touch, stroke*	To examine with the fingers and hands Examination with the fingers and hands
sphygmomanometer	**SFIG**-moh-mah-**NOM**-ih-ter	S/ R/CF R/CF	-meter *instrument to measure* sphygm/o- *pulse* -man/o- *pressure*	Instrument for measuring arterial blood pressure
stethoscope	**STETH**-oh-skope	S/ R/CF	-scope *instrument to examine* steth/o- *chest*	Instrument for listening to respiratory and cardiac sounds
vena cava venae cavae (pl)	**VEE**-nah **KAY**-vah **VEE**-nee **KAY**-vee	R/CF R/	ven/a *vein* cava *cave*	One of the two largest veins in the body The two largest veins in the body (superior and inferior venae cavae)
venule	**VEN**-yule or **VEEN**-yule	S/ R/	-ule *small* ven- *vein*	Small vein leading from the capillary network

EXERCISES

A. Build *your knowledge of the elements and terms that make up the language of the cardiovascular system. Fill in the blanks.* **LO 6.2 and 6.6**

1. A small vein leading away from a capillary network: ______________________________.
2. To examine with the fingers and hands: ______________________________
3. To disseminate or spread out: ______________________________
4. State of equilibrium in the body is called ______________________________.
5. The two largest veins in the body are collectively called ______________________________.

B. Construct *the correct medical term to match the definition. If the term does not have a particular element, insert N/A. Fill in the blanks.* **LO 6.1, 6.2, and 6.7**

1. minute blood vessel between the arterial and venous systems:

______________ / ______________ / ______________
P R/CF S

2. instrument for listening to respiratory and cardiac sounds:

______________ / ______________ / ______________
P R/CF S

3. pertaining to the arm:

______________ / ______________ / ______________
P R/CF S

4. instrument for measuring arterial blood pressure:

______________ / ______________ / ______________
R/CF R/CF S

5. small terminal artery leading into the capillary network:

______________ / ______________ / ______________
P R/CF S

Lesson 6.3 (cont'd)

Keynote

- **All the disorders of the systemic arterial and venous systems are grouped under the term peripheral vascular disease (PVD).**

Abbreviations

CAD	coronary artery disease
DVT	deep vein thrombosis
PVD	peripherial vascular disease

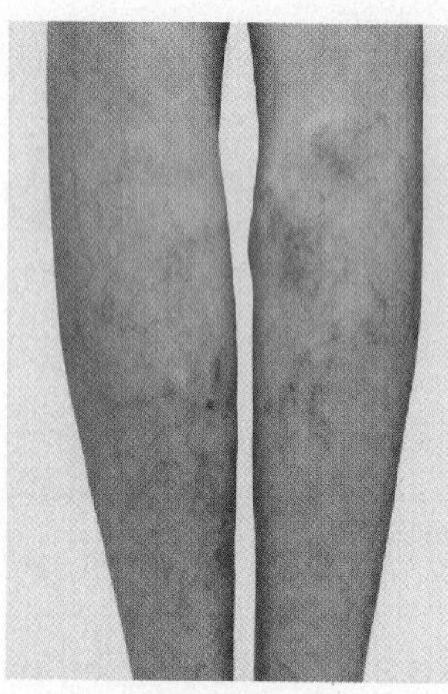

▲ **FIGURE 6.20**
Varicose Veins of the Leg.
Marina113/Getty Images

Case Report 6.3 *(continued)*

Mrs. Martha Jones, who had been referred to Dr. Bannerjee's cardiovascular clinic, has several circulatory problems related to her diabetes and obesity. She was diagnosed previously with hypertension, **CAD**, and diabetic retinopathy. She now has severe pain in her legs when walking. Doppler studies and angiograms showed significant blockage of blood flow due to arteriosclerosis of the large arteries in her legs. This blockage produces the pain when walking (intermittent claudication) and is part of her peripheral vascular disease **(PVD).**

The ulcers on the edges of her big toes are a result of thickening capillary walls and arterioles; this has led to poor circulation in her feet. Mrs. Jones' diabetes has caused these problems.

In addition, in her left leg's venous (vein) system, the tender cord-like lesion is due to **thrombophlebitis** of a superficial vein. A venogram showed a deep vein thrombosis **(DVT).**

Disorders of Veins (LO 6.2 and 6.6)

Our veins and arteries can be prone to certain disorders, like the DVT experienced by Mrs. Jones in the preceding case report.

Thrombophlebitis is an inflammation of the lining of a vein, allowing clots (thrombi) to form.

Deep vein thrombosis (DVT) is a thrombus formation in a deep vein. The increased pressure in the capillaries due to back pressure from the blocked blood flow in the veins creates a collection of fluid in the tissues called **edema.**

A major complication of thrombus (clot) formation is that a piece of the clot can break off **(embolus)** and be carried in the bloodstream to another organ where it can block blood flow. It often lodges in the lungs, causing a pulmonary embolus or mass *(see Chapter 8).*

Varicose veins are superficial veins that have lost their elasticity and appear swollen and tortuous *(Figure 6.20).* Their valves become incompetent, and blood flows backward and pools. Smaller, more superficial varicose veins are called spider veins. Treatments offered include laser technology and **sclerotherapy,** in which solutions that scar the veins are injected into them. **Collateral** circulations develop to take the blood through alternative routes.

A phlebotomist is a technician who draws blood (phlebotomy).

Disorders of Arteries (LO 6.2 and 6.6)

An **aneurysm** is a localized **dilation** of an artery, and this commonly occurs in the abdominal aorta *(Figure 6.21).* Aneurysms can **rupture,** leading to severe bleeding and hypovolemic shock. Surgical repair consists of excision of the aneurysm and replacement with a **synthetic** graft.

Intracranial aneurysms are an important cause of bleeds into the cranial cavity and brain tissue.

Thromboangiitis obliterans (Buerger disease) is an inflammatory disease of the arteries with clot formation, usually in the legs. The occlusion of arteries and impaired circulation lead to intermittent pain when walking, and a person will often limp to compensate.

Raynaud disease is episodes of spasm (following exposure to cold) of the small arteries supplying the fingers, hands, and feet. It can be associated with connective tissue disorders like scleroderma and lupus.

Carotid artery disease affects the carotid arteries–the two major arteries supplying the brain. They can be involved in arteriosclerosis and the deposition of plaque. This puts the patient at risk for a stroke. A carotid **endarterectomy** can be performed to surgically remove the plaque.

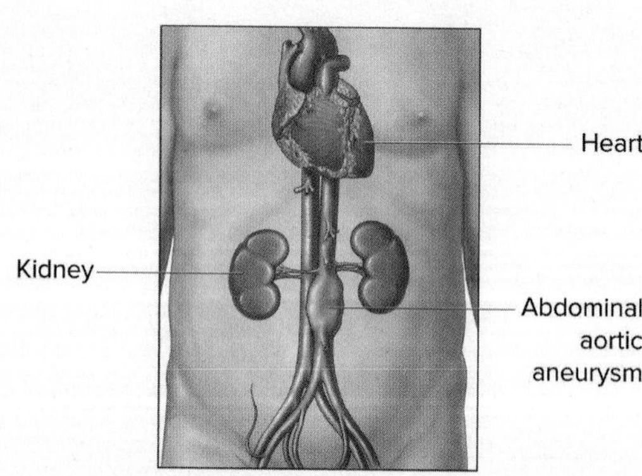

▲ **FIGURE 6.21**
Diagram of an Abdominal Aortic Aneurysm.

Word Analysis and Definition

S = Suffix P = Prefix R = Root R/CF = Combining Form

WORD	PRONUNCIATION	ELEMENTS		DEFINITION
aneurysm	**AN**-yur-izm		Greek *dilation*	Circumscribed dilation of an artery or cardiac chamber
claudication	klaw-dih-**KAY**-shun	S/ R/	-ation *process* claudic- *limping*	Intermittent leg pain and limping
collateral	koh-**LAT**-er-al	S/ P/ R/	-al *pertaining to* col- *before* -later- *at the side*	Situated at the side, often to bypass an obstruction
edema edematous (adj) pitting edema	ee-**DEE**-mah ee-**DEM**-ah-tus **PIT**-ing ee-**DEE**-mah	 S/ R/	Greek *swelling* -tous *pertaining to* edema- *swelling, edema*	Excessive accumulation of fluid in cells and tissues Pertaining to or marked by edema Edema that maintains indentations made by applying pressure to the area for a time
embolus emboli (pl)	**EM**-boh-lus		Greek *plug, stopped*	Detached piece of thrombus, a mass of bacteria, quantity of air, or foreign body that blocks a blood vessel
peripheral	peh-**RIF**-er-al	S/ R/	-al *pertaining to* peripher- *outer part*	Pertaining to the periphery or an external boundary
phlebitis	fleh-**BIE**-tis	S/ R/	-itis *inflammation* phleb- *vein*	Inflammation of a vein
thromboembolism	**THROM**-boh-**EM**-boh-lizm	S/ R/CF R/	-ism *condition* thromb/o- *clot* -embol- *plug*	A piece of detached blood clot (embolus) blocking a distant blood vessel
thrombophlebitis	**THROM**-boh-fleh-**BIE**-tis	S/ R/CF R/	-itis *inflammation* thromb/o- *clot* -phleb- *vein*	Inflammation of a vein with clot formation
thrombus thrombosis	**THROM**-bus throm-**BOH**-sis	S/ R/ S/	-us *pertaining to* thromb- *clot* -osis *condition*	A clot attached to a diseased blood vessel or heart lining Formation of a thrombus

EXERCISES

A. Apply *the language of the cardiovascular system. Select the best answer to complete each statement.* **LO 6.1 and 6.6**

1. The suffix tells you that **thrombophlebitis** is a(n)
   a. puncture **b.** inflammation **c.** excision **d.** vein
2. **Collateral** means
   a. at the front **b.** in the middle **c.** at the side
3. The combining form *phleb/o-* means
   a. artery **b.** vein **c.** capillary
4. The combining form *scler/o-* describes a
   a. softening **b.** clotting **c.** hardening **d.** constriction
5. The symptom of **edema** is a
   a. rash **b.** swelling **c.** lesion
6. **Aneurysm** describes a blood vessel that is
   a. dilated **b.** constricted **c.** collapsed **d.** obstructed
7. The roots tell you that **thromboembolism** is a(n)
   a. clot or plug **b.** tear or rupture **c.** swelling or lesion **d.** vein or artery
8. The combining form *thromb/o-* means
   a. clot **b.** lump **c.** plug **d.** vein

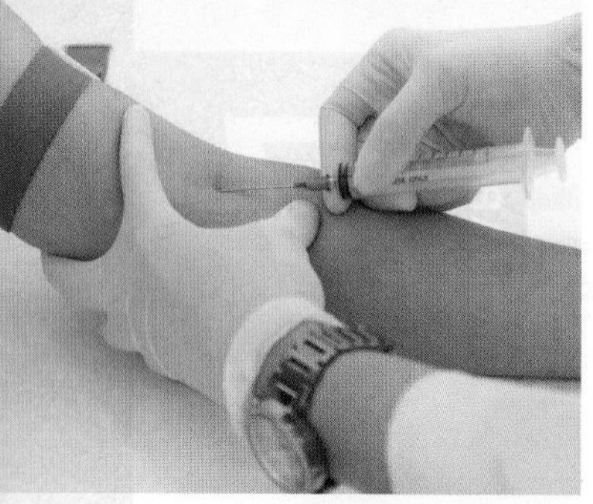

mikumistock/Shutterstock

Objectives

The average-sized adult carries about 5 liters (10 pints) of blood in the body at all times. The information in this lesson relates to the composition, functions, and uses of blood, and enables you to use correct medical terminology to:

7.1.1 Identify the components of blood.

7.1.2 Describe plasma and its functions.

7.1.3 Explain the functions of blood.

Keynote

- **Serum is identical to plasma except for the absence of clotting proteins.**

Abbreviations

Hct	hematocrit
RBC	red blood cell
WBC	white blood cell

The health professionals involved in the diagnosis and treatment of problems with the blood, lymphatic, and immune systems include the following:

- **Hematologists** are physicians who specialize in the diagnosis, treatment, and prevention of blood and bone marrow diseases.
- **Immunologists and allergists** are physicians who specialize in immune system disorders, such as allergies, asthma, and immunodeficiency and autoimmune diseases.
- **Epidemiologists** are medical scientists involved in the study of epidemic diseases and how they are transmitted and controlled.
- **Medical or clinical laboratory technicians** perform routine testing procedures on body fluids, blood, and other tissues using microscopes, computers, and other laboratory equipment.
- **Immunology technicians** are certified laboratory technicians with a special interest in immunology who generally work alongside medical researchers.
- **Transfusion technicians** are certified technicians who deal with all phases of blood transfusions.
- **Phlebotomists** assist physicians by drawing patient blood samples for laboratory testing.

Lesson 7.1

Components and Functions of Blood

Components of Blood (LO 7.3 and 7.4)

The study of the blood and its disorders—the red and white blood cells within the blood, their proportions, and overall cell health—is called **hematology.** A **hematologist** is a medical specialist who is trained in this area.

Blood is a type of connective tissue that consists of cells contained in a liquid **matrix.** If a blood specimen is collected in a tube and centrifuged, the cells of the blood separate out and fill the bottom 45% of the tube *(see Figure 7.1)*. Ninety-nine percent of these cells are red blood cells **(RBCs);** white blood cells **(WBCs)** and **platelets** make up the remainder of this sample. The **hematocrit (Hct)** is the percentage of total blood volume composed of red blood cells.

Plasma—a clear, yellowish liquid that is 91% water—makes up the remaining 55% of the blood sample in the tube. Plasma is a **colloid,** a liquid that contains floating particles, most of which are plasma proteins. **Nutrients,** waste products, hormones, and enzymes are dissolved in plasma for transportation. When blood clots, and the solid clot is removed, **serum** remains. Serum is a clear, yellowish fluid that contains all the blood proteins not used in clotting and all the electrolytes, antibodies, antigens, and hormones that are carried in blood.

FIGURE 7.1
Components of Blood.

(Components of blood): Eric Wise; (Adult male body - anterior view): Joe DeGrandis/McGraw-Hill Education

Word Analysis and Definition

S = Suffix P = Prefix R = Root R/CF = Combining Form

WORD	PRONUNCIATION	ELEMENTS		DEFINITION
allergist	**AL**-er-jist	S/ R/ R/	-ist *specialist* all- *other, strange* -erg- *work*	Specialist in hypersensitivity reactions
anemia **anemic (adj)**	ah-**NEE**-me-ah ah-**NEE**-mik	P/ R/ S/	an- *without* -emia *a blood condition* -emic *pertaining to a condition of the blood*	Decreased number of red blood cells Pertaining to or suffering from anemia
colloid	**COLL**-oyd	S/ R/	-oid *resembling* coll- *glue*	Liquid containing suspended particles
hematocrit (Hct)	he-**MAT**-oh-krit	S/ R/CF	-crit *to separate* hemat/o- *blood*	Percentage of red blood cells in the blood
hematology **hematologist**	he-mah-**TOL**-oh-jee he-mah-**TOL**-oh-jist	S/ R/CF S/	-logy *study of* hemat/o- *blood* -logist *one who studies, specialist*	Medical specialty of the blood and its disorders Specialist in hematology
matrix	**MAY**-triks		Latin mater *mother*	Substance that surrounds and protects cells, is manufactured by the cells, and holds cells together
nutrient **nutrition** **nutritionist**	**NYU**-tree-ent nyu-**TRISH**-un nyu-**TRISH**-un-ist	 S/ R/ S/	Latin *to nourish* -ion *action, condition* nutrit- *nourishment* -ist *specialist*	Constituent of food necessary for the body to function normally The study of food and liquid requirements for normal function of the human body A person who specializes in the study of food and liquid requirements for normal function of the human body
plasma	**PLAZ**-mah		Greek *something formed*	Fluid, noncellular component of blood
platelet (*Also called* **thrombocyte.**)	**PLAYT**-let	S/ R/	-let *little, small* plate- *flat*	Small particle involved in the clotting process
serum	**SEER**-um		Latin *whey*	Fluid remaining after removal of blood cells and the formation of a clot
vitamin (**Note:** *The duplicate letter "a" is omitted. It was originally thought that all vitamins were amines.*)	**VYE**-tah-min	S/ R/	-amin(e) *nitrogen-containing substance* vita- *life*	Essential organic substance necessary in small amounts for normal cell function

EXERCISE

A. Review *Case Report 7.1. Select the answer that correctly completes the statement or answers the question.* **LO 7.4, 7.9, and 7.14**

1. The lab results showed an abnormality in Ms. Sosin's:

a. platelets **b.** albumin **c.** red blood cells **d.** white blood cells **e.** plasma

2. How might have Ms. Sosin described her fatigue?

a. "My heart beats very rapidly."
b. "I feel tired all of the time."
c. "It is difficult to breathe."
d. "I have episodes of dizziness."

3. The diagnostic test that Dr. Lee ordered was:

a. computed tomogram **b.** sonography **c.** electrocardiography **d.** blood work **e.** bone marrow biopsy

4. What is your role in Ms. Sosin's care?

a. proper documentation
b. drawing the blood for testing
c. diagnosing her condition
d. filling her prescription

B. Match *the definition in column 1 with the correct medical term in column 2. Fill in the blanks.* **LO 7.4 and 7.5**

_____ **1.** decreased number of RBCs — **a.** platelet
_____ **2.** study of blood disorders — **b.** plasma
_____ **3.** fluid remaining after removal of clot — **c.** anemia
_____ **4.** fluid noncellular component of blood — **d.** hematology
_____ **5.** also called a thrombocyte — **e.** serum

Lesson 7.1 (cont'd)

Keynotes

- RBCs are unable to move themselves and are dependent on the heart pump and blood flow to move them around the body.
- The average life span of an RBC is 120 days, during which time the cell circulates through the body about 75,000 times.
- Anemia produces pallor (pale color) because of the deficiency of the red-colored oxyhemoglobin, the combination of oxygen and hemoglobin.
- Hemolysis liberates hemoglobin from RBCs.

Abbreviations

CO_2	carbon dioxide
Hb or Hgb	hemoglobin
NO	nitric oxide
O_2	oxygen
PA	pernicious anemia
SOB	short(ness) of breath

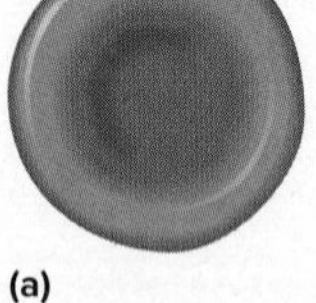

(a)

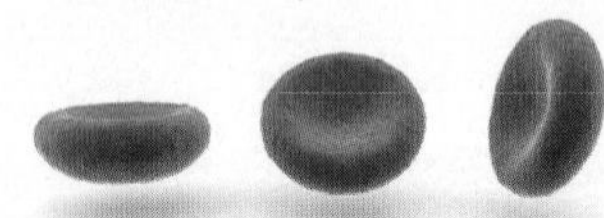

(b)

▲ **FIGURE 7.2**
Red Blood Cells.
(a) Top view. (b) Side view.

7.2b: ClaudioVentrella/Getty Images

Functions of Blood (LO 7.4)

Your blood travels throughout your body while performing a number of important functions. Your blood:

1. **Maintains your body's homeostasis** *(see Chapter 2).*
2. **Transports nutrients, vitamins, and minerals** from your digestive system and storage areas to your organs and cells. Examples of nutrients are glucose and amino acids *(see Chapter 9).*
3. **Transports waste products** from your cells and tissues to your liver and kidney for excretion. These waste products include creatinine, urea, bilirubin, and lactic acid.
4. **Transports hormones,** like insulin and thyroxine *(see Chapter 12),* from your endocrine glands to target cells.
5. **Transports gases,** like oxygen and carbon dioxide *(see Chapter 8),* to and from your lungs and cells.
6. **Protects against foreign substances, including microorganisms and toxins.** Cells and chemicals in your blood are an important part of your immune system's protective properties.
7. **Forms clots.** Clots provide protection against blood loss. Clotting is the first step in tissue repair and restoration of normal function.

Structure, Functions, and Disorders of Red Blood Cells (Erythrocytes) (LO 7.5)

Structure of RBCs (Erythrocytes) (LO 7.5)

Each RBC is a disk with edges that are thicker than and raised above the flattened center *(Figure 7.2).* This biconcave surface area enables a more rapid flow of gases into and out of the disk.

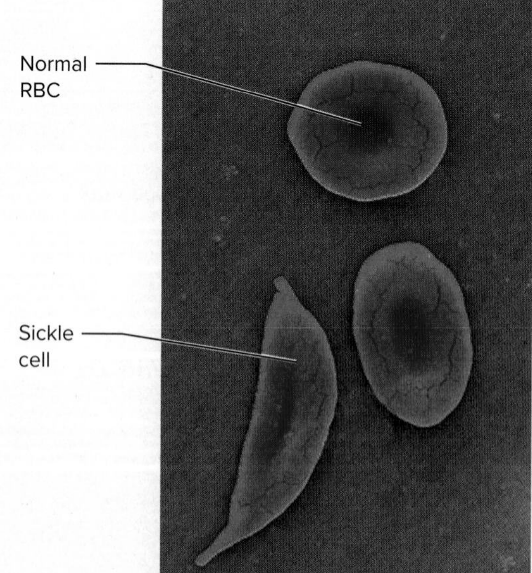

► **FIGURE 7.3**
Sickle Cell Disease.

ClaudioVentrella/Getty Images

The main component of RBCs is **hemoglobin (Hb),** which gives the cells and blood their red color. Hb is composed of the iron-containing pigment **heme** bound to a protein called **globin.** The rest of the red blood cell consists of the cell membrane, water, electrolytes, and enzymes. Mature RBCs do not have a nucleus.

Functions of RBCs (Erythrocytes) (LO 7.3 and 7.5)

The functions of the RBCs are to:

1. **Transport oxygen (O_2),** in combination with hemoglobin, throughout the body, from the lungs to the cells;
2. **Transport carbon dioxide (CO_2)** from the tissue cells to the lungs for excretion; and
3. **Transport nitric oxide (NO),** a gas produced by the lining cells of blood vessels that signals smooth muscle to relax, throughout the body.

Disorders of Red Blood Cells (LO 7.3 and 7.5)

Anemia is a red blood cell condition where the number of RBCs or amount of hemoglobin contained in each RBC is reduced. Both of these conditions reduce the blood's oxygen-carrying capacity, producing shortness of breath **(SOB)** and fatigue.

The different types of anemia include:

- **Iron-deficiency anemia** is the diagnosis for Ms. Sosin *(Case Report 7.1).* The cause was chronic bleeding from her gastrointestinal tract due to the aspirin and other painkillers she was taking. Her stools were positive for **occult blood.** Other causes of iron-deficiency anemia can be heavy menstrual bleeds or a diet deficient in iron.
- **Pernicious anemia (PA)** is due to vitamin B_{12} deficiency. It is caused by a shortage of intrinsic factor, which is normally secreted by cells in the stomach lining *(see Chapter 9)* and binds with B_{12}. This complex is absorbed into the bloodstream. Without B_{12}, hemoglobin cannot form. The number of red cells decreases, hemoglobin concentration decreases, and the size of the red cells increases.
- **Sickle cell anemia** is a genetic disorder found most commonly in African Americans. Here, the production of abnormal hemoglobin causes the RBCs to form a rigid sickle shape *(Figure 7.3).* The abnormal cells **agglutinate** (clump together) and block small capillaries. This creates intense pain in the **hypoxic** tissues (a sickle cell crisis) and can lead to stroke, kidney failure, and heart failure. **Sickle cell trait** is a minor form of this disease and rarely has any symptoms.

Word Analysis and Definition

S = Suffix P = Prefix R = Root R/CF = Combining Form

WORD	PRONUNCIATION	ELEMENTS		DEFINITION
agglutinate (verb)	ah-**GLUE**-tin-ate	S/ P/ R/	**-ate** *composed of, pertaining to* **ag- (ad-)** *to* **-glutin-** *stick*	Stick together to form clumps
erythrocyte	eh-**RITH**-roh-site	S/ R/CF	**-cyte** *cell* **erythr/o-** *red*	Red blood cell (RBC)
heme	**HEEM**		Greek *blood*	The iron-based component of hemoglobin that carries oxygen
hemoglobin **oxyhemoglobin** **hemoglobinopathy**	**HE**-moh-**GLOW**-bin **OCK**-see-he-moh-**GLOW**-bin **HE**-moh-**GLOW**-bin-**OP**-ah-thee	R/CF R/ R/ S/ R/CF R/CF	**hem/o-** *blood* **-globin** *protein* **oxy-** *oxygen* **-pathy** *disease* **hem/o-** *blood* **-globin/o-** *protein*	Red-pigmented protein that is the main component of red blood cells Combination of hemoglobin and oxygen Disease caused by the presence of an abnormal hemoglobin in red blood cells
hypoxia (**Note:** *The duplicate letter "o" is omitted.*) **hypoxic (adj)**	high-**POCK**-see-ah high-**POCK**-sik	S/ P/ R/ S/	**-ia** *condition* **hypo-** *below, deficient* **-ox-** *oxygen* **-ic** *pertaining to*	Below-normal levels of oxygen in tissues, gases, or blood Deficient in oxygen
occult blood	oh-**KULT BLUD**		occult Latin *to hide*	Blood that cannot be seen in the stool but is positive on a fecal occult blood test
pallor	**PAL**-or		Latin *paleness*	Paleness of the skin
pernicious anemia	per-**NISH**-us ah-**NEE**-me-ah	S/ P/ R/ P/ R/	**-ous** *pertaining to* **per-** *through* **-nici-** *lethal* **an-** *without* **-emia** *a blood condition*	Chronic anemia due to lack of vitamin B_{12}
polycythemia	**POL**-ee-sigh-**THEE**-me-ah	S/ P/ R/	**-hemia** *blood condition* **poly-** *many, much* **-cyt-** *cell*	A disease of bone marrow, excess production of RBCs
trait	**TRAYT**		Latin *an extension*	A discrete characteristic that has a known quality

EXERCISES

A. Identify *the meanings of the word elements that construct medical terms. Select the correct answer.* **LO 7.1**

1. The suffix in the term hypoxia means:

a. blood **b.** oxygen **c.** deficient **d.** condition

2. The combining form in the term erythrocyte means:

a. red **b.** white **c.** cell **d.** disc

3. The suffix in the term hemoglobinopathy means:

a. pertaining to **b.** condition of **c.** disease **d.** protein

4. The prefix in the term polycythemia means:

a. cell **b.** blood condition **c.** many **d.** through

5. The root in the term pernicious means:

a. lethal **b.** cell **c.** small **d.** crescent

B. Fill *in the correct disorder that matches the description.* **LO 7.2, 7.3, and 7.5**

1. numbers of RBCs reduced ____________________

2. bone marrow produces an excess of erythrocytes ____________________

3. genetic disorder found most commonly in African Americans ____________________

4. disease caused by the presence of an abnormal hemoglobin in red blood cells ____________________

5. disorder caused by vitamin B_{12} deficiency ____________________

Keynote

- Leukocytosis is too many white blood cells and often indicates the presence of an infection.

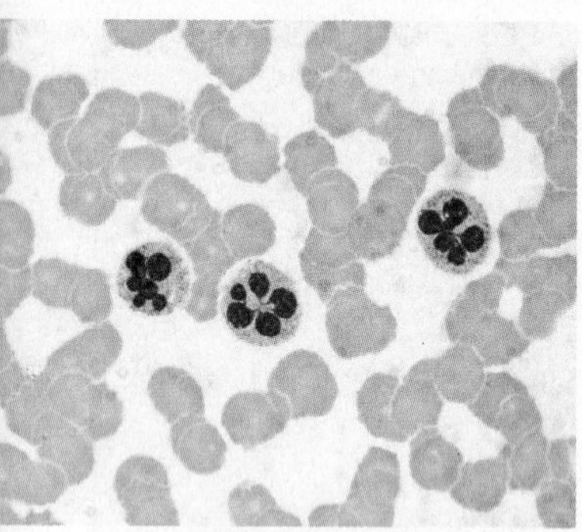

▲ FIGURE 7.4
Neutrophils Are Granulocytes.

Jose Luis Calvo Martin & Jose Enrique Garcia-Maurino/Getty Images

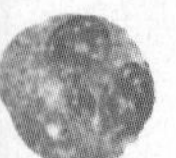
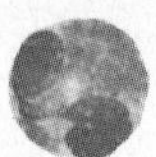
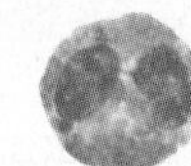

▲ FIGURE 7.5
Eosinophils Are Granulocytes.

toeytoey2530/Getty Images

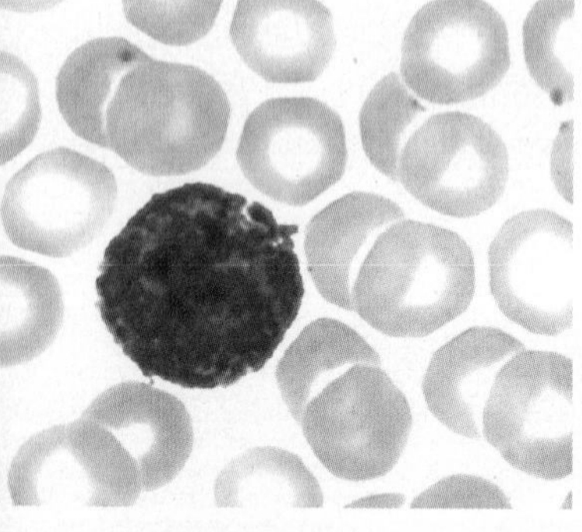

▲ FIGURE 7.6
Basophils Are Granulocytes.

Alvin Telser/McGraw-Hill Education

Abbreviations

DIFF	differential white blood cell count
Ig	immunoglobulin
PMNL	polymorphonuclear leukocyte

Disorders of Red Blood Cells *(continued)*

- **Hemolytic anemia** is caused by excessive destruction of normal and abnormal RBCs. **Hemolysis** (the destruction of RBCs) can result from toxic substances, such as snake and spider venoms, mushroom toxins, and overdoses of drugs, entering the bloodstream. Trauma to RBCs by hemodialysis or heart-lung machines, or an incompatible blood transfusion, can also cause hemolysis.
- **Aplastic anemia** is a condition in which the bone marrow is unable to produce sufficient new cells of all types–red cells, white cells, and platelets. It can be associated with exposure to radiation, benzene, and certain drugs.
- **Polycythemia** is an overproduction of RBCs by the bone marrow. The cause is unknown.

Types and Functions of White Blood Cells (Leukocytes) (LO 7.3 and 7.6)

The types of white blood cells **(WBCs)** can be categorized as **granulocytes** or **agranulocytes.** Granulocytes contain a granular cytoplasm, made up of granules, which are sites for enzyme and chemical production. Agranulocytes do not contain cytoplasmic granules.

Granulocytes (LO 7.3 and 7.6)

1. **Neutrophils** *(Figure 7.4),* also called **polymorphonuclear leukocytes (PMNLs),** are normally 55% to 65% of the total WBC count. These cells ingest bacteria, fungi, and some viruses. In **neutropenia,** the number of neutrophils is decreased. In **neutrophilia,** the number is increased.
2. **Eosinophils** *(Figure 7.5)* are normally 2% to 4% of the total WBC count. They leave the bloodstream to enter tissue that is undergoing an allergic response. In allergic reactions, the number and percentage of eosinophils increase.
3. **Basophils** *(Figure 7.6)* are normally less than 1% of the total WBC count. Basophils migrate to damaged tissues to release histamine (which increases blood flow) and heparin (which prevents blood clotting).

Agranulocytes (LO 7.3 and 7.6)

4. **Monocytes** *(Figure 7.7)* are the largest blood cells and are normally 3% to 8% of the total WBC count. Monocytes leave the bloodstream and become **macrophages** that ingest bacteria, dead neutrophils, and dead cells in the tissues.
5. **Lymphocytes** *(Figure 7.8)* are the smallest white blood cells and comprise 25% to 35% of the total WBC count. Lymphocytes are produced in red bone marrow and migrate through the bloodstream to lymphatic tissues–lymph nodes, tonsils, spleen, and thymus–where they multiply.
   There are two main types of lymphocytes:
   a. **B cells** differentiate into plasma cells, which are stimulated by bacteria or toxins to produce antibodies or immunoglobulins **(Ig)**.
   b. **T cells** attach directly to foreign antigen-bearing cells like bacteria, which they kill with toxins they secrete.

In a laboratory report, a **differential white blood cell count (DIFF)** lists the percentages of the different leukocytes in a blood sample.

Disorders of White Blood Cells (LO 7.3 and 7.6)

A normal cubic millimeter (mm^3) of blood contains 5,000 to 10,000 white blood cells. In **leukocytosis,** the total WBC count exceeds 10,000 per cubic millimeter. Other conditions that increase the WBC count beyond the normal range include:

- Allergic reactions, which increase the number of eosinophils;
- Typhoid fever, malaria, and tuberculosis, which increase the number of monocytes; and
- Whooping cough and infectious mononucleosis, which increase the number of lymphocytes.

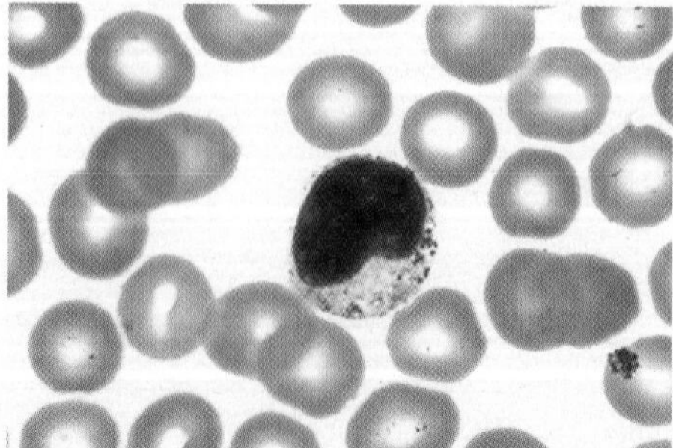

▲ FIGURE 7.7
Monocytes Are Agranulocytes.

Al Telser/McGraw-Hill Education

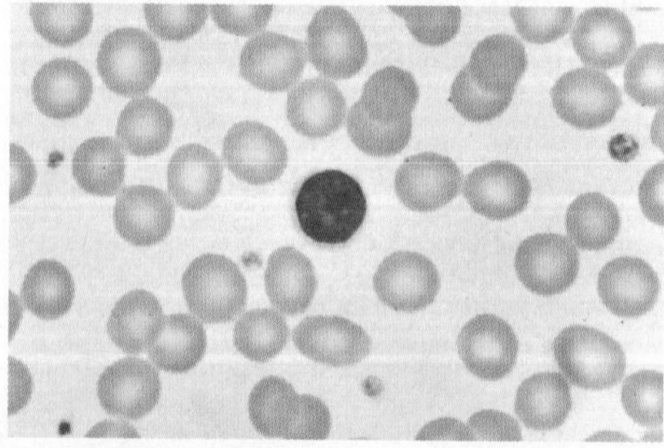

▲ FIGURE 7.8
Lymphocytes Are Agranulocytes.

jarun011/Getty Images

Word Analysis and Definition

S = Suffix P = Prefix R = Root R/CF = Combining Form

WORD	PRONUNCIATION	ELEMENTS		DEFINITION
agranulocyte	a-**GRAN**-you-loh-site	S/ P/ R/CF	-cyte *cell* a- *without, not* -granul/o- *granule*	A white blood cell without any granules in its cytoplasm
aplastic anemia	a-**PLAS**-tik ah-**NEE**-me-ah	S/ P/ R/ P/ R/	-tic *pertaining to* a- *without* -plas- *formation* an- *without* -emia *blood condition*	Condition in which the bone marrow is unable to produce sufficient red cells, white cells, and platelets
basophil	**BAY**-so-fill	S/ R/CF	-phil *attraction* bas/o- *base*	A basophil's granules attract a basic blue stain in the laboratory
eosinophil	ee-oh-**SIN**-oh-fill	S/ R/CF	-phil *attraction* eosin/o- *dawn*	An eosinophil's granules attract a rosy-red color on staining
granulocyte	**GRAN**-you-loh-site	S/ R/CF	-cyte *cell* granul/o- *small grain*	A white blood cell that contains multiple small granules in its cytoplasm
leukocyte **leucocyte (syn)** **(Note:** *Either spelling is acceptable.*) **leukocytosis**	**LOO**-koh-site **LOO**-koh-sigh-**TOE**-sis	S/ R/CF S/	-cyte *cell* leuk/o- *white* -osis *condition*	Another term for a white blood cell An excessive number of white blood cells
lymphocyte	**LIM**-foh-site	R/ R/CF	-cyte *cell* lymph/o- *lymph*	Small white blood cell with a large nucleus
hemolysis **hemolytic (adj)**	he-**MOL**-ih-sis he-moh-**LIT**-ik	S/ R/CF S/ R/	-lysis *destruction* hem/o- *blood* -ic *pertaining to* -lyt- *destroy*	Destruction of red blood cells so that hemoglobin is liberated Pertaining to the destruction of red blood cells
monocyte	**MON**-oh-site	R/ P/	-cyte *cell* mono- *single*	Large white blood cell with a single nucleus
mononucleosis	**MON**-oh-nyu-klee-**OH**-sis	S/ P/ R/	-osis *condition* mono- *single* -nucle- *nucleus*	Presence of large numbers of specific, diagnostic mononuclear leukocytes
neutrophil **neutropenia** **neutrophilia**	**NEW**-troh-fill **NEW**-troh-**PEE**-nee-ah **NEW**-troh-**FILL**-ee-ah	S/ R/CF S/ S/	-phil *attraction* neutr/o- *neutral* -penia *deficiency* -philia *attraction*	Neutrophils' granules take up purple stain equally, whether the stain is acid or alkaline A deficiency of neutrophils An increase in neutrophils
polymorphonuclear	**POL**-ee-more-foh-**NEW**-klee-ar	S/ P/ R/CF R/	-ar *pertaining to* poly- *many* -morph/o- *shape* -nucle- *nucleus*	White blood cell with a multilobed nucleus

EXERCISES

A. Using the medical terms *related to of white blood cells, match the correct term in column one to its meaning in column two. Fill in the blanks.* **LO 7.6**

______	**1.** eosinophil	**a.** largest blood cells
______	**2.** leucocyte	**b.** white blood cell with a multilobed nucleus
______	**3.** basophil	**c.** white blood cell
______	**4.** monocyte	**d.** releases histamine in damaged tissues
______	**5.** polymorphonuclear	**e.** involved in an allergic response

B. Provide the abbreviation *for each given definition. Fill in the blanks.* **LO 7.3 and 7.6**

1. A group of cells that include those that fight infection, produce antibodies, or respond to allergens: _______

2. A lab test that reports the percentage of each type white blood cell: ________

3. Proteins that are produced by B cells: ________

4. Type of leukocyte that ingest bacteria ________

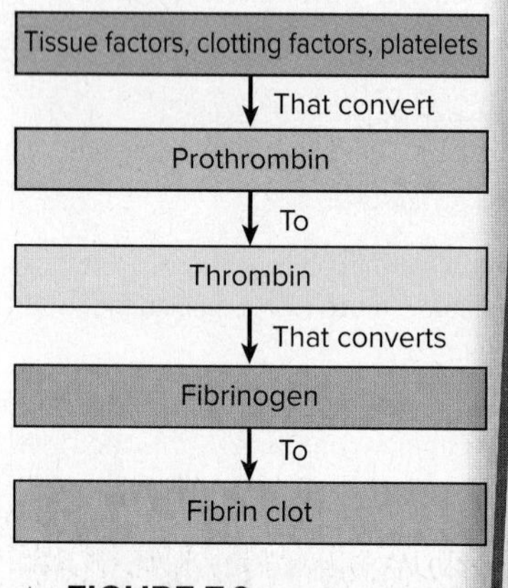

▲ **FIGURE 7.9**
Blood Coagulation.

CASE REPORT 7.2

You are . . .

. . . an emergency medical technician (EMT) working in the Fulwood Medical Center Emergency Department.

You are communicating with . . .

. . . Janis Tierney, a 17-year-old high school student who presents with fainting at school. She is pale. Her pulse is 90 and her blood pressure is 100/60. She tells you that she is having a menstrual period with excessive bleeding. Her physical examination is otherwise unremarkable. She has a past history of easy bruising and recurrent nosebleeds, and an episode of severe bleeding after a tooth extraction. Janis has a deficiency of **von Willebrand factor (vWF).** Her platelets are unable to stick together, and a platelet plug cannot form in the lining of her uterus to help end her menstrual flow.

Disorders of White Blood Cells *(continued)*

Infectious mononucleosis occurs in the 15- to 25-year-old population. Its cause—the **Epstein-Barr virus (EBV)**—is a very common virus and a member of the herpes family. The EBV is transmitted by an exchange of saliva, such as a kiss.

Leukemia is cancer of the blood-forming tissues and produces a high number of leukocytes and their precursors. The **leukemic** cells multiply, taking over the bone marrow and causing a deficiency of normal red blood cells, white blood cells, and platelets. This makes the patient anemic and vulnerable to infection and bleeding.

In **leukopenia,** the WBC count drops below 5,000 cells per cubic millimeter of blood. Leukopenia is seen in viral infections like measles, mumps, chickenpox, poliomyelitis, and AIDS.

In **pancytopenia,** the erythrocytes (red blood cells), leukocytes (white blood cells), and thrombocytes (platelets) in the circulating blood are all noticeably reduced. This can occur with cancer chemotherapy.

Hemostasis (LO 7.3 and 7.7)

Hemostasis, the control of bleeding, is a vital issue in maintaining **homeostasis,** the state of the body's equilibrium. Uncontrolled bleeding can offset the body's balance by decreasing blood volume and lowering blood pressure.

Platelets (also called **thrombocytes**) play a key role in hemostasis. They are minute fragments of large bone marrow cells and consist of a small amount of granular cytoplasm surrounded by a plasma membrane. They have no nucleus.

Hemostasis is achieved through a three-step process:

1. **Vascular spasm,** an immediate but temporary constriction of the injured blood vessels.
2. **Platelet plug formation,** an accumulation of platelets that bind themselves together and adhere to surrounding tissues. The binding and adhesion of platelets are mediated through **von Willebrand factor (vWF),** a protein produced by the cells lining the blood vessels.
3. **Blood coagulation** is the process of going through **prothrombin** and **thrombin** to the formation of a blood clot that traps blood cells, platelets, and tissue fluid in a network of **fibrin** *(Figure 7.9).*

After a blood clot forms, platelets adhere to strands of fibrin and contract to pull the fibers and the edges of the broken blood vessel together. **Fibroblasts** invade the clot to produce a fibrous connective tissue that seals the blood vessel.

Disorders of Coagulation (Coagulopathies) (LO 7.3 and 7.7)

There are several disorders that can prevent the blood from clotting properly, and these can lead to further health problems.

- **Hemophilia,** in its classical form (hemophilia A), is a disease males inherit from their mothers. It results from a deficiency of the coagulation factor named **factor VIII.**
- **Von Willebrand disease (vWD)**—the most common hereditary bleeding disorder—is a protein deficiency of the factor VIII complex **(vWF)** that is different from the factor deficiency involved in hemophilia.

Abbreviations

DIC	disseminated intravascular coagulation
EBV	Epstein-Barr virus
ITP	idiopathic thrombocytopenic purpura
vWD	von Willebrand disease
vWF	von Willebrand factor

Word Analysis and Definition

S = Suffix P = Prefix R = Root R/CF = Combining Form

WORD	PRONUNCIATION	ELEMENTS		DEFINITION
coagulant	koh-**AG**-you-lant	S/ R/	**-ant** *forming, pertaining to* **coagul-** *clot, clump*	Substance that causes clotting
coagulation **anticoagulant**	koh-ag-you-**LAY**-shun **AN**-tee-koh-**AG**-you-lant	S/ P/	**-ation** *process* **anti-** *against*	Process of blood clotting Substance that prevents clotting
fibrin	**FIE**-brin		Latin *fiber*	Stringy protein fiber that is a component of a blood clot
fibroblast	**FIE**-broh-blast	S/ R/CF	**-blast** *immature cell* **fibr/o-** *fiber*	Cell that forms collagen fibers
hematoma (*also called* bruise)	he-mah-**TOE**-mah	S/ R/	**-oma** *mass, tumor* **hemat-** *blood*	Collection of blood that has escaped from vessels into surrounding tissues
hemophilia	he-moh-**FILL**-ee-ah	S/ R/CF	**-philia** *attraction* **hem/o-** *blood*	An inherited disease from a deficiency of clotting factor VIII
hemostasis (**Note:** *Homeostasis has a very different meaning.*)	he-moh-**STAY**-sis	S/ R/CF	**-stasis** *control, stop* **hem/o-** *blood*	Control of or stopping bleeding
leukemia **leukemic (adj)** **leukopenia**	loo-**KEE**-mee-ah loo-**KEE**-mik loo-koh-**PEE**-nee-ah	S/ R/ S/ S/	**-emia** *a blood condition* **leuk-** *white* **-emic** *pertaining to a blood condition* **-penia** *deficiency*	Disease when the blood is taken over by white blood cells and their precursors Pertaining to or affected by leukemia A deficient number of white blood cells
pancytopenia	**PAN**-site-oh-**PEE**-nee-ah	S/ P/ R/CF	**-penia** *deficiency* **pan-** *all* **-cyt/o-** *cell*	Deficiency of all types of blood cells
prothrombin	pro-**THROM**-bin	S/ P/ R/	**-in** *substance* **pro-** *before* **-thromb-** *blood clot*	Protein formed by the liver and converted to thrombin in the blood-clotting mechanism
thrombocyte (*also called* platelet) **thrombocytopenia**	**THROM**-boh-site **THROM**-boh-site-oh-**PEE**-nee-uh	S/ R/CF S/ R/CF	**-cyte** *cell* **thromb/o-** *blood clot* **-penia** *deficiency* **-cyt/o-** *cell*	Another name for a platelet Deficiency of platelets in circulating blood
von Willebrand	VON **WILL**-eh-brand		E.A. von Willebrand, Finnish physician, 1870–1949	

EXERCISES

A. Review *Case Report 7.2 to answer the following questions. Select the correct answer to each question.* **LO 7.7, 7.13, and 7.14**

1. Why is Janis Tierney in the Emergency Department at Fulwood Medical Center?

a. bruising, tachycardia **b.** menstrual period with excessive bleeding **c.** pallor and nosebleeds **d.** fainting at school

2. What is causing her blood-related issues?

a. deficiency of von Willebrand factor **c.** lack of oxygen in the blood

b. excessive white blood cells **d.** deficient number of platelets

3. Which of the following are Janis Tierney's symptoms?

a. fatigue **b.** menstrual period with excessive bleeding **c.** palpitations **d.** increased pain with activity

4. What blood-related issues does she have in her past medical history? (choose all that apply)

a. she is pale **b.** easy bruising **c.** recurrent nosebleeds **d.** fainting **e.** hypertension

5. Translate into medical language: "her blood clotting cells are unable to stick together"

a. thrombocytopenia **b.** anemia **c.** inability to coagulate **d.** pancytopenia

B. A suffix *completes a medical term. The element* leuk *or* leuk/o *remains the same in each term below. Fill in the blanks.* **LO 7.1 and 7.6**

penia **cyte** **cytosis** **emia** **ic**

1. An excessive number of white blood cells is: ____________________

2. The disease when the blood is taken over by the WBCs is: ____________________

3. Another term for a white blood cell is: ____________________

4. A deficient number of white blood cells is: ____________________

5. Pertaining to leukemia: ____________________

Keynote

- All blood groups are inherited.

Abbreviations

Ab	antibody
ABO	blood group system
Rh	Rhesus

CASE REPORT 7.3

You are . . .

. . . an emergency medical technician–paramedic (EMT-P) working in the Level One Trauma Unit at Fulwood Medical Center.

You are communicating with . . .

. . . Ms. Joanne Rodi, an 18-year-old student, who has been admitted to the unit from the operating room. Ms. Rodi has had surgery for multiple fractures sustained in a car accident. She is receiving a blood **transfusion.** You document that her temperature has risen to 102.8°F, her respirations have risen to 24 per minute, and she has chills. You take her blood pressure, and it has fallen to 90/60. What is your next step?

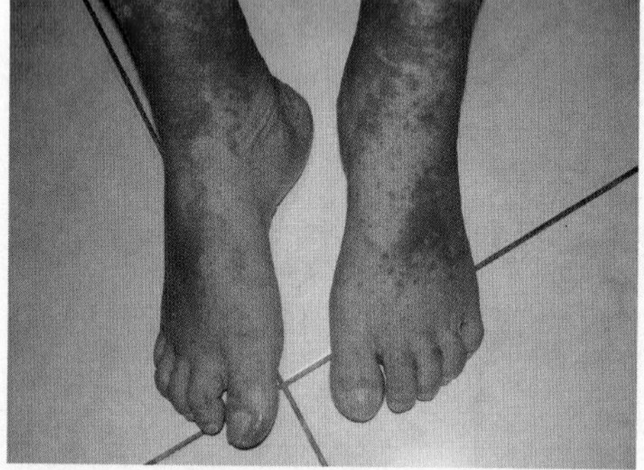

(b)

▲ **FIGURE 7.10**
Subsurface Bleeding.
(a) Purpura. (b) Petechiae.

7.10a: LoyFah4158/Shutterstock; 7.10b: TisforThan/Shutterstock

Disorders of Coagulation (Coagulopathies) *(continued)*

- **Disseminated intravascular coagulation (DIC)** occurs when a severe bacterial infection activates the clotting mechanism simultaneously throughout the cardiovascular system. Small clots form and obstruct blood flow into tissues and organs, particularly the kidney, leading to renal failure.
- **Thrombus** formation **(thrombosis)** is a clot that forms attached to a diseased or damaged area on the walls of blood vessels or the heart. If part of the thrombus breaks loose and moves through the circulation, it is called an **embolus.**
- **Thrombocytopenia** is a deficiency of platelets.
- **Purpura** is bleeding into the skin from small arterioles that produces a larger individual lesion than the tiny red spots or **petechiae** from capillary bleeds *(Figure 7.10a and b).* **Bruises** (or **hematomas**) are leaks of blood from all types of blood vessels.
- **Idiopathic thrombocytic purpura (ITP)** occurs when the immune system destroys the body's platelets. An acute, self-limiting form of the disease occurs in children; a chronic form affects adults.

Blood Groups and Transfusions (LO 7.3 and 7.8)

Red Cell Antigens (LO 7.3 and 7.8)

Antigens are molecules that exist on the surfaces of red blood cells. **Antibodies** are present in the plasma. Each antibody can combine with only a specific antigen. If the plasma antibodies combine with another red cell antigen, bridges form to connect these red cells together. This is called **agglutination,** or clumping, of the cells. Hemolysis (destruction) of the cells also occurs.

The antigens on the surfaces of the cells have been categorized into groups. Two of these groups—the **ABO** and **Rh** blood groups—are the most important.

Case Report 7.3 *(continued)*

In Joanne Rodi's case, she has type A blood and by mistake received type AB blood, the red cells of which agglutinated in the presence of her anti-B antibodies. Your immediate response is to stop the transfusion, replace it with a saline **infusion,** call your supervisor, and notify the doctor.

Word Analysis and Definition

S = Suffix P = Prefix R = Root R/CF = Combining Form

WORD	PRONUNCIATION	ELEMENTS		DEFINITION
agglutination (noun)	ah-glue-tih-**NAY**-shun	S/ P/ R/	-ation *process* ag- *to (same as ad-)* -glutin- *glue*	Process by which cells or other particles adhere to each other to form clumps
antibody antibodies (pl)	AN-tee-body	P/ R/	anti- *against* -body *substance, body*	Protein produced in response to an antigen
antigen	**AN**-tee-gen	P/ R/	anti- *against* -gen *produce, create*	Substance capable of triggering an immune response
autologous	awe-**TOL**-oh-gus	P/ R/	auto- *self, same* -logous *relation*	Blood transfusion with the same person as donor and recipient—self-transfusion
embolus	**EM**-boh-lus		Greek *plug, stopper*	Detached piece of thrombus, a mass of bacteria, quantity of air, or foreign body that blocks a blood vessel
infusion	in-**FYU**-zhun	P/ R/	in- *in* -fusion *to pour*	Introduction intravenously of a substance other than blood
petechia petechiae (pl)	peh-**TEE**-kee-ah peh-**TEE**-kee-ie		Latin *spot on the skin*	Pinpoint capillary hemorrhagic spot in the skin
purpura	**PUR**-pyu-rah		Greek *purple*	Skin hemorrhages that are red initially and then turn purple
Rhesus factor	**REE**-sus **FAK**-tor		Greek *mythical king of Thrace*	Antigen on surface of red blood cells of Rh+ individuals; it was first identified in Rhesus monkeys
transfusion	trans-**FYU**-zhun	P/ R/	trans- *across* -fusion *to pour*	Transfer of blood or a blood component from donor to recipient

EXERCISES

A. Select *the correct term in bold that completes each statement* **LO 7.3 and 7.8**

1. It is the ______________________ on the erythrocyte that determines a person's blood type.

   antigen **antibody**

2. It is ______________________ that contains antibodies that seek out antigens.

   red blood cells **plasma**

3. Dr. Schnick ordered a(n) ______________________ of packed red blood cells .

   infusion **transfusion**

4. The aspirin inhibited ______________________, leading to an increased loss of blood.

   thrombus **thrombosis**

5. The ______________________ of normal saline increased the patient's blood volume.

   infusion **transfusion**

B. Fill in the blanks *with the correct medical term related to the disorders of coagulation.* **LO 7.2, 7.3, and 7.8**

1. A decrease in the number of thrombocytes in the circulating blood: ____________
2. A thrombus that has detached and lodged in another blood vessel: ____________
3. A pinpoint hemorrhage: ______________
4. Multiple pinpoint hemorrhages: ______________
5. Skin hemorrhages that at first appear red and then turn purple: ______________

C. Review *Fill in the blanks.* **LO 7.1 and 7.8**

_____ **1.** trans **a.** to pour

_____ **2.** anti **b.** glue

_____ **3.** fusion **c.** against

_____ **4.** glutin **d.** across

_____ **5.** gen **e.** produce

Lesson 7.1 (cont'd) Blood Groups and Transfusions (continued)

Keynote

- **Rh factor is an antigen on the surface of a red blood cell. Its presence or absence is inherited.**

Abbreviations

HDN	hemolytic disease of the newborn
Rh	rhesus
RhoGAM	Rhesus immune globulin

ABO Blood Group (LO 7.3 and 7.8)

The two major antigens on the cell surface are antigen A and antigen B.

A person with only antigen A has *type A* blood.

A person with only antigen B has *type B* blood.

A person with both antigen A and antigen B has *type AB* blood.

A person with neither antigen has *type O* blood and is a universal donor, able to give blood to any other person.

Specific antibodies are synthesized in the plasma during the first 8 months after birth:

- Whenever antigen A is absent, anti-A antibody is produced.
- Whenever antigen B is absent, anti-B antibody is produced.

Figure 7.11 shows the different combinations of antigens and antibodies in the different blood types.

A **transfusion** of blood or packed red blood cells replaces lost red blood cells to restore the blood's oxygen-carrying capacity. **Autologous** donation and transfusion occur when people donate their own blood ahead of time to be given back to them if necessary during a surgical procedure.

Rh Blood Group (LO 7.3 and 7.8)

If an Rh antigen is present on the red cell surface, the blood is said to be Rh-positive (Rh+). This is common, as about 85% of people are Rh-positive. If there is no Rh antigen on the surface, the blood is Rh-negative (Rh−), which is the case for the other 15% of the population.

If an Rh-negative person receives a transfusion of Rh-positive blood, anti-Rh antibodies will be produced. This can cause RBC clumping (agglutination) and destruction (hemolysis).

If an Rh-negative woman and an Rh-positive man conceive an Rh-positive child *(Figure 7.12a),* the placenta normally prevents **maternal** and **fetal** blood from mixing. However, at birth or during a **miscarriage,** fetal cells can enter the mother's bloodstream. These Rh-positive cells stimulate the mother's tissues to produce Rh antibodies *(Figure 7.12b).*

If the mother becomes pregnant with a second Rh-positive fetus, her Rh antibodies can cross the **placenta** and agglutinate and hemolyze the fetal red cells *(Figure 7.12c).* This causes hemolytic disease of the newborn **(HDN,** or **erythroblastosis fetalis).**

Hemolytic disease of the newborn due to Rh incompatibility can be prevented. The Rh-negative mother giving birth to an Rh-positive child should be given Rh-immune globulin **(RhoGAM).**

Other causes of hemolytic disease in newborns include ABO **incompatibility,** incompatibility in other blood group systems, hereditary **spherocytosis,** and infections acquired before birth.

Red blood cell
Antibody anti-B
Antigen A

(a)

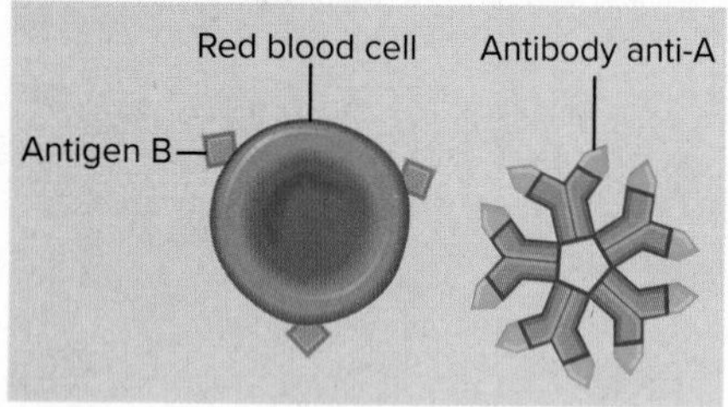

(b)

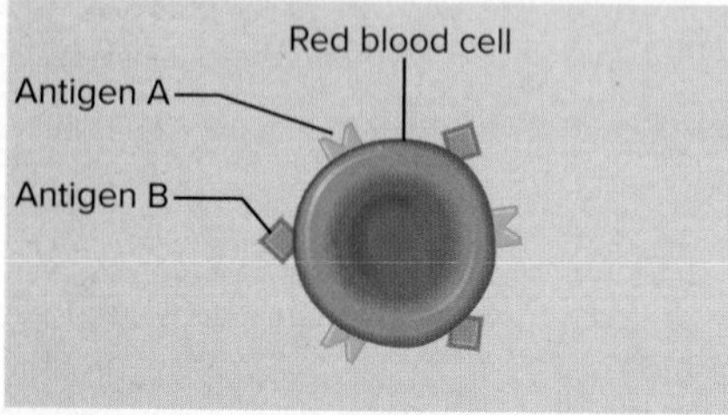

(c)

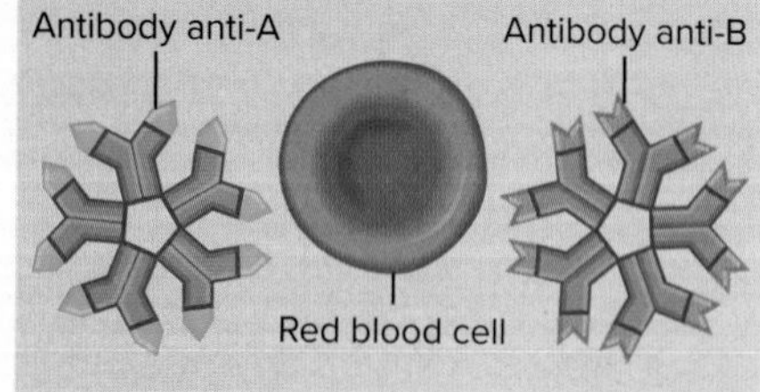

(d)

▲ **FIGURE 7.11**
(a) Type A blood.
(b) Type B blood.
(c) Type AB blood.
(d) Type O blood.

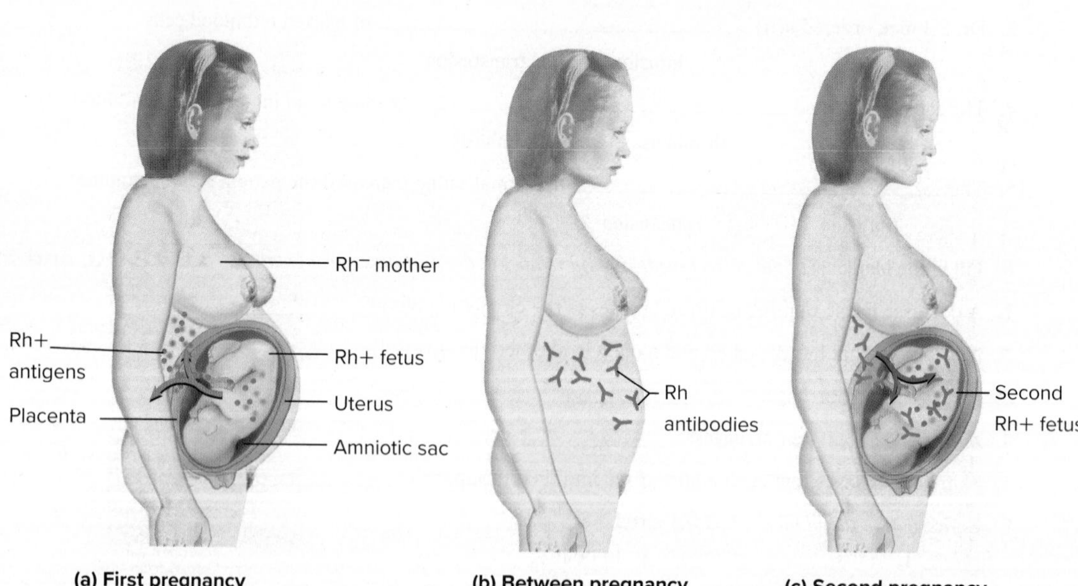

▲ **FIGURE 7.12**
Hemolytic Disease of the Newborn.
(a) First pregnancy. (b) Between pregnancies. (c) Second pregnancy.

Word Analysis and Definition

S = Suffix P = Prefix R = Root R/CF = Combining Form

WORD	PRONUNCIATION	ELEMENTS		DEFINITION
erythroblastosis fetalis	eh-**RITH**-roh-blast-**OH**-sis fee-**TAH**-lis	S/ R/CF R/ S/ R/	-osis *condition* erythr/o- *red* -blast- *immature cell* -is *belonging to* fetal- *fetus*	Erythroblastosis fetalis is a hemolytic disease of the newborn (HDN)
fetus	**FEE**-tus		Latin *offspring*	Human organism from the end of the eighth week after conception to birth
fetal (adj)	**FEE**-tal	S/ R/	-al *pertaining to* fet- *fetus*	Pertaining to the fetus
incompatible	in-kom-**PAT**-ih-bul	S/ P/ R/	-ible *can do* in- *not* -compat- *tolerate*	Substances that interfere with each other physiologically
incompatibility	in-kom-**PAT**-ih-bil-i-tee	S/	-ibility *able to do*	The quality of being incompatible
maternal	mah-**TER**-nal	S/ R/	-al *pertaining to* matern- *mother*	Pertaining to or derived from the mother
miscarriage	mis-**KAR**-aj	P/	mis- *not, incorrect* -carriage Old English *to carry*	Spontaneous expulsion of the products of pregnancy before fetal viability
placenta	plah-**SEN**-tah		Latin *a cake*	Organ that allows metabolic exchange between the mother and the fetus
spherocyte	**SFEAR**-oh-site	R/CF R/	spher/o- *sphere* -cyte *cell*	A spherical cell
spherocytosis	**SFEAR**-oh-site-**OH**-sis	S/	-osis *condition*	Presence of spherocytes in blood

EXERCISES

A. Test *your knowledge of blood, blood groups, and Rh factor by selecting the correct answer to the following questions.* **LO 7.1 and 7.8**

1. A person with both antigen A and antigen B will have
   a. blood type O   b. blood type A   c. blood type B   d. blood type AB
2. Blood is said to be Rh-positive if the
   a. Rh antigen is present on the RBC surface
   b. Rh antibody is present in the blood type
   c. Rh antibody is present in the plasma
   d. Rh antigen is present on the WBCs
   e. blood type is AB
3. A person with type B blood has B ______.
   a. antigens   b. antibodies
4. A person with type A blood has ____.
   a. anti-A antibodies   b. anti-B antibodies   c. no antigens

B. Explain the disorder erythroblastosis fetalis. *Select the correct answer to complete the statement or answer the quesion.* **LO 7.3 and 7.8**

1. In the medical term **erythroblastosis fetalis**, the condition affects which component of the blood?
   a. white blood cells   b. plasma   c. coagulation   d. red blood cells
2. In the medical condition **erythroblastosis fetalis**, who is harmed: the mother or the baby?
   a. mother   b. baby
3. In order for **erythroblastosis fetalis** to occur, the mother must have blood that is:
   a. type A   b. type B   c. type O   d. Rh-   e. Rh+
4. The trigger for **erythroblastosis fetalis** to occur is a baby with blood that is:
   a. type A   b. type B   c. type O   d. Rh-   e. Rh+
5. It is impossible for the first child to have this condition.
   a. True   b. False

C. Use your knowledge *of medical terminology to answer the following questions. Fill in the blanks.* **LO 7.2 and 7.8**

1. What is the medical term for *red blood cells clumping together?* ______________________
2. What is more common: being Rh+ or Rh- ? ______________________
3. The abbreviation for erythroblastosis fetalis is: ______________________.
4. Transferring of blood from donor to recipient: ______________________
5. The abbreviation for the Rhesus immune globulin given to mothers to prevent erythroblastosis fetalis: ______________________

Abbreviations

CBC	complete blood count
ITP	idiopathic thrombocytic purpura
MCV	mean corpuscular volume
PT	prothrombin time
PTT	partial thromboplastin time
TPA	tissue plasminogen activator

Diagnostic Procedures for Blood Disorders

(LO 7.3, 7.4, 7.5, 7.6, 7.7, and 7.9)

The patient's medical and family histories and physical examination are most important tools in diagnosing blood disorders.

- A **complete blood count (CBC)** gives important information about the types and numbers of cells in the blood, enabling diagnosis of the cause of such symptoms as weakness, fatigue, and bruising. Included in the CBC is the number of red blood cells; if the count is low, anemia could be present, and if the count is high, polycythemia can be the diagnosis. If the total amount of **hemoglobin** in the blood and the **hematocrit** are both low in the CBC, anemia is present. A red blood cell **index,** the **mean corpuscular volume (MCV),** shows the average size of the red blood cells. If the cells are small **(microcytic),** the most common cause is an iron-deficiency anemia. If the cells are large **(macrocytic),** a possible cause is pernicious anemia.
- A **white blood cell (WBC) count** is usually included in a CBC along with the numbers and types of the different WBCs, a **WBC differential.** These tests give the pathologists and clinicians who read the tests critical information about the body's response to infection, **toxic** medicines, chemicals, and allergens and show many other conditions, such as leukemia.
- Also included in a CBC is the number of platelets. A low platelet count can indicate **idiopathic thrombocytopenic purpura (ITP).** There are more than a dozen **coagulopathies** (bleeding disorders), and the diagnostic procedures to determine the cause of a patient's abnormal bleeding include the CBC, a **bleeding time, prothrombin time (PT), and partial thromboplastin time (PTT),** which help define where deficiencies might lie in the clotting process. The combination of all these tests is called a **coagulation panel.**
- Other diagnostic procedures for blood disorders include a **blood smear,** in which a drop of blood is smeared on a slide, stained, and examined under a microscope to determine the size and shape of RBCs, WBCs, and platelets. A **bone marrow aspiration (biopsy)** is a procedure used to define the production of the different blood cells. In disorders of the lymphatic system, the essential diagnostic procedure is biopsy of an enlarged lymph node. This can be followed by X-rays, CT scans, and MRI scans to determine the spread of a disease such as lymphoma.

Therapeutic Procedures for Blood Disorders

(LO 7.4, 7.5, 7.6, 7.7, and 7.9)

In anemia, treatment consists of replacing any deficiency in the production of hemoglobin, such as iron or vitamin B_{12}. For hemolytic and aplastic anemias, the treatment is to define and remove the toxin, drug, or radiation source that is causing the destruction of, or inability of the bone marrow to produce, red cells. A **bone marrow transplant** is the transfer of bone marrow from a healthy, compatible donor to a patient with aplastic anemia, leukemia, lymphoma, or other disease.

Word Analysis and Definition

S = Suffix P = Prefix R = Root R/CF = Combining Form

WORD	PRONUNCIATION	ELEMENTS		DEFINITION
aspiration	as-pih-**RAY**-shun	S/ R/	-ion *process* aspirat- *to breathe on*	Removal by suction of fluid or gas from a body cavity
coagulopathy **coagulopathies (pl)**	koh-ag-you-**LOP**-ah-thee	S/ R/CF	-pathy *disease* coagul/o *clotting*	Disorder of blood clotting
corpuscle **corpuscular (adj)**	**KOR**-pus-ul kor-**PUS**-kyu-lar	S/ R/ S/	-cle *small* corpus- *body* -ar *pertaining to*	A red blood cell Pertaining to a red blood cell
index **indices (pl)**	**IN**-deks **IN**-dih-seez		Latin *one that points out*	A standard indicator of measurement
macrocyte **macrocytic (adj)**	**MACK**-roh-site mack-roh-**SIT**-ik	P/ S/ S/	macro- *large* -cyte *cell* -ic *pertaining to*	Large red blood cell Pertaining to a large red blood cell
microcyte **microcytic (adj)**	**MY**-kroh-site my-kroh-**SIT**-ik	P/ R/ S/	micro- *small* -cyte *cell* -ic *pertaining to*	Small red blood cell Pertaining to a small red blood cell
parenteral	pah-**REN**-ter-al	S/ P/ R/	-al *pertaining to* par- *beside, abnormal* -enter- *intestine*	Administering medication by any other means than the GI tract
transplant	**TRANZ**-plant	P/ R/	trans- *across* -plant *insert, plant*	To transfer from one tissue or organ to another

EXERCISES

A. Interpret abbreviations. *Given the abbreviation, choose what the diagnostic test is measuring.* Select the correct answer to complete each statement. **LO 7.3, 7.4, 7.5, 7.6, and 7.9**

1. WBC differential

a. number of leukocytes **b.** measure of inflammation **c.** types of leukocytes **d.** average red blood cell size

2. PT

a. evaluates bleeding and clotting disorders
b. hemoglobin amount per erythrocyte
c. counts the number of platelets
d. determines presence of bone cancer

3. MCV

a. measures amount of iron in the blood
b. determines amount of hemoglobin per erythrocyte
c. reports the average size of red blood cells
d. used to monitor anticoagulation therapies

B. Deconstruct *the following terms into their elements. If a term does not have a particular element, insert N/A.* **LO 7.1 and 7.2**

1. parenteral __________ / __________ / __________
P R/CF S

2. coagulopathy __________ / __________ / __________
P R/CF S

3. corpuscular: __________ / __________ / __________
P R/CF S

4. transplant: __________ / __________ / __________
P R/CF S

5. aspiration: __________ / __________ / __________
P R/CF S

Pharmacology for Blood Disorders (LO 7.3, 7.4, 7.5, 7.6, 7.7, and 7.9)

Anticoagulants used to reduce or prevent blood clotting include:

- **Aspirin,** which reduces platelet **adherence** and is used in small 81 mg doses to reduce the incidence of heart attack.
- **Heparin,** which prevents prothrombin and fibrin formation and is given **parenterally**; its dose is monitored by **activated partial thromboplastin time** (aPTT).
- **Warfarin** ***(Coumadin),*** which inhibits the synthesis of prothrombin and others to act as an anticoagulant. It is given by mouth and its dose is monitored by **prothrombin times** (PTs), which are reported as an **International Normalized Ratio** (INR).
- **Dabigatran etexilate** ***(Pradaxa)*** and **rivaroxaban** ***(Xarelto),*** which inhibit the **synthesis** of thrombin and are given by mouth to reduce the risk of **embolism** and stroke in patients with nonvalvular atrial fibrillation *(see Chapter 10).* **Idarucizumab** ***(Praxbind injection)*** is available for patients using *Pradaxa* when reversal of its anticoagulant effects is needed for emergency surgery, for urgent procedures, or in life-threatening or uncontrolled bleeding.
- **Streptokinase**, derived from hemolytic streptococci, which dissolves the fibrin in blood clots. Given intravenously within 3 to 4 hours of a heart attack, it is often effective in dissolving a clot that has caused the heart attack.

Recombinant Factor VIII, developed through **recombinant DNA** technology, is the main medication used to treat hemophilia A. It is given intravenously through a vein in the arm or a port in the chest. **Desmopressin acetate** *(DDAVP)* is a synthetic version of **vasopressin** that helps stop bleeding in patients with mild hemophilia.

Pernicious anemia is treated initially with injections of vitamin B_{12}, and then the vitamin B_{12} can be given through a nasal gel.

Eltrombopag ***(Promacta)*** is available for pediatric patients with idiopathic thrombocytopenic purpura (ITP) who have not responded to corticosteroids, immunoglobulins, or splenectomy.

Most **leukemias** in both adults and children are treated with **chemotherapy**, often with added radiation therapy and a stem cell transplant.

Word Analysis and Definition

S = Suffix P = Prefix R = Root R/CF = Combining Form

WORD	PRONUNCIATION	ELEMENTS		DEFINITION
adhere adherence	add-**HEER** add-**HEER**-ents	 S/ R/	Latin *to stick to* -ence *forming, quality of* adher- *stick to*	To stick to something The act of sticking to something
chemotherapy	**KEE**-moh-**THAIR**-ah-pee	R/CF R/	chem/o- *chemical* therapy *treatment*	Treatment using chemical agents
embolism	**EM**-boh-lizm		Greek *a plug or patch*	A plug of tissue or air from afar that obstructs a blood vessel
parenteral	pah-**REN**-ter-al	S/ P/ R/	-al *pertaining to* par- *abnormal* -enter- *intestine*	Administering medication by any means other than the GI tract
recombinant DNA	ree-**KOM**-bin-ant **DEE**-en-a	S/ P/ R/	-ant *forming* re- *again* -combin- *combine*	Deoxyribonucleic acid (DNA) altered by inserting a new sequence of DNA into the chain
streptokinase	strep-toh-**KIE**-nase	P/ R/	strepto- *curved* -kinase *enzyme*	An enzyme that dissolves clots
vasopressin (also called antidiuretic hormone)	vay-soh-**PRESS**-in	S/ R/CF R/	-in *chemical compound* vas/o *blood vessel* -press- *close, press*	Pituitary hormone that constricts blood vessels and decreases urinary output

EXERCISES

A. Describe the action of medications as they relate to hematology. *Place the anticoagulant with the action it uses to prevent or reduce the formation of clots.* **LO 7.2 and 7.9**

Pradaxa **aspirin** ***Coumadin*** **streptokinase** ***Xarelto*** **heparin (has two actions, use the term twice)**

Dissolves fibrin in blood clots	Decreases platelet adherence	Inhibits synthesis of prothrombin	Inhibits synthesis of thrombin
1.	2.	3.	5.
		4.	6.
			7.

B. Match the therapy In the first column to the disorder it treats in the second column. *Fill in the blanks.* **LO 7.5, 7.7, and 7.9**

_____ **1.** Vitamin B_{12} — **a.** idiopathic thrombocytopenic purpura

_____ **2.** *Promacta* (eltrombopag) — **b.** mild hemophilia

_____ **3.** desmopressin acetate — **c.** pernicious anemia

_____ **4.** Recombinant Factor VIII — **d.** hemophilia A

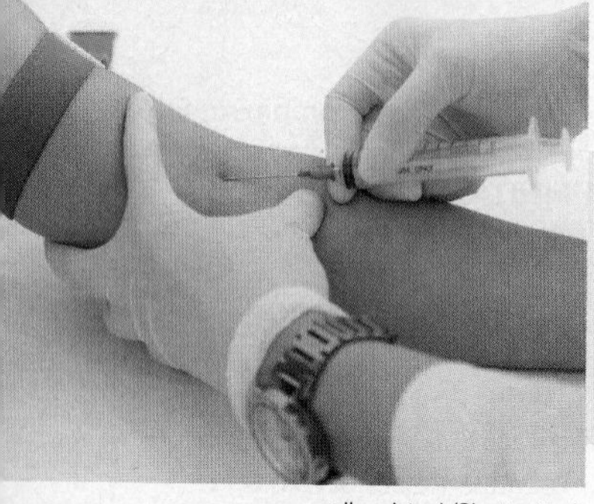
mikumistock/Shutterstock

Lesson 7.2

Lymphatic System

Objectives

As part of your body's defense mechanisms, the lymphatic system and its fluid provide surveillance and protection against foreign materials. In this lesson, the information provided will enable you to use correct medical terminology to:

7.2.1 Detail the anatomy of the **lymphatic** system.

7.2.2 Define the functions of the lymphatic system.

7.2.3 Identify the major cells of the lymphatic system and their functions.

7.2.4 Distinguish the anatomy and functions of the **lymph nodes, tonsils, thymus,** and **spleen.**

7.2.5 Recognize the common disorders of the lymphatic system.

Abbreviation

Ab antibody

CASE REPORT 7.4

You are . . .

. . . a medical assistant working with Susan Lee, MD, in her primary care clinic.

You are communicating with . . .

. . . Ms. Anna Clemons, a 20-year-old waitress, who is a new patient. She has noticed a lump in the left side of her neck. On questioning, you learn that Ms. Clemons has lost about 8 pounds in the past couple of months, has felt tired, and has had some night sweats. Her vital signs are normal. There are two firm, enlarged **lymph nodes** in her left neck in front of the **sternocleidomastoid** muscle (the long muscle in the side of the neck that extends up to the base of the skull behind the ear). Physical examination is otherwise unremarkable.

Lymphatic System (LO 7.10)

You live in a world that surrounds you with chemicals and disease-causing organisms waiting for a chance to enter your body and harm you. Your body has three lines of defense mechanisms against foreign organisms **(pathogens),** cells (cancer), or molecules **(pollutants** and **allergens).**

1. **Physical defense mechanisms** include your skin and mucous membranes; chemicals in your perspiration, saliva, and tears; hairs in your nostrils; and cilia and mucus to protect your lungs. The physical defense mechanisms are further discussed in the individual body system chapters.
2. **Humoral defense mechanisms** *(see Lesson 7.3),* based on antibodies **(Abs).** These are found in body fluids and bind to bacteria, toxins, and extracellular viruses, tagging them for destruction.
3. **Cellular defense mechanisms,** based on defensive cells **(lymphocytes).** These directly attack suspicious cells like cancer cells, transplanted tissue cells, or cells infected with viruses or parasites.

The lymphatic system has three functions:

1. **Absorb** excess **interstitial** fluid and return it to the bloodstream;
2. **Remove** foreign chemicals, cells, and debris from the tissues; and
3. **Absorb** dietary lipids from the small intestines *(see Chapter 9).*

Word Analysis and Definition

S = Suffix P = Prefix R = Root R/CF = Combining Form

WORD	PRONUNCIATION		ELEMENTS	DEFINITION
absorb	ab-**SORB**		Latin *to swallow*	To take in
allergen **(Note:** *The duplicate letter "g" is omitted.***)**	**AL**-er-jen	S/ R/ R/	-gen *create* all- *other, strange* -erg- *work*	Substance creating a hypersensitivity (allergic) reaction
allergic (adj) allergy	ah-**LER**-jik **AL**-er-jee	S/ S/	-ic *pertaining to* -ergy *process of working*	Pertaining to or suffering from an allergy Hypersensitivity to a particular allergen
interstitial	in-ter-**STISH**-al	S/ R/	-al *pertaining to* interstiti- *space between cells*	Pertaining to spaces between cells in an organ or tissue
lymph	LIMF		Latin *clear, spring water*	A clear fluid collected from tissues and transported by lymph vessels to the venous circulation
lymphatic (adj)	lim-**FAT**-ik	S/ R/	-atic *pertaining to* lymph- *lymph*	Pertaining to lymph or the lymphatic system
lymphoid (adj)	**LIM**-foyd	S/	-oid *resembling*	Resembling lymphatic tissue
node	NOHD		Latin *a knot*	A circumscribed mass of tissue
pathogen	**PATH**-oh-jen	S/ R/CF	-gen *produce, create, form* path/o- *disease*	A disease-causing microorganism
pollutant	poh-**LOO**-tant	S/ R/	-ant *pertaining to* pollut- *unclean*	Substance that makes an environment unclean or impure
sternocleidomastoid	**STER**-no-kly-doe-**MAS**-toyd	S/ R/CF R/CF R/	-oid *pertaining to* stern/o *breastbone* cleid/o *clavicle* mast *breast*	Long muscle in the side of the neck that extends up to the base of the skull behind the ear

EXERCISES

A. Review *Case Report 7.4 to answer the following questions. Select the correct answer to complete each statement or answer each question.* **LO 7.3, 7.10, and 7.13**

1. Which of the following are Ms. Clemons' symptoms? (choose all that apply)
   a. weight loss **b.** night sweats **c.** hypertension **d.** muscular pain **e.** ear ache
2. What is present on physical examination of the patient?
   a. tenderness on the left side of her neck
   b. swelling on the left side of the neck
   c. two firm, enlarged lymph nodes in the left side of her neck
   d. bulging of the sternocleidomastoid muscle
3. Where is the sternocleidomastoid muscle?
   a. on the side of the neck in front of the ear
   b. on the side of the neck and attaching to the mandible
   c. on the side of the neck, extending up to the base of the skull, behind the ear
   d. on the side of the neck, extending up to the base of the skull, in front of the ear
4. What was the status of the patient's VS?
   a. below normal **b.** above normal **c.** normal **d.** not recorded
5. What is the best description of a node?
   a. enlarged lymph gland **b.** cancerous growth **c.** circumscribed mass of tissue **d.** benign growth **e.** thickened fluid

B. Construct *the correct medical terms that match the definitions given. If a term does not have a particular element, insert N/A for that blank. Fill in the blanks.* **LO 7.1 and 7.10**

1. substance that makes the environment unclean or impure:
   ______ / ______ / ______
   P R/CF S
2. substance creating a hypersensitivity reaction:
   ______ / ______ / ______
   R/CF R/CF S
3. resembling lymphatic tissue:
   ______ / ______ / ______
   P R/CF S
4. a disease-causing microorganism:
   ______ / ______ / ______
   P R/CF S
5. hypersensitivity to a particular allergen:
   ______ / ______ / ______
   R/CF R/CF S

Keynote

- **Tissues that are the first line of defense against pathogens–for example, the airway passages–have lymphatic tissue in the submucous layers to help protect against invasion.**

Lymphatic System (continued) (LO 7.2 and 7.10)

The lymphatic system *(Figure 7.13)* has three components:

1. A network of thin **lymphatic capillaries and vessels,** similar to blood vessels, that penetrates the **interstitial spaces** (the spaces between tissues) of nearly every tissue in the body except cartilage, bone, red bone marrow, and the CNS;
2. A group of tissues and organs that produce **immune cells;** and
3. **Lymph,** a clear colorless fluid similar to blood plasma but with a composition that varies throughout the body. It flows through the network of lymphatic capillaries and vessels.

The **lymphatic network** begins with lymphatic capillaries that are closed-ended tubes nestled among **blood capillary networks** *(Figure 7.14).* The lymphatic capillaries are designed to let interstitial fluid enter so it can become lymph. In addition, bacteria, viruses, cellular debris, and traveling cancer cells can enter the lymphatic capillaries with the interstitial fluid. The lymphatic capillaries converge to form the larger **lymphatic collecting vessels,** which resemble small veins and have one-way valves. They travel alongside veins and arteries.

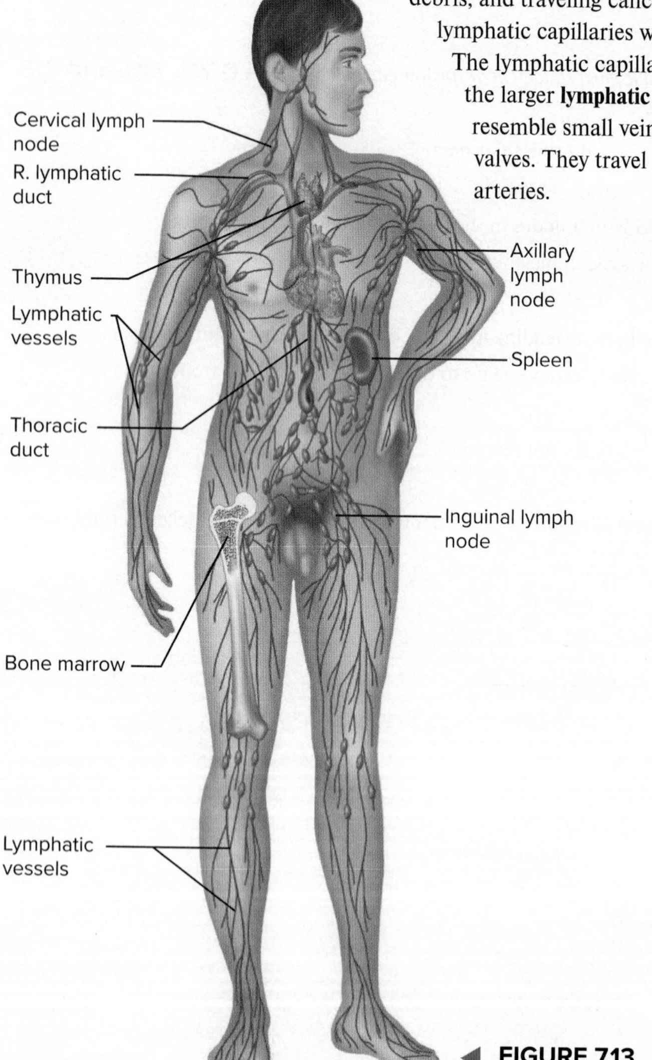

FIGURE 7.13
The Lymphatic System.

Lymph Nodes (LO 7.2 and 7.10)

At irregular intervals, the collecting vessels mentioned above enter into the lymph nodes *(Figure 7.15).* There are hundreds of lymph nodes stationed all over the body *(Figure 7.13).* They are concentrated in the neck, axilla, and groin. Their functions are to filter impurities from the lymph and alert the immune system to the presence of pathogens.

The lymph moves slowly through the nodes, which filter the lymph and remove any foreign matter. Macrophages in the lymph nodes ingest and break down foreign matter and display its fragments to T cells. This alerts the immune system to the presence of an invader. Lymph leaves the nodes when it enters into the **efferent** collecting vessels. All these lymph vessels move lymph toward the thoracic cavity.

Collecting vessels merge into **lymphatic trunks** that drain lymph from a major body region. These lymphatic trunks then merge into two large **lymphatic ducts**–the thoracic duct on the left and the right lymphatic duct, which empty into the veins beneath the collarbone, the subclavian veins *(Figure 7.13).*

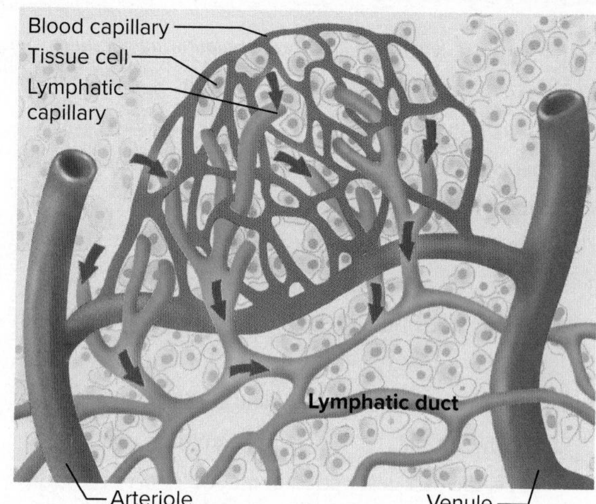

FIGURE 7.14
Lymphatic Flow.

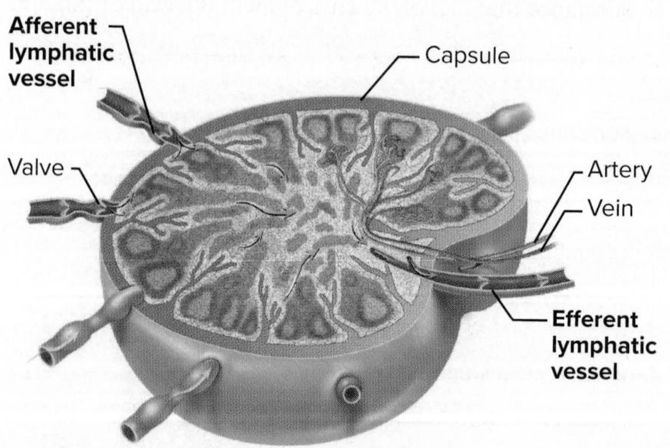

FIGURE 7.15
Lymph Node.

Word Analysis and Definition

S = Suffix P = Prefix R = Root R/CF = Combining Form

WORD	PRONUNCIATION	ELEMENTS		DEFINITION
efferent	**EFF**-eh-rent	S/ R/	**-ent** *end result, pertaining to* **effer-** *move away from the center*	Moving away from a center
afferent (**Note:** *These are opposite terms.*)	**AFF**-eh-rent	R/	**affer-** *move toward the center*	Moving toward a center
immune	im-**YUNE**		Latin *protected from*	Protected from an infectious disease
immunity	im-**YUNE**-ih-tee	S/ R/	-ity *condition* **immun-** *immune*	State of being protected
immunology	im-you-**NOL**-oh-jee	S/ R/CF	**-logy** *study of* **immun/o-** *immune*	The science and practice of immunity and allergy
immunologist	im-you-**NOL**-oh-jist	S/	**-logist** *one who studies, specialist*	Medical specialist in immunology
immunize (verb)	**IM**-you-nize	S/ R/	**-ize** *affect in a specific way* **immun-** *immune*	To cause to be resistant to an infectious disease
immunization (noun)	**IM**-you-nih-**ZAY**-shun	S/	**-ization** *process of inserting or creating*	Administration of an agent to provide immunity

Exercises

A. Precision *in usage is important if you want to communicate correct information. These six terms all contain a common root/combining form. Insert the correct term in each sentence.* **LO 7.2, 7.10, and 7.11**

immune **immunology** **immunity** **immunologist** **immunization** **immunize**

1. One who specializes in (the study of the science of immunity and allergy) ______________________ is termed an (type of specialist) ______________________.

2. The ______________________ system is a group of specialized cells in different parts of the body that recognize foreign substances and neutralize them.

3. We need to ______________________ young children before they start school.

4. A prior (injection) ______________________ obtained before she went overseas boosted her (status of being immune) ______________________ to the disease.

B. Demonstrate *your understanding of anatomy and function of the lymphatic system. Select the correct answer to each question.* **LO 7.11**

1. Where are the interstitial spaces located?
   a. in the capillary bed **b.** between blood vessels **c.** between tissues **d.** between cells
   e. within the blood vessels

2. Lymph is similar to what other body fluid?
   a. spinal fluid **b.** sputum **c.** urine **d.** blood plasma

3. Which of the following are functions of the lymphatic system? (choose all that apply)
   a. eliminate excess bilirubin from the blood
   b. absorb interstitial fluid and return it to the bloodstream
   c. remove foreign chemicals, cells, and debris from tissues
   d. absorb dietary lipids from the small intestine

4. Which of the following tissues lack lymphatic capillaries and vessels in the interstitial spaces? (select all that apply)
   a. cartilage **b.** bone **c.** pancreas **d.** central nervous system
   e. red bone marrow

5. Where in the body are the major concentrations of lymph nodes?
   a. neck, chest, groin **b.** axilla, chest, abdomen **c.** neck, axilla, abdomen **d.** neck, axilla, groin
   e. chest, abdomen, groin

6. What substance enters lymphatic capillaries to become lymph?
   a. blood plasma **b.** interstitial fluid **c.** red bone marrow **d.** lymphocytes **e.** mucus

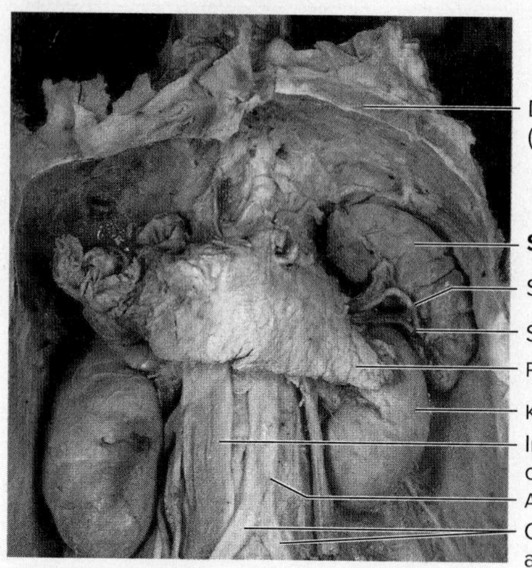

▲ **FIGURE 7.16**
Position of Spleen.

Dennis Strete/McGraw-Hill Education

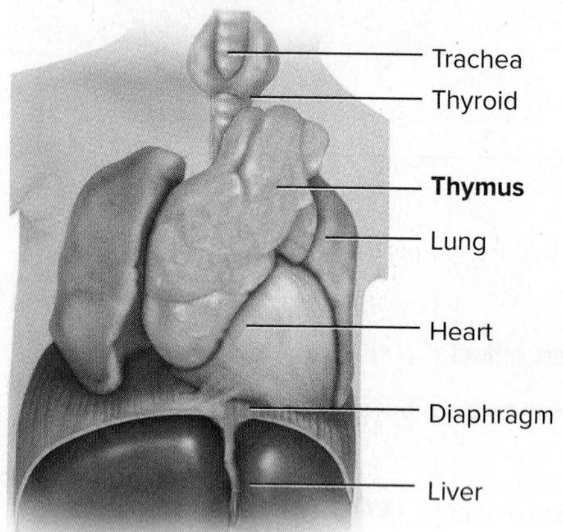

(a)

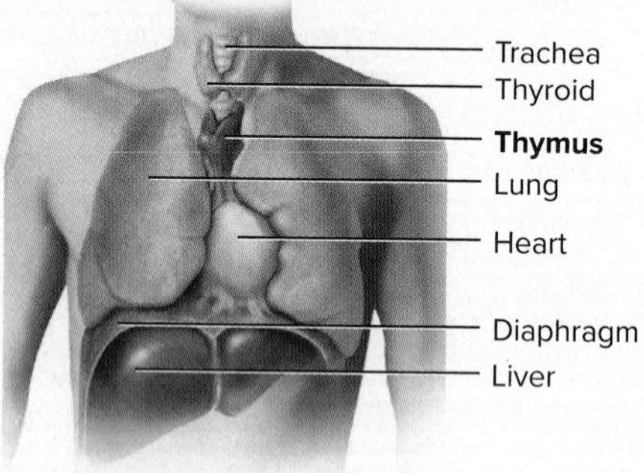

(b)

▲ **FIGURE 7.17**
Thymus.
(a) Large thymus in infant.
(b) Adult thymus.

Abbreviation

Ig immunoglobulin

Lymphatic Tissues and Cells (LO 7.2 and 7.10)

In some organs, lymphocytes and other cells form dense clusters called lymphatic **follicles.** These are constant features in the lymph nodes, the tonsils, and the ileum (a part of the small intestine).

Lymphatic tissues are composed of a variety of cells that include:

- **T lymphocytes (T cells):** The "T" stands for thymus, which is where these cells develop and mature. T lymphocytes make up 75% to 85% of body lymphocytes.
- **B lymphocytes (B cells):** These cells mature in the bone marrow. B lymphocytes make up 15% to 25% of lymphocytes. They respond to a specific antigen and become plasma cells to produce antibodies **(immunoglobulins, Ig)** that immobilize, neutralize, and prepare the specific antigen for destruction. Macrophages that have developed from monocytes ingest and destroy antigens, tissue debris, **bacteria,** and other foreign matter (phagocytosis).

Lymphatic Organs (LO 7.2 and 7.10)

Spleen (LO 7.2 and 7.10)

The **spleen,** a highly vascular and spongy organ, is the largest lymphatic organ. It is located in the left upper quadrant of the abdomen, below the diaphragm and lateral to the kidney *(Figure 7.16).*

The functions of the spleen are to:

- **Phagocytose (consume)** bacteria and other foreign materials.
- **Initiate an immune response** when antigens are found in the blood.
- **Phagocytose old, defective erythrocytes** and platelets.
- **Serve as a reservoir** for erythrocytes and platelets.

Tonsils and Adenoids (LO 7.2 and 7.10)

The **tonsils** *(see Chapter 8)* are two masses of lymphatic tissue located at the entrance to the upper part of the throat (the oropharynx) that entrap inhaled and ingested pathogens. **Adenoids** are similar tissues on the posterior wall of the upper pharynx or nasopharynx *(see Chapter 8).* The tonsils and adenoids form lymphocytes and antibodies, trap bacteria and viruses, and drain them into the tonsillar lymph nodes for elimination. Both the tonsils and the adenoids can also become infected.

Thymus (LO 7.2 and 7.10)

The thymus, a small organ of the immune system located in the center of the upper chest, has both endocrine *(see Chapter 12)* and lymphatic functions. T lymphocytes develop and mature in the thymus and are released into the bloodstream. The thymus is largest in infancy *(Figure 7.17a)* and reaches its maximum size at puberty. It then shrinks *(Figure 7.17b)* and is eventually replaced by fibrous and fatty (adipose) tissue.

Word Analysis and Definition

S = Suffix P = Prefix R = Root R/CF = Combining Form

WORD	PRONUNCIATION		ELEMENTS	DEFINITION
antecubital	an-teh-**KYU**-bit-al	S/ P/ R/	**-al** *pertaining to* **ante-** *in front of, before* **-cubit-** *elbow*	In front of the elbow
autoimmune	awe-toe-im-**YUNE**	P/ R/	**auto-** *self, same* **-immune** *protected*	Immune reaction directed against a person's own tissue
discrimination	**DIS**-krim-ih-**NAY**-shun	S/ P/ R/	**-ation** *process* **dis-** *away from* **-crimin-** *distinguish*	Ability to distinguish between different things
gurney	**GURR**-knee		Scottish *to grimace in pain*	A stretcher on wheels used to transport hospital patients
mutation	myu-**TAY**-shun		Latin *to change*	Change in the chemistry of a gene
specific **specificity** **(Note:** *Has two suffixes.***)**	speh-**SIF**-ik spes-ih-**FIS**-ih-tee	S/ R/ S/	**-ic** *pertaining to* **specif-** *species* **-ity** *condition, state*	Relating to a particular entity State of having a specific, fixed relation to a particular entity
toxin **toxicity**	**TOK**-sin toks-**ISS**-ih-tee	 S/ R/	Greek *poison* **-ity** *state, condition* **toxic-** *poison*	Poisonous substance formed by a cell or organism The state of being poisonous

Exercises

A. Analyze *Case Report 7.5 and select the correct answer to complete each statement.* **LO 7.11 and 7.13**

1. What is the purpose of flushing the wound?

a. Hydrate the skin **b.** Replace any lost blood **c.** Remove pathogens from the wound **d.** Water is a natural antibiotic

2. Mr. Cowan's high fever is most likely due to:

a. an infection **b.** heatstroke **c.** an allergic reaction **d.** cardiac arrest

3. If you have been exposed to a pathogen, your body will react to it by creating:

a. haptens **b.** erythrocytes **c.** mutations **d.** antibodies

B. Decide *if the statement is true or false. Select T if the statement is true. Select F if the statement is false.* **LO 7.11**

1. Opportunistic infections occur when the immune system is strong. T F

2. The immune system is composed of specific organs that fight infections. T F

3. An autoimmune disorder develops when a person's immune system recognizes an agent as "self." T F

4. Immunity to one pathogen grants immunity to others. T F

5. A bacterium or virus develops resistance when a person's immune system is weakened. T F

C. Each of these questions *requires a one-word answer. Think carefully before writing the answers.* **LO 7.2, 7.11, and 7.13**

1. Ability to distinguish between different things: ____________________

2. Change in the chemistry of a gene produces a: ____________________.

3. A molecule that triggers a response: ____________________

Keynotes

- **Antibodies do not actively destroy an antigen. They render it harmless and mark it for destruction by phagocytes.**
- **The immune system is thought to be able to produce some 2 million different antibodies.**

Immunity (LO 7.11)

Immunity is the state of being able to resist a specific infectious disease. It is classified biologically into two types, although these often respond to the same antigen:

1. **Cellular (cell-mediated) immunity:** This is a direct form of defense based on the actions of lymphocytes to attack foreign and diseased cells and destroy them. The many different types of T cells, B cells, and macrophages described in the previous lesson of this chapter are involved in this style of attack *(Figure 7.19).*
2. **Humoral (antibody-mediated) immunity:** This is an indirect form of attack that employs antibodies produced by plasma cells, which have been developed from B cells. The antibodies bind to an antigen and tag it for destruction. These antibodies are called **immunoglobulins,** present in blood plasma and body secretions.

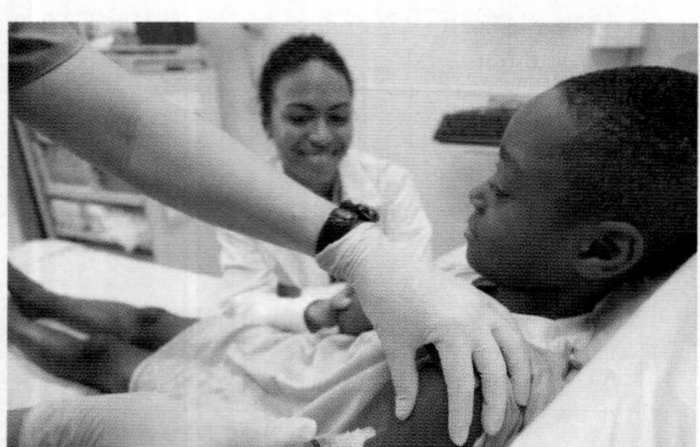

ERproductions Ltd/Blend Images LLC

Complement Fixation (LO 7.2 and 7.11)

The complement system is a group of 20 or more proteins continually present in blood plasma. Immunoglobulins bind to foreign cells, initiating the binding of **complement** to the cell and leading to its destruction.

Immunization (LO 7.2 and 7.11)

Immunization is the preventive method of stimulating the immune system without exposing the body to an infection. An agent **(vaccine)** composed of the antigenic components of a killed or **attenuated** microorganism or its inactivated toxins is injected into the body. **Vaccination** is a crucial step in keeping our population healthy. For example, vaccination has eradicated smallpox worldwide. However, if we stop vaccinating against smallpox, our population will again be susceptible to smallpox outbreaks. The same concept applies to the diseases in childhood immunizations *(Table 7.1).*

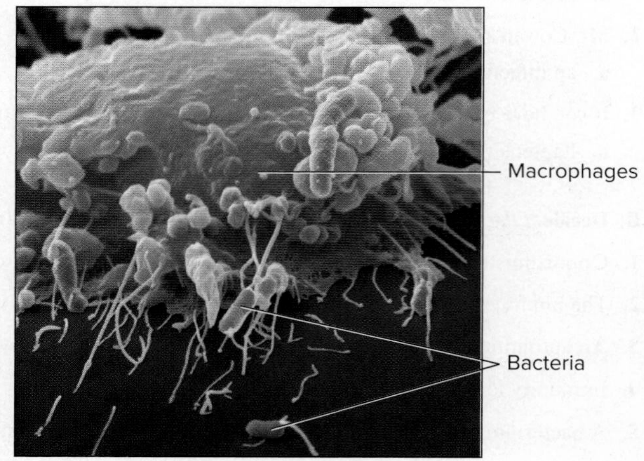

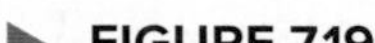

FIGURE 7.19
Macrophage Phagocytoses Bacteria. Filamentous extensions of a macrophage cell snare the bacteria and draw them to the surface of the cell where they are engulfed into the macrophage.

Eye of Science/Science Source

TABLE 7.1
RECOMMENDED IMMUNIZATIONS FOR PERSONS AGED 0 TO 6 YEARS

Hepatitis A (HepA)	Hepatitis B (HepB)
Rotavirus (RV)	Influenza (Yearly)
Inactivated poliovirus (IPV)	Varicella (chickenpox)
Diphtheria, tetanus, pertussis (DTaP)	Pneumococcal (PCV)
Measles, mumps, rubella (MMR)	
Hemophilus influenza type b (Hib)	

Source: Centers for Disease Control and Prevention, 2014.

Word Analysis and Definition

S = Suffix P = Prefix R = Root R/CF = Combining Form

WORD	PRONUNCIATION		ELEMENTS	DEFINITION
attenuate attenuated (adj)	ah-**TEN**-you-ate ah-**TEN**-you-a-ted	S/ R/ S/	-ate *composed of, pertaining to* attenu- *weaken* -ated *pertaining to a condition*	Weaken the ability of an organism to produce disease Weakened
complement	**KOM**-pleh-ment		Latin *that which completes*	Group of proteins in serum that finish off the work of antibodies to destroy bacteria and other cells
humoral immunity	**HYU**-mor-al im-**YUNE**-ih-tee	S/ R/ S/ R/	-al *pertaining to* humor- *fluid* -ity *condition* immun- *immune*	Defense mechanism arising from antibodies in the blood
vaccinate (verb) vaccination vaccine	**VAK**-sin-ate vak-sih-**NAY**-shun **VAK**-seen	S/ R/ S/	-ate *pertaining to, composed of* vaccin- *vaccine, giving a vaccine* -ation *process* Latin *related to a cow*	To administer a vaccine Administration of a vaccine Preparation to generate active immunity

EXERCISES

A. Patient Education. Select the statement that correctly explains functions of immunity. **LO 7.11 and 7.14**

1. Explain to your patient how immunization works to protect the body.

- **a.** "An immunization contains live microorganisms that cause you to develop the infection so that components of the immune system prevent repeated infections."
- **b.** "An immunization contains killed microorganisms or toxins that do not cause infection but stimulate components of the immune system to protect you from repeat infections."
- **c.** "An immunization is a type of medication that heightens the awareness of the immune system for foreign invaders."
- **d.** "An immunization is a type of medication that strengthens the immune system so that it can do its job more effectively."

2. Explain what the complement system does for the body.

- **a.** "Complement is a type of cell-mediated immunity involving lymphocytes that attack foreign and diseased cells and destroy them."
- **b.** "Complement is a type of immunization to protect a person against infection."
- **c.** "Complement refers to a group of 20 or more immunoglobulins that are present in a vaccine."
- **d.** "Complement is a group of 20 or more proteins that bind to foreign cells, leading to their destruction."

3. Your patient has asked you what agglutinate means. How would you explain the concept to your patient?

- **a.** "Agglutinate refers to the destruction of foreign cells."
- **b.** "Agglutinate refers to cells sticking together to form clumps."
- **c.** "Agglutinate refers to the clumping together of platelets due to an allergic reaction"
- **d.** "Agglutinate refers to destruction of microorganisms following an immunization."

B. Identify the meanings of the word elements. *Select the answer that correctly completes each statement.* **LO 7.1**

1. The root attenu- means:

a. clumping **b.** inject **c.** fluid **d.** weaken

2. The suffix -ity means:

a. source **b.** process **c.** condition **d.** pertaining to

3. The suffix -ation means:

a. weaken **b.** process **c.** condition **d.** pertaining to

Lesson 7.3 (cont'd)

Keynotes

- **Common food and drug allergens are peanuts, milk, eggs, wheat, shellfish, penicillin and related antibiotics, and sulfa drugs.**
- **HIV is found in blood, semen, vaginal secretions, saliva, tears, and breast milk of infected mothers.**
- **The most common means of transmission of HIV are:**
  - **Sexual intercourse (vaginal, oral, anal).**
  - **Shared needles for drug use.**
  - **Contaminated blood products. (All donated blood is now tested for HIV.)**
  - **Transplacental transmission, from an infected mother to her fetus.**

Abbreviations

AIDS	acquired immunodeficiency syndrome
HIV	human immunodeficiency virus

Men 70%

Women 30%

(a)

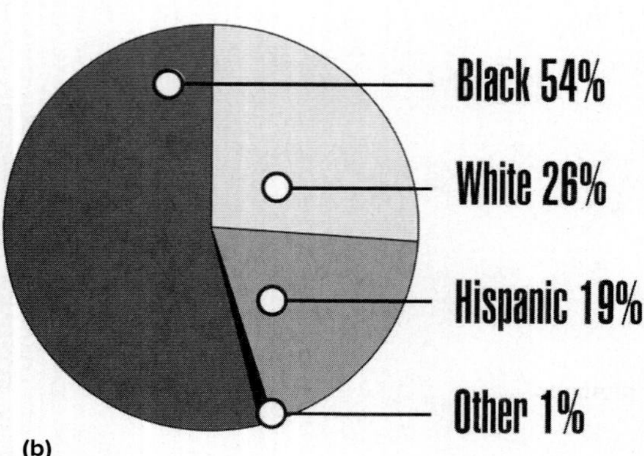

▲ **FIGURE 7.20**
New HIV Infections Each Year in the United States.
(a) by gender (b) by race.

Disorders of the Immune System (LO 7.11)

The immune system is prone to very serious disorders, from allergic reactions to life-threatening infections.

Hypersensitivity is an excessive immune response to an antigen that would normally be tolerated. In most allergic (hypersensitivity) reactions, allergens (antigens) stimulate the cells to produce **histamine.** The symptoms produced by these changes include edema, mucus hypersecretion and congestion, watery eyes, and hives **(urticaria).**

Hypersensitivity includes:

- **Allergies**—reactions to environmental antigens like pollens, molds, dusts, foods, and drugs.
- **Autoimmune disorders**—abnormal reactions to your own tissues.
- **Alloimmune disorders**—reactions to tissues transplanted from another person.

Anaphylaxis is an acute, immediate, and severe allergic reaction, which can be relieved by **antihistamines.**

Anaphylactic shock is more severe and is characterized by difficulty in breathing **(dyspnea)** due to bronchiole constriction, circulatory shock, and even death. It is a life-threatening medical emergency.

Asthma is triggered by allergens, listed above, and by air pollutants, drugs, and emotions. Bronchioles constrict spasmodically **(bronchospasm),** leading to the wheezing and coughing of asthma.

Autoimmune disorders are an over-vigorous response of the immune system. Here, the immune system fails to distinguish self-antigens from foreign antigens. These self-antigens produce autoantibodies that attack the body's own tissues. This type of response occurs, for example, in lupus erythematosus, type 1 diabetes, multiple sclerosis, rheumatoid arthritis, and psoriasis.

Immunodeficiency disorders are a deficient response of the immune system where it fails to respond vigorously enough. These disorders are classified into three categories:

1. **Congenital (inborn) disorders** are caused by a genetic abnormality that is often sex-linked, with boys affected more often than girls. An example is **inherited combined immunodeficiency disease,** characterized by an absence of both T cells and B cells *(Figure 7.20).* These children are very susceptible to **opportunistic** infections and must live in protective sterile enclosures.
2. **Immunosuppression** is a common side effect of corticosteroids used in treatment to prevent transplant rejection and in chemotherapy treatment for cancer.
3. **Acquired immunodeficiency** results from diseases like **acquired immunodeficiency syndrome (AIDS),** which involves a severely depressed immune system from infection with the human immunodeficiency virus **(HIV).**

HIV and AIDS (LO 7.11)

HIV is one of a group of viruses known as **retroviruses.** Like other viruses, it can replicate only inside a living host cell and it invades helper T cells and cells in the upper respiratory tract and CNS. Inside the cell, the virus can stay **dormant** for months or years. When it is activated (AIDS), the new viruses emerge from the dying host cell and attack more cells. This dormant phase **(incubation)** can range from a few months to 12 years.

As the virus destroys more and more cells, the body cannot produce antibodies. Symptoms appear, including chills, fever, night sweats, fatigue, weight loss, and lymphadenitis. Opportunistic infections by bacteria, viruses, and fungi can occur. These infections include toxoplasmosis, pneumocystitis, tuberculosis, herpes simplex, cytomegalovirus, and candidiasis. Cancers can also invade, and a form of skin cancer called **Kaposi sarcoma** *(Figure 7.21)* is common.

HIV survives poorly outside the human body. It is destroyed by laundering, dishwashing, chlorination, and the use of disinfectants, alcohol, and germicidal skin cleansers.

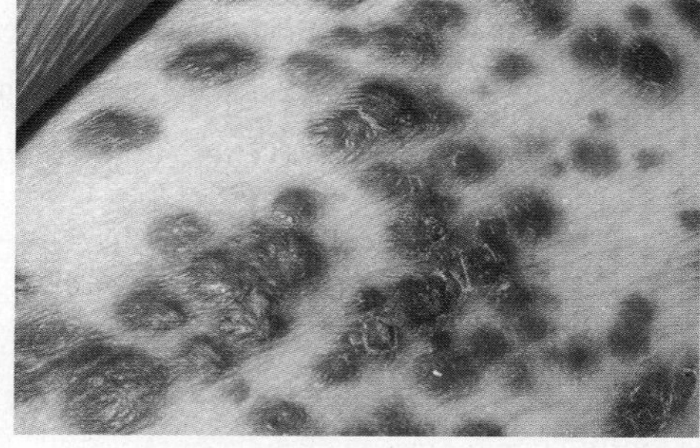

▲ **FIGURE 7.21**
Lesions of Kaposi Sarcoma, a Malignancy that Is a Complication of AIDS.

National Institutes of Health/Stocktrek Images/Getty Images

Word Analysis and Definition

S = Suffix P = Prefix R = Root R/CF = Combining Form

WORD	PRONUNCIATION		ELEMENTS	DEFINITION
alloimmune	**AL**-oh-im-**YUNE**	P/ R/	**all/o-** *other, strange* **-immune** *immunity*	Immune reaction directed against foreign tissue
anaphylaxis	**AN**-ah-fih-**LAK**-sis	P/ R/	**ana-** *excessive* **-phylaxis** *protection*	Immediate severe allergic response
anaphylactic (adj)	**AN**-ah-fih-**LAK**-tik	S/ R/	**-tic** *pertaining to* **-phylac-** *protect*	Pertaining to anaphylaxis
asthma	**AZ**-mah		Greek *asthma*	Episodes of breathing difficulty due to narrowed or obstructed airways.
asthmatic (adj)	az-**MAT**-ik	S/ R/	**-atic** *pertaining to* **asthm-** *asthma*	Suffering from or pertaining to asthma.
dormant	**DOR**-mant	S/ R/	**-ant** *forming* **dorm-** *sleep*	Inactive
histamine	**HISS**-tah-mean	R/ R/	**hist-** *derived from histidine* **-amine** *nitrogen- containing substance*	Compound liberated in tissues as a result of injury or an immune response
antihistamine	**AN**-tih-**HISS**-tah-mean	P/	**anti –** *against*	Drug used to treat allergic symptoms because of its action antagonistic to histamine
hypersensitivity	**HIGH**-per-sen-sih-**TIV**-ih-tee	S/ P/ R/	**-ity** *condition* **hyper-** *excessive* **-sensitiv-** *feeling*	Exaggerated abnormal reaction to an allergen
immunodeficiency	**IM**-you-noh-dee-**FISH**-en-see	S/ R/CF R/	**-ency** *quality, state of* **immun/o-** *immune response* **-defici-** *failure, lacking*	Failure of the immune system
immunosuppression	**IM**-you-noh-suh-**PRESH**-un	S/ R/	**-ion** *action, condition* **-suppress-** *press under*	Failure of the immune system caused by an outside agent
incubation	in-kyu-**BAY**-shun	S/ R/	**-ation** *process* **incub-** *lie on, hatch*	Process to develop an infection
Kaposi sarcoma	Kah-**POH**-see sar-**KOH**-mah		Moritz Kaposi, Hungarian dermatologist, 1837–1902	A skin cancer often seen in AIDS patients
opportunistic	**OP**-or-tyu-**NIS**-tik	S/ R/	**-istic** *pertaining to* **opportun-** *take advantage of*	An organism or a disease in a host with lowered resistance
retrovirus	**REH**-troh-**VIE**-rus	P/ R/	**retro-** *backward* **-virus** *poison*	Virus with an RNA core
urticaria	ur-tee-**KARE**-ee-ah		Latin *nettle*	Rash of itchy wheals (hives)

Exercises

A. Build *more medical vocabulary for the language of immunology. Complete the construction of each term by using the following elements to fill in the blanks. There are more answers than you need.* **LO 7.1 and 7.11**

defici allo suppress sensitiv ion hyper incub osis phylaxis ic ency dorm

1. exaggerated, abnormal reaction to an allergen: _______/_______/ity
2. inactive: ________/ant
3. process to develop an infection: _______/ation
4. failure of the immune system: immuno /________/_______
5. immune reaction toward a foreign tissue: ______/immune

B. Identify the meaning of the word elements. *Given the term, identify the correct definition of the indicated word element.* **LO 7.1 and 7.11**

1. In the term retrovirus, the root means:
   a. poison **b.** cancer **c.** process **d.** nettle
2. In the term hypersensitivity, the root means:
   a. condition **b.** allergen **c.** feeling **d.** inflammation
3. In the term dormant, the suffix means:
   a. forming **b.** take advantage **c.** pertaining to **d.** sleep
4. In the term opportunistic, the root means:
   a. forming **b.** take advantage of **c.** press **d.** backward

Keynote

- When viruses spread from person to person, they are said to be contagious.
- Viral diseases do not respond to antibiotics.
- Nosocomial infections (hospital-acquired infections) are becoming increasingly common and lethal.
- Handwashing is the most important factor in preventing the transmission of infections.

Abbreviations

CA-MRSA	community-associated methicillin-resistant *Staphylococcus aureus*
CDC	Centers for Disease Control and Prevention
CRE	carbapenem-resistant *Enterobacteriaceae*
MRSA	methicillin-resistant *Staphylococcus aureus*
SARS	severe acute respiratory syndrome
WNV	West Nile virus

Infection (LO 7.12)

Microbes (microorganisms) are everywhere–in the air, water, and soil and all over our bodies, where they are called **normal flora.** These normal microorganisms are found on your skin, in your nose and respiratory tract, and in your mouth and digestive tract. Your brain and cardiovascular system, however, are microbe-free **(sterile).**

If microorganisms other than the normal flora invade the body, they become pathogens, which cause an **infection.** Pathogens include bacteria, viruses, fungi, and parasites. If the infection harms the body, it creates an **infectious disease.** Bacterial, viral, fungal, and parasitic infections are all caused by pathogens.

Bacterial Infections (LO 7.12)

Thousands of different bacteria can cause infections. Bacteria are single-celled microorganisms that reproduce by dividing. Frequently seen bacteria include:

- **Staphylococcus ("staph"),** which can be harmless when present on the skin's surface but causes infections in wounds or other normally sterile places, like in a joint or the peritoneum;
- **Streptococcus ("strep"),** which is a cause of sore throats;
- **Pneumococcus,** which is a cause of pneumonia; and
- **Coliform** bacteria that normally live in the GI tract but cause infections elsewhere, such as the urinary tract.

In addition, methicillin-resistant *Staphylococcus aureus* **(MRSA)** is a type of bacteria that is resistant to the antibiotics normally used to treat staph infections. MRSA infections occur most frequently in hospitals **(nosocomial** infection), but are now being seen in community health care facilities as community-associated MRSA **(CA-MRSA).**

Clostridium difficile (C.diff) infection is a growing problem in health care facilities, and the infection kills 14,000 people in America alone each year. When **broad-spectrum** antibiotics, such as **clindamycin,** have destroyed normal gut flora, *C.diff* can take over the gut and release toxins, causing severe diarrhea and abdominal pain that can be difficult to treat and can be life threatening or fatal.

Carbapenem-resistant Enterobacteriaceae **(CRE)** is a lethal "superbug" occuring in American hospitals and responsible for about 9,300 infections and 610 deaths every year. The antibiotic carbapenem is considered a last-resort antibiotic for bacteria that have not responded to other antibiotics. In several cases, the CRE has been found in duodenoscopes, the complex design of which makes them difficult to clean and sterilize.

Viral Infections (LO 7.12)

Viruses are the smallest of the microorganisms. They cannot be seen under an ordinary light **microscope** but are visible through an electron **microscope.** Viruses spread from person to person through coughs, sneezes, and unwashed hands.

Viruses cause specific childhood diseases like measles (rubeola), German measles (rubella), chickenpox (varicella), and mumps. They cause upper respiratory infections *(see Chapter 8),* including modern respiratory infections like **severe acute respiratory syndrome (SARS), avian influenza** (bird flu), and **West Nile virus (WNV).** WNV is a seasonal **epidemic** in North America that flares up in the summer and fall.

Fungal Infections (LO 7.12)

Many fungi are "good fungi," for example, the mushrooms that you eat and the yeasts that ferment beer and bread. Penicillin is derived from a fungus. The most common pathogenic fungi are those that cause skin infections *(see Chapter 3).*

Opportunistic fungi are normally harmless, but like their name, they pounce on any opportunity to cause disease. People who are on prolonged doses of antibiotics, are receiving chemotherapy or immunosuppressive therapy, or have diabetes mellitus or AIDS are especially susceptible.

Parasitic Infections (LO 7.12)

Parasites are organisms that live on or in another organism and steal nourishment from their host. In many rural areas of the world, parasites are **endemic. Malaria** is caused by a parasite that is transmitted from person to person by a single mosquito bite.

Pinworms are the most common parasite in America. Pinworm eggs are introduced into the body through the mouth and hatch in the intestine. The young worms migrate to the anus, where the female deposits her eggs. These eggs can be transferred unknowingly by the fingers from the anus or from infected bedding, to the mouth of the same child or to another child.

Word Analysis and Definition

S = Suffix P = Prefix R = Root R/CF = Combining Form

WORD	PRONUNCIATION		ELEMENTS	DEFINITION
broad-spectrum	broad-**SPECK**-trum		broad Latin *wide* spectrum Latin *image*	An antibiotic with a wide range of activity against a variety of organisms
Clostridium difficile **(also known as** ***Clostridiodes difficile*****)**	klah-**STRID**-ee-um **DIFF**-ih-seal	S/ R/	-ium *structure* clostrid- *spindle*	Gram-positive spore-forming bacteria that causes antibiotic-associated diarrhea.
contagious	kon-**TAY**-jus	S/ P/ R/	-ious *pertaining to* con- *with, together* -tag- *touch*	Infection can be transmitted from person to person or from a person to a surface to a person
endemic	en-**DEM**-ik	S/ P/ R/	-ic *pertaining to* en- *in* -dem- *the people*	Pertaining to a disease always present in a community
epidemic	ep-ih-**DEM**-ik	P/	epi- *above, upon*	Pertaining to an outbreak in a community of a disease or a health-related behavior
pandemic	pan-**DEM**-ik	P/	pan- *all*	Pertaining to a disease attacking the population of a very large area
flora	**FLO**-rah		Latin *flower*	Microorganisms covering the exterior and interior surfaces of a healthy animal
infect (verb) **infection (noun)** **infectious (adj)**	in-**FEKT** in-**FEK**-shun in-**FEK**-shus	 S/ R/ S/	Latin *invade internally* -ion *condition, action* infect- *internal invasion* -ious *pertaining to*	To invade an organism by a microorganism Invasion of the body by disease-producing microorganisms Capable of being transmitted to a person; or a disease caused by the action of a microorganism
microbe **microorganism**	**MY**-krohb **MY**-kroh-**OR**-gan-izm	P/ R/ S/ R/	micro- *small* -be *life* -ism *process* -organ- *organ, instrument*	Short for microorganism Any organism too small to be seen by the naked eye
microscope **microscopic** **microscopy**	**MY**-kroh-skope **MY**-kroh-**SKOP**-ik my-**CROSS**-koh-pee	P/ S/ S/ S/	micro- *small* -scope *instrument for viewing* -ic *pertaining to* -scopy *to examine, to view*	Instrument for viewing something small that cannot be seen in detail by the naked eye Visible only with the aid of a microscope Investigation of minute objects through a microscope
nosocomial	noh-soh-**KOH**-mee-al	S/ R/CF R/	-ial *pertaining to* nos/o- *disease* -com- *take care of*	Acquired while in the hospital

EXERCISES

A. Correct usage *of the appropriate grammatical form of a medical term is the mark of an educated professional. Practice your language of immunology in the following sentences. Fill in the blanks.* **LO 7.2 and 7.12**

1. infect infection infectious

This patient has a rarely seen (a) ____________. Please refer her to the (b) ____________ disease specialist.

2. bacterium bacteria bacterial

The (a) ____________ streptococcus causes (b) ____________ infections in the throat.

3. sterile sterility sterilize

An autoclave is used to (a) ____________ instruments.

If the (b) ____________ of an instrument is in question, it should not be used.

The term (c) ____________ can also mean *unable* to *reproduce*.

B. Use the language of immunology *and select the best answer.* **LO 7.2 and 7.12**

1. What agent causes infections in wounds and joints?

a. staph **b.** pneumococcus **c.** heme

2. What term is the same as "microbe free"?

a. opportunistic **b.** anemic **c.** sterile

3. MRSA occurs most frequently in:

a. prisons **b.** schools **c.** hospitals

4. Another name for microbes is:

a. normal flora **b.** bacteria **c.** pollutants

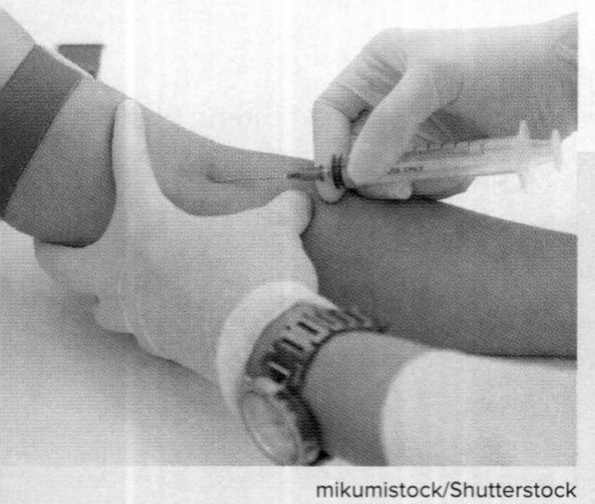
mikumistock/Shutterstock

Lesson 7.4

Diagnostic and Therapeutic Procedures and Pharmacology for the Immune System

Objectives

Immunoassays rely on the ability of an antibody to recognize and bind to a specific antigen and produce a measurable response. In some cases they can use an antigen to detect for the presence of antibodies, and again produce a measurable response. A wide range of medical tests are immunoassays:

7.4.1 Identify immunodiagnostic tests that involve an antigen-antibody reaction.

7.4.2 Define the mechanism of agglutination tests.

7.4.3 Recognize diagnostic tests used for allergies.

Diagnostic Procedures (LO 7.9)

Immunodiagnostics uses an antigen-antibody reaction as a diagnostic tool; an antigen is used to detect antibodies to a **pathogen;** an antibody is used to detect an antigen of a pathogen in a patient's specimen. Very small amounts of biochemical substances can be detected when antibodies specific for a desired antigen are **conjugated** with a radiolabel, fluorescent label, or a color-forming enzyme and used as a "probe" to detect it.

Applications include pregnancy testing, dipsticks, and **enzyme-linked immunosorbent assay (ELISA).** ELISA uses antibodies and enzymes linked to color-changing dyes to detect specific antibodies and chemicals. ELISA is used to diagnose HIV, West Nile virus, malaria, tuberculosis, and rotavirus in feces, as well as in drug screening.

In **agglutination tests,** a particle such as a latex bead or a **bacterium** is coupled to a **reagent** antigen or antibody and the resulting particle **complex** is mixed with the specimen (e.g., serum or CSF). If the target antibody or antigen is present in the specimen, it attaches to the particle complex and produces agglutination.

A **complement fixation** test measures the amount of an antibody in the serum or CSF to viral and fungal infections such as **coccidioidomycosis.**

Diagnostic tests for allergies include:

- **nasal smears** to check the amount of eosinophils in the nose.
- **skin tests** to measure the level of IgE antibodies in response to allergens that are injected under the skin or applied with a small scratch. A reaction appears as a small red area.
- **blood tests** measure IgE antibodies to specific allergens in the blood. A **radioallergosorbent test (RAST)** uses a **radioimmunoassay** to detect the specific IgE antibodies, but is now little used.
- **Challenge testing** is performed by an allergist, who administers a very small amount of an allergen orally or by inhalation and monitors its effect.

High blood levels of IgA are found in multiple myeloma, autoimmune diseases such as rheumatoid arthritis and systemic lupus erythematosus *(see Chapter 3),* and cirrhosis of the liver *(see Chapter 9).* Low levels of IgA occur in some types of leukemia and in nephrotic syndrome *(see Chapter 13).*

High blood levels of IgG can indicate a chronic infection, such as HIV and in chronic hepatitis and multiple sclerosis. Low levels are found in some types of leukemia and in nephrotic syndrome.

High blood levels of IgE are also found in patients with parasitic infections.

Word Analysis and Definition

S = Suffix **P = Prefix** R = Root R/CF = Combining Form

WORD	PRONUNCIATION		ELEMENTS	DEFINITION
bacterium **bacteria (pl)**	bak-**TEER**-ee-um bak-**TEER**-ee-ah		Greek *a staff*	A unicellular microorganism that multiplies by cell division
complex	**KOM**-pleks		Latin *woven together*	A stable combination of two or more compounds in the body
conjugate	**KON**-joo-gate	S/ P/ R/	-ate *composed of, pertaining to* con- *together* jug- *yoke*	To join together, usually in pairs.
immunoassay	**IM**-you-no-**ASS**-ay	R/CF R/	immun/o- *immune* -assay *evaluate*	Biochemical test that uses the reaction of an antibody to its antigen to measure the amount of a substance in a liquid
immunodiagnostics	**IM**-you-no-die-ag-**NOSS**-tiks	S/ R/CF R/	-ics *pertaining to* immun/o- *immune* -diagnost- *decision*	A diagnostic process using antigen-antibody reactions
radioallergosorbent	**RAY**-dee-oh-ah-**LUR**-go-**SOAR**-bent	S/ R/CF R/CF R/	-ent *end result* radi/o- *radiation* -allerg/o- *allergy* -sorb- *suck in*	A radioimmunoassay to detect IgE-bound allergens responsible for tissue hypersensitivity
radioimmunoassay	**RAY**-dee-oh-im-you-no-**ASS**-ay	R/CF R/	-immun/o *immune* -assay *evaluate*	Immunoassay of a substance that has been radioactively labeled

EXERCISES

A. Immunoglobulin (Ig) levels are used to support the diagnosis of lymphatic system disorders. Match the Ig levels in the first column with the condition it is associated with in the second column. **LO 7.3 and 7.9**

______ **1.** increased IgE antibodies **a.** HIV infection

______ **2.** increased IgG antibodies **b.** leukemia

______ **3.** decreased IgG antibodies **c.** parasitic infections

B. Choose the correct test used in the diagnosis of conditions caused by immune system disorders. LO 7.3 and 7.9

1. The test used to detect the presence of HIV infection:

a. ELISA **b.** RAST **c.** challenge testing **d.** Ig levels

2. Patient inhales allergens to see if they cause an allergic reaction:

a. skin test **b.** blood test **c.** challenge testing **d.** agglutination testing

3. Measures the amount of antibody present in cerebrospinal fluid or serum:

a. RAST **b.** complement fixation test **c.** ELISA **d.** challenge testing

Therapeutic Procedures and Pharmacology for the Immune System (LO 7.9)

Immunotherapy, also called **biologic therapy,** is designed to boost the body's natural defenses against cancer by using substances either made in the laboratory or made by the body to enhance or restore immune system function. This form of therapy can stop or slow the growth of cancer cells, and stop cancer from metastasizing.

The types of immunotherapy include:

- **Monoclonal antibodies,** made in the laboratory, can attach to cancer cells to flag them so that macrophages in the body's immune system can recognize and destroy them. Two pathways inside cells that cancers use to evade the immune system have been identified and named PD-1/PD-L1 and CTLA-4. These pathways can be blocked with antibodies called **immune checkpoint inhibitors** to allow the body's immune system to respond to the cancer. Immune checkpoint inhibitors ipilimumab *(Yervoy),* nivolumab *(Opdivo),* and pembrolizumab *(Keytruda)* have been shown to improve overall patient survival in advanced melanoma.
- **Interferons** are a nonspecific immunotherapy mostly given at the same time as other cancer treatments such as chemotherapy or radiation therapy. An interferon called **interferon alpha** made in a laboratory is the most common type of interferon used in cancer treatment.
- **Interleukins** are also a nonspecific immunotherapy used to treat kidney and skin cancers, including melanoma.

Human immunoglobulins are given by injection to confer passive (temporary) immunity that provides immediate protection lasting several weeks. There are two types:

- **Human normal immunoglobulin (HNIG)** made from the plasma of about 1,000 unselected donors to provide antibodies against hepatitis A, rubella, measles, and other viruses found in the general population.
- **Hyperimmune specific immunoglobulins** are made from selected donors and provide antibodies individually against hepatitis B, varicella zoster, rabies, tetanus, and cytomegalovirus.

Immunosuppressant Drugs (LO 7.9)

Immunosuppressant drugs inhibit or prevent activity of the immune system and are used to prevent the rejection of transplanted organs and tissues, treat autoimmune diseases, and help control long-term allergic asthma. There are four main types of immunosuppressant drugs:

- **Glucocorticoids,** which suppress cell-mediated immunity and protect through T-cells and macrophages, and by stimulating cells to secrete **cytokines**.
- **Cytostatics,** which inhibit cell division. Cyclophosphamide *(Cytoxan),* a nitrogen mustard **alkylating** agent, is probably the most potent immunosuppressant. Methotrexate, an **antimetabolite,** interferes with the **synthesis** of nucleic acids and is used in the treatment of autoimmune diseases. Azathioprine (*Imuran*) is the main immunosuppressive **cytotoxic** substance and is used to control transplant rejection reactions.
- **Antibodies** can be used as quick immunosuppressive therapy and are described above in sections on monoclonal antibodies and immunoglobulins.
- **Calcineurin** is a phosphatase that stimulates the growth and differentiation of T-cells. **Calcineurin inhibitors** such as ciclosporin *(Sandimmune),* tacrolimus *(Prograf),* and sirolimus *(Rapamune)* are used in the prevention and treatment of transplant rejection reactions.

Alcohol, marijuana, and illicit drugs have been shown to depress the immune system.

Word Analysis and Definition

S = Suffix P = Prefix R = Root R/CF = Combining Form

WORD	PRONUNCIATION		ELEMENTS	DEFINITION
alkylation	al-kih-**LAY**-shun	S/ R/	-ation *process* alkyl- *alkali*	Introduction of a side chain into a compound
antimetabolite	**AN**-tih-meh-**TAB**- oh-lite	S/ P/ R/	-ite *resembling* anti- *against* -metabol- *change*	A substance that antagonizes another substance
biologic	**BI**-oh-**LOJ**-ik	S/ R/CF R/	-ic *pertaining to* bio- *life* -log- *study of*	Pertaining to the study of life and living organisms
calcineurin	kal-see-**NYUR**-in	S/ R/CF R/	-in *chemical* calc/i *calcium* -neur- *nerve*	A chemical that stimulates the growth and differentiation of T-cells
cytokine	**SIGH**-toh-kine	S/ R/CF	-kine *movement* cyt/o- *cell*	A hormone-like protein that regulates the intensity of an immune response
cytostatic	**SIGH**-toh-**STAT**-ik	S/ R/CF R/	-ic *pertaining to* cyt/o *cell* -stat- *stop*	Inhibiting cell division
cytotoxic	**SIGH**-toh-**TOK**-sik	S/	-toxic *able to kill*	Destructive to cells
immunoglobulin	**IM**-you-noh-**GLOB**-you-lin	S/ R/CF R/	-in *chemical* immun/o *immune response* -globul- *protein*	Specific protein (antibody) generated by an antigen
immunotherapy	**IM**-you-noh-**THAIR**-ah-pee	R/ R/CF	immun/o *immune response* -therapy *treatment*	Treatment to boost immune system function
inhibitor	in-**HIB**-ih-tor	S/ R/	-or *that which does* inhibit- *restrain*	An agent that restrains a chemical action
interferon	in-ter-**FEER**-on	S/ P/ R/	-on *on* inter- *between* -fer- *to strike*	A small protein produced by T-cells in response to infection
interleukin	**IN**-ter-**LOO**-kin	S/ P/ R/	-in *chemical* inter- *between* leuk- *white*	A group of cytokines synthesized by white blood cells
monoclonal	**MON**-oh-**KLOH**-nal	S/ P/ R/	-al *pertaining to* mono- *one* -clon- *cutting used for propagation*	Derived in the laboratory from a protein from a single colony of cells

Exercises

A. Identify the action of the drug based on a word element that it contains. *Being able to pick out and define word elements can help you determine the meaning of the word. Select the answer that correctly completes each statement.* **LO 7.9**

1. A medication that would provide antibodies to persons to prevent viral infections:

a. cytostatic **b.** glucocorticoid **c.** human normal immunoglobulin **d.** monoclonal antibodies

2. A medication that would inhibit cell division:

a. cytostatic **b.** calcineurin **c.** interleukin **d.** interferon

B. Categorize medications of immunotherapy. *Match the medication in the first column with the disorder it is used to treat in the second column.* **LO 7.9**

_____ **1.** interleukin — **a.** treat kidney and skin cancers

_____ **2.** interferons — **b.** flag cancer cells for macrophages

_____ **3.** monoclonal antibodies — **c.** given alongside chemotherapy and radiation therapy

C. Categorize immunosuppressant drugs. *Match the medication in the first column with the disorder it is used to treat in the second column.* **LO 7.9**

_____ **1.** methotrexate — **a.** interferes with nucleic acids as a means to treat autoimmune diseases

_____ **2.** tacrolimus (*Prograf*) — **b.** most potent immunosuppressant

_____ **3.** glucocorticoid — **c.** suppresses cell-mediated immunity

_____ **4.** cyclophosphamide (*Cytoxan*) — **d.** prevents and treats transplant rejection reactions

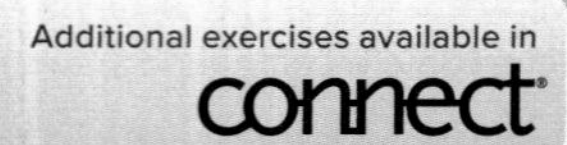

Chapter Review exercises, along with additional practice items, are available in Connect!

The Respiratory System

The Essentials of the Language of Pulmonology

CHAPTER 8

Rick Brady/McGraw-Hill Education

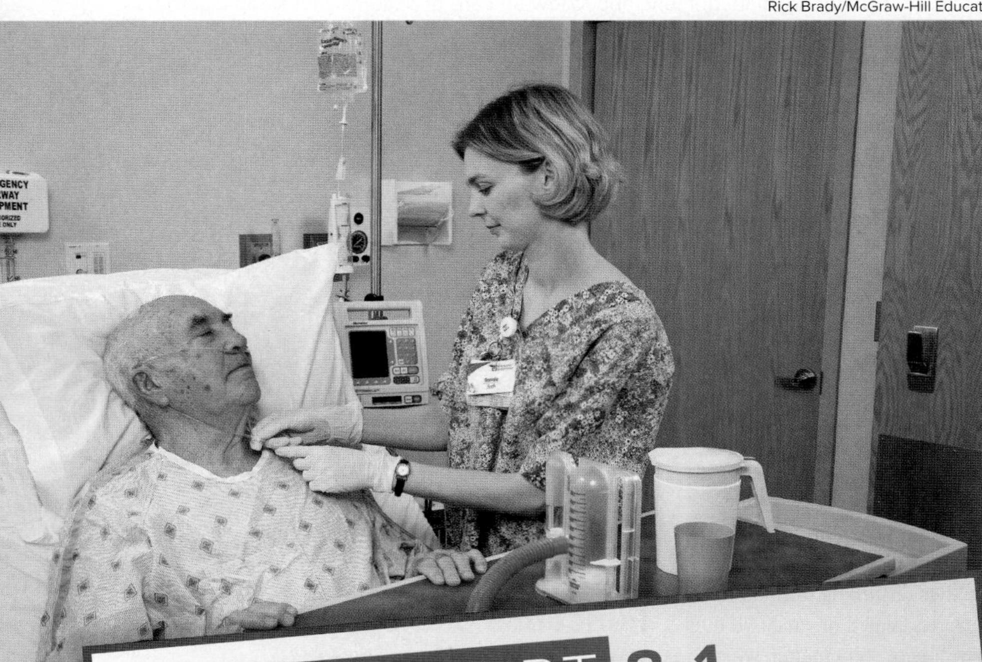

CASE REPORT 8.1

You are . . .

. . . an advanced-level **registered respiratory therapist (RRT)** working with **pulmonologist** Tavis Senko, MD, in the Acute Respiratory Care unit of Fulwood Medical Center.

You are communicating with . . .

. . . Mr. Jude Jacobs, a 68-year-old white, retired, mail carrier, who has chronic obstructive pulmonary disease **(COPD)** and is on continual **oxygen (O_2)** by nasal prongs. He has smoked two packs of cigarettes per day throughout his adult life.

Last night, he was unable to sleep because of increased shortness of breath **(SOB)** and cough. He had to sit upright in bed in order to breathe. His cough produces yellow **sputum.**

Mr. Jacobs' vital signs are temperature **(T)** of 101.6°, pulse **(P)** of 98, respirations **(R)** of 36, and blood pressure **(BP)** 150/90. On examination, he is **cyanotic** and frightened, and he is on oxygen by nasal prongs. Air entry is diminished in both lungs, and there are **rales** (crackles) at the bases of both lungs.

You have been ordered to draw blood for arterial blood gases **(ABGs)** and to measure the amount of air entering and leaving his lungs by using **spirometry.**

Learning Outcomes

In order to provide optimal care to Mr. Jacobs, determine what is causing his symptoms and signs, and communicate with the other health professionals involved in his care, you need to be able to:

LO 8.1 **Use roots, combining forms, suffixes, and prefixes to construct and analyze (deconstruct) medical terms related to the respiratory system.**

LO 8.2 **Spell and pronounce correctly medical terms related to the respiratory system in order to communicate with accuracy and precision in any health care setting.**

LO 8.3 **Define accepted abbreviations related to the respiratory system.**

LO 8.4 **Relate the structures of the anatomical elements of the upper respiratory tract to their functions and signs and symptoms of respiratory disorders.**

LO 8.5 **Use the structures of the elements of the lower respiratory tract to explain the mechanics of respiration and the functions and disorders of the lower respiratory tract.**

LO 8.6 **Explain the diagnostic and therapeutic procedures and pharmacologic agents used for disorders of the respiratory system.**

LO 8.7 **Apply your knowledge of the medical terms of the respiratory system to documentation, medical records, and medical reports.**

LO 8.8 **Translate the medical terms of the respiratory system into everyday language in order to communicate clearly with patients and their families.**

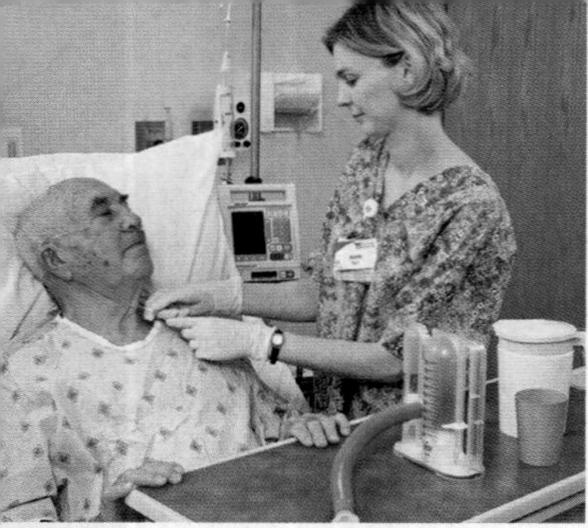

Rick Brady/McGraw-Hill Education

In your future career, being able to communicate comfortably, accurately, and effectively with the health professionals involved in the diagnosis and treatment of respiratory problems is key. You may work directly and/or indirectly with one or more of the following:

- **Pulmonologists** are physicians who specialize in the diagnosis and treatment of lung/pulmonary conditions.
- **Registered respiratory therapists (RRT) or respiratory care practitioners** assist physicians in evaluating, treating, and caring for patients who have respiratory disorders. They also supervise RT technicians.
- **Respiratory therapy (RT) technicians** assist physicians and RRTs in evaluating, monitoring, and treating patients with respiratory disorders.
- **Sleep technologists** are trained in sleep technology and sleep medicine. These technologists assist sleep specialists in the assessment, monitoring, management, and follow-up care of patients with sleep disorders.

Objectives

*Your **upper respiratory tract** consists of your nose, pharynx, and trachea. It is the first site that brings air and its pollutants inside your body. The information in this lesson will enable you to use correct medical terminology to:*

8.1.1 Trace the flow of air from the nose through the pharynx and larynx.

8.1.2 Define the protective mechanisms of the upper respiratory tract.

8.1.3 Describe how sound is produced.

8.1.4 List the functions of the respiratory system.

Abbreviations

ABG	arterial blood gas
COPD	chronic obstructive pulmonary disease
O_2	oxygen
RRT	registered respiratory therapist

Lesson 8.1

Introduction to the Respiratory System (LO 8.4 and 8.5)

Communication (LO 8.2)

It sounds like a good scheme. Humans and animals breathe in **oxygen** and breathe out **carbon dioxide,** while plants and trees breathe in carbon dioxide and breathe out oxygen. Unfortunately, we continue to generate increasing amounts of carbon dioxide in the air by burning coal, oil, and natural gas, and cutting down forests, thus disturbing this natural balance. In addition, humans have created organic and inorganic chemicals and small particles of solid matter, which float through the air and enter our bodies as we breathe. These **pollutants** can damage our respiratory tracts and cause cancer, brain damage, and birth defects.

The Respiratory Tract (LO 8.4 and 8.5)

The **respiratory tract** *(Figure 8.1)* has six connected elements:

1. **Nose**
2. **Pharynx**
3. **Larynx**
4. **Trachea**
5. **Bronchi** and **bronchioles**
6. **Alveoli**

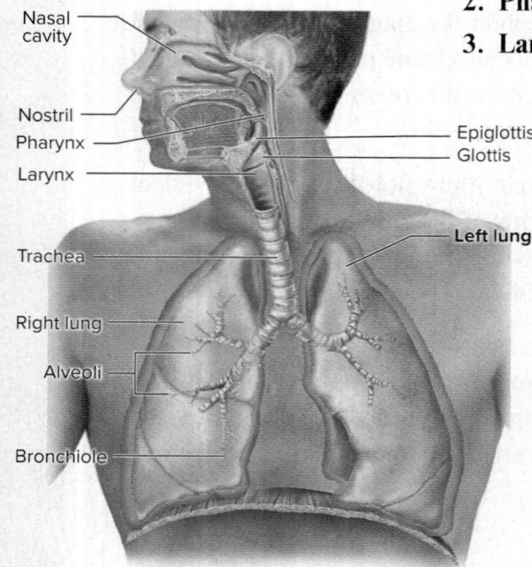

▲ **FIGURE 8.1**
The Respiratory System.

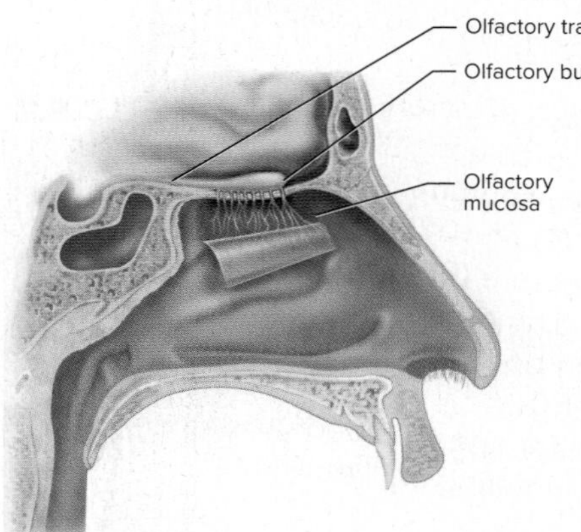

▲ **FIGURE 8.2**
Olfactory Region of the Nose.

Respiration has two components:

- **Ventilation,** which is the movement of air and its gases into **(inspiration)** and out of **(expiration)** the lungs; and
- The **exchange of gases** between air and blood, and between blood and interstitial fluids.

Functions of the Respiratory System (LO 8.4 and 8.5)

Your respiratory system is responsible for the following key functions:

1. **Exchange of gases:** All of your body cells need oxygen and produce carbon dioxide. Your respiratory system allows oxygen from the air to enter the blood and carbon dioxide to leave the blood and enter the air.
2. **Regulation of blood pH:** Regulation occurs by changing carbon dioxide levels in the blood.
3. **Protection:** The respiratory system protects against foreign bodies and against some microorganisms.
4. **Voice production:** Movement of air across the vocal cords makes voice and sound possible.
5. **Olfaction:** The 12 million receptor cells for smell are in a quarter-sized patch of epithelium. These are located in the **olfactory region** *(Figure 8.2),* the extreme superior region of the nasal cavity. Each cell has 10 to 20 hair-like structures called **cilia** that project into the nasal cavity in a thin mucous film.

Because the olfactory region is right at the top of your nose, you often have to sniff deeply to stimulate the sense of smell. Because dogs have 4 billion receptor cells in their noses, they can be trained to sniff for drugs, explosives, or human scent.

Word Analysis and Definition

S = Suffix P = Prefix R = Root R/CF = Combining Form

WORD	PRONUNCIATION	ELEMENTS		DEFINITION
alveolus **alveoli (pl)** **alveolar (adj)**	al-**VEE**-oh-lus al-**VEE**-oh-lee al-**VEE**-oh-lar	 S/ R/	Latin *hollow sac* **-ar** *pertaining to* **alveol-** *air sac*	Terminal element of respiratory tract where gas exchange occurs Pertaining to the alveoli
bronchus **bronchi (pl)** **bronchiole**	**BRONG**-kuss **BRONG**-key **BRONG**-key-ole	 S/ R/CF	Greek *windpipe* **-ole** *small* **bronch/i-** *bronchus*	One of two subdivisions of the trachea Increasingly smaller subdivisions of bronchi
cilium **cilia (pl)**	**SILL**-ee-um **SILL**-ee-ah		Latin *eyelash*	Hairlike motile projection from the surface of a cell
expiration (**Note:** *The "s" is deleted from the root* spirat *because the prefix* ex *already has the "s" sound.*)	**EKS**-pih-**RAY**-shun	S/ P/ R/	**-ion** *action, condition, process of* **ex-** *out* **-spirat-** *breathe*	Breathe out
inspiration (**Note:** *The opposite of expiration*)	in-spih-**RAY**-shun	S/ P/ R/	**-ion** *action, condition, process of* **in-** *into* **-spirat-** *breathe*	Breathe in
olfaction **olfactory (adj)**	ol-**FAK**-shun ol-**FAK**-toh-ree	S/ S/ R/	**-ion** *action, condition, process of* **-ory** *having the function of* **olfact-** *smell*	Sense of smell Relating to the sense of smell
oxygen	**OCK**-si-jen	S/ R/	**-gen** *create* **oxy-** *oxygen*	The gas essential for life
pharynx **pharyngeal (adj)**	**FAH**-rinks fah-**RIN**-jee-al	 S/ R/	Greek *throat* **-eal** *pertaining to* **pharyng-** *pharynx*	Tube from the back of the nose to the larynx. Pertaining to the pharynx
pulmonary **pulmonology** **pulmonologist**	**PULL**-moh-**NAR**-ee **PULL**-moh-**NOL**-oh-jee **PULL**-moh-**NOL**-oh-jist	S/ R/ S/ R/CF S/	**-ary** *pertaining to* **pulmon-** *lung* **-logy** *study of* **pulmon/o-** *lung* **-logist** *one who studies, specialist*	Pertaining to the lungs Study of the lungs, or the medical specialty of disorders of the lungs Specialist in treating disorders of the lungs
rale **rales (pl)**	RAHL RAHLS		French *rattle*	Crackle heard through a stethoscope when air bubbles through liquid in the lungs
respiration **respirator** **respiratory (adj)**	**RES**-pih-**RAY**-shun **RES**-pih-**RAY**-tor **RES**-pih-rah-tor-ee	S/ P/ R/ S/ S/	**-ation** *a process, formed from* **re-** *again* **-spir-** *to breathe* **-ator** *person or thing that does something* **-atory** *pertaining to, produced by*	Process of breathing; fundamental process of life used to exchange oxygen and carbon dioxide Another name for ventilator Pertaining to respiration
sputum	**SPYU**-tum		Latin *to spit*	Matter coughed up and spat out by individuals with respiratory disorders
trachea **trachealis (adj)**	**TRAY**-kee-ah tray-kee-**AY**-lis	 S/ R/	Greek *windpipe* **-alis** *pertaining to* **trache-** *trachea*	Air tube from the larynx to the bronchi Pertaining to the trachea

EXERCISES

A. Review *Case Report 8.1 before answering the questions. Fill in the blanks.* **LO 8.2, 8.4, and 8.5**

1. In Case Report 8.1, the type of physician that is responsible for Mr. Jacobs's care is a: ______________________.

2. The device that is delivering oxygen therapy to Mr. Jacobs is: ______________________

3. The device that measures that amount of air entering and leaving Mr. Jacobs's lungs is a: ______________________

4. Which test ordered for Mr. Jacobs involves drawing his blood? (Provide the abbreviation) ______________________

5. The material that Mr. Jacobs brought up from is lung is termed: ______________________

6. The medical term in Case Report 8.1 that indicates that is skin has a blue color is: ______________________

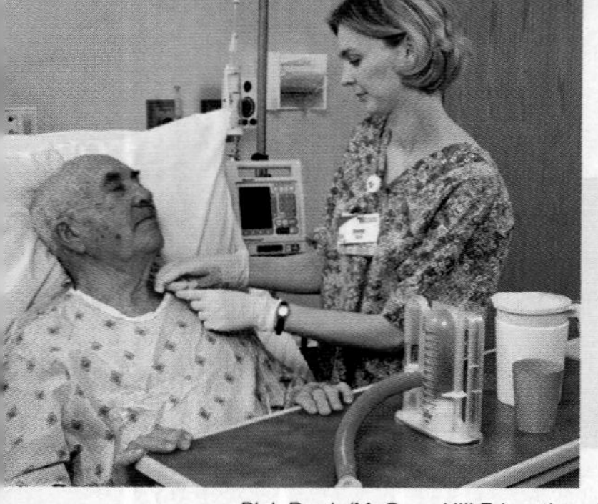

Rick Brady/McGraw-Hill Education

Lesson 8.2

Upper Respiratory Tract

Objectives

8.2.1 Identify the functions of the nose.

8.2.2 Describe disorders of the nose.

The Nose (LO 8.4)

When you breathe in air through your nose, the air goes through the nostrils **(nares)** into the **nasal cavity.** Internal hairs guard the nares to prevent large particles from entering your body.

The nasal **septum** divides the nasal cavity into right and left compartments. The **palate** forms the floor of the nose *(Figure 8.3).* The **paranasal frontal** and **maxillary sinuses** *(Chapter 4)* open into the nose.

Functions of the Nose (LO 8.4)

The nose serves as an important part of the respiratory system in several ways:

1. **Passageway for air** to enter or leave the body.
2. **Air cleanser:** The nasal hairs and the mucus (secreted by the nasal mucous membrane) trap particles of dust and solid pollutants.
3. **Air moisturizer:** It adds moisture to the air. Moisture is secreted by the nasal mucosa (mucous membrane) and from tears that drain into the nasal cavity through the nasal lacrimal duct *(see Chapter 11).*
4. **Air warmer:** The blood flowing through the nasal cavity beneath the mucous membrane lining also warms the air. This prevents damage from cold to the more fragile lower respiratory passages.
5. **Sense of smell (olfaction):** The olfactory region recognizes some 4,000 separate smells *(see previous pages).*

Abbreviation

URI upper respiratory infection

Disorders of the Nose (LO 8.4)

A **common cold** is a viral upper respiratory infection **(URI).** It is contagious and easily transmitted in airborne droplets through coughing and sneezing. There is no proven effective treatment.

Rhinitis, also called **coryza,** is an inflammation of the nasal mucosa, which is usually viral.

Allergic rhinitis affects 15% to 20% of the population. The mucous membranes of the nose, pharynx, and sinuses swell and produce a clear, watery discharge. Treatment entails defining and removing the allergy-causing agent.

Sinusitis is an infection of the paranasal sinuses, often following a viral upper respiratory tract infection. It can also be part of an allergic response. It can be treated with **antibiotics** and **decongestants.**

A **deviated nasal septum** occurs when the partition between the two nostrils is pushed to one side, leading to a partially obstructed airway in one nostril. Treatment is by surgery.

Nasal polyps are benign growths arising from the mucosa of the nasal cavity or a sinus. These can be surgically removed.

Epistaxis (a nosebleed) is bleeding from the septum of the nose, usually as a result of trauma.

Most nose bleeds can be treated at home by pinching the soft part of the nose for 15 to 20 minutes. If this fails, medical treatment can consist of **cauterization,** or nasal packing with gauze strips.

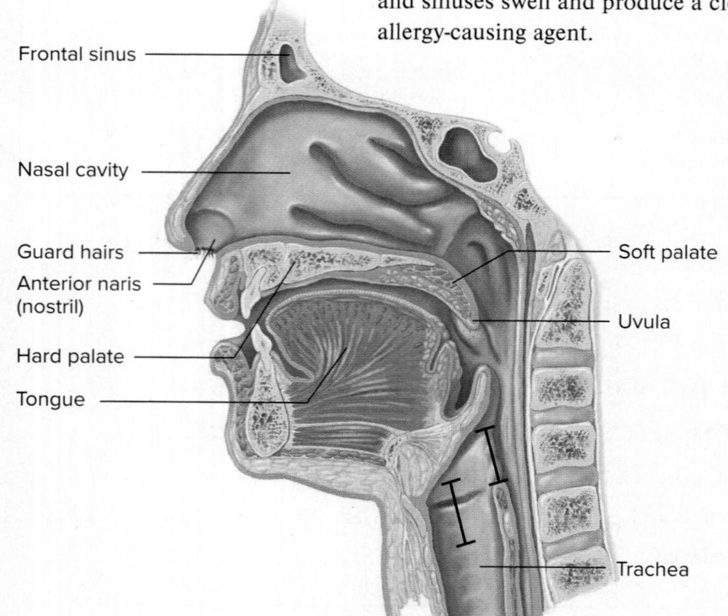

FIGURE 8.3
Upper Respiratory Tract.

Word Analysis and Definition

S = Suffix P = Prefix R = Root R/CF = Combining Form

WORD	PRONUNCIATION		ELEMENTS	DEFINITION
cautery **cauterize** **cauterization**	**KAW**-ter-ee **KAW**-ter-ize **KAW**-ter-eye-**ZAY**-shun	S/ R/ S/	Greek *branding iron* **-ize** *action* **cauter-** *to burn* **ation** *a process*	A device to scar, burn, or cut a tissue To apply a cautery The act of cauterizing
coryza (*also called* **rhinitis**)	koh-**RYE**-zah		Greek *catarrh*	Acute inflammation of the mucous membrane of the nose
decongestant	dee-con-**JESS**-tant	S/ P/ R/	**-ant** *pertaining to* **de-** *take away, remove* **-congest-** *accumulation of fluid*	Agent that reduces the swelling and fluid in the nose and sinuses
epistaxis	ep-ih-**STAK**-sis	S/ P/ R/	**-is** *pertaining to* **epi-** *above, upon* **-stax-** *fall in drops*	Nosebleed
naris **nares (pl)** **nasal**	**NAH**-ris **NAH**-rees **NAY**-zal	S/ R/	Latin *nostril* **-al** *pertaining to* **nas-** *nose*	Nostril Pertaining to the nose
palate	**PAL**-at		Latin *palate*	Roof of the mouth, floor of the nose
paranasal	**PAR**-ah-**NAY**-zal	S/ P/ R/	**-al** *pertaining to* **para-** *adjacent to* **-nas-** *nose*	Adjacent to the nose
polyp	**POL**-ip		Latin *many feet*	Any mass of tissue that projects outward
rhinitis (*also called* **coryza**)	rye-**NIE**-tis	S/ R/	**-itis** *inflammation* **rhin-** *nose*	Acute inflammation of the nasal mucosa
septum **septa (pl)**	**SEP**-tum **SEP**-tah		Latin *partition*	Thin wall separating two cavities or tissue masses
sinus **sinusitis**	**SIGH**-nus sigh-nu-**SIGH**-tis	R/ S/	Latin *cavity* **sinus-** *sinus* **-itis** *inflammation*	Cavity or hollow space in a bone or other tissue Inflammation of the lining of a sinus

EXERCISES

A. Elements: *Work with elements to build your knowledge of the language of pulmonology. One element in each of the following medical terms is boldfaced. Identify the type of element (P, R, CF, or S) in column 2; then provide the meaning of that element in column 3.* **LO 8.1**

Medical Term	Type of Element	Meaning of Element
1. **nas**al	________________	________________
2. decongest**ant**	________________	________________
3. **rhin**itis	________________	________________
4. epi**stax**is	________________	________________
5. **para**nasal	________________	________________
6. sinus**itis**	________________	________________

B. Greek and Latin terms. *Not all terms can be deconstructed into word parts. Identify the definitions of the following terms related to the language of pulmonology.* **LO 8.4**

_____ **1.** septum **a.** branding iron

_____ **2.** sinus **b.** partition

_____ **3.** polyp **c.** nostril

_____ **4.** cautery **d.** many feet

_____ **5.** naris **e.** cavity

CASE REPORT 8.2

You are . . .

. . . a sleep technologist in the Sleep Disorders Clinic at Fulwood Medical Center. You are about to position the electrodes on your patient for an overnight **polysomnography** (sleep study).

You are communicating with . . .

. . . Mr. Tye Gawlinski, a 29-year-old professional football player, and his wife. Mrs. Helen Gawlinski states that her husband snores loudly and has 40 or 50 periods in the night when he stops breathing. The snoring is so loud that she cannot sleep, even in the adjoining bedroom. Mr. Gawlinski complains of being tired all day and not having the energy he needs for his job. The sleep study is being performed to confirm a diagnosis of obstructive sleep **apnea.**

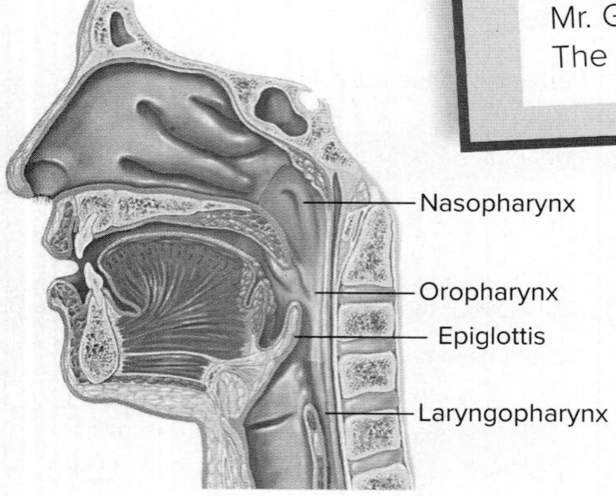

▲ **FIGURE 8.4**
Regions of the Pharynx.

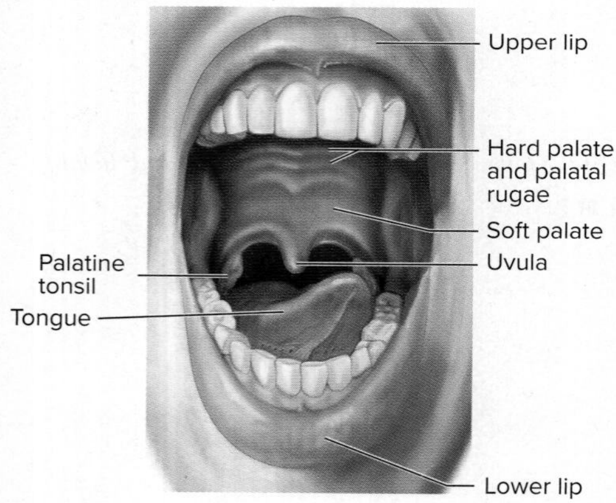

▲ **FIGURE 8.5**
Soft Tissues at the Back of the Mouth.

The Pharynx (LO 8.4)

Your pharynx is a muscular funnel that receives air from the nasal cavity, and food and drink from the oral cavity. It is divided into three regions *(Figure 8.4):*

1. **Nasopharynx:** Located at the back of the nose and above the soft palate and uvula. The posterior surface contains the pharyngeal **tonsil (adenoid).** Only air moves through this region;
2. **Oropharynx:** Located at the back of the mouth, and below the soft palate and above the epiglottis. It contains two sets of tonsils called the palatine and lingual tonsils. Air, food, and drink all pass through this region; and
3. **Laryngopharynx:** Located below the tip of the epiglottis. It is the pathway to the esophagus. Only food and drink pass through the laryngopharynx.

Disorders of the Pharynx (LO 8.4)

Snoring occurs regularly in 25% of normal adults and is most common in overweight males. It worsens with age. Snoring noises are made at the back of the mouth and nose where the tongue and upper pharynx meet the soft palate and uvula *(Figure 8.5).*

Obstructive sleep apnea is the condition Mr. Gawlinski has. Bulky neck tissue from his football training causes an obstruction by the soft tissues at the back of his nose and mouth. This leads to frequent episodes of gasping for breath, followed by complete cessation of breathing **(apnea).** These episodes reduce the level of oxygen in the blood **(hypoxemia),** making his heart pump harder. If this problem goes untreated for several years, it can cause hypertension and cardiac enlargement.

Pharyngitis is an acute or chronic infection involving the pharynx, tonsils, and uvula. It is usually viral in children. Increasing air humidity and getting extra rest are effective treatments.

Tonsillitis is usually a viral infection of the tonsils in the oropharynx. In less than 20% of cases, this infection is caused by a streptococcus. A rapid strep test and throat culture are used to identify the strep sore throat or pharyngitis.

Nasopharyngeal carcinoma is a rare form of cancer that occurs mostly in males between the ages of 50 and 60. Treatment includes radiation and chemotherapy.

Case Report 8.2 *(continued)*

Initially, Mr. Gawlinski was instructed to sleep on his side and to use a device that, through a mask over his nose and mouth, produces a continuous positive airway pressure **(CPAP)** in his airways. He found this very uncomfortable, and it kept him awake. Instead, he chose to have the pillar procedure, in which three tiny pillars were placed in the back of his throat to support the tissues. Subsequently, Mr. Gawlinski has stopped snoring and Mrs. Gawlinski is back in the same bed.

Abbreviation

CPAP	continuous positive airway pressure

Word Analysis and Definition

S = Suffix P = Prefix R = Root R/CF = Combining Form

WORD	PRONUNCIATION	ELEMENTS		DEFINITION
adenoid	**ADD**-eh-noyd	S/ R/	**-oid** *resembling* **aden-** *gland*	Single mass of lymphoid tissue in the midline at the back of the throat
apnea	**AP**-nee-ah	P/ R/	**a-** *without* **-pnea** *breathe*	Absence of spontaneous respiration
hypoxemia	high-pock-**SEE**-me-ah	S/ P/ R/	**-emia** *condition of the blood* **hyp-** *below* **-ox-** *oxygen*	Low oxygen level in arterial blood
hypoxia (noun)	high-**POCK**-see-ah	S/	**-ia** *condition*	Decreased below normal levels of oxygen in tissues, gases, or blood
hypoxic (adj)	high-**POCK**-sik	S/	**-ic** *pertaining to*	Deficient in oxygen
laryngopharynx	lah-**RIN**-go-**FAH**-rinks	R/CF R/	**laryng/o-** *larynx* **-pharynx** *pharynx, throat*	Region of the pharynx below the epiglottis that includes the larynx
nasopharynx	**NAY**-zoh-**FAH**-rinks	R/CF R/	**nas/o-** *nose* **-pharynx** *pharynx, throat*	Region of the pharynx at the back of the nose and above the soft palate
nasopharyngeal (adj)	**NAY**-zoh-fah-**RIN**-jee-al	S/ R/CF	**-eal** *pertaining to* **-pharyng-** *pharynx, throat*	Pertaining to the nasopharynx
oropharynx	**OR**-oh-fah-rinks	R/CF R/	**or/o-** *mouth* **-pharynx** *pharynx, throat*	Region at the back of the mouth between the soft palate and the tip of the epiglottis.
oropharyngeal (adj)	**OR**-oh-fah-**RIN**-jee-al	S/ R	**-eal** *pertaining to* **-pharyng-** *pharynx, throat*	Pertaining to the oropharynx
pharyngitis	fair-in-**JIE**-tis	S/ R/	**-itis** *inflammation* **pharyng-** *pharynx, throat*	Inflammation of the pharynx
polysomnography	**POLL**-ee-som-**NOG**-rah-fee	S/ P/ R/CF	**-graphy** *process of recording* **poly-** *many* **-somn/o-** *sleep*	Test to monitor brain waves, muscle tension, eye movement, and oxygen levels in the blood as the patient sleeps
tonsil	**TON**-sill		Latin *tonsil*	Mass of lymphoid tissue on either side of the throat at the back of the tongue
tonsillitis (**Note:** *double "ll"*)	ton-sih-**LIE**-tis	S/ R/	**-itis** *inflammation* **tonsill-** *tonsil*	Inflammation of the tonsils
tonsillectomy	ton-sih-**LEK**-toh-me	S/	**-ectomy** *surgical excision*	Surgical removal of the tonsils

Exercises

A. After reading Case Report 8.2, *answer the following questions.* **LO 8.6 and 8.7**

1. What are Mr. Gawlinski's symptoms? (Choose all that apply)
   a. daytime sleepiness **b.** sore throat **c.** lack of energy **d.** runny nose
2. Mr. Gawlinski underwent the diagnostic procedure of:
   a. tonsillectomy **b.** endoscopy **c.** polysomnography **d.** sonogram
3. The first therapy Mr. Gawlinski used to treat his sleep apnea:
   a. PFTs **b.** CPAP **c.** tonsillectomy **d.** hypoxemia
4. Why is polysomnography done overnight?
   a. The test requires at least 8 hours of monitoring.
   b. The technicians are only hired for the night shift.
   c. Sleep apnea only occurs in the nighttime hours.
   d. The test requires monitoring of a typical night's sleep.

B. Use the medical terms *relating to the pharynx and its disorders.* **LO 8.2, 8.6, and 8.8**

1. Inflammation of the tonsils: ____________.
2. Low oxygen level in the arterial blood: ____________.
3. The medical term for a common sore throat is ____________.
4. Surgical excision of the tonsils is ____________.
5. Absence of spontaneous respiration: ____________.
6. Condition in which the body is deficient in oxygen: ____________.

Keynotes

- **On December 14, 1799, President George Washington died of an obstructed airway due to acute epiglottitis.**
- **Croup occurs in children aged 3 months to 5 years.**
- **Heavy smokers and drinkers have a 200 times greater risk of developing cancer of the larynx.**

The Larynx (LO 8.4)

The flow of inhaled air moves on from your pharynx to your **larynx.** The upper opening into the larynx from the oropharynx is called the **glottis.** The spoon-shaped **epiglottis** guards the glottis. When you swallow food, your tongue pushes down the epiglottis to close the glottis and direct the food into the esophagus behind it *(Figure 8.6).* The **thyroid** cartilage, or the Adam's apple, forms the anterior and lateral walls of the larynx. Inside the larynx, two pairs of horizontal ligaments–your **vocal** cords *(Figures 8.7 and 8.8)*–stretch across the lateral walls and enable sounds to be made as air passes between them.

Functions of the Larynx (LO 8.4)

Two major roles of your larynx are:

1. Maintaining an open passage for the movement of air to and from the trachea *(Figure 8.7)* and
2. Producing sounds through the vocal cords.

Sound Production Air moving past the vocal cords makes them vibrate to produce sound. The force of the air moving past the vocal cords determines the loudness of the sound. Muscles in the cords pull them closer together with varying degrees of tautness *(Figure 8.8).* A high-pitched sound is produced by taut cords, and a low-pitched sound is made by more relaxed cords. Males' vocal cords are longer and thicker than those of females. They vibrate more slowly and produce lower-pitched sounds.

The crude sounds produced by the larynx are transformed into words by the actions of the pharynx, tongue, teeth, and lips.

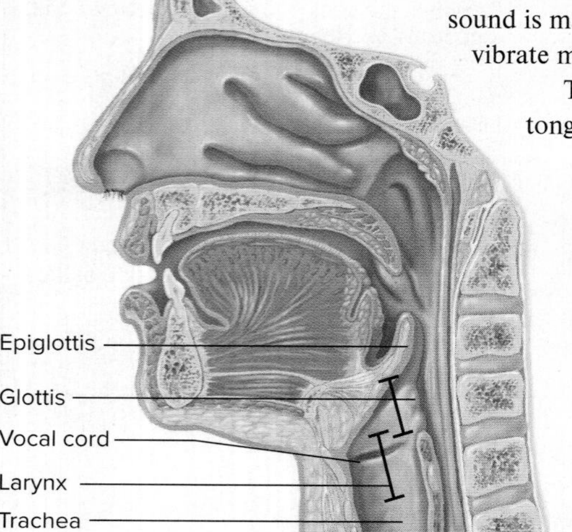

▲ **FIGURE 8.6**
Larynx Location.

Disorders of the Larynx (LO 8.4 and 8.6)

Laryngitis is an inflammation of the mucosal lining of the larynx, which produces hoarseness and sometimes progresses to a loss of voice.

Epiglottitis is an inflammation of the epiglottis. **Acute epiglottitis** is seen most commonly in children between the ages of 2 and 7 years. It can cause acute airway obstruction, which requires a tube to be inserted into the windpipe **(intubation).** It is preventable by vaccine.

Croup (laryngotracheobronchitis) is a group of viral diseases causing an inflammation and obstruction of the upper airway. It's most common in children between the ages of 3 months and 5 years. In severe cases, a child makes a high-pitched, squeaky, inspiratory noise called **stridor.** Humidity is the initial treatment.

Papillomas or polyps are benign tumors of the larynx due to overuse or irritation. These are surgically removed using a **laryngoscope.**

Carcinoma of the larynx produces a persistent hoarseness. Its incidence peaks among people in their 50s and 60s. Treatment can be radiation and/or chemotherapy.

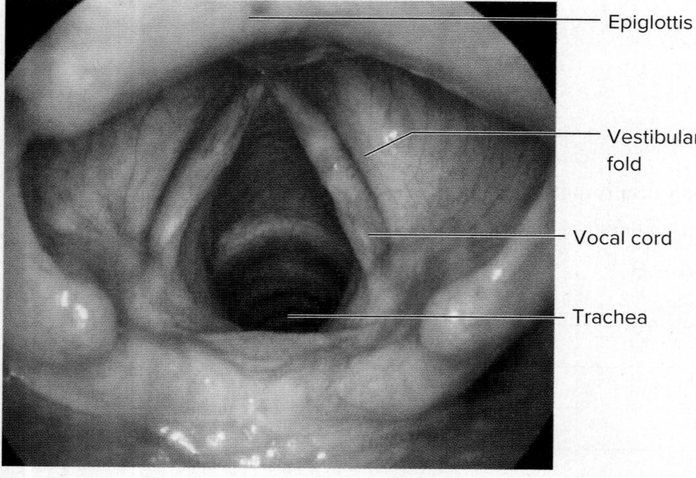

▲ **FIGURE 8.7**
View of Larynx Using a Laryngoscope.

CNRI/Science Source

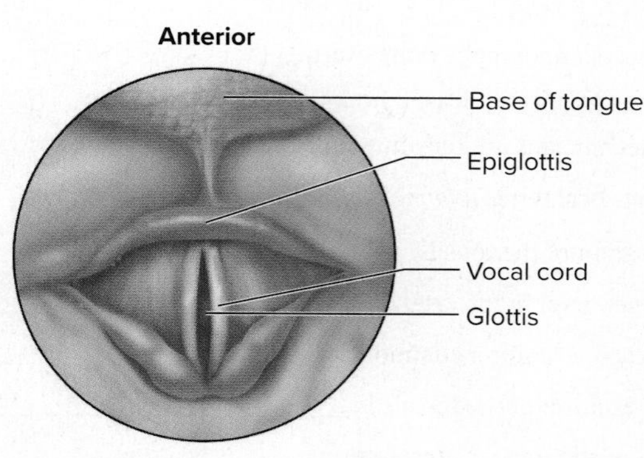

▲ **FIGURE 8.8**
Vocal Cords Pulled Close and Taut.

Word Analysis and Definition

S = Suffix P = Prefix R = Root R/CF = Combining Form

WORD	PRONUNCIATION	ELEMENTS		DEFINITION
croup (*also called* **laryngotracheobronchitis**)	**KROOP**		Old English *to cry out loud*	Infection of the upper airways in children characterized by a barking cough
epiglottis **epiglottitis** **glottis**	ep-ih-**GLOT**-is ep-ih-glot-**EYE**-tis **GLOT**-is	P/ R/ S/ R/	**epi-** *above* **-glottis** *mouth of windpipe* **-itis** *inflammation* **-glott-** *mouth of windpipe* Greek *opening of larynx*	Leaf-shaped plate of cartilage that shuts off the larynx during swallowing Inflammation of the epiglottis The opening from the oropharynx into the larynx
intubation	**IN**-tyu-**BAY**-shun	S/ P/ R/	**-ation** *a process* **in-** *in* **-tub-** *tube*	Insertion of a tube into the trachea
laryngotracheobronchitis (*also called* **croup**)	lah-**RING**-oh-**TRAY**-kee-oh-brong-**KIE**-tis	S/ R/CF R/CF R/	**-itis** *inflammation* **laryng/o-** *larynx* **-trache/o** *-trachea* **-bronch-** *bronchus*	Inflammation of the larynx, trachea, and bronchi
larynx **laryngeal (adj)** **laryngitis** **laryngoscope**	**LAH**-rinks lah-**RIN**-jee-al lah-rin-**JEYE**-tis lah-**RING**-oh-skope	S/ R/ S/ R/CF S/	Greek *larynx* **-eal** *pertaining to* **laryng-** *larynx* **-itis** *inflammation* **laryng/o-** *larynx* **-scope** *instrument for viewing*	Organ of sound production Pertaining to the larynx Inflammation of the larynx Hollow tube with a light and camera used to visualize or operate on the larynx
papilla **papillae (pl)** **papilloma**	pah-**PILL**-ah pah-**PILL**-ee pap-ih-**LOH**-mah	S/ R/CF	Latin *small pimple* **-oma** *tumor, mass* **papill/o-** *pimple*	Any small projection Benign projection of epithelial cells
stridor	**STRY**-door		Latin *a harsh, creaking sound*	High-pitched noise made when there is a respiratory obstruction in the larynx or trachea
vocal	**VOH**-kal	S/ R/	**-al** *pertaining to* **voc-** *voice*	Pertaining to the voice

Study Hint

Whether the term is 24 letters long or 5 letters long, *the principle is the same:* Know the meaning of the elements, and you will know the meaning of the term!

EXERCISES

A. Deconstruction: *For long or short medical terms, deconstruction into word elements is your key to solving the meaning of the term. Follow the directions and fill in the blanks.* **LO 8.1**

1. *laryngotracheobronchitis* ________ / ________ / ________
2. *epiglottis* ________ / ________ / ________
3. *vocal* ________ / ________ / ________

B. Apply *the language of pulmonology to answer the following questions correctly.* **LO 8.2, 8.4, and 8.6**

1. What is another term meaning *croup?* ________
2. What body parts are involved in speech production? ________
3. What is the squeaky noise on *inspiration* termed? ________
4. What is the medical term for a benign tumor of the *larynx?* ________
5. What is the name of the device used to view the larynx? ________

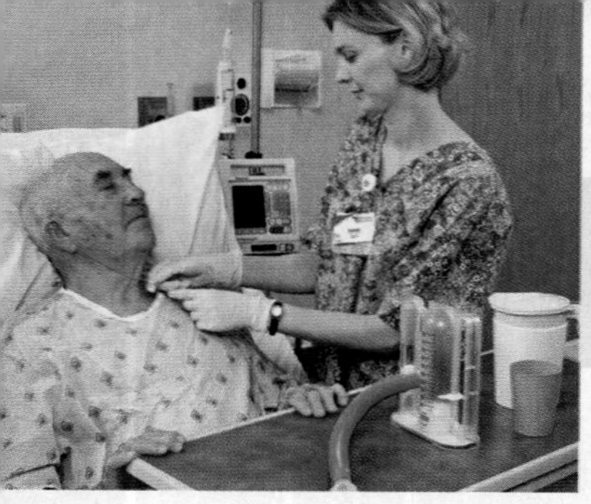
Rick Brady/McGraw-Hill Education

Lesson 8.3

Lower Respiratory Tract

Objectives

Once the air you inhale has passed through the upper airway and many of the pollutants and impurities have been filtered out, the major needs still remain: to get oxygen (O_2) into the blood and remove carbon dioxide (CO_2) from the blood. To make this possible, the inhaled air has to travel into the alveoli of the lungs, where these exchanges can occur. In this lesson, you will learn to use correct medical terminology to:

8.3.1 Trace the passage of air from the larynx into the alveoli and back.

8.3.2 Describe the mechanics of ventilation.

8.3.3 Integrate the functions of the different elements of the lower airway with their structures.

8.3.4 Discuss the effects of common disorders of the lungs on health.

Abbreviations

CO_2 carbon dioxide
O_2 oxygen

Trachea (LO 8.5)

The flow of inhaled air now moves into your trachea (windpipe). This is a rigid tube that descends from the larynx and divides into the two main **bronchi** *(Figure 8.9),* which serve as airways going to your right and left lungs.

The Lungs (LO 8.5)

Your two lungs are the main organs of respiration and are located in the thoracic cavity. Each lung is a soft, spongy, cone-shaped organ with its **base** resting on the **diaphragm** and its top **(apex)** above and behind the clavicle. Its outer convex, costal surface presses against the **rib cage.** Its inner concave surface presses against the chest region **(mediastinum).**

The right lung has three **lobes:** superior, middle, and inferior. The left lung has two lobes; superior and inferior *(Figure 8.9a).* Each lobe is separated from the others by **fissures.**

Tracheobronchial Tree (LO 8.5)

The tracheobronchial tree is an upside-down, tree-like structure that conducts air in your chest. It is comprised of the trachea, bronchi, and bronchial tubes. As inhaled air continues down the respiratory tract, the main bronchi divide into a **secondary (lobar)** bronchus for each lobe. Each secondary bronchus then divides into tertiary (third) bronchi that supply **segments** of each lobe *(Figure 8.10).* These divisions create branch-like airways.

Bronchioles and Alveoli (LO 8.5)

These tertiary bronchi further divide into **bronchioles,** which in turn divide into several thin-walled **alveoli.** Each **alveolus** is a thin-walled sac supported by a thin **respiratory membrane.** This membrane allows the exchange of gases with the surrounding pulmonary capillary network.

The Pleura (LO 8.5)

The **pleura** is a double-layered serous membrane that covers the surface of both lungs. The space between these two layers is called the **pleural cavity,** which contains a thin film of lubricant fluid. This lubricant enables the lungs to expand (inspiration) and deflate (expiration) with minimal friction.

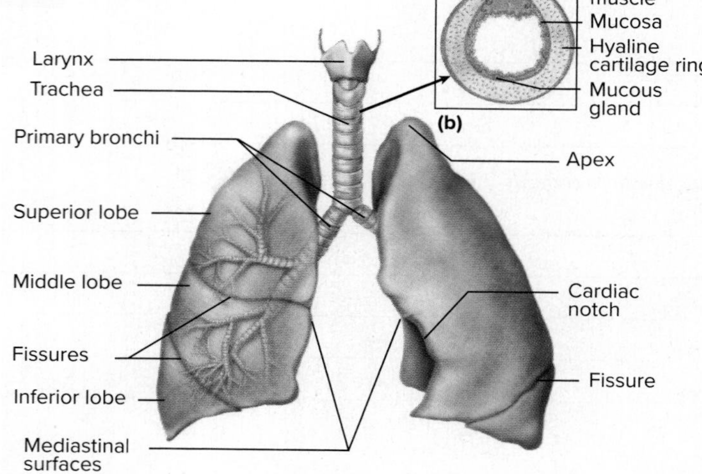

FIGURE 8.9 **Lower Respiratory Tract.**
(a) Gross anatomy.
(b) C-shaped tracheal cartilage.

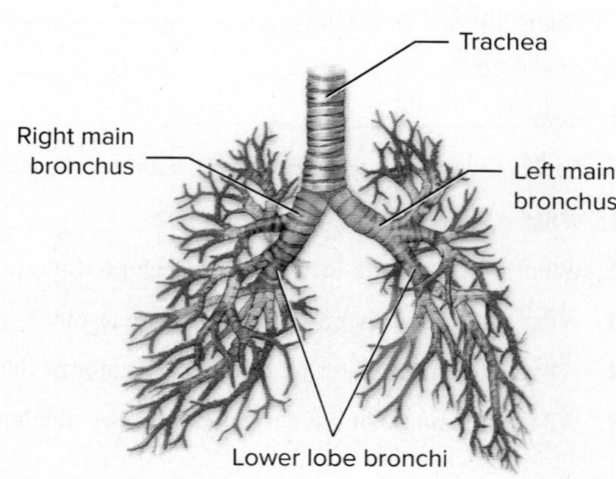

FIGURE 8.10 **Latex Cast of the Tracheobronchial Tree.**

Word Analysis and Definition

S = Suffix P = Prefix R = Root R/CF = Combining Form

WORD	PRONUNCIATION	ELEMENTS		DEFINITION
diaphragm	**DIE**-ah-fram		Greek *diaphragm*	The muscular sheet separating the abdominal and thoracic cavities
diaphragmatic (adj)	**DIE**-ah-frag-**MAT**-ik	S/ R/CF	-tic *pertaining to* diaphragm/a- *diaphragm*	Pertaining to the diaphragm
fissure fissures (pl)	**FISH**-ur	S/ R/	-ure *process, result of* fiss- *split*	Deep furrow or cleft
lobe	**LOBE**		Greek *lobe*	Subdivision of an organ or other part
lobar (adj)	**LOW**-bar	S/ R/	-ar *pertaining to* lob- *lobe*	Pertaining to a lobe
lobectomy	low-**BECK**-toe-me	S/	-ectomy *surgical excision*	Surgical removal of a lobe
mediastinum	**ME**-dee-ass-**TIE**-num	S/ P/ R/	-um *structure* media- *middle* -stin- *partition*	Area between the lungs containing the heart, aorta, venae cavae, esophagus, and trachea
mediastinal (adj)	**ME**-dee-ass-**TIE**-nal	S/	-al *pertaining to*	Pertaining to the mediastinum
pleura pleurae (pl)	**PLUR**-ah **PLUR**-ee		Greek *rib*	Membrane covering the lungs and lining the ribs in the thoracic cavity
pleural (adj)	**PLUR**-al	S/ R/	-al *pertaining to* pleur- *pleura*	Pertaining to the pleura
pleurisy	**PLUR**-ih-see	S/	-isy *inflammation*	Inflammation of the pleura
segment	**SEG**-ment		Latin *to cut*	A section of an organ or structure

Exercises

A. Precision in communication *means using the correct form of the medical term, as well as the correct spelling. Test your knowledge of plurals, adjectives, and spelling with this exercise. Select the correct choice.* **LO 8.2, 8.5, and 8.7**

1. The area between the lungs containing the heart, aorta, venae cavae, esophagus, and trachea is the

   a. mediastenum **b.** medisternum **c.** mediastinum **d.** midiasternum

2. The patient was diagnosed with ____________ pneumonia.

   a. lobe **b.** lobular **c.** lobar **d.** lumbar

3. Is the term for the functional cells of an organ.

   a. perenchyma **b.** parenchyma **c.** perinchkima **d.** perenkima

4. Because there is a hilum in each lung, collectively they are referred to as the

   a. hilla **b.** hila **c.** hilia **d.** hilea

5. The muscle separating the abdominal and thoracic cavities is the

   a. diaphram **b.** diaphragm **c.** diahragm **d.** diapragm

6. Removal of a lobe of a lung would be a

   a. lobotomy **b.** lobectomy **c.** lobarectomy **d.** lobarotomy

Study Hint

Frequent errors are made on test questions regarding the term *pleural*, meaning *pertaining to the pleura*. It is not spelled "plural," which means *more than one*. Be especially careful when dealing with this term, and always check your spelling. Both terms sound alike, are spelled differently, and have very different meanings. *The right answer (pleural) is wrong if it is spelled "plural."* Don't lose points on a test because of carelessness.

B. Provide the term *being described using the language of pulmonology.* **LO 8.2 and 8.5**

1. The top of the lung is termed the: ____________
2. The bottom of the lung is termed the: ____________
3. Which lung has three lobes, the right or the left? ____________
4. Each lung lobe is separated by a: ____________
5. The serous membrane that covers the surface of the lungs is called the: ____________
6. The medical term that means inflammation of the pleura: ____________
7. The procedure that removes a lobe of the lung: ____________

Mechanics of Respiration (LO 8.5)

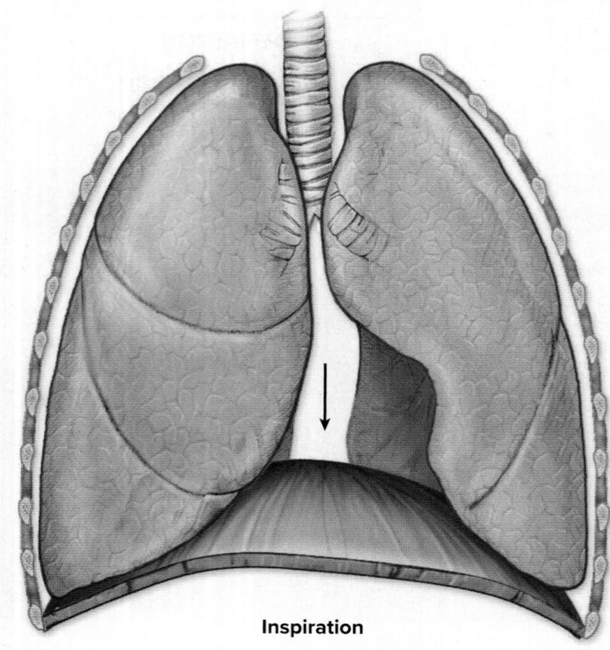

Diaphragm contracts; vertical dimensions of thoracic cavity increase.

(a)

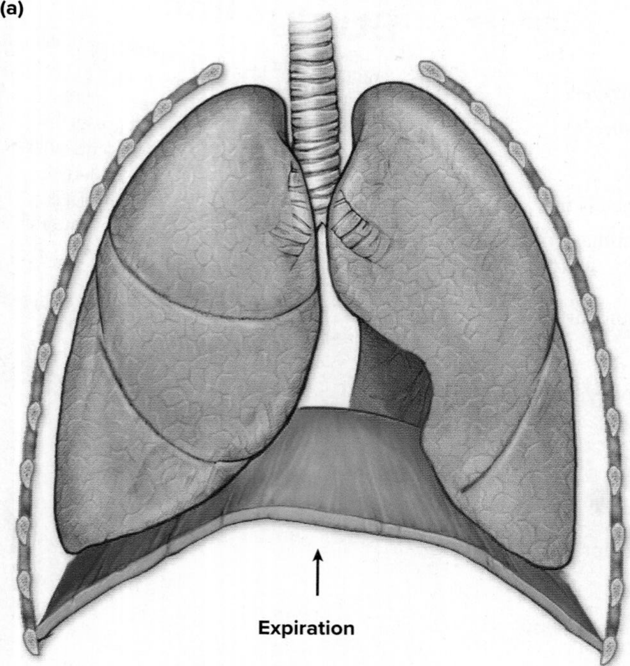

Diaphragm relaxes; vertical dimensions of thoracic cavity decrease.

(b)

▲ **FIGURE 8.11**
Inspiration and Expiration.

Abbreviation

DOB Difficulty of Breathing

A resting adult breathes 10 to 15 times per minute and **inhales** about 500 mL of air during inspiration and **exhales** it during expiration. The mission is to get air into and out of the alveoli so that oxygen can enter the bloodstream and carbon dioxide can exit.

Your diaphragm does most of the work. In inspiration, it drops down and flattens to expand the thoracic cavity and reduce the pressure in the airways. The external intercostal muscles also help by lifting the chest wall up and out to further expand the thoracic cavity *(Figure 8.11a).*

Expiration is a process of letting go. The diaphragm and the intercostal muscles relax, and the thoracic cavity springs back to its original size *(Figure 8.11b).*

Common Signs and Symptoms of Respiratory Disorders (LO 8.4 and 8.5)

The common signs and symptoms of respiratory disorders are often visible and audible, and they include the following:

1. **Cough** is triggered by irritants in the respiratory tract. Irritants include cigarette smoke (as with Mr. Jacobs), infection, or tumors, as in lung cancer. A productive cough produces **sputum,** which can be swallowed or **expectorated.** Bloody sputum is called **hemoptysis.** Thick, yellow **(purulent)** sputum indicates infection. A **nonproductive** cough is dry and hacking.
   Abnormal amounts of mucus arising from the upper respiratory tract and expectorated or coughed up are called **phlegm.**

2. **Dyspnea,** or difficult breathing **(DOB),** can occur from exertion or, in severe disorders, during rest when all the respiratory muscles are used to exchange only a small volume of air.

3. **Cyanosis** is seen when the blood has increased levels of **unoxygenated hemoglobin** and has a characteristic dark red-blue color.

4. **Changes in the rate of breathing** may occur. **Eupnea** is the normal, easy respiration (around 15 breaths per minute) in a resting adult. Both **tachypnea** (rapid rate of breathing) and **hyperpnea** (breathing deeper and more rapidly than normal) are signs of respiratory difficulty, as is **bradypnea** (slow breathing).

5. **Sneezing** is caused by irritants in the nasal cavity.

6. **Hiccups** are reflex spasms of the diaphragm. The etiology is unknown, and there is no specific medical cure.

7. **Yawning** is a reflex that originates in the brainstem in response to hypoxia, boredom, or sleepiness. The exact mechanisms are not known.

Word Analysis and Definition

S = Suffix P = Prefix R = Root R/CF = Combining Form

WORD	PRONUNCIATION	ELEMENTS		DEFINITION
bradypnea (*opposite of* **tachypnea**)	brad-ip-**NEE**-ah	P/ R/	**brady-** *slow* **-pnea** *breathe*	Slow breathing
cyanosis **cyanotic (adj)**	sigh-ah-**NO**-sis sigh-ah-**NOT**-ik	S/ R/ S/ R/CF	**-osis** *condition* **cyan-** *dark blue* **-tic** *pertaining to* **cyan/o** *dark blue*	Blue discoloration of the skin, lips, and nail beds due to low levels of oxygen in the blood Pertaining to or marked by cyanosis
dyspnea	disp-**NEE**-ah	P/ R/	**dys-** *bad, difficult* **-pnea** *breathe*	Difficult breathing
eupnea	yoop-**NEE**-ah	P/ R/	**eu-** *normal, good* **-pnea** *breathe*	Normal breathing
exhale	**EKS**-hail	P/ R/	**ex-** *out* **-hale** *breathe*	Breathe out
expectorate	ek-**SPEK**-toh-rate	S/ P/ R/	**-ate** *pertaining to* **ex-** *out* **-pector-** *chest*	Cough up and spit out mucus from the respiratory tract
hemoptysis	he-**MOP**-tih-sis	R/CF S/	**hem/o-** *blood* **-ptysis** *spit*	Bloody sputum
hyperpnea	high-perp-**NEE**-ah	P/ R/	**hyper-** *excessive* **-pnea** *breathe*	Deeper and more rapid breathing than normal
inhale	**IN**-hail	P/ R/	**in-** *in* **-hale** *breathe*	Breathe in
phlegm	**FLEM**		Greek *flame*	Abnormal amounts of mucus expectorated from the respiratory tract
tachypnea (*opposite of* **bradypnea**)	tak-ip-**NEE**-ah	P/ R/	**tachy-** *rapid* **-pnea** *breathe*	Rapid breathing

Study Hint

The English word *breath* is a noun and is the air you inhale and exhale. ("Take a deep breath.") The English word *breathe* has an "e" on the end of it and is the verb meaning to *inhale and exhale*. ("She was unable to breathe.")

Exercises

A. Construct terms: *Knowing just one element will enable you to build more terms with the addition of other elements. Practice building your pulmonology terms with the following root and various prefixes. Fill in the blanks.* **LO 8.1, 8.2, and 8.5**

1. The root *pnea* means ______________________________.

Add the following prefixes to the root pnea *to form the new terms.*

tachy brady dys eu hyper

2. difficult breathing ____________ / pnea

3. deeper breathing than normal ____________ / pnea

4. slow breathing ____________ / pnea

5. normal breathing ____________ / pnea

6. rapid breathing ____________ / pnea

B. Translate everyday language *to medical terms. Use the provided terms below to complete each sentence. Not all terms will be used. Fill in the blanks.* **LO 8.2, 8.5, and 8.8**

cyanotic **cyanosis** **exhale** **expectorate** **hemoptysis** **inhale** **phlegm**

Mrs. Mortimer has arrived to the Emergency Department. Her skin appears **(1)** __________ (blue in color). She is immediately brought back to a bed. After giving her oxygen via nasal prongs, she states that she is unable to **(2)** _______ (breathe in) deeply. She is able to **(3)** _________ (cough up) large amounts of thick green **(4)** ________ (mucus coughed up from the respiratory tract). She denies **(5)** ________ (bloody sputum).

Lesson 8.3 (cont'd)

Keynotes

- **Worldwide, 65 million people are affected by moderate to severe COPD.**
- **In 2019, 16 million Americans are affected by moderate to severe COPD.**
- **Alabama, Tennessee, Kentucky, and West Virginia have the highest incidence of COPD.**

Abbreviations

CAO	chronic airway obstruction
CF	cystic fibrosis
CHF	congestive heart failure
COPD	chronic obstructive pulmonary disease

Disorders of the Lower Respiratory Tract

(LO 8.3 and 8.5)

There are a number of disorders that are specific to your lower respiratory tract. These disorders are described below.

Acute bronchitis can be viral or bacterial, leading to the production of excess mucus with some obstruction of airflow. It resolves without significant residual damage to the airway.

Chronic bronchitis is the most common obstructive disease, caused by cigarette smoking or repeated episodes of acute bronchitis. Along with excess mucus production, cilia are destroyed. A pattern develops, involving chronic cough, dyspnea, and recurrent acute infections.

In advanced chronic bronchitis, hypoxia and **hypercapnia** (excess carbon dioxide) are produced and heart failure follows.

Bronchiolitis is a viral inflammation of the small airway bronchioles. It occurs in adults as the early and often unrecognized start of airway changes in cigarette smokers or in those exposed to "secondhand smoke." Bronchiolitis also affects children under the age of 2 because their small airways become blocked very easily. In severe cases, this disease can cause noticeable respiratory distress.

Pulmonary emphysema is a disease of the respiratory bronchioles and alveoli. These airways become enlarged, and the septa between the alveoli are destroyed, forming large sacs of air **(bullae).** There is a loss of surface area for gas exchange.

Chronic airway obstruction (CAO) is also called **chronic obstructive pulmonary disease (COPD).** It is a progressive disease, as Mr. Jacobs' history shows. It involves both chronic bronchitis and emphysema. A history of heavy cigarette smoking *(Figure 8.12),* with chronic cough and sputum production, is followed by increasing dyspnea and need for oxygen. Right-sided heart failure (cor pulmonale, *see Chapter 6*) is the end result, due to pulmonary hypertension and backup of blood into the right ventricle.

Bronchiectasis is the abnormal dilation of the small bronchioles due to repeated infections. The damaged, dilated bronchi are unable to clear secretions, making them prone to further infections and increased damage.

Bronchial asthma is a disorder with recurrent acute episodes of bronchial obstruction. This results from a constriction of bronchioles **(bronchoconstriction),** a **hypersecretion** of mucus, and an inflammatory swelling of the bronchiolar lining. Between attacks, breathing can be normal. The etiology of asthma is an allergic response to substances like pollen, animal dander, or the feces of dust mites.

Cystic fibrosis (CF) is a genetic disorder caused by an increased **viscosity** (thickness and stickiness) of secretions from the pancreas, salivary glands, liver, intestine, and lungs. In the lungs, a very thick mucus obstructs the airways and causes repeated infections. Many CF patients die before the age of 30 from respiratory failure.

Pulmonary edema is the collection of fluid in the lung tissues and alveoli. It commonly results from left ventricular failure or mitral valve disease with congestive heart failure **(CHF).**

During **auscultation** (examination by stethoscope) of the chest, the air bubbling through abnormal fluid in the alveoli and small bronchioles, as in pulmonary edema, produces a noise called **rales.** When the bronchi are partly obstructed and air is being forced past the obstruction, a high-pitched noise called a **rhonchus** is heard.

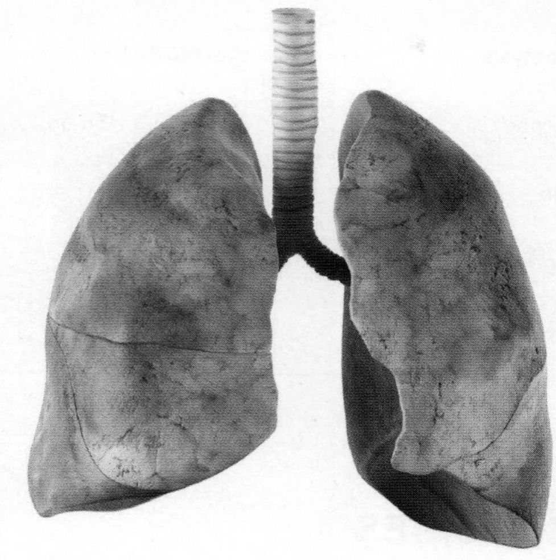

(a)

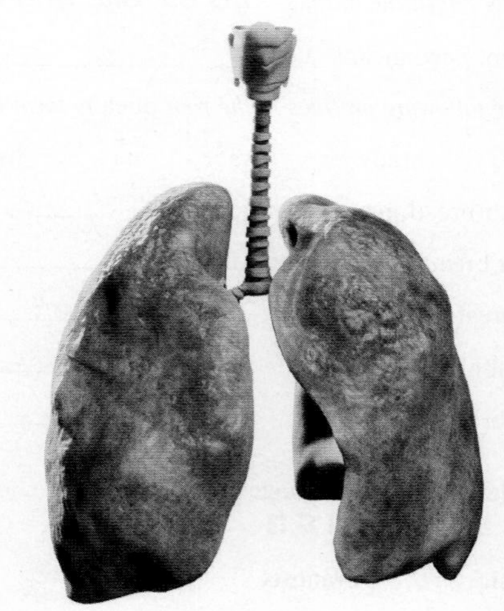

(b)

▲ **FIGURE 8.12**

Whole Lungs.

(a) Lungs of a Non-smoker. (b) Lungs of a Smoker.

Word Analysis and Definition

S = Suffix P = Prefix R = Root R/CF = Combining Form

WORD	PRONUNCIATION	ELEMENTS		DEFINITION
asthma	**AZ**-mah		Greek *asthma*	Episodes of breathing difficulty due to narrowed or obstructed airways
asthmatic (adj)	az-**MAT**-ik	S/ R/	**-atic** *pertaining to* **asthm-** *asthma*	Pertaining to or suffering from asthma
auscultation	aws-kul-**TAY**-shun	S/ R/	**-ation** *a process* **auscult-** *listen to*	Diagnostic method of listening to body sounds with a stethoscope
bronchiectasis	brong-key-**ECK**-tah-sis	S/ R/CF	**-ectasis** *dilation* **bronch/i-** *bronchus*	Chronic dilation of the bronchi following inflammatory disease and obstruction
bronchiolitis	brong-key-oh-**LYE**-tis	S/ R/CF	**-itis** *inflammation* **bronchiol/o** *bronchus*	Inflammation of the small bronchioles
bronchitis	brong-**KI**-tis	S/ R/	**-itis** *inflammation* **bronch-** *bronchus*	Inflammation of the bronchi
bronchoconstriction	**BRONG**-koh-kon-**STRIK**-shun	S/ R/CF R/	**-ion** *action, condition* **bronch/o-** *bronchus* **-constrict-** *to narrow*	Reduction in diameter of a bronchus
bulla **bullae (pl)**	**BULL**-ah **BULL**-ee		Latin *bubble*	Bubble-like dilated structure
cystic fibrosis	**SIS**-tik fie-**BRO**-sis	S/ R/ S/ R/	**-ic** *pertaining to* **cyst-** *cyst* **-osis** *abnormal condition* **fibr-** *fiber*	Genetic disease in which excessive viscid mucus obstructs passages, including bronchi
emphysema	em-fih-**SEE**-mah	P/ R/	**em-** *in, into* **-physema** *blowing*	Dilation of respiratory bronchioles and alveoli
hypercapnia	**HIGH**-per-**KAP**-nee-ah	S/ P/ R/	**-ia** *condition* **hyper-** *excessive* **-capn-** *carbon dioxide*	Abnormal increase of carbon dioxide in the arterial bloodstream
hypersecretion	**HIGH**-per-seh-**KREE**-shun	S/ P/ R/	**-ion** *action, condition* **hyper-** *excessive* **-secret-** *secrete*	Excessive secretion of mucus (or enzymes or waste products)
rhonchus **rhonchi** (pl)	**RONG**-kuss **RONG**-key		Greek *snoring*	Wheezing sound heard on auscultation of the lungs; made by air passing through a constricted lumen
viscosity **viscous (adj)** (*cf.* **viscus**, *any internal organ*)	viss-**KOS**-ih-tee **VISS**-kus	S/ R/	**-ity** *condition* **viscos-** *viscous, sticky*	The resistance of a fluid to flow Sticky fluid that is resistant to flow

EXERCISES

A. Elements. *The elements below all appear in the language of pulmonology. Match the word element in the first column with its correct meaning in the second column.* **LO 8.1, 8.4, and 8.5**

_____ **1.** ectasis	**a.** listen to
_____ **2.** capn	**b.** sticky
_____ **3.** physema	**c.** carbon dioxide
_____ **4.** viscos	**d.** blowing
_____ **5.** auscult	**e.** small
_____ **6.** ole	**f.** dilation

B. Apply *the language of pulmonology to answer the following questions correctly.* **LO 8.2, 8.5, and 8.7**

1. A sticky fluid that is resistant to flow is said to be: ____________________

2. More than one bubble-like dilated structure: ____________________

3. *Hypercapnia* is excessive ____________________.

4. *Hypoxia* is deficient ____________________.

Disorders of the Lower Respiratory Tract (continued)

(LO 8.3 and 8.5)

Pneumonia *(Figure 8.13)* is an acute infection of the alveoli and lung **parenchyma** (functional cells of the lung). Pneumonia is mostly caused by bacteria or viruses. The alveoli become filled with inflammatory fluid, decreasing the exchange of oxygen and carbon dioxide. **Lobar pneumonia** is an infection limited to one lung lobe. **Bronchopneumonia** is an infection in the bronchioles that spreads to the alveoli.

When an area of the lung **(segment)** or a lobe becomes airless as a result of the infection, the lung is **consolidated.** When an area of the lung collapses as a result of bronchial obstruction, this is called **atelectasis.**

Pleurisy, an inflammation of the pleurae, can be a complication of pneumonia. This condition makes breathing painful because the parietal pleura is very pain-sensitive. The inflammation often leads to fluid accumulating in the pleural cavity. This is a **pleural effusion.** If the pleural effusion contains pus, the condition is called **empyema.** If it contains blood, the condition is called **hemothorax.** When pleural fluid is drawn off for therapeutic reasons or for laboratory analysis, the procedure is **aspiration** or **thoracentesis.**

Lung abscess can be a complication of bacterial pneumonia or cancer. Long-term antibiotics are used, and partial surgical excision of the abscess may be necessary.

Pneumothorax is the entry of air into the pleural cavity *(Figure 8.14)*. The cause can be unknown, called a **spontaneous pneumothorax,** but it often results from trauma when a fractured rib, knife blade, or bullet lacerates the pleura.

Adult respiratory distress syndrome (ARDS) is sudden, life-threatening lung failure caused by a variety of underlying conditions from major trauma to sepsis. The alveoli fill with fluid and collapse, shutting down gas exchange. Hypoxia results. **Mechanical ventilation** is mandatory. The mortality rate is 35% to 50%.

Neonatal respiratory distress syndrome (NRDS) is seen in premature babies whose lungs have not matured enough to produce surfactant, a substance secreted in the lungs. The alveoli collapse, and mechanical ventilation is needed to keep them open.

Chronic infections of the lung parenchyma are the result of prolonged exposure to infection or to occupational irritant dusts or droplets. These disorders are called **pneumoconioses.** Levels of dust inhalation overwhelm the airways' particle-clearing abilities. The dust particles accumulate in the alveoli and parenchyma, leading to fibrosis. **Asbestosis** results from inhaling asbestos particles and can lead to a cancer in the pleura called **mesothelioma. Silicosis** from silica particles is called "stonecutters' disease." **Anthracosis** from coal dust particles is called "coal miners' disease." **(Anthrax** is a different disease, caused by toxins produced by the anthrax bacillus.) **Sarcoidosis** produces lesions and is a fibrotic (scarring) disorder of the lung parenchyma.

Pulmonary tuberculosis is a chronic, infectious disease of the lungs.

Lung cancer, related to tobacco use, was once only a male disease. Now, fatalities in women from lung cancer exceed those from breast cancer. Ninety percent of lung cancers arise in the mucous membranes of the larger bronchi and are called **bronchogenic carcinomas.** A subgroup of bronchogenic carcinomas called **adenocarcinoma** accounts for 30% to 50% of all lung cancers and is the most common in women. The lung cancer obstructs the bronchus, spreads into the surrounding lung tissues, and metastasizes to the lymph nodes, liver, brain, and bone. This disease is associated with cigarette smoking.

Abbreviations

ARDS	adult respiratory distress syndrome
NRDS	neonatal respiratory distress syndrome

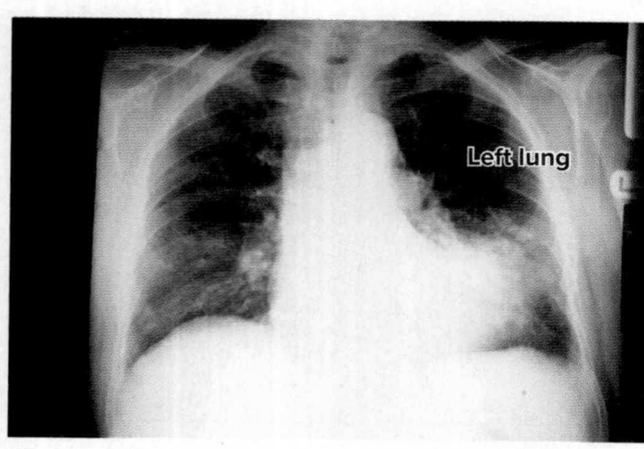

▲ **FIGURE 8.13**
Chest X-ray of Patient with Pneumonia in the Lower Lobe of the Left Lung.

Anthony Ricci/Shutterstock

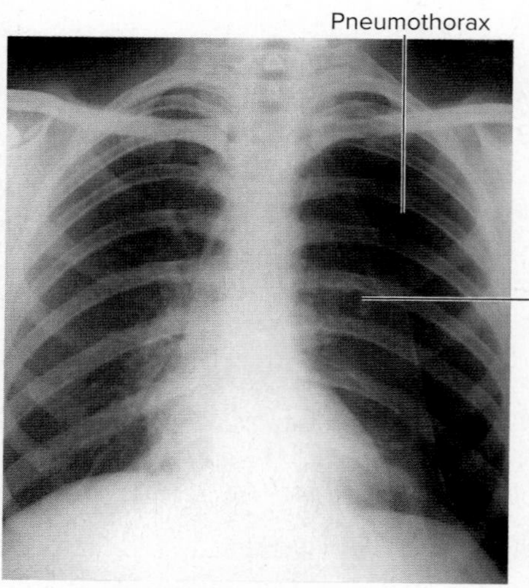

▲ **FIGURE 8.14**
Left Pneumothorax.
There are no lung markings seen in the area of the pneumothorax.

Zephyr/Science Source

Word Analysis and Definition

S = Suffix P = Prefix R = Root R/CF = Combining Form

WORD	PRONUNCIATION	ELEMENTS		DEFINITION
adenocarcinoma	**ADD**-eh-noh-kar-sih-**NOH**-mah	S/ R/CF R/	-oma *tumor* aden/o- *gland* -carcin- *cancer*	A cancer arising from glandular epithelial cells
anthracosis	an-thra-**KOH**-sis	S/ R/	-osis *condition* anthrac- *coal*	Lung disease caused by the inhalation of coal dust
anthrax	**AN**-thraks		Greek *carbuncle*	A severe, malignant infectious disease
asbestosis	as-bes-**TOE**-sis	S/ R/	-osis *condition* asbest- *asbestos*	Lung disease caused by the inhalation of asbestos particles
aspiration	as-pih-**RAY**-shun	S/ R/	-ion *process* aspirat- *to breathe on*	Removal by suction of fluid or gas from a body cavity
atelectasis	at-el-**ECK**-tah-sis	S/ R/	-ectasis *dilation* atel- *incomplete*	Collapse of part of a lung
bronchogenic	**BRONG**-koh-**JEN**-ik	S/ R/CF	-genic *creation* bronch/o- *bronchus*	Arising from a bronchus
bronchopneumonia	**BRONG**-koh-new-**MOH**-nee-ah	S/ R/CF R/	-ia *condition* bronch/o- *bronchus* -pneumon- *air, lung*	Acute inflammation of the walls of smaller bronchioles with spread to lung parenchyma
empyema	**EM**-pie-**EE**-mah	S/ P/ R/	-ema *quality of, quantity of* em- *in, into* -py- *pus*	Pus in a body cavity, particularly in the pleural cavity
hemothorax	he-moh-**THOR**-ax	R/CF R/	hem/o- *blood* -thorax *chest*	Blood in the pleural cavity
parenchyma	pah-**REN**-ki-mah		Greek *to pour in*	The specific functional cells of a gland or organ (e.g., the lung) that are supported by the connective tissue framework
pneumoconiosis pneumoconioses (pl)	new-moh-koh-nee-**OH**-sis new-moh-koh-nee-**OH**-seez	S/ R/CF R/	-osis *condition* pneum/o- *lung, air* -coni- *dust*	Fibrotic lung disease caused by the inhalation of different dusts
pneumonia pneumonitis (*same as* **pneumonia**)	new-**MOH**-nee-ah new-moh-**NI**-tis	S/ R/ S/	-ia *condition* pneumon- *lung, air* -itis *inflammation*	Inflammation of the lung parenchyma (tissue)
pneumothorax	new-moh-**THOR**-ax	R/CF R/	pneum/o- *air, lung* -thorax *chest*	Air in the pleural cavity
sarcoidosis (**Note:** *Two suffixes*)	sar-koy-**DOH**-sis	S/ S/ R/	-osis *condition* -oid- *resembling* sarc- *flesh*	Granulomatous lesions of the lungs and other organs; cause is unknown
silicosis	sil-ih-**KOH**-sis	S/ R/	-osis *condition* silic- *silicon, glass*	Fibrotic lung disease from inhaling silica particles
thoracentesis (*same as* **pleural tap**)	**THOR**-ah-sen-**TEE**-sis	S/ R/	-centesis *to puncture* thora- *chest*	Insertion of a needle into the pleural cavity to withdraw fluid or air
tuberculosis	too-**BER**-kyu-**LOW**-sis	S/ R/	-osis *condition* tubercul- *nodule, swelling, tuberculosis*	Infectious disease that can infect any organ or tissue

EXERCISE

A. Suffixes: *Confirm your knowledge of suffixes by filling in the chart with the correct meaning for the element.* **LO 8.1 and 8.2**

Term	Suffix	Meaning of the Suffix
thoracentesis	**1.**	**2.**
tuberculosis	**3.**	**4.**
bronchogenic	**5.**	**6.**
atelectasis	**7.**	**8.**

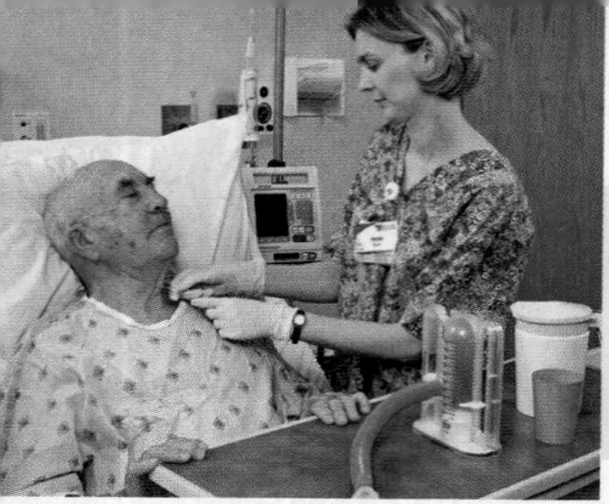

Rick Brady/McGraw-Hill Education

Lesson 8.4

Diagnostic and Therapeutic Procedures and Pharmacology

Objectives

Specific diagnostic and therapeutic procedures, as well as a wide range of pharmacologic agents, are available to help patients with lung diseases. In this lesson, the information will enable you to use correct medical terminology to:

8.4.1 Identify specific pulmonary function tests (PFTs) and other diagnostic procedures.

8.4.2 Describe common therapeutic procedures.

8.4.3 List different classes of pharmacologic agents and their effects on the lungs.

Keynotes

- **Measure pulmonary function with a spirometer, a peak flow meter, and arterial blood gases.**
- **Bronchoscopy is a procedure for inserting a fiber optic tube into the bronchial tubes to visually examine the tubes, take a tissue biopsy, or do a washing for secretions.**
- **Mediastinoscopy is used to stage lung cancer and diagnose mediastinal masses. The mediastinoscope is inserted through an incision in the suprasternal notch.**
- **Thoracentesis is the insertion of a needle through an intercostal space to remove fluid from a pleural effusion for laboratory study or to relieve pressure. The procedure is also called a pleural tap.**

Case Report 8.1 *(continued)*

Mr. Jacobs' forced expiratory volume was only 40% of normal because the fibrotic (scarring) effects of his repeated lung infections had reduced the volume of his airways. When he was off oxygen, his arterial oxygen levels were below 50% of normal. Even with nasal prongs and oxygen, his arterial oxygen levels were still only 75% of normal.

Diagnostic Procedures (LO 8.4, 8.5, and 8.6)

Pulmonary Function Tests (PFTs) (LO 8.4, 8.5, and 8.6)

Pulmonary function can be measured by the following PFTs to estimate the quality of a patient's respiratory function. A **spirometer** is a device for measuring the volume of air that patients move in and out of their respiratory systems. The volume of air expired at the end of the test is the patient's **forced expiratory vital capacity (FVC).** The spirometer also measures **firstflow rates.** For example, the **forced expiratory volume in 1 second (FEV1)** is the amount of air expired in the second of the test.

A **peak flow meter** records the greatest flow of air that can be sustained for 10 milliseconds on forced expiration, the **peak expiratory flow rate (PEFR).** This test is valuable in following the course of asthma, and in postoperative care to monitor the return of lung function after anesthesia.

Arterial blood gases, the measurement of oxygen and carbon dioxide levels in the blood, are good indicators of respiratory function.

A **pulse oximeter** is a sensor placed on the finger to measure the oxygen saturation of the blood.

Other Diagnostic Procedures (LO 8.4, 8.5, and 8.6)

Chest X-ray (CXR) is a radiographic image of the chest taken in **anteroposterior (AP), posteroanterior (PA),** lateral, and sometimes oblique and lateral decubitus positions.

Computed tomography (CT), angiography of the pulmonary circulation using contrast materials, **magnetic resonance angiography (MRA)** to define emboli in the pulmonary arteries, and **ultrasonography** of the pleural space are chest-imaging techniques in modern use. **Positron emission tomography (PET)** can sometimes distinguish benign from malignant lesions.

Tracheal aspiration uses a soft catheter that allows brushings and washings to be performed to remove cells and secretions from the trachea and main bronchi. The catheter can be passed through a tracheostomy or **endotracheal** (windpipe) tube, or through the mouth and nose.

Percutaneous transthoracic needle aspiration is the insertion of a needle with a cutting chamber through an intercostal space (between the ribs) to take a specimen of parietal pleura for examination.

Thoracotomy is used to obtain an open biopsy of tissue from the lung, hilum, pleura, or mediastinum. It is performed through an intercostal incision under general anesthesia.

Abbreviations

AP	anteroposterior
CT	computed tomography
CXR	chest X-ray
FEV1	forced expiratory volume in 1 second
FVC	forced vital capacity
MRA	magnetic resonance angiography
PA	posteroanterior
PEFR	peak expiratory flow rate
PET	positron emission tomography
PFTs	pulmonary function tests

Word Analysis and Definition

S = Suffix P = Prefix R = Root R/CF = Combining Form

WORD	PRONUNCIATION	ELEMENTS		DEFINITION
bronchoscopy bronchoscope	brong-**KOS**-koh-pee **BRONG**-koh-skope	S/ R/CF S/	-scopy *to examine, view* bronch/o *bronchus* -scope *instrument for viewing*	Examination of the interior of the tracheobronchial tree with an endoscope Endoscope used for bronchoscopy
endotracheal	en-doh-**TRAY**-kee-al	S/ P/ R/	-al *pertaining to* endo- *inside* -trache- *trachea*	Pertaining to being inside the trachea
mediastinoscopy	**ME**-dee-ass-tih-**NOS**-koh-pee	S/ R/CF	-scopy *to examine, view* mediastin/o *mediastinum*	Examination of the mediastinum using an endoscope
spirometer spirometry	spy-**ROM**-eh-ter spy-**ROM**-eh-tree	S/ R/CF S/	-meter *measure* spir/o- *to breathe* -metry *process of measuring*	An instrument used to measure respiratory volumes Use of a spirometer
thoracotomy	thor-ah-**KOT**-oh-me	S/ R/CF	-tomy *surgical incision* thorac/o *chest*	Incision through the chest wall
tomography	toe-**MOG**-rah-fee	S/ R/CF	-graphy *process of recording* tom/o- *cut, slice, layer*	Radiographic image of a selected slice of tissue
transthoracic	tranz-thor-**ASS**-ik	S/ P/ R/	-ic *pertaining to* trans- *across* -thorac- *chest*	Going through the chest wall
ultrasonography	**UL**-trah-soh-**NOG**-rah-fee	S/ P/ R/CF	-graphy *process of recording* ultra- *beyond* -son/o- *sound*	Delineation of deep structures using sound waves

EXERCISES

A. Provide the abbreviation *that each statement is describing. Fill in the blanks.* **LO 8.3 and 8.6**

1. X-ray of the chest:______

2. A group of diagnostic tests that measures flow rates, the amount of air brought into and out of the lungs:______

3. An X-ray that passes first through the front of the chest.______

4. A diagnostic test that provides high-resolution images of blood vessels. This test does not use radiation to create the image: ______

B. Identify the meaning *of the word elements of pulmonary diagnostic terms. Select the correct answer.* **LO 8.1, 8.2, and 8.6**

1. The root in the term spirometer means:

a. surgical incision **b.** to breathe **c.** chest **d.** measure

2. The root in the term ultrasonography means:

a. beyond **b.** cut, slice, layer **c.** sound **d.** process of recording

3. The suffix in the term bronchoscopy means:

a. to view **b.** across **c.** instrument for viewing **d.** lung

4. The prefix in the term transthoracic means:

a. through **b.** across **c.** chest **d.** pertaining to

5. The prefix in the term endoscope means:

a. process of recording **b.** to view **c.** inside **d.** surgical incision

Therapeutic Procedures (LO 8.6)

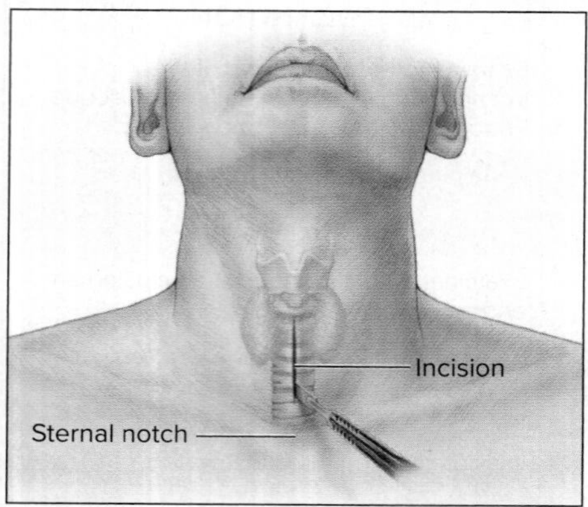

(1) Tracheotomy incision is made superior to sternal notch.

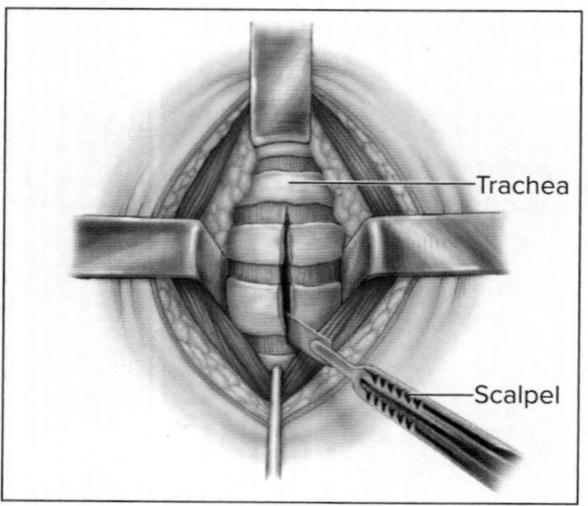

(2) Retractors separate the tissue, and an incision is made through the third and fourth tracheal rings.

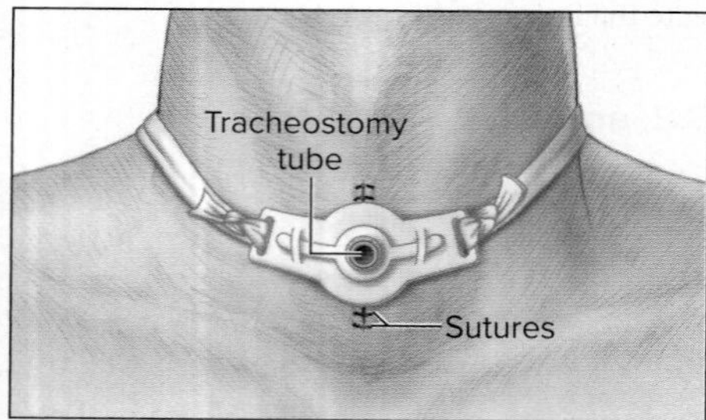

(3) A tracheostomy tube is inserted, and the remaining incision is sutured closed.

▲ **FIGURE 8.15**
Tracheostomy Procedure.

Many effective therapeutic procedures are available for successfully treating pulmonary function disorders. These procedures are outlined below.

Pulmonary rehabilitation includes education, breathing exercises and retraining, exercises for the upper and lower extremities, and psychosocial support.

Nutritional support is critical for patients who have difficulty breathing, or who need to lose or have lost a lot of weight.

Immunizations are available against influenza and the pneumococcus bacterium–the most common cause of bacterial pneumonia.

Postural drainage therapy (PDT) uses gravity (by positioning and tilting the patient) to promote the drainage of secretions from lung segments. Chest **percussion** (tapping) on the chest wall can help loosen, mobilize, and drain any retained secretions. These two procedures are part of **chest physiotherapy.**

Constant positive airway pressure (CPAP) is an attempt to keep alveoli open by maintaining a positive pressure in the airways. A mask is fitted over the patient's nose and mouth and attached to a **ventilator.** This can be used at night when sleeping or for acute situations in COPD.

Positive end expiratory pressure (PEEP) is a ventilation technique to keep the alveoli from collapsing in ARDS and neonatal respiratory distress syndrome.

An **oropharyngeal airway** is used in the unconscious patient during bag and mask ventilation to maintain an open airway. A tube is inserted to prevent the tongue from falling back and obstructing the airway and to facilitate suctioning the airway. An **endotracheal intubation** involves the placement of a tube into the trachea. This allows the patient to be placed on a ventilator so his or her breathing can be controlled.

Pulmonary resection is the surgical removal of lung tissue.

- **Wedge resection** is the removal of a small, localized area of diseased lung.
- **Segmental resection** is the removal of lung tissue attached to a bronchiole.
- **Lobectomy** is the removal of a lobe.
- **Pneumonectomy** is the removal of an entire lung.

Tracheotomy is an incision made into the trachea (windpipe) so that a temporary or permanent opening into the windpipe, called a **tracheostomy,** is created *(Figure 8.15).* A tube is placed into the opening to provide an airway. A tracheostomy is used to maintain an airway when there is obstruction or paralysis in the respiratory structures above it.

Mechanical ventilation is a process involving the movement of gases into and out of the lungs via a device programmed to meet the patient's respiratory requirements. A tracheostomy or endotracheal tube must be attached to the mechanical device **(ventilator).** This procedure can augment or replace the patient's own **ventilatory** efforts.

Pulmonary Pharmacology (LO 8.6)

- **Bronchodilators** relax the smooth muscles of the bronchioles. Examples are theophylline, beta2-agonists such as salbutamol and terbutaline, and anticholinergics such as ipratropium bromide.
- **Anti-inflammatory** drugs, such as corticosteroids, are best given by inhalation, but can be used orally or intravenously in acute episodes of asthma or COPD.
- **Mucolytics** are agents that attempt to break up mucus so it can be cleared more effectively from the airways. Examples are guaifenesin (common in over-the-counter cough medications), potassium iodide, and N-acetylcysteine taken through a **nebulizer.**
- **Antibiotics** are used when a bacterial infection is present. Penicillin, erythromycin, cefotaxime, and flucloxacillin are frequently used.
- **Oxygen** is used in hypoxemia and can be given by nasal **cannula** or by mask and intubation. Patients with severe, chronic COPD can be attached to a portable oxygen cylinder.

Abbreviations

CPAP	continuous positive airway pressure
PDT	postural drainage therapy
PEEP	positive end expiratory pressure

Word Analysis and Definition

S = Suffix P = Prefix R = Root R/CF = Combining Form

WORD	PRONUNCIATION	ELEMENTS		DEFINITION
bronchodilator	**BRONG**-koh-die-**LAY**-tor	S/ R/CF R/	**-or** *one who does, that which does something* **bronch/o-** *bronchus* **-dilat-** *expand, open up*	Agent that increases the diameter of a bronchus
cannula	**KAN**-you-lah		Latin *reed*	Tube inserted into a blood vessel or cavity as a channel for fluid or gas
immunization	im-you-nih-**ZAY**-shun	S/ R/	**-ation** *process* **immuniz-** *make immune*	Administration of an agent to provide immunity
mucolytic	**MYU**-koh-**LIT**-ik	S/ R/CF R/	**-ic** *pertaining to* **muc/o-** *mucus* **-lyt-** *dissolve*	Agent capable of dissolving or liquefying mucus
nebulizer	**NEB**-you-liz-er	S/ R/	**-izer** *line of action, affects in a particular way* **nebul-** *cloud*	Device used to deliver liquid medicine in a fine mist
pneumonectomy	**NEW**-moh-**NECK**-toe-me	S/ R/	**-ectomy** *surgical excision* **pneumon-** *lung, air*	Surgical removal of a lung
resection resect (verb)	ree-**SEK**-shun ree-**SEKT**	S/ P/ R/	**-ion** *action, condition* **re-** *back* **-sect-** *cut off*	Removal of a specific part of an organ or structure
tracheostomy tracheotomy	tray-kee-**OST**-oh-me tray-kee-**OT**-oh-me	S/ R/CF S/	**-stomy** *new opening* **trache/o-** *trachea* *-tomy surgical incision*	Insertion of a tube into the windpipe to assist breathing Incision made into the trachea to create a tracheostomy
ventilation ventilator	ven-tih-**LAY**-shun **VEN**-tih-lay-tor	S/ R/ S/	**-ation** *a process* **ventil-** *wind* **-ator** *person or thing that does something*	Movement of gases into and out of the lungs Device that breathes for the patient

EXERCISES

A. Deconstruct: *Define the elements related to therapeutic procedures used to treat pulmonary disorders. Fill in the blanks.* **LO 8.1 and 8.6**

Medical Term	Meaning of Root/CF	Meaning of Suffix
immunization	**1.**	**2.**
nebulizer	**3.**	**4.**
tracheostomy	**5.**	**6.**
tracheotomy	**7.**	**8.**

B. Meet lesson and chapter objectives *by applying the language of pulmonology to answer the following questions correctly.* **LO 8.2, 8.6, and 8.7**

1. A person who has trouble expectorating thick mucus may benefit from this type of drug: ____________________

2. A device that breathes for the patient: ____________________

3. The removal of a small piece of the lung is termed a ________________ resection.

4. An airway that is placed in the mouth and pharynx is termed an ________________ airway.

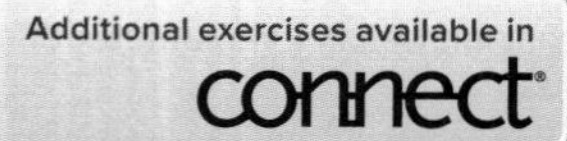

Chapter Review exercises, along with additional practice items, are available in Connect!

The Digestive System

The Essentials of the Language of Gastroenterology

Rick Brady/McGraw-Hill Education

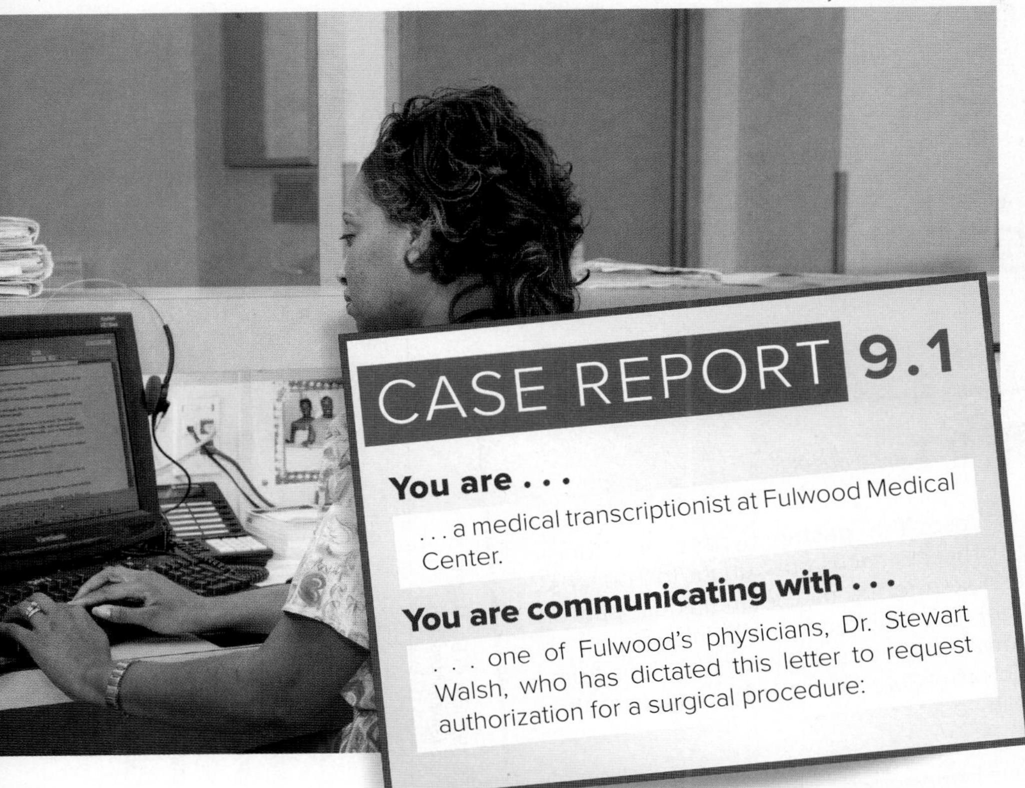

CASE REPORT 9.1

You are . . .

. . . a medical transcriptionist at Fulwood Medical Center.

You are communicating with . . .

. . . one of Fulwood's physicians, Dr. Stewart Walsh, who has dictated this letter to request authorization for a surgical procedure:

Fulwood Medical Center
3333 Medical Parkway, Fulwood, MI 01234
555-247-6100

Center for Bariatric Surgery

Charles Leavenworth, MD
Medical Director
Lombard Insurance Company
One Lombard Place
Haverson, MI 01233

10/06/11
Request for authorization of surgery
Mrs. Martha Jones Subscriber ID: 056437

Dear Doctor Leavenworth,

Mrs. Jones is a 52-year-old former waitress, recently divorced. She is 5 feet 4 inches tall and weighs 275 pounds. She has type 2 diabetes with frequent episodes of hypoglycemia and also ketoacidosis, requiring three different hospitalizations. She now has diabetic retinopathy and peripheral vasculitis. Complicating this are hypertension (185/110), coronary artery disease, and pulmonary edema. In spite of monthly meetings with our nutritionist, she has gained 25 pounds in the past six months.

To reduce and control her weight, I am proposing to perform a gastric bypass using a laparoscopic approach. We will need to admit her two days prior to surgery to control her blood sugar and cardiovascular problems, and we anticipate that she will remain in the hospital for two days after surgery, barring any complications. She is also very aware of the necessary follow-up to the procedure and the counseling required for a new lifestyle.

We believe not only that this is an essential procedure medically but that it will reduce in the long term the financial burden of her multiple therapies and improve the quality of the patient's life. Enclosed is supportive documentation of her current history and medical problems.

Your company has designated our hospital as a Center of Excellence for bariatric surgery, and I look forward to your prompt agreement with this approach for this patient.

Sincerely,

Stewart Walsh, MD, FACS
Chief of Surgery

Learning Outcomes

As a medical transcriptionist (MT), your job is to accurately transcribe the voice-recorded reports of physicians and any other health care professionals into readable text. To ensure that Mrs. Jones receives the best possible care, you and the health care professionals directly and indirectly involved with her care, need to be able to:

LO 9.1 **Use roots, combining forms, suffixes, and prefixes to construct and analyze medical terms related to the digestive system.**

LO 9.2 **Spell and pronounce correctly medical terms related to the digestive system in order to communicate them with accuracy and precision in any health care setting.**

LO 9.3 **Define accepted abbreviations related to the digestive system.**

LO 9.4 **Relate the overall anatomy of the alimentary canal to the actions and functions of digestion.**

LO 9.5 **Describe the anatomy of the mouth, pharynx, and esophagus; their roles in mastication and swallowing; and their disorders.**

LO 9.6 **Relate the anatomy of the stomach and small intestine to the digestion that takes place therein and their disorders.**

LO 9.7 **Explain the anatomy and roles of the liver, gallbladder, and pancreas in digestion and their disorders related to digestion.**

LO 9.8 **Describe the overall process of digestion and the malabsorption syndromes.**

LO 9.9 **Relate the anatomy of the large intestine to its functions and disorders.**

LO 9.10 **Describe the diagnostic and therapeutic procedures and pharmacologic agents used for disorders of the digestive system.**

LO 9.11 **Apply your knowledge of the medical terms of the digestive system to documentation, medical records, and medical reports.**

LO 9.12 **Translate the medical terms of the digestive system into everyday language in order to communicate clearly with patients and their families.**

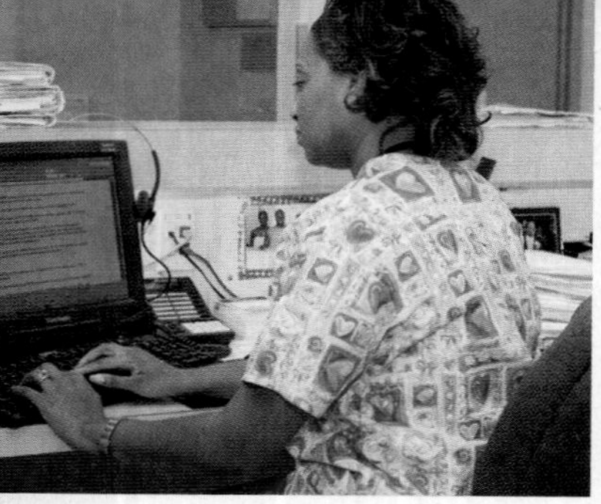

Rick Brady/McGraw-Hill Education

In your future career, being able to communicate comfortably, accurately, and effectively with the health professionals involved in the diagnosis and treatment of problems in the **gastroenterological** system is key. You may work directly and/or indirectly with one or more of the following:

- **Gastroenterologists** are medical specialists in the field of gastroenterology.
- **Proctologists** are surgical specialists in diseases of the anus and rectum.
- **Dentists** are qualified practitioners in the anatomy, physiology, and pathology of the oral-facial complex.
- **Periodontists** are specialists in disorders of the tissues surrounding the teeth.
- **Nutritionists** are professionals who prevent and treat illness by promoting healthy eating habits.
- **Dietitians** manage food services systems and promote sound eating habits.

Objectives

There are basic terms and elements of medical terminology that apply throughout the different parts of the digestive system. Understanding these basic terms and elements of the digestive system will enable you to use correct medical terminology to:

9.1.1 Name the health professionals involved in gastroenterology.

9.1.2 List the organs and accessory organs of the digestive system.

9.1.3 Identify the components of the alimentary canal.

9.1.4 Describe the structure and functions of the digestive system.

Lesson 9.1

The Digestive System

Case Report 9.1 *(continued)*

In Mrs. Jones's case, the **gastric** bypass procedure reduced the size of her stomach from 2 quarts to 2 ounces. The bypass was taken to the mid-ileum (middle part of the small intestine). This resulted in her being able to eat less and to absorb less. She had no complications from the **laparoscopic** procedure and lost 15 pounds in the 2 months that followed.

Alimentary Canal and Accessory Organs (LO 9.4)

Every cell in your body requires a constant supply of nourishment in a form that can be absorbed across its cell membrane. The **digestive system** breaks down the **nutrients** in food into elements that can be transported to the cells via the blood and lymphatics.

The digestive system consists of the **alimentary canal,** or digestive tract, which extends from the mouth to the **anus,** and **accessory organs** connected to the canal to assist in digestion.

Gastroenterology is the study of the digestive system.

The **alimentary canal** *(Figure 9.1)* includes the:

- **Mouth**
- **Pharynx**
- **Esophagus**
- **Stomach**
- **Small intestine**
- **Large intestine**

The **accessory organs** of digestion include the:

- **Teeth**
- **Tongue**
- **Salivary glands**
- **Liver**
- **Gallbladder**
- **Pancreas**

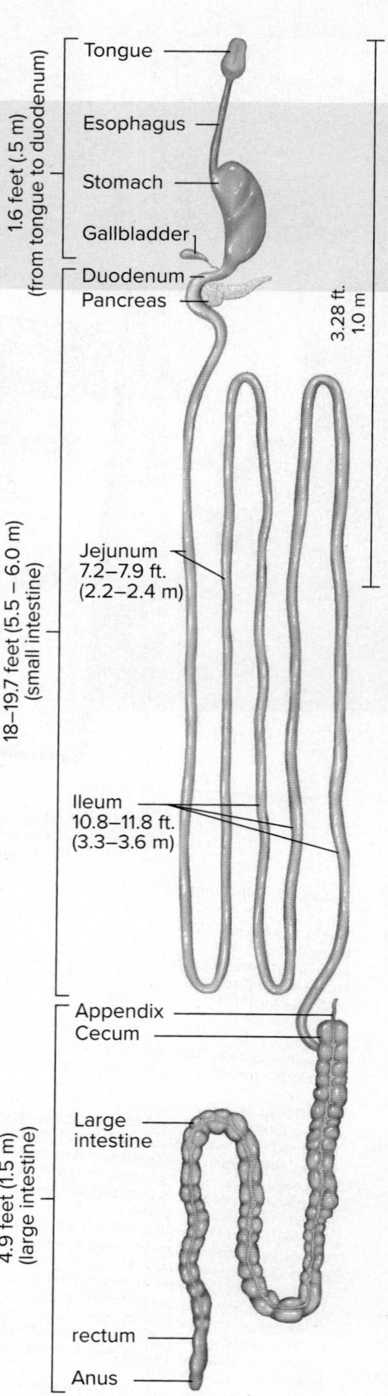

▲ **FIGURE 9.1** Alimentary Canal.

Word Analysis and Definition

S = Suffix   P = Prefix   R = Root   R/CF = Combining Form

WORD	PRONUNCIATION	ELEMENTS		DEFINITION
alimentary alimentary canal	al-ih-**MEN**-tar-ee kah-**NAL**	S/ R/	-ary *pertaining to* aliment- *nourishment, food* canal, Latin *a duct or channel*	Pertaining to the digestive tract Digestive tract
anus anal (adj)	**A**-nus **A**-nal	 S/ R/	Latin *a ring* -al *pertaining to* an- *anus*	Terminal opening of the digestive tract through which feces are discharged Pertaining to the anus
bariatric	bar-ee-**AT**-rik	S/ R/	-atric *treatment* bari- *weight*	Treatment of obesity
digestion digestive (adj)	die-**JESS**-chun die-**JEST**-iv	S/ R/ S/	-ion *action* digest- *to break down food* -ive *nature of, quality of*	Breakdown of food into elements suitable for cell metabolism Pertaining to digestion
esophagus	ee-**SOF**-ah-gus		Greek *gullet*	Tube linking the pharynx and the stomach
gastric (adj) gastroenterology gastroenterologist gastrointestinal	**GAS**-trik **GAS**-troh-en-ter-**OL**-oh-gee **GAS**-troh-en-ter-**OL**-oh-jist **GAS**-troh-in-**TESS**-tin-al	S/ R/ S/ R/CF R/CF S/ S/ R/CF R/	-ic *pertaining to* gastr- *stomach* -logy *study of* gastr/o- *stomach* -enter/o- *intestine* -logist *one who studies, specialist* -al *pertaining to* gastr/o- *stomach* intestin- *gut, intestine*	Pertaining to the stomach Medical specialty of the stomach and intestines Medical specialist in gastroenterology Pertaining to the stomach and intestines
intestine intestinal (adj)	in-**TESS**-tin in-**TESS**-tin-al	 S/ R/	Latin *intestine, gut* -al *pertaining to* intestin- *gut, intestine*	The digestive tube from stomach to anus Pertaining to the intestines
laparoscopy laparoscope laparoscopic (adj)	lap-ah-**ROS**-koh-pee **LAP**-ah-roh-skope **LAP**-ah-roh-**SKOP**-ik	S/ R/CF S/ S/	-scopy *to view, to examine* lapar/o- *abdomen in general* -scope *instrument for viewing* -ic *pertaining to*	Examination of contents of abdomen using an endoscope Instrument (endoscope) used for viewing abdominal contents Pertaining to laparoscopy
nutrient nutritive (adj) nutrition nutritionist	**NYU**-tree-ent **NYU**-trih-tiv nyu-**TRISH**-un nyu-**TRISH**-un-ist	 S/ R/ S/ S/	Latin *to nourish* -ive *nature of, pertaining to* nutrit- *nourishment* -ion- *action, condition* -ist *specialist in*	A substance in food required for normal physiologic function Providing nourishment The study of food and liquid requirements for normal function of the human body Certified professional in nutrition science

EXERCISES

A. Review *Case Report 9.1, the Request for authorization of surgery document, and Case Report. 9.1 (continued). Then provide the correct term that answers each question. Fill in the blanks.* **LO 9.2, 9.4, 9.10, and 9.11**

1. What is the term for the type of surgery being proposed for Mrs. Jones? ______
2. What method of surgery will be used to perform the procedure? ______
3. What disease has previously caused Mrs. Jones to be hospitalized? ______
4. What type of specialist has worked with Dr. Walsh to explain the procedure to Ms. Jones? ______
5. What type of specialist attempted to help Ms. Jone with her diet? ______

B. Analyzing *the elements can help you determine the meaning of a medical term. Use the terms provided below to complete each sentence. Fill in the blanks.* **LO 9.1, 9.4, and 9.10**

gastric **gastroenterology** **gastrointestinal** **gastroenterologist** **gastroscope**

1. After completion of his training, the physicians assistant chose to work in the field of ______.
2. After eating a large amount of fatty and sugary food, the patient experienced ______ upset.
3. Due to chronic pain the the digestive tract, the family practice physician referred the patient to a ______.
4. The ______ is used to view the inside of the stomach.
5. The patient is complaining of intense burning pain in the stomach; you document this as ______ pain.

Lesson 9.1 (cont'd)

Keynotes

- **Digestion is both mechanical and chemical.**
- **Water liquefies the food to make it easier to digest and absorb.**
- **Enzymes break down the food.**

Actions and Functions of the Digestive System (LO 9.4)

The actions and functions of your digestive system have these five components:

1. **Propulsion:** The mechanical movement of food from the mouth to the anus *(Figure 9.2)*. Normally, this takes 24 to 36 hours.

2. **Digestion:** The breakdown of foods into forms that can be transported to cells and absorbed into these cells. This process has two parts:

   a. **Mechanical digestion** breaks larger pieces of food into smaller ones without altering their chemical composition. **Mastication** (chewing) breaks down the food into smaller particles so that digestive **enzymes** have a larger surface area with which to interact. **Deglutition** (swallowing) moves the **bolus** (mass or lump) of food from the mouth into the esophagus. **Peristalsis** (waves of contraction and relaxation) moves food material through most of the alimentary canal.

   b. **Chemical digestion** breaks down large molecules of food into smaller and simpler chemicals by way of digestive enzymes (made by the salivary glands, stomach, small intestine, and pancreas). The digestive enzymes have three main groups:

   - **Amylases,** which digest carbohydrates
   - **Lipases,** which digest fats
   - **Proteases,** which digest proteins

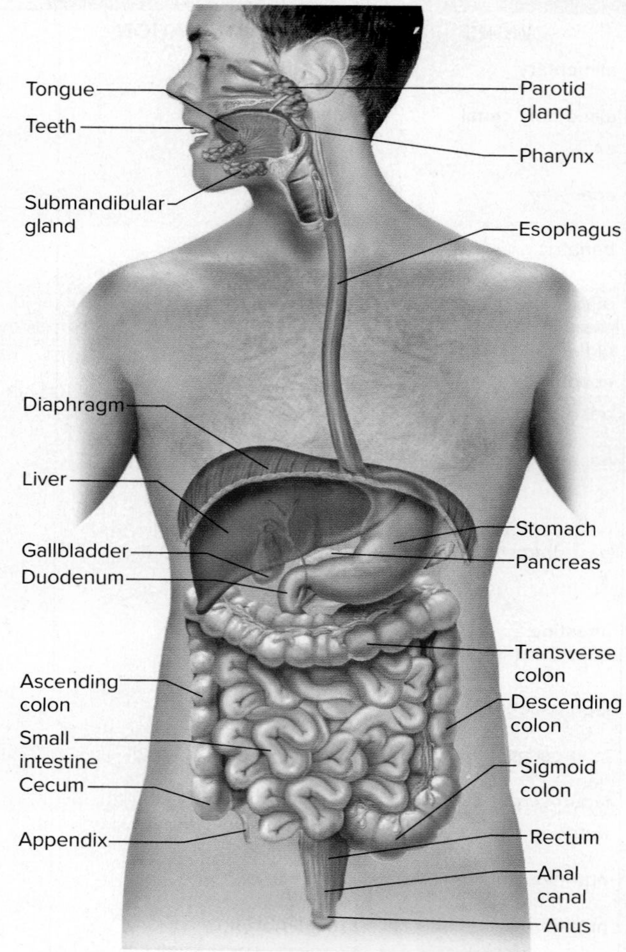

▲ **FIGURE 9.2**
The Digestive System.

3. **Secretion:** The addition of secretions like mucus that lubricate, liquefy, and digest food throughout the digestive tract, while also keeping the tract's lining lubricated.

4. **Absorption:** The movement of nutrient molecules out of the digestive tract, through the epithelial cells lining the tract, and into the blood or lymph for transportation to body cells.

5. **Elimination:** The process by which the body removes undigested food residue.

Word Analysis and Definition

S = Suffix P = Prefix R = Root R/CF = Combining Form

WORD	PRONUNCIATION	ELEMENTS		DEFINITION
amylase	**AM**-ih-laze	S/ R/	-ase *enzyme* **amyl-** *starch*	One of a group of enzymes that breaks down starch
bolus	**BOH**-lus		Greek *lump*	A single mass of a substance
deglutition	dee-glue-**TISH**-un	S/ R/	-ion *action, condition* **deglutit-** *to swallow*	The act of swallowing
elimination	ee-lim-ih-**NAY**-shun	S/ R/	-ation *process* **elimin-** *throw away*	Removal of waste material from the digestive tract
enzyme	**EN**-zime	P/ R/	**en-** *in* **-zyme** *fermenting*	Protein that induces changes in other substances
lipase	**LIE**-paze	S/ R/	-ase *enzyme* **lip-** *fat*	Enzyme that breaks down fat
masticate (verb) **mastication (noun)**	**MAS**-tih-kate mas-tih-**KAY**-shun	S/ R/ S/	-ate *pertaining to, composed of* **mastic-** *chew* -ation *process*	To chew The process of chewing
peristalsis	per-ih-**STAL**-sis	P/ R/	**peri-** *around* **-stalsis** *constrict*	Waves of alternate contraction and relaxation of the intestinal wall to move food along the digestive tract
protease	**PRO**-tee-aze	S/ R/CF	-ase *enzyme* **prot/e-** *protein*	Group of enzymes that breaks down protein

EXERCISES

A. Match *the correct medical term in column 2 to the definition in column 1. The body process, or action, is described for you below. Fill in the blanks.* **LO 9.4 and 9.8**

_____ **1.** swallowing — **a.** mastication

_____ **2.** intestinal muscle contractions — **b.** elimination

_____ **3.** chewing — **c.** deglutition

_____ **4.** removal of waste material — **d.** peristalsis

B. Review *the text to obtain answers to the following questions. Fill in the blanks.* **LO 9.4 and 9.8**

1. What is the mechanical movement of food from mouth to anus called? ____________________

2. Which enzyme helps to break down protein? ____________________

3. What lubricates the food in the digestive tract? ____________________

4. Which enzyme breaks down fat? ____________________

5. Which enzyme breaks down starch? ____________________

6. What is the medical term used to describe the lump of food that is moved from the mouth to esophagus? ____________________

C. Build *the medical terms by filling in their missing elements. Fill in the blanks.* **LO 9.1 and 9.4**

1. The process of chewing: ______________ / ______________

2. Removal of waste material from the digestive tract: ______________ / ______________

3. The act of swallowing: ______________ / ______________

4. To chew: ______________ / ______________

5. Waves that move food in intestines: ______________ / ______________

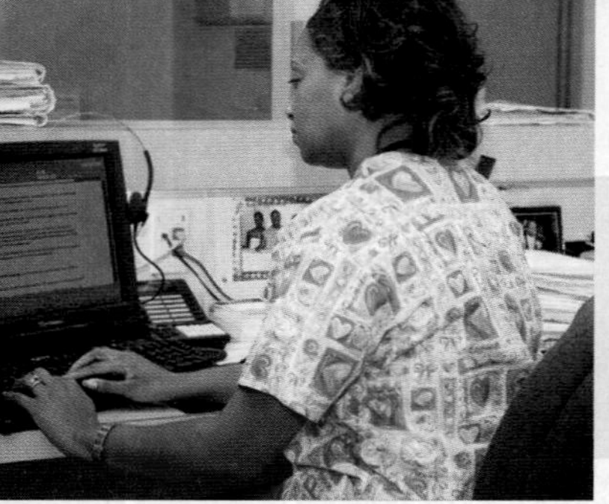

Rick Brady/McGraw-Hill Education

Lesson 9.2

Mouth, Pharynx, and Esophagus

Objectives

When you pop a piece of chicken and some vegetables into your mouth, you start a cascade of digestive tract events that will occur during the next 24 to 36 hours. In this chapter, you will follow the food as it moves through the digestive tract. And in this lesson, you will become familiar with the first stages in the cascade of events, when the food is in the mouth and then swallowed. The information in this lesson will enable you to use correct medical terminology to:

9.2.1 Identify the structures and functions of the teeth, tongue, and salivary glands.

9.2.2 Document the processes and outcomes of mastication and deglutition.

9.2.3 Describe the structures, functions, and disorders of the mouth, pharynx, and esophagus.

The Mouth and Mastication (LO 9.5)

Your **mouth** *(Figure 9.3)* is the gateway to your digestive tract. It's the first site of mechanical digestion, through mastication (chewing), and of chemical digestion, through an **enzyme** in your **saliva.**

The roof of your mouth is called the **palate,** and its anterior two-thirds is the bony **hard palate.** The posterior one-third is the muscular **soft palate.** The skeletal muscle of the soft palate has a projection or flap called the **uvula,** which closes off the **nasopharynx** (upper pharynx) when swallowing.

Your **tongue** moves food around your mouth and helps the cheeks, lips, and gums hold food in place while you chew it. Small, rough, raised areas on the tongue, called **papillae,** contain some 4,000 taste buds that react to the chemical nature of food to give you different taste sensations *(Figure 9.4).* A taste-bud cell lives for 7 to 10 days before it's replaced.

Adult Teeth (LO 9.5)

The average adult has 32 teeth—16 rooted in the upper jaw (maxilla) and 16 in the lower jaw (mandible) *(Figure 9.3).* The bulk of a tooth is composed of **dentine** (also spelled *dentin*), a substance like bone but harder, that is covered in **enamel.** The dentine surrounds a central **pulp** cavity, containing blood vessels, nerves, and connective tissue. The blood vessels and nerves reach this cavity from the jaw through tubular root canals.

Salivary Glands (LO 9.5)

Salivary glands secrete saliva. The two **parotid** glands (beside the ears), the two **submandibular** glands (beneath the mandible), the two **sublingual** glands (beneath the tongue) *(Figure 9.5),* and numerous minor salivary glands scattered in the mucosa of the tongue and cheeks secrete more than a quart of saliva daily.

Saliva is 95% water, and its major functions are to begin the digestion of starch and fat and to lubricate food so it's easier to swallow. Imagine you are eating a piece of chicken and some vegetables. By **mastication,** the chicken has been torn and ground into small pieces by your teeth, and its fat has begun to be digested by the lipase in your saliva. The vegetables have also been ground into small pieces, and their starch has begun to be digested by the amylase in your saliva.

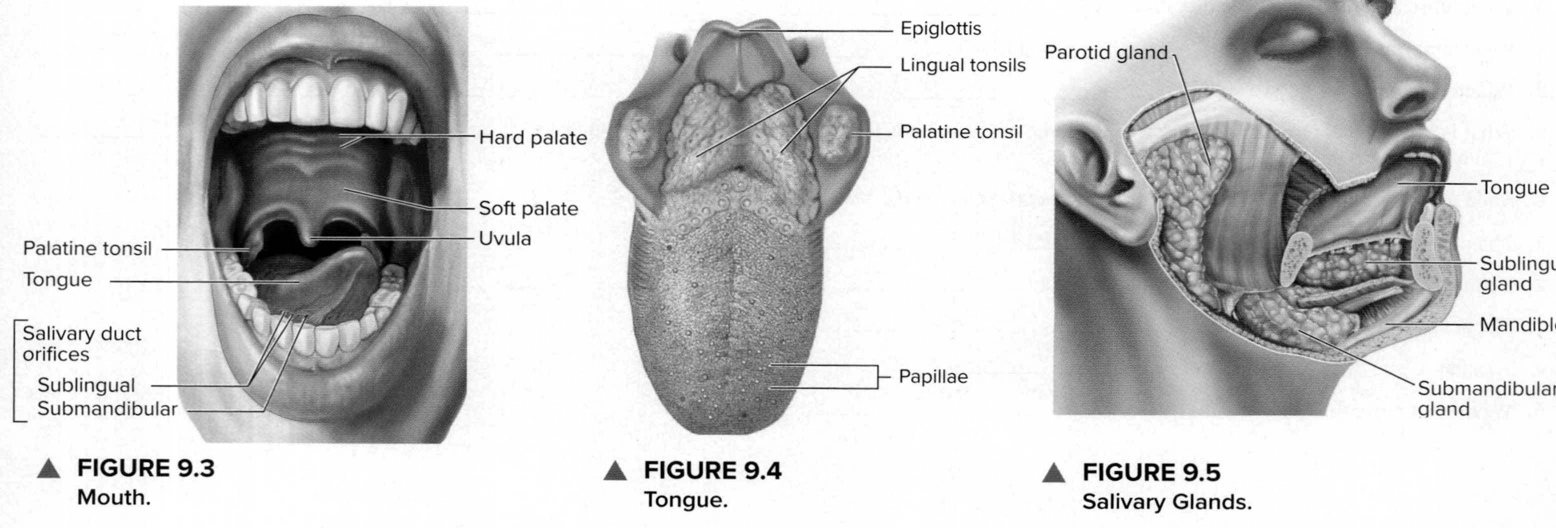

▲ **FIGURE 9.3** Mouth.

▲ **FIGURE 9.4** Tongue.

▲ **FIGURE 9.5** Salivary Glands.

Word Analysis and Definition

S = Suffix P = Prefix R = Root R/CF = Combining Form

WORD	PRONUNCIATION	ELEMENTS		DEFINITION
dentine (*also spelled* **dentin**)	**DEN**-tin	S/ R/	**-ine** *pertaining to, substance* **dent-** *tooth*	Dense, ivory-like substance located under the enamel in a tooth
dentist	**DEN**-tist	S/ R/	**-ist** *specialist* **dent-** *tooth*	A qualified practitioner in the anatomy, physiology, and pathology of the oral-facial complex
enamel	ee-**NAM**-el		French *enamel*	Hard substance covering a tooth
mouth	**MOWTH**		Old English *mouth*	External opening of a cavity or canal
nasopharynx	**NAY**-zoh-**FAIR**-inks	R/CF R/	**nas/o-** *nose* **-pharynx** *throat*	Region of the pharynx at the back of the nose and above the soft palate
oral	**OR**-al	S/ R/	**-al** *pertaining to* **or- (os)** *mouth*	Pertaining to the mouth
palate	**PAL**-at		Latin *palate*	Roof of the mouth
papilla **papillae (pl)**	pah-**PILL**-ah pah-**PILL**-ee		Latin *small pimple*	Any small projection
parotid	pah-**ROT**-id	S/ P/ R/	**-id** *having a particular quality* **par-** *beside* **-ot-** *ear*	The parotid gland is the salivary gland beside the ear
pulp	**PULP**		Latin *flesh*	Dental pulp is the connective tissue in the cavity in the center of the tooth
saliva (noun) **salivary (adj)**	sa-**LIE**-vah **SAL**-ih-var-ee	 S/ R/	Latin *spit* **-ary** *pertaining to* **saliv-** *saliva*	Secretion in mouth from salivary glands Pertaining to saliva
sublingual	sub-**LING**-wal	S/ P/ R/	**-al** *pertaining to* **sub-** *underneath* **-lingu-** *tongue*	Underneath the tongue
submandibular	sub-man-**DIB**-you-lar	S/ P/ R/	**-ar** *pertaining to* **sub-** *underneath* **-mandibul-** *mandible*	Underneath the mandible
tongue	**TUNG**		Latin *tongue*	Mobile muscle mass in the mouth; bears the taste buds
uvula	**YOU**-vyu-lah		Latin *grape*	Fleshy projection of the soft palate

Exercises

A. Apply *your knowledge of the same elements to various terms, and increase your medical vocabulary. Focus on what is the same and what is different about the following terms. Fill in the chart.* **LO 9.1, 9.2, and 9.5**

Medical Term	Meaning of Prefix	Meaning of Root	Meaning of Suffix
submandibular	1.	2.	3.
sublingual	4.	5.	6.
parotid	7.	8.	9.

B. Use *medical terms relating to the mouth and mastication to correctly complete each sentence. Fill in the blanks.* **LO 9.5**

1. The roof of the mouth is termed the ______________________.

2. During swallowing, the ______________________ covers the entrance to the nose from the back of the throat.

3. Taste buds are located on the sides of the tongue's ______________________.

4. The ______________________ moves food around in the mouth during mastication.

Lesson 9.2 (cont'd)

Keynotes

- **Cleft palate is a congenital fissure in the median line of the palate. It is often associated with a cleft lip.**
- **Glossodynia is a painful, burning sensation of the tongue. It occurs in postmenopausal women. Its etiology is unknown. There is no successful treatment.**
- **Periodontal disease is thought to be associated with coronary artery disease, but no causal relationship has been established.**

Abbreviation

HSV-1 Herpes simplex virus, type 1

Disorders of the Mouth

(LO 9.5)

The human mouth is the entrance to the digestive system, and since so many elements pass through it, the human mouth is prone to tooth disorders and a host of other conditions.

A buildup of **dental plaque** (a collection of oral microorganisms and their products), or **tartar** (calcified deposits at the margin of the teeth along the gums), is a precursor to invasion by dental disease-causing bacteria.

Dental caries, which are tooth decay and cavity formation, are erosions of the tooth surface caused by bacteria *(Figure 9.6).* If untreated, it can lead to an abscess at the root of the tooth. **Gingivitis** is an infection of the gums. **Periodontal disease** occurs when the gums and the jawbone are involved in a disease process. In **periodontitis,** infection causes the gums to pull away from the teeth, forming pockets that become sources of infection that can spread to underlying bone. Infection of the gums with a purulent or pus-like discharge is called **pyorrhea.**

The term **stomatitis** is used for any infection of the mouth, including:

- **Mouth ulcers,** also called **canker** sores, are erosions of the mucous membrane lining the mouth. **Aphthous** ulcers are the most common and occur in clusters of small ulcers that last for 3 or 4 days. These are usually stress- or illness-related but can also be caused by trauma.
- **Cold sores,** or fever blisters *(Figure 9.7),* are recurrent blisters on the lips, lining of the mouth, and gums due to infection with the virus **herpes simplex type 1 (HSV-1).** These blisters usually clear up spontaneously.
- **Thrush** *(Figure 9.8)* is an infection occurring anywhere in the mouth that is caused by the fungus *Candida albicans.* This fungus is normally found in the mouth, but it can multiply out of control as a result of prolonged antibiotic or steroid treatment, cancer chemotherapy, or diabetes. Newborn babies can acquire oral thrush from the mother's vaginal yeast infection during the birth process. Treatment with antifungal agents is usually successful.
- **Oral cancer** occurs most often on the lip, but it can also occur on the tongue. Eighty percent of oral cancers are associated with smoking or chewing tobacco. Metastasis occurs to lymph nodes, bones, lungs, and liver.

Halitosis is the medical term for bad breath, which occurs in association with any of the above mouth disorders.

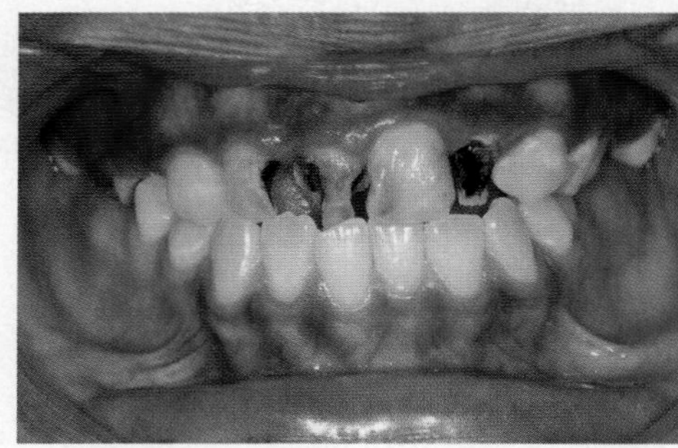

▲ **FIGURE 9.6**
Dental Caries.

watanyou/Getty Images

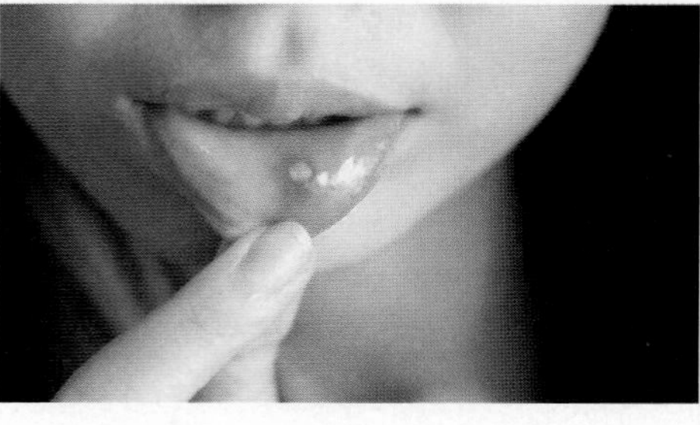

▲ **FIGURE 9.7**
Cold Sores on the inside of the Lower Lip.

C.PIPAT/Shutterstock

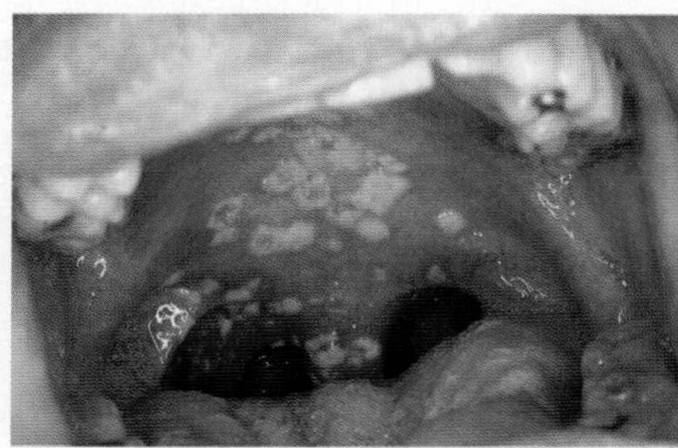

▲ **FIGURE 9.8**
Oral Thrush.

Dr. Sol Silverman, Jr., DDS/CDC

Word Analysis and Definition

S = Suffix P = Prefix R = Root R/CF = Combining Form

WORD	PRONUNCIATION		ELEMENTS	DEFINITION
aphthous	**AF**-thus		Greek *ulcer*	Painful small oral ulcers (canker sores)
canker	**KANG**-ker		Latin *crab*	Nonmedical term for aphthous ulcer
caries	**KARE**-eez		Latin *dry rot*	Bacterial destruction of teeth
gingiva **gingival (adj)** **gingivitis** **gingivectomy**	**JIN**-jih-vah **JIN**-jih-val jin-jih-**VI**-tis jin-jih-**VEC**-toe-me	 S/ R/ S/ S/	Latin *gum* **-al** *pertaining to* **gingiv-** *gum* **-itis** *inflammation* **-ectomy** *surgical excision*	Tissue surrounding the teeth and covering the jaw Pertaining to the gums Inflammation of the gums Surgical removal of diseased gum tissue
glossodynia	gloss-oh-**DIN**-ee-ah	S/ R/CF	**-dynia** *pain* **gloss/o-** *tongue*	Painful, burning tongue
halitosis	hal-ih-**TOE**-sis	S/ R/	**-osis** *condition* **halit-** *breath*	Bad odor of the breath
periodontal **periodontics** **periodontist** **periodontitis**	**PER**-ee-oh-**DON**-tal **PER**-ee-oh-**DON**-tiks **PER**-ee-oh-**DON**-tist **PER**-ee-oh-don-**TIE**-tis	S/ P/ R/ S/ S/ S/	**-al** *pertaining to* **peri-** *around* **-odont-** *tooth* **-ics** *knowledge* **-ist** *specialist* **-itis** *inflammation*	Around a tooth Branch of dentistry specializing in disorders of tissues around the teeth Specialist in periodontics Inflammation of tissues around a tooth
plaque	PLAK		French *plate*	Patch of abnormal tissue
pyorrhea	pie-oh-**REE**-ah	R/ R/CF	**-rrhea** *flow* **py/o-** *pus*	Purulent discharge
stomatitis	**STOE**-mah-**TI**-tis	S/ R/CF	**-itis** *inflammation* **stomat/i-** *oral cavity, mouth*	Inflammation of the mucous membrane in the mouth
tartar	**TAR**-tar		Latin *crust on wine casks*	Calcified deposit at the gingival margin of the teeth
thrush	**THRUSH**		Root unknown	Infection with *Candida albicans*

EXERCISES

A. Suffixes: *Find the correct suffix to complete the medical terms. Fill in the blanks.* **LO 9.1 and 9.5**

ist itis ectomy rrhea osis al ics

1. inflammation of the gums gingiv/ ____________________
2. specialized branch of dentistry periodont/ ____________________
3. around a tooth periodont/ ____________________
4. bad breath halit/ ____________________
5. surgical removal of diseased gum tissue gingiv/ ____________________
6. specialist in periodontics periodont/ ____________________
7. purulent discharge pyo/ ____________________

B. Identify *the following medical terms that have their origin in Greek, Latin, or French. Fill in the blanks.* **LO 9.2 and 9.5**

1. patch of abnormal tissue ____________________
2. canker sores ____________________
3. pertaining to the gums ____________________
4. nonmedical term for a mouth ulcer ____________________
5. bacterial destruction of teeth ____________________

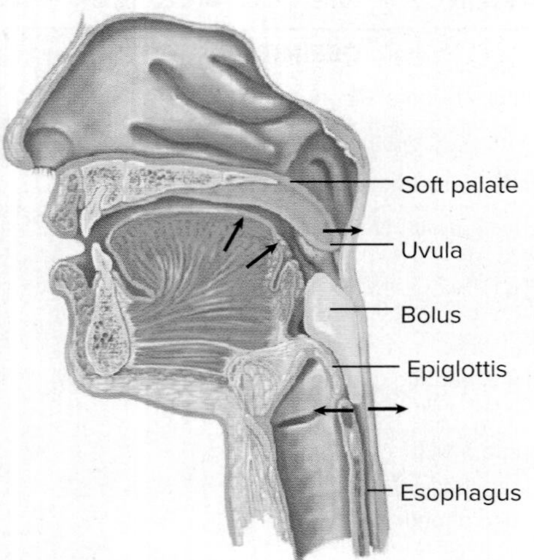

▲ **FIGURE 9.9**
Swallowing.
The bolus of food is in the oropharynx.

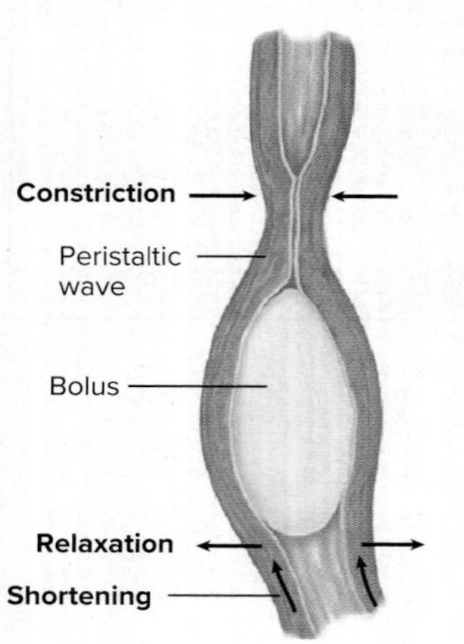

▲ **FIGURE 9.10**
Swallowing.
The bolus of food is in the esophagus.

Esophagus (LO 9.5)

The chicken and vegetables that you ingested earlier have now been sliced and ground into small particles by the teeth. These particles are partly digested and lubricated by saliva, and rolled into a bolus between the tongue and the hard palate, the bony roof of the mouth. The bolus is now ready to be swallowed down the oropharynx (upper part of the throat) *(Figure 9.9)* into the **esophagus.**

The bolus enters the esophagus from the lower end of the pharynx. In the esophagus, peristaltic, or wavelike, contractions of the esophageal wall muscles move it downward *(Figure 9.10).* At the lower end of the esophagus, the **cardiac sphincter** relaxes to allow the bolus to enter the stomach.

The **esophagus** *(Figure 9.11)* is a tube 9 to 10 inches long. It pierces the diaphragm at the esophageal **hiatus** to go from the thoracic cavity to the abdominal cavity *(Figure 9.11).*

Disorders of the Esophagus (LO 9.5)

Just like the mouth, the esophagus, too, can be prone to illness. **Esophagitis** is an inflammation of the lining of the esophagus, producing a burning chest pain **(heartburn)** after eating, pain on swallowing, and occasional vomiting of blood **(hematemesis).** The most common cause is **reflux** of the stomach's acid contents into the esophagus, also known as **gastroesophageal reflux disease (GERD).**

Hiatal hernia occurs when a portion of the stomach protrudes through the diaphragm alongside the esophagus at the esophageal hiatus *(Figure 9.12).* Surgical repair—a hiatal **herniorrhaphy**—may be necessary.

Esophageal varices are varicose veins of the esophagus. They are **asymptomatic** until they rupture, causing massive bleeding and hematemesis. They are a complication of cirrhosis of the liver *(see later in this chapter).*

Cancer of the esophagus arises from the tube's lining. Symptoms are **dysphagia** (difficulty swallowing), a burning sensation in the chest, and weight loss. Risk factors include cigarettes, alcohol, betel-nut chewing, and esophageal reflux. The cancer metastasizes to the liver, bones, and lungs.

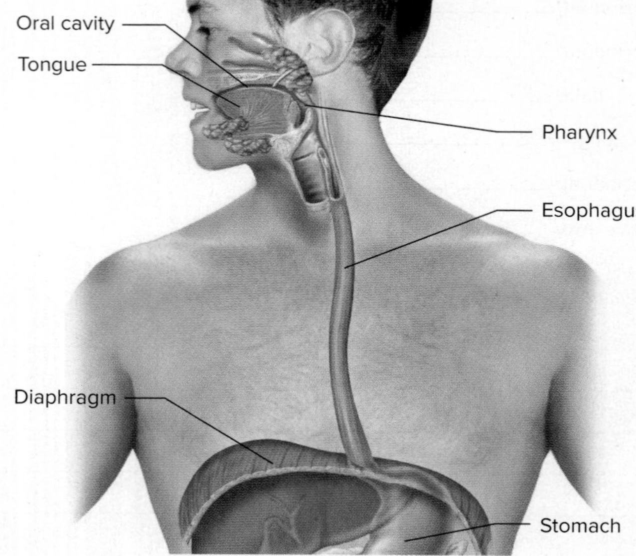

▶ **FIGURE 9.11**
Esophagus.

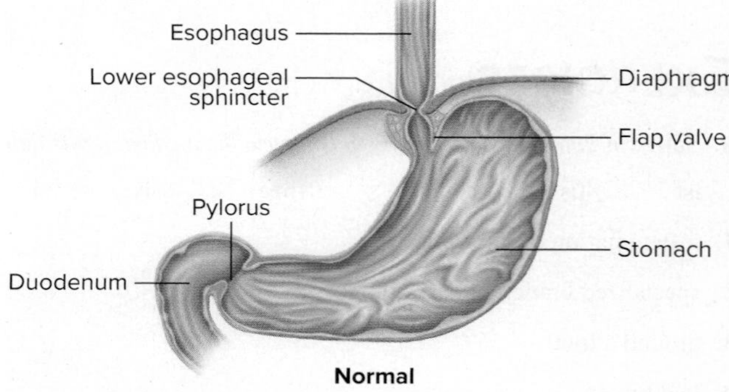

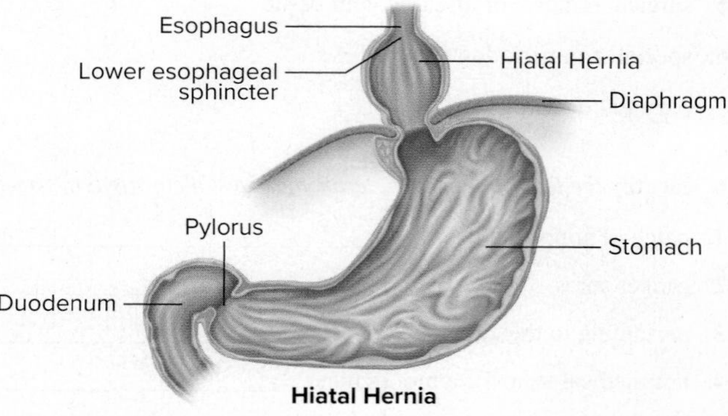

▲ **FIGURE 9.12**
Hiatal Hernia.

Word Analysis and Definition

S = Suffix P = Prefix R = Root R/CF = Combining Form

WORD	PRONUNCIATION		ELEMENTS	DEFINITION
asymptomatic **symptomatic** (*with* **symptoms**)	**A**-simp-toe-**MAT**-ik simp-toe-**MAT**-ik	S/ P/ R/	-ic *pertaining to* a- *without* symptomat- *symptom*	Without any symptoms or abnormalities experienced by the patient Pertaining to the symptoms of a disease
dysphagia	dis-**FAY**-jee-ah	P/ R/	dys- *difficulty* -phagia *swallowing*	Difficulty in swallowing
emesis **hematemesis**	**EM**-eh-sis he-mah-**TEM**-eh-sis	 R/ R/	Greek *to vomit* hemat- *blood* -emesis *to vomit*	Vomit Vomiting of red blood
esophagus **esophageal (adj)** **esophagitis**	ee-**SOF**-ah-gus ee-**SOF**-ah-**JEE**-al ee-**SOF**-ah-**JI**-tis	 S/ R/ S/	Greek *gullet* -eal *pertaining to* esophag- *esophagus* -itis *inflammation*	Tube linking pharynx to stomach Pertaining to the esophagus Inflammation of the lining of the esophagus
hernia **herniorrhaphy**	**HER**-nee-ah **HER**-nee-**OR**-ah-fee	 S/ R/CF	Latin *rupture* -rrhaphy *suture* herni/o- *hernia*	Protrusion of a structure through the tissue that normally contains it Repair of a hernia
hiatus (noun) **hiatal (adj)**	high-**AY**-tus high-**AY**-tal	 S/ R/	Latin *an aperture* -al *pertaining to* hiat- *opening*	An opening through a structure Pertaining to a hiatus
reflux	**REE**-fluks	P/ R/	re- *back* -flux *flow*	Backward flow
sphincter	**SFINK**-ter		Greek *a band*	A band of muscle that encircles an opening; when it contracts, the opening squeezes closed
varix **varices (pl)** **varicose (adj)**	**VAIR**-iks **VAIR**-ih-seez **VAIR**-ih-kose	 S/ R/	Latin *dilated vein* -ose *full of* varic- *varicosity; dilated, tortuous vein*	Dilated, tortuous vein Characterized by or affected with varices

Exercises

A. Knowledge *of elements is your best tool for increasing your medical vocabulary. Each of the following terms has an element in bold. Identify that element and give its meaning. Fill in the chart.* **LO 9.1 and 9.5**

Medical Term	Identity of Element (P, R, CF, or S)	Meaning of Element
***re*flux**	**1.**	**2.**
dys*phagia*	**3.**	**4.**
hernio*rrhaphy*	**5.**	**6.**
hemat*emesis*	**7.**	**8.**
***a*symptomatic**	**9.**	**10.**

B. Apply *the language of gastroenterology and fill in the blanks.* **LO 9.2 and 9.5**

1. What is another term for *varicose veins* of the esophagus? ______
2. What is the medical term for inflammation of the lining of the esophagus? ______
3. What structure does the esophagus travel through from the *thoracic cavity* to the abdominal cavity? ______
4. What is burning chest pain called? ______
5. What are you vomiting in *hematemesis?* ______

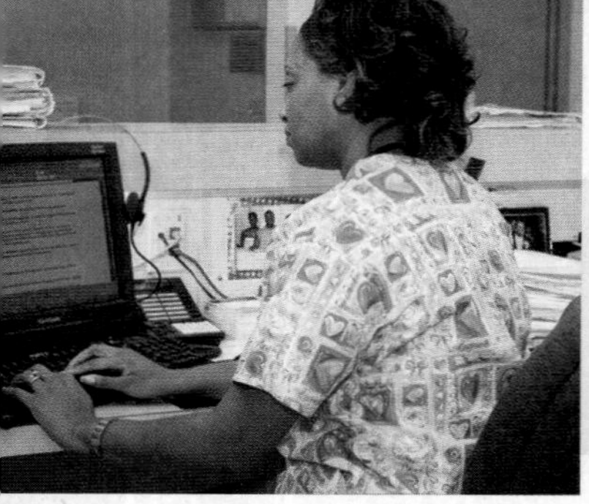
Rick Brady/McGraw-Hill Education

Lesson 9.3

Digestion—Stomach and Small Intestine

Objectives

The bolus of food that you swallowed has now passed down your esophagus and into your stomach. The process of digestion begins in earnest. The stomach continues the mechanical breakdown of the food particles and initiates the chemical digestion of protein and fats. The small intestine is where the greatest amount of food digestion and absorption occurs. The information in this lesson will enable you to use correct medical terminology to:

9.3.1 Define the functions of the stomach and small intestine in digestion.

9.3.2 Explain how food is propelled through the stomach and small intestine.

9.3.3 Describe the process of digestion in the stomach and small intestine.

Abbreviations

HCl	hydrochloric acid
ml	milliliter

CASE REPORT 9.2

You are . . .

. . . a medical interpreter working in Fulwood Medical Center.

You are communicating with . . .

. . . Mr. Xavier Ramirez, a 45-year-old farm worker, who has come to Dr. Susan Lee's primary care clinic. Mr. Ramirez complains of experiencing persistent, burning epigastric pain for several months. He has been a chain-smoker since the age of 14. His pain is eased by antacids but quickly returns. He has been taking aspirin because of joint pain in his fingers while he works. Dr. Lee has decided to refer him to a gastroenterologist for a gastroscopy. Your role is to explain the procedure to Mr. Ramirez and ensure that he keeps his appointments.

Digestion: The Stomach (LO 9.6)

Your stomach's peristaltic contractions mix different boluses of food together and push these contents toward the **pylorus** (the stomach opening that leads to the bowel) *(Figure 9.13)* to produce a mixture of semi-digested food called **chyme.**

The cells of your stomach's lining secrete *(Figure 9.14)*:

1. **Mucus,** which lubricates food and protects the stomach lining;
2. **Hydrochloric acid (HCl),** which breaks up the connective tissue of meat and the cell walls of vegetables (think of the chicken-and-vegetables meal you ate earlier);
3. **Pepsin** (an active enzyme), which digests chicken and vegetable proteins;
4. **Intrinsic factor,** which is essential for vitamin B_{12} absorption in the small intestine; and
5. **Gastrin** (a chemical), which stimulates HCl and **pepsinogen** production, and encourages the stomach's peristaltic contractions.

A typical meal like chicken and vegetables takes 3 to 4 hours to exit the stomach as **chyme.** Peristaltic waves squirt 2 to 3 milliliters **(ml)** of this chyme at a time through the **pyloric sphincter** into the **duodenum** (the first part of the small intestine) *(Figure 9.13).*

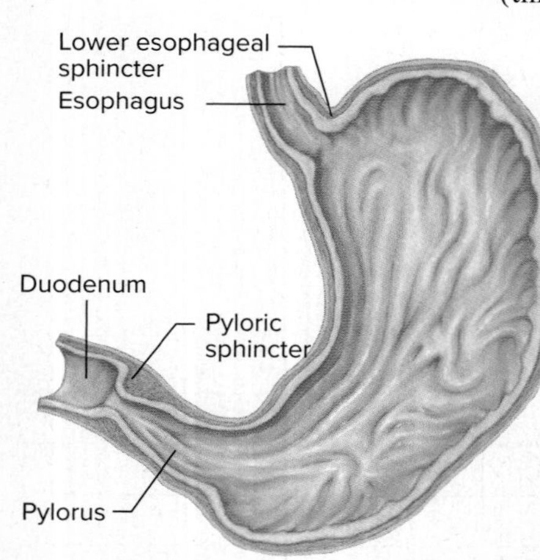

▲ **FIGURE 9.13**
Stomach.

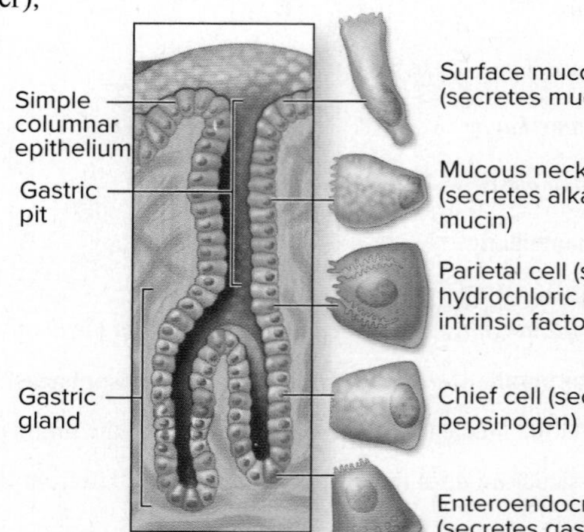

▲ **FIGURE 9.14**
Gastric Cells and Their Secretions.

Word Analysis and Definition

S = Suffix P = Prefix R = Root R/CF = Combining Form

WORD	PRONUNCIATION	ELEMENTS		DEFINITION
chyme	**KYME**		Greek *juice*	Semifluid, partially digested food passed from the stomach into the duodenum
duodenum **duodenal (adj)**	du-oh-**DEE**-num du-oh-**DEE**-nal	S/ R/ S/	-um *structure* duoden- *twelve* -al *pertaining to*	The first part of the small intestine; approximately twelve finger-breadths (9 to 10 inches) in length Pertaining to the duodenum
gastrin	**GAS**-trin	S/ R/	-in *substance, chemical compound* gastr- *stomach*	Hormone secreted in the stomach that stimulates secretion of HCl and increases gastric motility
hydrochloric acid (HCl)	high-droh-**KLOR**-ik **ASS**-id	S/ R/CF R/	-ic *pertaining to* hydr/o- *water* -chlor- *green*	The acid of gastric juice
intrinsic factor	in-**TRIN**-sik **FAK**-tor	S/ R/ R/	-ic *pertaining to* intrins- *on the inside* factor *maker*	Makes the absorption of vitamin B_{12} happen
mucus (noun) **mucous (adj)** **mucin**	**MYU**-kus **MYU**-kus **MYU**-sin		Latin *slime*	Sticky secretion of cells in mucous membranes Relating to mucus or the mucosa Protein element of mucus
pepsin **pepsinogen**	**PEP**-sin pep-**SIN**-oh-jen	 S/ R/CF	Greek *to digest* -gen *produce* pepsin/o- *pepsin*	Enzyme produced by the stomach that breaks down protein Converted by HCl in the stomach to pepsin
pylorus **pyloric (adj)**	pie-**LOR**-us pie-**LOR**-ik	S/ R/ S/	-us *pertaining to* pylor- *gate, pylorus* -ic *pertaining to*	Exit area of the stomach Pertaining to the pylorus

EXERCISES

A. Use Case Report 9.2 *to answer the following questions. Select the correct answer that completes each statement.* **LO 9.6, 9.10, and 9.11**

1. Mr. Ramirez complains of pain:

a. in his abdomen **c.** above his stomach

b. in his mouth **d.** of his tongue

2. The doctor that he has been referred to is a specialist in the treatment of:

a. stomach and intestines **c.** blood and cancer

b. heart and blood vessels **d.** ear, nose, and throat

3. Mr. Ramirez takes antacids to treat his:

a. cough **c.** joint pain

b. stomach pain **d.** nausea

B. Define the actions of the secretions of the stomach. *Match the secretion in the first column with its function listed in the second column. Fill in the blanks.* **LO 9.6**

_____ **1.** intrinsic factor **a.** protects the lining of the stomach

_____ **2.** pepsin **b.** breaks up cell walls of plants

_____ **3.** mucus **c.** allows for absorption of vitamin B_{12}

_____ **4.** hydrochloric acid **d.** enzyme that breaks down protein

Keynote

- **Difficulty in swallowing is called dysphagia.**

Abbreviations

GERD	Gastroesophageal reflux disease
NSAID	Nonsteroidal anti-inflammatory drug

Disorders of the Stomach (LO 9.6)

Case Report 9.2 *(continued)*

A **gastroscopy** on Mr. Ramirez reveals a gastric ulcer.

Gastroesophageal reflux disease (GERD) refers to the regurgitation of stomach contents back into the esophagus. The acidity of regurgitated food can irritate and ulcerate the esophageal lining and cause bleeding. Scar tissue can cause an esophageal **stricture** and **dysphagia.**

Vomiting can result from overexpansion or irritation of any part of the digestive tract. The muscles of the diaphragm and abdominal wall forcefully contract and expel the stomach contents upward into the esophagus and mouth.

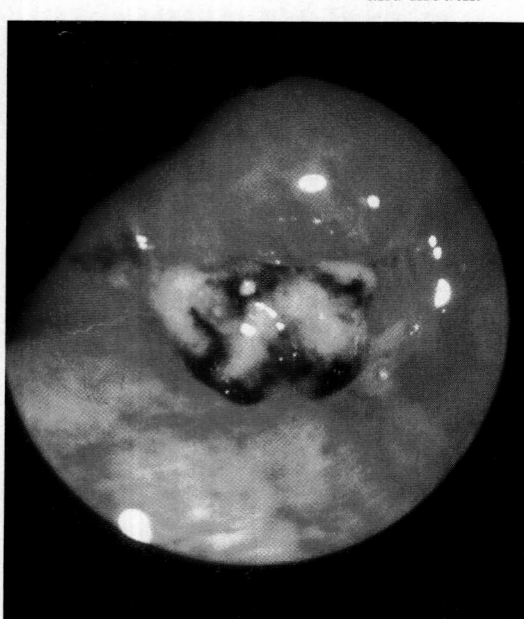

▲ FIGURE 9.15
Bleeding Peptic Ulcer.

Gastritis is an inflammation of the stomach lining, producing symptoms of epigastric pain, feeling of fullness, nausea, and occasional bleeding. It can be acute or chronic, and is caused by common medications like aspirin and **NSAIDs,** by radiotherapy and chemotherapy, and by alcohol and smoking. Treatment involves removing the factors causing the gastritis, acid neutralization, and suppression of gastric acid.

Peptic ulcers occur in the stomach and duodenum when the mucosal lining breaks down *(Figure 9.15).* Most peptic ulcers are caused by the bacterium *Helicobacter pylori (H. pylori),* which produces enzymes that weaken the protective mucus. These ulcers respond to antibiotics. **Dyspepsia** (epigastric pain with bloating and nausea) is the most common symptom.

Gastric ulcers are peptic ulcers that occur in the stomach. If a blood vessel erodes, bleeding may also be present. If untreated, the ulcer can eat into the entire wall, causing a **perforation.**

Gastric cancer can be asymptomatic for a long period and then cause **indigestion, anorexia,** abdominal pain, and weight loss. It affects men twice as often as women. It metastasizes to the lymph nodes, liver, peritoneum, chest, and brain. It is usually treated with surgery and chemotherapy.

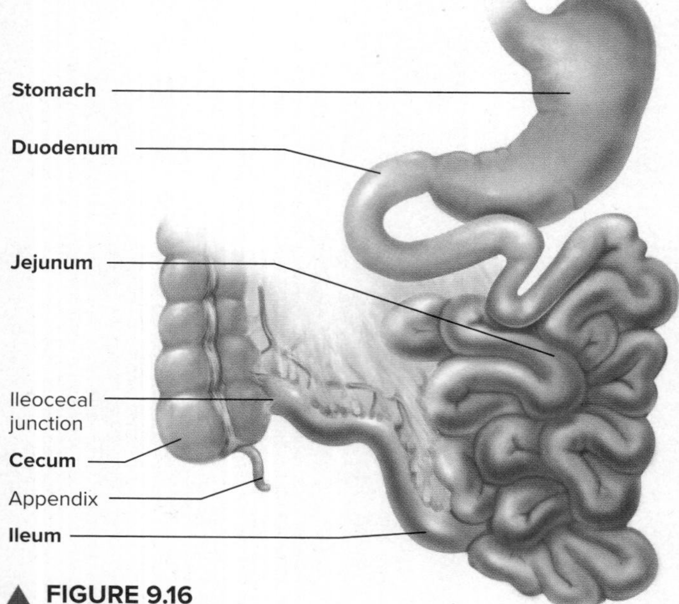

▲ FIGURE 9.16
Small Intestine.

Small Intestine (LO 9.6)

The small intestine, called *small* because of its diameter, completes the chemical digestion process. It is responsible for the **absorption** of most of the nutrients. The small intestine extends from the pylorus of the stomach to the beginning of the large intestine, and it has three segments *(Figure 9.16),* as listed below:

1. The **duodenum** is the first 9 to 10 inches of the small intestine. It receives chyme from the stomach, together with pancreatic juices and bile;
2. The **jejunum** makes up about 40% of the small intestine's length. It is the primary region for chemical digestion and nutrient absorption; and
3. The **ileum** makes up about 55% of the small intestine's length. It ends at the **ileocecal** valve, a **sphincter** that controls entry into the large intestine.

Digestion in the Small Intestine (LO 9.6)

After leaving the stomach as chyme, food spends 3 to 5 hours in the small intestine.

Anywhere from 4 to 6 hours after consuming the chicken and vegetables mentioned earlier, the food has passed through the small intestine and is ready to be passed into the large intestine. While in the small intestine, the protein, carbohydrates, and fats have been broken down by enzymes and absorbed into the bloodstream.

Word Analysis and Definition

S = Suffix P = Prefix R = Root R/CF = Combining Form

WORD	PRONUNCIATION	ELEMENTS		DEFINITION
absorption	ab-**SORP**-shun	S/ R/	**-ion** *action, condition* **absorpt-** *to swallow*	Uptake of nutrients and water by cells in the GI tract
anorexia	an-oh-**RECK**-see-ah	S/ P/ R/	**-ia** *condition* **an-** *without* **-orex-** *appetite*	Without an appetite; or an aversion to food
cecum (noun) **cecal (adj)**	**SEE**-kum **SEE**-kal	 S/ R/	Latin *blind* **-al** *pertaining to* **cec-** *cecum*	Blind pouch that is the first part of the large intestine Pertaining to the cecum
dyspepsia	dis-**PEP**-see-ah	S/ P/ R/	**-ia** *condition* **dys-** *difficult, bad* **-peps-** *digestion*	"Upset stomach," epigastric pain, nausea, and gas
gastritis	gas-**TRY**-tis	S/ R/	**-itis** *inflammation* **gastr-** *stomach*	Inflammation of the lining of the stomach
gastroesophageal	**GAS**-troh-ee-sof-ah-**JEE**-al	S/ R/CF R/CF	**-al** *pertaining to* **gastr/o-** *stomach* **-esophag/e-** *esophagus*	Pertaining to the stomach and esophagus
gastroscope **gastroscopy**	**GAS**-troh-skope gas-**TROS**-koh-pee	S/ R/CF S/	**-scope** *instrument for viewing* **gastr/o-** *stomach* **-scopy** *to examine, to view*	Endoscope for examining the inside of the stomach Endoscopic examination of the stomach
ileum **ileocecal**	**ILL**-ee-um **ILL**-ee-oh-**SEE**-cal	S/ R/ S/ R/CF R/	**-um** *structure* **ile-** *ileum* **-al** *pertaining to* **ile/o-** *ileum* **cec-** *cecum*	Third portion of small intestine Pertaining to the junction of the ileum and cecum
indigestion	in-dih-**JESS**-chun	S/ P/ R/	**-ion** *action, condition* **in-** *in, not* **-digest-** *to break down*	Symptoms resulting from difficulty in digesting food
jejunum (noun) **jejunal (adj)**	je-**JEW**-num je-**JEW**-nal	 S/ R/	Latin *empty* **-al** *pertaining to* **jejun-** *jejunum*	Segment of small intestine between the duodenum and the ileum Pertaining to the jejunum
peptic	**PEP**-tik	S/ R/	**-ic** *pertaining to* **pept-** *digest*	Relating to the stomach and duodenum
perforation	per-foh-**RAY**-shun	S/ R/	**-ion** *action, condition* **perforat-** *bore through*	A hole through the wall of a structure
stricture	**STRICK**-shur		Latin *draw tight*	Narrowing of a tube

Exercises

A. The definitions *of the elements will help you understand the meaning of the term. Select the correct answer that completes each statement.* **LO 9.1 and 9.6**

1. The meaning of the prefix in the medical term **dyspepsia** is:
   - **a.** digestion **c.** difficult
   - **b.** condition **d.** stomach
2. The meaning of the root in the medical term **peptic** is:
   - **a.** pump **c.** ulcer
   - **b.** digest **d.** digest
3. The meaning of the suffix in the medical term **perforation** is:
   - **a.** structure **c.** pertaining to
   - **b.** condition **d.** inflammation
4. The meaning of the root in the medical term **anorexia** is:
   - **a.** digestion **c.** without
   - **b.** stomach **d.** appetite

B. Fill in the blanks *with the medical term being described.* **LO 9.2, 9.3, and 9.6**

1. This condition can be caused by *Helicobacter pylori:* ______________________ ulcer
2. Inflammation of the lining of the stomach: ______________________
3. Regurgitation of the stomach contents back into the esophagus (provide the abbreviation): ______________________

Disorders of the Small Intestine (LO 9.6)

The absorption of nutrients occurs primarily through the small intestine. **Impairment of absorption,** including Crohn disease and lactose intolerance, is covered in *Lesson 9.5* of this chapter.

- **Infections** of the small intestine are common and are caused by a variety of agents.
- **Gastroenteritis,** or inflammation of the stomach and small intestine, can result in acute vomiting and diarrhea. It can be caused by a variety of viruses and bacteria (including, occasionally, the parasite ***Giardia lamblia***) and is initiated by contact with contaminated food (food poisoning) and water.
- **Bleeding** from the small intestine is usually caused by a duodenal ulcer.
- **Celiac disease** is an allergy to gluten, which is a protein contained in wheat, rye, barley, and other grains. Celiac disease *(Figure 9.17)* damages the lining of the small intestine and can cause abdominal swelling, gas, pain, weight loss, fatigue, and weakness. Treatment is a strict gluten-free diet.
- The symptoms of **irritable bowel syndrome (IBS)** are chronic abdominal pain, bloating, and either diarrhea or constipation or an alternating pattern of the two. X-rays, scans, and endoscopies of patients with IBS show no abnormality. Treatment is difficult and often unsuccessful.
- An **intussusception** *(Figure 9.18)* occurs when a part of the small intestine slides into a neighboring portion of the small intestine–much like the way that parts of a collapsible telescope slide into each other. Eighty percent of intussusceptions can be cured with an enema; the remaining 20% require surgical intervention.
- **Ileus** is a disruption of the normal peristaltic ability of the small intestine. It can be caused by a bowel obstruction or by intestinal paralysis. Risk factors for **paralytic ileus** include GI surgery, diabetic ketoacidosis *(see Chapter 12),* peritonitis, and medications, such as opiates.
- **Cancer** of the small intestine occurs infrequently compared with tumors in other parts of the GI tract. An **adenocarcinoma** is the most common malignant tumor of the small bowel.

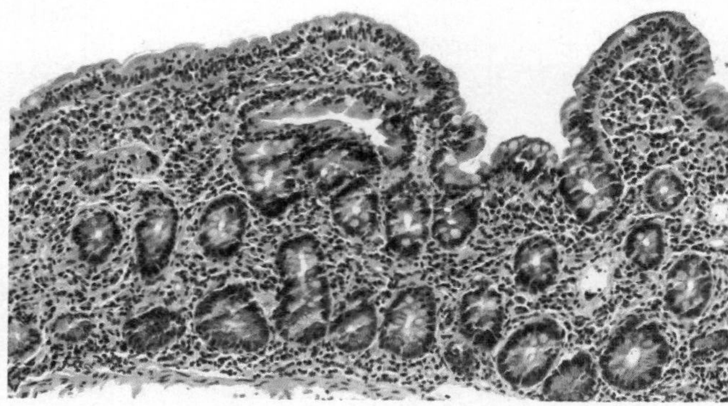

▲ **FIGURE 9.17**
Celiac Disease of the Small Bowel showing atrophy of the villi on the surface of the intestinal lining.
David Litman/Shutterstock

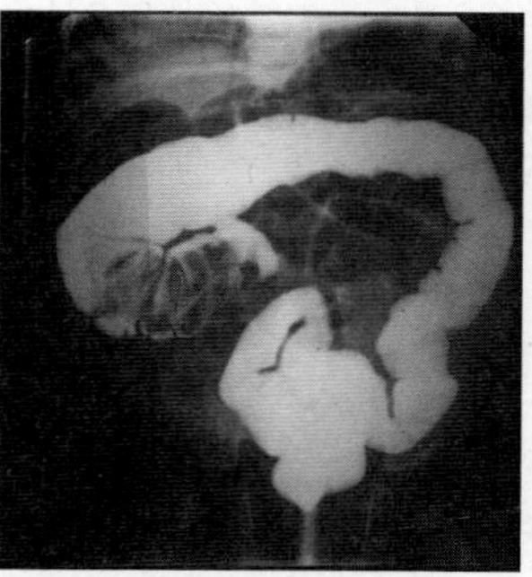

▲ **FIGURE 9.18**
Abdominal X-ray showing intussusception of the intestines.
CNRI/Science Source

Word Analysis and Definition

S = Suffix P = Prefix R = Root R/CF = Combining Form

WORD	PRONUNCIATION	ELEMENTS		DEFINITION
celiac	**SEE**-lee-ack	S/ R/	-ac *pertaining to* celi- *abdomen*	Relating to the abdominal cavity
celiac disease	**SEE**-lee-ack diz-**EEZ**	P/ R/	dis- *apart* -ease *normal function*	Disease caused by a sensitivity to gluten
gastroenteritis	**GAS**-troh-en-ter-**I**-tis	S/ R/CF R/	-itis *inflammation* gastr/o- *stomach* -enter- *intestine*	Inflammation of the stomach and intestines
Giardia	jee-**AR**-dee-ah		Alfred Giard, 1846–1908 French biologist	Parasite that can affect the small intestine
gluten	**GLU**-ten		Latin *glue*	Insoluble protein found in wheat, barley, and rye
ileus	**ILL**-ee-us		Greek *intestinal colic*	Dynamic or mechanical obstruction of the small intestine
intussusception	**IN**-tuss-sus-**SEP**-shun	S/ P/ R/	-ion *action* intus- *within* -suscept- *to take up*	The slippage of one part of the bowel inside another, causing obstruction

Exercises

A. Match *the disorder of the small intestine in column 1 with the correct statement describing it in column 2.* **LO 9.3 and 9.6**

_____ **1.** ileus **a.** Parasite that causes gastroenteritis

_____ **2.** IBS **b.** Part of the small intestine slides into a neighboring part

_____ **3.** celiac disease **c.** Disruption of the normal peristalsis of the small intestine

_____ **4.** *Giardia lamblia* **d.** Treatment is difficult and often unsuccessful

_____ **5.** intussusception **e.** Allergy to gluten

B. Use your knowledge *of the small intestine and answer the questions. Select T if the statement is true. Select F if the statement is false.* **LO 9.3 and 9.6**

1. The absorption of nutrients occurs primarily through the small intestine. T F

2. Gastroenteritis can result in acute vomiting and diarrhea. T F

3. Bleeding from the small intestine is usually from an infection. T F

4. Chronic abdominal pain, bloating, and either diarrhea or constipation can be signs of IBS. T F

5. Risk factors for paralytic ileus include GI surgery, diabetic ketoacidosis, and medicines such as opiates. T F

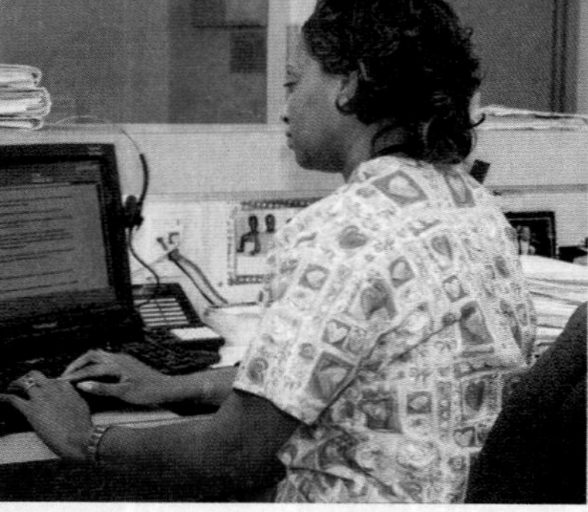

Rick Brady/McGraw-Hill Education

Lesson 9.4

Digestion—Liver, Gallbladder, and Pancreas

Objectives

Your liver and pancreas secrete enzymes that are responsible for the majority of digestion occurring in the small intestine. You will need to be able to use correct medical terminology to:

9.4.1 Describe the digestive functions and common disorders of the liver, gallbladder, bile ducts, and pancreas.

Keynotes

- **Only the production of bile relates the liver to digestion.**
- **Vaccines are available to prevent hepatitis A and B.**

Abbreviations

HAV	hepatitis A virus
HBV	hepatitis B virus
HCV	hepatitis C virus

CASE REPORT 9.3

You are . . .

. . . a coder in the Health Information Management department at Fulwood Medical Center.

You are communicating with . . .

. . . Dr. Susan Lee, and you are questioning the documentation of Mrs. Sandra Jacobs's care. Mrs. Jacobs, a 46-year-old mother of four, presented in Dr. Lee's primary care clinic with episodes of cramping pain in her upper abdomen associated with nausea and vomiting. A physical examination reveals an obese white woman with tenderness over her gallbladder. Her BP is 170/90 and she has slight **pedal** edema. A **provisional diagnosis** of gallstones has been made. She has been referred for an ultrasound examination and an appointment has been made to see Dr. Walsh in the surgery department.

The Liver (LO 9.7)

Your **liver** is your largest internal organ. It is a complex structure located under your right ribs just below your diaphragm *(Figure 9.19).*

As a complex organ, your liver's multiple functions include:

- Manufacturing and excreting **bile;**
- Removing **bilirubin** (a rust-colored pigment) from the bloodstream;
- Storing excess sugar as **glycogen;** and
- Manufacturing blood proteins, including those needed for clotting *(see Chapter 7).*

▲ **FIGURE 9.19**
Location of Liver.

Disorders of the Liver (LO 9.7)

Hepatitis is an inflammation of the liver causing **jaundice,** where the skin and sometimes the eyes have a yellowish hue. Viral hepatitis is the most common cause of hepatitis and is related to three major types of virus:

1. **Hepatitis A virus (HAV)** is highly contagious and causes a mild to severe infection. It is transmitted by contaminated food.
2. **Hepatitis B virus (HBV),** or serum hepatitis, is transmitted through contact with blood, semen, vaginal secretions, or saliva, as well as by a needle prick and the sharing of contaminated needles. Vaccines are available to prevent hepatitis A and B.
3. **Hepatitis C virus (HCV)** is the most common blood-borne infection in the United States, occurring mostly through injections given with contaminated syringes and needles. The disease can vary in severity from a mild illness lasting a few weeks to a serious, lifelong condition that can lead to cirrhosis of the liver or liver cancer. More than 3 million Americans are chronically infected with hepatitis C virus. Combination antiviral drugs are used, and new therapeutic agents are being licensed. There is no vaccine yet available.

In addition, **hepatitis D** can occur in association with hepatitis B, making the infection worse. **Hepatitis E** is similar to hepatitis A and occurs mostly in under-developed countries.

Chronic hepatitis occurs when the acute hepatitis is not healed after 6 months. It progresses slowly, can last for years, and is difficult to treat.

Cirrhosis of the liver is a chronic irreversible disease, replacing normal liver cells with hard, fibrous scar tissue. Its most common cause is alcoholism. There is no known cure.

Cancer of the liver as a primary cancer usually arises in patients with chronic liver disease, often from HBV infection.

Word Analysis and Definition

S = Suffix P = Prefix R = Root R/CF = Combining Form

WORD	PRONUNCIATION		ELEMENTS	DEFINITION
bile bile acids biliary (adj)	BILE **BILE AH**-sids **BILL**-ee-air-ee	 S/ R/CF	Latin *bile* -ary *pertaining to* bil/i- *bile*	Fluid secreted by the liver into the duodenum Steroids synthesized from cholesterol Pertaining to bile or the biliary tract
bilirubin	bill-ee-**RU**-bin	S/ R/CF	-rubin *rust colored* bil/i- *bile*	Bile pigment formed in the liver from hemoglobin
cirrhosis	sir-**ROE**-sis	S/ R/	-osis *condition* cirrh- *yellow*	Extensive fibrotic liver disease
glycogen	**GLYE**-koh-gen	S/ R/CF	-gen *produce, create* glyc/o- *sugar, glycogen*	The body's principal carbohydrate reserve, stored in the liver and skeletal muscle
hepatic hepatitis	hep-**AT**-ik hep-ah-**TIE**-tis	S/ R/ S/	-ic *pertaining to* hepat- *liver* -itis *inflammation*	Pertaining to the liver Inflammation of the liver
jaundice	**JAWN**-dis		French *yellow*	Yellow staining of tissues with bile pigments, including bilirubin
liver	**LIV**-er		Old English *liver*	Body's largest organ, located in the right upper quadrant of the abdomen
pedal	**PEED**-al	S/ R/	-al *pertaining to* ped- *foot*	Pertaining to the foot
provisional diagnosis (*also called* **preliminary diagnosis**)	pro-**VIZH**-un-al die-ag-**NO**-sis	S/ R/ P/ R/	-al *pertaining to* provision- *provide* dia- *complete* -gnosis *knowledge of an abnormal condition*	A temporary diagnosis pending further examination or testing The determination of the cause of a disease

EXERCISES

A. Refer *to Case Report 9.3. Then select the choice that correctly completes each statement or answers each question.* **LO 9.7, 9.10, and 9.11**

1. A provisional diagnosis means that the diagnosis is:
   - **a.** confirmed
   - **b.** unsupported
   - **c.** temporary
2. Aside from pain in her abdomen, Ms. Jacobs also has:
   - **a.** swelling in her feet
   - **b.** pain in her calf
   - **c.** yellow-colored skin
   - **d.** low blood pressure
3. The pain in Mrs. Jacobs' abdomen is thought to be due to:
   - **a.** viral infection of digestive tract
   - **b.** gallstones
   - **c.** cancer in the liver
   - **d.** inflammation of the pancreas
4. What additional diagnostic procedure is she scheduled for?
   - **a.** sigmoidoscopy
   - **b.** cholecystectomy
   - **c.** barium enema
   - **d.** ultrasound

B. Elements: *Select the answer that correctly completes each statement.* **LO 9.1**

1. In the term *hepatic,* the root means:
   - **a.** pancreas
   - **b.** stomach
   - **c.** liver
2. The suffix in *cirrhosis* indicates this is:
   - **a.** a condition
   - **b.** surgical excision
   - **c.** a structure
3. *Bilirubin* is the color of:
   - **a.** coal
   - **b.** milk
   - **c.** rust
4. The root in *cirrhosis* indicates a:
   - **a.** color
   - **b.** size
   - **c.** location

Lesson 9.4 (cont'd)

Gallbladder, Biliary Tract, and Pancreas (LO 9.7)

Gallbladder and Biliary Tract (LO 9.7)

On the underside of your liver is your **gallbladder (GB),** which stores and concentrates the bile produced by the liver. The **cystic duct** from the gallbladder joins with the **hepatic duct** to form the **common bile duct.** This duct system, which moves the bile from the liver to the duodenum, is called the **biliary tract** *(Figure 9.20a and b).*

Keynotes

- **Between meals, the gallbladder absorbs water and electrolytes from the bile and concentrates it 10 to 20 times.**
- **Jaundice is caused by deposits of bilirubin in the tissues.**
- **The pancreas is the only organ that is both an endocrine and an exocrine gland.**

Abbreviations

CF	cystic fibrosis
GB	gallbladder

Disorders of the Gallbladder (LO 9.7)

Gallstones (cholelithiasis) can form in the gallbladder from excess cholesterol, bile salts, and bile pigment *(Figure 9.21).* The stones can vary in size and number. Risk factors are obesity, high-cholesterol diets, multiple pregnancies, and rapid weight loss.

Case Report 9.3 *(continued)*

Mrs. Jacobs presented with the classic gallstone symptoms of severe waves of right upper quadrant pain (biliary colic), nausea, and vomiting.

Choledocholithiasis occurs when small stones become impacted in the common bile duct. This can cause biliary colic and jaundice *(see below).*

Cholecystitis is an acute or chronic inflammation of the gallbladder, usually associated with cholelithiasis and obstruction of the cystic duct with a stone.

Jaundice (icterus) is a symptom of many different diseases in the biliary tract and liver. It is a yellow discoloration of the skin and sclera of the eyes caused by deposits of bilirubin just below the skin's outer layers.

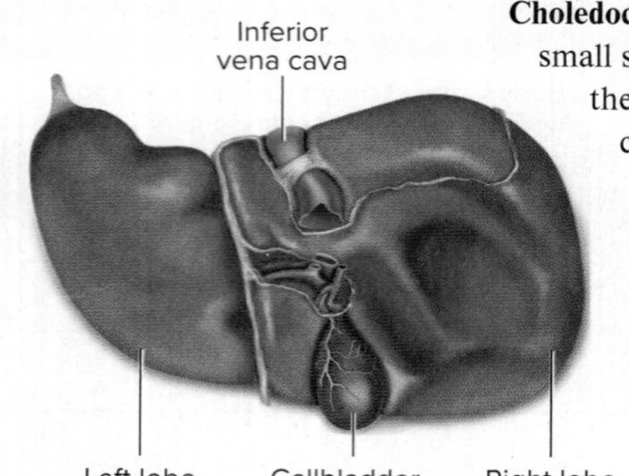
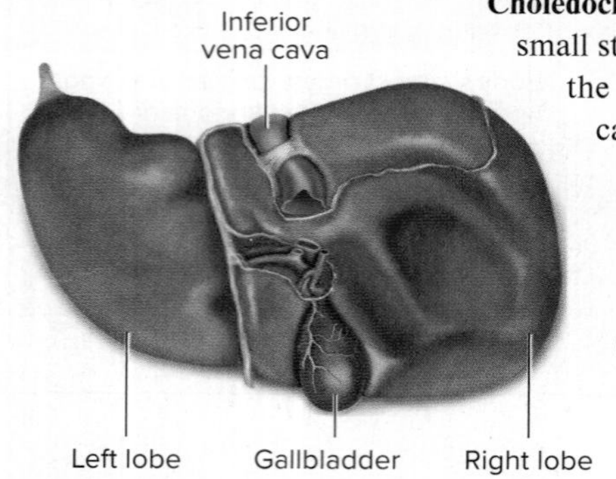

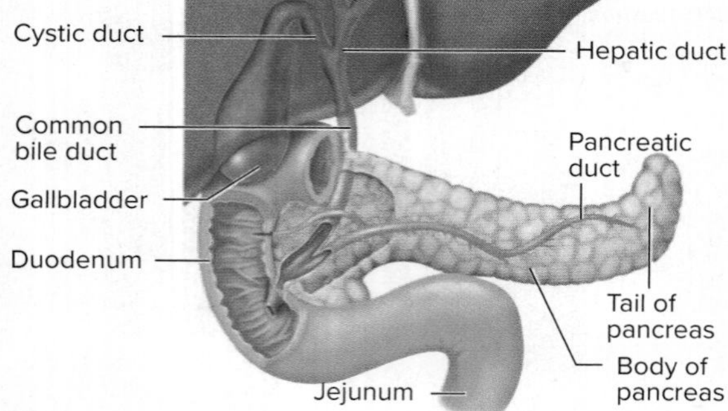

▲ **FIGURE 9.20**
(a) Underside of liver.
(b) Anatomy of gallbladder, pancreas, and biliary tract.

The Pancreas (LO 9.7)

Your **pancreas** is a spongy, exocrine gland. **Exocrine** glands secrete fluids. In fact, many of the glands in your body are exocrine glands, including your sweat glands, mammary glands, and other digestive enzyme-releasing glands. The majority of the pancreas secretes digestive juices, but smaller areas of **pancreatic islet cells** secrete the hormones **insulin** and **glucagon** *(see Chapter 12).*

The pancreas produces pancreatic digestive juices that are excreted through the pancreatic duct. This duct joins the common bile duct shortly before it opens into the duodenum *(Figure 9.20b),* which encircles the top or head of the pancreas *(Figure 9.20b).* Pancreatic and bile juices then enter the duodenum.

Other pancreatic cells secrete insulin and glucagon, which go directly into the bloodstream. This part of the pancreas is an **endocrine** (hormone-secreting) gland.

Pancreatic juices contain alkaline electrolytes, which help neutralize the acid chyme as it comes from the stomach, and enzymes, which break down starches, fats, and proteins into simpler elements.

Disorders of the Pancreas (LO 9.7)

Pancreatitis is an inflammation of the pancreas. The acute disease ranges from a mild, self-limiting episode to an acute life-threatening emergency. In the chronic form, there is a progressive destruction of pancreatic tissue leading to malabsorption and diabetes.

Pancreatic cancer is the fourth leading cause of cancer-related death. Early diagnosis is difficult because the presenting symptoms are very vague. Treatment is surgical resection of the cancer. The prognosis is poor.

Cystic fibrosis (CF) is an inherited disease that becomes apparent in infancy or childhood. With CF, the pancreas, liver, intestines, sweat glands, and lungs all produce abnormally thick mucous secretions. The malabsorption of fat and protein leads to large, bulky, foul-smelling stools. Problems with thick mucous secretions in the lungs lead to chronic lung disease.

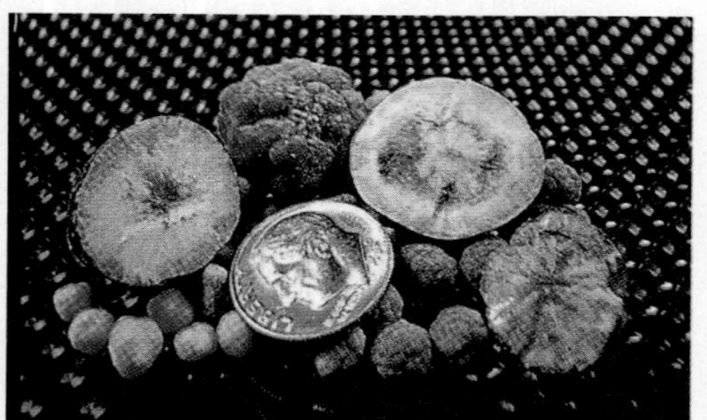

◀ **FIGURE 9.21**
Gallstones.
The dime is included to illustrate the relative size of the gallstones.

Southern Illinois University/Science Source

Word Analysis and Definition

S = Suffix P = Prefix R = Root R/CF = Combining Form

WORD	PRONUNCIATION	ELEMENTS		DEFINITION
cholecystitis	**KOH**-leh-sis-**TIE**-tis	S/ R/CF R/	-itis *inflammation* chol/e- *bile* -cyst- *bladder*	Inflammation of the gallbladder
cholecystectomy	**KOH**-leh-sis-**TECK**-toe-me	S/	-ectomy *surgical excision*	Surgical removal of the gallbladder
choledocholithiasis	koh-leh-**DOH**-koh-lih-**THIGH**-ah-sis	S/ R/CF R/	-iasis *condition* choledoch/o- *common bile duct* -lith- *stone*	Presence of a gallstone in the common bile duct
cholelithiasis	**KOH**-leh-lih-**THIGH**-ah-sis	S/ R/CF R/CF	-iasis *condition* chol/e- *bile* -lith/o- *stone*	Condition of having bile stones (gallstones)
cholelithotomy	**KOH**-leh-lih-**THOT**-oh-me	S/	-tomy *surgical incision*	Surgical removal of a gallstone(s)
endocrine	**EN**-doh-krin	P/ R/	endo- *within, inside* -crine *secrete*	A gland that produces an internal or hormonal substance and secretes it into the bloodstream
exocrine	**EK**-soh-krin	P/	exo- *outward, outside*	A gland that secretes substances outwardly through excretory ducts
gallstone	**GAWL**-stone	R/ R/	gall- *bitter* -stone *pebble*	Hard mass of cholesterol, calcium, and bilirubin that can be formed in the gallbladder and bile duct
gallbladder	**GAWL**-blad-er		bladder, Old English *receptacle*	Receptacle on the inferior surface of the liver for storing bile
glucagon	**GLU**-kah-gon	R/ R/	gluc- *glucose, sugar* -agon *to fight*	Hormone that mobilizes glucose from body storage
insulin	**IN**-syu-lin	S/ R/	-in *chemical compound* insul- *island*	Pancreatic hormone that suppresses blood glucose levels and transports glucose into cells
pancreas	**PAN**-kree-as		Greek *sweetbread*	Lobulated gland, the head of which is tucked into the curve of the duodenum
pancreatic (adj)	pan-kree-**AT**-ik	S/ R/	-ic *pertaining to* pancreat- *pancreas*	Pertaining to the pancreas
pancreatitis	**PAN**-kree-ah-**TIE**-tis	S/	-itis *inflammation*	Inflammation of the pancreas

EXERCISES

A. Define *the elements chol/e and choledoch/o. Fill in the blanks.* **LO 9.2 and 9.7**

1. The element chol/e means ______________________________.

2. The element choledoch/o means ______________________________.

B. Construct *terms related to the gallbladder. Use this group of elements, in addition to* chol/e *and* choledoch/o *to form the medical terms that are defined. Some elements you will use more than once; some elements you will not use at all. Fill in the blanks.* **LO 9.1 and 9.7**

lith iasis chole ectomy osis cyst tomy cyst/o itis choledoch/o

1. condition of gallstones: ______________ / ______________ / ______________

2. surgical removal of gallbladder: ______________ / ______________ / ______________

3. gallstone in the common bile duct: ______________ / ______________ / ______________

4. surgical incision into gallbladder to remove gallstones: ______________ / ______________ / ______________

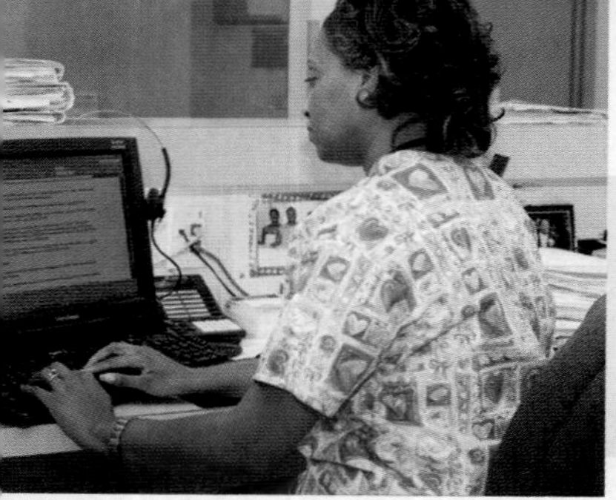

Rick Brady/McGraw-Hill Education

Lesson 9.5

Absorption and Malabsorption

Objectives

In the previous lessons in this chapter, you learned about the digestive secretions of the different segments of the digestive tract, liver, and pancreas. This information can now be brought together to review the overall process of digestion so that you will be able to use correct medical terminology to:

9.5.1 Explain the chemical digestion and absorption of proteins, carbohydrates, and fats.

9.5.2 Describe disorders of chemical digestion, absorption, and **malabsorption.**

CASE REPORT 9.4

You are . . .

. . . a dietitian working at Fulwood Medical Center.

You are communicating with . . .

. . . Mrs. Jan Stark, a 36-year-old pottery maker, and her husband, Mr. Tom Stark. From her medical record, you see that Mrs. Stark has been referred to you by Dr. Cameron Grabowski, a gastroenterologist.

For the past 10 years, Mrs. Stark has had spasmodic episodes of **diarrhea** and **flatulence** associated with severe headaches and fatigue. During those episodes, her stools were greasy and pale. She has seen several physicians who have recommended low-fat, high-carbohydrate diets, but she has had no relief. Dr. Grabowski has performed an intestinal biopsy through an oral **endoscopy** and diagnosed **celiac disease.** This condition is a sensitivity to the protein **gluten** that is found in wheat, rye, barley, and oats. Dr. Grabowski has asked you to ensure that Mrs. Stark accepts a diet free of gluten-containing foods like breads, cereals, cookies, and beer.

Chemical Digestion, Absorption, and Transport (LO 9.6 and 9.9)

Carbohydrates (LO 9.6 and 9.9)

In your small intestine, carbohydrates like **starches** are broken down into simple sugars–glucose and fructose–which are absorbed by the lining cells and transferred to the capillaries of the **villi** *(Figure 9.22).* The most commonly consumed carbohydrates are bread, soft drinks, cookies, cakes, doughnuts, syrups, jams, potatoes, and rice. From the capillaries of the villi, the simple sugars are carried by the **portal vein** to the liver, where the non-glucose sugars are converted to glucose. Glucose is the major source of energy for all cells.

Glycogen, the storage form of carbohydrate, is found in the liver and skeletal muscle. Glycogen in muscles supplies glucose during high-intensity and endurance exercise.

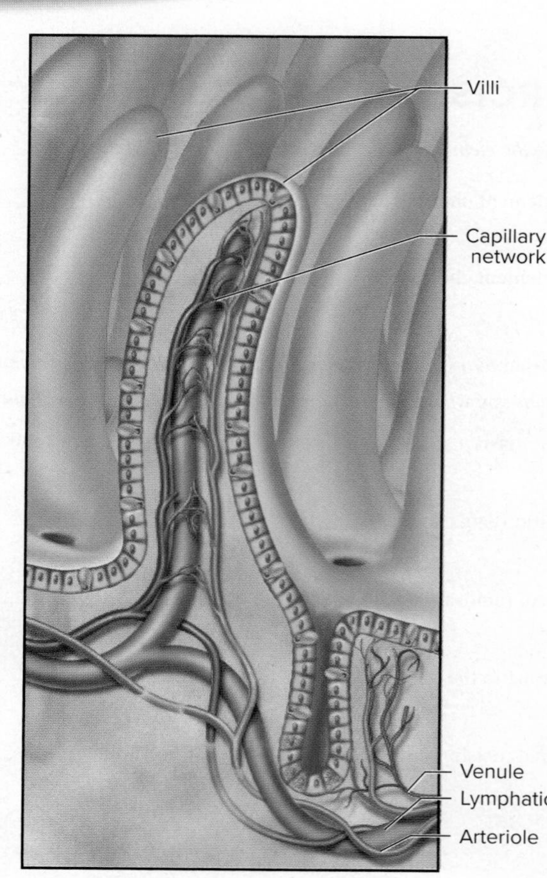

FIGURE 9.22 Intestinal Villi.

Word Analysis and Definition

S = Suffix P = Prefix R = Root R/CF = Combining Form

WORD	PRONUNCIATION	ELEMENTS		DEFINITION
celiac disease	**SEE**-lee-ack diz-**EEZ**	S/ R/ P/ R/	-ac *pertaining to* celi- *abdomen* dis- *apart* -ease *normal function*	Disease caused by sensitivity to gluten
diarrhea	die-ah-**REE**-ah	P/ R/	dia- *complete* -rrhea *flow, discharge*	Abnormally frequent and loose stools
endoscopy endoscope	en-**DOS**-koh-pee **EN**-doh-skope	P/ S/ R/	endo- *inside, within* -scopy *to examine, view* -scope *instrument for viewing*	The use of an endoscope Instrument used to examine the interior of a tubular or hollow organ
flatulence flatus	**FLAT**-you-lents **FLAY**-tus	S/ R/	-ence *forming* flatul- *excessive gas, flatus* Latin *blowing*	Excessive amount of gas in the stomach and intestines Gas or air expelled through the anus
glycogen	**GLYE**-koh-jen	S/ R/CF	-gen *to produce* glyc/o- *sugar/glucose*	The body's principal carbohydrate reserve, stored in the liver and skeletal muscle
malabsorption	mal-ab-**SORP**-shun	S/ P/ R/	-ion *action, condition* mal- *bad, difficult* -absorpt- *swallow, take in*	Inadequate gastrointestinal absorption of nutrients
portal vein	**POR**-tal **VANE**		portal, Latin *gate* vein, Latin *vein*	The vein that carries blood from the intestines to the liver
starch	**STARCH**		Anglo-Saxon *stiffen*	Complex carbohydrate made of multiple units of glucose attached together
villus villi (pl)	**VILL**-us **VILL**-eye		Latin *shaggy hair*	Thin, hairlike projection, particularly of a mucous membrane lining a cavity

EXERCISES

A. Review *Case Report 9.4. Select the correct answer to complete each statement.* **LO 9.10 and 9.11**

1. The endoscope was inserted through Mrs. Stark's:

a. mouth **c.** abdominal incision
b. rectum

2. Mrs. Stark's discomfort is due to:

a. smoking **c.** drinking alcohol
b. diet **d.** lack of exercise

3. Dr. Grabowski is a specialist in the treatment of disorders of the:

a. mouth **c.** stomach only
b. stomach and intestines **d.** liver

> **Study Hint**
>
> *Endoscope* is a generic (general) term that means any instrument *(scope)* used to examine the inside *(endo)* of a tubular or hollow organ. The instrument obtains its specific name from the organ it is used to examine. Thus, an instrument used to view a stomach is a gastroscope specifically, but it is also an endoscope in general.

B. Construct *the correct medical term to match the definitions. If a term does not have a particular element, insert N/A. Fill in the blanks.* **LO 9.1, 9.6, 9.9, and 9.10**

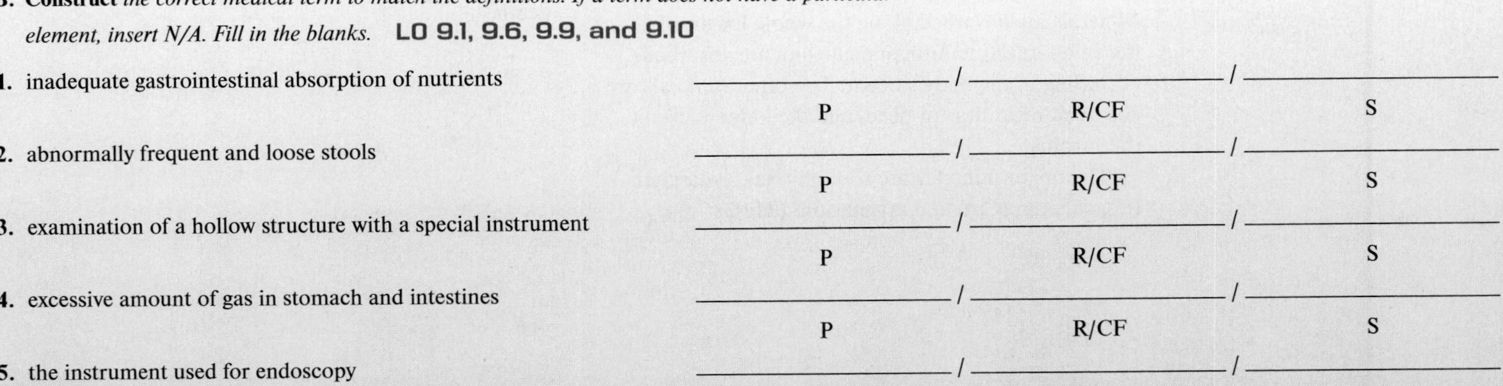

1. inadequate gastrointestinal absorption of nutrients _______ / _______ / _______
P R/CF S

2. abnormally frequent and loose stools _______ / _______ / _______
P R/CF S

3. examination of a hollow structure with a special instrument _______ / _______ / _______
P R/CF S

4. excessive amount of gas in stomach and intestines _______ / _______ / _______
P R/CF S

5. the instrument used for endoscopy _______ / _______ / _______
P R/CF S

Keynotes

- **Proteins are broken down into amino acids.**
- **Minerals are electrolytes.**
- **In malnutrition, the body breaks down its own tissues to meet its nutritional and metabolic needs.**
- **Milk sugar is lactose. The enzyme lactase breaks down lactose into glucose.**
- **Diarrhea is caused by irritation of the intestinal lining that causes feces to pass through the intestine too quickly for adequate amounts of water to be reabsorbed.**

Abbreviations

Ca	calcium
ED	emergency department
K	potassium
Mg	magnesium
Na	sodium

Chemical Digestion, Absorption, and Transport (continued)

Proteins (LO 9.8)

Proteins are only 10 to 20% digested when they arrive in the duodenum and small intestine. Enzymes produced by cells in the small intestine, and the pancreatic enzyme trypsin, break down the remaining proteins into **amino acids.**

The amino acids are carried away in the blood and are transported to cells all over the body to be used as building blocks for new tissue formation.

Lipids (LO 9.8)

Lipids (fats) enter the duodenum and small intestine as large globules. These have to be **emulsified** by the bile salts into smaller droplets so that pancreatic **lipase** (fat-reducing enzymes) can digest them into very small droplets of free **fatty acids** and **monoglycerides.**

These small droplets are taken up by the **lacteals** (lymphatic vessels) inside the villi and then move into the lymphatic system. The droplets now comprise a milky, fatty lymphatic fluid called **chyle,** which eventually reaches the thoracic duct and moves into the bloodstream *(see Chapter 7).* Chyle is stored in adipose tissue. The fat-soluble vitamins A, D, E, and K are absorbed with the lipids.

Water (LO 9.8)

Water has no caloric value and makes up approximately 60% of your body weight (about 10 gallons). Your small intestine absorbs 92% of your body's water, which is taken into the bloodstream through the capillaries in the villi. Water-soluble vitamins, C and the B complex, are absorbed with water except for B_{12}.

You can survive 6 to 8 weeks without food, but only a few days without water.

Minerals (LO 9.8)

Minerals are absorbed along the whole length of the small intestine. Iron and calcium are absorbed according to the body's needs. The other minerals are absorbed regardless of need, and the kidneys excrete the surplus.

The major minerals are sodium **(Na),** potassium **(K),** calcium **(Ca),** and magnesium **(Mg).**

Disorders of Malabsorption (LO 9.8)

The term **malabsorption syndromes** refers to a group of diseases in which intestinal absorption of nutrients is impaired.

Malnutrition can arise from malabsorption, but can also result from a lack of food, as with famine and poverty. Malnutrition can also result from a loss of appetite in people with cancer or a terminal illness.

Lactose intolerance occurs when the small intestine is not producing enough of the enzyme **lactase** to break down the milk sugar lactose. The result is diarrhea and cramps. Lactase can be taken in pill form before eating dairy products, and milk products can be avoided.

Crohn disease (or **regional enteritis**) is an inflammation of the small intestine, frequently in the ileum and occasionally also in the large intestine. The symptoms are abdominal pain, diarrhea, fatigue, and weight loss. There is no cure.

Celiac disease is an autoimmune disease that damages the villi of the small intestine and interferes with the absorption of nutrients. It is due to an **intolerance** to a protein, **gluten,** found in wheat, barley, and rye products. It affects about 1% of the population in the United States. In addition, there is a nonceliac sensitivity (allergy) to gluten products that affects about 4% of the population.

Constipation occurs when fecal movement through the large intestine is slow and thus too much water is reabsorbed by the large intestine. The feces become hardened. Constipation can be caused by lack of dietary fiber, lack of exercise, and emotional upset.

Gastroenteritis (stomach "flu") is an infection of the stomach and intestine that can be caused by a large number of bacteria and viruses. It causes vomiting, diarrhea, and fever. An outbreak of gastroenteritis can sometimes be traced to contaminated food or water.

Dysentery is a severe form of bacterial gastroenteritis with blood and mucus in frequent, watery stools.

Malnutrition, malabsorption, and severe forms of diarrhea and vomiting can cause dehydration and an electrolyte imbalance, possibly leading to coma and death.

Word Analysis and Definition

S = Suffix P = Prefix R = Root R/CF = Combining Form

WORD	PRONUNCIATION	ELEMENTS		DEFINITION
amino acid	ah-**ME**-no ASS-id	R/CF	amin/o- *nitrogen containing* acid, Latin *sour*	The basic building block for protein
chyle	KYLE		Greek *juice*	A milky fluid that results from the digestion and absorption of fats in the small intestine
Crohn disease	**KRONE** diz-**EEZ**		Burrill Crohn, New York gastroenterologist 1884–1983	Narrowing and thickening of terminal small intestine
dysentery	**DISS**-en-tare-ee	P/ R/	dys- *bad, difficult* -entery *condition of the small intestine*	Disease with diarrhea, bowel spasms, fever and dehydration
emulsify emulsion (noun)	ee-**MUL**-sih-fye ee-**MUL**-shun	S/ R/ S/	-ify *to become* emuls- *suspend in a liquid* -ion *condition, action*	Break up into very small droplets to suspend in a solution (emulsion) The system that contains small droplets suspended in a liquid
gastroenteritis	**GAS**-troh-en-ter-**EYE**-tis	S/ R/ R/CF	-itis *inflammation* -enter- *intestine* gastr/o *stomach*	Inflammation of the stomach and small intestine
lacteal	**LAK**-tee-al	S/ R/CF	-eal *pertaining to* lact- *milk*	A lymphatic vessel carrying chyle away from the intestine
lactose lactase	**LAK**-toes **LAK**-tase	S/ R/	Latin *milk sugar* -ase *enzyme* lact- *milk*	The disaccharide in cow's milk Enzyme that breaks down lactose to glucose
lipase	**LIE**-paze	S/ R/	-ase *enzyme* lip- *fat*	Enzyme that breaks down fat
lipid	**LIP**-id		Greek *fat*	General term for all types of fatty compounds; e.g., cholesterol, triglycerides, and fatty acids
mineral	**MIN**-er-al	S/ R/	-al *pertaining to* miner- *mines*	Inorganic compound usually found in the earth's crust

EXERCISES

A. Identify *the meaning of word elements. Select the correct answer that completes each statement.* **LO 9.1 and 9.8**

1. The suffix that is used to form the names of enzymes is

 a. -ic **b.** -al **c.** -ase **d.** -ous **e.** -ion

2. The medical term that has an element that means **milk**:

 a. lipid **b.** chyme **c.** protease **d.** chyle **e.** lacteal

3. The medical term that has an element that means **mines**:

 a. chyle **b.** fats **c.** lipids **d.** minerals **e.** emulsify

4. The root **enter** means:

 a. blood **b.** to begin **c.** water **d.** small intestine **e.** bile

B. Provide *the correct terms being described below. Fill in the blanks.* **LO 9.2, 9.8, and 9.11**

1. Lymphatic vessel that carries chyle away from the intestine: ____________________
2. Inorganic compounds found in the earth's crust: ____________________
3. Condition of hardened fecal matter: ____________________
4. Condition caused by severe bacterial infection resulting in frequent watery stools containing blood and mucus: ____________________
5. Crohn disease is also known as: ____________________

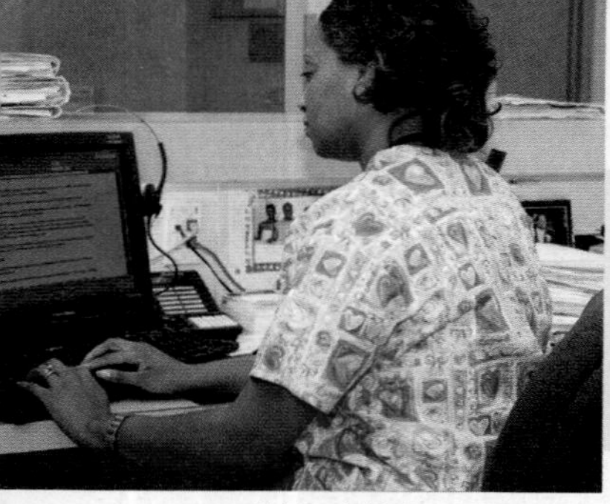

Rick Brady/McGraw-Hill Education

Lesson 9.6

The Large Intestine and Elimination

Objectives

Once your small intestine has digested and absorbed the nutrients, the residual materials must be prepared in your large intestine so they can be eliminated from your body. The information in this lesson will enable you to use correct medical terminology to:

9.6.1 Describe the structure and functions of the large intestine.

9.6.2 Outline disorders of the large intestine.

Keynotes

- **A sphincter is a ring of smooth muscle that forms a one-way valve.**
- **Colon: Ascending to transverse to descending to sigmoid to rectum to anus.**

Structure and Functions of the Large Intestine (LO 9.9)

Structure of the Large Intestine (LO 9.9)

Your **large intestine** is so named because its diameter is much greater than that of your small intestine. In your abdominal cavity, the large intestine forms a perimeter around the central mass of the small intestine.

At the junction between the small and large intestines, a ring of smooth muscle called the **ileocecal sphincter** forms a one-way valve. This allows chyme to pass into the large intestine and prevents the large intestine's contents from backing into the ileum.

The **cecum** is located at the beginning of the large intestine. It is a pouch in the abdomen's right lower quadrant. A narrow tube with a closed end (the **vermiform appendix**) projects downward from the cecum *(Figure 9.23a and b).* The function of the appendix is not known.

The ascending **colon** begins at the cecum and extends upward to underneath the liver. Here, it makes a sharp turn at the hepatic **flexure** and becomes the transverse colon. At the left side of the abdomen, near the spleen at the splenic flexure, the transverse colon turns downward to form the descending colon. At the pelvic brim, the descending colon forms an S-shaped curve called the **sigmoid** colon. This descends in the pelvis to become the rectum and then the **anal canal.**

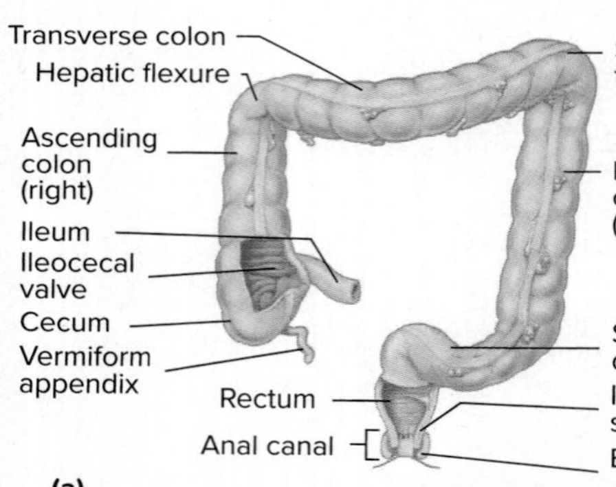

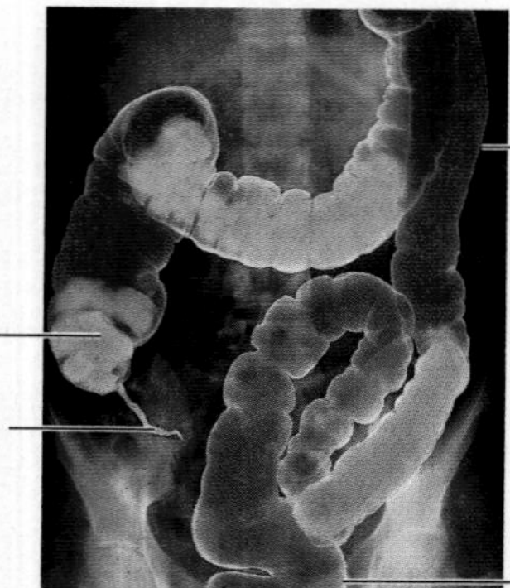

FIGURE 9.23 Large Intestine. (a) Surface anatomy. (b) X-ray of large intestine following barium enema.

CNRI/Science Photo Library/Science source

The **rectum** has three transverse folds–rectal valves that enable it to retain **feces** while passing gas (flatus).

The anal canal *(Figure 9.24)* is the last 1 to 2 inches of the large intestine, opening to the outside as the **anus.** An internal anal sphincter, composed of smooth muscle from the intestinal wall, and an external anal sphincter, composed of skeletal muscle that can be controlled voluntarily, guard the exit of the anus.

Functions of the Large Intestine (LO 9.9)

Your large intestine has the following key functions:

- **Absorption** of water and electrolytes. The large intestine receives more than 1 liter (1,000 ml) of chyme each day from the small intestine. It reabsorbs water and electrolytes to reduce the volume of chyme to 100 to 150 ml of feces, which are eliminated by **defecation;**
- **Secretion** of mucus that protects the intestinal wall and holds particles of fecal matter together;
- **Digestion** (by the bacteria that inhabit the large intestine) of any food remnants that have escaped the small intestine's digestive enzymes;
- **Peristalsis** happens a few times a day in the large intestine to produce mass movements toward the rectum; and
- **Elimination** of materials that were not digested or absorbed.

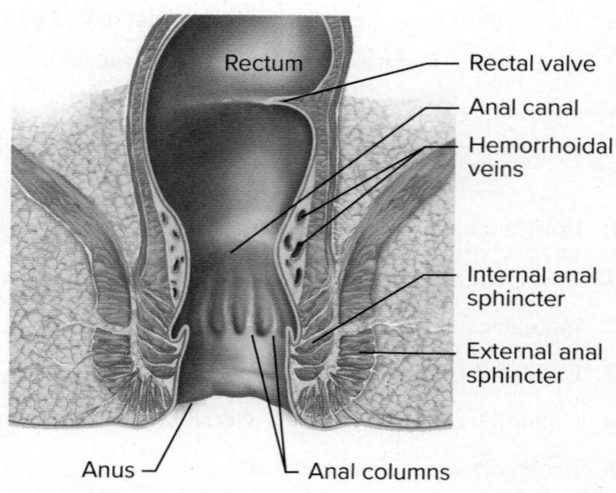

FIGURE 9.24 Anal Canal.

Word Analysis and Definition

S = Suffix P = Prefix R = Root R/CF = Combining Form

WORD	PRONUNCIATION	ELEMENTS		DEFINITION
anus	**A**-nus		Latin *ring*	Terminal opening of the digestive tract through which feces are discharged
anal (adj)	**A**-nal	S/ R/CF	-al *pertaining to* an/o- *anus*	Pertaining to the anus
anorectal junction	**A**-no-**RECK**-tal **JUNK**-shun	R/ S/ R/	-rect- *rectum* -ion *condition, action* junct- *joining together*	The junction between the anus and rectum
appendix	ah-**PEN**-dicks		Latin *appendage*	Small blind projection from the pouch of the cecum
appendicitis	ah-pen-dih-**SIGH**-tis	S/ R/	-itis *inflammation* appendic- *appendix*	Inflammation of the appendix
appendectomy (**Note:** *elimination of "ic" prior to "ec" of* **-ectomy**)	ah-pen-**DEK**-toe-me	S/	-ectomy *surgical excision*	Surgical removal of the appendix
colon	**KOH**-lon		Greek *colon*	The large intestine, extending from the cecum to the rectum
colic (adj)	**KOL**-ik	S/ R/	-ic *pertaining to* col- *colon*	Spasmodic, crampy pains in the abdomen
colitis	koh-**LIE**-tis	S/	-itis *inflammation*	Inflammation of the colon
feces	**FEE**-seez		Latin *dregs*	Undigested, waste material discharged from the bowel
fecal (adj)	**FEE**-kal	S/ R/	-al *pertaining to* fec- *feces*	Pertaining to feces
defecation	def-eh-**KAY**-shun	S/ P/	-ation *process* de- *removal*	Evacuation of feces from rectum and anus
flexure	**FLEK**-shur		Latin *bend*	A bend in a structure
ileum	**ILL**-ee-um		Latin *roll up, twist*	Third portion of the small intestine
ileocecal sphincter	**ILL**-ee-oh-**SEE**-cal **SFINK**-ter	S/ R/CF R/	-al *pertaining to* ile/o- *ileum* -cec- *cecum* sphincter, Greek *band*	Band of muscle that encircles the junction of ileum and cecum
rectum	**RECK**-tum		Latin *straight*	Terminal part of the colon from the sigmoid to the anal canal
rectal (adj)	**RECK**-tal	S/ R/	-al *pertaining to* rect- *rectum*	Pertaining to the rectum
sigmoid	**SIG**-moyd		Greek *letter "S"*	Sigmoid colon is shaped like an "S"

EXERCISES

A. Apply *the language of the digestive system and answer the following questions. Fill in the blanks.* **LO 9.2, 9.9, and 9.11**

1. What part of the digestive system contains both an internal and external sphincter? ____________________
2. What body part has no known use or function? ____________________
3. What is a ring of smooth muscle that forms a one-way valve called? ____________________
4. What is the name of the area of the colon that is shaped like an "S"? ____________________
5. What is the name of the procedure where the appendix is removed? ____________________
6. The *hepatic flexure* is near what major body organ? ____________________

B. Deconstruct: *Break down these terms into their elements to define the word. Know the meaning of the elements = know the meaning of the term. If a term does not have a particular word element, insert N/A. Fill in the chart.* **LO 9.1, 9.9, and 9.11**

Medical Term	Meaning of Prefix	Meaning of Root/CF	Meaning of Suffix
colitis	**1.**	**2.**	**3.**
defecation	**4.**	**5.**	**6.**
appendicitis	**7.**	**8.**	**9.**
junction	**10.**	**11.**	**12.**

Lesson 9.6 (cont'd)

Keynotes

- **A proctologist is a surgical specialist in diseases of the anus and rectum.**
- **Fissures are tears; fistulas are abnormal passages.**
- **Consuming black licorice, Pepto-Bismol, or blueberries can produce black stools.**

Abbreviations

BM	bowel movement
IBS	irritable bowel syndrome

Disorders of the Large Intestine and Anal Canal (LO 9.9)

Disorders of the Large Intestine (LO 9.9)

Appendicitis is the most common cause of acute abdominal pain in the right lower quadrant. If neglected, the inflamed appendix can rupture, leading to **peritonitis.** Appendicitis is treated with a surgical appendectomy, usually performed through laparoscopy.

Diverticulosis is the presence of small pouches (**diverticula**) bulging outward through weak spots in the large intestine's lining *(Figure 9.25)*. The pouches are asymptomatic until they become infected and inflamed, a condition called **diverticulitis.** The most likely cause of **diverticular disease** (diverticulosis and diverticulitis) is a low-fiber diet.

Ulcerative colitis is an extensive inflammation and ulceration of the large intestine's lining. It produces bouts of bloody diarrhea, crampy pain, weight loss, and an electrolyte imbalance.

Irritable bowel syndrome (IBS) is an increasingly common large-bowel disorder presenting with crampy pain, gas, and changes in bowel habits to either constipation or diarrhea. There are no anatomical changes seen in the bowel. The cause is unknown.

Polyps, which vary in size and shape, are masses of tissue arising from the large intestine's wall and protruding into the bowel lumen. Although most polyps are benign, an endoscopic biopsy can determine if they are precancerous or cancerous.

Colon and rectal cancers are the second cause of cancer deaths after lung cancer. The majority of these cancers occur in the rectum and sigmoid colon. They can spread through the bowel wall, extend down the lumen, and metastasize to regional lymph nodes and to liver, lungs, bones, and brain through the bloodstream.

Obstruction of the large bowel can be caused by cancers, large polyps, or diverticulitis.

Proctitis is an inflammation of the rectum's lining, often associated with ulcerative colitis, Crohn disease, or radiation therapy.

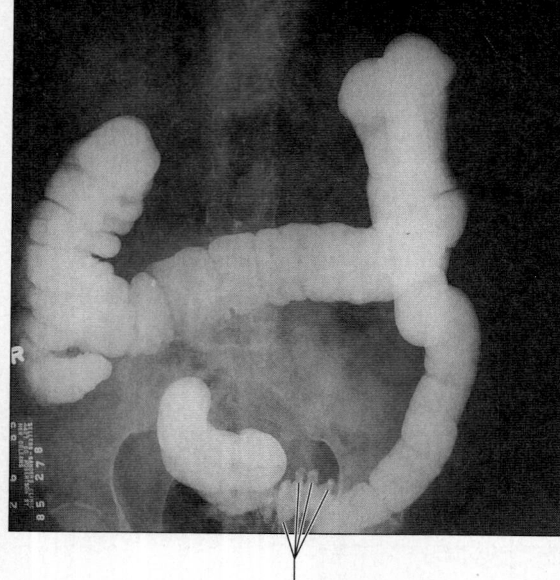

▲ **FIGURE 9.25**
Barium Enema Showing Diverticulosis.

Susan Leavine/Science Source

Disorders of the Anal Canal (LO 9.9)

Hemorrhoids are dilated veins in the submucosa (connective tissue layer) of the anal canal, often associated with pregnancy, chronic constipation, diarrhea, or aging. They protrude into the anal canal **(internal)** or bulge out along the edge of the anus **(external)** *(Figure 9.26),* producing pain and bright red blood from the anus. A **thrombosed** hemorrhoid, in which blood has clotted, is very painful.

Anal fissures are tears in the anal canal's lining, perhaps from difficult bowel movements **(BMs). Anal fistulas** occur following abscesses in the anal glands and are an abnormal passage (fistula) between the anal canal and the skin outside the anus. Surgical procedures–a **fistulectomy** and a **fistulotomy**–are used to treat anal fistulas.

Gastrointestinal (GI) Bleeding (LO 9.6 and 9.9)

GI tract bleeding can have a variety of causes, which are not always easy to recognize. Sometimes, the bleeding can be internal and painless. It can present in different ways, however, to provide a clue as to the site of bleeding:

- **Hematemesis** is the vomiting of bright red blood, which indicates an upper GI source of bleeding (esophagus, stomach, duodenum) that is brisk.
- **Vomiting of "coffee grounds"** occurs when bleeding from an upper GI source has slowed or stopped.
- **Melena,** the passage of black, tarry stools, usually indicates upper GI bleeding.
- **Occult blood** cannot be seen in the stool, but when a chemical fecal occult blood test **(Hemoccult)** is positive, the source of the bleeding can be anywhere in the GI tract.

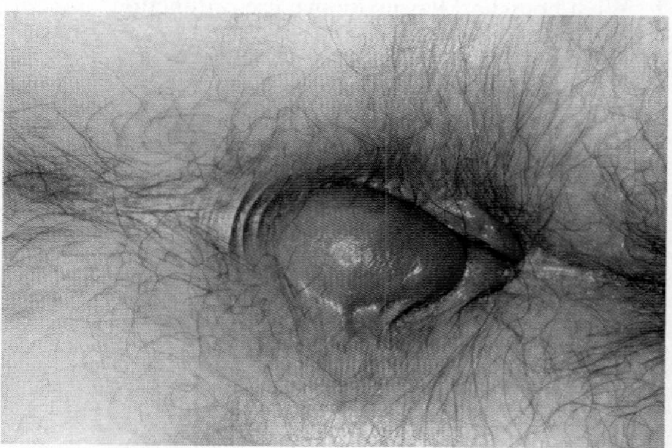

▲ **FIGURE 9.26**
External Hemorrhoid.

Dr P. Marazzi/Science Source

Word Analysis and Definition

S = Suffix P = Prefix R = Root R/CF = Combining Form

WORD	PRONUNCIATION	ELEMENTS		DEFINITION
bowel	**BOUGH**-el		Latin *sausage*	Another name for intestine
diverticulum diverticula (pl) diverticulosis diverticulitis	die-ver-**TICK**-you-lum di-ver-**TICK**-you-lah **DIE**-ver-tick-you-**LOW**-sis **DIE**-ver-tick-you-**LIE**-tis	S/ R/ S/ S/	-um *tissue, structure* **diverticul-** *byroad* -osis *condition* -itis *inflammation*	A pouchlike opening or sac from a tubular structure (e.g., intestine) Presence of a number of small pouches in the wall of the large intestine Inflammation of the diverticula
fissure	**FISH**-ur		Latin *slit*	Deep furrow or cleft
fistula	**FIS**-tyu-lah		Latin *pipe, tube*	Abnormal passage
hemorrhoid hemorrhoids (pl) hemorrhoidectomy (**Note:** *This term has two suffixes.*)	**HEM-oh-royd** **HEM**-oh-royd-**EK**-toh-me	S/ R/CF S/	-rrhoid *flow* **hem/o-** *blood* -ectomy *surgical excision*	Dilated rectal vein producing painful anal swelling Surgical removal of hemorrhoids
melena	mel-**EN**-ah		Greek *black*	The passage of black, tarry stools
occult blood Hemoccult test	oh-**KULT BLUD** **HEEM**-o-kult **TEST**		occult, Latin *to hide*	Blood that cannot be seen in the stool but is positive on a fecal occult blood test Trade name for a fecal occult blood test
peritoneum peritoneal (adj) peritonitis	per-ih-toe-**NEE**-um **PER**-ih-toe-**NEE**-al **PER**-ih-toe-**NIE**-tis	S/ R/CF S/ S/	-um *tissue* **periton/e-** *stretch over* -al *pertaining to* -itis *inflammation*	Membrane that lines the abdominal cavity Pertaining to the peritoneum Inflammation of the peritoneum
polyp polyposis polypectomy	**POL**-ip pol-ih-**POH**-sis pol-ip-**ECK**-toh-mee	 S/ R/ S/	Latin *foot* -osis *condition* **polyp-** *polyp* -ectomy *surgical excision*	Mass of tissue that projects into the lumen of the bowel Presence of several polyps Excision or removal of a polyp
proctitis proctologist	prok-**TIE**-tis prok-**TOL**-oh-jist	S/ R/ S/ R/CF	-itis *inflammation* **proct-** *anus, rectum* -logist *specialist* **proct/o-** *anus, rectum*	Inflammation of the lining of the rectum A surgical specialist in diseases of the anus and rectum

EXERCISES

A. Suffixes: *Insert the correct suffix to complete the term. There are more suffixes than you need. Fill in the blanks.* **LO 9.1, 9.4, 9.9, and 9.10**

osis ectomy um itis al ion

1. excision or removal of a polyp polyp/ ______
2. inflammation of the diverticula diverticul/ ______
3. membranous structure lining the abdominal cavity peritone/ ______
4. condition of having multiple polyps polyp/ ______
5. pertaining to the peritoneum peritone/ ______

B. Singular and plural terms. *Insert the correct medical terms in the blanks; watch for spelling. Fill in the blanks.* **LO 9.2, 9.9, and 9.11**

diverticulitis diverticulum diverticulosis diverticula

1. What starts out as a single ______ can be followed by many other ______. The condition of having a number of these small pouches in the wall of the intestine is known as ______. Should these pouches become inflamed, ______ will result.

polypectomy polyps polyposis polyp

2. The first ______ was found on sigmoidoscopy. A follow-up colonoscopy 6 months later found several more ______ in the large intestine. Diagnosis is ______. Proposed treatment is ______.

peritoneum peritonitis peritoneal

3. The ______ laceration sliced completely through the ______. Because of an infection in the wound, the patient developed ______.

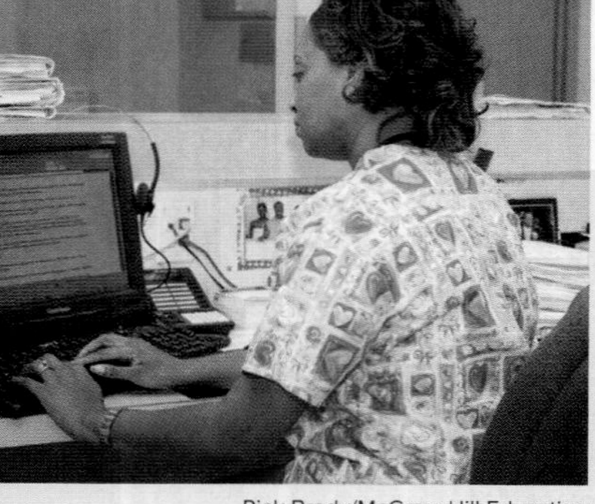

Rick Brady/McGraw-Hill Education

Lesson 9.7

Diagnostic and Therapeutic Procedures and Pharmacology of the Digestive System

Lesson Objectives

The information provided in this lesson will enable you to:

9.7.1 Describe the diagnostic procedures used in gastronterology.

9.7.2 Explain the therapeutic procedures used in gastroenterology.

9.7.3 Discuss the pharmacologic agents used in gastroenterology.

Diagnostic Procedures (LO 9.10)

Nasogastric aspiration and lavage are used to detect upper GI bleeding. The presence of bright red blood in the lavage material indicates active upper GI bleeding; "coffee grounds" indicate the bleeding has slowed or stopped.

Enteroscopy uses an oral, flexible **endoscope** containing light-transmitting fibers or a video transmitter to visualize and biopsy tumors and ulcers and to control bleeding from the esophagus, stomach, and duodenum. Visualization of the stomach is called **gastroscopy**; visualization of the esophagus, stomach, and duodenum is called **panendoscopy**.

Capsule endoscopy enables examination of the entire small intestine by ingesting a pill-sized video capsule with its own camera and light source that sends images to a data recorder worn on the patient's belt.

Double balloon endoscopy uses two balloons at the tip of the endoscope that are inflated sequentially to move the endoscope further into the small intestine than with a usual endoscope.

Upper GI tract barium X-rays (barium swallow) use barium sulfate, a contrast material, to study the distal esophagus, the stomach, and duodenum. They are less accurate than enteroscopy at identifying bleeding lesions.

Angiography uses injected dye to highlight blood vessels and is used to detect the site of bleeding in the GI tract.

In a **digital rectal examination** the physician palpates the rectum and prostate gland with a gloved, lubricated index finger to determine the presence of lesions.

Proctoscopy is procedure performed with a proctoscope that allows for the visual examination of the anus, rectum, and sigmoid colon to look for diseases, causes of rectal bleeding or check on abnormal results seen during a barium enema.

Fecal occult blood test (Hemoccult) is used to detect the presence in the stool of blood not visible to the naked eye. It is a good first screening test for cancer of the large intestine.

Anoscopy is an examination of the anus and lower rectum using a rigid instrument. Flexible **sigmoidoscopy** examines the rectum and sigmoid colon and **flexible colonoscopy** examines the whole length of the colon.

In a **barium swallow,** the patient ingests barium sulfate, a contrast material, to show details of the pharynx and esophagus on X-rays.

In a **barium meal,** barium sulfate is used to study the distal esophagus, stomach, and duodenum on X-rays *(Figure 9.27).*

Barium enema uses the contrast material barium sulfate, which is injected into the large intestine as an enema and X-ray films are taken *(Figure 9.28).*

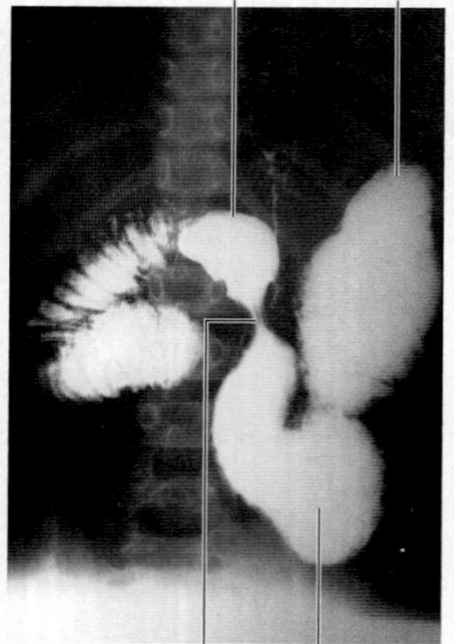

▲ **FIGURE 9.27** Barium Meal Showing Pylorus and Duodenum.

Medicimage/UIG/Shutterstock

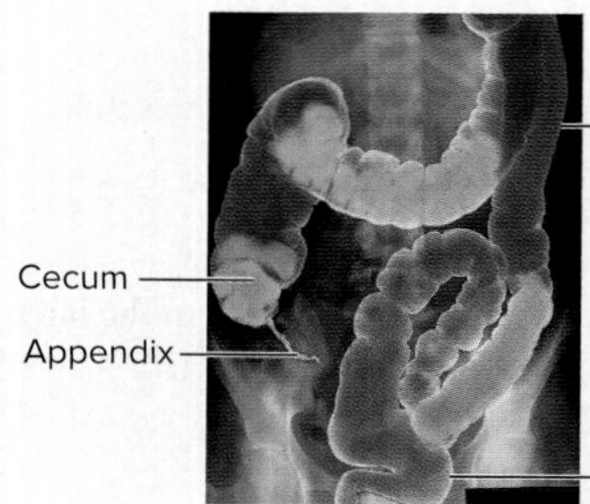

▲ **FIGURE 9.28** Barium Enema of the Large Intestine.

CNRI/Science Photo Library/Science source

LO 9.7 Liver Function Tests

Liver function tests (LFTs) are a group of tests to show how well your liver is functioning. They are divided into four categories:

1. **Measuring liver proteins in blood serum**
   - Measuring proteins, albumin, and globulin *(see Chapter 7),* which are low when there is liver damage.
2. **Measuring liver enzymes in blood serum**
   - Measuring enzymes made in the liver, known as **transaminases,** including **alanine aminotransferase (ALT**; also known as **serum glutamic-pyruvic transaminase,** or **SGPT**) and **aspartate aminotransferase (AST**; also known as **serum glutamic oxaloacetic acid transaminase,** or **SGOT**). Elevated levels of these enzymes in the blood indicate liver damage.
3. **Measuring cholestatic liver enzymes in the blood serum**
   - Measuring **alkaline phosphatase (ALP),** which metabolizes phosphorus and makes energy available for the body. Elevated blood levels are found in liver and biliary tract disorders.
   - Measuring **gamma-glutamyl transpeptidase (GGT),** which is elevated in liver disease.
4. **Measuring bilirubin in the bloodstream**
   - **Bilirubin** is formed in the liver from hemoglobin and secreted into the biliary system. If the liver is damaged, bilirubin can leak out into the bloodstream, producing elevated levels and jaundice.

Word Analysis and Definition

S = Suffix P = Prefix R = Root R/CF = Combining Form

WORD	PRONUNCIATION		ELEMENTS	DEFINITION
angiography	an-jee-**OG**-rah-fee	S/ R/CF	-graphy *process of recording* angio- *blood vessel*	Process of recording the image of blood vessels after injection of contrast material
anoscopy	**A**-nos-koh-pee	S/ R/CF	-scopy *to examine* an/o- *anus*	Endoscopic examination of the anus
aspiration	**AS**-pih-**RAY**-shun	S/ R/CF	-ion *process* aspirat- *to breathe on*	Removal by suction of fluid or gas from a body cavity
cholangiography	**KOH**-lan-jee-**OG**-rah-fee	S/ R/ R/CF	-graphy *process of recording* chol- *bile* -angi/o- *blood vessel, lymph vessel*	X-ray of the bile ducts after injection or ingestion of a contrast medium
colonoscopy	koh-lon-**OSS**-koh-pee	S/ R/CF	-scopy *to examine* colon/o *colon*	Endoscopic examination of the colon
digital	**DIJ**-ih-tal	S/ R/	-al *pertaining to* digit- *finger or toe*	Pertaining to a finger or toe
endoscope **endoscopic (adj)** **endoscopy**	**EN**-doh-skope **EN**-doh-**SKOP**-ik en-**DOSS**-koh-pee	P/ R/ S/ S/	endo- *within, inside* -scope *instrument for viewing* -ic *pertaining to* -scopy *to examine*	Instrument to examine the inside of a tubular or hollow organ Pertaining to the use of an endoscope The use of an endoscope
enema	**EN**-eh-mah		Greek *injection*	An injection of fluid into the rectum
enteroscopy	en-ter-**OSS**-koh-pee	S/ R/CF	-scopy *to examine, to view* enter/o- *intestine*	The examination of the lining of the digestive tract
gastroscope **gastroscopy**	**GAS**-troh-skope gas-**TROS**-koh-pee	S/ R/CF S/	-scope *instrument for viewing* gastr/o *stomach* -scopy *to examine*	Instrument to view the inside of the stomach Endoscopic examination of the stomach
ileoscopy	ill-ee-**OS**-koh-pee	S/ R/CF	-scopy *to examine* ile/o- *ileum*	Endoscopic examination of the ileum
lavage	lah-**VAHZH**		Latin *to wash*	Washing out of a hollow cavity, tube, or organ
panendoscopy	pan-en-**DOS**-koh-pee	S/ P/ P/	-scopy *to examine* pan *all* -endo- *inside*	Endoscopic examination of the esophagus, stomach, and duodenum
proctoscopy	prok-**TOSS**-koh-pee	S/ R/CF	-scopy *to examine* proct/o- *anus and rectum*	Examination of the inside of the anus and the rectum by procto-scope or rectoscope
resection **resect (verb)**	ree-**SEK**-shun	S/ P/ R/	-ion *action, condition* re- *back* -sect- *cut off*	Removal of a specific part of an organ or structure
sigmoidoscopy	sig-moi-**DOS**-koh-pee	S/ R/CF	-scopy *to examine* sigmoid/o- *sigmoid colon*	Endoscopic examination of the sigmoid colon

EXERCISES

A. Use *the correct terms for patient documentation. Using the terms provided below, fill in the blanks with the correct term. Not all terms will be used. Fill in the blanks.* **LO 9.9, 9.10, and 9.11**

endoscopy proctoscopy colonoscopy enema gastroenterologist sigmoidoscopy barium angiography

A patient is complaining of blood in his stool. The physician requested that you schedule a **(1)**____________________ **(2)**____________________ with the radiology department. One week later, the test results came back and were inconclusive.
The physician decided that further tests were needed, and therefore wished to view the inside of the large intestines. Because the physician believed the source of the bleeding was in the large intestine, she ordered a **(3)**__________. The medical assistant called the hospital's **(4)**____________ department to schedule the procedure.

Lesson 9.7 (cont'd) Therapeutic Procedures (LO 9.10)

Many of the diagnostic procedures in the previous section can also be used as therapeutic procedures. For example, endoscopy can be used to remove polyps, biopsy suspicious lesions, stop bleeding, and be used as screening procedures for cancer.

Alternatively, food can be inserted directly into the stomach via a **nasogastric** or stomach tube, when medically indicated.

Laparoscopy uses a thin, lighted tube inserted through an **incision** in the abdominal wall to examine abdominal and pelvic organs. Biopsy samples can be taken through the **laparoscope,** and in many cases surgery can be performed instead of using a much larger incision. Laparoscopy is done to check for and remove abnormal tumors; **ligate** Fallopian tubes; fix **hiatal** and **inguinal hernias**; and remove such organs as the uterus, spleen, gallbladder, ovaries, or appendix. **Resection** of the colon can also be performed **laparoscopically.**

Intestinal resections are used to surgically remove diseased portions of the intestine. The remaining portions of the intestine can be joined back together through an **anastomosis** *(Figure 9.29a).* If there is insufficient bowel remaining for an anastomosis, an **ostomy** *(Figure 9.29b)* can be performed, where the end of the bowel opens onto the skin at a **stoma**. **Ileostomy** and **colostomy** are two such procedures.

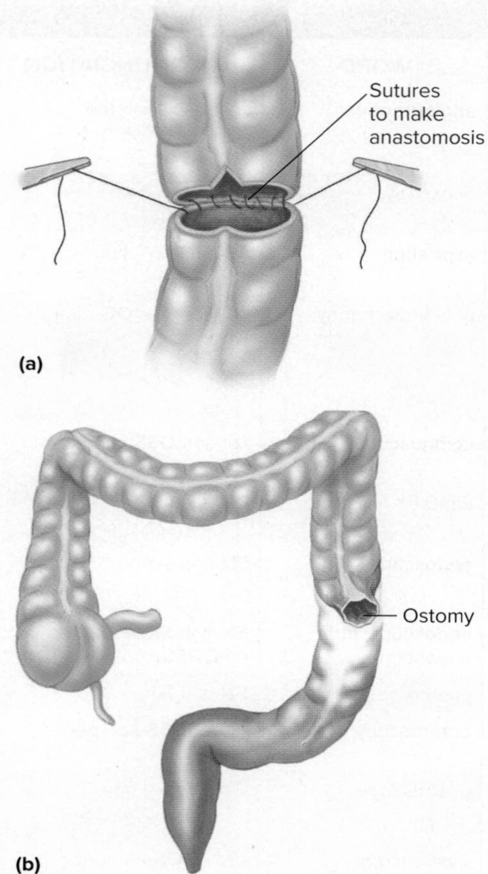

▲ **FIGURE 9.29** Intestinal Resections.

Abbreviations

ERCP	endoscopic retrograde cholangiopancreatography
EUS	endoscopic ultrasound

Endoscopic retrograde cholangiopancreatography (ERCP) is used to diagnose and treat problems in the biliary ductal system. Through an endoscope, the physician can see the inside of the duodenum and inject radiographic contrast dye into the biliary tract ducts. Gallstones and cancer can be treated with this technique.

Pancreas endoscopic ultrasound (EUS) is a type of endoscopic examination that enables detailed imaging and analysis of the pancreas. A thin tube tipped with an ultrasound probe is inserted through the mouth down into the stomach and the first part of the small intestine. The probe emits sound waves that bounce off surrounding structures, and these sound waves are recaptured by the probe and converted to black and white images that can be interpreted by the physician. EUS is of great value in assessing pancreatic tumors and cysts and acute and chronic pancreatitis.

Gastric cancer is usually treated with **resection** and chemotherapy.

Word Analysis and Definition

S = Suffix P = Prefix R = Root R/CF = Combining Form

WORD	PRONUNCIATION		ELEMENTS	DEFINITION
appendectomy	ah-pen-**DEK**-toh-mee	S/ R/	-ectomy *surgical excision* append- *appendix*	Surgical removal of the appendix
anastomosis **anastomoses** (pl)	ah-**NAS**-to-**MOH**-sis ah-**NAS**-to-**MOH**-seez	S/ R/	-osis *condition* anastom- *join together*	A surgically made union between two tubular structures
cholecystectomy	**KOH**-leh-sis-**TEK**-toh-mee	S/ R/CF R/	-ectomy *surgical excision* chol/e- *bile* -cyst- *bladder*	Surgical removal of the gallbladder
cholelithotomy	**KOH**-leh-lih-**THOT**-oh-mee	S/ R/	-otomy *surgical incision* -lith- *stone*	Surgical incision to remove a gallstone(s)
hernia	**HER**-nee-ah		Latin *rupture*	Protrusion of a structure through the tissue that normally contains it
hiatal	high-**AY**-tal	S/ R/	-al *pertaining to* hiat- *aperture*	Pertaining to an opening through a structure
inguinal	**IN**-gwin-al	S/ R/	-al *pertaining to* inguin- *groin*	Pertaining to the groin
ostomy (Note: an "s" is removed for the purpose of spelling)	**OS**-toh-mee	S/ R/	-stomy *new opening* os- *mouth*	Surgery to create an artificial opening into a tubular structure
colostomy	ko-**LOS**-toh-mee	R/	col- *colon*	Artificial opening from the colon to the outside of the body
ileostomy	ill-ee-**OS**-toh-mee	R/	ile- *ileum*	Artificial opening from the ileum to the outside of the body
pancreatography	**PAN**-kree-ah-**TOG**-raff-ee	S/ R/CF	-graphy *process of recording* pancreat/o *pancreas*	Process of recording the structure of the pancreas
retrograde	**RET**-roh-grade	P/ R/	retro- *backward* -grade *going*	Reversal of a normal flow
stoma	**STOH**-mah		Greek *mouth*	Artificial opening
ultrasound	**UL**-trah-sownd	P/ R/	ultra- *higher* -sound *noise*	Very-high-frequency sound waves

Exercises

A. Use *word elements to build medical terms. Given the definition of the procedure, provide the correct word element to create the medical term. Fill in the blanks.* **LO 9.1 and 9.10**

1. Surgical incision to remove a gallstone: cholelitho/______________________________
2. Surgical removal of the appendix: ___________________________ /ectomy
3. Surgery to create an opening from a tubular structure to the outside: _______________________ /tomy
4. Surgical removal of the gallbladder: chole/_____________________ /ectomy
5. Artificial opening from the ileum to the outside of the body: ile/___________________ /tomy

B. Deconstruct *medical terms to determine their meanings. Select the correct answer for each question.* **LO 9.1, 9.3, 9.9, and 9.10**

1. In the procedure ERCP, the "E" stands for
   a. enteric **b.** echo **c.** endoscopic **d.** electrical
2. In the procedure of inserting a nasogastric tube, the practitioner first inserts the tube through the
   a. nose **b.** mouth **c.** stomach **d.** rectum
3. In the procedure ERCP, the "C" tells you that the structure being treated is the
   a. stomach **b.** pancreas **c.** biliary ducts **d.** duodenum
4. In an anastomosis, the root means
   a. removal **b.** creation of an opening **c.** join together **d.** incision

Gastrointestinal Drugs (LO 9.10)

Drugs to Treat Excess Gastric Acid

Antacids, which are taken orally, neutralize gastric acid and relieve heartburn and acid indigestion. Examples of antacids include:

- aluminum hydroxide and magnesium hydroxide (*Maalox, Mylanta*)
- magnesium hydroxide (*Milk of Magnesia*)
- calcium carbonate (*Tums, Rolaids*)

Histamine-2 receptor antagonists (H_2-blockers) block signals that tell the stomach cells to produce acid. They are used to treat gastroesophageal reflux (GERD) and esophagitis *(see Lesson 9.2)*. Examples include:

- cimetidine (*Tagamet*)
- famotidine (*Pepcid*)
- ranitidine (*Zantac*)
- nizatidine (*Axid*)

Less potent OTC variants of these drugs are also available.

Proton pump inhibitors (PPIs) suppress gastric acid secretion in the lining of the stomach by blocking the secretion of gastric acid from the cells into the lumen of the stomach. Examples include:

- omeprazole (*Prilosec*)
- lansoprazole (*Prevacid*)
- esomeprazole (*Nexium*)

A new form of PPI called imidazopyridine (*Tenatoprazole*) appears to be extremely effective in reducing gastric acid.

Misoprostol (*Cytotec*) inhibits the secretion of gastric acid and is approved for the prevention of **nonsteroidal anti-inflammatory drug (NSAID)**–induced gastric acid.

Sucralfate (*Carafate*) reacts with gastric acid (hydrogen chloride **[HCl]**) to form a paste that binds to stomach mucosal cells and inhibits the **diffusion** of acid into the stomach lumen. It also forms a protective barrier on the surface of an ulcer. Its main use is in the **prophylaxis** of stress ulcers.

Anti–*H. pylori* therapy for the treatment of peptic ulcer and chronic gastritis is given with a combination of two antibiotics (for example, amoxicillin [generic] and clarithromycin [generic]) and a proton pump inhibitor.

Drugs to Treat Nausea and Vomiting

Antiemetics, drugs that are effective against vomiting and nausea, are used to treat motion sickness and the side effects of opioid analgesics, general anesthetics, and chemotherapy. The types of antiemetics include:

- **Serotonin antagonists,** which block serotonin receptors in the CNS and GI tract. They are used to treat postoperative and chemotherapy nausea and vomiting. Examples include dolasetron (*Anzemet*), granisetron (*Kytril*), and ondansetron (*Zofran*).
- **Dopamine antagonists,** which act in the brain. They are inexpensive but have an extensive side-effect profile and have been replaced by serotonin antagonists. Examples include chlorpromazine (*Thorazine*) and prochlorperazine (*Compazine*).
- **Antihistamines**, which are used to treat motion sickness, morning sickness in pregnancy, and opioid nausea. Examples include diphenhydramine (*Benadryl*) and promethazine (*Phenergan*).
- **Cannabinoids,** which are used in patients with **cachexia** or who are unresponsive to other antiemetics. Examples include cannabis (medical marijuana) and dronabinol (*Marinol*).

Abbreviations

H_2-blocker	histamine-2 receptor antagonist
PPI	proton pump vinhibitor

Drugs to Treat Constipation

Laxative drugs are used to treat chronic constipation:

- If increased water and fiber are unsuccessful, OTC forms of magnesium hydroxide are the first-line agents to be used.
- Lubiprostone (*Resolor*) has received FDA approval; it acts on the epithelial cells of the GI tract to produce a chloride-rich fluid that softens the **stool** and increases bowel **motility**.

Drugs to Treat Diarrhea

Antidiarrheal drugs are widely available OTC. Examples include loperamide (*Imodium A-D, Maalox*), which reduces bowel motility; bismuth subsalicylate (*Pepto-Bismol*), which decreases the secretion of fluid into the intestine; and attapulgite (*Kaopectate*), which pulls diarrhea-causing substances away from the GI tract; as well as enzymes and nutrients. A combination of diphenyloxylate and atropine (*Lomotil*), a Schedule V drug, reduces bowel motility.

Word Analysis and Definition

S = Suffix   P = Prefix   R = Root   R/CF = Combining Form

WORD	PRONUNCIATION	ELEMENTS		DEFINITION
antidiarrheal	**AN**-tee-die-ah-**REE**-al	S/ P/ P/ R/	-al *pertaining to* **anti-** *against* **-dia-** *complete, through* **-rrhea** *flow, discharge*	Drug that prevents abnormally frequent and loose stools
antiemetic	**AN**-tee-eh-**MEH**-tik	P/ R/	**anti-** *against* **-emetic** *causing vomiting*	Agent that prevents vomiting
antihistamine	an-tee-HISS-tah-meen	P/ R/ R/CF	**anti-** *against* **-hist-** *tissue* **-amine** *nitrogen compound*	Drug that can be used to treat allergic symptoms or prevent vomiting
cachexia	kah-**KEK**-see-ah	P/ R/	**cach-** *bad* **-exia** *condition of body*	A general weight loss and wasting of the body
cannabinoid	can-**AH**-bi-noyd	S/ R/	**-oid** *resembling* **cannabin-** *hemp*	A group of chemical compounds, some of which increase appetite and others treat nausea and vomiting
laxative	**LAK**-sah-tiv	S/ R/CF	**-tive** *pertaining to* **lax/a-** *looseness*	An oral agent that promotes the expulsion of feces
motility	moh-**TILL**-ih-tee	S/ R/	**-ility** *condition, state of* **mot-** *to move*	The ability for spontaneous movement
proton pump inhibitor (PPI)	**PROH**-ton PUMP in-**HIB**-ih-tor	R/ R/ S/ R/	**proton** *first* **pump** *pump* **-or** *a doer* **inhibit-** *repress*	Agent that blocks production of gastric acid
stool	STOOL		Old English ***a seat***	The matter discharged in one movement of the bowels

EXERCISE

A. Match *the definition in the first column with the correct medication it is describing in the second column.* **LO 9.10**

_____	**1.** inhibits proton pumps in the stomach	**a.** Maalox
_____	**2.** treats motion sickness	**b.** Imodium
_____	**3.** neutralizes gastric acid and relieves heartburn	**c.** Tagamet
_____	**4.** used for treatment of chemotherapy nausea	**d.** Nexium
_____	**5.** antidiarrheal drug	**e.** Benadryl
_____	**6.** histamine blocker used to treat GERD	**f.** Zofran

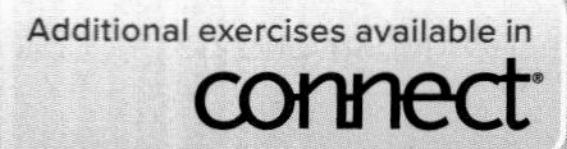

Chapter Review exercises, along with additional practice items, are available in Connect!

The Nervous System and Mental Health

CHAPTER 10

The Essentials of the Languages of Neurology and Psychiatry

Rick Brady/McGraw-Hill Education

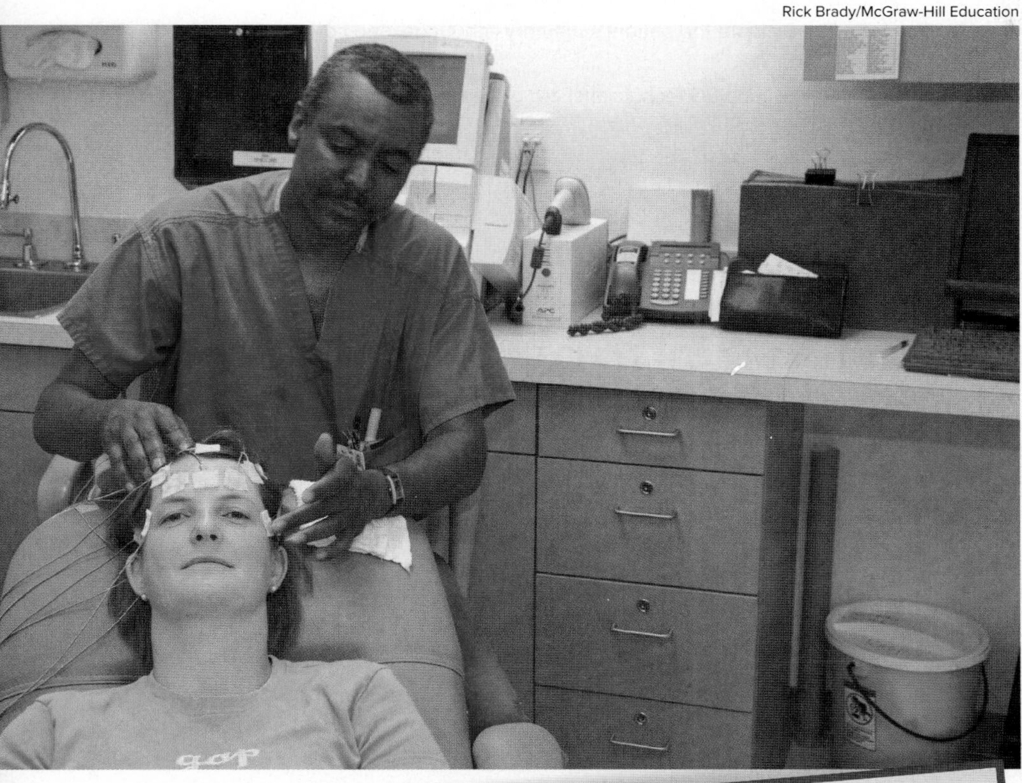

Learning Outcomes

Your roles are to perform electroneurodiagnostic evaluations, communicate with Ms. Gaston and her parents, communicate with other health professionals, and maintain and document Ms. Gaston's history and care. To perform these roles, you must be able to:

LO 10.1 **Use roots, combining forms, suffixes, and prefixes to construct and analyze (deconstruct) medical terms related to the nervous system and mental health.**

LO 10.2 **Spell and pronounce correctly medical terms related to the nervous system and mental health to communicate them with accuracy and precision in any health care setting.**

LO 10.3 **Define accepted abbreviations related to the nervous system and mental health.**

LO 10.4 **Relate the structures of the brain, cranial nerves, spinal cord, peripheral nerves, and meninges to their functions.**

LO 10.5 **Identify the medical terms used in disorders of the brain, cranial nerves, spinal cord, and meninges, and in the management of pain.**

LO 10.6 **Describe the diagnostic procedures, therapeutic methods, and pharmacologic agents used in treating disorders of the nervous system and mental health.**

LO 10.7 **Define mental health, the difference between psychiatry and psychology, and the different types of common mental health disorders.**

LO 10.8 **Apply your knowledge of medical terms relating to the nervous system and mental health to documentation, medical records, and medical reports.**

LO 10.9 **Translate the medical terms relating to the nervous system and mental health into everyday language in order to communicate clearly with patients and their families.**

CASE REPORT 10.1

You are . . .

. . . an **electroneurodiagnostic** technologist working with Gregory Solis, MD, a **neurosurgeon** at Fulwood Medical Center.

You are communicating with . . .

. . . Ms. Roberta Gaston, a 39-year-old woman, who has been referred by Raul Cardenas, MD, a **neurologist,** for evaluation for possible **neurosurgery.** Ms. Gaston has had **epileptic** seizures since the age of 16. She also has daily minor spells in which she stops interacting and blinks rhythmically for about 20 seconds, after which she returns to normal. She is unable to work and is cared for by her parents. Her **neurologic** examination is normal. Her **electroencephalogram (EEG)** shows diffuse epileptic discharges in the left frontal region. Her CT scan is normal. An MRI shows a 20-mm-diameter mass adjacent to her left ventricle.

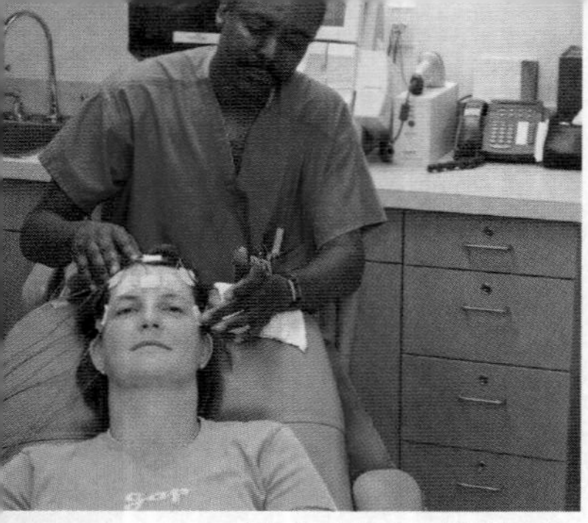

Rick Brady/McGraw-Hill Education

Objectives

The trillions of cells in your body must communicate and work together for you to function effectively. This communication is done through your ***nervous system,*** *so it is essential that you understand how this system operates. In this lesson, you will learn to use correct medical terminology to:*

10.1.1 Describe the structure of the nervous system.

10.1.2 Relate the functions of the nervous system to the structures of its components.

10.1.3 List the subdivisions of the nervous system, their different functions, and their basic cells.

Abbreviations

ANS	autonomic nervous system
CNS	central nervous system
CT	computed tomography
EEG	electroencephalogram
MRI	magnetic resonance imaging
PNS	peripheral nervous system

The health professionals involved in the diagnosis and treatment of problems with the neurological system and mental health include the following:

- **Neurologists** are medical doctors who specialize in disorders of the nervous system.
- **Neurosurgeons** are medical doctors who perform surgical procedures on the nervous system.
- **Psychiatrists** are medical doctors who are licensed in the diagnosis and treatment of mental disorders.
- **Anesthesiologists** are medical doctors who are certified to administer anesthetics and can also be responsible for pain management.
- **Psychologists** are professionals who are licensed in the science concerned with the behavior of the human mind.
- **Neuropsychologists** are individuals who evaluate the patient's memory, language, and cognitive functions, and develop appropriate treatment plans.
- **Electroneurodiagnostic technicians** (also called EEG technicians) are professionals who operate specialized equipment that measures the electrical activity of the brain, peripheral nervous system, and spinal cord.

Lesson 10.1

Structure and Functions of the Nervous System

Structure of the Nervous System (LO 10.2 and 10.4)

The nervous system *(Figure 10.1)* has two major anatomical subdivisions.

1. The **central nervous system (CNS),** consisting of the brain and spinal cord; and
2. The **peripheral nervous system (PNS),** consisting of all the neurons and nerves outside the central nervous system. It includes 12 pairs of cranial nerves originating from the brain and 31 pairs of spinal nerves originating from the spinal cord.

The peripheral nervous system is further subdivided into:

i. The **sensory division,** in which sensory nerves (**afferent** nerves) carry messages toward the spinal cord and brain from sense organs; and

ii. The **motor division,** in which motor nerves (**efferent** nerves) carry messages away from the brain and spinal cord to muscles and organs.

a. The **visceral motor division** is called the **autonomic nervous system (ANS).** It carries signals to glands and to cardiac and smooth muscle. It operates at a subconscious level outside your voluntary control, and it has two subdivisions:

- The **sympathetic division** arouses the body for action by increasing the heart and respiratory rates to increase oxygen supply to the brain and muscles.
- The **parasympathetic division** calms the body, slowing down the heartbeat but stimulating digestion.

b. The **somatic motor division** carries signals to the skeletal muscles and is within your voluntary control.

FIGURE 10.1
Components of the Nervous System.

Word Analysis and Definition

S = Suffix P = Prefix R = Root R/CF = Combining Form

WORD	PRONUNCIATION	ELEMENTS		DEFINITION
afferent (**Note:** *Also called sensory; opposite of efferent*)	**AFF**-eh-rent		Latin *to bring to*	Moving toward a center; for example, nerve fibers conducting *impulses to the spinal cord and brain*
efferent (**Note:** *Also called motor; opposite of afferent*)	**EFF**-eh-rent		Latin *to bring away from*	Moving away from a center; for example, conducting nerve impulses away *from the brain or spinal cord*
electroencephalogram (EEG)	ee-**LEK**-troh-en-**SEF**-ah-low-gram	S/ R/CF R/CF	-gram *recording* electr/o- *electricity* -encephal/o- *brain*	Record of the electrical activity of the brain
electroencephalograph	ee-**LEK**-troh-en-**SEF**-ah-low-graf	S/	-graph *to write, record*	Device used to record the electrical activity of the brain
electroencephalography	ee-**LEK**-troh-en-**SEF**-ah-LOG-rah-fee	S/	-graphy *process of recording*	The process of recording the electrical activity of the brain
electroneurodiagnostic (adj)	ee-**LEK**-troh-**NYUR**-oh-die-ag-**NOS**-tik	S/ R/CF R/CF R/	-ic *pertaining to* electr/o- *electricity* -neur/o- *nerve* -diagnost- *decision*	Pertaining to the use of electricity in the diagnosis of a neurologic disorder
epilepsy	**EP**-ih-**LEP**-see		Greek *seizure*	Chronic brain disorder due to paroxysmal excessive neuronal discharges
epileptic (adj) (**Note:** *An epileptic episode is called a* seizure.)	**EP**-ih-**LEP**-tik **SEE**-zhur	S/ R/	-ic *pertaining to* epilept- *seizure*	Pertaining to or suffering from epilepsy
motor	**MOH**-tor		Latin *to move*	Structures of the nervous system that send impulses out to cause muscles to contract or glands to secrete
nerve	NERV		Latin *nerve*	A cord of nerve fibers bound together by connective tissue
nervous system	**NER**-vus **SIS**-tem	S/ R/	-ous *pertaining to* nerv- *nerve* system, Greek *an organized whole*	The whole, integrated nerve apparatus
neurology	nyu-**ROL**-oh-jee	S/ R/CF	-logy *study of* neur/o- *nerve*	Medical specialty of disorders of the nervous system
neurologist	nyu-**ROL**-oh-jist	S/	-logist *one who studies, specialist*	Medical specialist in disorders of the nervous system
neurologic (adj)	**NYU**-roh-**LOJ**-ik	S/ R/	-ic *pertaining to* -log- *to study*	Pertaining to the nervous system
neurosurgeon	**NYU**-roh-**SUR**-jun	S/ R/	-eon *one who does* -surg- *operate*	One who performs surgery on the nervous system
neurosurgery	**NYU**-roh-**SUR**-jer-ee	S/	-ery *process of*	Operating surgically on the nervous system
parasympathetic (**Note:** *This term contains two prefixes.*)	par-ah-sim-pah-**THET**-ik	S/ P/ P/ R/	-ic *pertaining to* para- *beside* -sym- *together* -pathet- *suffering*	Division of the autonomic nervous system; has opposite effects to the sympathetic division
sensory	**SEN**-soh-ree	S/ R/	-ory *having the function of* sens- *feel*	Pertaining to sensation; structures of the nervous system that carry impulses to the brain
somatic	soh-**MAT**-ik	S/ R/	-ic *pertaining to* somat- *body*	A division of the peripheral nervous system serving the skeletal muscles OR relating to the body in general
sympathetic	sim-pah-**THET**-ik	S/ P/ R/	-ic *pertaining to* sym- *together* -pathet- *suffering*	Division of the autonomic nervous system operating at an unconscious level
visceral (adj)	**VISS**-er-al	S/ R/	-al *pertaining to* viscer- internal organs	Pertaining to the internal organs
viscus **viscera (pl)**	**VISS**-kus **VISS**-er-ah		Latin an internal organ	Any single internal organ

EXERCISE

A. Documentation: *Fill in the following paragraph with the appropriate language of neurology. Review Case Report 10.1 to assist you in completing this exercise. Fill in the blanks.* **LO 10.2, 10.3, 10.5, and 10.6**

electroencephalography **electroneurodiagnostic** **epilepsy** **electroencephalograph**
neurologist **electroencephalogram** **neurosurgeon**

Roberta Gaston and her parents were sent to this office by her (1) ____________________.

Dr. Solis has ordered some (2) ____________________ tests because of her (3) ____________________.

The particular type of test is an (4) ____________________, which will produce an EEG on the (device) (5) ____________________.

After the results of the (6) ____________________, if Ms. Gaston needs surgery, it will be performed by a(n) (7) ____________________.

Structure of the Nervous System (continued)

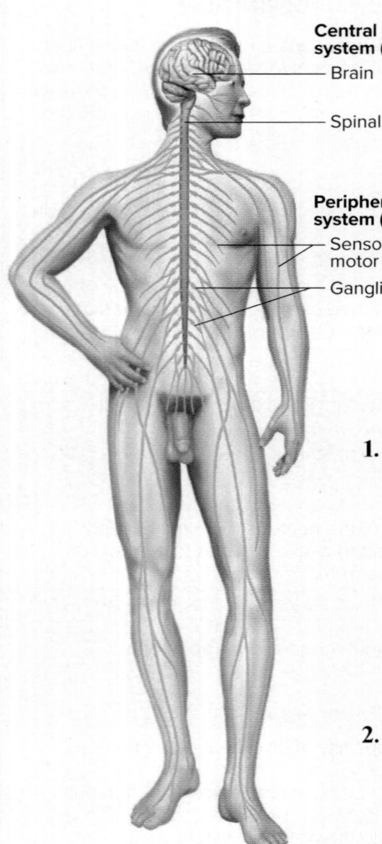

FIGURE 10.2 The Nervous System.

Functions of the Nervous System

(LO 10.2 and 10.4)

Optimal communication between your nervous system and all the cells in your body requires that the following five functions are always working smoothly:

1. **Sensory input** to the brain comes from receptors all over your body at both the conscious and subconscious levels. You are conscious of external stimuli that you receive from your body as it interacts with your environment. Inside your body, internal stimuli concerning the amount of oxygen and carbon dioxide in your blood, and other homeostatic variables like your body temperature, are being processed continually at the subconscious level.
2. **Motor output** from your brain stimulates the skeletal muscles to contract, which enables you to move. Your nervous system controls the production of sweat, saliva, and digestive enzymes without active input from you.
3. **Evaluation and integration** occur in your brain and spinal cord to process the **sensory** input, initiate a response, and store the event in memory.
4. **Homeostasis** is maintained by your nervous system taking in internal sensory input and responding to it. For example, the nervous system responds by stimulating the heart to deliver the correct volume of blood to ensure oxygenation of and removal of waste products from cells.
5. **Mental activity** occurs in your brain so that you can think, feel, understand, respond, and remember.

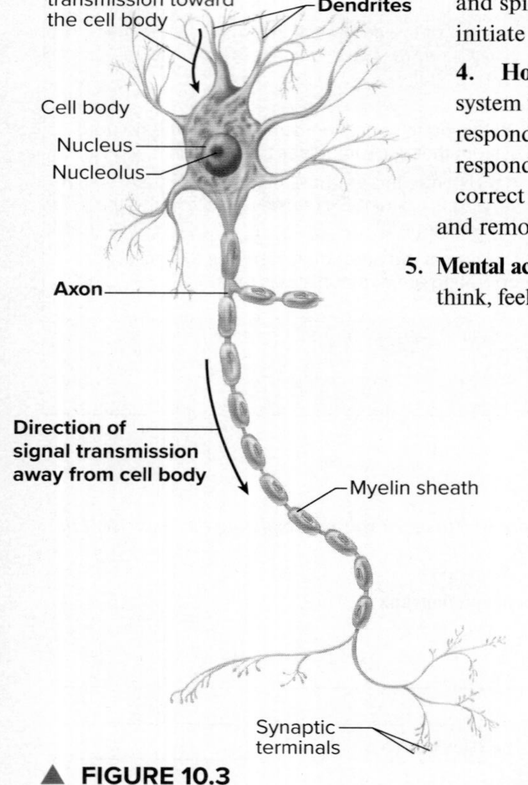

FIGURE 10.3 Neuron.

Cells of the Nervous System

(LO 10.2 and 10.4)

Neurons (nerve cells) receive stimuli and transmit impulses to other neurons or to organ receptors. Each neuron consists of a cell body and two types of processes or extensions, called **axons** and **dendrites** *(Figure 10.3).*

Dendrites are short, multiple, highly branched extensions of the neuron's cell body. They direct impulses toward the cell body. A single axon, or nerve fiber, arises from the cell body, is covered in a fatty **myelin** sheath, and carries the impulse away from the cell body. Each axon measures a few millimeters to a meter in length.

Bundles of axons appear white in color and create the **white matter** of the brain and spinal cord. Neuron cell bodies, dendrites, and synapses appear gray and create the **gray matter.**

The axon terminates in a network of small branches that ends at a **synapse** (junction) with a dendrite from another neuron, or with a receptor on a muscle cell or gland cell *(Figure 10.4).* **Neurotransmitters** cross the synapse to stimulate or inhibit another neuron or the cell of a muscle or gland. Examples of neurotransmitters are norepinephrine, serotonin, and **dopamine.**

Groups of cell bodies cluster together to form ganglia, and groups of cell bodies and axons collect together to form nerves.

The trillion neurons in the nervous system are outnumbered 50 to 1 by the supportive **glial** cells **(neuroglia).**

The blood-brain barrier is a physical barrier—composed of glial cells and the capillary blood vessel walls—that prevents foreign substances, toxins, and infections from leaving the bloodstream and affecting the brain cells.

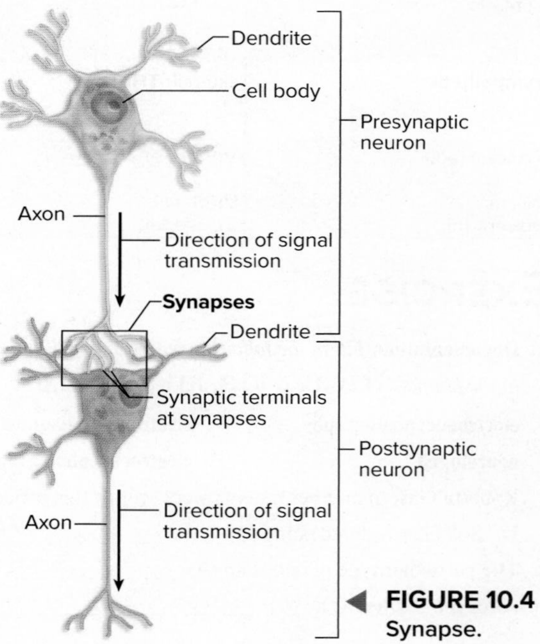

FIGURE 10.4 Synapse.

Word Analysis and Definition

S = Suffix P = Prefix R = Root R/CF = Combining Form

WORD	PRONUNCIATION		ELEMENTS	DEFINITION
autonomic	awe-toh-**NOM**-ik	S/ P/ R/	-ic *pertaining to* **auto-** *self* -nom- *law*	Self-governing visceral motor division of the peripheral nervous system
axon	**ACK**-son		Greek *axis*	Single process of a nerve cell carrying nervous impulses away from the cell body
dendrite	**DEN**-dright		Greek *looking like a tree*	Branched extension of the nerve cell body that receives nervous stimuli
dopamine	**DOH**-pah-meen		Precursor of norepinephrine	Neurotransmitter in some specific small areas of the brain
glia **glial (adj)** **neuroglia**	**GLEE**-ah **GLEE**-al nyu-roh-**GLEE**-ah	 S/ R/ R/CF	Greek *glue* -al *pertaining to* -glia *glue* neur/o- *nerve*	Connective tissue that holds a structure together Pertaining to glia or neuroglia Connective tissue holding nervous tissue together
myelin	**MY**-eh-lin	S/ R/	-in *substance, chemical compound* myel- *spinal cord*	Material of the sheath around the axon of a nerve
neuron	**NYUR**-on		Greek *nerve*	Technical term for a nerve cell; consists of cell body with its dendrites and axons
neurotransmitter **(Note:** Transmit *is a word itself, so the prefix trans is in the middle of the overall word.*)	**NYUR**-oh-trans-**MIT**-er	S/ R/CF P/ R/	-er *agent* neur/o- *nerve* -trans- *across* -mitt- *send*	Chemical agent that relays messages from one nerve cell to the next
synapse	**SIN**-aps	P/ R/	syn- *together* -apse *clasp*	Junction between two nerve cells, or a nerve fiber and its target cell, where electrical impulses are transmitted between the cells

EXERCISES

A. Elements: *Solid knowledge of elements is the key to learning medical terminology. Match each element in first column with its correct meaning in second column.* **LO 10.1**

_____ **1.** ic	**a.** self
_____ **2.** syn	**b.** pertaining to
_____ **3.** viscer	**c.** spinal cord
_____ **4.** auto	**d.** together
_____ **5.** myel	**e.** internal organ
_____ **6.** glia	**f.** glue

B. Deconstruct *the following terms into their elements.* **LO 10.1**

1. neurotransmitter ______________/ ______________/ ______________/ ______________

2. nueroglia ______________/ ______________/ ______________/ ______________

3. autonomic ______________/ ______________/ ______________/ ______________

4. synapse ______________/ ______________/ ______________

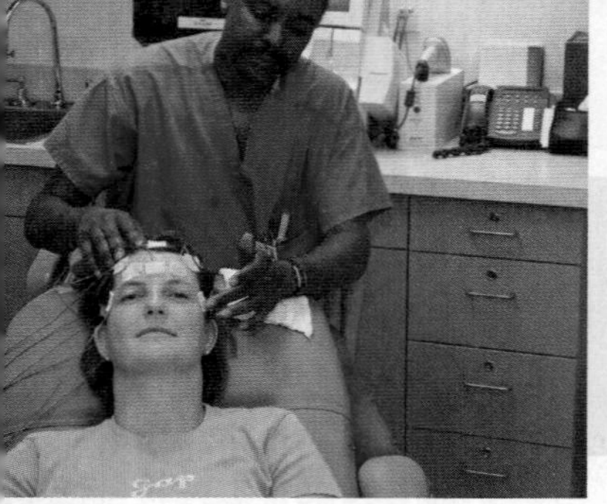

Rick Brady/McGraw-Hill Education

Lesson 10.2

The Brain and Cranial Nerves

Objectives

The sensations of smelling the roses, seeing them, and touching them are recognized and interpreted in your brain, as are all sensations. The actions of kneeling down, cutting the rose stem, walking into the house, and placing it in a vase originate in your brain, as do all your voluntary actions. The information in this lesson will enable you to use correct medical terminology to:

10.2.1 Describe the essential structures of the brain and spinal cord.

10.2.2 Identify the major sensory and motor areas of the brain.

10.2.3 Explain how the brain and spinal cord are protected and supported.

Abbreviation

CSF cerebrospinal fluid

The Brain (LO 10.4)

Your adult brain weighs about 3 pounds. Its size and weight are proportional to your body size, not your intelligence. Your brain is divided into three major regions: the **cerebrum,** the **brain stem,** and the **cerebellum.**

Cerebrum (LO 10.4)

The cerebrum makes up about 80% of your brain. It consists of two **cerebral** hemispheres, which are mirror images of each other. These hemispheres are separated by a deep longitudinal fissure, and at the bottom of this, they are connected by a bridge of nerve fibers (the **corpus callosum**).

On the surface of the cerebrum, numerous ridges, **gyri,** are separated by fissures called **sulci** *(Figure 10.5)*. The cerebral hemispheres are covered by a thin layer of gray matter (nerve cells and dendrites) called the cerebral **cortex.** It is folded into the gyri, and sulci, and contains 70% of all the neurons in the nervous system. Below the cerebral cortex is a mass of white matter, in which bundles of myelinated nerve fibers connect the neurons of the cortex to the rest of the nervous system.

Functional Cerebral Regions (LO 10.4)

Each cerebral hemisphere is divided into four lobes:

1. The **frontal lobe,** located behind the forehead, forms the anterior part of the hemisphere. This lobe is responsible for intellect, planning, problem solving, and the voluntary motor control of muscles.
2. The **parietal lobe** is posterior to the frontal lobe. This lobe receives and interprets sensory information, like spoken words.
3. The **temporal lobe** is below the frontal and parietal lobes. This lobe interprets sensory experiences.
4. The **occipital lobe** forms the posterior part of the hemisphere. This lobe interprets visual images and written words.

Deep inside each cerebral hemisphere are spaces called ventricles, which contain watery **cerebrospinal fluid (CSF).** CSF circulates through the ventricles and around the brain and spinal cord. It helps to protect, cushion, and provide nutrition for the brain and spinal cord.

Located beneath the cerebral hemispheres and ventricles are the:

- **Thalamus,** which receives all sensory impulses and channels them to the appropriate region of the cortex for interpretation; and
- **Hypothalamus,** *Figure 10.6* which regulates blood pressure, body temperature, water, and electrolyte balance.

Brainstem and Cerebellum (LO 10.4)

The **brainstem** relays sensory impulses from peripheral nerves to higher brain centers. It also controls vital cardiovascular and respiratory activities.

The **cerebellum,** the most posterior area of the brain, coordinates skeletal muscle activity to maintain the body's posture and balance.

▼ **FIGURE 10.5** Brain. (a) View from the left side. (b) View from above.

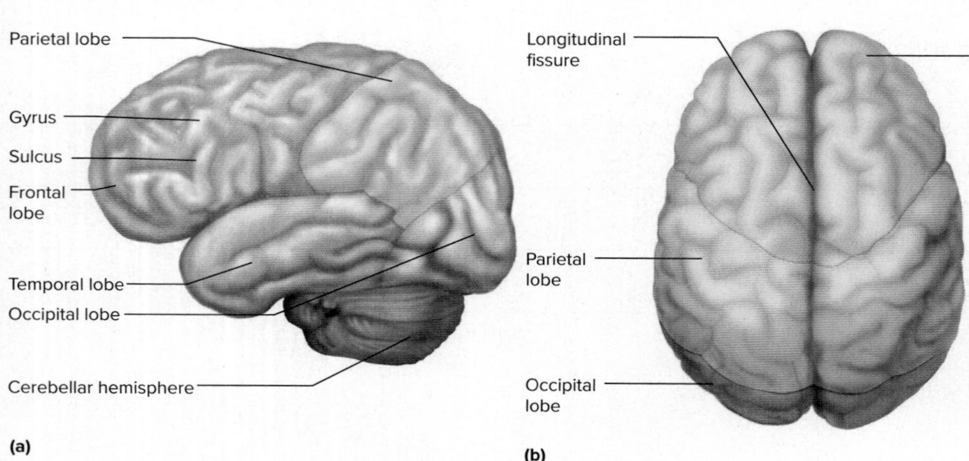

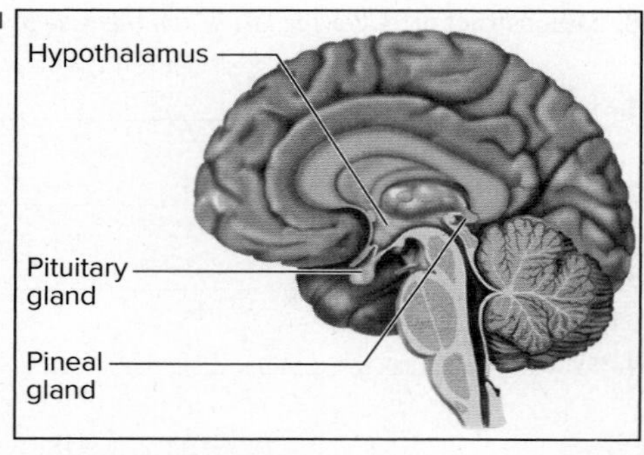

▲ **FIGURE 10.6** Hypothalamus, Pituitary Gland, and Pineal Gland.

Word Analysis and Definition

S = Suffix P = Prefix R = Root R/CF = Combining Form

WORD	PRONUNCIATION	ELEMENTS		DEFINITION
cerebellum	ser-eh-**BELL**-um	S/ R/	**-um** *structure* **cerebell-** *little brain*	The most posterior area of the brain located between the midbrain and the cerebral hemispheres
cerebrospinal (adj) **cerebrospinal fluid (CSF)**	**SER**-ee-broh-**SPY**-nal	S/ R/CF R/	**-al** *pertaining to* **cerebr/o-** *brain* **-spin-** *spinal cord*	Pertaining to the brain and spinal cord Fluid formed in the ventricles of the brain; surrounds the brain and spinal cord
cerebrum **cerebral (adj)**	**SER**-ee-brum **SER**-ee-bral	 S/ R/	Latin *brain* **-al** *pertaining to* **cerebr-** *cerebrum*	Cerebral hemispheres Pertaining to the cerebral hemispheres of the brain
corpus callosum	**KOR**-pus kah-**LOW**-sum	R/ S/ R/	**corpus** *body* **-um** *structure* **callos-** *thickening*	Bridge of nerve fibers connecting the two cerebral hemispheres
frontal lobe	**FRUNT**-al **LOBE**	S/ R/	**-al** *pertaining to* **front-** *front of*	Front area of the cerebral hemisphere
gyrus **gyri (pl)**	**JI**-rus **JI**-ree		Greek *circle*	Rounded elevation on the surface of the cerebral hemispheres
hypothalamus **hypothalamic (adj)**	high-poh-**THAL**-ah-muss high-poh-thah-**LAM**-ik	P/ S/ S/ R/	**hypo-** *below* **-us** *pertaining to* **-ic** *pertaining to* **-thalam-** *thalamus*	An endocrine gland in the floor and wall of the third ventricle of the brain Pertaining to the hypothalamus
occipital lobe	ock-**SIP**-it-al **LOBE**	S/ R/	**-al** *pertaining to* **occipit-** *back of head*	Posterior area of the cerebral hemisphere
parietal lobe	pah-**RYE**-eh-tal **LOBE**	S/ R/	**-al** *pertaining to* **pariet-** *wall*	Area of the brain under the parietal bone
sulcus **sulci (pl)**	**SUL**-cuss **SUL**-sigh		Latin *furrow, ditch*	Groove on the surface of the cerebral hemispheres that separates gyri
temporal lobe	**TEM**-pore-al **LOBE**	S/ R/	**-al** *pertaining to* **tempor-** *time, temple*	Posterior two-thirds of the cerebral hemispheres
thalamus	**THAL**-ah-mus		Greek *inner room*	Mass of gray matter under the ventricle in each cerebral hemisphere

EXERCISES

A. Roots. *The lobes of the cerebral hemispheres share a common suffix -al, meaning pertaining to. It is the root that describes the exact location of the lobe in the cerebral hemispheres. Use your knowledge of roots to understand the anatomical location of the lobes. Fill in the blanks.* **LO 10.1, 10.2, and 10.4**

1. The cerebral lobe located above the ear: ____________________/al. The root means ____________________.

2. The cerebral lobe located behind the forehead: ____________________/al. The root means ____________________.

3. The most posterior cerebral lobe: ____________________/al. The root means: ____________________.

B. Describe the structure of the cerebrum. *Identify the cerebral structures being described. Fill in the blanks.* **LO 10.1, 10.2, and 10.4**

1. Elevation or "ridge" of the cerebrum:

singular form ____

plural form ____________________.

2. Gray covering of the cerebrum: ____________________.

3. Shallow indention of the cerebrum:

singular form ____________________

plural form ____________________.

Cranial Nerves, Spinal Cord, and Meninges (LO 10.4)

Cranial Nerves (LO 10.4)

Your brain communicates with the rest of your body through the cranial nerves and spinal cord. The cranial nerves are part of the peripheral nervous system. They originate on the lower or inferior surface of the brain and are identified by names and numbers, the latter written in Roman numerals *(Figure 10.7)*.

The cranial nerves provide sensory and motor functions for your head and neck areas except for the vagus nerve, which supplies your thorax and abdomen.

Oh	(olfactory-I)
once	(optic-II)
one	(oculomotor-III)
takes	(trochlear-IV)
the	(trigeminal-V)
anatomy	(abducens-VI)
final	(facial-VII)
very	(vestibulocochlear-VIII)
good	(glossopharyngeal-IX)
vacations	(vagus-X)
are	(accessory-XI)
heavenly!	(hypoglossal-XII)

▲ **FIGURE 10.7**
Cranial Nerves
This mnemonic device will help you remember the cranial nerves. Use the sentence in column one (read down) to help you remember the correct order and names of the cranial nerves.

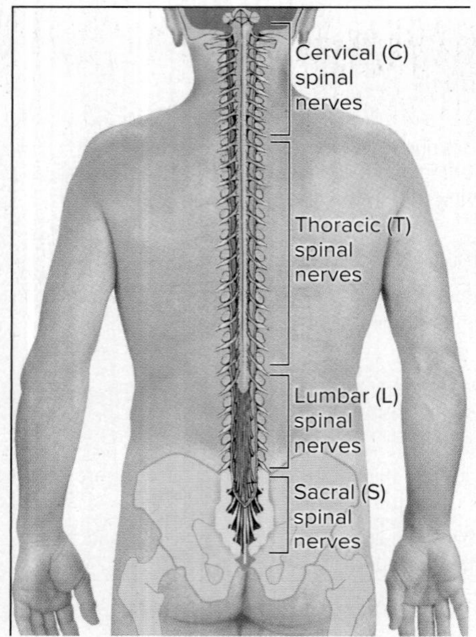

▲ **FIGURE 10.8**
Spinal Cord Regions.

Spinal Cord (LO 10.4)

Your spinal cord lies within, and is protected by, the vertebral canal of the spinal column. It has 31 segments, each of which gives rise to a pair of spinal nerves *(Figure 10.8)*. These are the major link between the brain and the peripheral nervous system, and are the pathway for sensory and motor impulses.

Your spinal cord is divided into four regions *(Figure 10.8)*:

1. The **cervical** region is continuous with the brain stem (lower part of the brain). It contains the motor neurons that supply the neck, shoulders, and upper limbs through 8 pairs of cervical spinal nerves (C1–C8);
2. The **thoracic** region contains the motor neurons that supply the thoracic cage, rib movement, vertebral column movement, and postural back muscles through 12 pairs of thoracic spinal nerves (T1–T12);
3. The **lumbar** region supplies the hips and the front of the lower limbs through 5 pairs of lumbar nerves (L1–L5); and
4. The **sacral** region supplies the buttocks, genitalia, and backs of the lower limbs through 5 sacral nerves (S1–S5) and 1 coccygeal nerve, relative to the small bone at the base of the spine.

Meninges (LO 10.4)

Your brain and spinal cord are protected by the cranium and the vertebrae, cushioned by the CSF, and covered by the **meninges** *(Figure 10.9)*. The meninges have three layers.

1. The **dura mater** is the outermost layer of tough connective tissue attached to the cranium's inner surface. Within the vertebral canal the dura mater splits into two sheets, separated by the **epidural space,** into which epidural injections of medication are given to produce **analgesia** during childbirth or for the treatment of low back pain.
2. The **arachnoid mater** is a thin web over the brain and spinal cord. The CSF is contained in the **subarachnoid space** between the arachnoid and pia mater. It is into this space that a needle is introduced to obtain CSF for testing or to place medication in spinal **anesthesia.**
3. The **pia mater** is the innermost layer of the meninges, attached to the surface of the brain and spinal cord. It supplies nerves and blood vessels that nourish the outer cells of the brain and spinal cord.

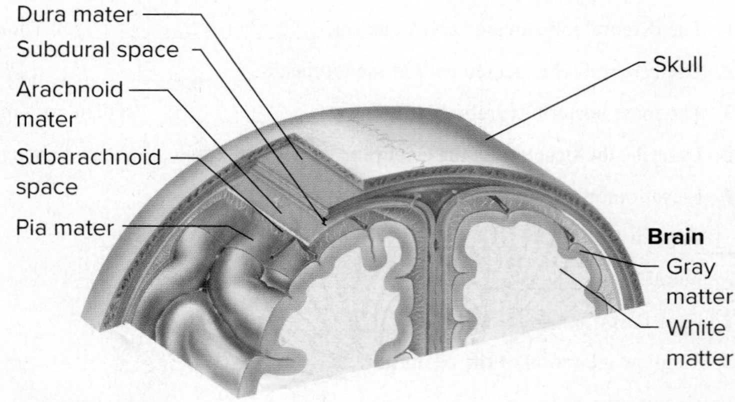

▲ **FIGURE 10.9**
Meninges of Brain.

Word Analysis and Definition

S = Suffix P = Prefix R = Root R/CF = Combining Form

WORD	PRONUNCIATION	ELEMENTS		DEFINITION
analgesia	an-al-**JEE**-zee-ah	S/ P/ R/	-ia *condition* an- *without* -alges- *sensation of pain*	State in which pain is reduced
anesthesia	an-es-**THEE**-zee-ah	S/ P/ R/CF	-ia *condition* an- *without* -esthes- *feeling*	Complete loss of sensation
arachnoid mater	ah-**RACK**-noyd **MAY**-ter	S/ R/ R/	-oid *resembling* arachn- *cobweb, spider* mater *mother*	Weblike middle layer of the three meninges
dura mater (**Note:** *Both terms are stand-alone roots.*)	**DYU**-rah **MAY**-ter	R/ R/	dura *hard* mater *mother*	Hard, fibrous outer layer of the meninges
epidural **epidural space**	ep-ih-**DYU**-ral	S/ P/ R/	-al *pertaining to* epi- *above* -dur- *dura*	Above the dura Space between the dura mater and the wall of the vertebral canal
meninges **meningitis**	meh-**NIN**-jeez men-in-**JIE**-tis	 S/ R/	Greek *membrane* -itis *inflammation* mening- *meninges*	Three-layered covering of the brain and spinal cord Inflammation of the meninges
pia mater *(stand-alone roots)*	**PEE**-ah **MAY**-ter	R/ R/	pia *delicate* mater *mother*	Delicate inner layer of the meninges
subarachnoid space	sub-ah-**RACK**-noyd **SPASE**	S/ P/ R/	-oid *resembling* sub- *under* -arachn *-cobweb, spider*	Space between the pia mater and the arachnoid membrane

Exercises

A. Construct the following *medical terms by filling in the missing elements. Fill in the blanks.* **LO 10.1 and 10.4**

1. under the arachnoid mater: ____________________ /arachn/oid
2. inflammation of the meninges: mening/____________________
3. weblike middle layer of meninges: ____________________/____________________/oid mater
4. pertaining to above the dura: ____________________ /dur/al
5. hard, fibrous outer layer of meninges: ____________________ ____________________

B. Place the meninges in order from superficial to deep. *Place a "1" in the blank for the most superficial layer and "3" for the deepest layer. Fill in the blanks.* **LO 10.4**

__________ arachnoid mater

__________ pia mater

__________ dura mater

C. Deconstruct the terms into their basic elements. *Select the correct answer that completes each sentence.* **LO 10.1 and 10.4**

1. The term that has an element that means below:

   a. epidural **b.** analgesia **c.** subarachnoid **d.** meningitis

2. The term that has an element that means without:

   a. epidural **b.** analgesia **c.** pia mater **d.** meningitis

3. The term that has an element that means hard:

   a. dura mater **b.** analgesia **c.** subarachnoid **d.** pia mater

4. The term that has an element that means delicate:

   a. dura mater **b.** analgesia **c.** subarachnoid **d.** pia mater

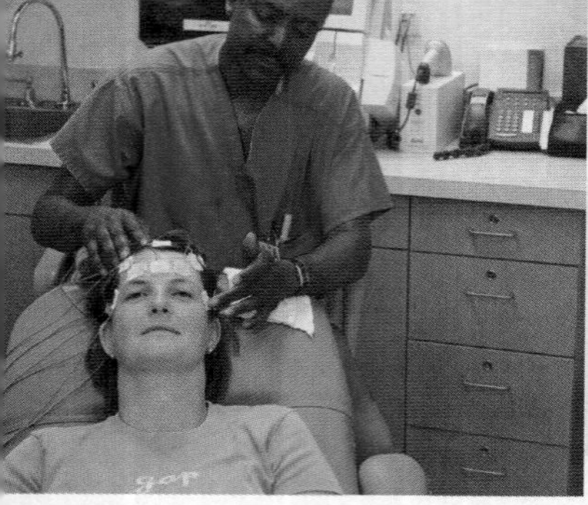

Rick Brady/McGraw-Hill Education

Lesson 10.3

Disorders of the Brain, Cranial Nerves, and Meninges

Objectives

An invaluable benefit of working with patients as a health professional is the opportunity for ongoing learning. By routinely communicating with patients, your education and knowledge of various disorders will continue to be enhanced and reinforced. Information in this lesson will enable you to use correct medical terminology to:

10.3.1 Describe common disorders of the brain, cranial nerves, and meninges.

10.3.2 Communicate about the brain, cranial nerves, and meninges and their disorders with physicians and other health professionals.

Abbreviations

AMS	altered mental state
CVA	cerebrovascular accident
FTD	frontotemporal dementia

CASE REPORT 10.2

You are . . .

. . . a medical assistant working with Dr. Raul Cardenas, a neurologist at Fulwood Medical Center.

You are communicating with . . .

. . . Mr. Lester Rood, a 75-year-old man who was diagnosed with **dementia** a year ago. He lives with his daughter, Judy, and she is with him today.

Patient Interview:

Mr. Rood: "How am I feeling? Scared stiff. Sometimes I don't know where I am. I get so messed up. I can't cook anymore. I forget what I'm doing, can't get things straight. I find myself in the street and don't know how I got there. Judy has to help me shower and remind me to go to the bathroom. And it's only going to get worse. I don't want to be a burden. I used to have 100 people working for me. It's so frustrating, so frightening."

Disorders of the Brain (LO 10.2 and 10.5)

Dementia (LO 10.2 and 10.5)

Your **empathy** allowed Mr. Rood to talk comfortably without interruption. His condition made clear again the specific symptoms of **dementia.** These include an irreversible short-term memory loss, the inability to solve problems, and confusion. Inappropriate behavior, like wandering away, and impaired intellectual function that interferes with normal activities and relationships are also key signs of dementia. Dementia requires a lot of **sympathy** from family and caregivers.

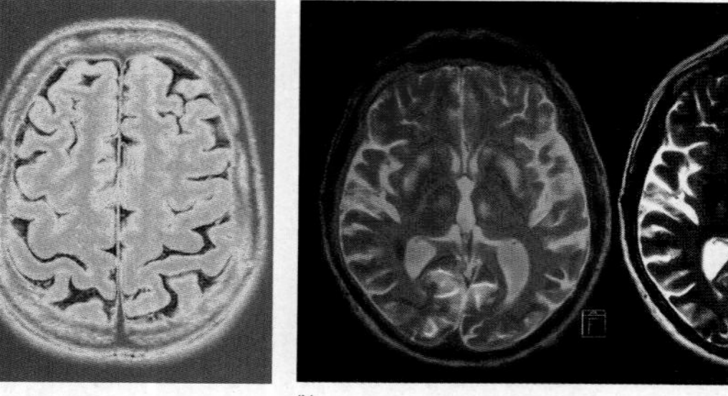

▲ **FIGURE 10.10**
Brain Sections.
(a) MRI scan, normal brain.
(b) MRI scan of Alzheimer disease, showing cerebral atrophy (yellow).

10.10a: PEYROUX/age fotostock;
10.10b: Semnic/Shutterstock

- **Senile dementia** is not a normal part of aging and is not a specific disease. It is a term used for a collection of symptoms that can be caused by a number of disorders affecting the brain.
- **Alzheimer disease** *(Figure 10.10)*–the most common form of dementia–affects 10% of the population over 65, and 50% of the population over 85. Nerve cells in the areas of the brain associated with memory and **cognition** are replaced by abnormal protein clumps and tangles.
- **Vascular dementia**–the second most common form of dementia–can come on gradually when arteries supplying the brain become arteriosclerotic (narrowed or blocked), depriving the brain of oxygen. It can also occur suddenly after a **stroke** *(see later in this chapter).*
- **Frontotemporal dementia (FTD)** is caused by progressive cell degeneration in the brain's frontal and temporal lobes, which control planning and judgment, emotions, speaking and understanding speech, and certain types of movement. It accounts for 10% to 15% of all dementias, but it is more common in those younger than 65.

Word Analysis and Definition

S = Suffix P = Prefix R = Root R/CF = Combining Form

WORD	PRONUNCIATION	ELEMENTS		DEFINITION
Alzheimer disease	**AWLZ**-high-mer diz-**EEZ**		Dr. Alois Alzheimer, German physician, 1864–1915	Common form of dementia
cognition	kog-**NIH**-shun		Latin *knowledge*	Process of acquiring knowledge through thinking, learning, and memory
confusion	kon-**FEW**-zhun	S/ R/	-ion *condition, action* confus- *bewildered*	Mental state in which environmental stimuli are not processed appropriately
delirium	de-**LIR**-ee-um	S/ R/	-um *structure* deliri- *disorientation, confusion*	Acute altered state of consciousness with agitation and disorientation
dementia	dee-**MEN**-she-ah	S/ P/ R/	-ia *condition* de- *removal, without* -ment- *mind*	Chronic, progressive, irreversible loss of the mind's cognitive, and intellectual functions
empathy **sympathy**	**EM**-pah-thee **SIM**-pah-thee	P/ R/ P/ R/	em- *into* -pathy *emotion, disease* sym- *together* -pathy *emotion, disease*	Ability to place yourself into the feelings, emotions, and reactions of another person Appreciation and concern for another person's mental and emotional state
sedative **sedation**	**SED**-ah-tiv seh-**DAY**-shun	S/ R/ S/	-ive *pertaining to, quality of* sedat- *to calm* -ion *condition, action*	Agent that calms nervous excitement State of being calmed
senile	**SEE**-nile	S/ R/	-ile *pertaining to* sen- *old age*	Characteristic of old age
stroke (same as **cerebrovascular accident, CVA)**	STROHK		Old English *to strike*	Acute clinical event caused by impaired cerebral circulation

Exercises

A. Disorders of the brain. *Match each disorder in the first column with its correct description in the second column. Fill in the blanks.* **LO 10.5**

______	**1.** delirium	**a.** common form of dementia due to protein clumps and tangles
______	**2.** Alzheimer disease	**b.** dementia due to decreased blood flow to the brain
______	**3.** confusion	**c.** altered state of consciousness with agitation and disorientation
______	**4.** vascular dementia	**d.** condition in which a person cannot properly process information

B. Identify *the elements in each medical term, and unlock the meaning of the word. Fill in the chart.* **LO 10.1, 10.5, and 10.8**

Medical Term	Meaning of Prefix	Meaning of Root/CF	Meaning of Suffix
dementia	**1.**	**2.**	**3.**
sympathy	**4.**	**5.**	**6.**
delirium	**7.**	**8.**	**9.**
confusion	**10.**	**11.**	**12.**
empathy	**13.**	**14.**	**15.**
sedation	**16.**	**17.**	**18.**

Disorders of the Brain (continued)

Keynotes

- **Epilepsy affects 1 in 200 people, and 50% of cases develop before age 10.**
- **Status epilepticus is a medical emergency and requires maintenance of the airway, breathing, and circulation and intravenous administration of anticonvulsant drugs.**
- **The first-aid treatment during a seizure is to place the person in a reclining position, cushion the head, and turn the person on his or her side. Do not try to hold down the person's arms or legs or restrain the tongue.**
- **There is no cure for tic disorders, but they can be treated pharmacologically with haloperidol or clonidine.**

Dementia *(continued)* (LO 10.5)

Other conditions causing dementia include reactions to medications, like **sedatives** and antiarthritics; depression in the elderly; and infections, such as AIDS or encephalitis.

Confusion is used to describe people who cannot process information normally. They cannot answer questions appropriately, understand where they are, or remember important facts, like their name and address.

Delirium is an altered mental state **(AMS),** characterized by the sudden onset of disorientation, an inability to think clearly or pay attention. The level of consciousness varies from increased wakefulness to drowsiness. It is not a disease, it is reversible, and it can be part of dementia or a stroke.

Case Report 10.1 *(continued from the chapter opening)*

For Ms. Roberta Gaston, who was seen in Dr. Solis's neurosurgery clinic, the EEG did not pinpoint an epileptic source. In order to further investigate the source, Dr. Solis inserted deep brain electrodes into the region of the suspicious mass that showed on the MRI. Seizures were recorded arising in the mass itself. Dr. Solis performed a surgical resection of the mass, which was a **glioma**. Ms Gaston has been seizure-free since the surgery a year ago.

Epilepsy (LO 10.5)

Epilepsy is a chronic disorder in which clusters of neurons (nerve cells) discharge their electrical signals in an abnormal rhythm. This disturbed electrical activity (a **seizure** or a **convulsion**) can cause strange sensations and behavior, convulsions, and loss of consciousness. The causes of epilepsy are numerous, from abnormal brain development to brain damage.

The International League Against Epilepsy created the following classification system for seizures:

1. **Partial seizures** occur when the epileptic activity is in one localized area of the brain only, causing, for example, involuntary jerking movements of a single limb.
2. **Generalized seizures** can be categorized into one of the following three types:
   a. **Absence seizures,** previously known as **"petit mal,"** which begin between ages 5 and 10. The child stares vacantly for a few seconds and may be accused of daydreaming.
   b. **Tonic-clonic seizures,** previously called **"grand mal,"** which are dramatic. The person experiences a **loss of consciousness (LOC),** breathing stops, the eyes roll up, and the jaw is clenched. This "tonic" phase lasts for 30 to 60 seconds. It is followed by the "clonic" phase, in which the whole body shakes with a series of violent, rhythmic jerkings of the limbs. The seizures last for a couple of minutes, and then consciousness returns.
   c. **Febrile seizures,** which are triggered by a fever in infants and toddlers aged 6 months to 5 years. Very few of these children go on to develop epilepsy.

Status epilepticus is considered to be a medical emergency. It is defined as having one continuous seizure or recurrent seizures without regaining consciousness for 30 minutes or more.

Any seizure may be followed by a period of diminished function in the area of the brain surrounding the seizure's main origin. This temporary neurologic deficit is called a **postictal** state.

Tourette syndrome and other **tic** disorders are characterized by episodes of involuntary, rapid, repetitive, fixed movements of individual muscle groups in the face or the limbs. They are associated with meaningless vocal sounds or meaningful words and phrases. The tics may be genetic.

Narcolepsy is a chronic disorder in which patients fall asleep during the day—from a few seconds up to an hour. There is no cure.

Case Report 10.1 *(continued)*

Ms. Gaston suffered from both **absence** and **tonic-clonic** seizures.

Word Analysis and Definition

S = Suffix P = Prefix R = Root R/CF = Combining Form

WORD	PRONUNCIATION	ELEMENTS		DEFINITION
grand mal	**GRAHN** MAL	R/ R/	grand *big* mal *bad*	Previous name for generalized tonic-clonic seizure
narcolepsy	**NAR**-koh-lep-see	S/ R/CF	-lepsy *seizure* narc/o- *stupor*	Involuntary falling asleep
petit mal	peh-**TEE** MAL	R/ R/	petit *small* mal *bad*	Previous name for absence seizures
postictal (adj)	post-**IK**-tal	S/ P/ R/	-al *pertaining to* post- *after* -ict- *seizure*	Transient neurologic deficit after a seizure
ictal (adj)	**IK**-tal	S/	-al *pertaining to*	Pertaining to, or a condition caused by, a stroke or epilepsy
tic	TIK		French *tic*	Sudden, involuntary, repeated contraction of muscles
tonic	**TON**-ik	S/ R/	-ic *pertaining to* ton- *pressure, tension*	State of muscular contraction
tonic-clonic seizure	**TON**-ik-**KLON**-ik **SEE**-zhur	R/ S/ R/	clon- *tumult* -ure *process* seiz- *to grab*	The body alternates between excessive muscular rigidity (tonic) and jerking muscular contractions (clonic)
Tourette syndrome	tur-**ET SIN**-drome		Gilles de la Tourette, French neurologist, 1857–1904	Disorder of multiple motor and vocal tics

EXERCISES

A. Refer to Case Report 10.1 (continued from the chapter opening) *to correctly complete each statement and answer the question. Fill in the blanks.* **LO 10.2, 10.3, 10.5, and 10.8**

1. Provide the medical term (not the abbreviation) for the diagnostic test that can determine the the electrical activity of the brain: _________
2. Provide the medical term (not the abbreviation) for the diagnostic test that provided an image of the mass: ______
3. The cause of Ms. Gaston's seizures is a(n):_________
4. Provide the therapeutic procedure written in the Case Report that Dr. Solis performed:_________
5. Did the therapeutic procedure correct Ms. Gaston's neurological disorder? (yes or no) ______

B. In practice, *you will find that some people will use the new terms for seizures, and some will use the older traditional terms. It is important that you know both. Fill in the blanks with the correct term.* **LO 10.2 and 10.5**

1. A tonic-clonic seizure is traditionally known as a ______ mal seizure.
2. An absence seizure is traditionally known as a ______ mal seizure.

C. Signs of brain disorders. *Match the sign of the brain disorder in the first column with its corresponding condition in the second column. Fill in the blanks.* **LO 10.5**

______	**1.** multiple seizures for 30 minutes without regaining consciousness	**a.** absence seizure
______	**2.** infant with high fever	**b.** narcolepsy
______	**3.** child appears to be daydreaming	**c.** febrile seizure
______	**4.** transient neurologic deficit after a seizure	**d.** Tourette syndrome
______	**5.** person suddenly falls asleep	**e.** status epilepticus
______	**6.** a tic disorder	**f.** postictal state

Lesson 10.3 (cont'd) Disorders of the Brain (continued)

Keynotes

- **Risk factors for ischemic strokes are hypertension, diabetes mellitus, high cholesterol levels, cigarettes, and obesity.**
- **Risk factors for hemorrhagic strokes are hypertension, cerebral arteriovenous malformations, and cerebral aneurysms.**
- **One-third of people with TIAs have subsequent TIAs, and one-third have a subsequent full-blown stroke.**

Abbreviations

ASD	autism spectrum disorder
BSE	bovine spongiform encephalopathy
CJD	Creutzfeldt-Jakob disease
CVA	cerebrovascular accident
TIA	transient ischemic attack
tPA	tissue plasminogen activator

Cerebrovascular Accidents (CVAs) or Strokes (LO 10.3 and 10.5)

A stroke (also known as a cerebrovascular accident or CVA) occurs when the blood supply to a part of the brain is suddenly interrupted, depriving the brain cells of oxygen. Some cells die; others are badly damaged. With timely treatment, the damaged cells can be saved. There are two types of stroke:

1. **Ischemic strokes** account for 90% of all strokes and are caused by:
   a. **Atherosclerosis:** Plaque in the wall of a cerebral artery *(Figure 10.11a);* or
   b. **Embolism:** A blood clot in a cerebral artery originating from elsewhere in the body *(Figure 10.11b).*

   Treatment of ischemic strokes is by thrombolysis together with clot busters like **tissue plasminogen activator (tPA).** This must occur within 3½ hours of the stroke, using supportive measures followed by rehabilitation.

2. **Hemorrhagic strokes (intracranial hemorrhage)** occur when a blood vessel in the brain bursts or when a cerebral **aneurysm** ruptures.

   Cerebral arteriography can determine the site of bleeding in hemorrhagic stroke. A surgical procedure can be performed to stop the bleed or clip off the aneurysm.

Transient Ischemic Attack (TIA) (LO 10.3 and 10.5)

Transient ischemic attacks **(TIAs)** are small, short-term strokes with symptoms lasting for less than 24 hours. If neurologic symptoms persist for more than 24 hours, the condition is a full-blown stroke with brain cell damage and death.

The most frequent cause of TIAs is a small embolus that occludes (blocks) a small artery in the brain. Often, the embolus arises from a clot in the atrium in atrial fibrillation or from an atherosclerotic plaque in a carotid artery. Treatment is directed at the underlying cause. A **carotid endarterectomy** may be necessary if a carotid artery is significantly blocked with plaque.

Other Brain Disorders (LO 10.3 and 10.5)

Parkinson disease is caused by the degeneration of neurons in the basal ganglia that produce a neurotransmitter called dopamine. Motor symptoms of abnormal movements, **tremor** of the hands, rigidity, a shuffling gait, and weak voice appear, and gradually become more and more severe. There is no cure.

Creutzfeld-Jakob disease (CJD) produces a rapid deterioration of mental function, with difficulty in muscle movement coordination. Some cases are linked to the consumption of beef from cattle with mad cow disease **(bovine spongiform encephalopathy, BSE).**

Syncope (fainting or passing out) is a temporary loss of consciousness and posture. It is usually due to hypotension and the associated deficient oxygen supply (hypoxia) to the brain.

Migraine produces an intense throbbing, pulsating pain in one area of the head, often with nausea and vomiting. It can be preceded by an aura, visual disturbances like flashing lights, or temporary loss of vision. Prevention is difficult.

Encephalitis, an inflammation of the parenchyma (tissue) of the brain, is often caused by a virus such as HIV, West Nile virus, herpes simplex, or childhood measles, mumps, chickenpox, and rubella.

Brain abscess is usually a direct spread of infection from sinusitis, otitis media (middle ear infection), or mastoiditis (an infection in the skull bone behind the ear). It can also result from blood-borne pathogens arising from lung or dental infections.

Brain tumors are often secondary tumors that have metastasized from cancers in the lung, breast, skin, or kidney. Primary brain tumors arise from any of the glial cells and are called gliomas. In Case Report 10.1, Ms. Gaston has a glioma.

Autism spectrum disorder (ASD) is a range of complex developmental disorders characterized by communication difficulties, impaired social interactions, and rigid or repetitive patterns of behavior. It is estimated that more than 1% of children aged eight will have an ASD, and it is four times as likely to occur in males than females. It occurs in all ethnic and socioeconomic groups. Twenty to 30% of children with an ASD develop epilepsy before reaching adulthood. Treatment is with highly structured educational and behavioral interventions. Medications can be used to treat autism-related symptoms, such as depression and seizures.

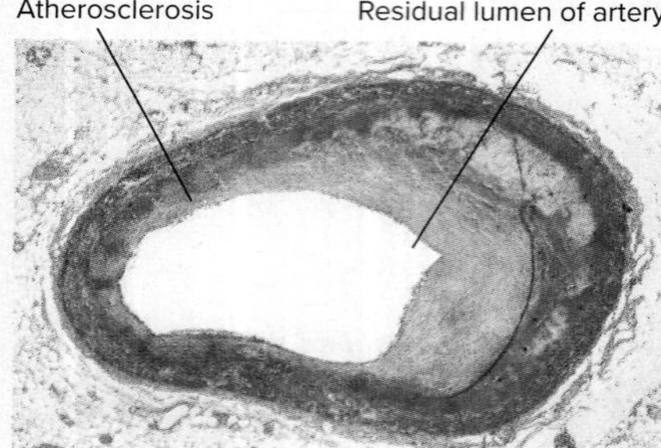

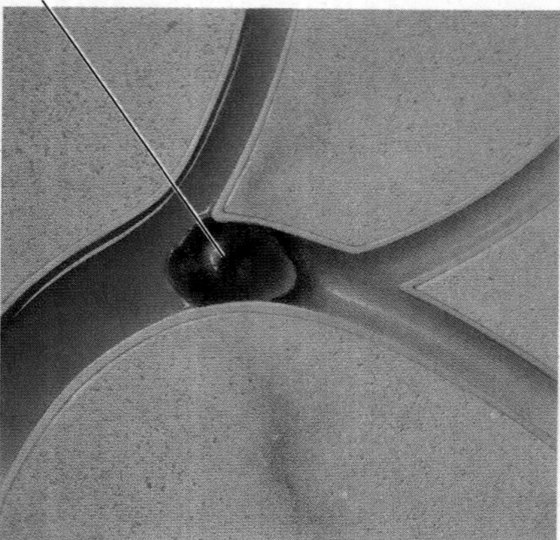

FIGURE 10.11
Causes of Ischemic Strokes.
(a) Atherosclerosis in a cerebral artery, leaving a small, residual lumen.
(b) Embolus blocking an artery. Healthy tissue is on the left (pink) and blood-starved tissue is on the right (blue).

10.11a: Kateryna Kon/Shutterstock

Word Analysis and Definition

S = Suffix P = Prefix R = Root R/CF = Combining Form

WORD	PRONUNCIATION	ELEMENTS		DEFINITION
aneurysm	**AN**-yur-izm		Greek *dilation*	Small, circumscribed dilation of an artery or cardiac chamber
arteriography	ar-teer-ee-**OG**-rah-fee	S/ R/CF	-graphy *recording* arteri/o- *artery*	X-ray visualization of an artery after injection of contrast material
autism	**AWE**-tizm		Greek *self*	A disorder with severely abnormal social and communication skills
autistic	awe-**TIS**-tik	S/ R/	-tic *pertaining to* autis- *autism*	Pertaining to autism
bovine spongiform encephalopathy (BSE)	**BO**-vine **SPON**-jee-form en-sef-ah-**LOP**-ah-thee	S/ R/ S/ R/CF S/ R/CF	-ine *pertaining to* bov- *cattle* -form *appearance of* spong/i- *sponge* -pathy *disease* encephal/o- *head*	Disease of cattle ("mad cow disease") that can be transmitted to humans, causing Creutzfeldt-Jakob disease
carotid endarterectomy	kah-**ROT**-id **END**-ar-ter-**EK**-toe-me	 S/ P/ R/	carotid, Greek *large neck artery* -ectomy *surgical excision* end- *inside* -arter- *artery*	Surgical removal of diseased lining from the carotid artery to leave a smooth lining and restore blood flow
Creutzfeldt-Jakob disease (CJD)	**KROITS**-felt **YAK**-op **DIZ**-eez		Hans Creutzfeldt, 1885–1964, and Alfons Jakob, 1884–1931, German psychiatrists	Progressive, incurable, neurologic disease caused by infectious prions
encephalitis	en-**SEF**-ah-**LIE**-tis	S/ R/	-itis *inflammation* encephal- *brain*	Inflammation of brain cells and tissues
migraine	**MY**-grain	P/ R/	mi- *derived from hemi, half* -graine *head pain*	Paroxysmal severe headache confined to one side of the head
Parkinson disease	**PAR**-kin-son diz-**EEZ**		James Parkinson, British physician, 1755–1824	Disease of muscular rigidity, tremors, and a mask-like facial expression
prion	**PREE**-on		Latin *protein*	Small, infectious protein particle
syncope	**SIN**-koh-pee		Greek *cutting short*	Temporary loss of consciousness and postural tone due to diminished cerebral blood flow
tremor	**TREM**-or		Latin *to shake*	Small, shaking, involuntary, repetitive movements of hands, extremities, neck, or jaw

EXERCISES

A. Diagnosis: *Patient documentation is given to you below. Select the correct language of neurology for the diagnosis.* **LO 10.5 and 10.8**

1. Patient is experiencing shaking, involuntary movements of her extremities.
   Diagnosis: **a.** *syncope* **b.** *prion* **c.** *tremor*
2. Radiologic studies show a small, circumscribed dilation of the cerebral artery.
   Diagnosis: **a.** *Parkinson disease* **b.** *aneurysm* **c.** *migraine*
3. The patient's paroxysmal headache is confined to the left temporal region.
   Diagnosis: **a.** *syncope* **b.** *tremor* **c.** *migraine*
4. Tests and studies have confirmed inflammation of the brain cells and tissues to make this diagnosis.
   Diagnosis: **a.** *meningitis* **b.** *fasciitis* **c.** *encephalitis*
5. This patient has experienced loss of consciousness due to diminished cerebral blood flow.
   Diagnosis: **a.** *syncope* **b.** *tremor* **c.** *migraine*

B. Provide the abbreviation *for the described condition. Fill in the blanks.* **LO 10.3, 10.5, and 10.8**

1. Short episodes of low oxygen delivery to the brain usually due to an embolus: ____________________
2. An embolus in a cerebral artery that is stopping the delivery of oxygen to an area of the brain: ____________________
3. Rapid deterioration of mental function, some of which are caused by BSE: ____________________
4. General term that describes a condition that has a range of developmental disorders including physical repetitive movements: ____________________

Lesson 10.3 (cont'd)

Traumatic Brain Injury (TBI) (LO 10.3 and 10.5)

Keynote

- **About 5.3 million Americans (2% of the population) are living with disabilities from TBI.**

Traumatic brain injury (TBI) results from any one of many types of injuries to the head, from a bad fall on a hard surface to a car accident to war injuries. Every year, physicians treat over 1 million patients who have experienced TBI; as many as 10% of these have long-term damage affecting their normal **activities of daily living (ADLs).**

Imagine driving your car along the highway at 50 miles per hour. Suddenly, you are hit head-on by another driver. Your brain goes from 50 miles per hour to zero—instantly. Your soft brain is propelled forward and squished against the front of your hard skull **(coup).** Next, you rebound backward, and your brain slams against the back of your skull **(contrecoup).** Your brain now has at least one bruise or **contusion,** if not worse damage.

A mild head injury **(concussion)** may leave you feeling dazed, confused, or unable to recall the event that caused your concussion. Repeated concussions, like those experienced by famous boxer Muhammad Ali, have a cumulative effect, leading to a reduced mental ability and reaction time, and/or trauma-induced Parkinson's disease.

A severe injury may include torn blood vessels that bleed into the brain. The brain may also tear, or swell within the hard, inflexible skull, cutting off important signals and connections.

Shaken baby syndrome (SBS) is a type of TBI produced when a baby is violently shaken. A baby has weak neck muscles and a heavy head. Shaking makes the brain bounce back and forth in the skull, leading to severe brain damage.

Posttraumatic stress disorder is discussed later in this chapter, in Lesson 10.6 Mental Health.

Disorders of the Meninges (LO 10.5)

Meningitis is an inflammation of the membranes (meninges) covering the brain and spinal cord. Viral meningitis—the most common form—can occur at any age. Bacterial meningitis predominantly affects the very young or very old. **Meningococcal** meningitis is contagious, transmitted through a simple cough or sneeze. It is most commonly passed among people who live in close quarters—such as students in college dormitories. Vaccines are available to prevent most types of meningitis.

A **subdural hematoma** is bleeding into the subdural space below the dura mater, which is frequently associated with closed-head injuries and bleeding from broken veins caused by violent head rotations.

An **epidural hematoma** is a pooling of blood in the epidural space between the skull and the dura mater, often associated with a fractured skull and bleeding from an artery within the meninges.

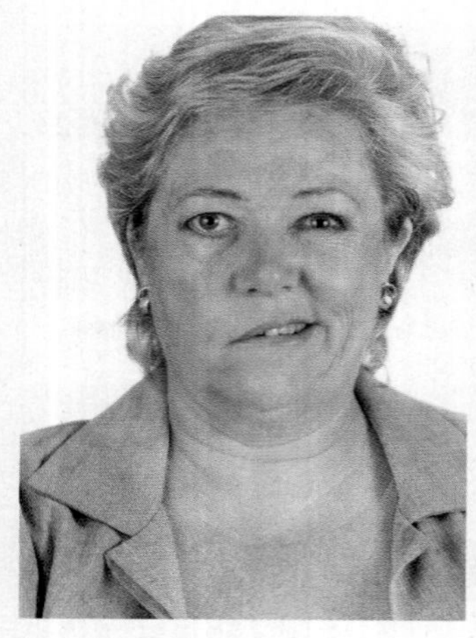

▲ **FIGURE 10.12** Bell Palsy of Left Side of Face.

Jo Ann Snover/Shutterstock

Disorders of the Cranial Nerves (LO 10.5)

Bell palsy is a facial nerve (vii) disorder characterized by a sudden weakness or paralysis of muscles on one side of the face. The inability to smile or whistle, the uncontrollable drooping of the mouth and drooling of saliva, and an inability to close the eye *(Figure 10.12)* are common symptoms. The use of steroids in the early stages can prevent the paralysis from becoming permanent.

Trigeminal neuralgia (TN), **tic douloureux,** is an extremely painful chronic disorder of the trigeminal (v) cranial nerve caused by nerve injury or compression of the nerve by a blood vessel. The facial pain can be constant or sporadic and is very intense. The anticonvulsant carbamazepine (Tegretol) is the first-line treatment, and opiates can be prescribed for pain. The evidence for a good result from surgical treatment is poor.

An **acoustic neuroma** is a benign, slow-growing tumor on the vestibulocochlear (viii) nerve that causes hearing loss, tinnitus, and dizziness. Treatment is with surgery and/or radiation.

Pain Management (LO 10.5)

It's estimated that more than 6 million Americans are affected by the acute or chronic pain of **fibromyalgia,** 5 million are disabled by back pain, and 40 million suffer from recurrent headaches. Interventional procedures (such as nerve blocks or trigger point injections) can target the tissue or the organ causing pain, and physical medicine and rehabilitation **(physiatry)** can use physical techniques such as heat, electrotherapy, therapeutic exercises, and biofeedback techniques. Pain management practitioners include anesthesiologists, physiatrists, physiotherapists, occupational therapists, and chiropractors.

Medications prescribed based on the severity of the pain include:

- **Analgesics** (such as acetaminophen) and nonsteroidal anti-inflammatory drugs (NSAIDs) for mild pain;
- **Opiods** (codeine, hydrocodone, and oxycodone) in combination with analgesics for moderate pain; and
- Higher doses of opiates for severe pain. These are often used on their own, and include **morphine** and fentanyl.

Abbreviations

ADL	activity of daily living
NSAID	nonsteroidal anti-inflammatory drug
SBS	shaken baby syndrome
TBI	traumatic brain injury
TN	trigeminal neuralgia

Word Analysis and Definition

S = Suffix P = Prefix R = Root R/CF = Combining Form

WORD	PRONUNCIATION	ELEMENTS		DEFINITION
acoustic	ah-**KYU**-stik		Greek *hearing*	Pertaining to hearing
analgesia **analgesic (adj)**	an-al-**JEE**-zee-ah an-al-**JEE**-zik	S/ P/ R/ S/	**-ia** *condition* **an-** *without* **-alges-** *sensation of pain* **-ic** *pertaining to*	State in which pain is reduced Substance that produces analgesia
Bell palsy	BELL **PAWL**-zee		Charles Bell, Scottish -surgeon, 1774–1842	Paresis, or paralysis, of one side of the face
concussion	kon-**KUSH**-un	S/ R/	**-ion** *action, condition* **concuss-** *shake or jar violently*	Mild brain injury
contrecoup	**KON**-treh-koo		French *counterblow*	Injury to the brain at a point directly opposite the point of contact
contusion	kon-**TOO**-zhun	S/ R/	**-ion** *action, condition* **contus-** *bruise*	Hemorrhage into a tissue (bruising), including the brain
coup	KOO		French *a blow*	Injury to the brain directly under the skull at the point of contact
fibromyalgia	fie-broh-my-**AL**-jee-ah	S/ R/CF R/	**-algia** *pain* **fibr/o-** *fiber* **-my-** *muscle*	Pain in the muscle fibers
meningococcal	meh-nin-goh-**KOK**-al	S/ R/CF R/	**-al** *pertaining to* **mening/o-** *meninges* **-cocc-** *round bacterium*	Pertaining to the meningococcus bacterium
neuroma	nyu-**ROH**-mah	S/ R/	**-oma** *tumor* **neur-** *nerve*	Any tumor arising from cells in the nervous system
subdural space	sub-**DYU**-ral SPASE	S/ P/ R/	**-al** *pertaining to* **sub-** *below* **-dur-** *dura, hard*	Space between the arachnoid and dura mater layers of the meninges
trauma **traumatic**	**TRAW**-mah traw-**MAT**-ik	 S/ R/	Greek *wound* **-tic** *pertaining to* **trauma-** *injury*	A physical or mental injury Pertaining to or caused by trauma
trigeminal **neuralgia**	try-**GEM**-in-al nyu-**RAL**-jee-ah	S/ P/ R/ S/ R/	**-al** *pertaining to* **tri-** *three* **-gemin-** *double* **-algia** *pain* **neur-** *nerve*	Fifth (v) cranial nerve with three branches supplying the face Trigeminal neuralgia; painful facial muscles supplied by the trigeminal nerve
tic douloureux	TIK duh-luh-**RUE**		**douloureux** French *painful tic*	Synonym for trigeminal neuralgia

EXERCISE

A. Diseases and disorders. *Are you familiar enough with their terminology and symptoms to match the correct disease or disorder with the appropriate statement for each patient? Select the correct answer that completes each sentence.* **LO 10.5**

1. The patient has a slow-growing tumor tumor on the vestibulochochlear nerve:

a. acoustic neuroma **b.** tic douloureaux **c.** intracranial hemorrhage

2. Patient has inflammation of the coverings of the brain:

a. meningitis **b.** encephalitis **c.** vasculitis

3. Brain injury occurred after the patient was hit head-on while driving his truck:

a. acoustic neuroma **b.** Bell palsy **c.** countrecoup

4. Patient complains of intermittent, shooting pain in the area of the face and head:

a. trigeminal neuralgia **b.** peripheral neuropathy **c.** neuritis

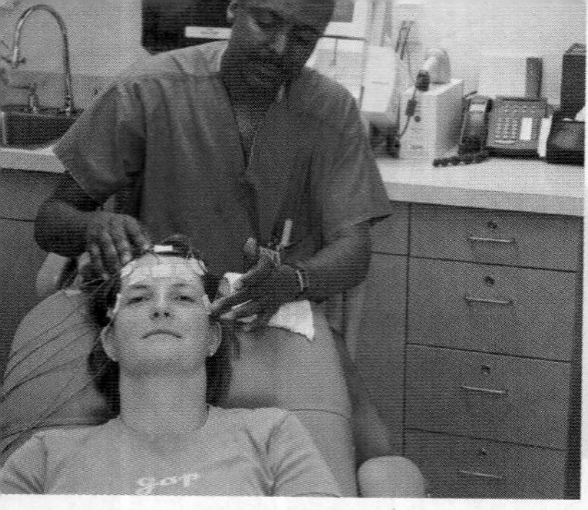

Rick Brady/McGraw-Hill Education

Lesson 10.4

Disorders of the Spinal Cord and Peripheral Nerves

Objectives

Many disorders of the nervous system can affect the spinal cord and the peripheral nerves without affecting the brain. In this lesson, the information will enable you to use correct medical terminology to:

10.4.1 Discuss disorders of the spinal cord and peripheral nerves.

10.4.2 Communicate about the nervous system and its disorders with patients and other health professionals.

10.4.3 Name common congenital disorders of the nervous system.

CASE REPORT 10.3

You are . . .

. . . Tanisha Colis, an electroneurodiagnostic technologist working for Raul Cardenas, MD, a neurologist at Fulwood Medical Center.

You are communicating with . . .

. . . Mrs. Suzanne Kalish, a 42-year-old social worker employed by the medical center. Mrs. Kalish has recently had an exacerbation of her symptoms due to **multiple sclerosis (MS)**. She is going to have a visual evoked potential **(VEP)** test, followed by an MRI of her brain and spinal cord.

Patient Interview:

Tanisha: "Good morning, Mrs. Kalish. I'm Tanisha Colis, the technologist who'll be performing your visual evoked potential test. How are you feeling?"

Mrs. Kalish: "I've been doing OK for the last 4 or 5 years. Then, a few weeks ago, I started dragging my right foot like a wounded witch. I've got to hang onto the walls to stay vertical. I'm tired out, can't come to work. It's a struggle to walk the few yards just to pick up the mail."

Tanisha: "The MRI you are going to have today will give us a lot of information about what's going on."

Mrs. Kalish: "My mind is going 'wheelchair, wheelchair, wheelchair.' Especially since in the last couple of days the vision in my right eye has gotten all blurred."

Tanisha: "That's the reason you are having the visual evoked potential test."

Mrs. Kalish: "I hate this disease. If I had cancer, I've got a chance. I'd fight it to the end, whatever that would be. Nobody's ever beat MS. You can only lose. It can be kind and leave you for a while, but it's never far away."

Tanisha: "Let me help you up, and we'll go get this test done."

Mrs. Kalish: "I can manage, thank you."

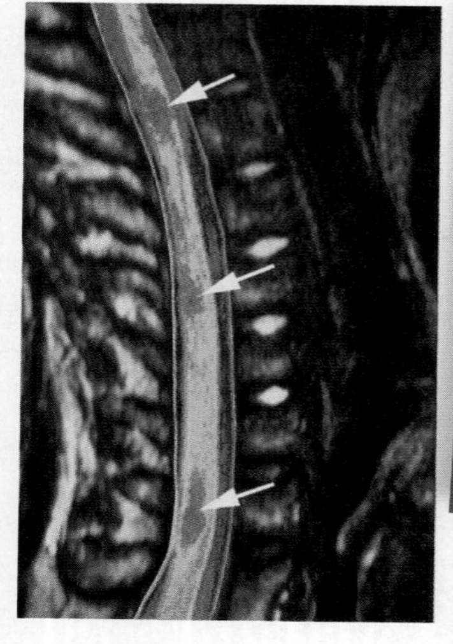

▲ **FIGURE 10.13**
Multiple Sclerosis of the Spinal Cord.
Areas of demyelination are arrowed and shown in red.

Source: CAVALLINI JAMES/BSIP/age fotostock

Abbreviations

MS	multiple sclerosis
PNS	peripheral nervous system
VEP	visual evoked potential

Disorders of the Myelin Sheath of Nerve Fibers (LO 10.5)

When the myelin sheath surrounding nerve fibers is damaged, nerves do not conduct impulses normally. In newborns, many of their nerves have immature myelin sheaths, which is why some of their movements are jerky and uncoordinated.

Demyelination, the destruction of an area of the myelin sheath, can occur in the PNS and be caused by inflammation, vitamin B_{12} deficiency, poisons, and some medications.

Multiple sclerosis (MS), a chronic, progressive disorder, is the most common condition in which demyelination of nerve fibers in the brain, spinal cord, and optic nerves can occur *(Figure 10.13).* **Intermittent** myelin damage and scarring slow nerve impulses. This leads to muscle weakness, pain, abnormal sensations **(paresthesias),** numbness, and vision loss. Because different nerve fibers are affected at different times, MS symptoms often worsen **(exacerbations)** or show partial or complete reduction **(remissions).** Suzanne Kalish is now in an exacerbation.

Word Analysis and Definition

S = Suffix P = Prefix R = Root R/CF = Combining Form

WORD	PRONUNCIATION		ELEMENTS	DEFINITION
demyelination	dee-**MY**-eh-lin-A-shun	S/ P/ R/	-ation *process* de- *without* -myelin- *myelin*	Process of losing the myelin sheath of a nerve fiber
exacerbation (contrast **remission**)	ek-zas-er-**BAY**-shun	S/ R/	-ion *condition, action* exacerbat- *increase, aggravate*	Period when there is an increase in the severity of a disease
intermittent	IN-ter-**MIT**-ent	S/ P/ R/	-ent *end result* inter- *between* -mitt- *send*	Alternately ceasing and beginning again
modify	**MOD**-ih-fie		Latin *to limit*	Change the form or qualities of something; here, the pathology of MS
paresthesia **paresthesias (pl)** (**Note:** the "a" following the "r" in *para* is dropped for ease of pronunciation.)	par-es-**THEE**-ze-ah	S/ P/ R/	-ia *condition* par(a)- *abnormal* -esthes- *sensation*	Abnormal sensation; e.g., tingling, burning, pricking
remission (contrast **exacerbation**)	ree-**MISH**-un	S/ P/ R/	-ion *condition, action* re- *back* -miss- *send*	Period when there is a lessening or absence of the symptoms of a disease
sclerosis	skleh-**ROH**-sis	S/ R/CF	-sis *abnormal condition* scler/o- *hardness*	Thickening and hardening of a tissue; in the nervous system, hardening of nervous tissue by fibrous and glial connective tissue

EXERCISES

A. Review Case Report 10.3. *Select the answer that answers the question or completes the statement.* **LO 10.3, 10.5, 10.8, and 10.9**

1. Why did Dr. Cardenas order the VEP for Mrs. Kalish?
   a. she has trouble standing **b.** she has blurred vision **c.** her energy level has decreased
2. Mrs. Kalish states that her condition will "...leave you for a while, but it's never far away." The medical term for her statement is:
   a. exacerbation **b.** acute **c.** remission
3. Which disorder does Mrs. Kalish have?
   a. peripheral neuritis **b.** fibromyalgia **c.** multiple sclerosis
4. The focus of Dr. Cadenas's speciality is to:
   a. treat autoimmune diseases **c.** medically treat neurological disorders
   b. surgically treat neurological disorders **d.** counsel patients on psychological disorders

B. Test yourself *on the elements and terms related to neurologic disorders. Select the correct answer.* **LO 10.1 and 10.5**

1. The term *intermittent* contains:
   a. prefix, root, and suffix **b.** prefix and root **c.** combining form and suffix
2. *Remission* is the opposite of:
   a. intermittent **b.** exacerbation **c.** demyelination
3. *To modify* something is to:
   a. dispose of it **b.** change it **c.** renew it
4. In the term *demyelination* the prefix means:
   a. without **b.** in front of **c.** half
5. If a disease is *exacerbated,* it:
   a. is more severe **b.** has not changed **c.** is less severe

Lesson **10.4** (cont'd)

Keynote

- **Approximately half a million people in the United States have spinal cord injuries (SCIs). There are approximately 8,000 new injuries each year, of which 82% involve males between the ages of 16 and 30.**

Abbreviations

SCI	spinal cord injury
PPS	Postpolio syndrome
ALS	Amyotrophic lateral sclerosis
POLIO	Poliomyelitis

▼ FIGURE 10.14
Spinal Cord Injuries.
(a) Severed spinal cord from fracture-dislocation of vertebra.
(b) Compressed spinal cord with vertebral fracture.

10.14a: Richman Photo/Shutterstock
10.14b: Suttha Burawonk/Shutterstock

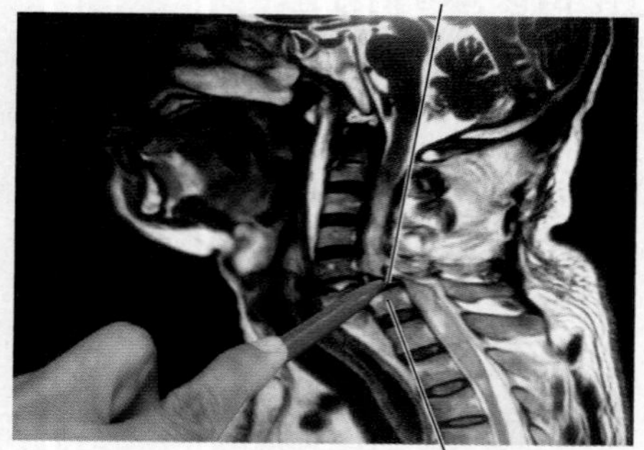

(a)

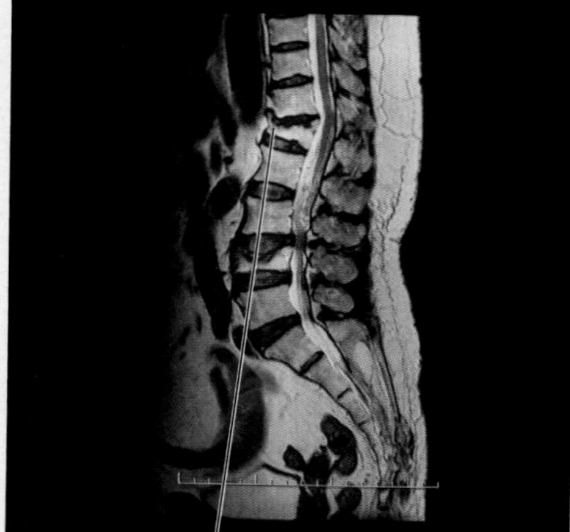

(b)

Disorders of the Myelin Sheath of Nerve Fibers (continued) (LO 10.5)

MS, most common in women, has an average age of onset between 18 and 35 years. Its cause is unknown, but it is thought to be an autoimmune disease. There is no known cure for MS, but currently there are 10 medications that help to slow the disease's progress. For people with relapsing MS, like Mrs. Kalish, high doses of corticosteroids are used to treat severe exacerbations, and three oral and four injectable medications are available for less severe exacerbations. Other drugs are in the research pipeline. Rehabilitation programs that focus on function are also of value.

Disorders of the Spinal Cord (LO 10.5)

Trauma (LO 10.5)

The spinal cord can be injured in three ways:

1. **Severed,** by a fractured vertebra *(Figure 10.14a);*
2. **Contused,** as in a sudden, violent jolt to the spine; and
3. **Compressed,** by a dislocated vertebra, bleeding, or swelling *(Figure 10.14b).*

Because of its anatomy—with nerve fibers and tracts going up and down, to and from the brain—a spinal cord injury results in a loss of function below the injury site. For example, if the cord is injured in the thoracic region, the arms function normally but the legs can be **paralyzed.** Both muscle control and sensation are lost. **Paresis** is partial paralysis.

If the spinal cord is severed, the loss of function is permanent. Contusions can cause temporary loss, lasting days, weeks, or months.

Compression of the cord can also occur from a tumor in the cord or spine or from a **herniated disc.** The intervertebral disc *(see Lesson 4.2 of Chapter 4)* can move out of place (herniate, slip) or break open (rupture) from injury or strain. This causes pressure on the spinal nerves leading to pain, numbness, and/or weakness. Cancer or osteoporosis can cause a vertebra to collapse and also compress the cord.

Other Disorders of the Spinal Cord (LO 10.5)

Acute transverse myelitis is a localized spinal cord disorder that blocks the transmission of impulses up and down the spinal cord.

Subacute combined degeneration of the spinal cord is due to a deficiency of vitamin B_{12}. The spinal cord's sensory nerve fibers degenerate, producing weakness, clumsiness, tingling, and a sensory loss as to the position of the limbs. Treatment involves vitamin B_{12} injections.

In **syringomyelia,** fluid-filled cavities form in the spinal cord and compress nerves that detect pain and temperature. There is no specific cure.

Poliomyelitis (POLIO) is an acute infectious disease, occurring mostly in children, due to the poliovirus. The virus destroys motor neurons. It is preventable by vaccination and has almost been eradicated worldwide.

Postpolio syndrome (PPS) is when people develop tired, painful, and weak muscles many years after recovery from polio.

Amyotrophic lateral sclerosis (ALS), or "Lou Gehrig's disease," occurs when motor nerves in the spinal cord progressively deteriorate. There is no cure.

Disorders of Peripheral Nerves (LO 10.5)

Peripheral neuropathy is used here as any disorder affecting one or more peripheral nerves. **Mononeuropathy** is damage to a single peripheral nerve. Examples are:

- **Carpal tunnel syndrome,** in which the median nerve at the wrist is compressed between the wrist bones and a strong overlying ligament.
- **Ulnar nerve palsy,** which results from nerve damage as the forearm's ulnar nerve crosses close to the surface over the humerus at the back of the elbow.
- **Peroneal nerve palsy,** which arises from nerve damage as the peroneal or lower leg bone nerve passes close to the surface near the back of the knee. Compression of this nerve occurs in people who are bedridden or strapped in a wheelchair.

Polyneuropathy is damage to, and the simultaneous malfunction of, many motor and/or sensory peripheral nerves throughout the body. There are many causes of peripheral polyneuropathy; diabetes is a common cause. Symptoms include numbness, pain, tingling sensations, and weakness. Treatment is aimed at the underlying problem and pain reduction.

Herpes zoster, or **shingles,** is an infection of peripheral nerves arising from a reactivation of the dormant childhood chickenpox (varicella) virus.

Word Analysis and Definition

S = Suffix P = Prefix R = Root R/CF = Combining Form

WORD	PRONUNCIATION	ELEMENTS		DEFINITION
amyotrophic	a-my-oh-**TROH**-fik	S/ P/ R/CF R/	-ic *pertaining to* a- *without* -my/o- *muscle* -troph- *nourishment, development*	Pertaining to muscular atrophy
compression	kom-**PRESH**-un	S/ P/ R/	-ion *action, condition* com- *together* -press- *squeeze*	Squeeze together to increase density and/or decrease a dimension of a structure
herniation **hernia (noun)** **herniate (verb)**	her-nee-**AY**-shun **HER**-nee-ah **HER**-nee-ate	S/ R/ S/	-ation *process* herni- *rupture* -ate *composed of*	Protrusion of an anatomical structure from its normal location Protrusion of a structure through the tissue that normally contains it
myelitis	**MY**-eh-**LIE**-tis	S/ R/	-itis *inflammation* myel- *spinal cord*	Inflammation of the spinal cord
neuropathy **mononeuropathy** **polyneuropathy**	nyu-**ROP**-ah-thee **MON**-oh-nyu-**ROP**-ah-thee **POL**-ee-nyu-**ROP**-ah-thee	S/ R/CF P/ P/	-pathy *disease* neur/o- *nerve* mono- *one* poly- *many*	Any disorder of the nervous system Disorder affecting a single nerve Disorder affecting many nerves
paralyze (verb) **paralysis (noun)** **paralytic (adj)**	**PAR**-ah-lyze pah-**RAL**-ih-sis par-ah-**LYT**-ik	P/ R/ R/ S/ R/	para- *beside, abnormal* -lyze *destroy* -lysis *destruction* -ic *pertaining to* -lyt- *destroy*	To make incapable of movement Loss of voluntary movement Suffering from paralysis
paresis **hemiparesis**	par-**EE**-sis **HEM**-ee-pah-**REE**-sis	 P/ R/	Greek *weakness* hemi- *half* -paresis *weakness*	Partial paralysis (weakness) Weakness of one side of the body
poliomyelitis **(Note: abbreviated as polio)** **postpolio syndrome (PPS)**	**POE**-lee-oh-**MY**-eh-lie-tis post-**POE**-lee-oh **SIN**-drome	S/ R/ R/ P/ R/ P/ R/	-itis *inflammation* polio- *gray matter* -myel- *spinal cord* post- *after* -polio *gray matter* syn- *together* -drome *running*	Inflammation of the gray matter of the spinal cord, leading to paralysis of the limbs and muscles of respiration Progressive muscle weakness in a person previously affected by polio
syringomyelia	sih-**RING**-oh-my-**EE**-lee-ah	S R/CF R/	-ia *condition* syring/o- *tube, pipe* -myel- *spinal cord*	Abnormal longitudinal cavities in the spinal cord that cause paresthesias and muscle weakness
trauma **traumatic**	**TRAW**-mah traw-**MAT**-ik	 S/ R/	Greek *wound* -tic *pertaining to* trauma- *injury*	A physical or mental injury Pertaining to or caused by trauma

EXERCISES

A. Abbreviations *are common in medical documentation. Provide the abbreviation each statement is describing. Fill in the blanks.* **LO 10.3 and 10.5**

1. The muscle weakness the occurs after having poliomyelitis: ____________

2. Injury to the spinal cord: ____________

3. Another name for Lou Gehrig's disease: ____________

4. Inflammation of the gray matter of the spinal cord due to virus: ____________

B. Identify the element, *and give its meaning. Fill in the chart.* **LO 10.1 and 10.5**

Element	Element Identity (P, R, CF, or S)	Meaning of Element
myo	**1.**	**2.**
herni	**3.**	**4.**
pathy	**5.**	**6.**
syringo	**7.**	**8.**

Lesson 10.4 (cont'd)

Congenital Anomalies of the Nervous System (LO 10.5)

Keynote

- **Classification of CP by number of limbs impaired:**
  - **Quadriplegia: All four limbs are affected.**
  - **Paraplegia: Both lower extremities are affected.**
  - **Hemiplegia: The arm and leg of one side of the body are affected.**
  - **Monoplegia: Only one limb is affected, usually an arm.**

Some of the most devastating congenital neurologic abnormalities develop in the first 8 to 10 weeks of pregnancy, when the nervous system is in its early stages of formation. These malformations can be detected using ultrasonography and amniocentesis *(see Chapter 15)*. Many of these can be prevented by the mother taking 4 mg/day of folic acid before conception and during early pregnancy.

A **teratogen** is an agent that can cause **anomalies** of an embryo or fetus *(see Chapter 15)*. It can be a chemical, a virus, or radiation. Some teratogens found in the workplace include textile dyes, photographic chemicals, semiconductor materials, and the metals lead, mercury, and cadmium.

Anencephaly is the absence of the cerebral hemispheres and is incompatible with life. **Microcephaly,** decreased head size, is associated with small cerebral hemispheres and moderate to severe motor and mental retardation.

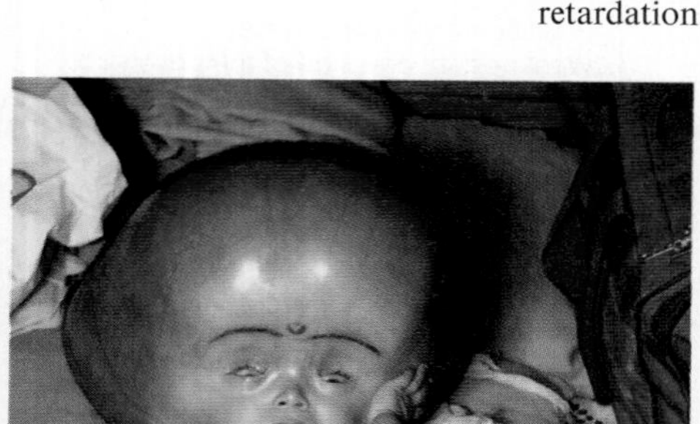

▲ **FIGURE 10.15**
Infant with Hydrocephalus.

Indian Photo Agency/Shutterstock

Hydrocephalus *(Figure 10.15)* is ventricular enlargement in the cerebral hemispheres with excessive CSF; it is usually due to a blockage that prevents the CSF from exiting the ventricles to circulate around the spinal cord. Treatment involves placing a tube (shunt) into the ventricle to divert the excess fluid into the abdominal cavity or a neck vein.

Spina bifida (neural tube defect) occurs mostly in the lumbar and sacral regions. It is variable in its presentation and symptoms. **Spina bifida occulta** has a small partial defect in the vertebral arch. The spinal cord or meninges do not protrude. Often the only sign is a tuft of hair on the skin overlying the defect.

In **spina bifida cystica** there is no vertebral arch formed. The spinal cord and meninges protrude through the opening and may or may not be covered with a thin layer of skin *(Figure 10.16a and b)*. Protrusion of only the meninges is called a **meningocele.** Protrusion of the meninges and spinal cord is called a **meningomyelocele** (myelomeningomyelocele). The lower limbs may be paralyzed.

Fetal alcohol syndrome (FAS) can occur when a pregnant woman drinks alcohol. A child born with FAS has a small head, narrow eyes, and a flat face and nose. Intellect and growth are impaired. FAS is the third most common cause of mental retardation in newborns.

Abbreviations

CP	cerebral palsy
FAS	fetal alcohol syndrome

Cerebral Palsy (LO 10.5)

Cerebral palsy (CP) is the term used to describe the motor impairment resulting from brain damage in an infant or young child. It is not hereditary. In congenital CP, the cause is often unknown but can be a brain malformation or maternal use of cocaine. CP developed at birth or in the neonatal period is usually related to an incident causing hypoxia of the brain.

Cerebral palsy causes delay in the development of normal milestones in infancy and childhood. The affected limbs can be **spastic** (muscles are tight and resistant to stretch) and may show **athetoid** movements, where the limbs involuntarily writhe and constantly move. A poor sense of balance and coordination may also be present, leading to **ataxia.**

A rehabilitation program focused on function is the key component in treatment of cerebral palsy.

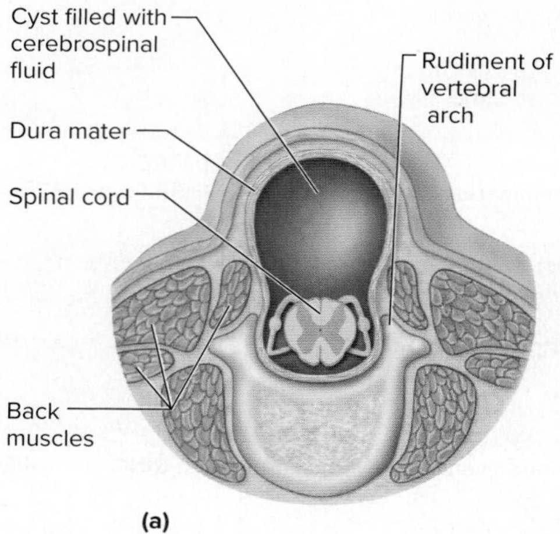

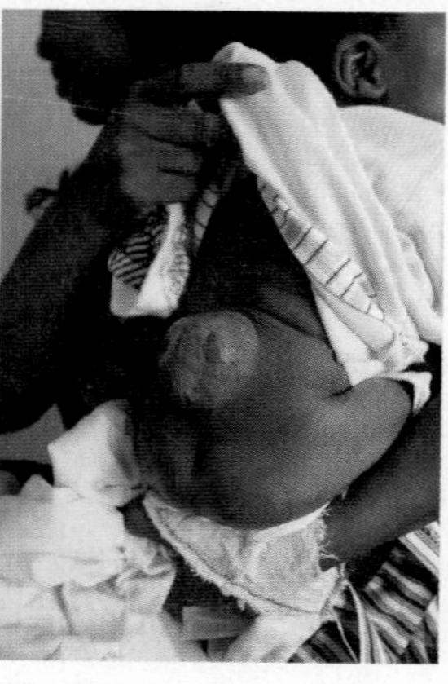

▲ **FIGURE 10.16**
Spina Bifida Cystica.
(a) Cross section of a spinal meningocele.
(b) Child with spina bifida cystica.

10.16b: BSIP/UIG/Getty Images

Word Analysis and Definition

S = Suffix P = Prefix R = Root R/CF = Combining Form

WORD	PRONUNCIATION	ELEMENTS		DEFINITION
anencephaly	**AN**-en-**SEF**-ah-lee	S/ P/ R/	-aly *condition* an- *without* **-enceph-** *brain*	Born without cerebral hemispheres
microcephaly	**MY**-kroh-**SEF**-ah-lee	P/ R/	micro- *small* **-ceph-** *head*	An abnormally small head
ataxia	a-**TAK**-see-ah	S/ P/ R/	-ia *condition* a- *without* **-tax-** *coordination*	Inability to coordinate muscle activity, leading to jerky movements
ataxic (adj)	a-**TAK**-sik	S/	-ic *pertaining to*	Pertaining to or suffering from ataxia
athetosis	ath-eh-**TOE**-sis	S/ R/	-osis *condition* **athet-** *without position, uncontrolled*	Slow, writhing involuntary movements
athetoid (adj)	**ATH**-eh-toyd	S/	-oid *resembling*	Resembling or suffering from athetosis
hemiplegia	hem-ee-**PLEE**-jee-ah	S/ P/ R/	-ia *condition* hemi- *half* **-pleg-** *paralysis*	Paralysis of one side of the body
hemiplegic (adj)	hem-ee-**PLEE**-jik	S/	-ic *pertaining to*	Pertaining to or suffering from hemiplegia
hemiparesis	**HEM**-ee-pah-**REE**-sis	R/	**-paresis** *weakness*	Weakness of one side of the body
meningocele	meh-**NIN**-goh-seal	S/ R/CF	-cele *hernia* **mening/o-** *meninges*	Protrusion of the meninges from the spinal cord or brain through a defect in the vertebral column or cranium
meningomyelocele	meh-nin-goh-**MY**-el-oh-seal	S/ R/CF	-cele *hernia* **-myel/o-** *spinal cord*	Protrusion of the spinal cord and meninges through a defect in the vertebral arch of one or more vertebrae
monoplegia	**MON**-oh-**PLEE**-jee-ah	S/ P/ R/	-ia *condition* mono- *one* **-pleg-** *paralysis*	Paralysis of one limb
monoplegic (adj)	**MON**-oh-**PLEE**-jik	S/	-ic *pertaining to*	Pertaining to or suffering from monoplegia
palsy	**PAWL**-zee		Latin *paralysis*	Paralysis or paresis from brain damage
paraplegia	par-ah-**PLEE**-jee-ah	S/ P/ R/	-ia *condition* para- *abnormal* **-pleg-** *paralysis*	Paralysis of both lower extremities
paraplegic (adj)	par-ah-**PLEE**-jik	S/	-ic *pertaining to*	Pertaining to or suffering from paraplegia
quadriplegia	kwad-rih-**PLEE**-jee-ah	S/ P/ R/	-ia *condition* quadri- *four* **-pleg-** *paralysis*	Paralysis of all four limbs
quadriplegic (adj)	kwad-rih-**PLEE**-jik	S/	-ic *pertaining to*	Pertaining to or suffering from quadriplegia
spina bifida	**SPY**-nah **BIH**-fih-dah	R/CF P/ R/	**spin/a** *spine* bi- *two* **-fida** *split*	Failure of one or more vertebral arches to close during fetal development
spina bifida cystica	**SIS**-tik-ah	S/ R/	-ica *pertaining to* **cyst-** *cyst*	Meninges and spinal cord protruding through the absent vertebral arch and having the appearance of a cyst
spina bifida occulta	**OH**-kul-tah	R/CF	**occult/a** *hidden*	The deformity of the vertebral arch is not apparent from the surface
teratogen	**TER**-ah-toe-gen	S/ R/CF	**-gen** *create, produce* **terat/o-** *monster, malformed fetus*	Agent that produces fetal deformities

EXERCISE

A. Search and find *the correct term for the element you are given. Select the correct answer.* **LO 10.1 and 10.5**

1. Find the term with the prefix meaning *without:*
   a. hydrocephalus **b.** anencephaly **c.** bifida
2. Find the term with the suffix meaning *hernia:*
   a. meningocele **b.** cystica **c.** teratogen
3. Find the term with the root meaning *hidden:*
   a. spina bifida **b.** spina bifida cystica **c.** spina bifida occulta
4. Find the term with the root meaning *coordination:*
   a. monoplegia **b.** athetosis **c.** ataxia

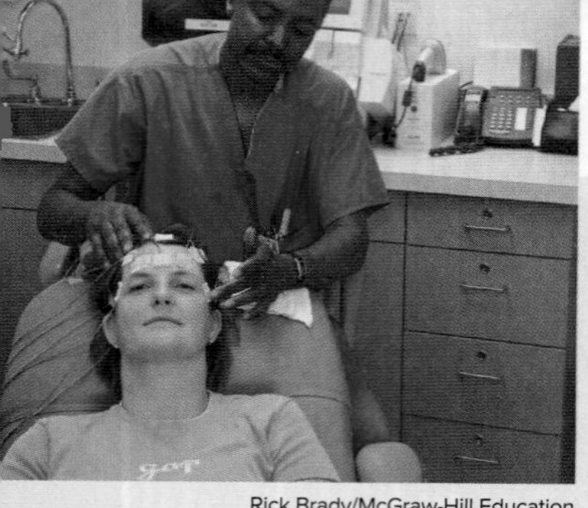

Rick Brady/McGraw-Hill Education

Lesson 10.5

Diagnostic and Therapeutic Procedures and Pharmacology of the Nervous System

Objectives

Many new medical terms are being produced in neurology, particularly in the areas of improved diagnostic measures and in new and/or improved treatments. The information in this lesson will enable you to:

10.5.1 Understand the procedures used in the diagnosis of neurological disorders.

10.5.2 Explain the therapeutic procedures used for neurological disorders.

10.5.3 Describe the pharmacological agents used to treat neurological disorders.

Abbreviations

CT	computed tomography
EMG	electromyography
LP	lumbar puncture
MRI	magnetic resonance imaging
PET	positron emission tomography

Diagnostic Procedures in Neurology (LO 10.5)

To obtain a specimen of CSF, a **lumbar puncture (LP)** or **spinal tap** is performed *(Figure 10.17)*. A needle is inserted through the skin, back muscles, spinal ligaments of an intervertebral space, epidural space, dura mater, and arachnoid mater into the subarachnoid space. The CSF is then aspirated. Laboratory examination of the CSF that shows white blood cells suggests meningitis. High protein levels indicate meningitis or damage to the brain or spinal cord. Blood suggests a brain hemorrhage or a traumatic tap.

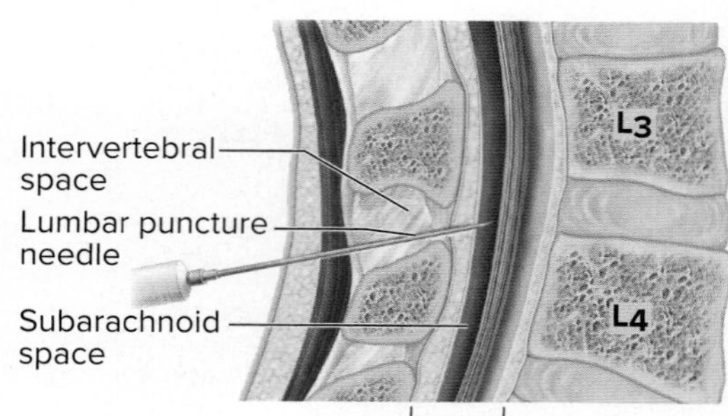

▲ **FIGURE 10.17**
Lumbar Puncture (spinal tap).

Electroencephalography records the brain's electrical activity and helps identify seizure disorders, sleep disturbances, degenerative brain disorders, and brain damage.

Computed tomography (CT), a computer-enhanced X-ray technique, generates images of slices of the brain and can detect a wide range of brain and spinal cord disorders, including tumors, areas of dead brain tissue due to stroke, and birth defects.

Magnetic resonance imaging (MRI) produces highly detailed anatomical images of most neurologic disorders, including strokes, brain tumors, and myelin sheath damage.

Magnetic resonance angiography uses an injection of a radiopaque dye to produce images of blood vessels of the head and neck during MRI.

Cerebral angiography is an invasive procedure in which a radiopaque dye is injected into the blood vessels of the neck and brain. It can detect blood vessels that are partially or completely blocked, aneurysms, or arteriovenous malformations.

Cerebral arteriography can determine the site of bleeding in hemorrhagic strokes.

Color Doppler ultrasonography uses high-frequency sound (ultrasound) waves to show different rates of blood flow through the arteries of the neck or the base of the brain. This evaluates TIAs and the risk of a full-blown stroke.

Echoencephalography uses ultrasound waves to produce an image of the brain in children under the age of 2 because their skulls are thin enough for the waves to pass through them.

Positron emission tomography (PET) involves attaching radioactive molecules onto a substance necessary for brain function (for example, the sugar glucose). As the molecules circulate in the brain, the radioactive labels give off positively charged signals that can be recorded *(Figure 10.18)*.

Myelography is the use of X-rays of the spinal cord that are taken after a radiopaque dye has been injected into the CSF by spinal tap. It has been replaced by MRI when that is available.

Evoked responses are a procedure in which stimuli for vision, sound, and touch are used to activate specific areas of the brain and their responses are measured with EEG or PET scans. This provides information about how that specific area of the brain is functioning in disorders such as MS.

Electromyography (**EMG**) involves placing small needles into a muscle to record its electrical activity at rest and during contraction. It is used to provide information in disorders of muscles, peripheral nerves, and the **neuromuscular** junction.

Nerve conduction studies measure the speed at which motor or sensory nerves conduct impulses. The studies exclude disorders of the brain, spinal cord, and muscles and focus on the peripheral nerves.

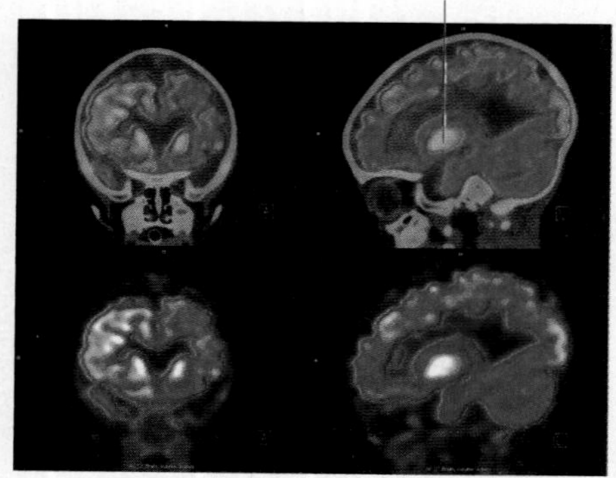

▲ **FIGURE 10.18**
PET Scan of the Brain Showing the Motor Cortex. ©Marcus E. Raichle

wenht/Getty Images

Word Analysis and Definition

S = Suffix **P = Prefix** R = Root R/CF = Combining Form

WORD	PRONUNCIATION	ELEMENTS		DEFINITION
angiography	an-jee-**OG**-rah-fee	S/ R/CF	**-graphy** *process of recording* **angi/o-** *blood vessel*	Process of recording the image of blood vessels after injection of contrast material
arteriography	ar-teer-ee-**OG**-rah-fee	S/ R/CF	**-graphy** *process of recording* **arteri/o-** *artery*	X-ray visualization of an artery after injection of contrast material
Doppler	**DOP**-ler		Johann Christian Doppler, 1803–1853, Austrian mathematician and physicist	Diagnostic instrument that sends an ultrasonic beam into the body
Doppler ultrasonography	**DOP**-ler **UL**-trah-soh-**NOG**-rah-fee	S/ P/ R/CF	**-graphy** *process of recording* **ultra-** *beyond* **-son/o-** *sound*	Imaging that detects direction, velocity, and turbulence of blood flow; used in workup of stroke patients
color Doppler ultrasonography				Computer-generated color image to show directions of blood flow
echoencephalography	**EK**-oh-en-sef-ah-**LOG**-rah-fee	S/ R/CF R/CF	**-graphy** *process of recording* **ech/o-** *sound wave* **-encephal/o-** *brain*	Use of ultrasound in the diagnosis of intracranial lesions
electroencephalogram (EEG)	ee-**LEK**-troh-en-**SEF**-ah-loh-gram	S/ R/CF R/CF	**-gram** *recording* **electr/o-** *electricity* **-encephal/o-** *brain*	Record of the electrical activity of the brain
electroencephalograph	ee-**LEK**-troh-en-**SEF**-ah-loh-graf	S/	**-graph** *to write, record*	Device used to record the electrical activity of the brain
electroencephalography	ee-**LEK**-troh-en-**SEF**-ah-**LOG**-rah-fee	S/	**-graphy** *process of recording*	The process of recording the electrical activity of the brain
electromyogram **electromyography**	ee-**LECK**-troh-**MY**-oh-gram ee-**LEK**-troh-my-**OG**-rah-fee	S/ S/ R/CF R/CF	**-gram** *record, recording* **-graphy** *process of recording* **electr/o-** *electricity* **-my/o-** *muscle*	Record of the electrical activity of a muscle. Recording of electrical activity in muscle
myelography	my-eh-**LOG**-rah-fee	S/ R/CF	**-graphy** *process of recording* **myel/o-** *spinal cord*	Radiography of the spinal cord and nerve roots after injection of contrast medium into the subarachnoid space
nerve conduction study	NERV kon-**DUK**-shun **STUD**-ee	R/ S/ P/ R/ R/	**nerve** *nerve* **-ion** *action* **con-** *with, together* **-duct-** *lead* **study** *inquiry*	Procedure to measure the speed at which an electrical impulse travels along a nerve

Exercise

A. **Construct medical terms common to diagnostic procedures in neurology.** *Given the definition, complete the medical term it is defining using word elements related to diagnostic terms in neurology. Fill in the blanks.* **LO 10.1, 10.5, and 10.6**

1. The machine that creates the record of the electrical activity of the brain. electro/encephalo/____________________
2. The process of recording arteries. arterio/____________________
3. The use of high-fequency sound waves to view blood flow. Doppler ultra/____________________/graphy
4. Process of recording the spinal cord. ____________________/graphy
5. Process of recording the electrical activity of the muscle. electr/o/____________________/graphy

Lesson 10.5 (cont'd) Therapeutic Procedures (LO 10.5 and 10.6)

Craniotomy is the surgical removal of part of a skull bone (the bone flap) to expose the brain for surgery.

Cranioplasty is the repair of a bone defect in the skull, often the result of craniotomy.

Deep brain stimulation is the surgical placement of electrodes deep into specific areas of the brain to deliver electrical stimulations to treat the tremors of Parkinson disease, essential tremor, or multiple sclerosis.

Endoscopic pituitary surgery utilizes an approach through the inside of the nose to remove pituitary tumors.

Endovascular coiling blocks the blood flow to an aneurysm.

Flow diversion uses **stents** placed via a catheter to maintain blood flow through a blood vessel where blockage or an aneurysm has occurred.

Treatment of many acute ischemic strokes is by **thrombolysis** using clotbusters such as **tissue plasminogen activator (tPA)** within 4½ hours of the stroke, with supportive measures followed by rehabilitation.

Treatment for TIA is directed at the underlying cause. **Carotid endarterectomy** may be necessary if a carotid artery is significantly occluded with plaque.

Treatment of Cerebral Palsy

A multidisciplinary team of health professionals is required to develop an individualized treatment plan and to involve the patients, families, teachers, and caregivers in decision making and planning.

Physical therapy is designed to prevent muscles from becoming weak or rigidly fixed with **contractures**, to improve motor development, and to facilitate independence. Speech therapy and psychotherapy complement physical therapy.

Muscle relaxants, such as diazepam, can reduce **spasticity** for short periods of time, and a variety of devices and mechanical aids ranging from muscle braces to motorized wheelchairs help overcome physical limitations.

Treatment of Gliomas

Treatment is a combination of surgery, radiotherapy, and chemotherapy. The combination is necessary because even if you remove 99% of a tumor, there will be up to 1 billion cells remaining. A more recent therapy, **brachytherapy**, implants small radioactive pellets directly into the tumor. The radiation is released over time.

Word Analysis and Definition

S = Suffix **P = Prefix** R = Root R/CF = Combining Form

WORD	PRONUNCIATION	ELEMENTS		DEFINITION
Botox	**BOH**-tox		Botulinum toxin	Neurotoxin injected into muscles to prevent the muscles from contracting
brachytherapy	brah-kee-**THAIR**-ah-pee	P/ R/	**brachy-** *short* **-therapy** *medical treatment*	Radiation therapy in which the source of irradiation is implanted in the tissue to be treated
cranium **cranioplasty** **craniotomy**	**KRAY**-nee-um **KRAY**-nee-oh-**PLASTY** **KRAY**-nee-**OT**-oh-mee	 S/ R/CF S/	Greek *skull* **-plasty** *surgical repair* **crani/o-** *skull* **-tomy** *surgical incision*	The bony container of the brain, excluding the face Repair of a bone defect in the skull Surgical removal of part of a skull bone to expose the brain for surgery
endovascular	**END**-oh-**VAS**-kyu-lar	S/ P/ R/	**-ar** *pertaining to* **endo-** *inside* **-vascul-** *blood vessel*	Relating to the inside of a blood vessel

EXERCISE

A. **Demonstrate understanding of word elements in medical terms.** *This will make short work of answer questions in this course and interpreting patient medical records in clinical practice. This exercise uses layman's terms and asks you to replace those words the medical term they are describing. Fill in the blanks.* **LO 10.5 and 10.8**

A 27 year old male is brought to the emergency department by paramedics. The male is unconscious. The paramedics report that he was involved in an altercation at a bar when he was struck in the head with a barstool. He was immediately brought to the operating room where the (1) *surgical expert in the treatment of neurological conditions* performed a (2) *procedure in which part of the skull was removed.* A large clot was removed from the subdural space. The wound was closed and the patient was admitted to the surgical ICU.The injury to skull shattered several areas of the (3) *bones that cover the brain*, and therefore the patient will require a (4) *repair of defect of the skull* at a later date when he becomes medically stable.

1. The medical term that replaces the italicized words: ____________________

2. The medical term that replaces the italicized words: ____________________

3. The medical term that replaces the italicized words: ____________________

4. The medical term that replaces the italicized words: ____________________

Lesson 10.5 (cont'd) Pharmacology of the Nervous System (LO 10.6)

Abbreviations

LSD lysergic acid diethylamide
MDMA methylenedioxymethamphetamine (ecstasy)
PCP phencyclidine (angel dust)
THC tetrahydrocannabinol (marijuana)

The transmission of impulses from one neuron to another and from a neuron to a cell is achieved by neurotransmitters at synaptic connections. Drugs that affect the nervous system, called *psychoactive drugs,* target this synaptic mechanism.

Psychoactive drugs are able to change mood, behavior, cognition, and anxiety. They can be classified into several families:

1. **Stimulants**—caffeine, nicotine, amphetamines, and cocaine—enhance the **stimulation** provided by the sympathetic nervous system. They cause the level of dopamine to rise in the synapses, leading to the pleasurable effects associated with these drugs.
2. **Sedatives**—ethanol (beverage alcohol), barbiturates, and meprobamate—decrease the sensitivity of the postsynaptic neurons to quiet the nervous excitement. They also act on the sleep centers to induce sleep.
3. Inhaled anesthetics such as isoflurane act similarly to, but are more powerful than, sedatives.
4. Opiates—morphine, codeine, heroin, methadone, and oxycodone—depress nerve transmission in the synapses of sensory pathways of the brain and spinal cord. They also inhibit centers in the brain controlling coughing, breathing, and intestinal motility. Codeine is used in cough medicines. Constipation is a side effect of all these drugs. Opiates are **addictive** because they produce tolerance and physical dependence.
5. Opiate **antagonists**, such as naloxone and naltrexone, prevent opiates from acting in the synapses. They can be used in drug overdoses and to help recovering heroin addicts stay drug-free.
6. **Tranquilizers**, such as chlorpromazine, haloperidol, and the benzodiazepines (*Librium, Valium, Xanax*), act like sedatives but without their sleep-inducing effect.
7. Antidepressants all increase the amount of serotonin at the synapses, where it is a neurotransmitter. *Zoloft* and *Prozac* are examples.
8. **Antiepileptics** act in different ways on the synaptic junction to keep stimuli from passing across the synapse. Phenytoin and carbamazepine are examples.
9. **Psychedelics** distort sensory perceptions, particularly sight and sound. They can be natural plant products, such as mescaline, psilocybin, and dimethyltryptamine. They also can be synthetic, such as **lysergic acid diethylamide (LSD), methylenedioxymethamphetamine** (**MDMA** or "ecstasy"), and **phencyclidine** (**PCP** or "angel dust"). They increase the amount of serotonin in the synaptic junctions, and some have an additional amphetamine stimulation.
10. **Marijuana** has the active ingredient **tetrahydrocannabinol (THC).** It produces the drowsiness of sedatives like alcohol, the dulling of pain like opiates, and, in high doses, the perception distortions of the psychedelics. Unlike the case with opiates or sedatives, **tolerance** does not occur.

Word Analysis and Definition

S = Suffix **P = Prefix** R = Root R/CF = Combining Form

WORD	PRONUNCIATION		ELEMENTS	DEFINITION
addict	**AD**-ikt	P/ R/	**ad-** *to* **-dict** *consent, surrender*	Person with a psychologic or physical dependence on a substance or practice
addiction	ah-**DIK**-shun	S/	**-ion** *condition, action*	Habitual psychologic and physiologic dependence on a substance or practice
addictive	ah-**DIK**-tiv	S/	**-ive** *quality of, pertaining to*	Pertaining to or causing addiction
anesthetic	an-ees-**THET**-ic	P/ R/ S/	**an-** *without, lack of* **-esthet** *sensation, perception* **-ic** *pertaining to*	agent that causes absence of feeling sensation
antagonism	an-**TAG**-oh-nizm	S/ P/ R/	**-ism** *process, action* **ant-** *against* **-agon-** *contest against*	Situation of opposing
antagonist	an-**TAG**-oh-nist	S/	**-ist** *agent*	An opposing structure, agent, disease, or process
antidepressant	**AN**-teh-dee-**PRESS**-ant	S/ P/ P/ R/	**-ant** *against* **anti-** *against* **de-** *without* **-press-** *press close, press down*	An agent to suppress the symptoms of depression
antiepileptic	**AN**-tee-eh-pih-**LEP**-tik	S/ P/ R/	**-tic** *pertaining to* **anti-** *against* **-epilep-** *seizure*	A pharmacologic agent capable of preventing or arresting epilepsy
psychedelic	sigh-keh-**DEL**-ik	S/ R/CF R/	**-ic** *pertaining to* **psych/e-** *mind, soul* **-del-** *visible*	Agent that intensifies sensory perception
psychoactive	sigh-koh-**AK**-tiv	S/ R/CF R/	**-ive** *quality of, pertaining to* **psych/o-** *mind, soul* **-act-** *to do*	Able to alter mood, behavior, and/or cognition
sedative	**SED**-ah-tiv	S/ R/	**-ive** *quality of, pertaining to* **sedat-** *to calm*	Agent that calms nervous excitement
sedation	seh-**DAY**-shun	S/	**-ion** *condition, action*	State of being calmed
stimulant **stimulate (verb)** **stimulation**	**STIM**-you-lant **STIM**-you-late stim-you-**LAY**-shun	S/ R/ S/	**-ant** *forming* **stimul-** *excite, strengthen* **-ation** *process*	Agent that excites or strengthens functional activity Arousal to increased functional activity
tolerance	**TOL**-er-ants	S/ R/	**-ance** *state of, condition* **toler-** *endure*	The capacity to become accustomed to a stimulus or drug
tranquilizer	**TRANG**-kwih-lie-zer	S/ R/	**-izer** *affects in a particular way* **tranquil-** *calm*	Agent that calms without sedating or depressing

EXERCISE

A. **Deconstruct this *language of neurology* into its basic elements to help understand the meaning of the term.** *Write the elements between the slashes. The first one is done for you. Every term does not need every element, so you will have some blanks.* **LO 10.1 and 10.6**

1. antagonist ____ant____ / ____agon____ / ____ist____
2. addict ________ / ________ / ________
3. tranquilizer ________ / ________ / ________
4. stimulant ________ / ________ / ________
5. psychedelic ________ / ________ / ________
6. tolerance ________ / ________ / ________
7. psychoactive ________ / ________ / ________

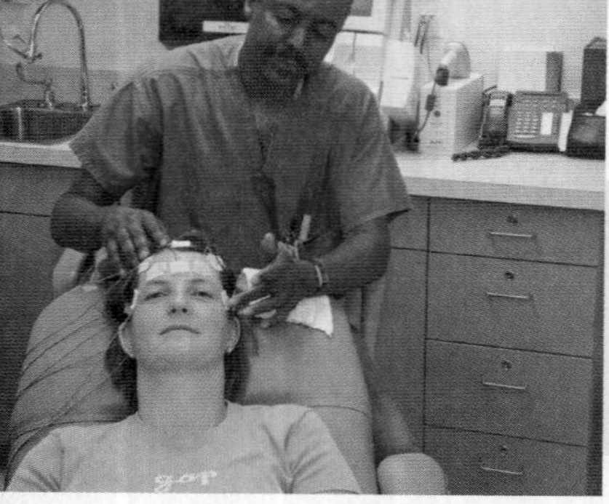

Rick Brady/McGraw-Hill Education

Lesson 10.6
Mental Health

CASE REPORT 10.4

You are . . .

. . . a **psychiatric technician** employed in the Psychiatric Department of Fulwood Medical Center. Your patient has been referred from the Emergency Department, where he was seen earlier this morning.

Your patient is . . .

. . . Mr. Dante Costello, a 21-year-old homeless man, brought in by the police after he was found sitting immobile in the middle of a main street (**catatonia**).

Mr. Costello's explanation is "the voices told me to do it." He has heard voices (**hallucinations**) telling him to do things for the past year. The voices often comment on his behavior. He has isolated himself from other people because "they are not who they say they are, and they are trying to get me" (**delusions**). He is taking no drugs or medications, and he denies any **suicidal** or **homicidal** intent.

Mr. Costello is dirty and disheveled, with poor hygiene. He can give no home or family address. His **affect** is **congruent,** though expressionless. His speech is slow, and his thoughts are disorganized and confused.

The most probable diagnosis is **schizophrenia.** He needs to be admitted to the hospital because he is a danger to himself and other people.

Objectives

To be an effective member of the mental health team that will be responsible for Mr. Costello's care, you will need to be able to:

10.6.1 Define mental health, and differentiate between psychiatry and psychology.
10.6.2 Discuss psychosis and schizophrenia.
10.6.3 Review common mood disorders.
10.6.4 Describe the major types of anxiety disorders.
10.6.5 Identify personality disorders.
10.6.6 Explain the effects of common psychoactive drugs.

Keynotes

- **A specialist in psychiatry is a physician called a psychiatrist, who is licensed to prescribe medications.**
- **A specialist in psychology is a psychologist, who is not licensed to prescribe medications.**
- **Insanity is a legal term for a severe mental illness that impairs a defendant's ability to understand the moral wrong of the act he/she committed. It is not a medical diagnosis.**

Mental Health Definitions
(LO 10.7 and 10.8)

- **Mental health** is defined by the World Health Organization (**WHO**) as "a state of wellbeing in which the individual realizes his or her own abilities, can cope with the normal stresses of life, can work productively and fruitfully, and is able to make a contribution to the community."
- **Psychology** is the scientific study of behavior–talking, reading, sleeping, interacting with others–and mental processes–thinking, feeling, remembering, and dreaming.
- **Psychiatry** is the medical specialty concerned with the origin, diagnosis, prevention, and treatment of mental, emotional, and behavioral disorders.
- **Mental health disorders** are of different types and will be considered in this chapter under the headings Psychosis and Schizophrenia, Mood Disorders, Anxiety Disorders, Personality Disorders, and Substance Abuse and Chemical Dependence.

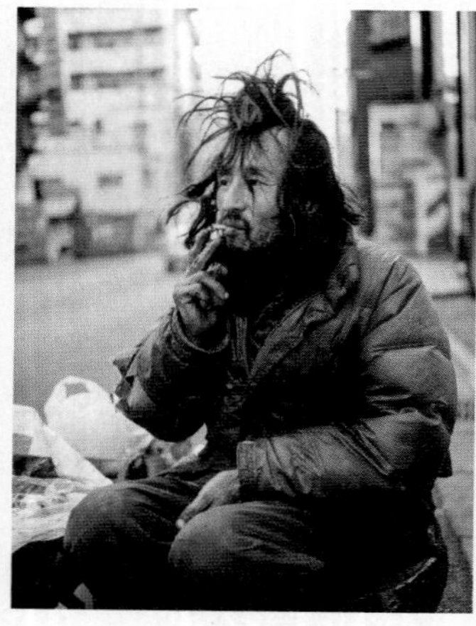

FIGURE 10.19
Homeless Schizophrenic Man on the Street.
RichLegg/Getty Images

Psychosis and Schizophrenia
(LO 10.7)

Psychosis is an abnormal mental state in which the individual has a loss of contact with reality. People suffering from psychosis are described as **psychotic.**

Schizophrenia is a form of psychosis in which the individual loses contact with reality. People with schizophrenia do *not* have a "split personality," but their perceptions are separated from reality, their words are separated from their meanings, and their behaviors are separated from their thought processes. They perceive things without stimulation (**hallucinations**). They suffer from mistaken beliefs that are contrary to facts (**delusions**). The delusions can be **paranoid,** with pervasive distrust and suspicion of others. Their speech is disorganized and can be incoherent, and they may refuse or be unable to speak (**mute**) *(Figure 10.19).* In the Case Report above, Mr. Costello showed all of these symptoms.

Word Analysis and Definition

S = Suffix P = Prefix R = Root R/CF = Combining Form

WORD	PRONUNCIATION	ELEMENTS		DEFINITION
affect	**AFF**-ekt		Latin *state of mind*	External display of feelings, emotions, and thoughts
congruent	**KON**-gru-ent	S/ P/ R/	-ent *end result* **con-** *with* **-gru-** *to move*	Coinciding or agreeing with
delusion	dee-**LOO**-zhun	S/ R/	-ion *condition* **delus-** *deceive*	Fixed, unyielding false belief despite strong evidence to the contrary
hallucination	hah-loo-sih-**NAY**-shun	S/ R/	-ation *condition* **hallucin-** *imagination*	Perception of an object or event when there is no such thing present
homicide	**HOM**-ih-side	S/ R/CF	**-cide** *to kill* **hom/i** *man*	Killing of one human by another
homicidal	hom-ih-**SIDE**-al	S/	**-cidal** *pertaining to*	Having the tendency to commit homicide
mute	MYUT		Latin *silent*	Unable or unwilling to speak
paranoia	par-ah-**NOY**-ah	P/ R/	**para-** *abnormal* **-noia** *to think*	Presence of persecutory delusions
paranoid	**PAR**-ah-noyd	S/	**-oid** *resembling*	Having persecutory delusions
psychiatry	sigh-**KIGH**-ah-tree	S/ R/	**iatry-** *treatment* **psych-** *mind*	Diagnosis and treatment of mental disorders
psychiatrist	sigh-**KIGH**-ah-trist	S/	**-iatrist** *one who treats*	Licensed medical specialist in psychiatry
psychology	sigh-**KOL**-oh-jee	S/ R/CF	**-logy** *study of* **psych/o-** *mind*	Science concerned with the behavior of the human mind
psychologist	sigh-**KOL**-oh-jist	S/	**-logist** *one who treats*	Licensed specialist in psychology
psychosis	sigh-**KOH**-sis	S/ R/	**-osis** *condition* **psych-** *mind*	Disorder with loss of contact with reality
psychotic	sigh-**KOT**-ik	S/ R/CF	**-tic** *pertaining to* **psych/o-** *mind*	Affected by psychosis
schizophrenia	skitz-oh-**FREE**-nee-ah	S/ R/CF R/	**-ia** *condition* **schiz/o-** *to split* **-phren-** *mind*	Disorder of perception and behavior with loss of reality
schizophrenic	skitz-oh-**FREN**-ik	S/	**-ic** *pertaining to*	Suffering from schizophrenia
suicide	**SOO**-ih-side	R/CF R/CF	**su/i-** *self* **-cid/e** *kill*	The act of killing oneself
suicidal	**SOO**-ih-SIGH-dal	S/	**-al** *pertaining to*	Wanting to kill oneself

EXERCISES

A. After reading Case Report 10.4, *select the correct answer to complete each statement.* **LO 10.7**

1. The term that means wanting to kill oneself:

a. homicidal **b.** schizophrenic **c.** suicidal **d.** psychotic

2. Mr. Costello's inappropriate behavior is due to:

a. homicidal thoughts **b.** poor hygiene **c.** hearing voices **d.** homelessness

3. In the statement "His affect is congruent, though expressionless," the term **congruent** means:

a. the behavior matches his appearance

b. he is not speaking

c. he believes people are out to get him

d. his behavior points to hurting other people

4. His behavior of sitting in the street for long periods of time describes which condition?

a. paranoia **b.** mutism **c.** homicidal **d.** catatonia

B. Reinforce *your learning of the languages of psychology and psychiatry by providing the term that is being defined. Fill in the blanks.* **LO 10.2, 10.7, 10.8, and 10.9**

1. A medical doctor who specializes in the origin, diagnosis, prevention, and treatment of mental, emotional, and behavioral disorders: ___________

2. A front-line worker who directly cares for those with mental illnesses and/or developmental disabilities: ___________ technician.

3. The general term for a licensed specialist in psychology: ___________

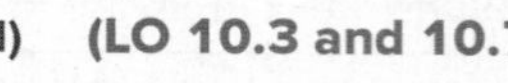

Lesson 10.6 (cont'd) Mood Disorders

(LO 10.3 and 10.7)

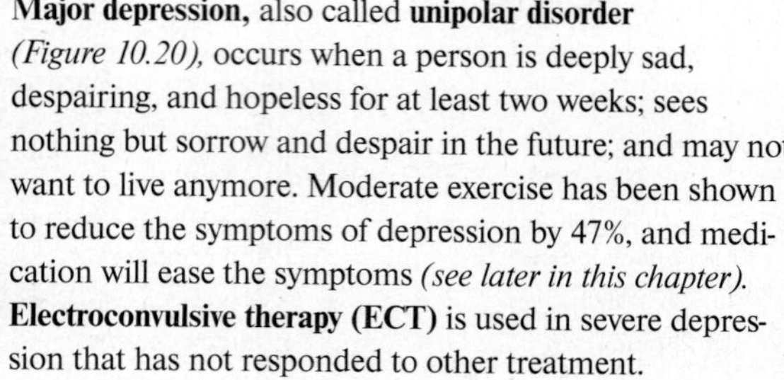

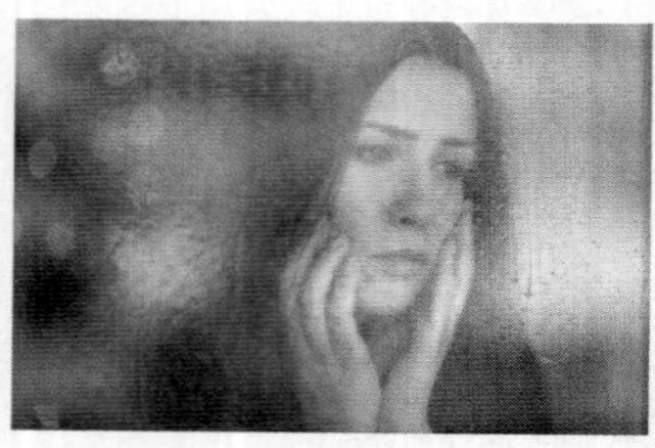

▲ **FIGURE 10.20** Depressed Woman at a Window.

Bojan Kontrec/Getty Images

Major depression, also called **unipolar disorder** *(Figure 10.20),* occurs when a person is deeply sad, despairing, and hopeless for at least two weeks; sees nothing but sorrow and despair in the future; and may not want to live anymore. Moderate exercise has been shown to reduce the symptoms of depression by 47%, and medication will ease the symptoms *(see later in this chapter).* **Electroconvulsive therapy (ECT)** is used in severe depression that has not responded to other treatment.

- **Bipolar disorder,** which used to be called **manic-depressive disorder,** is the alternation of major episodes of depression with periods of excessive overexcitement, impulsive behavior, **insomnia,** and lack of fatigue, called **mania.** Untreated mixed (manic and depressive) episodes usually last around four to five months.
- **Dysphoric mania** combines the frenetic energy of mania with dark thoughts and paranoid delusions. It may be the cause of some mass shootings.
- **Seasonal affective disorder (SAD)** has episodes of depression that occur in the fall and winter months. It appears to be related to a lack of sunshine causing increased melatonin production by the pineal gland *(see Chapter 12).* It can be helped by **phototherapy** with bright white fluorescent lights and by antidepressant medications.

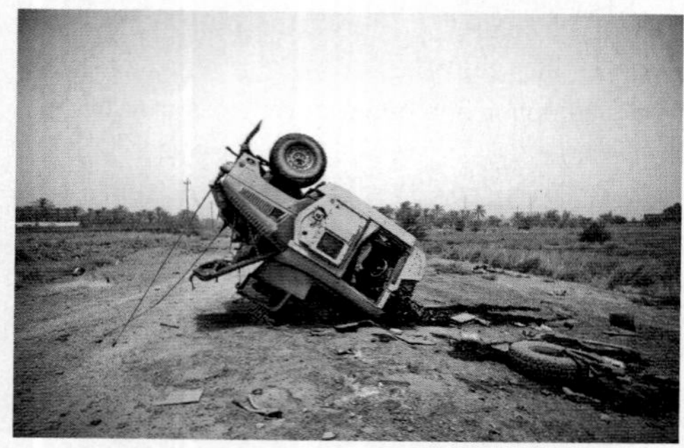

▲ **FIGURE 10.21** The remains of an American Humvee, one of four that were disabled by massive IEDs, lies on a dirt road on August 4, 2007, in Hawr Rajab, Iraq.

Benjamin Lowy/Getty Images

Abbreviations

CBT	cognitive behavioral therapy
CPT	cognitive processing therapy
GAD	generalized anxiety disorder
ECT	electroconvulsive therapy
IED	improvised explosive device
OCD	obsessive-compulsive disorder
PTSD	posttraumatic stress disorder
SAD	seasonal affective disorder
SSRI	selective serotonin reuptake inhibitor

Anxiety Disorders

(LO 10.2, 10.3, and 10.7)

Anxiety disorders are the most common category of mental disorder found in the United States. They are characterized by an unreasonable anxiety and fear so intense and persistent that it disrupts the person's life. There are five categories of anxiety disorders:

1. **Generalized anxiety disorder (GAD)** consists of uncontrollable anxiety not focused on one situation or event that has lasted for six months or more. People with the disorder develop physical fear reactions, including palpitations, insomnia, difficulty concentrating, and irritability.
2. **Posttraumatic stress disorder (PTSD)** affects about 7.7 million American adults. It arises after significant trauma, such as a life-threatening incident, loss of a loved one, abuse, torture or combat in war, or a high level of stress in daily life *(Figure 10.21).* Symptoms include flashbacks of the traumatic event, nightmares, intense physical reactions to reminders of the event, feeling emotionally numb, irritability, outbursts of anger, and difficulty concentrating. Alcohol and drug abuse are common. Treatment is with **cognitive behavioral therapy (CBT),** in which the traumatic experiences are relived and worked through; **cognitive processing therapy (CPT),** in which the thoughts and beliefs generated by the trauma are explored and reframed; and antidepressants.
3. **Panic disorder** is characterized by sudden, brief attacks of intense fear that cause physical symptoms, occur often for no reason, and peak in 10 minutes or less. Treatment is with CBT and medication with benzodiazepines or selective serotonin reuptake inhibitors (**SSRI**) *(see later in this lesson).*
4. **Phobias** differ from panic attacks in that a *specific* situation or event brings on the strong fear response. There are two categories of phobias:
   - **Situational phobias** involve a fear of specific situations. Examples are **acrophobia** (fear of heights), **agoraphobia** (fear of crowded places), and **claustrophobia** (fear of confined spaces).
   - **Social phobias** involve a fear of being embarrassed in social situations. The most common are fear of public speaking and fear of eating in public.
5. In **obsessive-compulsive disorder (OCD),** most patients have both **obsessions** and **compulsions.** Obsessions are recurrent thoughts, fears, doubts, images, or impulses. Compulsions are recurrent, irresistible impulses to perform actions such as counting, hand washing, checking, and systematically arranging things. Treatment is with CBT and/or an SSRI.

Psychosomatic disorder is a real physical illness in which anxiety and stress play a causative role. Examples are tension headaches and low back pain. Treatment is with **biofeedback** and relaxation techniques *(Figure 10.22).*

A person called a **hypochondriac** has **hypochondriasis** and interprets some minor symptom such as a cough or a bruise as a sign of serious disease, and cannot believe normal physical examinations and reassurances.

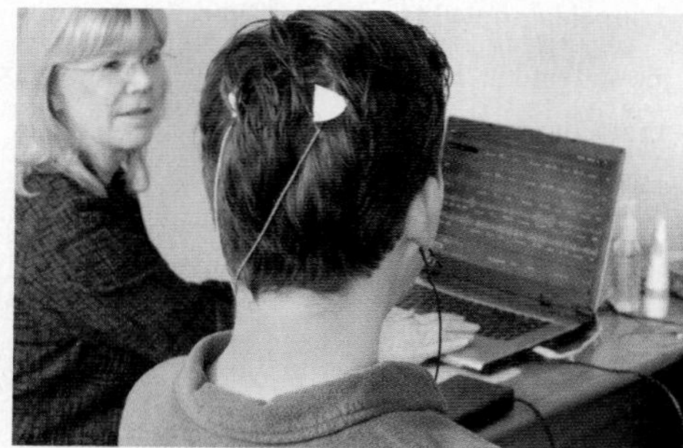

▲ **FIGURE 10.22** Person Undergoing Biofeedback.

leezsnow/Getty Images

Word Analysis and Definition

S = Suffix P = Prefix R = Root R/CF = Combining Form

WORD	PRONUNCIATION	ELEMENTS		DEFINITION
acrophobia	ak-roh-**FOH**-be-ah	S/ R/CF	**-phobia** *fear* **acr/o-** *peak, highest point*	Pathologic fear of heights
agoraphobia	ah-gor-ah-**FOH**-be-ah	S/ R/CF	**-phobia** *fear* **agor/a-** *marketplace*	Pathologic fear of being trapped in a public place
anxiety	ang-**ZI**-eh-tee		Greek *distress, anxiety*	Distress caused by fear
biofeedback **(Note:** *This term has no prefix or suffix.)*	bi-oh-**FEED**-back	R/CF R/ R/	**bi/o-** *life* **-feed-** *to give food, nourish* **-back** *back, return*	Training techniques to achieve voluntary control of responses to stimuli
bipolar disorder	bi-**POH**-lar dis-**OR**-der	S/ P/ R/	**-ar** *pertaining to* **bi-** *two* **-pol-** *pole*	A mood disorder with alternating episodes of depression and mania
claustrophobia	klaw-stroh-**FOH**-be-ah	S/ R/CF	**-phobia** *fear* **claustr/o-** *confined space*	Pathologic fear of being trapped in a confined space
cognitive	**KOG**-nih-tiv	S/ R/	**-ive** *quality of* **cognit-** *thinking*	Pertaining to the mental activities of thinking and learning
cognitive behavioral therapy (CBT) **(Note:** Behavioral *has two suffixes to make the word flow.)*	**KOG**-nih-tiv be-**HAYV**-yur-al **THAIR**-ah-pee	S/ R/ S/ S/ R/ R/	**-ive** *quality of* **cognit-** *thinking* **-al** *pertaining to* **-ior-** *pertaining to* **behav-** *mental activity* **therapy** *medical treatment*	Psychotherapy that emphasizes thoughts and attitudes in one's behavior
cognitive processing therapy (CPT)	**KOG**-nih-tiv **PROS**-es-ing **THAIR**-ah-pee	S/ R/ S/ P/ R/	**-ive** *quality of* **cognit-** *thinking* **-ing** *doing* **pro-** *before* **-cess-** *going forward*	Psychotherapy to build skills to deal with effects of trauma in other areas of life
compulsion	kom-**PULL**-shun	S/ R/	**-ion** *action, condition* **compuls-** *drive, compel*	Uncontrollable impulses to perform an act repetitively
compulsive (adj)	kom-**PULL**-siv	S/	**-ive** *nature of, quality of*	Possessing uncontrollable impulses to perform an act repetitively
depression	de-**PRESH**-un	S/ R/	**-ion** *condition, process* **depress-** *press down*	Mental disorder with feelings of deep sadness and despair
electroconvulsive therapy	ee-**LEK**-troh-kon-**VUL**-siv **THAIR**-ah-pee	S/ R/CF P/ R/	**-ive** *quality of* **electr/o-** *electricity* **-con-** *with* **-vuls-** *tear, pull*	Passage of electric current through the brain to produce convulsions and treat persistent depression, mania, and other disorders
hypochondriac	high-poh-**KON**-dree-ack	S/ P/ R/	**-iac** *pertaining to* **hypo-** *below* **-chondr-** *cartilage*	A person who exaggerates the significance of symptoms
hypochondriasis	**HIGH**-poh-kon-**DRY**-ah-sis	S/	**-iasis** *condition, state of*	Belief that a minor symptom indicates a severe disease
insomnia	in-**SOM**-nee-ah	S/ P/ R/	**-ia** *condition* **in-** *not* **-somn-** *sleep*	Inability to sleep
mania	**MAY**-nee-ah		Greek *frenzy*	Mood disorder with hyperactivity, irritability, and rapid speech
manic	**MAN**-ik	S/ R/	**-ic** *pertaining to* **man-** *mania*	Pertaining to or characterized by mania
manic-depressive disorder	**MAN**-ik-de-**PRESS**-iv dis-**OR**-der	S/ R/	**-ive** *quality of* **depress-** *press down*	An outdated name for bipolar disorder
obsession	ob-**SESH**-un	S/ R/	**-ion** *action, condition* **obsess-** *besieged by thoughts*	Persistent, recurrent, uncontrollable thoughts or impulses
obsessive (adj)	ob-**SES**-iv	S/	**-ive** *nature of, quality of*	Possessing persistent, recurrent, uncontrollable thoughts or impulses
phobia	**FOH**-be-ah		Greek *fear*	Pathologic fear or dread
posttraumatic	post-traw-**MAT**-ik	S/ P/ R/	**-ic** *pertaining to* **post-** *after* **-traumat-** *wound*	Occurring after and caused by trauma
psychosomatic	sigh-koh-soh-**MAT**-ik	S/ R/CF R/	**-tic** *pertaining to* **psych/o-** *mind* **-soma-** *body*	Pertaining to disorders of the body usually resulting from disturbances of the mind
unipolar disorder	you-nih-**POLE**-ar dis-**OR**-der	S/ P/ R/	**-ar** *pertaining to* **uni-** *one* **-pol-** *pole (at the pole of depression)*	Depression

EXERCISE

A. Match *the term in the first column to its correct definition in the second column. Pay close attention to the word elements to assist you in choosing the correct definition for each term.* **LO 10.2, 10.3, and 10.7**

	Term		Definition
______	**1.** psychosomatic	**a.**	fear of being trapped in a public space
______	**2.** acrophobia	**b.**	fear of heights
______	**3.** obsessive	**c.**	inability to sleep
______	**4.** hypochondriasis	**d.**	disorder of body due to disturbance of the mind
______	**5.** insomnia	**e.**	belief that a minor symptom indicates a severe disease
______	**6.** agoraphobia	**f.**	uncontrollable impulses to perform acts repetitively
______	**7.** compulsion	**g.**	persistent, recurrent, uncontrollable thoughts

Lesson 10.6 (cont'd) Personality Disorders

(LO 10.3 and 10.7)

Personality is defined as an individual's unique and stable patterns of thoughts, feelings, and behaviors. When these patterns become rigid and inflexible in response to different situations, they can cause impairment of the individual's ability to deal with other people (i.e., to function socially).

- **Borderline personality disorder (BPD)** is a frequent diagnosis in people who are impulsive, unstable in mood, and manipulative. They can be exciting, charming, and friendly one moment and angry, irritable, and sarcastic the next. Their identity is fragile and insecure, their self-worth low. They can be promiscuous and self-destructive; for example, with **self-mutilation (self-injury)** *(Figure 10.23)* or suicide. People with **narcissistic personality disorder** have an exaggerated sense of self-importance and seek constant attention.
- **Antisocial personality disorder,** used interchangeably with the terms **sociopath** and **psychopath,** describes people who lie, cheat, steal, and have no sense of responsibility and no anxiety or guilt about their behavior. Psychopaths have these characteristics but tend to be more violent and anger easily.
- **Schizoid** and **paranoid personality disorders** describe people who are absorbed with themselves, untrusting, and fearful of closeness with others.
- Treatment for personality disorders is not successful.

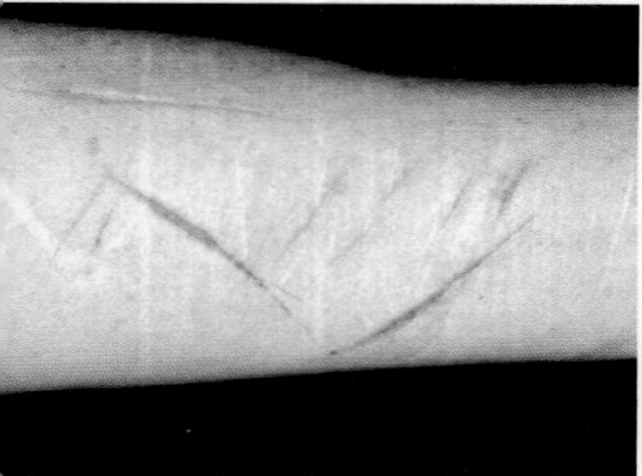

▲ **FIGURE 10.23** Self-Mutilated Arm.

Science Photo Library/Alamy Images

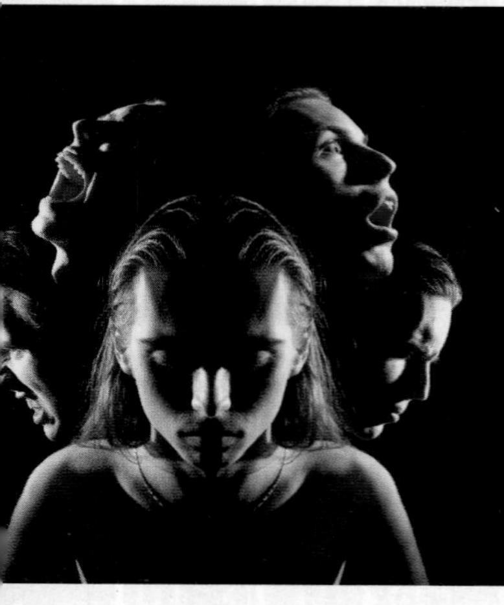

▲ **FIGURE 10.24** Dissociative Identity Disorder (Multiple Personality Disorder).

Stepan Kapl/Shutterstock

Dissociative Disorders

(LO 10.3 and 10.7)

Dissociative disorders involve a disassociation (splitting apart) of past experiences from present memory or consciousness. The development of distinctly separate personalities is called **dissociative identity disorder (DID).** It was formerly called **multiple personality disorder (MPD).** Two or more distinct personalities, each with its own memories and behaviors, inhabit the same person at the same time *(Figure 10.24).* The basic origin of all these disorders is the need to escape, usually from extreme trauma, and most often from sexual, emotional, or physical abuse in childhood. Treatment is with psychotherapy.

Impulse Control Disorders

(LO 10.3 and 10.7)

Impulse control disorders involve an inability to resist an impulse to perform an action that is harmful to the individual or to others. These disorders include:

- **Kleptomania,** which is characterized by stealing—not for gain but to satisfy an irresistible urge to steal. Behavior therapy can help, and SSRIs appear to be of value.
- **Trichotillomania (TTM),** which is characterized by the repeated urge to pull out one's own scalp, beard, pubic, and other body hair.
- **Pyromania,** which is repeated fire setting with no motive other than a fascination with fire and fire engines. Some pyromaniacs end up as volunteer firefighters.

Treatment with behavior therapy is sometimes successful.

Abbreviations

BPD	borderline personality disorder
DID	dissociative identity disorder
MPD	multiple personality disorder
TTM	trichotillomania

Substance Abuse and Chemical Dependence

(LO 10.3 and 10.7)

Substance abuse involves a person's continued use of psychoactive drugs, including alcohol and illicit drugs, despite having significant problems or distress related to their use. This continued use can lead to a **dependence** syndrome, which includes the strong need to take the drug, persistence in its use despite harmful consequences to the user and others, daily priority given to drug use, and increased **tolerance.** Tolerance is the process by which the body continually adapts to a substance and requires increasingly larger amounts to achieve the original effects.

- **Addiction** includes dependence syndrome, but it refers to not only psychoactive drugs but also such entities as exercise addiction, food addiction, computer addiction, and gambling. The patterns of behavior and habits of use associated with an addiction are characterized by immediate gratification coupled with the long-term harmful effects, which include changes in the structure and function of the brain.
- **Abused substances** include tobacco, alcohol, marijuana, cocaine, heroin, methamphetamines, Ecstasy, LSD, and PCP. In addition, prescription drug abuse is increasing dramatically. The three classes of prescription drugs being abused are:
  1. **Opioids,** which include oxycodone (Oxycontin), hydrocodone (Vicodin), meperidine (Demerol), hydromorphone (Dilaudid), and fentanyl (Duragesic and others).
  2. **CNS depressants** such as the benzodiazepines Xanax and Valium.
  3. **CNS stimulants** such as Adderall and Ritalin.

Abuse of prescription drugs now ranks second to marijuana among illicit drug users, and the number of fatal poisonings from prescription opioid analgesics outnumbers total deaths from heroin and cocaine.

Word Analysis and Definition

S = Suffix P = Prefix R = Root R/CF = Combining Form

WORD	PRONUNCIATION	ELEMENTS		DEFINITION
addict addiction	**ADD**-ikt ah-**DIK**-shun	P/ R/ S/	**ad-** *toward* **-dict** *surrender* **-ion** *condition, action*	Person with a psychologic or physical dependence on a substance or practice Habitual psychologic and physiologic dependence on a substance or practice
antisocial personality disorder	**AN**-tee-**SOH**-shal per-son-**AL**-ih-tee dis-**OR**-der	S/ P/ R/ S/ S/ R/	**-al** *pertaining to* **anti-** *against* **-soci-** *partner, ally, community* **-ity** *condition, state* **-al-** *pertaining to* **person-** *person*	Disorder of people who lie, cheat, steal, and have no guilt about their behavior
dissociative identity disorder	di-**SO**-see-ah-tiv eye-**DEN**-tih-tee dis-**OR**-der	S/ P/ R/	**-ative** *quality of* **dis-** *apart, away from* **-soci-** *partner, ally, community*	Mental disorder in which part of an individual's personality is separated from the rest, leading to multiple personalities
kleptomania	klep-toe-**MAY**-nee-ah	S/ R/CF	**-mania** *frenzy* **klept/o-** *to steal*	Uncontrollable need to steal
narcissism narcissistic (adj)	**NAR**-sih-sizm **NAR**-sih-**SIS**-tik	 S/ S/ R/	Greek mythical character, Narcissus, who was in love with his own reflection in water **-ism** *a process* **-istic** *pertaining to* **narciss-** *self-love*	Self-love; person interprets everything purely in relation to himself or herself Relating everything to oneself
pathologic gambling	path-oh-**LOJ**-ik **GAM**-bling	S/ R/CF R/	**-ic** *pertaining to* **path/o-** *disease* **-log-** *study of*	Morbid, constant, uncontrollable, destructive gambling
psychopath	**SIGH**-koh-path	S/ R/CF	**-path** *disease* **psych/o-** *mind*	Person with antisocial personality disorder
pyromania	pie-roh-**MAY**-nee-ah	S/ R/CF	**-mania** *frenzy* **pyr/o-** *fire*	Morbid impulse to set fires
schizoid	**SKITZ**-oyd	S/ R/	**-oid** *resemble* **schiz-** *split*	Withdrawn, socially isolated
self-mutilation	self-myu-tih-**LAY**-shun	S/ R/ R/	**-ation** *process* **self-** *own individual* **-mutil-** *to maim*	Injury or disfigurement made to one's own body
sociopath	**SO**-see-oh-path	S/ R/CF	**-path** *disease* **soci/o-** *partner, ally, community*	Person with antisocial personality disorder

EXERCISE

A. Use the correct abbreviation *for personality disorders. Read the description of the personality disorder and give the correct abbreviation for which it is describing. Fill in the blanks.* **LO 10.3 and 10.7**

1. A person who pulls the hairs from the eyebrows and eyelids: ____________________

2. The current title for a condition in which a person states that he or she has two separate and distinct personalities: ____________________

3. The older abbreviation for a person with two separate and distinct personalities: __________

4. This person is known to be manipulative, yet charming. His or her moods are unstable and behavior is impulsive: __________

▼ TABLE 10.1

PSYCHOACTIVE DRUGS (LO 10.6 AND 10.7)

Type/Mode of Action	Name	Common Effects	Effects of Abuse
Stimulants ("uppers") Speed up activity in the CNS	Caffeine	Wakefulness, shorter reaction time, alertness	Restlessness, insomnia, heartbeat irregularities
	Nicotine	Varies from alertness to calmness, appetite for carbohydrates decreases	Heart disease; high blood pressure; vasoconstriction; bronchitis; emphysema; lung, throat, mouth cancer
	Amphetamines	Wakefulness, alertness, increased metabolism, decreased appetite	Nervousness, high blood pressure, delusions, psychosis, convulsions, death
	Cocaine	**Euphoria,** high energy, illusions of power	Excitability, paranoia, anxiety, panic, depression, heart failure, death
Depressants ("downers") Slow down activity in the CNS	Alcohol	1–2 drinks—reduced inhibitions and anxiety	Blackouts, mental and neurologic impairment, psychosis, cirrhosis of liver, death
		Many drinks—slow reaction time, poor coordination and memory	
	Barbiturates and **tranquilizers**	Reduced anxiety and tension, sedation	Impaired motor and sensory functions, amnesia, loss of consciousness, death
Narcotics Mimic the actions of natural **endorphins**	Codeine, opium, morphine, heroin	Euphoria, pleasure, relief of pain	High tolerance of pain, nausea, vomiting, constipation, convulsions, coma, death
Psychedelics Disrupt normal thought processes	Marijuana	Relaxation, euphoria, increased appetite, pain relief	Sensory distortion, hallucinations, paranoia, throat and lung damage
	LSD, mescaline, MDMA (Ecstasy)	Exhilaration, euphoria, hallucinations, insightful experiences	Panic, extreme delusions, bad trips, paranoia, psychosis
Antidepressants Affect the neurotransmitters serotonin, norepinephrine, and dopamine	Selective serotonin reuptake inhibitors (SSRIs)—Prozac, Paxil, Zoloft	Enhanced mental clarity, improved sleep, diminished depression	Anxiety, decreased sex drive, insomnia, restlessness, fatigue, headaches
	Serotonin and norepinphrine reuptake inhibitors (SNRIs)—Effexor XR, Pristiq, Cymbalta	Diminished depression, pain relief	Raised blood pressure, liver and kidney failure, fatal outcome with overdose
	Tricyclic antidepressants (TCAs)—amitriptyline, Tofranil	Effective relief of depression but numerous side effects	Decreased sex drive and outcomes, difficulty urinating, sedation, weight gain, dry mouth, fatal outcome with overdose
Anxiolytics (anti-anxiety) Affect inhibitory neurotransmitters and their synaptic receptors	Benzodiazepines—Librium, Valium, Xanax	Relief of anxiety and panic disorder in the short term with rapid action	Habit forming, addiction tendencies, drowsiness, dizziness, worsen the effects of alcohol
	Selective serotonin reuptake inhibitors (SSRIs) (see above)	Used because they are not addictive	Fatigue, nausea, depression, insomnia
	Azaspirones—BuSpar	Effective in mild to moderate anxiety—takes 2–4 weeks to have effect; not addictive	Overdose leads to unconsciousness
	Beta blockers—Inderal, Tenormin *(see Chapter 6)*	Greatly reduce certain anxiety symptoms, such as shaking, palpitations, and sweating	Nausea, diarrhea, bronchospasm, bradycardia, insomnia, erectile dysfunction
Antiepileptic drugs (AEDs) (anticonvulsants) Do not cure epilepsy, but suppress seizures while medications are in the body	Broad-spectrum AEDs—Depakote, Lamictal, Topamax, Keppra	Effective for a wide range of all types of seizures	Weight gain, tremor, hair loss, osteoporosis, low blood count, memory problems
	Narrow-spectrum AEDs—phenobarbital, Dilantin, Tegretol, Lyrica	Effective for specific types of seizures	GI upset, weight gain, blurred vision, low blood counts, fatigue

Word Analysis and Definition

S = Suffix P = Prefix R = Root R/CF = Combining Form

WORD	PRONUNCIATION	ELEMENTS		DEFINITION
antiepileptic	**AN**-tih-epi-**LEP**-tik	S/ P/ R/	-ic *pertaining to* **anti-** *against* **-epilept-** *seizure*	An agent to suppress seizures
anxiolytic	**ANG**-zee-oh-**LIT**-ik	S/ R/CF	-lytic *soluble* **anxi/o** *anxiety*	An agent that reduces the symptoms of anxiety
dependence	dee-**PEN**-dense		Latin *to hang from*	State of needing someone or something
depressant **antidepressant**	dee-**PRESS**-ant **AN**-tih-dee-**PRESS**-ant	S/ R/ P/	-ant *agent* **depress-** *press down* **anti-** *against*	Substance that diminishes activity, sensation, or tone An agent to suppress the symptoms of depression
endorphin	en-**DOR**-fin	P/ R/	**end-** *within* **-orphin** *morphine*	Natural substance in the brain that has the same effect as opium
euphoria	yoo-**FOR**-ee-ah	S/ P/ R/	-ia *condition* **eu-** *normal* **-phor-** *bear, carry*	Exaggerated feeling of well-being
narcotic	nar-**KOT**-ik	S/ R/CF	-tic *pertaining to* **narc/o-** *sleep, stupor*	Drug derived from opium or a synthetic drug with similar effects
psychedelic	sigh-keh-**DEL**-ik	S/ R/ R/	-ic *pertaining to* **psyche-** *mind, soul* **-del-** *manifest, visible*	Agent that intensifies sensory perception
psychoactive	sigh-koh-**AK**-tiv	S/ R/CF R/	-ive *quality of, nature of* **psych/o-** *mind, soul* **-act-** *performance*	Able to alter mood, behavior, and/or cognition
stimulant	**STIM**-you-lant	S/ R/	-ant *agent* **stimul-** *excite*	Agent that excites or strengthens functional activity
tolerance	**TOL**-er-ans	S/ R/	-ance *condition, state of* **toler-** *endure*	The capacity to become accustomed to a stimulus or drug
tranquilizer	**TRANG**-kwih-lie-zer	S/ R/	-izer *affect in a particular way* **tranquil-** *calm*	Agent that calms without sedating or depressing

EXERCISE

A. Deconstruct *each medical term into its basic elements to better understand the meaning of the term. If the term does not have a particular element, leave it blank. Fill in the blanks.* **LO 10.1, 10.6, and 10.7**

1. psychoactive __________/__________/__________
P R, R/CF S

2. psychedelic __________/__________/__________
P R, R/CF S

3. euphoria __________/__________/__________
P R, R/CF S

4. antidepressant __________/__________/__________
P R, R/CF S

5. tranquilizer __________/__________/__________
P R, R/CF S

Additional exercises available in connect

Chapter Review exercises, along with additional practice items, are available in Connect!

Special Senses of the Eye and Ear

CHAPTER 11

The Essentials of the Languages of Ophthalmology and Otology

Rick Brady/McGraw-Hill Education

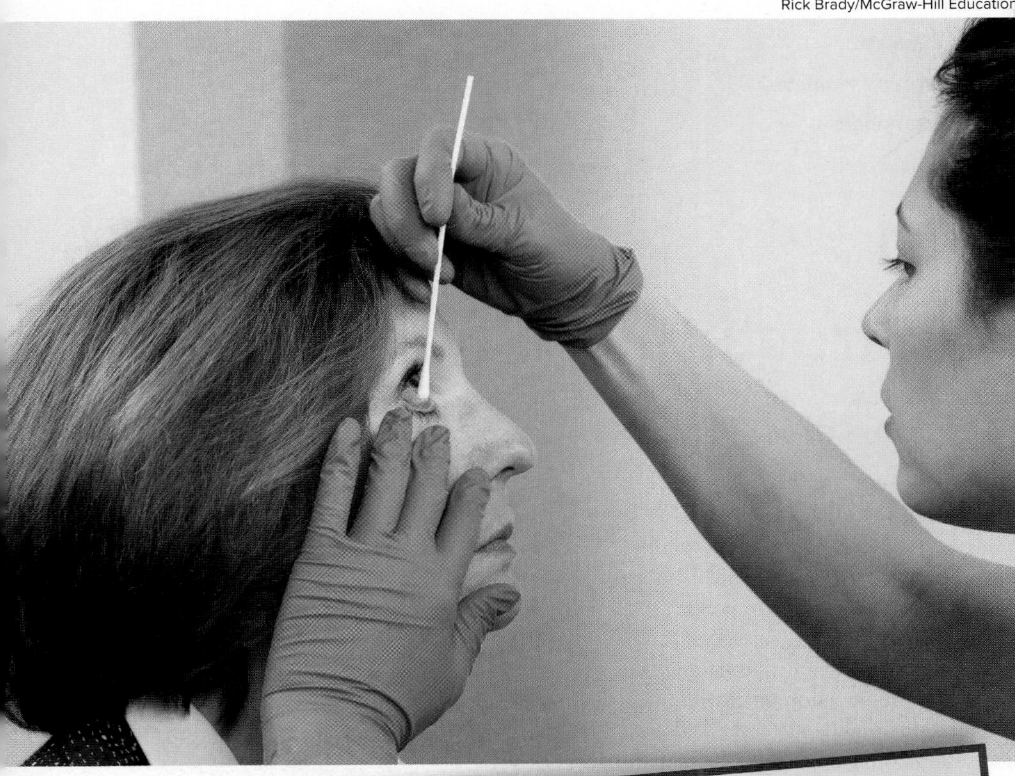

Learning Outcomes

In order to make correct decisions in situations like Mrs. Hughes' case, to communicate with Dr. Chun about the patient, to participate in patient education, and to document the patient's care, you need to be able to:

LO 11.1 **Use roots, combining forms, suffixes, and prefixes to construct and analyze (deconstruct) medical terms related to the eye and ear.**

LO 11.2 **Spell and pronounce correctly medical terms related to the eye and ear in order to communicate them with accuracy and precision in any health care setting.**

LO 11.3 **Define accepted abbreviations related to the eye and ear.**

LO 11.4 **Relate the position and anatomy of the accessory structures and extrinsic muscles of the eye to their functions, disorders, and treatments.**

NOTE: The sense of smell is discussed as an integral part of the respiratory system; the sense of taste, as an integral part of the digestive system; and the sense of touch, as an integral part of the nervous system.

CASE REPORT 11.1

You are . . .

. . . an **ophthalmic** technician (OT) working in the office of **ophthalmologist** Angela Chun, MD, a member of the Fulwood Medical Group.

You are communicating with . . .

. . . Mrs. Jenny Hughes, a 30-year-old computer software consultant. She walked into the office with painful, red, swollen eyelids and a sticky, purulent discharge from both eyes. The administrative medical assistant did not hold her in the reception area but brought her directly to you. Mrs. Hughes complains of headache and **photophobia,** and says her eyelids were stuck together when she woke up this morning. She tells you that a couple of days earlier, she had gone into a small business office to install software at the firm's 10 workstations. One of the employees was absent with **pink eye.** Mrs. Hughes wants to know if she could have contracted the disease from that employee's keyboard, and how to prevent her husband and two children from getting it. In your hand, you have a pen and clipboard with the office Notice of Privacy Practices and sign-in sheet for her to sign. How do you proceed?

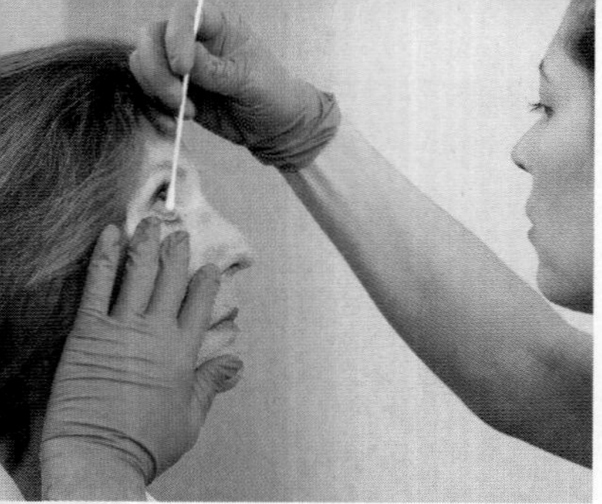

Rick Brady/McGraw-Hill Education

Objectives

*Mrs. Jenny Hughes' **"pink eye"** involved her **conjunctiva** and eyelids–two of the **periorbital** accessory structures of the eye, located around the **orbit** and in front of the eyeball. All the accessory structures support and protect the exposed front surface of the eyes.*

The information in this lesson will enable you to use correct medical terminology to:

11.1.1 Describe the accessory structures of the eye.

11.1.2 Link the anatomy of each of the accessory structures to its functions.

11.1.3 Discuss disorders of the accessory structures.

11.1.4 Explain the effects of disorders of the extrinsic muscles on the eye.

In your future career, you may work directly and/or indirectly with one or more of the following:

- **Ophthalmologists** are medical specialists in the diagnosis and treatment of diseases of the eye.
- **Optometrists** are professionals skilled in the measurement of vision.

The health professionals listed below perform specific assigned procedures and support ophthalmologists according to the depth of their training:

- **Certified ophthalmic medical technicians**
- **Certified ophthalmic assistants**
- **Certified ophthalmic technicians**
- **Certified ophthalmic technologists**
- **Registered ophthalmic ultrasound biometrists**
- **Diagnostic ophthalmic sonographers**

Lesson 11.1

Accessory Structures of the Eye (LO 11.2 and 11.4)

A beam of light travels to the eye at 186,000 miles per second, or 671 million miles per hour. Before it can reach the eyeball, it passes through external accessory structures, which have important functions that support and protect the exposed front surface of the eye.

The **eyebrows** *(Figure 11.1)* keep sweat from running into the eyes and function in nonverbal communication to show how you're feeling in response to certain stimuli.

The **eyelids** protect the eyes from foreign objects. They blink to move tears across the eyes' surface and sweep debris away. They close in sleep to keep out visual stimuli. They are the body's thinnest layer of skin.

The **eyelashes** are strong hairs that help keep debris out of the eyes. They arise from hair follicles with their sebaceous glands on the edge of the lids.

Eyelashes
Eyebrow
Pupil
Upper eyelid
Lower eyelid
Conjunctiva

▲ **FIGURE 11.1**
External Anatomy of the Eye.

Joe DeGrandis/McGraw-Hill Education

The **conjunctiva** is a transparent mucous membrane that lines the inside of both eyelids. It moves freely over the eyeball and covers the front of the eye but not the central portion (the **cornea**). In the conjunctiva, numerous goblet cells secrete a thin film of mucin (a complex protein) that keeps the eyeball moist. It has numerous small blood vessels and is richly supplied with nerve endings that make it very sensitive to pain.

The **lacrimal apparatus** *(Figure 11.2)* consists of the **lacrimal (tear) gland** located in the superolateral corner of the orbit. This gland secretes tears, and short ducts carry the tears to the conjunctiva's surface. After washing across the conjunctiva, the tears leave the eye at its medial corner by draining into the **lacrimal sac.** They then flow into the **nasolacrimal duct,** which carries the tears into the nose, from where they are swallowed.

The functions of tears are to:

- **Clean and lubricate** the surface of the eyes;
- **Deliver** nutrients and oxygen to the conjunctiva; and
- **Prevent infection** through bactericidal (bacteria-killing) enzymes.

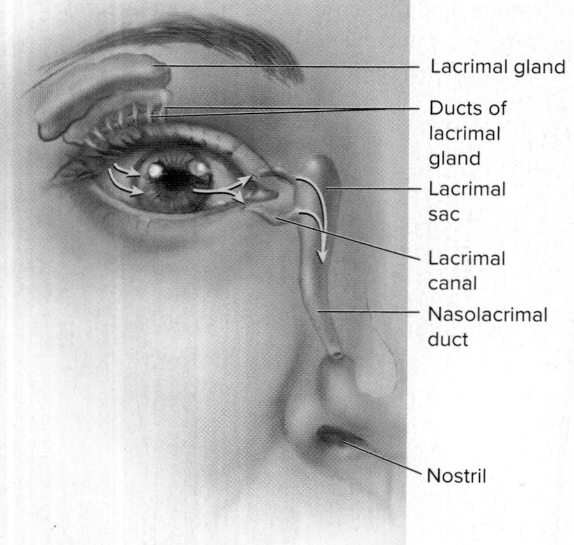

▲ **FIGURE 11.2**
Lacrimal Apparatus.

Word Analysis and Definition

S = Suffix P = Prefix R = Root R/CF = Combining Form

WORD	PRONUNCIATION		ELEMENTS	DEFINITION
conjunctiva **conjunctival (adj)** **conjunctivitis** **"pink eye"**	kon-junk-**TIE**-vah kon-junk-**TIE**-val kon-junk-tih-**VI**-tis	 S/ R/ S/	Latin *inner lining of eyelids* **-al** *pertaining to* **conjunctiv-** *conjunctiva* **-itis** *inflammation* Lay term for conjunctivitis	Inner lining of eyelids Pertaining to the conjunctiva Inflammation of the conjunctiva Conjunctivitis
cornea **corneal (adj)**	**KOR**-nee-ah **KOR**-nee-al	 S/ R/	Latin *web, tunic* **-al** *pertaining to* **corne-** *cornea*	The central, transparent part of the outer coat of the eye covering the iris and pupil Pertaining to the cornea
lacrimal **nasolacrimal duct**	**LAK**-rim-al **NAY**-zoh-**LAK**-rim-al DUKT	S/ R/ R/CF R/	**-al** *pertaining to* **lacrim-** *tear* **nas/o-** *nose* **duct** *to lead*	Pertaining to tears and the tear apparatus Passage from the lacrimal sac to the nose
ophthalmology **ophthalmologist** **ophthalmic (adj)**	off-thal-**MALL**-oh-jee off-thal-**MALL**-oh-jist off-**THAL**-mik	S/ R/CF S/ S/ R/	**-logy** *study of* **ophthalm/o-** *eye* **-logist** *one who studies, specialist* **-ic** *pertaining to* **ophthalm-** *eye*	Diagnosis and treatment of diseases of the eye Medical specialist in ophthalmology Pertaining to the eye
orbit **orbital (adj)** **periorbital**	**OR**-bit **OR**-bit-al per-ee-**OR**-bit-al	 S/ R/ P/	Latin *circle* **-al** *pertaining to* **orbit-** *orbit* **peri-** *around*	The bony socket that holds the eyeball Pertaining to the orbit Pertaining to tissues around the orbit
photophobia **photophobic (adj)**	foh-toe-**FOH**-bee-ah foh-toe-**FOH**-bik	S/ R/CF R/ S/	**-ia** *condition* **phot/o-** *light* **-phob-** *fear* **-ic** *pertaining to*	Abnormal sensitivity to light due to pain in the eyes Pertaining to or suffering from photophobia

Exercises

A. Build *your medical vocabulary. If the term does not have an element, insert N/A. The first one has been done for you. Fill in the chart.* **LO 11.1**

Medical Term	Prefix	Meaning of Prefix	Root(s)/CF(s)	Meaning of R/CF	Suffix	Meaning of Suffix
corneal	**1. N/A**	**2. N/A**	**3. corne-**	**4. cornea**	**5. -al**	**6. pertaining to**
conjunctivitis	**7.**	**8.**	**9.**	**10.**	**11.**	**12.**
periorbital	**13.**	**14.**	**15.**	**16.**	**17.**	**18.**
ophthalmologist	**19.**	**20.**	**21.**	**22.**	**23.**	**24.**
ophthalmology	**25.**	**26.**	**27.**	**28.**	**29.**	**30.**

B. Read Case Report 11.1 *and content related to accessory structures of the eye to correctly complete each statement. Select the correct answer to complete each statement.* **LO 11.4 and 11.10**

1. What words could Jenny Hughes likely use to describe her condition of **photophobia**:

a. "It hurts to blink my eye."
b. "My eye is dry and scratchy."
c. "My eyelids are painful."
d. "The light hurts my eye."

2. The medical term that is used to document the condition **pink eye** is:

a. conjuctivitis **b.** corneal abrasion **c.** blepharitis **d.** ptosis

3. Dr. Chun's specialty is described as a:

a. specialist in the measurements of vision
b. technician that fits patients with prescription eyeware
c. medical doctor specializing in the diagnosis and treatment of eye disorders.
d. technician that assists optometrists

Lesson 11.1 (cont'd) Disorders of the Accessory Glands

(LO 11.4)

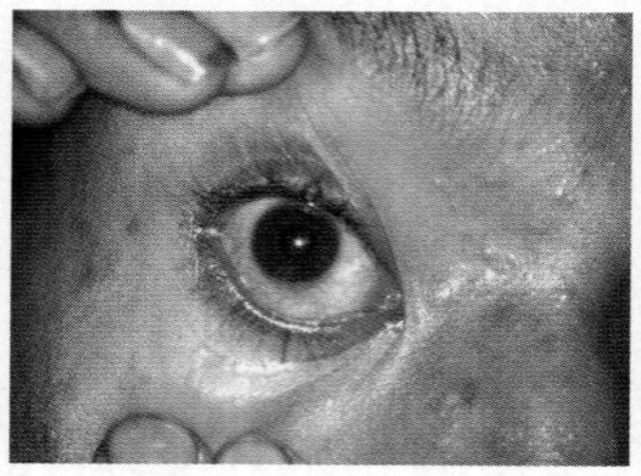

▲ **FIGURE 11.3**
Conjunctivitis.
Centers for Disease Control

The accessory glands of the eyes can be affected by a number of different disorders, most of which cause noticeable discomfort.

Conjunctivitis *(Figure 11.3)*, an inflammation of the conjunctiva, is more commonly viral than bacterial; it can also be caused by irritants like chlorine, soaps, fumes, and smoke.

Eyelid edema, a generalized swelling of the eyelids, is often produced by an allergic reaction *(see Chapter 8)* from cosmetics, pollen in the air, or insect stings and bites.

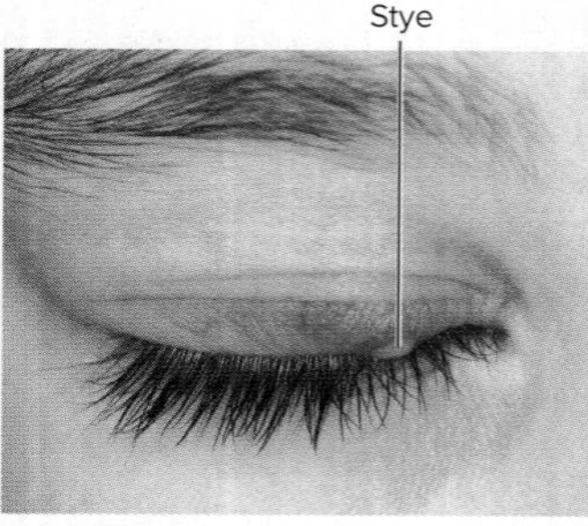

▲ **FIGURE 11.4**
Stye Showing Pus-Filled Cyst.
ElRoi/Shutterstock

A **stye** or **hordeolum** is an infection of an eyelash follicle that produces an abscess *(Figure 11.4)*, with localized pain, swelling, redness, and pus at the edge of the eyelid.

Blepharitis occurs when multiple eyelash follicles become infected. The eyelid's margin shows persistent redness and crusting and may become ulcerated *(Figure 11.5)*.

Ptosis, in which the upper eyelid is constantly drooped over the eye, is due to **paresis** of the muscle that raises the upper lid *(Figure 11.6)*. The term **blepharoptosis** defines the sagging of the eyelids from excess skin. The plastic surgery procedure of **blepharoplasty** is used to repair the eyelid.

Dry eye disease (dysfunctional tear syndrome) is due to decreased tear production by the lacrimal glands. It leads to ocular discomfort and potential damage to the conjunctiva and cornea. Some cases are due to **Sjogren's syndrome,** in which the lacrimal glands are affected by autoimmune processes. Dry eye is more common in females and the elderly, and in people who wear contact lenses.

Case Report 11.1 *(continued)*

Mrs. Hughes' pink eye is called acute **contagious** conjunctivitis ***(Figure 11.3)***. It responds well to **antibiotic** eyedrops. Her hands were **contaminated** from the keyboard of the employee who had left work and gone home with pink eye. She transmitted the infection to her eye by touching or rubbing it.

Your documentation of Mrs. Hughes' office visit could read:

Progress Note: 04/10/19

Mrs. Jenny Hughes was brought directly into the clinical area at 1030 hrs with what appeared to be conjunctivitis, "pink eye." Both eyelids were red and swollen with a **purulent discharge.** She complained of headache and photophobia. Dr. Chun prescribed three drops q4h of Neosporin eyedrops and sent a swab of the discharge to the laboratory. I instructed and watched Mrs. Hughes wash her hands and use an alcohol-based hand gel. I then had her sign in and sign our Notice of Privacy Practices. I instructed her in the use of the eyedrops and emphasized home care and hand care measures to prevent the infection from spreading to her family. She was given a return appointment in 1 week and told to call the office if the eyedrops do not help.

—Daphne Butras, OT, 1055 hrs.

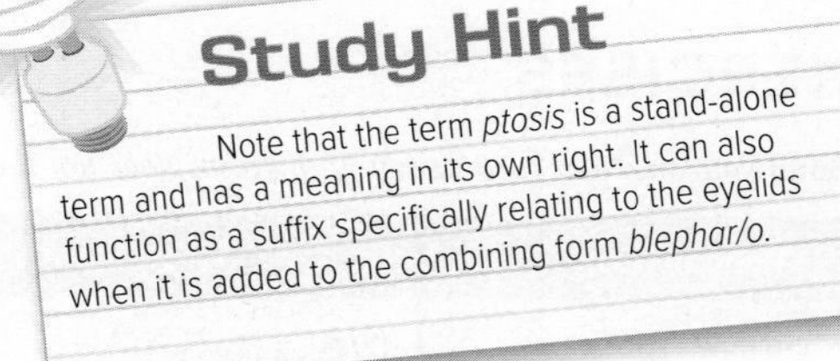

Study Hint

Note that the term *ptosis* is a stand-alone term and has a meaning in its own right. It can also function as a suffix specifically relating to the eyelids when it is added to the combining form *blephar/o*.

Abbreviation

q4h	Every four hours.

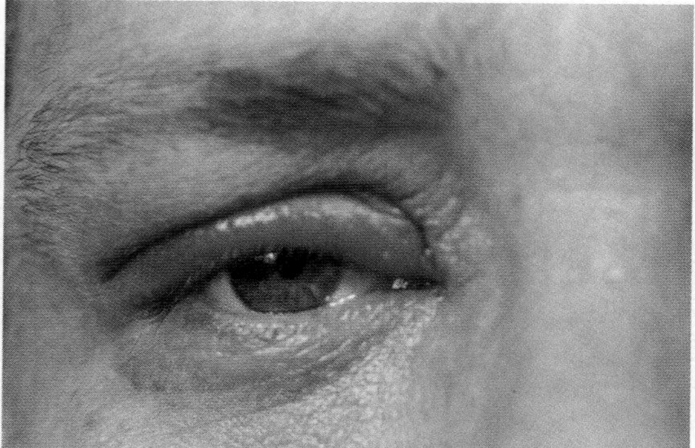

▲ **FIGURE 11.5**
Blepharitis of the Upper Lid.
Images By Kenny / Alamy Stock Photo

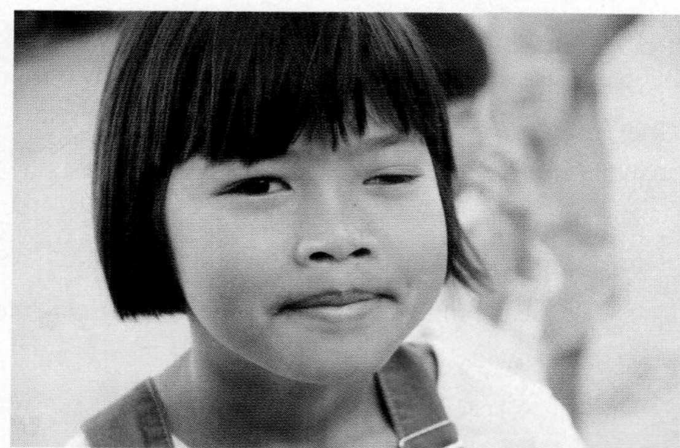

▲ **FIGURE 11.6**
Ptosis of Left Eyelid.
Richman Photo/Shutterstock

Word Analysis and Definition

S = Suffix P = Prefix R = Root R/CF = Combining Form

WORD	PRONUNCIATION	ELEMENTS		DEFINITION
antibiotic	**AN**-tih-bye-**OT**-ik	S/ P/ R/	-tic *pertaining to* **anti-** *against* -bio- *life*	A substance that has the capacity to inhibit the growth of or destroy bacteria and other microorganisms
blepharitis	blef-ah-**RYE**-tis	S/ R/	-itis *inflammation* **blephar-** *eyelid*	Inflammation of the eyelid
blepharoptosis	**BLEF**-ah-**ROP**-toe-sis	S/ R/CF	-ptosis *drooping* **blephar/o-** *eyelid*	Drooping of the upper eyelid
blepharoplasty	**BLEF**-ah-roh-plas-tee	S/	-plasty *surgical repair*	Surgical repair of the eyelid
conjunctivitis		S/ R/	-itis *inflammation* **conjunctiv-** *conjunctiva*	Inflammation of the conjunctiva
contagious	kon-**TAY**-jus		Latin *touch closely*	Infection can be transmitted from person to person or from a person to a surface to a person
contaminate (verb)	kon-**TAM**-in-ate	S/ P/ R/	-ate *composed of, pertaining to* **con-** *together* -tamin- *touch*	To cause the presence of an infectious agent to be on any surface
contamination (noun)	**KON**-tam-ih-**NAY**-shun	S/	-ation *process*	The presence of an infectious agent on any surface
hordeolum (*also called* **stye)**	hor-**DEE**-oh-lum		Latin *stye in the eye*	Abscess in an eyelash follicle
paresis	par-**EE**-sis		Greek *paralysis*	Partial paralysis
ptosis (**Notes:** *When a word begins with two consonants, the first is silent.* **Ptosis** *can also be used as a suffix.*)	**TOE**-sis		Greek *drooping*	Drooping down of the upper eyelid or an organ
purulent	**PURE**-you-lent	S/ R/	-ulent *abounding in* **pur-** *pus*	Showing or containing a lot of pus

EXERCISES

A. Disorders: The accessory structures of the eye have their own disorders. *The patient conditions are described in the first column; match the condition with the correct medical term in the second column from this lesson.* **LO 11.4**

______	**1.** inflammation of the conjunctiva	**a.** paresis
______	**2.** drooping of upper eyelid	**b.** hordeolum
______	**3.** partial paralysis	**c.** blepharoptosis
______	**4.** red, crusted, and ulcerated eyelid	**d.** blepharitis
______	**5.** abscess in an eyelash follicle	**e.** conjuctivitis

B. There are three medical terms below that need to be translated *for Mrs. Hughes so she can understand her condition and treatment. Select the answer that will correctly complete each statement.* **LO 11.4, 11.5, and 11.10**

Mrs. Hughes has **conjunctivitis(1)** of both eyes. It is important that she wash her hands before touching things, because this condition is **contagious (2)**. Instruct her to instill one drop of **antibiotic (3)** eye drops into the eyes two times per day.

1. Mrs. Hughes, you have a(n)

a. inflammation of the inner lining of the eyelid.
b. infection of the tear duct.
c. partial paralysis of the eyelid.
d. abscess in an eyelash follicle.

2. This condition

a. can cause a fever.
b. is an infection that can be given to other people.
c. can lead to paralysis.
d. remains in your body for up to one year.

3. The medication in the eye drops

a. relieves your dry eyes. **b.** fights off allergens. **c.** dilates your pupils. **d.** kills the bacterial infection.

CASE REPORT 11.2

You are . . .

. . . an ophthalmic technician employed by Angela Chun, MD, an ophthalmologist at Fulwood Medical Center.

You are communicating with . . .

. . . Mrs. Jenny Hughes, the mother of Sam Hughes, a 2½-year-old boy, who has been referred by his pediatrician to Dr. Chun.

Mrs. Hughes states that for the past couple of months, Sam's right eye has turned in. The only visual difficulty she has noticed is that he sometimes misses a Cheerio when he tries to grab it.

You are responsible for documenting Sam's diagnostic and therapeutic procedures and explaining their significance to his mother.

Extrinsic Muscles of the Eye (LO 11.2 and 11.4)

Humans have two eyes positioned on the face, one on either side of the nose facing forward, which work closely together. This eye configuration gives us very good three-dimensional perception **(stereopsis)** and hand-eye coordination. Stereopsis depends on an accurate alignment of the two eyes.

Six coordinated **extrinsic** eye muscles in each eye—attached to the inner wall of the orbit and outer surface of the eyeball—keep the eyes properly aligned, and move the eyes in all directions.

When there is a muscle imbalance in one eye, the alignment breaks down and **strabismus** *(Figure 11.7),* also known as a "cross-eyed" condition, results. It can be cured by vision therapy or surgery.

Esotropia is a condition where the eye is turned in toward the nose. In congenital or infantile esotropia, both eyes look in toward the nose—the right eye looks to the left and the left eye looks to the right *(Figure 11.8).* Children with this condition require surgery.

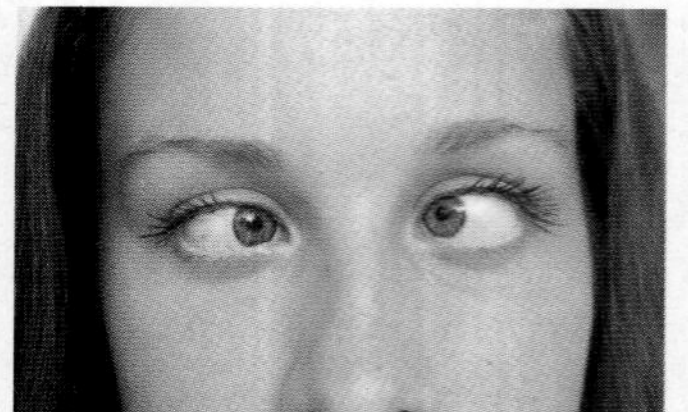

▲ **FIGURE 11.7**
Strabismus.
sruilk/Shutterstock

Accomodative esotropia is an inward eye turn, usually noticed around age 2 in 1 to 2% of children. Sam Hughes had an accommodative esotropia in one eye. Wearing glasses and perhaps a patch over the stronger eye will help to correct Sam's problem.

Exotropia, an outward eye turn, is noticed in children around ages 2 to 4. It will often respond to vision therapy, which includes eye exercises and glasses, from an **optometrist.** Eye muscle surgery can establish good **ocular** alignment.

Amblyopia, or "lazy eye," occurs in children when vision in one eye has not developed as well as vision in the other. Instead, it occurs because the eye and the brain won't cooperate for the affected eye. Amblyopia is treated with a patch over the stronger eye in order to develop the vision in the weaker eye.

Nystagmus is a term to describe fast, uncontrollable movements of the eye that may be side to side (horizontal nystagmus), up and down (vertical nystagmus), or **rotary** (rotary nystagmus). The condition can be congenital or acquired from head injury, inner ear disorders *(see the section on the Ear in this chapter),* stroke, or drugs, such as excess alcohol, sedatives, or anti-epilepsy drugs *(see Chapter 10).* There is no cure, but some cases improve spontaneously.

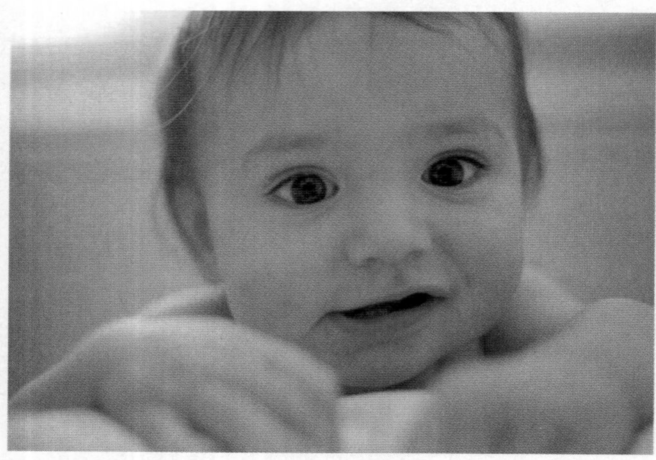

▲ **FIGURE 11.8**
Congenital Esotropia (both eyes are affected).
Matt Harris Photography/Alamy Images

Word Analysis and Definition

S = Suffix P = Prefix R = Root R/CF = Combining Form

WORD	PRONUNCIATION	ELEMENTS		DEFINITION
accommodation (noun) **accommodate (verb)** **accommodative (adj)**	ah-kom-oh-**DAY**-shun ah-**KOM**-oh-date ah-kom-oh-**DAY**-tiv	S/ P/ R/ S/ S/	**-ion** *action* **ac-** *toward* **-commodat-** *adjust* **-ate** *pertaining to, composed of* **-ive** *pertaining to*	The act of adjusting something to make it fit the needs; in this case, the lens of the eye adjusts itself To adapt to meet a need Pertaining to accommodation
amblyopia	am-blee-**OH**-pee-ah	P/ R/	**ambly-** *dull* **-opia** *sight*	Failure or incomplete development of the pathways of vision to the brain
esotropia **exotropia**	es-oh-**TROH**-pee-ah ek-soh-**TROH**-pee-ah	S/ P/ R/ P/	**-ia** *condition* **eso-** *inward* **-trop-** *turn* **exo-** *outward*	Turning the eye inward toward the nose Turning the eye outward away from the nose
extrinsic **intrinsic**	eks-**TRIN**-sik in-**TRIN**-sik		Latin *on the outer side* Latin *on the inner side*	Any muscle located entirely on the outside of the structure under consideration; e.g., the eye Any muscle located entirely within (inside) the structure under consideration; e.g., the eye
nystagmus	nis-**TAG**-muss		Greek *nodding*	Fast, uncontrollable movements of the eyeballs
ocular	**OCK**-you-lar	S/ R/	**-ar** *pertaining to* **ocul-** *eye*	Pertaining to the eye
optometrist **optometry**	op-**TOM**-eh-trist op-**TOM**-eh-tree	S/ R/CF S/	**-metrist** *skilled in measurement* **opt/o-** *vision* **-metry** *process of measuring*	Someone skilled in the measurement of vision but who cannot treat eye diseases or prescribe medication The profession of the measurement of vision
rotary	**ROW**-tah-ree		Latin *to revolve*	Circular movement
stereopsis	ster-ee-**OP**-sis	S/ R/	**-opsis** *vision* **stere-** *three-dimensional*	Three-dimensional vision
strabismus	strah-**BIZ**-mus	S/ R/	**-ismus** *take action* **strab-** *squint*	Turning of an eye away from its normal position

Exercises

A. Recognize *the definitions of disorders of the extrinsic muscles of the eye. Insert the disorder of the eye that is being described. Fill in the blanks.* **LO 11.2 and 11.4**

1. a turning of the eye outward away from the nose: __________
2. failure or incomplete development of the pathways of vision to the brain: __________
3. turning of the eye inward toward the nose: __________
4. a turning of an eye away from its normal position: __________
5. three-dimensional vision: __________
6. the adjustment of the lens by itself: __________

B. Deconstruct *the following medical terms into their elements. Complete the chart. If a term does not have an element, insert N/A. The first one has been done for you.* **LO 11.1**

Medical Term	Prefix	Root(s)/ Combining Form(s)	Suffix
exotropia	**1. exo-**	**2. -trop-**	**3. -ia**
optometrist	**4.**	**5.**	**6.**
esotropia	**7.**	**8.**	**9.**
amblyopia	**10.**	**11.**	**12.**
stereopsis	**13.**	**14.**	**15.**
ocular	**16.**	**17.**	**18.**

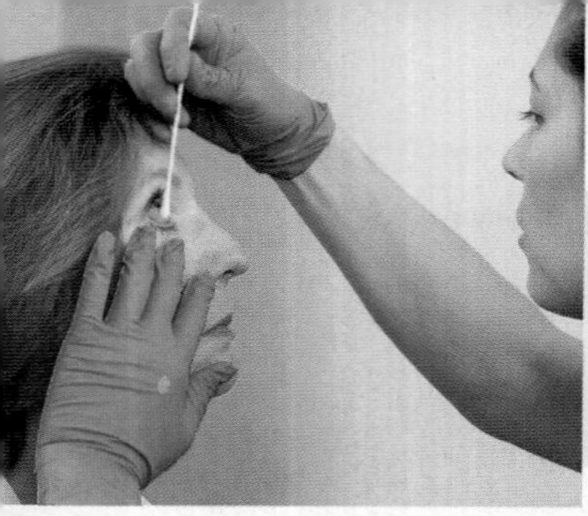
Rick Brady/McGraw-Hill Education

Lesson 11.2

The Eyeball and Seeing

Objectives

Although your eyeball may appear to be solid, it's actually a hollow sphere that measures around 1 inch in diameter. Knowledge of its terminology, structure, and function allows you to understand how we see and what major problems and disorders can arise with the eye. In this lesson, the information will enable you to use correct medical terminology to:

11.2.1 Identify the principal structures of the eyeball and their functions.

11.2.2 Explain the role of the cornea and the problems that can occur in that structure.

11.2.3 Describe the structures and functions of the lens and its associated structures.

11.2.4 Link the different components of the retina to their functions.

11.2.5 Discuss disorders of the eyeball.

Keynotes

- The cornea protects the eye and, by changing shape, provides about 60% of the eye's focusing power.
- The iris controls the amount of light entering the eye.
- The lens changes its shape to focus rays of light on the retina.
- Medical shorthand for a quick, normal eye examination can be **PERRLA: P**upils **E**qual, **R**ound, **R**eactive to **L**ight and **A**ccommodation.

The Eyeball (Globe)

(LO 11.5)

The functions of the eyeball are to continuously:

1. **Adjust** the amount of light it lets in to reach the retina;
2. **Focus** on near and distant objects; and
3. **Produce** images of those objects and instantly transmit them to the brain.

As shown earlier in this chapter, the front of the eyeball is covered by the conjunctiva. This thin layer of tissue lines the inside of the eyelids and curves over the eyeball to meet the **sclera** *(Figure 11.9)*, the tough, white outer layer of the eye.

At the center of the front of the eye is the **cornea,** a transparent, dome-shaped membrane. The cornea has no blood supply and obtains its nutrients from tears and from fluid in the anterior chamber behind it.

When light rays strike the eye, they pass through the cornea. Because of its dome curvature, those rays striking the edge of the cornea are bent toward its center. The light rays then go through the **pupil,** the black opening in the center of the colored area (the **iris**) in the front of the eye.

The iris controls the amount of light entering the eye. For example, when you're in the dark outside at night, the iris opens **(dilates)** to allow more light into the eye. When you're in bright sunlight or in a well-lit room, the iris closes **(constricts)** to allow less light into the eye.

After traveling through the pupil, the light rays pass through the transparent **lens.** This lens can become thicker and thinner, enabling it to bend light rays and focus them on the **retina** at the back of the eye. Accommodation is the process of changing focus, and **refraction** is the process of bending light rays.

The lens does not contain blood vessels **(avascular)** or nerves, and with increasing age, it loses its elasticity. Because of this reduced elasticity, when you reach your forties, your eyes may have difficulty focusing on near objects, a condition called **presbyopia.**

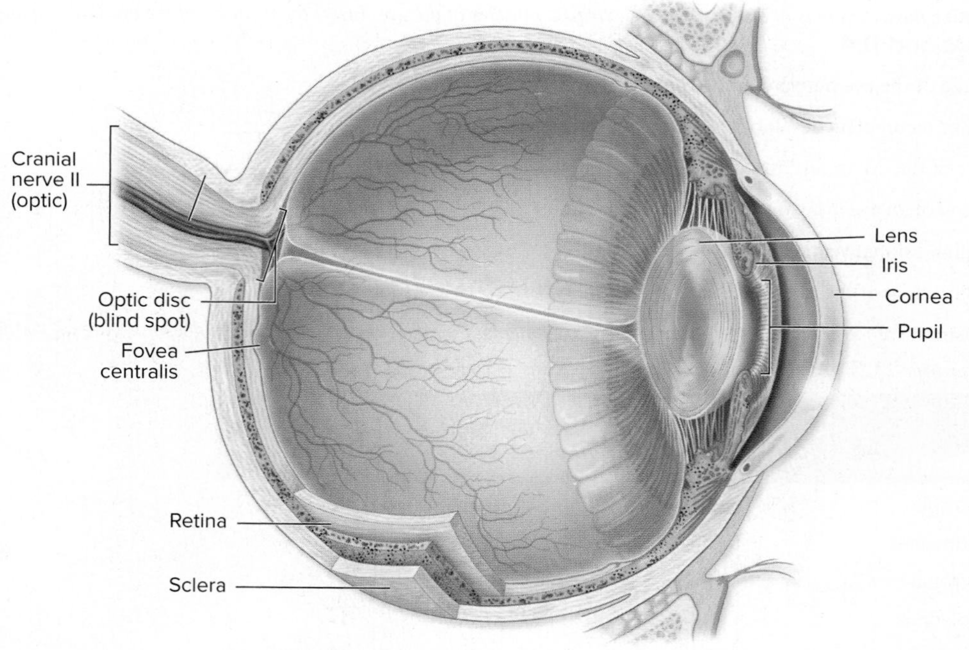

▲ **FIGURE 11.9**
Anatomy of the Eyeball.

Word Analysis and Definition

S = Suffix P = Prefix R = Root R/CF = Combining Form

WORD	PRONUNCIATION	ELEMENTS		DEFINITION
astigmatism	ah-**STIG**-maht-izm	S/ P/ R/	-ism *process* a- *without* -stigmat- *focus*	Inability to focus light rays that enter the eye in different planes
concave **convex**	kon-**KAVE** kon-**VEKS**		Latin concavus *arched* Latin convexus *vaulted*	Having a hollowed surface A surface that is evenly curved outward
foramen **foramina (pl)**	fo-**RAY**-men fo-**RAM**-ih-nah		Latin *hole*	An opening through a structure
myopia **(Note:** *One "op" is removed to allow the term to flow.*)	my-**OH**-pee-ah	R/ S/	**myop-** *to blink* -opia *sight*	Able to see close objects but unable to see distant objects
presbyopia	prez-bee-**OH**-pee-ah	R/ S/	**presby-** *old person* -opia *sight*	Difficulty in nearsighted vision occurring in middle and old age in both sexes

EXERCISES

A. Construct *the correct medical term to match the meaning given in the first column 1. Write each element in the correct column to form the complete term. Fill in the chart.* **LO 11.1 and 11.5**

Meaning of Medical Term	Prefix	Root(s)/Combining Form(s)	Suffix
inability to focus light rays	**1.**	**2.**	**3.**
able to see distant objects but not close ones	**4.**	**5.**	**6.**
able to see close objects but not distant ones	**7.**	**8.**	**9.**

B. Match *the disorder of refraction in the first column with the corrective lens in the second column.* **LO 11.5 and 11.6**

_____ **1.** astigmatism **a.** convex only

_____ **2.** myopia **b.** convex bifocals

_____ **3.** presbyopia **c.** cylindrical

_____ **4.** hyperopia **d.** concave

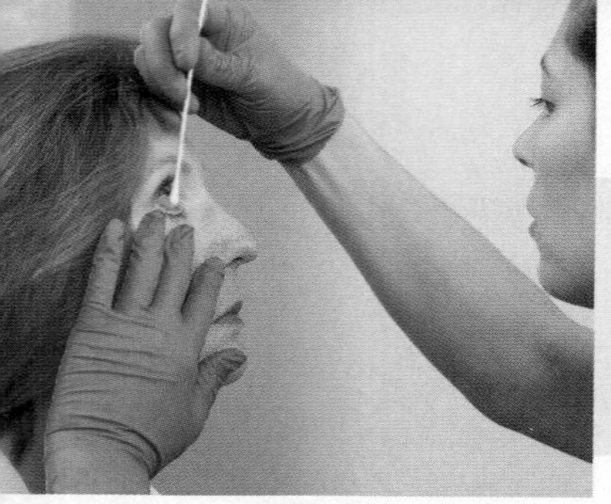

Rick Brady/McGraw-Hill Education

Lesson 11.3

Disorders of the Eye

Objectives

Many eye disorders can threaten a patient's vision, but if detected early, the majority of these conditions can be cured or treated to slow or prevent the progression of vision loss. Routine eye exams are important for early detection and prevention, and are recommended at different times throughout life. The information in this lesson will enable you to use correct medical terminology to:

11.3.1 Discuss common disorders of the eye and their effects on vision.

11.3.2 Describe common ophthalmic procedures performed in the doctor's office.

Disorders of the Anterior Eyeball (LO 11.5)

Conjunctivitis is the infectious, contagious, "bloodshot eyes"-causing condition that Mrs. Jenny Hughes had in the opening Case Report of this chapter. It can be caused by viruses and bacteria, and by organisms that cause sexually transmitted diseases (STDs) *(Chapter 15).* Four other types of conjunctivitis are:

- **Allergic conjunctivitis,** which can be part of seasonal hay fever or produced by year-round allergens like animal dander and dust mites *(Chapter 8);*
- **Irritant conjunctivitis,** which can be caused by air **pollutants** (smoke and fumes), chemicals like chlorine, and some ingredients found in soaps and cosmetics; and
- **Neonatal conjunctivitis (ophthalmia neonatorum),** which is specific to babies and can be caused by a blocked tear duct, by the antibiotic eye drops given routinely at birth, or by sexually transmitted bacteria from an infected mother's birth canal.
- **Keratoconjunctivitis** is a combined inflammation of the cornea and conjunctiva. It can be viral, bacterial, or allergic in origin.

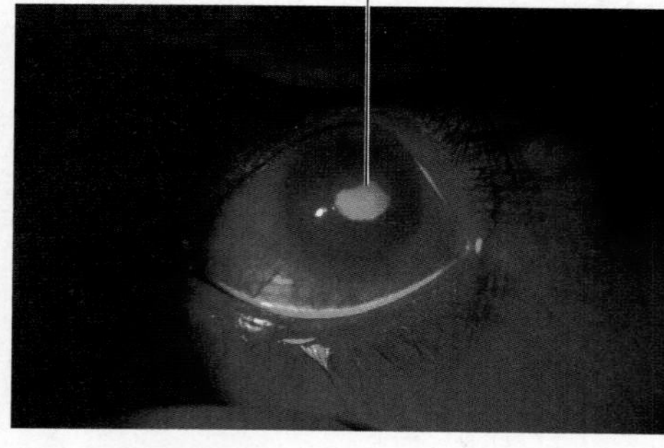

▲ **FIGURE 11.14**
Fluorescein-Stained Corneal Ulcer.

ARZTSAMUI/Shutterstock

Corneal abrasions are caused by foreign bodies, by direct trauma (like being poked by a fingernail), or by ill-fitting contact lenses. An abrasion can grow into an ulcer. This ulcer or lesion can be stained with drops of the dye **fluorescein** to make it more easily visible on examination *(Figure 11.14).*

Scleritis is an inflammation of the sclera (the white outer covering of the eyeball) that can affect one or both eyes.

Glaucoma results if fluid from inside the eyeball cannot escape from the eye into the bloodstream. The fluid continues to be produced and pressure builds up inside the eye. This pressure interferes with the blood supply to the retina, causing retinal cells to die and damage to the optic nerve fibers. Glaucoma is a major cause of blindness *(Figure 11.15).*

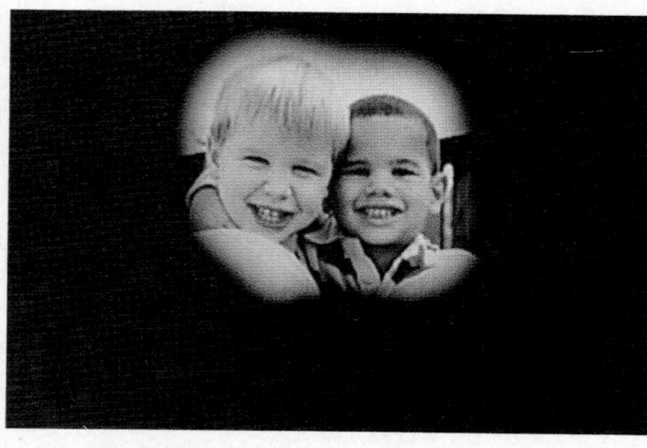

▲ **FIGURE 11.15**
Vision with Glaucoma.

Source: National Eye Institute, National Institutes of Health

A **cataract** is a cloudy or opaque area in the lens *(Figure 11.16).* It is caused by aging and may be associated with diabetes and cigarette smoke. Symptoms include blurred vision (*Figure 11.17*) and **photosensitivity.** A cataract may also be discovered during a routine eye exam. It is another major cause of blindness.

Congenital (present at birth) cataracts occur in less than 0.5% of newborns and can be unilateral (present in one eye) or bilateral (present in both eyes). They are treated in the same way as any other cataract.

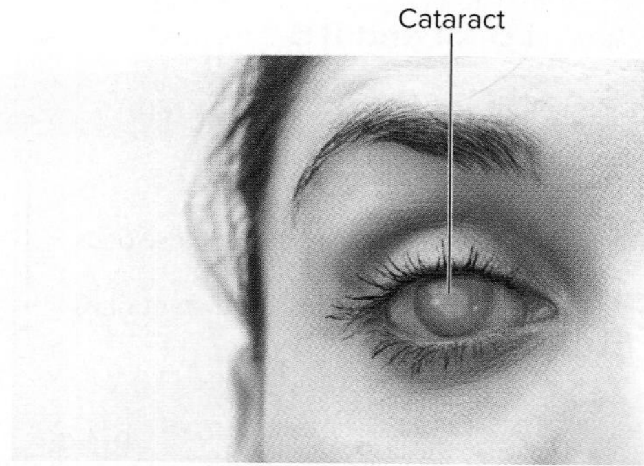

▲ **FIGURE 11.16**
Cataract.

sruilk/Shutterstock

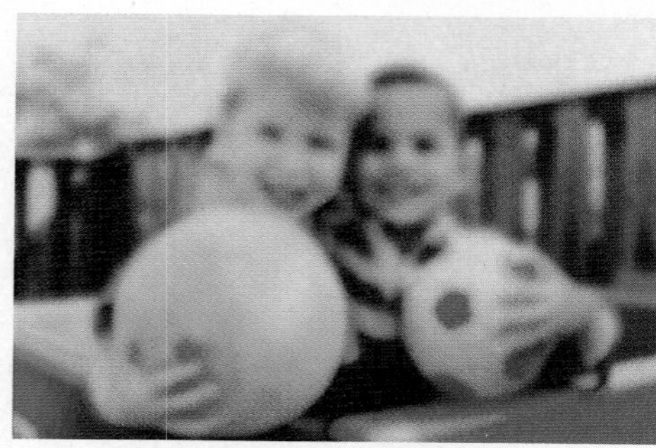

▲ **FIGURE 11.17**
Vision with Cataract.

National Eye Institute, National Institutes of Health

Word Analysis and Definition

S = Suffix P = Prefix R = Root R/CF = Combining Form

WORD	PRONUNCIATION	ELEMENTS	DEFINITION
abrasion	ah-**BRAY**-shun	S/ ion *action, condition, process* R/ abras- *scrape off*	Area of skin or mucous membrane that has been scraped off
cataract	**KAT**-ah-ract	Latin *to break down*	Complete or partial opacity of the lens
fluorescein	flor-**ESS**-ee-in	P/ **fluo-** *fluorine* R/ **-rescein** *resin*	Dye that produces a vivid green color under a blue light to diagnose corneal abrasions and foreign bodies
glaucoma	glau-**KOH**-mah	S/ -oma *mass, tumor* R/ glauc- *lens opacity*	Loss of vision due to increased intraocular pressure
keratoplasty	**KER**-ah-toh-**PLAS**-tee	S/ -plasty *repair* R/ kerat/o *cornea*	Corneal transplant or graft
keratoconjunctivitis	**KER**-ah-toh-con-junk-tih-**VI**-tis	S/ -itis *inflammation* R/ -conjunctiv- *conjunctiva*	Combined inflammation of the cornea and conjunctiva
ophthalmia neonatorum	off-**THAL**-me-ah ne-oh-nay-**TOR**-um	S/ -ia *condition* R/ ophthalm- *eye* S/ -orum *function of* P/ neo- *new* R/ -nat- *born*	Conjunctivitis of the newborn
photosensitivity	**FOH**-toe-sen-sih-**TIV**-ih-tee	S/ -ity *condition* R/CF phot/o- *light* R/ -sensitiv- *feeling*	When light produces pain in the eye
photosensitive (adj)	foh-toe-**SEN**-sih-tiv		Having a reaction to light
pollution	poh-**LOO**-shun	Latin *to defile*	Condition that is unclean, impure, and a danger to health
pollutant	poh-**LOO**-tant	S/ -ant *pertaining to* R/ pollut- *unclean*	Substance that makes an environment unclean or impure

EXERCISES

A. *Use the terms below to complete the following sentences. You may use a term only one time, but you will not use every term. Fill in the blanks.* **LO 11.2 and 11.5**

abrasion cataract fluorescein glaucoma photosensitive photosensitivity pollutants pollution

1. Loss of peripheral vision can be caused by ____________________.

2. Smoke and perfume are ____________________.

3. Scratching your eye with a tree branch can produce a(n) ____________________.

4. A clouding of the lens associated with aging is termed ____________________.

5. A person who states that light hurts theirs eyes is complaining of ____________________.

B. Deconstruct *the following medical terms into their elements.* **LO 11.1**

1. abrasion: ____________ / ____________
R S

2. glaucoma: ____________ / ____________
R S

3. ophthalmia: ____________ / ____________
R S

4. photosensitivity: ____________ / ____________ / ____________
R/CF R S

5. neonatorum: ____________ / ____________ / ____________
P R S

Lesson 11.3

(cont'd)

Disorders of the Retina (LO 11.5)

An impaired retina affects your ability to see in the same way that an injured leg affects your ability to walk. In either case, your level of functioning in normal, daily life is limited.

Macular Degeneration (LO 11.5)

Degeneration of the central macula results in a loss of visual acuity or sharpness, with a dark blurry area of vision loss in the center of the visual field *(Figure 11.18)*. Photoreceptor cell loss and bleeding with capillary proliferation and scar formation *(Figure 11.19)* also occur. Macular degeneration can progress to blindness. Most cases occur in people over 55.

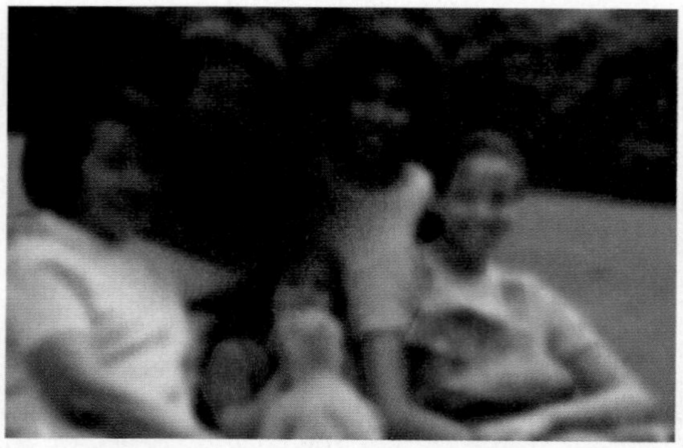

▲ **FIGURE 11.18**
Vision with Macular Degeneration.
Steve Mason/Getty Images

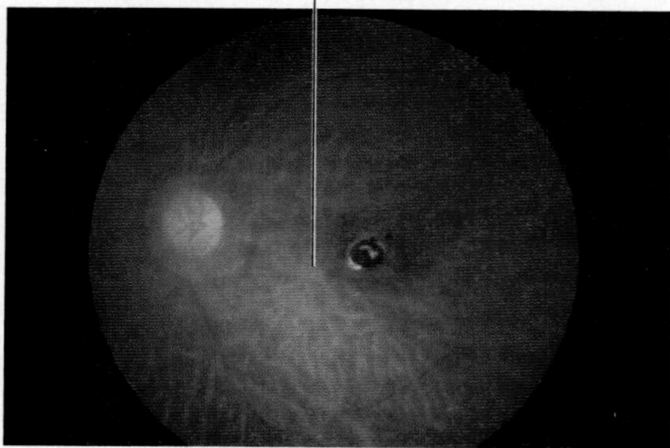

▲ **FIGURE 11.19**
Ophthalmoscopic View of Macular Degeneration.
memorisz/Shutterstock

Retinal Detachment (LO 11.5)

In retinal detachment, the retina may separate partially or completely from its underlying choroid layer, creating a retinal tear or hole. This detachment–visible on an **ophthalmoscopic** exam–can happen suddenly, without pain, but is considered a surgical emergency. The patient sees a dark shadow invading his or her peripheral vision.

Diabetic Retinopathy (LO 11.5)

Some 50% of diabetics have **retinopathy.** Patients may experience hemorrhages (bleeding), which can lead to the destruction of the photoreceptor cells (rods and cones) and visual difficulties (*Figure 11.20 and 11.21*).

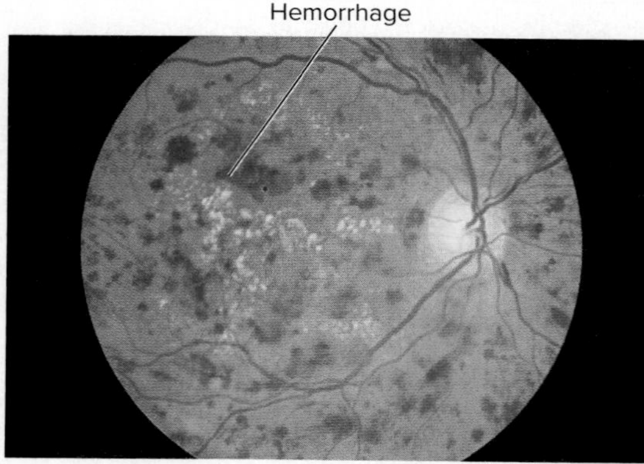

▲ **FIGURE 11.20**
Ophthalmoscopic View of Diabetic Retinopathy Showing Areas of Hemorrhage.
BSIP/UIG/Getty Images

Cancer of the Eye (LO 11.5)

Tumors of the skin of the eyelids include the **squamous cell** and basal cell carcinomas and melanoma described in Chapter 3.

Retinoblastoma is the most common cancer in children and is diagnosed most frequently around 18 months of age. Of those children affected, 20% have the cancer in both eyes. This condition can be hereditary. With early detection and aggressive chemotherapy and laser surgery treatment, 90% of these cases can be cured.

In adults, the most common eye cancers are metastases to the eye from lung cancer in men and breast cancer in women.

Night Blindness (LO 11.5)

Night blindness is the inability to see in poor light. It is a symptom of an underlying problem that can be:

- Uncorrected nearsightedness
- Cataracts
- Retinitis pigmentosa
- Vitamin A deficiency
- Glaucoma medications (such as pilocarpine) that constrict the pupil

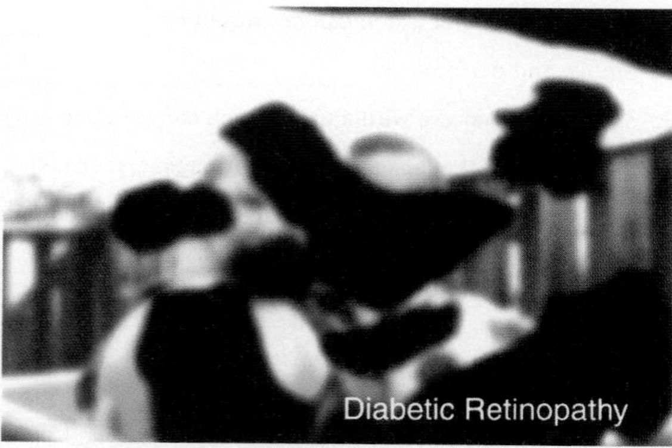

▲ **FIGURE 11.21**
Vision with Diabetic Retinopathy.
Source: Courtesy National Eye Institute, National Institutes of Health

Word Analysis and Definition

S = Suffix P = Prefix R = Root R/CF = Combining Form

WORD	PRONUNCIATION	ELEMENTS		DEFINITION
ophthalmoscope	off-**THAL**-moh-skope	S/ R/CF	-scope *instrument for viewing* ophthalm/o- *eye*	Instrument for viewing the retina
ophthalmoscopy ophthalmoscopic (adj)	**OFF**-thal-**MOS**-koh-pee **OFF**-thal-moh-**SCOP**-ik	S/ S/	-scopy *to view, examine* -ic *pertaining to*	The process of viewing the retina Pertaining to the use of an ophthalmoscope
retinoblastoma	**RET**-in-oh-blas-**TOE**-mah	S/ R/CF R/	-oma *tumor, mass* retin/o- *retina* -blast- *immature cell*	Malignant neoplasm of primitive retinal cells
retinopathy	ret-ih-**NOP**-ah-thee	S/	-pathy *disease*	Degenerative disease of the retina

Exercises

A. Elements *help build your knowledge of the language of ophthalmology. One element in each of the following medical terms is bolded and italicized. Identify the type of element (P, R/CF, S) in the second column, and then write the meaning of the element in the third column. Fill in the chart.* **LO 11.1 and 11.5**

Medical Term	P, R/CF, S	Meaning of Element
retino***blast***oma	**1.**	**2.**
ophthalmo***scope***	**3.**	**4.**
ophthalmoscop***ic***	**5.**	**6.**
ophthalmoscopy	**7.**	**8.**
retino***pathy***	**9.**	**10.**

B. Identify *the eye disorder being described. Fill in the blanks.* **LO 11.2 and 11.5**

1. This is a cancer of the eye. It is the most common cancer occurring in children: __________.

2. Inability to see in poor light: __________.

3. This condition can occur in diabetics and can lead to blindness. This condition is diabetic __________.

4. A loss of central vision due to the degeneration of the retina lateral to the optic disc: ___________degeneration.

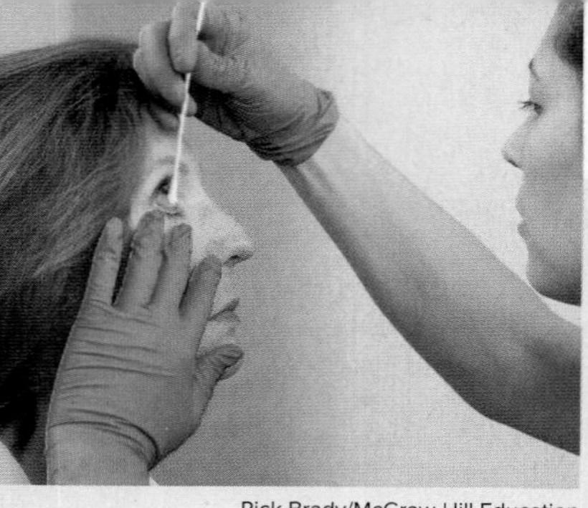

Rick Brady/McGraw-Hill Education

Lesson 11.4 Diagnostic and Therapeutic Procedures and Pharmacology for the Eye

Objectives

Diagnostic and therapeutic procedures and the application of medications to the external eye are performed by many different health professionals. The information in this lesson will enable you to:

11.4.1 Explain the diagnostic procedures used for disorders of the eye.

11.4.2 Discuss therapeutic procedures used for disorders of the eye.

11.4.3 Describe medications used for disorders of the eye.

Abbreviation

PERRLA pupils equal, round, reactive to light and accommodation

E 1

F P 2

T O Z 3

L P E D 4

P E C F D 5

E D F C Z P 6

F E L O P Z D 7

D E F P O T E C 8

L E F O D P C T 9

F D P L T C E O 10

P E Z O L C F T D 11

(a)

V = .50 D.

The fourteenth of August was the day fixed upon for the sailing of the brig Pilgrim, on her voyage from Boston round Cape Horn, to the western coast of North America. As she was to get under way early in the afternoon, I made my appearance on board at twelve o'clock in full sea-rig, and with my chest, containing an outfit for a two or three years voyage, which I had undertaken from a determination to cure, if possible, by an entire change of life, and by a long absence from books and study, a weakness of the eyes which had obliged me to give up my pursuits, and which no medical aid seemed likely to cure. The change from the tight dress coat, silk cap and kid gloves of an undergraduate at Cambridge, to the

V = .75 D.

loose duck trousers, checked shirt and tarpaulin hat of a sailor, though somewhat of a transformation, was soon made, and I supposed that I should pass very well for a Jack tar. But it is impossible to deceive the practiced eye in these matters; and while I supposed myself to be looking as salt as Neptune himself, I was, no doubt, known for a landsman by every one on board, as soon as I hove in sight. A sailor has a peculiar cut to his clothes, and a way of wear-

V = 1. D.

ing them which a green hand can never get. The trousers, tight around the hips, and thence hanging long and loose around the feet, a superabundance of checked shirt, a low-crowned, well-varnished black hat, worn on the back of the head, with half a fathom of black ribbon hanging over the left eye, and a peculiar tie to the black silk neckerchief, with sundry other *details*, are signs the want of which betray the beginner at once.

V = 1.25 D.

Beside the points in my dress which were out of the way, doubtless my complexion and hands would distinguish me from the regular *salt*, who, with a sun-browned cheek, wide step and rolling gait, swings his bronzed and toughened hands athwartships half open, as though just to ready to grasp a rope. "With all my imperfections

V = 1.50 D.

on my head," I joined the crew, and we hauled out into the stream and came to anchor for the night. The next day we were employed in preparation for sea, reeving and studding-sail gear, crossing royal yards, putting on chafing gear, and taking on board our powder. On the

(b)

▲ **FIGURE 11.22**

Visual Acuity Tests. (a) Snellen letter chart for distance vision. (b) Jaeger reading card.

Fig 11.22a: ©McGraw-Hill Education/Rick Brady, photographer. Fig 11.22b: Courtesy Good-Lite Company

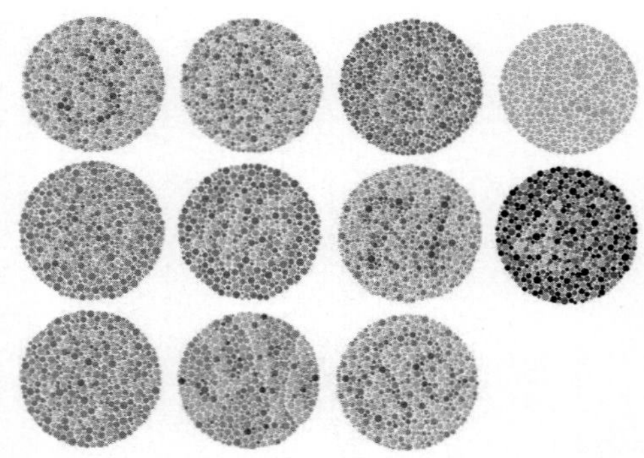

Complete **Ishihara** color test plates

▲ **FIGURE 11.23**

Test for Color Blindness. Reproduced with permission from *Ishihara's Tests for Color Deficiency*, published by Kanehara Trading Inc., Tokyo, Japan. Tests for color deficiency cannot be conducted with this figure. For accurate testing, the original plates should be used.

Alexander Kaludov/Alamy Stock Photo

Ophthalmic Diagnostic Procedures (LO 11.2, 11.5, and 11.6)

Examination of the eye includes evaluation of pupillary reaction. Medical shorthand for this quick normal eye examination can be **PERRLA,** which means ***p****upils* ***e****qual,* ***r****ound,* ***r****eactive to* ***l****ight and* ***a****ccommodation.*

Visual acuity, the sharpness and clearness of vision, is tested for each eye with the opposite eye covered with a solid object. For **distance vision**, patients look at a **Snellen letter chart** *(Figure 11.22a)* 20 feet away and vision is recorded as the smallest line in which the patient can read half of the letters. For **near vision**, the patient reads a standard **Jaeger reading card** *(Figure 11.22b)* at a distance of 14 inches.

Color vision is tested using the **Ishihara color system**. In the example shown in *Figure 11.23,* people with red-green color blindness would not be able to detect the number 74 among the colored dots.

Refractive error, the nature and degree to which light is bent by the eye, is measured with a **refractometer**.

Visual fields can be impaired by lesions anywhere in the neural visual pathway and in glaucoma, and can be assessed grossly by **direct confrontation**. The patient maintains a fixed gaze at the examiner's nose and a small object or finger is brought into the patient's visual periphery (**peripheral vision**) in each of the four visual quadrants. The patient indicates when the object is first seen. Each eye is tested separately.

Corneal examination uses **fluorescein** staining to reveal abrasions and ulcers.

Pupillary reaction to light is tested in each eye with a penlight as the patient looks into the distance.

Extrinsic muscles of the eyeball are tested by guiding the patient to look in 8 directions (up, up and right, right, down and right, down, down and left, left, left and up) with a moving finger or penlight.

Word Analysis and Definition

S = Suffix **P = Prefix** R = Root R/CF = Combining Form

WORD	PRONUNCIATION	ELEMENTS		DEFINITION
fluorescein	flor-**ESS**-ee-in	P/ R/	**fluo-** *fluorine* **-rescein** *resin*	Dye that produces a vivid green color under a blue light to diagnose corneal abrasions and foreign bodies in the eye
Ishihara color system	ish-ee-**HAR**-ah **KUH**-ler **SIS**-tem		Shinobu Ishihara, 1879–1963, Japanese ophthalmologist **color** Latin color **system** Greek to combine	Test for color vision defects
Jaeger reading cards	**YAY**-ger **REED**-ing CARDS	S/ R/	Edward Jaeger, 1818–1884, Austrian ophthalmologist **-ing** *quality of, doing* **read-** *advise, interpret, read* **card** Latin *leaf of papyrus*	Printed in different sizes of print for testing near vision
peripheral vision	peh-**RIF**-er-al **VIZH**-un	S/ R/	**-al** *pertaining to* **peripher-** *external boundary* **vision** Latin *to see*	Ability to see objects as they come into the outer edges of the visual field
refractometer	ree-frak-**TAH**-meh-tur	S/ R/CF	**-meter** *measure, instrument to measure* **refract/o-** *to bend (light)*	Device that measures refractive errors of the cornea
Snellen letter chart	**SNEL**-en **LET**-er CHART		Hermann Snellen, 1834–1908, Dutch ophthalmologist **letter** Latin *letter of the alphabet* **chart** Latin *piece of papyrus, document*	Test for acuity of distance vision

EXERCISE

A. The ophthalmic technician in Dr. Chun's office needs to be familiar with all these terms in order to communicate with Dr. Chun and her patients. *Show your understanding of the terms by selecting the correct answers.* **LO 11.6**

1. The test used to measure color blindness is

a. Snellen **b.** Jaeger **c.** Ishihara **d.** visual fields **e.** ophthalmoscope

2. Peripheral vision measures the outer edge of the

a. anterior segment **b.** vitreous body **c.** aqueous humor **d.** posterior segment **e.** visual field

3. A test for near vision is the

a. Snellen chart **b.** ophthalmoscope **c.** Jaeger card **d.** Ishihara **e.** visual fields

4. This is used to detect corneal abrasions or ulcers

a. ophthalmoscope **b.** refractometer **c.** tonometer **d.** fluorescein

Ophthalmic Diagnostic Procedures (continued)
(LO 11.2, 11.5, and 11.6)

Fundoscopy using an **ophthalmoscope** can detect lens opacities, retinal changes, and retinal vascular changes. The vascular changes can be areas of hemorrhage or changes in the retinal arteries indicating hypertension or arteriosclerosis. The retinal changes can show age-related macular degeneration, retinoblastoma, retinal detachment, signs of diabetes, signs of glaucoma, or signs of raised intracranial pressure (**papilledema**). Greater detail of the vessels of the eye can be seen with fluorescein **angiography**. Fluorescein is injected into the vein and pictures are taken as the dye passes through the retina revealing more details.

Slit-lamp examination focuses the height and width of a beam of light to give a **stereoscopic** view of the interior structures of the eyeball. It is used for identifying corneal foreign bodies and abrasions, and identifying retinal diseases.

Intraocular pressure is measured with a **tonometer,** which determines the eyeball's resistance to tension or indentation. There are several methods of **tonometry,** which include pneumatonometry and Goldmann tonometry.

Therapeutic Procedures for Diseases of the Eye
(LO 11.2, 11.5, and 11.6)

Photocoagulation therapy is used to reattach a torn or detached portion of the retina and to prevent further growth of abnormal blood vessels that can cause a detachment. A high-intensity, narrowly focused beam of light from the **argon laser** is absorbed by pigment in the retinal cells and converted into heat, which welds the edge of the retinal detachment against the underlying choroid. **Retinal cryopexy (cryotherapy)** uses intense cold to have the same effects as the heat of photocoagulation.

Photocoagulation therapy is also used to heal bleeding **microaneurysms** of small blood vessels in the early stages of **diabetic retinopathy,** and is used with **chemotherapy** in the treatment of **retinoblastoma**. It also can be used for wet age-related macular degeneration to destroy or seal off new blood vessels to prevent leakage, but the many small retinal scars it creates cause blind spots in the patient's visual field.

When a **cataract** is interfering with vision, the opaque lens is removed by **phacoemulsification** in which ultrasonic waves fragment the cataract to make its removal much easier. The lens is then replaced with an artificial **intraocular** lens, which becomes a permanent part of the eye.

Laser corneal surgery is a procedure that uses a laser to reshape the surface of the eye to change the curvature of the cornea. The surgical procedure **radial keratotomy** is used to treat myopia. Radial cuts, like the spokes of a wheel, flatten the cornea and enable it to refract the light rays to focus on the retina. In flattening the cornea, it can correct myopia (nearsightedness) and astigmatism (uneven curvature of the cornea) and alter the outer edges of the cornea to correct hypermetropia (farsightedness). These procedures are also called **refractive surgery** and **laser-assisted in situ keratomileusis (LASIK)**. An alternative to LASIK is **photorefractive keratectomy (PRK)**, in which spoke-like incisions are cut into the cornea to flatten its surface and correct nearsightedness.

Glaucoma is treated with a combination of eye drops *(see next section on ocular pharmacology),* pills, laser surgery, and traditional surgery with the goal of preventing loss of vision. The most commonly used laser procedure is **trabeculoplasty**, in which the eye's drainage system is changed by the laser beam to enable the aqueous humor fluid to drain out more easily into the blood stream. **Trabeculectomy** is the most common traditional surgical procedure, in which a passage is created in the sclera to allow excess fluid to drain out of the eye. More recently, a small silicone tube has been placed from the surface of the eye into the anterior chamber to allow drainage of the excess fluid.

If the cornea is scarred by trauma or infection and vision is impaired, a corneal transplant or graft (**keratoplasty**) from a deceased donor can be performed.

Abbreviation

LASIK laser-assisted in situ keratomileusis

Keynotes

- As the eye is heavily supplied with nerves, anesthesia is required for eye surgery and local anesthesia is most commonly used *(see the next section on ocular pharmacology).*
- Sterile precautions with the use of antiseptics, sterile drapes, gowns, and gloves are used in eye surgery to prevent infection.

Word Analysis and Definition

S = Suffix   P = Prefix   R = Root   R/CF = Combining Form

WORD	PRONUNCIATION		ELEMENTS	DEFINITION
argon laser	**AR**-gon **LAY**-zer		**argon** Greek *lazy* **laser** *acronym for **L**ight **A**mplification by **S**timulated **E**mission of **R**adiation*	Laser used for ophthalmic procedures consisting of photons in the blue and/or green spectrum
cryotherapy	**CRY**-oh-**THAIR**-ah-pee	S/ R/CF	**-therapy** *treatment* **cry/o-** *cold*	The use of cold in the treatment of disease
cryopexy	**CRY**-oh-**PEK**-see	S/	**-pexy** *fixation*	Repair of a detached retina by freezing it to surrounding tissue
fundus	**FUN**-dus		Latin *bottom*	Part farthest from the opening of a hollow organ
fundoscopy	fun-**DOS**-koh-pee	S/ R/CF	**-scopy** *to examine* **fund/o-** *fundus*	Examination of the fundus (retina) of the eye
fundoscopic (adj)	fun-doh-**SKOP**-ik	S/	**-ic** *pertaining to*	As a result of fundoscopy
in situ	IN **SIGH**-tyu		Latin *in its original place*	In the correct place
intraocular	in-trah-**OCK**-you-lar	S/ P/ R/	**-ar** *pertaining to* **intra-** *inside* **-ocul-** *eye*	Pertaining to the inside of the eye
keratectomy	**KER**-ah-**TEK**-toh-mee	S/ R/	**-ectomy** *excision* **kerat-** *cornea*	Surgery to remove corneal tissue
keratomileusis	**KER**-ah-toh-mie-**LOO**-sis	R/CF R/	**kerat/o-** *cornea* **-mileusis** *lathe*	A surgical procedure that involves cutting and shaping the cornea
keratoplasty	**KER**-ah-**TOT**-oh-mee **KER**-ah-toh-**PLAS**-tee	S/ R/	**-plasty** *repair* **kerat/o** *cornea*	Corneal transplant or graft
keratotomy		S/	**-tomy** *surgical incision*	Incision in the cornea
phacoemulsification	**FAK**-oh-ee-mul-sih-fih-**KAY**-shun	S/ R/CF R/	**-ation** *process* **phac/o-** *lens* **-emulsific-** *to milk out*	Technique used to fragment the center of the lens into very tiny pieces and suck them out of the eye
photocoagulation	foh-toh-koh-ah-you-**LAY**-shun	S/ R/CF R/	**-ation** *process* **phot/o-** *light* **-coagul-** *clot*	The use of light (laser beam) to form a clot
photoreactive	foh-toh-ree-**AK**-tiv	P/ R/	**-re-** *again* **-active** *movement*	Initiation by light of a process previously inactive
tonometer	toh-**NOM**-eh-ter	S/ R/CF	**-meter** *measure, instrument to measure* **ton/o-** *pressure, tension*	Instrument for determining intraocular pressure
tonometry	toh-**NOM**-eh-tree	S/	**-metry** *process of measuring*	The measurement of intraocular pressure
trabeculectomy	trah-**BEK**-you-**LEK**-toh-mee	S/ R/	**-ectomy** *excision* **trabecul-** *eye's fluid drainage system*	Surgical creation of passage in sclera to allow fluid to drain out of the eye
trabeculoplasty	trah-**BEK**-you-loh-plas-tee	S/ R/CF	**-plasty** *surgical repair* **trabecul/o-** *eye's fluid drainage system*	Laser repair of eye's fluid drainage system

EXERCISE

A. Identify the meaning of the word elements related to ophthalmology. *Match the element in the first column with its correct meaning in the second column.* **LO 11.1**

	Word Element	Meaning
______	**1.** *kerat-*	**a.** cold
______	**2.** *cry/o-*	**b.** light
______	**3.** *-ectomy*	**c.** surgical repair
______	**4.** *-plasty*	**d.** eye's fluid drainage system
______	**5.** *phot/o-*	**e.** cornea
______	**6.** *trabecul-*	**f.** excision

Lesson 11.4 (cont'd) Ocular Pharmacology (LO 11.2, 11.5, and 11.6)

There are a wide variety and number of medications placed directly into the conjunctival sac to treat different eye disorders or to help the clinician examine the eye more thoroughly and more easily.

- **Mydriatics** are drugs that cause the pupil to dilate and are mainly used to examine the eye fundus. **Mydriacil** *(Tropicamide)* takes 15 minutes for the eye to fully dilate and can last for 3 to 6 hours with blurred vision. Other dilating drops, for example, **atropine** and **homatropine,** are long acting, lasting 7 to 10 days.

- **Miotics** are drugs that constrict the pupil (**miosis**); for example **pilocarpine,** which can be part of a regimen for treating glaucoma.

- **Ocular topical anesthetics** temporarily block nerve conduction in the conjunctiva and cornea. They have a quick onset of 10 to 20 seconds and last for 10 to 20 minutes. They are used to assist with eye examinations and visual **acuity** testing and to help treat chemical burns, welding flash, and foreign bodies. Examples are **amethocaine,** 0.5% and 1%, and **oxybupricaine,** 0.4%.

- **Ocular diagnostic drops** stain conjunctival cells to improve diagnostic capabilities; for example, the presence of a foreign body or a corneal abrasion. Examples are **fluorescein** and **Lissamine Green.** The drops do not interfere with vision but are taken up by soft contact lenses, which should be removed prior to instillation of the drops.

- **Ocular lubricant drops** are used to replace tears, treat dry eyes, moisten hard contact lenses, protect the eye during eye surgical procedures, and help treat keratitis. Examples are *Visine, Refresh Optive,* and *Retaine.*

- **Anti-infective eye medications,** both drops and ointments, can be **antibacterial,** for example, **glatifloxacin** (*Zymaxid*) and **sulfacetamide** (*Klaron, Ovace*); **antifungal,** such as **natamycin** (*Natacyn*); and **antiviral,** for example, **idoxuridine** (*Herplex*) and **trifluridine** (*Viroptic*).

- **Anti-inflammatory eye medications** are used in allergic disorders, to prevent scarring and visual loss in inflammation of the eye, and to decrease postoperative eye inflammation and scarring. Examples are **corticosteroids** such as **dexamethasone** (*Decadron*) and **nonsteroidal anti-inflammatory agents** such as **flurbiprofen** (*Ocufen*) and **suprofen** (*Profenal*).

- In **glaucoma,** numerous eye medications are available and are used individually, in combinations, and/or with surgery *(see the previous section on eye therapeutic procedures).* **Miotics** decrease the size of the pupil and widen the trabecular network to enable fluid to escape more easily. **Beta-adrenergic blockers** decrease production of aqueous humor; examples are **timolol maleate** (*Timoptic*) and **betaxolol** (*Betoptic*). **Carbonic anhydrase inhibitors** reduce production of aqueous humor; examples are **acetazolamide sodium** (*Diamox*) and **dichlorphenamide** (*Daranide*); **alpha-adrenergic agents** increase the outflow of aqueous humor by unknown mechanisms; examples are **epinephrine** (*Epifrin*) and **phenylephrine** (*Neo-synephrine*).

Word Analysis and Definition

S = Suffix **P = Prefix** R = Root R/CF = Combining Form

WORD	PRONUNCIATION	ELEMENTS		DEFINITION
antibacterial	**AN**-teh-bak-**TEER**-ee-al	S/ P/ R/CF	**-al** *pertaining to* **anti-** *against* **-bacter/i-** *bacteria*	Destructive of or preventing the growth of bacteria
antifungal	**AN**-teh-**FUN**-gal	R/	**-fung-** *fungus*	Destructive of or preventing the growth of fungi
anti-infective	**AN**-teh-in-**FEK**-tiv	S/ R/	**-ive** *nature of* **-infect-** *taint*	Made incapable of transmitting an infection
anti-inflammatory	**AN**-teh-in-**FLAM**-ah-toh-ree	S/ P/ R/	**-ory** *having the function of* **-in-** *in* **-flammat-** *inflammation*	Reducing, removing, or preventing inflammation
antiviral	an-teh-**VIE**-ral	R/	**-vir-** *virus*	To weaken or abolish the action or replication of a virus
atropine	**AT**-roh-peen		Greek *belladonna*	Pharmacologic agent used to dilate pupils
inhibitor	in-**HIB**-ih-tor	S/ P/ R/	**-or** *one who does* **in-** *in* **-hibit-** *keep back*	An agent that restrains or retards physiologic, chemical, or enzymatic action
miosis	my-**OH**-sis		Greek *lessening*	Contraction of the pupil
miotic	my-**OT**-ik	S/ R/CF	**-tic** *pertaining to* **mi/o-** *less*	An agent that causes the pupil to contract
mydriasis	mih-**DRY**-ah-sis		Greek *dilation of the pupil*	Dilation of the pupil
mydriatic	mid-ree-**AT**-ik	S/ R/	**-atic** *pertaining to* **mydri-** *dilation of the pupil*	Pertaining to or an agent that causes dilation of the pupil

EXERCISE

A. Identify the medication that would treat each condition. *Match the medication on the left with its correct indicated use.* **LO 11.5 and 11.6**

_____ **1.** antibacterial — **a.** a treatment for glaucoma

_____ **2.** mydriatic — **b.** dry eyes

_____ **3.** anti-inflammatory — **c.** bacterial infection of the eye

_____ **4.** miotic — **d.** allergic disorder of the eye

_____ **5.** ocular topical anesthetic — **e.** dilate the pupil in order to view the eye fundus

_____ **6.** lubricant — **f.** chemical burn to the eyes

The Ear and Hearing

The Language of Otology

Rick Brady/McGraw-Hill Education

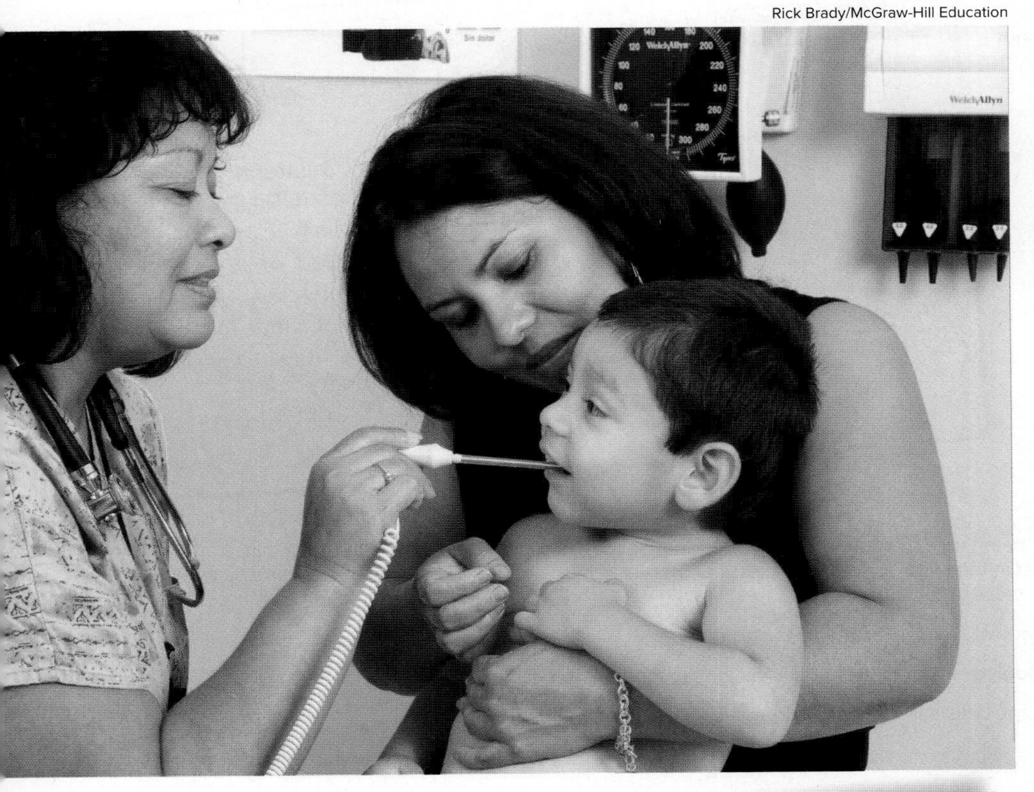

Learning Outcomes

In order to make correct decisions in situations like Mrs. Hughes' case, to communicate with Dr. Chun about the patient, to participate in patient education, and to document the patient's care, you need to be able to:

LO 11.5 **Relate the anatomy of the eyeball and retina to vision and refraction and their disorders and treatments.**

LO 11.6 **Explain the diagnostic and therapeutic procedures and the pharmacology used in the treatment of disorders of the eye.**

LO 11.7 **Describe the three chambers of the ear, their roles in hearing and balance, and their disorders and treatments.**

LO 11.8 **Explain the diagnostic and therapeutic procedures and the pharmacology used in the treatment of disorders of the ear.**

LO 11.9 **Apply your knowledge of medical terms relating to the eye and ear to documentation, medical records, and medical reports.**

LO 11.10 **Translate the medical terms relating to the eye and ear into everyday language in order to communicate clearly with patients and their families.**

NOTE: The sense of smell is discussed as an integral part of the respiratory system; the sense of taste, as an integral part of the digestive system; and the sense of touch, as an integral part of the nervous system.

CASE REPORT 11.3

You are . . .

. . . a medical assistant working for primary care physician Susan Lee, MD, of the Fulwood Medical Group.

You are communicating with . . .

. . . Mrs. Carmen Cardenas, who has brought in her 3-year-old son, Eddie. She tells you that Eddie has had a cold for a couple of days. Early this morning, he woke up screaming, felt hot, and was tugging his ears. She gave him **acetaminophen** with some orange juice, and he threw up. She also tells you this is the third similar episode in the past year, and, since the last time, she is concerned that he is not hearing normally. You see a worried mother and a restless toddler with a green nasal discharge. His oral temperature taken with an electronic digital thermometer is 102.4°F, and his pulse is 100. You tell Mrs. Cardenas that Dr. Lee will be in to see Eddie as soon as possible.

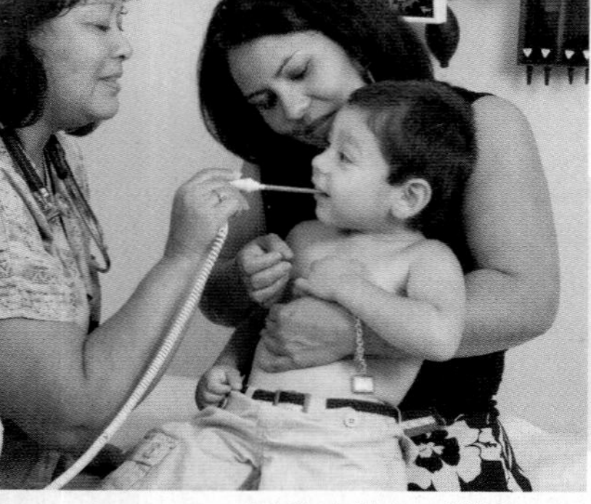

Rick Brady/McGraw-Hill Education

Lesson 11.5

The Ear and Hearing

Objectives

In order to understand and to address Eddie Cardenas' condition, you must be able to use correct medical terminology to:

11.5.1 Recognize the structures and functions of the three regions of the ear.

11.5.2 Explain how sound waves progress through the ear, are transferred to the brain, and are recognized as sounds.

11.5.3 Identify common diseases of the ear that interfere with the process of hearing.

11.5.4 Relate the appropriate structures of the ear to disorders of equilibrium and balance.

11.5.5 Recognize health professionals involved in the diagnosis and treatment of problems of the ear.

Abbreviations

BOM	bilateral otitis media
mg	milligram
OME	otitis media with effusion
p.r.n.	when necessary
q.i.d.	four times each day
URI	upper respiratory infection

Your ear has three major sections (*Figure 11.24*):

1. The external ear
2. The middle ear
3. The inner ear

Case Report 11.3 *(continued)*

Clinical Note. 05/10/18

Examination by Dr. Lee showed that Eddie has a **bilateral acute otitis media (BOM)** with an upper respiratory infection **(URI).** Dr. Lee is also concerned that Eddie has a **chronic** otitis media with **effusion (OME)** that is causing a hearing loss. She prescribed Amoxicillin 250 mg **q.i.d.** with acetaminophen 160 **mg p.r.n.** for 10 days, when she will see Eddie again. If, after the acute infection subsides, there remains an effusion with hearing loss, Dr. Lee may need to refer Eddie to an **otologist.** I explained this to Mrs. Cardenas.

—Luis Guittierez, CMA 1115 hrs.

In your future career, being able to communicate comfortably, accurately, and effectively with the health professionals involved in the diagnosis and treatment of problems of the ear is key. You may work directly and/or indirectly with one or more of the following:

- **Otologists** are medical specialists in diseases of the ear.
- **Otorhinolaryngologists** are medical specialists in diseases of the ear, nose, and throat.
- **Audiologists** are specialists in the evaluation of hearing function.

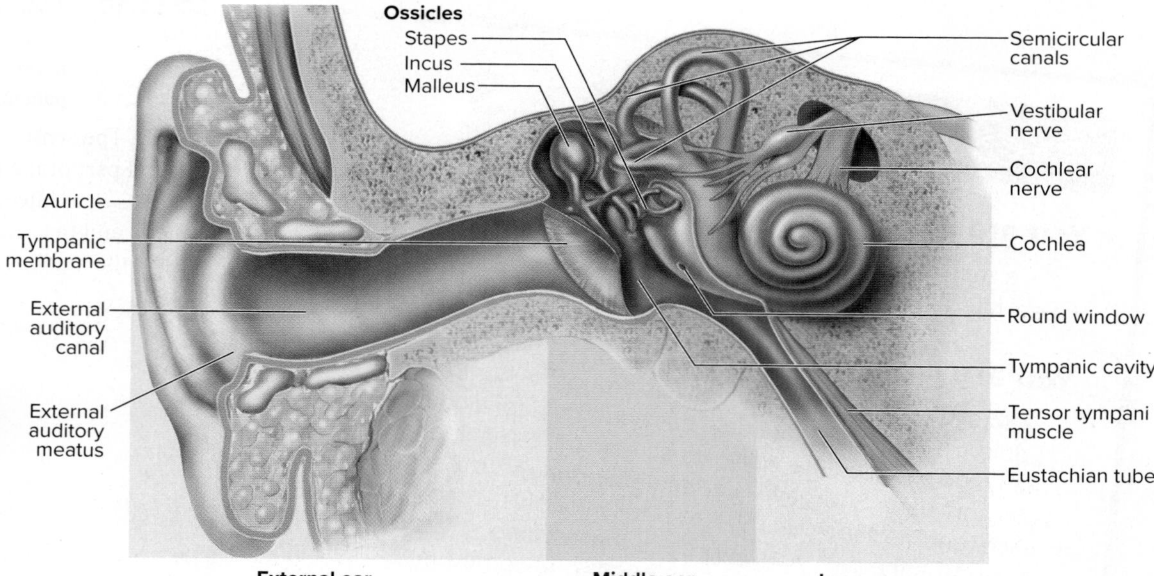

▲ **FIGURE 11.24**
Anatomical Regions of the Ear.

Word Analysis and Definition

S = Suffix P = Prefix R = Root R/CF = Combining Form

WORD	PRONUNCIATION		ELEMENTS	DEFINITION
acetaminophen	ah-seat-ah-**MIN**-oh-fen		Generic drug name	Medication that is an analgesic and antipyretic
acute	ah-**KYUT**		Latin *sharp*	Disease of sudden onset
audiology	aw-dee-**OL**-oh-jee	S/ R/CF	**-logy** *study of* **audi/o** *hearing*	Study of hearing disorders.
audiologist	aw-dee-**OL**-oh-jist	S/	**-logist** *one who studies*	Specialist in the evaluation of hearing function
bilateral	by-**LAT**-er-al	S/ P/ R/	**-al** *pertaining to* **bi-** *two* **-later-** *side*	On two sides; e.g., in both ears
chronic	**KRON**-ik		Greek *time*	A persistent, long-term disease
effusion	eh-**FYU**-shun		Latin *pouring out*	Collection of fluid that has escaped from blood vessels into a cavity or tissues
otitis media	oh-**TIE**-tis **ME**-dee-ah	S/ R/ R/	**-itis** *inflammation* **ot-** *ear* **media** *middle*	Inflammation of the middle ear
otologist	oh-**TOL**-oh-jist	S/ R/CF	**-logist** *specialist* **ot/o-** *ear*	Medical specialist in diseases of the ear
otology	oh-**TOL**-oh-jee	S/	**-logy** *study of*	Diagnosis and treatment of disorders of the ear
otorhinolaryngologist	oh-toe-rye-no-lah-rin-**GOL**-oh-jist	R/CF R/CF	**-rhin/o-** *nose* **-laryng/o-** *larynx*	Ear, nose, and throat medical specialist

EXERCISES

A. Construct medical terms. *Insert the missing word element that correctly completes the medical term being described. Fill in the blanks.* **LO 11.1**

1. One who specializes in the study of the ear: ______________/logist

2. Pertaining to both sides: ______________/later/al

3. Medical specialist in the treatment of the ear, nose, and throat: ot/o/rhino/______________ /logist

4. Infection of the middle ear: ot/______________ media

5. One who studies hearing: ______________/logist

B. Match *the abbreviation in the left column with its meaning in the right column. Fill in the blanks.* **LO 11.3**

______	**1.** URI	**a.** infection in both middle ears
______	**2.** mg	**b.** infection in both middle ears with a fluid collection
______	**3.** BOM	**c.** four times a day
______	**4.** OME	**d.** milligram
______	**5.** p.r.n.	**f.** when necessary
______	**6.** q.i.d.	**g.** upper respiratory infection

Lesson 11.5 (cont'd)

External Ear (LO 11.7)

The external ear comprises several structures that keep it functioning effectively.

The **auricle** or **pinna** is a wing-shaped structure that directs sound waves into the ear canal through the external **auditory meatus.** The external auditory canal ends at the very delicate **tympanic** membrane, otherwise known as the eardrum *(Figure 11.25).* When using an otoscope to examine the tympanic membrane, the pinna should be pulled up and out to straighten the external auditory canal.

The meatus and canal are lined with skin that contains many modified sweat glands called **ceruminous** glands, which secrete **cerumen.**

If a foreign body, like a small bead, gets into the auditory canal, or if cerumen becomes **impacted** in the canal, the result can be hearing loss.

Keynotes

- The **external auditory canal** is the only skin-lined cul-de-sac in the body.
- Cerumen combines with dead skin cells to form earwax.

Disorders of the External Ear (LO 11.7)

Some disorders of the external ear include infections and earwax buildup.

Otitis externa *(Figure 11.26)* is a bacterial or fungal infection of the external auditory canal lining. An **otoscopic** exam shows a painful, red, swollen ear canal, sometimes with a purulent drainage.

Swimmer's ear is a form of otitis externa resulting from swimming, particularly if the water is polluted.

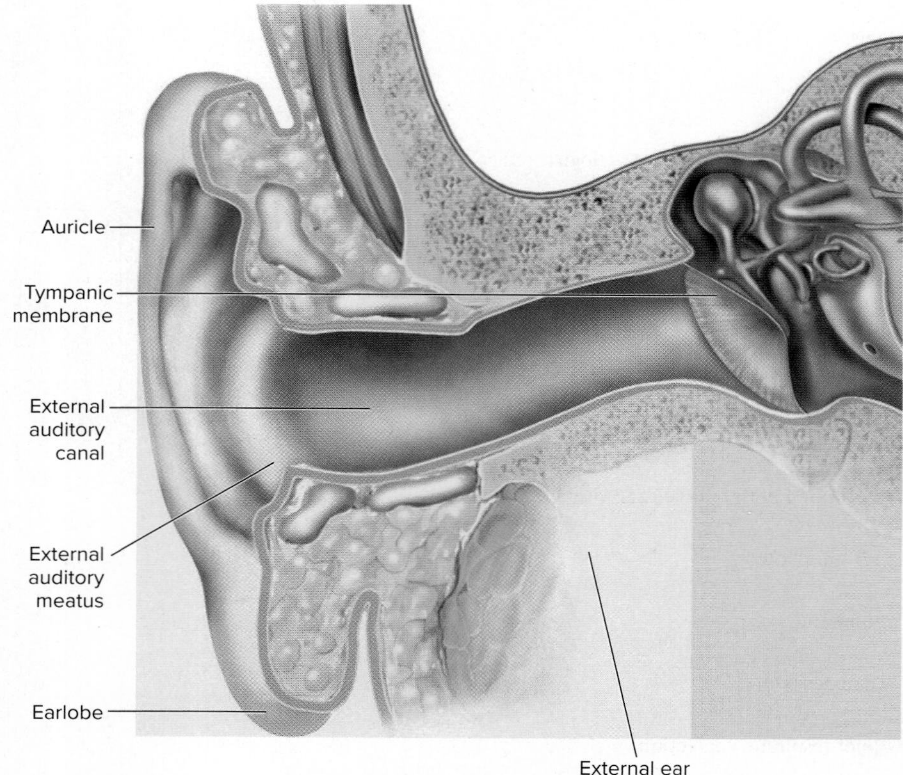

▲ **FIGURE 11.25**
External Ear.

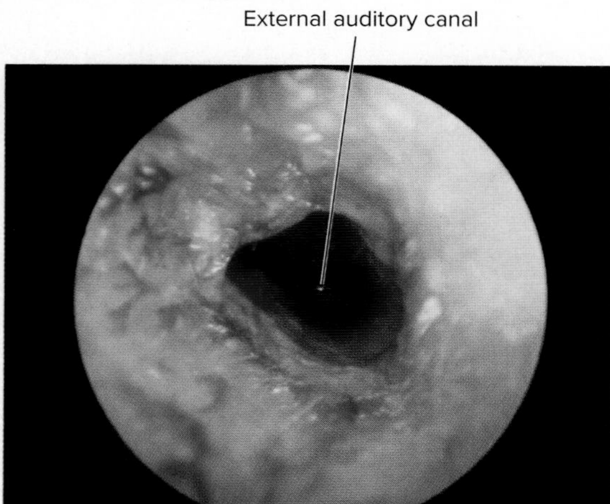

▲ **FIGURE 11.26**
Otoscopic View of Otitis Externa.

Richard Morton

Word Analysis and Definition

S = Suffix P = Prefix R = Root R/CF = Combining Form

WORD	PRONUNCIATION	ELEMENTS		DEFINITION
auditory (adj)	**AW**-dih-tor-ee		Latin *hearing*	Relating to hearing or the organs of hearing
auricle **(Note:** *same as* pinna)	**AW**-ri-kul		Latin *ear*	The shell-like external ear
cerumen **ceruminous (adj)**	seh-**ROO**-men seh-**ROO**-mih-nus	S/ R/	Latin *wax* **-ous** *pertaining to* **cerumin-** *cerumen*	Waxy secretion of glands of the external ear Pertaining to cerumen
impacted	im-**PAK**-ted		Latin *driven in*	Immovably wedged, as with earwax blocking the external canal
meatus **meatal (adj)**	me-**AY**-tus me-**AY**-tal		Latin *go through*	Passage or channel; also the external opening of a passage
pinna **pinnae (pl)**	**PIN**-ah **PIN**-ee		Latin *wing*	Another name for auricle
tympanic	tim-**PAN**-ik	S/ R/	**-ic** *pertaining to* **tympan-** *eardrum*	Pertaining to the tympanic membrane (eardrum) or tympanic cavity

EXERCISES

A. Test *your knowledge of the language of otology. Match the definition in the first column with its correct medical term in the second column. Fill in the blanks.* **LO 11.7**

________ **1.** pertaining to the eardrum — **a.** meatus

________ **2.** external opening of a passage — **b.** cerumen

________ **3.** shell-like external ear — **c.** tympanic

________ **4.** waxy secretion of the external ear — **d.** auricle

________ **5.** earwax that is wedged in the ear canal — **e.** impacted

B. Translate *medical terms into everyday language for your patients. Select the correct answer to each statement.* **LO 11.7, 11.8, and 11.10**

1. An otoscopic exam to look for cerumen impaction.

a. "The doctor will look in your ear to see if there is earwax lodged in the ear canal."

b. "The surgeon will cut a hole in the eardrum to release the fluid."

c. "The nurse will flush the ear canal to remove ear wax."

d. "You will need an X-ray of the skull to determine if you have a tumor in your ear."

2. Otitis externa

a. "The eardrum has a hole in it."

b. "Earwax in ear canal has hardened."

c. "Your outer ear is infected."

d. "The inner ear is filled with thick fluid."

3. Which of the following statements describes the **external auditory meatus?**

a. thin membrane at the end of the ear canal

b. outer area of the ear that directs sound waves into the ear canal

c. tube that leads to your eardrum

d. opening between the outermost area of the ear and the ear canal

Lesson 11.5 (cont'd) Middle Ear (LO 11.7)

Keynote

- The three ossicles amplify sound so that soft sounds can be heard. The stapes is the smallest bone in the body.

The middle ear has the following four components *(Figure 11.27).*

1. The **tympanic membrane** (eardrum) rests at the inner end of the external auditory canal. It vibrates freely as sound waves hit it. It has a good nerve supply and is very sensitive to pain. When examined through the otoscope, it is transparent and reflects light *(Figure 11.28).*
2. The **tympanic cavity** is immediately behind the tympanic membrane. It is filled with air that enters through the eustachian tube, and the cavity is continuous with the **mastoid** air cells in the bone behind it. The cavity contains small bones called **ossicles.**
3. The three **ossicles**—the **malleus, incus,** and **stapes**—work to amplify sounds and are attached to the tympanic cavity wall by tiny ligaments. The malleus is attached to the tympanic membrane and vibrates with the membrane when sound waves hit it. The malleus is also attached to the incus, which vibrates, too, and passes the vibrations onto the stapes. The stapes is attached to the oval window, an opening that transmits the vibrations to the inner ear.
4. The **eustachian (auditory) tube** connects the middle ear with the **nasopharynx** (throat), into which it opens near the pharyngeal **tonsils (adenoids)** *(Figure 11.29).* In children under 5 years of age, this tube is not fully developed. It is short and horizontal, and valve-like flaps in the throat that protect it are not yet developed.

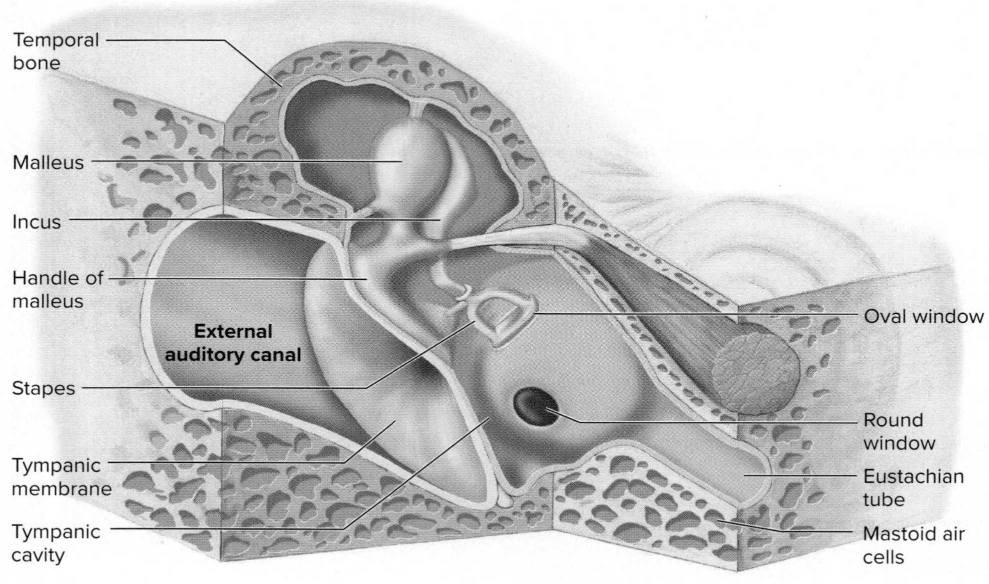

▲ **FIGURE 11.27**
Middle Ear.

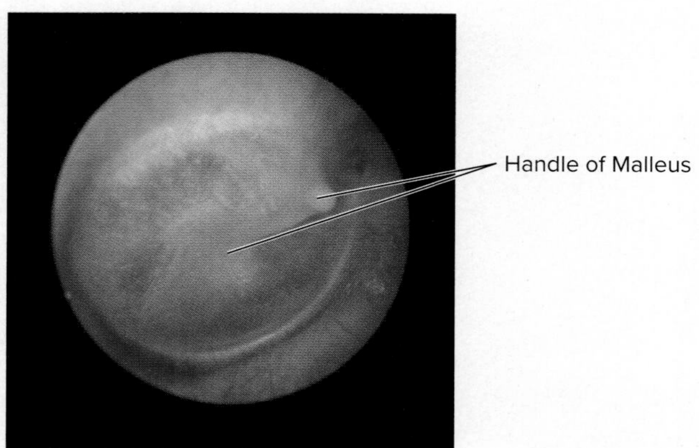

▲ **FIGURE 11.28**
Otoscopic View of Normal Tympanic Membrane.

Dr. G. Lacher/Science Source

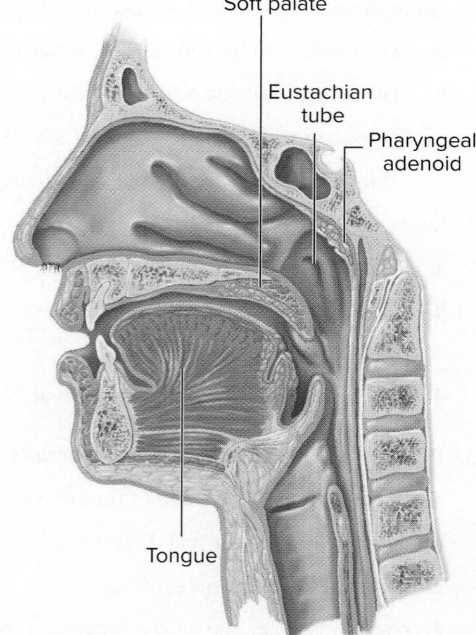

▲ **FIGURE 11.29**
Nasopharynx (Throat) showing the Eustachian tube.

Word Analysis and Definition

S = Suffix P = Prefix R = Root R/CF = Combining Form

WORD	PRONUNCIATION		ELEMENTS	DEFINITION
adenoid	**ADD**-eh-noyd	S/ R/	**-oid** *resembling* **aden-** *gland*	Single mass of lymphoid tissue in the midline at the back of the throat
eustachian tube (Note: *same as auditory tube)*	you-**STAY**-shun TYUB		Bartolomeo Eustachio, Italian anatomist, 1524–1574	Tube that connects the middle ear to the nasopharynx
incus	**IN**-cuss		Latin *anvil*	Middle one of the three ossicles in the middle ear; shaped like an anvil
malleus	**MAL**-ee-us		Latin *hammer*	Outer (lateral) one of the three ossicles in the middle ear; shaped like a hammer
mastoid	**MASS**-toyd	S/ R/	**-oid** *resembling* **mast-** *breast*	Small bony protrusion immediately behind the ear
nasopharynx **nasopharyngeal (adj)**	**NAY**-zoh-fair-inks **NAY**-zoh-fair-**RIN**-jee-al	R/CF R/ S/ R/	**nas/o-** *nose* **-pharynx** *throat* **-eal** *pertaining to* **-pharyng-** *pharynx*	Region of the pharynx at the back of the nose and above the soft palate Pertaining to the nasopharynx
ossicle	**OSS**-ih-kel	S/ R/CF	**-cle** *small* **oss/i-** *bone*	A small bone, particularly relating to the three bones in the middle ear
stapes	**STAY**-peez		Latin *stirrup*	Inner (medial) one of the three ossicles of the middle ear; shaped like a stirrup

EXERCISES

A. Review *the terms. Define the meanings of the word elements that construct medical terms. Select the correct answer that completes each statement.* **LO 11.1 and 11.7**

1. In the term *mastoid,* the suffix means:

   a. condition **b.** resembling **c.** inflammation

2. The element *mast* means:

   a. throat **b.** breast **c.** ear

3. The element *pharynx* means:

   a. throat **b.** nose **c.** tongue

4. The root in the term *ossicle* means:

   a. bone **b.** small **c.** stirrup

5. The root in the term *adenoid* means:

   a. resembling **b.** kidney **c.** gland

B. Employ *the language of otology and fill in the blanks with the correct term being described.* **LO 11.2 and 11.7**

1. List the ear ossicles in order from lateral to medial: ____________, ______________, ___________
2. The smallest bone in the body: ______________________________
3. Write the synonym for *eustachian tube.* ______________________________
4. What is the medical term for *eardrum?* ______________________________
5. The pharyngeal tonsils are the ______________________________.
6. What is the medical term for *throat?* ______________________________

Case Report 11.3 *(continued)*

Eddie Cardenas's ear problems began with his eustachian tube. His cold (upper respiratory infection, **URI,** or **coryza)** inflamed the mucous membranes of his throat and eustachian tube. Because he is so young, his eustachian tube is short and horizontal and so the inflammation spread easily from his throat into the middle ear, causing his acute otitis media **(AOM).** The inflammatory process produced fluid (effusion) in the middle ear. His tympanic membrane became inflamed and painful, which you could see through an otoscope *(Figure 11.30).*

Abbreviations

AOM	acute otitis media
PE tube	pressure-equalization tube
URI	upper respiratory infection

Disorders of the Middle Ear (LO 11.7)

The middle ear can be susceptible to the disorders outlined below.

- **Acute otitis media (AOM)** is the presence of pus in the middle ear with ear pain, fever, and redness of the tympanic membrane. AOM occurs most often in the first 2 to 4 years of age. If the infection is viral, it will go away on its own; if it's bacterial, oral antibiotics may be necessary.
- **Chronic otitis media** occurs when the acute infection subsides but the eustachian tube is blocked. The fluid in the middle ear caused by the infection cannot drain, and it gradually becomes stickier. This is called **chronic otitis media with effusion (OME)** and produces hearing loss because the sticky fluid prevents the ossicles from vibrating. You can see the fluid through the otoscope *(Figure 11.30).* Dr. Lee was concerned that this had happened to Eddie in his previous ear infection.
- A **perforated** tympanic membrane *(Figure 11.31)* can occur in acute otitis media **(AOM)** and chronic otitis media when pus in the middle ear cannot escape down the eustachian tube. The pus builds up pressure and punctures the eardrum. Most perforations will heal spontaneously in a month, leaving a small scar. Other perforation causes include a Q-tip puncture, an open-handed slap to the ear, or induced pressure as in scuba diving.
- **Cholesteatoma** is a complication of chronic otitis media with fluid or effusion (OME). Chronically inflamed middle ear cells multiply and collect into a tumor. They damage the ossicles and can spread to the inner ear. Surgical removal is required.
- **Otosclerosis** is a middle-ear disease that usually affects people between 18 and 35 years. It can impair one ear or both and produces a gradual hearing loss for low and soft sounds. Its etiology is unknown. Spongy bone forms around the junction of the oval window and stapes, preventing the stapes from conducting sound vibrations to the inner ear. The only treatment is to replace the stapes with a metal or plastic **prosthesis.**

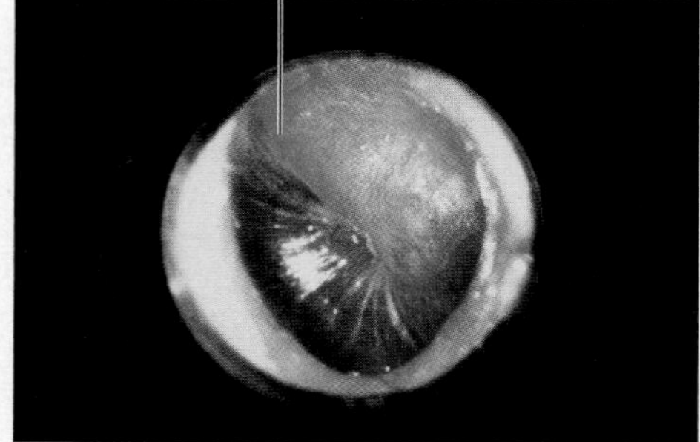

▲ **FIGURE 11.30**
Otoscopic View of Acute Otitis Media.

Lester V. Bergman/Corbis NX/Getty Images

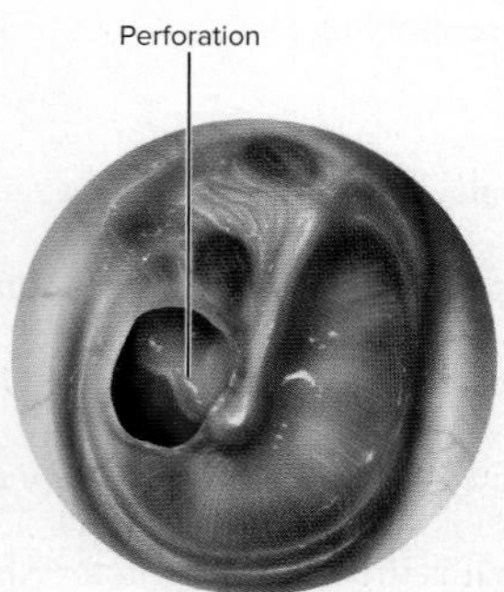

▲ **FIGURE 11.31**
Otoscopic View of Chronic Otitis Media with Perforation.

Bo Veisland/Science Source

Word Analysis and Definition

S = Suffix P = Prefix R = Root R/CF = Combining Form

WORD	PRONUNCIATION		ELEMENTS	DEFINITION
cholesteatoma	koh-less-tee-ah-**TOE**-mah	S/ R/CF R/	-oma *tumor, mass* chol/e- *bile* -steat- *fat*	Yellow, waxy tumor arising in the middle ear
coryza (Note: *same as acute rhinitis)*	koh-**RYE**-zah		Greek *catarrh*	Viral inflammation of the mucous membrane of the nose
otosclerosis	oh-toe-sklair-**OH**-sis	S/ R/CF R/CF	-sis *abnormal condition* ot/o- *ear* -scler/o- *hard*	Hardening at the junction of the stapes and oval window that causes loss of hearing
perforated **perforation**	**PER**-foh-ray-ted per-foh-**RAY**-shun	 S/ R/	Latin *to bore through* -ion *action* perforat- *bore through*	Punctured with one or more holes A hole through the wall of a structure
prosthesis	**PROS**-thee-sis		Greek *addition*	Manufactured substitute for a missing or diseased part of the body

EXERCISES

A. Build medical terms. *Fill in the blanks with the correct element to complete the terms.* **LO 11.1 and 11.7**

1. A hole through the wall of a structure: _______ /ion

2. Hardening at the junction of the stapes and oval window: oto/________ /sis

3. Yellow, waxy tumor in the middle ear: _______ /_______ /oma

B. Choose *the correct answer to each statement.* **LO 11.1 and 11.7**

1. The root in the term **perforation** means:

a. tumor **b.** bore through **c.** liquid **d.** bile **e.** blockage

2. In the term **cholesteatoma,** the word element that means fat is:

a. choles- **b.** -steat- **c.** -oma

3. In the term **otosclerosis,** the word element oto- means:

a. pertaining to **b.** hardening **c.** condition of **d.** ear

C. Match *the correct element in the first column to the correct meaning in the second column below. Fill in the blanks.* **LO 11.1 and 11.7**

_______ **1.** ion **a.** action

_______ **2.** scler/o **b.** fat

_______ **3.** oma **c.** tumor

_______ **4.** steat **d.** bile

_______ **5.** chol/e **e.** hard

Inner Ear for Hearing (LO 11.7)

The inner ear is a **labyrinth** *(Figure 11.32)* of complex, intricate systems of passages. The passages in the **cochlea**, a part of the labyrinth, contain receptors to translate vibrations into nerve impulses so that the brain can interpret them as different sounds.

The membrane of the oval window separates the middle ear from the **vestibule** of the inner ear. From the tympanic membrane *(① in Figure 11.33),* the stapes ② moves the oval membrane to generate pressure waves in the fluid inside the cochlea ③. The pressure waves cause **vestibular** and **basilar membranes** inside the cochlea to vibrate ④ and sway fine hair cells attached to the basilar membrane ⑤. The hair cells convert this motion into nerve impulses, which travel via the **cochlear nerve** to the brain. The excess pressure waves in the cochlea escape the inner ear via the round window ⑥.

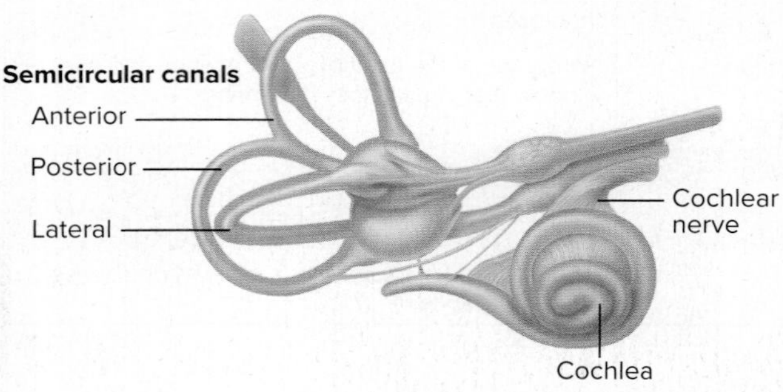

▲ **FIGURE 11.32**
Labyrinth of Inner Ear.

Hearing Disorders of the Inner Ear (LO 11.7)

Today, the most common cause of hearing loss is damage to the fine hairs in the cochlea by exposure to repeated loud noise, related either to work (for example, jack-hammers, leaf blowers) or to leisure activities (such as amplified music at concerts, personal listening devices, and motorcycles). This is a **sensorineural hearing loss**.

Hearing aids are becoming more sophisticated and smaller, but they do not help people with cochlear damage. **Cochlear implants** are used to bypass the damaged hair cells and directly stimulate cochlear nerve endings.

Keynotes

- Repeated exposure to loud noise causes hearing loss in young people as well as in older people.
- A **conductive hearing loss** occurs when sound is not conducted efficiently through the external auditory canal to the tympanic membrane and the ossicles. Causes include
  - Middle ear pathology, such as acute otitis media, otitis media with effusion, or a perforated eardrum.
  - Impacted cerumen.
  - An infected external auditory canal.
  - A foreign body in the external canal.

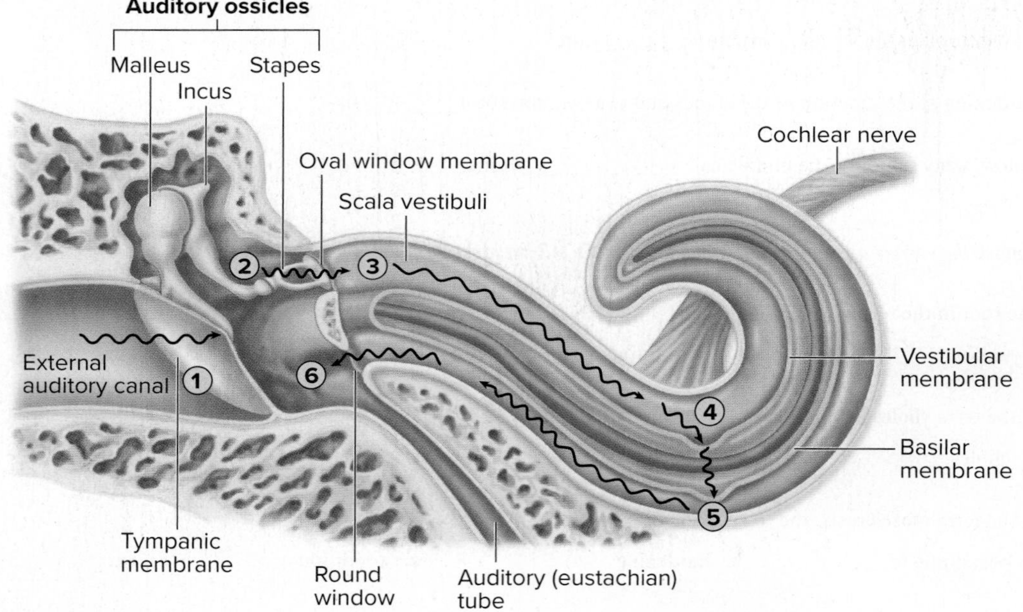

▲ **FIGURE 11.33**
Hearing Process in the Inner Ear.

Word Analysis and Definition

S = Suffix P = Prefix R = Root R/CF = Combining Form

WORD	PRONUNCIATION	ELEMENTS		DEFINITION
basilar	**BAS**-ih-lar	S/ R/	**-ar** *pertaining to* **basil-** *base, support*	Pertaining to the base of a structure
cochlea	**KOK**-lee-ah		Latin *snail shell*	An intricate combination of passages; used to describe the part of the inner ear used in hearing
cochlear (adj)	**KOK**-lee-ar	S/ R/	**-ar** *pertaining to* **cochle-** *cochlea*	Pertaining to the cochlea
conductive hearing loss	kon-**DUK**-tiv **HEER**-ing LOSS	 S/ R/	**conductive** Latin *to lead* **-ing** *quality of* **hear-** *to perceive sounds* **loss** Middle English *to lose*	Hearing loss caused by lesions in the outer ear or middle ear
labyrinth labyrinthitis	**LAB**-ih-rinth **LAB**-ih-rin-**THIE**-tis	 S/ R/	Greek *labyrinth* **-itis** *inflammation* **labyrinth-** *inner ear*	The inner ear Inflammation of the inner ear
sensorineural hearing loss	**SEN**-sor-ih-**NYUR**-al **HEER**-ing LOSS	S/ R/CF R/ S/ R/	**-al** *pertaining to* **sensor/i-** *sensory* **-neur-** *nerve* **-ing** *quality of* **hear-** *to perceive sounds* **loss** Middle English *to lose*	Hearing loss caused by lesions of the inner ear or the auditory nerve
vestibule vestibular (adj)	**VES**-tih-byul ves-**TIB**-you-lar	 S/ R/	Latin *entrance* **-ar** *pertaining to* **vestibul-** *vestibule of the inner ear*	Space at the entrance to a canal Pertaining to the vestibule of the inner ear

EXERCISE

A. Review *the material regarding the middle ear structures and their disorders; then choose the best answer.* **LO 11.1 and 11.7**

1. In the term **basilar,** ***basil-*** is a

   a. prefix **b.** root **c.** combining form

2. The **entrance to the inner ear** is the

   a. vestibule **b.** labyrinth **c.** cochlea **d.** aqueous **e.** choroid

3. Labyrinthitis is a(n)

   a. procedure **b.** symptom **c.** inflammation

4. The element ***neuro-*** means

   a. never **b.** nerve **c.** nose

5. Hearing loss caused by lesions of the outer ear is

   a. auditory **b.** basilar **c.** sensorineural **d.** aqueous

6. An **intricate combination of passages** in the ear is the

   a. cochlea **b.** vestibule **c.** labyrinth

7. The root meaning **inflammation** can be found in the word

   a. vestibule **b.** labyrinthitis **c.** otology

8. Hearing loss caused by lesions of the inner ear is called ________________ hearing loss.

   a. auditory **b.** basilar **c.** sensorineural

9. The suffix meaning **pertaining to** is found in the term

   a. vestibular **b.** labyrinthitis **c.** audiometer

Lesson 11.5 (cont'd)

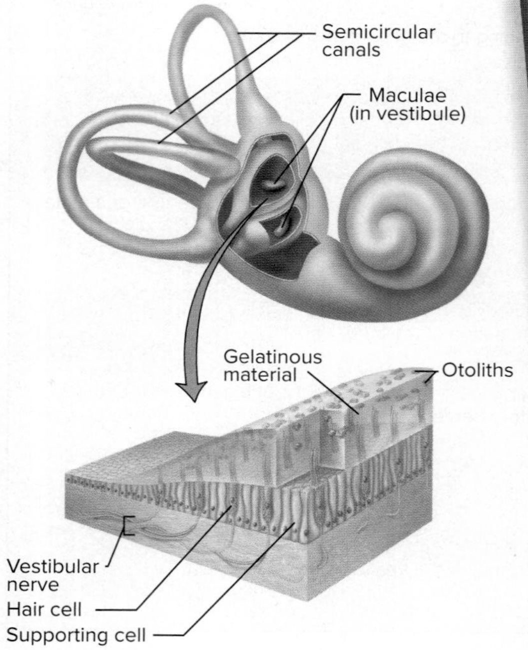

▲ **FIGURE 11.34**
Vestibule of the Inner Ear.

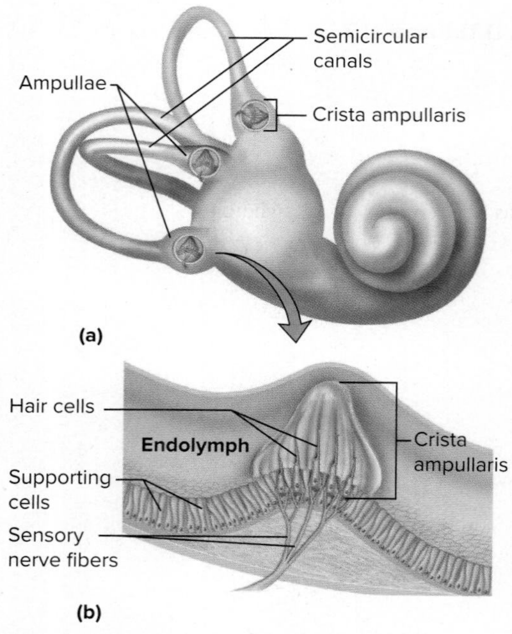

▲ **FIGURE 11.35**
Semicircular Canals (a) Anatomy (b) Histology.

Abbreviation

BPPV benign paroxysmal positional vertigo

CASE REPORT 11.4

You are . . .

. . . Sonia Ramos, a medical assistant working with Sylvia Thompson, MD, an otorhinolaryngologist at Fulwood Medical Center.

You are communicating with . . .

. . . Mr. Ernesto Santiago, a 44-year-old man who was referred to Dr. Thompson. Mr. Santiago complains of recurrent attacks of nausea, vomiting, a sense of spinning or whirling, and ringing in his ears. The attacks last about 24 hours and are getting more frequent. He has been having trouble hearing quiet speech on his left side. Your role is to document his examination, diagnosis, and care, and to act as translator between Mr. Santiago and Dr. Thompson.

Inner Ear for Equilibrium and Balance (LO 11.7)

The inner ear contains the organs in your body responsible for maintaining the true sense of balance. The **vestibule** and the three semicircular canals *(Figures 11.34 and 11.35)* in the inner ear maintain an individual's balance. These are the true organs of balance. Inside the fluid-filled vestibule are two raised, flat areas covered with hair cells and a jelly-like material. This gelatinous material contains calcium and protein crystals called **otoliths.** The position of the head alters the amount of pressure this gelatinous mass applies to the hair cells. The hair cells respond to horizontal and vertical changes and send impulses to the brain relating how the head is tilted.

Each of the three fluid-filled semicircular canals has a dilated end called an **ampulla.** The ampulla contains a mound of hair cells set in a gelatinous material that together are called the **crista ampullaris** *(Figure 11.36).* This detects rotational movements of the head that distort the hair cells and lead to stimulation of connected nerve cells. The nerve impulses travel through the vestibular nerve to the brain. From the brain, nerve impulses travel to the muscles to maintain **equilibrium** and balance.

Disorders of the Inner Ear for Balance (LO 11.7)

The sensation of spinning or whirling that Mr. Santiago experiences is called **vertigo,** often described by patients as dizziness. The ringing in his ears is called **tinnitus.** Both sensations arise in the inner ear. Tinnitus can also sound like hissing, buzzing, roaring, or clicking and may be associated with difficulty hearing, sleeping, or working. Treatment includes hearing aids, sound-masking devices, and learning ways to cope with the problem.

Benign paroxysmal positional vertigo (BPPV) is another type of intermittent vertigo caused by fragments of the otoliths in the vestibule migrating into the semicircular canals. The otolith fragments brush against the hair cells, sending conflicting signals to the brain. This produces vertigo.

Case Report 11.4 *(continued)*

The recurrent attacks that Mr. Santiago suffered are called **Ménière disease.** The disease involves the destruction of inner-ear hair cells, but the etiology is unknown and there is no cure. Dr. Thompson prescribed medication to control Mr. Santiago's nausea and vomiting.

Word Analysis and Definition

S = Suffix P = Prefix R = Root R/CF = Combining Form

WORD	PRONUNCIATION	ELEMENTS		DEFINITION
ampulla	am-**PULL**-ah		Latin *two-handled bottle*	Dilated portion of a canal or duct
crista ampullaris	**KRIS**-tah am-**PULL**-air-is	R/ S/ R/	**crista** *crest* **-aris** *pertaining to* **ampull-** *bottle-shaped*	Mound of hair cells and gelatinous material in the ampulla of a semicircular canal
equilibrium	ee-kwi-**LIB**-ree-um	P/ R/	**equi-** *equal* **-librium** *balance*	Being evenly balanced
Ménière disease	men-**YEAR** diz-**EEZ**		Prosper Ménière, French physician, 1799–1862	Disorder of the inner ear with acute attacks of tinnitus, vertigo, and hearing loss
otolith	**OH**-toe-lith	R/CF R/	**ot/o-** *ear* **-lith** *stone*	A calcium particle in the vestibule of the inner ear
paroxysmal	par-ock-**SIZ**-mal	S/ R/	**-al** *pertaining to* **paroxysm-** *sudden, sharp attack*	Occurring in sharp, spasmodic episodes
tinnitus	**TIN**-ih-tus		Latin *jingle*	Persistent ringing, whistling, clicking, or booming noise in the ears
vertigo	**VER**-tih-go		Latin *dizziness*	Sensation of spinning or whirling
vestibule vestibular (adj)	**VES**-tih-byul ves-**TIB**-you-lar	 S/ R/	Latin *entrance chamber* **-ar** *pertaining to* **vestibul-** *vestibule*	Space at the entrance to a canal Pertaining to the vestibule

EXERCISES

A. Review *Case Report 11.4 and 11.4 (continued). Insert the correct medical term to answer each question or complete the statement.* **LO 11.2, 11.7, and 11.9**

1. Which medical term is used in documentation for Mr. Santiago's "ringing in his ears?" __________

2. Which medical term is used in documentation for Mr. Santiago's "spinning or whirling?" __________

3. Because the attacks come and go, they can be be described as being: ____________

4. Will the medication correct the disorders of the inner ear? (yes or no) __________

B. Challenge *your knowledge of the ear by filling in the correct terms for the following definitions. Fill in the blanks.* **LO 11.2 and 11.7**

Definition	Medical Term
1. Persistent ringing in the ears	________________
2. Sensation of spinning or whirling	________________
3. Occurring in sharp, spasmodic episodes	________________
4. State of being evenly balanced	________________
5. Dilated portion of a canal or duct	________________
6. Calcium particle in the vestibule	________________
7. Mound of hair cells found in ampulla	________________

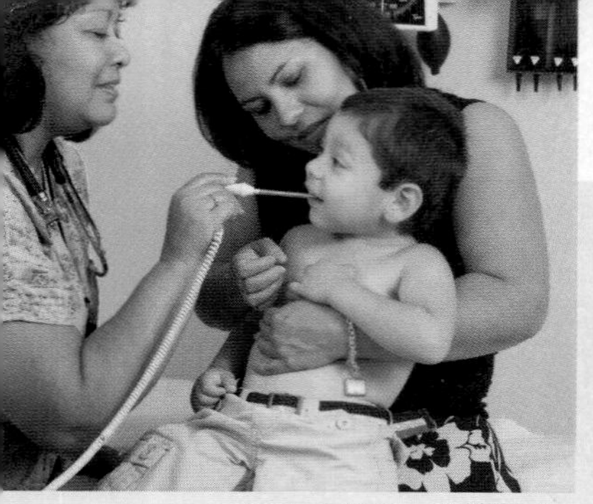

Rick Brady/McGraw-Hill Education

Lesson 11.6 Diagnostic and Therapeutic Procedures and Pharmacology for Disorders of the Ear

Objectives

Many of the diagnostic tests for hearing function and to determine diseases of the ear can be performed by technicians with physician overview. To communicate clearly and accurately, the terminology of these diagnostic procedures must be clearly understood by everyone involved. The information in this lesson will enable you to:

11.6.1 Describe the different tests that can be performed in a medical office.

11.6.2 Explain the uses of an otoscope.

11.6.3 Discuss the value of specialized tests for inner ear function.

11.6.4 Identify tests to measure the response of the nervous system to sound.

Abbreviations

ABR	auditory brainstem response
AD	right ear
AS	left ear
AU	both ears
CAT	computed axial tomography

Diagnostic Procedures for Diseases of the Ear (LO 11.8)

Basic hearing test procedures that can be performed in an office include:

- **Whispered speech testing**, which is a simple screening method in which one ear of the patient is covered and the patient is asked to identify whispered sounds.
- **Tuning fork screening tests**, which can identify on which side a hearing loss is located **(Weber test)** and whether the hearing loss is due to loss of bone or air conduction **(Rinne test)**.

An **audiometer** is an electronic device that generates sounds in different frequencies and intensities and prints out a graph (**audiogram**) of the patient's responses (*Figure 11.36*). **Audiometry** measures hearing function and is often performed by an **audiologist**. An audiologist is a specialist in **audiology**. **Tympanometry** helps detect problems between the tympanic membrane and the inner ear by using a small earpiece that generates pressure and sound in the ear canal to gather information (**tympanography**) about changes of pressure inside the ear.

When recording the results of hearing testing, **A.D.** is shorthand for the right ear, **A.S.** for the left ear, and **A.U.** for both ears.

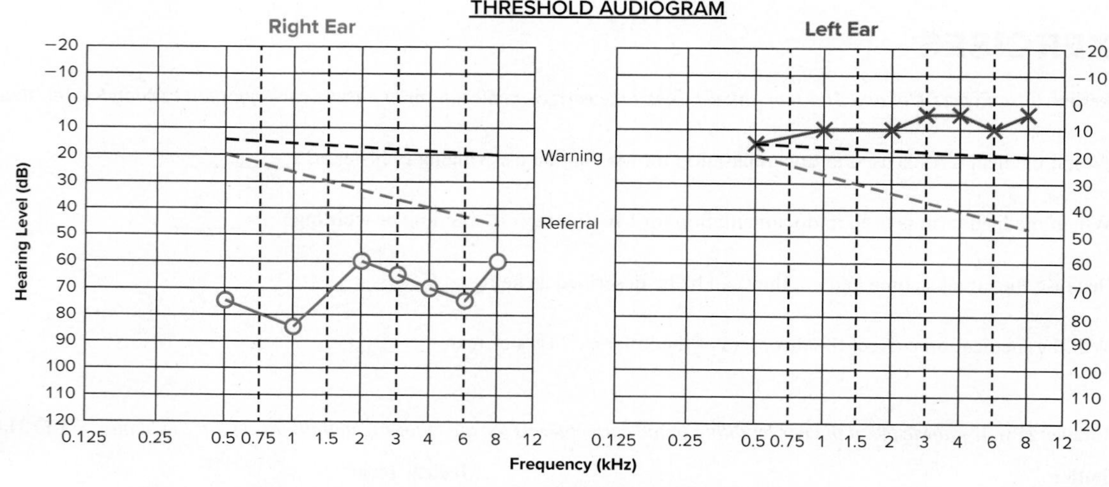

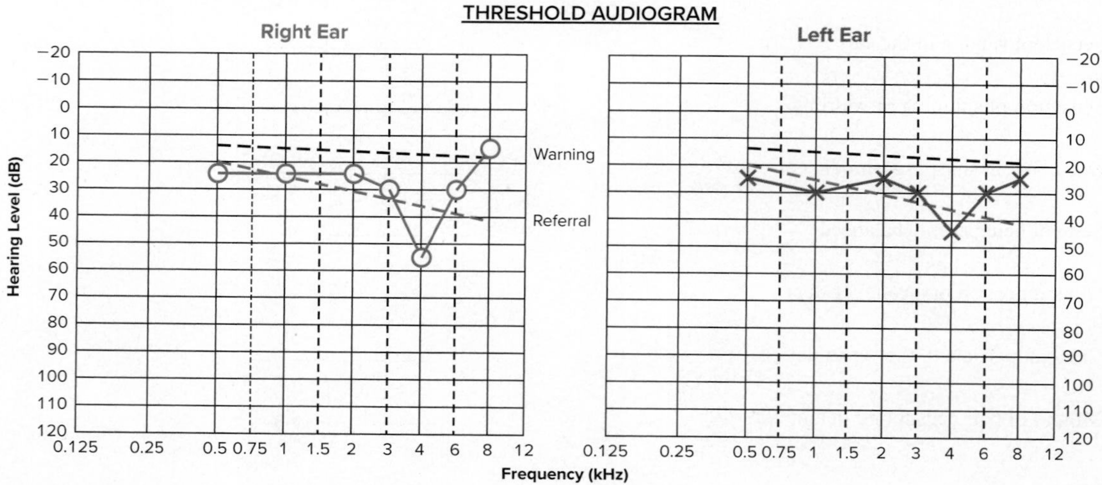

▲ **FIGURE 11.36**
Examples of Audiometry Results.

Word Analysis and Definition

S = Suffix P = Prefix R = Root R/CF = Combining Form

WORD	PRONUNCIATION	ELEMENTS		DEFINITION
audiology	aw-dee-**OL**-oh-jee	S/ R/CF	**-logy** *study of* **audi/o-** *hearing*	Study of hearing disorders
audiologist	aw-dee-**OL**-oh-jist	S/	**-logist** *specialist*	Specialist in evaluation of hearing function
audiometer	aw-dee-**OM**-eh-ter	R/CF R/	**audi/o-** *hearing* **-meter** *measure*	Instrument to measure hearing
audiometric (adj)	**AW**-dee-oh-**MET**-rik	S/ R/	**-ic** *pertaining to* **-metr-** *measure*	Pertaining to the measurement of hearing
audiometry	aw-dee-**OM**-eh-tree	S/	**-metry** *process of measuring*	The measurement of hearing
auditory	**AW**-dih-tor-ee	S/ R/	**-ory** *having the function of* **audit-** *hearing*	Pertaining to the sense of hearing or to the organs of hearing
Rinne test	**RIN**-eh TEST		Friedrich Rinne, 1819–1868, German otologist **test** Latin *earthen vessel*	Test for conductive hearing loss
tympanocentesis	**TIM**-pah-noh-sen-**TEE**-sis	S/ R/CF	**-centesis** *to puncture* **tympan/o-** *eardrum, tympanic membrane*	Puncture of the tympanic membrane with a needle
tympanography	**TIM**-pan-**OG**-rah-fee	S/	**-graphy** *process of recording*	Recording pressure changes inside the ear
tympanometry	**TIM**-pan-**OM**-eh-tree	S/	**-metry** *process of measuring*	Measurement of pressure changes between the middle and inner ears
Weber test	**VAY**-ber TEST		Ernst Weber, 1794–1878, German physiologist **test** Latin *earthen vessel*	Test for sensorineural hearing loss

Exercises

A. Define the different auditory diagnostic tests. *Match the test in the first column with its correct description in the second column. Fill in the blanks.* **LO 11.8**

______	**1.** tympanometry	**a.**	used to view the external ear and tympanic membrane
______	**2.** Rinne test	**b.**	test for conductive hearing loss
______	**3.** otoscopy	**c.**	test for sensorineural hearing loss
______	**4.** Weber test	**d.**	measures pressure changes between the middle and inner ears

B. Deconstruct medical terms relating to the diagnostic tests of the ear. *Fill in the blanks* **LO 11.1 and 11.8**

1. tympanometry: ______________________ / ______________________
CF S

2. tympanocentesis: ______________________ / ______________________
CF S

3. audiologist: ______________________ / ______________________
CF S

Lesson 11.6 (cont'd) Diagnostic Procedures for Diseases of the Ear (continued) (LO 11.8)

Abbreviations

CAT scan	computerized axial tomography
ECOG	electrocochleography
ENG	electronystagmography
MRI	magnetic resonance imaging
VNG	videonystagmography

The pinna (auricle) is examined visually and by touch. The external ear and the middle ear are examined via **otoscopy** with an **otoscope** (*Figure 11.37*). The pinna (auricle) of the ear is gently manipulated in order for a health care provider to obtain an **otoscopic** view of the external and middle ear. The otoscopic view enables the tympanic membrane and the ossicles behind it to be visualized.

A **pneumatic otoscope** pushes air into the ear and enables the examiner to see if the eardrum moves freely.

Electrocochleography (ECOG) measures the response to sound by the nervous system. A soft electrode is placed deeply in the external ear canal and other electrodes are placed on the forehead to measure responses to sound.

Auditory brainstem response test (ABR) also measures the nervous system response to sound with a setup and procedure similar to ECOG.

Magnetic resonance imaging (MRI) of structures in the inner ear can be helpful in the diagnosis of some vestibular disorders. **Computerized axial tomography (CAT scan)** can help diagnose problems in and around the inner ear.

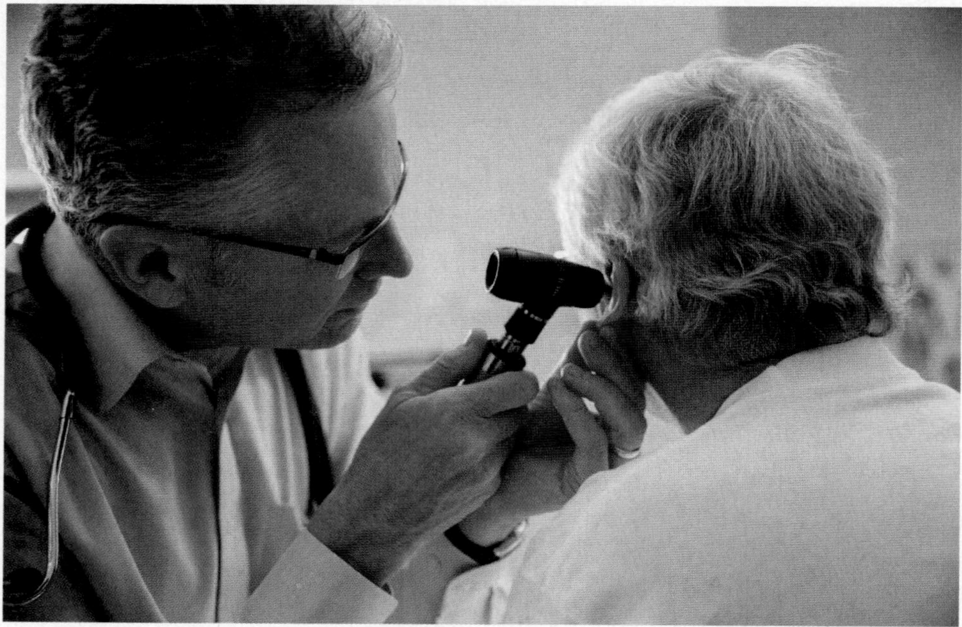

▲ **FIGURE 11.37**
Physician Using an Otoscope to Examine Patient's Ear.

Hero Images Inc./Alamy Images

Word Analysis and Definition

S = Suffix P = Prefix R = Root R/CF = Combining Form

WORD	PRONUNCIATION	ELEMENTS		DEFINITION
electrocochleography	ee-**LEK**-troh-kok-lee-**OG**-rah-fee	S/ R/CF R/CF	**-graphy** *process of recording* **electr/o-** *electric* **-cochle/o-** *cochlea*	Measurement of the electric potentials generated in the inner ear by sounds
otoscope otoscopic (adj) otoscopy	**OH**-toh-scope oh-toh-**SKOP**-ik oh-**TOS**-koh-pee	S/ R/CF S/ S/	**-scope** *instrument for viewing* **ot/o-** *ear* **-ic** *pertaining to* **-scopy** *to examine*	Instrument for examining the external and middle ears Pertaining to examination with an otoscope Examination of the ear
pneumatic	new-**MAT**-ik	S/ R/	**-ic** *pertaining to* **pneumat-** *structure filled with air*	Pertaining to a structure filled with air

EXERCISES

A. Use the following table *to list all the combining forms in the terms given and give their meaning:* **LO 11.1 and 11.8**

Terms	Combining Forms	Meaning of Combining Forms
otoscope		
electrocochleography		

B. Insert *the following terms to complete the medical documentation. Use each term only once; not all terms will be used. Fill in the blanks.* **LO 11.2, 11.8, and 11.9**

otoscope otoscopic otoscopy pneumatic

The patient was complaining of an earache. A(n) ________ (1) exam was necessary to quickly visualize the auditory canal and tympanic membrane. You hand Dr. Brown a(n) ________ (2) and she noticed that the membrane seemed to be abnormal. She used the ________ (3) attachment to see if the tympanic membrane moved freely.

C. Fill in the blanks *with the correct abbreviation being described.* **LO 11.3 and 11.8**

1. Use of goggles with a video camera to monitor eye movements as they follow different visual targets ______________

2. Records images of the structures of the inner ear without the use of radiation: ______________

3. Measures the nervous system's response to sound through the placement of electrodes in the ear canal and on the forehead: ______________

Lesson 11.6 (cont'd) Therapeutic Procedures for the Ear (LO 11.8)

Hearing

Ear clearing to equalize the pressure in the middle ear with the outside air pressure by making the ear(s) "pop" can be performed by yawning, swallowing, or using a method like a **Valsalva maneuver**, in which the nose is pinched, the mouth is closed, and attempts are made to breathe out through the nose.

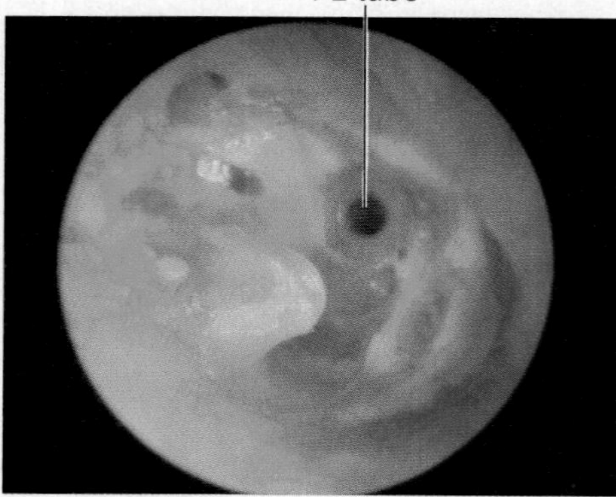

▲ **FIGURE 11.38**
Pressure Equalization (PE) Tube in Tympanic Membrane.

Yoav Levy/Diomedia/Medical Images

Ear wax blockage is removed by loosening it with oil, and then flushing, **curetting**, or suctioning out the softened wax.

Debridement is the removal of **necrotic** tissue and debris from the external ear canal in **otitis externa** using dry cotton wipes and/or suction. Mild otitis externa can then be treated with 2% acetic acid and hydrocortisone drops. Moderate infections require the addition of a **topical antibacterial suspension**, and severe infections require the insertion of an ear wick into the canal, wetted four times a day with a topical antibiotic or 5% aluminum acetate solution. Very severe infections may need systemic antibiotics. **Swimmer's ear** is a form of otitis externa and can be prevented by applying a few drops of a 1:1 mixture of rubbing alcohol and vinegar immediately after swimming.

Acute otitis media responds to an antibiotic such as amoxicillin, though some infections may subside spontaneously.

In **chronic otitis media with effusion**, when the sticky fluid persists in the middle ear, a **myringotomy** can be performed and a small, hollow plastic tube inserted through the tympanic membrane to allow the effusion to drain out. These tubes are called **tympanostomy tubes**, or **pressure equalization tubes** (**PE tubes**) (*Figure 11.38*). Surgical removal is required for a **cholesteatoma**.

Hearing aids can help a sensorineural hearing loss and an **audiologist** will recommend the type of device for each patient.

Cochlear implants can be used for a severe hearing loss. Unlike a hearing aid that amplifies sound and directs it through the ear canal, a cochlear implant compensates for damaged or nonworking elements in the cochlea. The devices pick up sound and **digitize** it, convert the digitized sound into electrical signals, and transmit those signals to electrodes embedded in the cochlea. The electrodes stimulate the cochlear nerve, sending signals to the brain.

Abbreviation

PE	pressure equalization (tubes)

Balance

Otolith repositioning procedures, performed by physical therapists with specialized training, are employed to return the tiny otolith granules to their correct resting place to resolve positional vertigo.

Exercises taught in a physical therapy setting can help with dizziness and vertigo to improve balance in different positions and activities.

Medications for the Ear (LO 11.8)

In the external ear canal, buildup of wax can be loosened with oil or with carbamide peroxide solution *(Debrox)*. Otitis externa can be treated with acetic acid drops to change the pH of the external canal or with drops containing an antibiotic or an antibiotic and steroid such as ciprofloxacin and dexamethazone *(Ciprodex)* or neomycin, polymycin, and hydrocortisone *(Corticosporin)*.

For infections of the middle ear, antibiotics such as penicillin, amoxicillin, and erythromycin are used.

For inner ear disorders, the antihistamine meclizine and the anti-anxiety medication diazepam *(Valium)* are used to diminish the vertigo of BPPV. The treatment of Ménière's disease has been revolutionized with the use of a single transtympanic injection of a low dose of gentamycin.

Word Analysis and Definition

S = Suffix P = Prefix R = Root R/CF = Combining Form

WORD	PRONUNCIATION	ELEMENTS		DEFINITION
curette **curettage** (Note: the final "e" of curette is dropped because the suffix "–age" begins with a vowel)	kyu-**RET** kyu-reh-**TAHZH**	S/ R/ S/	**-ette** *little* **cur-** *cleanse* **-age** *related to*	Scoop-shaped instrument for scraping the interior of a cavity or removing new growths Scraping the interior of a cavity or removing a new growth
debridement	day-**BREED**-mon	S/ P/ R/	**-ment** *resulting state* **de-** *take away* **-bride-** *rubbish*	The removal of necrotic or injured tissue
digitize	**DIJ**-ih-tize	S/ R/	**-ize** *affect in a specific way* **digit-** *finger, toe, number*	To change analog information into a numerical format to facilitate computer processing
maneuver	mah-**NYU**-ver		French *to work by hand*	A planned movement or procedure
myringotomy	mir-in-**GOT**-oh-mee	S/ R/CF	**-tomy** *surgical incision* **myring/o-** *tympanic membrane*	Incision in the tympanic membrane
necrosis necrotic (adj)	neh-**KROH**-sis neh-**KROT**-ik	S/ R/ S/ R/CF	**-osis** *condition* **necr-** *death* **-tic** *pertaining to* **necr/o-** *death*	Pathologic death of one or more cells Affected by necrosis
topical	**TOP**-ih-kal	S/ R/	**-al** *pertaining to* **topic-** *local*	Medication applied directly to obtain a local effect
tympanostomy	tim-pan-**OS**-toh-mee	S/ R/CF	**-stomy** *new opening* **tympan/o-** *eardrum, tympanic membrane*	Surgically created new opening in the tympanic membrane to allow fluid to drain from the middle ear
Valsalva	val-**SAL**-vah		Antonio Valsalva, 1666–1723, Italian physician	Any forced expiratory effort against a closed airway
irrigation	ih-rih-**GAY**-shun	S/ R/	**ation** *process* **irrig-** *to water*	Use of water; e.g., to remove wax from the external ear canal

EXERCISE

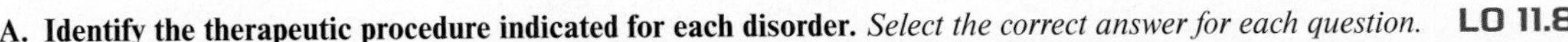

A. Identify the therapeutic procedure indicated for each disorder. *Select the correct answer for each question.* **LO 11.8**

1. Chronic otitis media may be treated with:

a. Valsalva maneuver **b.** tympanostomy tubes **c.** rubbing alcohol drops **d.** physical therapy

2. Acute otitis media is treated with:

a. myringotomy **b.** tympanostomy tubes **c.** oral antibiotics **d.** antihistamines

3. Positional vertigo can be treated with:

a. physical therapy **b.** anti-anxiety medications **c.** cochlear implants **d.** myringotomy

4. A treatment for excessive cerumen in the auditory canal:

a. alcohol and vinegar drops **b.** antibiotic drops **c.** myringotomy **d.** curettage

5. Cholesteatoma is treated with:

a. debridement **b.** excision **c.** acetic acid drops **d.** oral antibiotics

Additional exercises available in connect

Chapter Review exercises, along with additional practice items, are available in Connect!

The Endocrine System

The Essentials of the Language of Endocrinology

CHAPTER 12

Rick Brady/McGraw-Hill Education

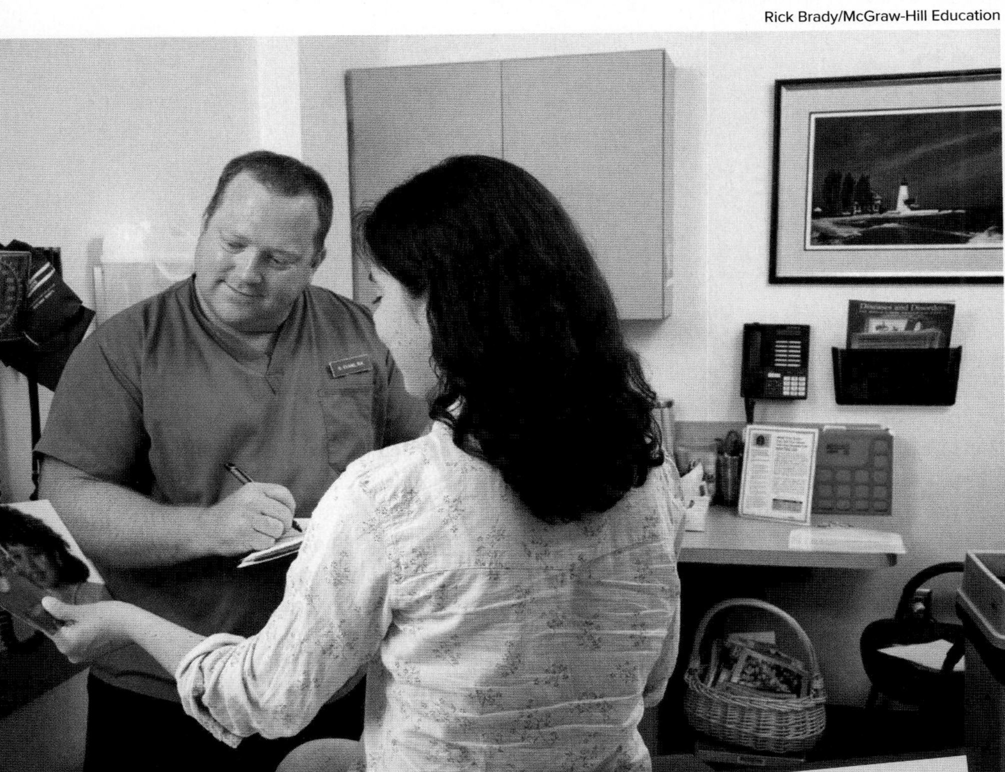

CASE REPORT 12.1

You are . . .

. . . a registered nurse working with **endocrinologist** Sabina Khalid, MD, in the Endocrinology Clinic at Fulwood Medical Center.

You are communicating with . . .

. . . Mrs. Gina Tacher, a 33-year-old schoolteacher. She complains of coarsening of her facial features and enlargement of the bones of her hands. Over the past 10 years, Mrs. Tacher's nose and jaw have increased in size and her voice has become husky. She has brought photos of herself at ages 9 and 16. She has no other health problems.

Learning Outcomes

The **endocrine** system is a communication system. The **hormones** produced by this system are blood-borne messengers secreted by endocrine glands; they circulate in the bloodstream, gaining access to all other body cells. They are distributed anywhere the blood travels, but only affect the target cells that have receptors for them. These hormones alter the metabolism of the target cells. The information in this chapter will enable you to:

- **LO 12.1** **Use roots, combining forms, suffixes, and prefixes to construct and analyze (deconstruct) medical terms related to the endocrine system.**
- **LO 12.2** **Spell and pronounce correctly medical terms related to the endocrine system in order to communicate them with accuracy and precision in any health care setting.**
- **LO 12.3** **Define accepted abbreviations related to the endocrine system.**
- **LO 12.4** **Identify the anatomical positions of the hypothalamus, pituitary, and pineal glands; the functions of the hormones they secrete; and their disorders and treatments.**
- **LO 12.5** **Describe the hormones secreted by the thyroid, parathyroid, and thymus glands; their functions; and their disorders and treatments.**
- **LO 12.6** **Compare the hormones secreted by the adrenal cortex and medulla, their functions, and their disorders and treatments.**
- **LO 12.7** **Relate the hormones secreted by the endocrine cells of the pancreas to the different types of diabetes mellitus and their symptoms, signs, and treatments.**
- **LO 12.8** **Explain the diagnostic and therapeutic procedures and the pharmacology for disorders of the endocrine glands.**
- **LO 12.9** **Apply your knowledge of medical terms relating to the endocrine system to documentation, medical records, and medical reports.**
- **LO 12.10** **Translate the medical terms relating to the endocrine system into everyday language in order to communicate clearly with patients and their families.**

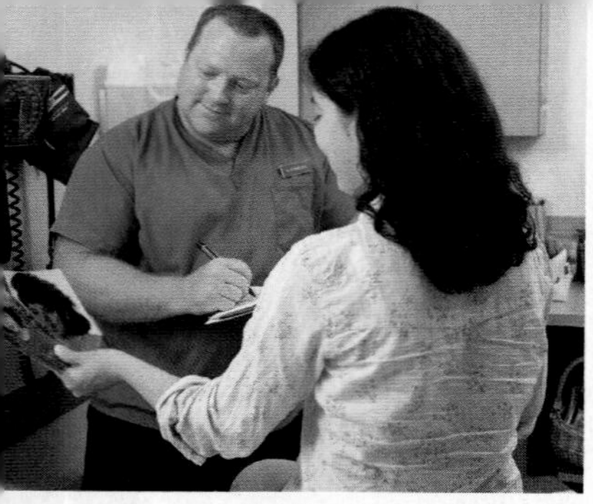

Rick Brady/McGraw-Hill Education

The health professionals involved in the diagnosis and treatment of problems with the endocrine system include:

- **Endocrinologists,** who are medical specialists concerned with the production and effects of hormones.
- **Endocrine physician assistants,** who work with endocrinologists to provide care and education to endocrine and diabetes patients.
- **Endocrine nurse practitioners,** who are registered nurses with specialized training in endocrinology.
- **Certified diabetic educators,** who are certified to possess specialized knowledge in diabetes self-management education and monitoring.

Objectives

Your endocrine system is a network of ductless glands whose cells secrete ***hormones*** *directly into your bloodstream. The information in this lesson will enable you to use correct medical terminology to:*

12.1.1 Name the glands that make up the endocrine system.
12.1.2 List the hormones produced by the hypothalamus and pituitary gland.
12.1.3 Identify the control that the hypothalamic and pituitary hormones exert over other endocrine glands.
12.1.4 Specify the roles of the pineal gland.
12.1.5 Describe disorders of the hypothalamus, pituitary, and pineal glands.

Keynotes

- **A hormone is secreted by an endocrine gland or cell and is carried by the bloodstream to act at distant target sites.**
- **The medical specialty concerned with the hormonal secretions of the endocrine glands is called endocrinology.**

Abbreviation

ADH antidiuretic hormone

Lesson 12.1

Endocrine System, Hypothalamus, and Pituitary and Pineal Glands

The Endocrine System (LO 12.4)

The endocrine system comprises several major organs *(Figures 12.1 and 12.2).* These organs, with their respective names and numbers in parentheses below, work together to ensure that this system operates smoothly:

- **Pituitary gland (1)** and the nearby **hypothalamus (1).**
- **Pineal gland (1).**
- **Thyroid gland (1).**
- **Parathyroid glands (4).**
- **Thymus gland (1).**
- **Adrenal glands (2).**
- **Pancreas (1).**
- **Gonads: testes (2) in the male; ovaries (2) in the female** (The male gonads are discussed in *Chapter 14* and the female in *Chapter 15.*)

In addition, endocrine cells found in tissues throughout the body secrete particular hormones. For example:

- **Cells in the upper GI tract** secrete hormones that include gastrin, which stimulates gastric secretions.
- **Cells in the kidney** secrete erythropoietin, which stimulates erythrocyte (red blood cell) production.
- **Fat cells** secrete leptin, which helps suppress appetite. Lack of leptin can lead to overeating and obesity.
- **Cells in tissues throughout the body** secrete **prostaglandins,** which act locally to dilate blood vessels, relax airways, stimulate uterine contractions in menstrual cramps or labor, and lower acid secretion in the stomach. When tissues are injured, prostaglandins promote an inflammatory response.

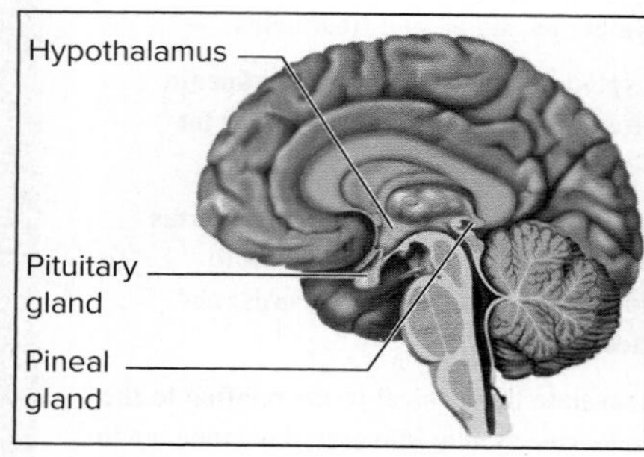

▲ **FIGURE 12.1**
Hypothalamus, Pituitary Gland, and Pineal Gland.

Hypothalamus (LO 12.2 and 12.4)

The hypothalamus, which is the size of an almond, is the part of the brain located just above the pituitary gland. It connects the brain to the endocrine system through blood vessels between the hypothalamus and the pituitary gland, thus enabling hypothalamic hormones to control pituitary hormone secretion. The hypothalamus secretes a total of eight hormones: four are releasing hormones that stimulate the secretion of hormones by the anterior lobe of the pituitary gland; two are inhibitory hormones that inhibit the secretion of anterior lobe pituitary gland hormones. These releasing and inhibitory hormones are named and described in the next section on the pituitary gland *and are shown there in italics.* The hypothalamus also produces two hormones–vasopressin and oxytocin–that travel directly to the posterior lobe of the pituitary, where they are stored. These two hormones are also described in the next section.

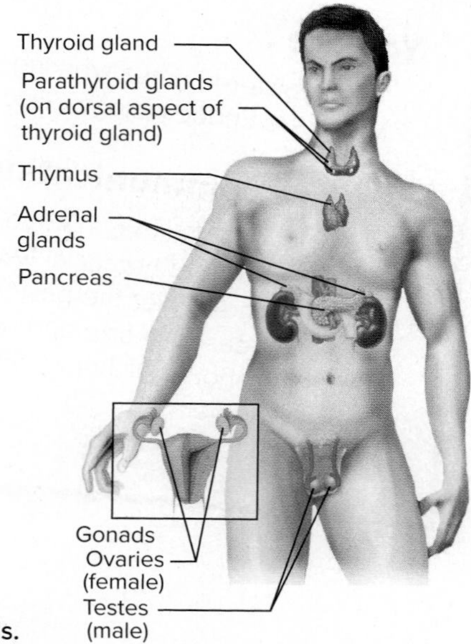

▶ **FIGURE 12.2**
Major Endocrine Glands.

Word Analysis and Definition

S = Suffix P = Prefix R = Root R/CF = Combining Form

WORD	PRONUNCIATION	ELEMENTS		DEFINITION
antidiuretic (**Note:** *Two prefixes*)	**AN**-tih-die-you-**RET**-ik	S/ P/ P/ R/	**-ic** *pertaining to* **anti-** *against* **-di-** *complete* **-uret-** *urination*	An agent that decreases urine production
endocrine	**EN**-doh-krin	P/ R/CF	**endo-** *within* **-crine** *secrete*	A gland that produces an internal or hormonal secretion
endocrinology (**Note:** *The "e" in* crine *changes to "o" for better flow.*)	**EN**-doh-krih-**NOL**-oh-jee	S/	**-logy** *study of*	Medical specialty concerned with the production and effects of hormones
endocrinologist	**EN**-doh-krih-**NOL**-oh-jist	S/	**-logist** *one who studies, specialist*	A medical specialist in endocrinology
hormone	**HOR**-mohn		Greek *to set in motion*	Chemical formed in one tissue or organ and carried by the bloodstream to stimulate or inhibit a function of another tissue or organ
hormonal (adj)	hor-**MOHN**-al	S/ R/	**-al** *pertaining to* **hormon-** *hormone*	Pertaining to hormones
hypothalamus	high-poh-**THAL**-ah-muss	S/ P/	**-us** *pertaining to* **hypo-** *below*	An endocrine gland in the floor and wall of the third ventricle of the brain
hypothalamic (adj)	high-poh-thal-**AM**-ik	S/ R/	**-ic** *pertaining to* **-thalam-** *thalamus*	Pertaining to the hypothalamus
melatonin	mel-ah-**TONE**-in	S/ R/ R/	**-in** *substance* **mela-** *black* **-ton-** *tension, pressure*	Hormone formed by the pineal gland
oxytocin	**OCK**-see-**TOE**-sin	S/ R/ R/	**-in** *substance* **oxy-** *oxygen* **-toc-** *labor and childbirth*	Pituitary hormone that stimulates the uterus to contract
pineal	**PIN**-ee-al		Latin *like a pine cone*	Pertaining to the pineal gland
pituitary	pih-**TYU**-ih-tary	S/ R/	**-ary** *pertaining to* **pituit-** *pituitary*	Pertaining to the pituitary gland
prostaglandin	**PROS**-tah-**GLAN**-din	S/ R/ R/	**-in** *chemical* **prosta-** *prostate* **-gland-** *gland*	Hormone present in many tissues, but first isolated from the prostate gland
serotonin	ser-oh-**TOE**-nin	S/ R/CF R/	**-in** *substance* **ser/o-** *serum* **-ton-** *tension, pressure*	Neurotransmitter in central and peripheral nervous systems

EXERCISES

A. Identify *organs, hormones, and functions of the hormones of the endocrine system. Fill in the blanks.* **LO 12.2 and 12.4**

1. The ____________________ is the connection between the brain and the endocrine system via blood vessels.

2. How many hormones does the hypothalamus secrete that control anterior pituitary gland hormone secretion? ____________________

3. The hormone secreted by fat cells that suppresses appetite: ____________________

4. The hormone that stimulates uterine contractions: ____________________

B. Elements *remain your best tool for understanding medical terms. The elements are listed in column 1. Identify the type of element in column 2, its meaning in column 3, and an example of a term related to the anatomy of the endocrine system containing that element in column 4. Fill in the chart.* **LO 12.1**

Element	Type of Element (P, R, CF, or S)	Meaning of Element	Medical Term Containing This Element
anti	**1.**	**2.**	**3.**
di	**4.**	**5.**	**6.**
ton	**7.**	**8.**	**9.**
hypo	**10.**	**11.**	**12.**
logy	**13.**	**14.**	**15.**
mela	**16.**	**17.**	**18.**

The Endocrine System (continued)

Abbreviations

ACTH	adrenocorticotropic hormone
ADH	antidiuretic hormone
CRH	cortico-releasing hormone
DI	diabetes insipidus
FSH	follicle-stimulating hormone
GH	growth hormone
GHRH	growth hormone-releasing hormone
GnRH	gonadotropin-releasing hormone
LH	luteinizing hormone
OT	oxytocin
PRL	prolactin
TRH	thyrotropin-releasing hormone
TSH	thyroid-stimulating hormone

Pineal Gland

(LO 12.2 and 12.4)

The pineal gland is located on the roof of the brain's third ventricle, posterior to the hypothalamus. It secretes the feel-good hormone **serotonin** by day, and at night, converts it to **melatonin,** which helps to regulate sleep and wake cycles. This gland reaches its maximum size in childhood and may regulate puberty's timing.

Case Report 12.1 *(continued)*

Dr. Khalid's examination of Mrs. Tacher shows a protruding mandible and an enlarged, deeply grooved tongue. Her feet and hands are enlarged, her ribs are thickened, and her heart is enlarged. X-rays show a thickened skull and enlarged nasal sinuses. Blood tests display high growth hormone levels. CT and MRI scans show a tumor in the **pituitary** gland, and as a result, Mrs. Tacher is scheduled for surgery to remove the tumor.

Pituitary Gland

(LO 12.2, 12.3, and 12.4)

Each hormone plays its part in maintaining the body's homeostasis, but the pituitary gland and hypothalamus work together and often influence hormone production in the other endocrine glands. The pituitary gland is suspended from the hypothalamus, and it has two components:

- A large anterior lobe; and
- A small posterior lobe.

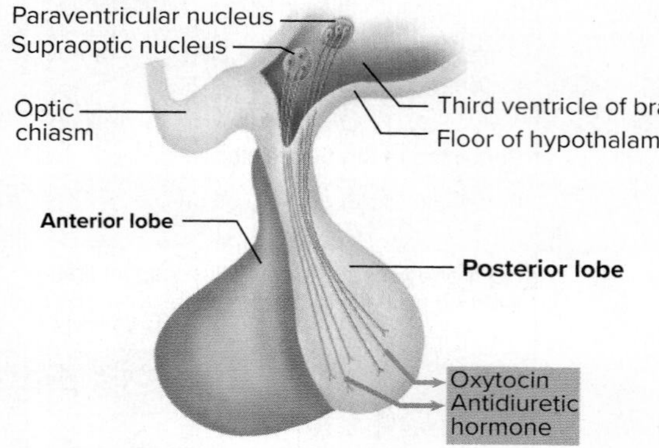

▲ **FIGURE 12.3** Hormones of the Posterior Lobe of the Pituitary Gland.

There are six **anterior-lobe hormones,** which are listed here with their functions:

1. **Follicle-stimulating hormone (FSH)** stimulates target cells in the ovaries to develop eggs, as well as sperm production in the testes.
2. **Luteinizing hormone (LH)** stimulates ovulation. It also encourages a corpus luteum (a yellow tissue mass) to form in the ovary *(see Chapter 15)* to secrete estrogen and progesterone. In the male, LH stimulates testosterone production *(see Chapter 14). Both FSH and LH production are stimulated by the* ***gonadotropin-releasing hormone (GnRH)*** *of the hypothalamus.*
3. **Thyroid-stimulating hormone (TSH),** or **thyrotropin,** stimulates the growth of the thyroid gland and the production of the chief thyroid hormone, thyroxine. *TSH production is stimulated by the* ***thyrotropin-releasing hormone (TRH)*** *of the hypothalamus.*
4. **Adrenocorticotropic hormone (ACTH),** or **corticotropin,** stimulates the adrenal glands to produce hormones called **corticosteroids,** including **hydrocortisone (cortisol)** and **cortisone.** *ACTH production is stimulated by the* ***cortico-releasing hormone (CRH)*** *of the hypothalamus.*
5. **Prolactin (PRL)** encourages the mammary glands to produce milk after pregnancy. In the male, it sensitizes the testes to LH, which enhances testosterone production. *Prolactin production is stimulated by the* ***thyrotropin-releasing hormone (TRH)*** *of the hypothalamus.*
6. **Growth hormone (GH),** or **somatotrophin,** stimulates cells to enlarge and divide. The body produces at least a thousand times more GH than any other pituitary hormone. *This production of growth hormone is stimulated by the* ***growth hormone-releasing hormone (GHRH)*** *of the hypothalamus.*

An **overproduction of growth hormone** in children produces gigantism. In adults, this overproduction produces **acromegaly,** the condition that Mrs. Tacher has. An **underproduction of growth hormone,** present at birth, leads to dwarfism.

Tropic hormones are hormones that stimulate other endocrine glands to produce their hormones. FSH and LH are called **gonadotropins** because they stimulate **gonadal** (reproductive organ) functions.

In addition to the six anterior-lobe hormones, there are the **posterior-lobe hormones.** These hormones are produced in the hypothalamus and stored and released in the pituitary posterior lobe *(Figure 12.3).* The two types of posterior-lobe hormones and their functions are:

1. **Oxytocin (OT)** in childbirth stimulates uterine contractions, and in lactation, it forces milk to flow down ducts to the nipple. In both sexes, its production increases during social interaction and sexual intercourse to help give the feelings of satisfaction and emotional bonding.
2. **Antidiuretic hormone (ADH),** also called **vasopressin,** reduces the volume of urine produced by the kidneys.

Diabetes insipidus (DI) (not diabetes mellitus) results from a decreased production of ADH. Symptoms of DI are excessive urine production leading to excessive thirst.

Word Analysis and Definition

S = Suffix P = Prefix R = Root R/CF = Combining Form

WORD	PRONUNCIATION	ELEMENTS		DEFINITION
acromegaly	ak-roe-**MEG**-ah-lee	S/ R/CF	**-megaly** *enlargement* **acr/o-** *peak, highest point*	Enlargement of head, face, hands, and feet due to excess growth hormone after growth plates have closed
adrenocorticotropic	ah-**DREE**-noh-**KOR**-tih-koh-**TROH**-pik	S/ R/CF R/CF	**-tropic** *a turning, change* **adren/o-** *adrenal gland* **-cortic/o-** *from the cortex*	Hormone of the anterior pituitary that stimulates the cortex of the adrenal gland to produce its own hormones
corticosteroid	**KOR**-tih-koh-**STAIR**-oyd	S/ R/CF	**-steroid** *steroid* **cortic/o-** *from the cortex*	A hormone produced by the adrenal cortex
corticotropin	**KOR**-tih-koh-**TROH**-pin	S/ R/CF	**-tropin** *stimulation* **cortic/o-** *from the cortex, cortex*	Pituitary hormone that stimulates the cortex of the adrenal gland to secrete cortisone
cortisone	**KOR**-tih-sohn	S/ R/	**-one** *hormone* **cortis-** *from the cortex*	A corticosteroid produced in small amounts by the adrenal cortex
diabetes insipidus (DI)	dye-ah-**BEE**-teez in-**SIP**-ih-dus	S/ P/ R/	diabetes, Greek *siphon* **-us** *pertaining to* **in-** *not* **-sipid-** *flavor*	Excretion of large amounts of dilute urine as a result of inadequate antidiuretic hormone production
gonadotropin	**GO**-nad-oh-**TROH**-pin	S/ R/CF	**-tropin** *stimulation* **gonad/o-** *testis, ovary*	Any hormone that stimulates gonadal function
gonad	**GO**-nad		gonad, Latin *seed*	An organ that produces sex cells; a testis or an ovary
hydrocortisone (also called **cortisol**)	high-droh-**KOR**-tih-sohn	S/ R/CF R/	**-one** *hormone* **hydr/o-** *water* **-cortis-** *from the cortex*	Potent glucocorticoid with antiinflammatory properties
prolactin	pro-**LAK**-tin	S/ P/ R/	**-in** *substance* **pro-** *before* **-lact-** *milk*	Pituitary hormone that stimulates the production of milk
somatotrophin (also called **growth hormone, GH**)	**SO**-mah-toh-**TROH**-fin	S/ R/CF	**-trophin** *stimulation* **somat/o-** *the body*	Hormone of the anterior pituitary that stimulates the growth of body tissues
thyrotropin	thigh-roe-**TROH**-pin	S/ R/CF	**-tropin** *stimulation* **thyr/o-** *thyroid*	Hormone from the anterior pituitary gland that stimulates function of the thyroid gland

EXERCISES

A. Identify *the meaning of the word element. Select the correct answer.* **LO 12.1 and 12.4**

1. The meaning of the suffix in the term cortisone:

a. before **b.** hormone **c.** seed **d.** cortex **e.** inflammation

2. The meaning of the suffix in the term gonadotropin:

a. thyroid **b.** hormone **c.** testis **d.** substance **e.** stimulation

3. The meaning of the combining form in the term somatotrophin:

a. body **b.** stimulation **c.** water **d.** growth **e.** hormone

B. Abbreviations *will be your answers in this matching exercise. Match the correct abbreviation to its description.* **LO 12.3 and 12.4**

_____ **1.** stimulates ovulation — **A.** LH

_____ **2.** stimulates production of corticosteroids — **B.** ADH

_____ **3.** stimulates uterine contractions — **C.** ACTH

_____ **4.** stimulates ovaries to develop eggs — **D.** TSH

_____ **5.** reduces volume of urine — **E.** OT

_____ **6.** stimulates production of thyroxin — **F.** FSH

Lesson 12.1 (cont'd) Pituitary Diagnostic Procedures (LO 12.8)

Visual field tests can show the presence of a **pituitary tumor** as the tumor presses on the **optic chiasma** causing loss of vision in the peripheral visual fields.

Levels of pituitary hormones in the blood and/or urine can be measured directly to show the presence of a hormone-producing pituitary **adenoma**.

Examples are the levels of **growth hormone** and **insulinlike growth factor-1** (IGF-1). When growth hormone levels are high, they cause the liver to produce more IGF-1. When both levels are very high, a pituitary tumor is the diagnosis. If the levels are only slightly increased, a **glucose suppression test** is performed. Ingestion of a large amount of sugar normally leads to a drop in growth hormone levels. If growth hormones remain high, a pituitary adenoma is the cause. High levels of growth hormone are found in gigantism, beginning in children, and acromegaly, beginning in adults.

Blood **prolactin** levels can be measured to check for a prolactinoma; **ACTH (corticotropin)** levels help distinguish ACTH-secreting pituitary tumors from adrenal gland tumors: **TSH (thyrotropin)** levels usually identify thyrotropin-secreting adenomas.

Diabetes insipidus, caused by failure in production of **ADH (antidiuretic hormone)** by the hypothalamus or by failure of the posterior pituitary to release it due to an adenoma, is diagnosed primarily by measurement of the amount of urine and its **osmolality**.

Magnetic resonance imaging (MRI) can show pituitary tumors greater than 3 mm across.

Biopsy of the tumor is sometimes needed to make a firm diagnosis. When pituitary tumors are removed surgically, they are always examined under a microscope to confirm the exact diagnosis.

Abbreviations

ACTH	adrenocorticotropic hormone, corticotropin
ADH	antidiuretic hormone
IGF-1	insulinlike growth factor-1
MRI	magnetic resonance imaging
TSH	thyroid-stimulating hormone, thyrotropin

Keynote

Pituitary tumors present with symptoms that lead to a complete medical history and physical examination, blood and urine tests, and X-rays.

Word Analysis and Definition

S = Suffix P = Prefix R = Root R/CF = Combining Form

WORD	PRONUNCIATION		ELEMENTS	DEFINITION
adenoma	**AD**-eh-**NOH**-mah	S/ R/	**-oma** *tumor* **aden-** *gland*	A benign neoplasm of epithelial tissue
biopsy (***Note:*** the extra "o" is dropped)	**BIE**-op-see	S/ R/	**-opsy** *to view* **bio-** *life*	Process of removing tissue from living patients for microscopic examination
chiasm **chiasma (alt)**	**KIE**-asm kie-**AZ**-mah		Greek *cross*	X-shaped crossing of the two optic nerves at the base of the brain
optic	**OP**-tik	S/ R/	**-ic** *pertaining to* **opt-** *vision*	Pertaining to the eye
osmolality	**OZ**-moh-**LAL**-ih-tee	S/ S/ R/	**-ity** *state* **-al-** *pertaining to* **osmol-** *concentration*	The concentration of a solution
tumor	**TOO**-mer		Latin *swelling*	Any abnormal swelling

Exercises

A. Given *the description, insert the abbreviation for the hormone. Fill in the blanks.* **LO 12.2 and 12.8**

1. Lack of this hormone would increase urine production. ____________________

2. This hormone will be increased with thyrotropin-secreting adenomas. ____________________

3. Helps distinguish corticotropin pituitary tumors from adrenal gland tumors. ____________________

B. Define the word elements to quickly decipher the meaning of the medical term. *Knowing the meaning of the word elements makes short work of defining medical terms. Identify the meaning of the element in the first column with its correct meaning in the second column. Fill in the blanks.* **LO 12.1 and 12.8**

_____ **1.** *osmol-* **a.** tumor

_____ **2.** *-oma* **b.** gland

_____ **3.** *bio-* **c.** to view

_____ **4.** *-opsy* **d.** concentration

_____ **5.** *aden-* **e.** life

Lesson 12.1 (cont'd) Pituitary Therapeutic Procedures (LO 12.8)

Surgical removal of a pituitary tumor is necessary if the tumor is pressing on the optic nerves or if it is overproducing hormones. In 99% of cases, this is performed by an **endoscopic transnasal transsphenoidal approach** in which the surgery is performed through the nose and sphenoid sinus using an **endoscope**. **Craniotomy**, in which a very large tumor is removed through the upper part of the skull, is occasionally necessary. The surgery can be made more efficient by using **image-guided stereotactic surgery** in which advanced computers create a three-dimensional image of the tumor to guide the surgeon.

Radiation therapy can be used alone, after surgery, or if the tumor persists or returns after surgery. Methods of radiation therapy include:

- **Gamma knife stereotactic radiosurgery**, which delivers a single high-dose radiation beam the size and shape of the tumor using special brain-imaging techniques.
- **Proton beam therapy**, which delivers positively charged ions (protons) rather than X-rays in beams that are finely controlled with minimal risk to surrounding healthy tissues.
- **External beam radiation**, which delivers X-rays in small increments, usually five times a week over a four- to six-week period. It may damage surrounding healthy pituitary and brain tissues.

Pituitary Medications and Hormone Replacement Therapy (LO 12.8)

Medications can help to block excessive hormone secretion and sometimes reduce pituitary tumor size:

- **Growth hormone-secreting tumors** have two types of drugs used if surgery has been unsuccessful in normalizing growth hormone production. **Somatostatin analogs** *(Sandostatin, Somatuline Depot)* cause a decrease in growth hormone production and are given by injection every four weeks. The second type, **pegvisomant** *(Somavert),* blocks the effect of excess growth hormone, is given by daily injection, and may cause liver damage.
- **Prolactin-secreting tumors (prolactinomas)** are treated with two drugs, **cabergoline** *(Dostinex)* and **bromocriptine** *(Parlodel),* that decrease prolactin secretion, but they can have serious side effects, including developing compulsive behaviors.

Pituitary hormone replacement therapy is needed after surgery or radiation therapy to maintain normal hormone levels. The medication taken depends on the hormones that need to be replaced, which include adrenocorticotropic hormone (ACTH), thyroxine, estrogen and progesterone, testosterone, antidiuretic hormone (ADH), and synthetic growth hormones.

Word Analysis and Definition

S = Suffix P = Prefix R = Root R/CF = Combining Form

WORD	PRONUNCIATION		ELEMENTS	DEFINITION
analog	**AN**-ah-log		Greek *proportionate*	A compound that resembles another in structure but not in function; analog is a means of the transmission of continuous information to our senses, in contrast with the digital transmission of only zeros and ones.
craniotomy	kray-nee-**OT**-oh-mee	S/ R/	-tomy *incision* crani/o *cranium*	Incision of the skull
endoscope	**EN**-doh-skope	P/ R/	endo- *inside* -scope *instrument for viewing*	Instrument for viewing the inside of a tubular or hollow organ
endoscopic	**EN**-doh-**SKOP**-ik	S/	-ic *pertaining to*	Pertaining to an endoscope.
gamma knife	**GAM**-ah NIFE		**gamma** *third letter in Greek alphabet* **knife** Old English *knife*	A minimally invasive radiosurgical system
proton	**PROH**-ton		Greek *first*	The positively charged unit of the nuclear mass
stereotactic	**STER**-ee-oh-**TAK**-tik	S/ R/CF R/	-ic *pertaining to* stere/o *three- dimensional* -tact- *orderly arrangement*	Pertaining to a precise three-dimensional method to locate a lesion or a tumor
transnasal	trans-**NAY**-zal	S/ P/ R/	-al *pertaining to* trans- *across, through* -nas- *nose*	Through the nose
transsphenoid	trans-**SFEE**-noyd	S/ P/ R/CF	-oid *resembling* trans- *through* sphen/o *wedge*	Through the sphenoid sinus

Exercises

A. Explain *the therapeutic procedures for disorders of the pituitary gland. Select the correct answer to complete the sentence or answer the question.* **LO 12.8**

1. Treatment of pituitary tumors is aimed at:

   a. shrinking or removing the tumor

   c. increasing pituitary hormone levels

   b. homone replacement therapy

   d. suppressing adrenal gland secretion

2. Large pituitary tumors may require a:

   a. Oral corticosteroids **b.** craniotomy **c.** lithotripsy **d.** lobectomy

3. After treatment of pituitary tumors, what type of therapy is often begun to maintain normal hormone levels?

   a. physical **b.** occupational **c.** radiation **d.** hormone-replacement

B. Identify *the word elements of medical terms will help you understand the purpose of the procedure. Choose the correct answer.* **LO 12.1 and 12.8**

1. The suffix of the term **endoscopic** means

   a. process of viewing **b.** use of a microscope **c.** across **d.** pertaining to

2. The suffix in the term **transsphenoid** means:

   a. pertaining to **b.** bony projection **c.** resembling **d.** across **e.** butterfly

3. The suffix in the term **craniotomy** means:

   a. incision into **b.** removal of **c.** skull **d.** treatment of **e.** covering

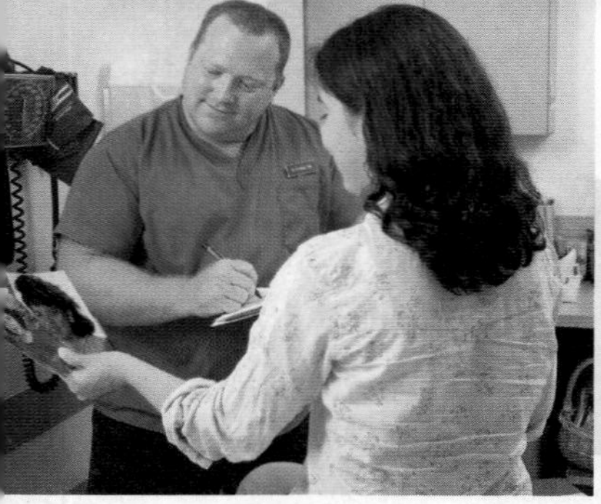

Rick Brady/McGraw-Hill Education

Lesson 12.2

Thyroid, Parathyroid, and Thymus Glands

Objectives

In order to understand what is happening to Ms. Norma Leary in the Case Report, to be able to help her, and to communicate about her situation with her parents and her physician, it's necessary to learn the correct medical terminology provided in this lesson to:

12.2.1 Describe the location and anatomy of the thyroid gland.

12.2.2 Explain how the three thyroid hormones are produced and secreted.

12.2.3 Specify the functions of the thyroid hormones.

12.2.4 Discuss common disorders of the thyroid gland.

12.2.5 Locate the positions of the parathyroid and thymus glands.

12.2.6 Name the hormones produced by the parathyroid and thymus glands and state their functions.

CASE REPORT 12.2

You are . . .

. . . an EMT working in the Emergency Department at Fulwood Medical Center at 0200 hours in the morning.

You are communicating with . . .

. . . the parents of Ms. Norma Leary, a 22-year-old college student who is living with her parents for the summer. Ms. Leary is **emaciated,** extremely agitated, and at times disoriented and confused. Her parents tell you that in the past 3 or 4 days she has been coughing and not feeling well. In the past 12 hours, she has become feverish and been complaining of a left-sided chest pain. Upon questioning, the parents reveal that prior to this acute illness, Ms. Leary had lost about 20 pounds in weight, although she was eating voraciously. Her **VS** are T 105.2, P 180 and irregular, R 24, BP 160/85.

You call for Dr. Hilinski, an emergency physician, STAT. On his initial examination, he believes that the patient is in thyroid storm, which is a medical emergency. There are no immediate laboratory tests that can confirm this diagnosis.

Thyroid Gland (LO 12.5)

Shaped like a bow tie and measuring about 2 inches wide, the **thyroid** gland lies just beneath the skin of the neck and below the thyroid cartilage ("Adam's apple"). Two lobes extend up on either side of the trachea (or windpipe) and are joined by an isthmus *(Figure 12.4).*

Cells in the thyroid gland secrete the two thyroid hormones **T3** and **T4.** The latter is known as **thyroxine.** The term **thyroid hormone** refers to T3 and T4 collectively, and it performs the following functions:

- **Stimulates** almost every tissue in the body to produce proteins;
- **Increases** the amount of oxygen that cells use; and
- **Controls** the speed of the body's chemical functions, known as the **metabolic rate.**

The thyroid also produces the hormone **calcitonin,** which promotes calcium deposition and bone formation.

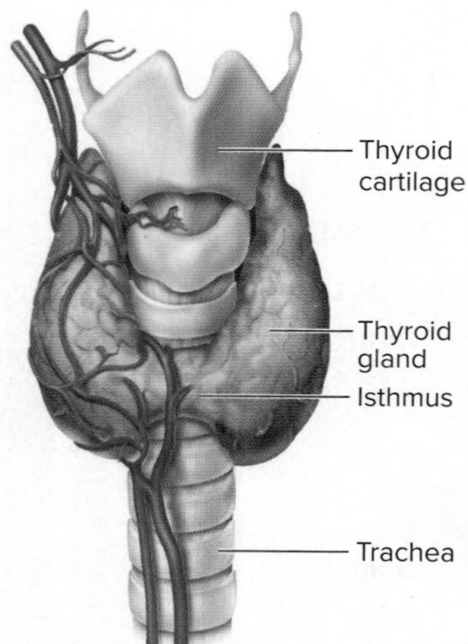

▲ **FIGURE 12.4** Anatomy of the Thyroid Gland.

Abbreviations

PTH	parathyroid hormone
T3	triiodothyronine
T4	tetraiodothyronine (thyroxine)
VS	vital signs: measurement of temperature (T), pulse (P), respiration (R), and blood pressure (BP)

Parathyroid Glands (LO 12.5)

Most people have four **parathyroid** glands, and these are partially embedded in the posterior surface of the thyroid gland. The parathyroid glands secrete **parathyroid hormone (PTH).** PTH stimulates bone resorption to bring calcium back into the blood, and calcitonin takes calcium from the blood to stimulate bone deposition *(see Chapter 4).*

Thymus Gland (LO 12.5)

The **thymus** gland is located in the mediastinum *(Figure 12.5).* This gland is large in children and over time, it decreases in size until it is mostly fibrous tissue in the elderly. It secretes a group of hormones that stimulate the production of T lymphocytes (see *Chapter 7*).

▶ **FIGURE 12.5** Position of the Thymus Gland.

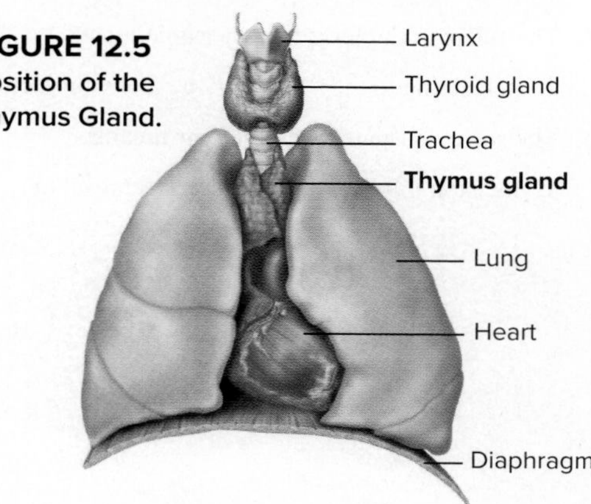

Word Analysis and Definition

S = Suffix P = Prefix R = Root R/CF = Combining Form

WORD	PRONUNCIATION		ELEMENTS	DEFINITION
calcitonin	kal-sih-**TONE**-in	S/ R/CF R/	-in *substance* calc/i- *calcium* -ton- *tension, pressure*	Hormone produced by the thyroid gland that moves calcium from blood to bones
emaciation **emaciated (adj)**	ee-may-see-**AY**-shun ee-may-see-**AY**-ted	S/ R/CF S/	-ation *process* emac/i- *make thin* -ated *pertaining to a condition*	Abnormal thinness Pertaining to or suffering from emaciation
parathyroid	par-ah-**THIGH**-royd	S/ P/ R/	-oid *resembling* para- *adjacent, beside* -thyr- *thyroid*	Endocrine glands embedded in the back of the thyroid gland
thymus	**THIGH**-mus		Greek *sweetbread*	Endocrine gland located in the mediastinum
thyroid	**THIGH**-royd		Greek *an oblong shield*	Endocrine gland in the neck; or a cartilage of the larynx
thyroxine	thigh-**ROCK**-sin	S/ R/ R/	-ine *pertaining to* thyr- *thyroid gland* -ox- *oxygen*	Thyroid hormone T4, tetraiodothyronine

EXERCISES

A. Review *Case Report 12.2, then select the correct answer that answers each question or completes the statement.* **LO 12.5 and 12.9**

1. What does the term **emaciated** mean?

a. exhausted **b.** anxious **c.** irritated **d.** thin

2. After reviewing her vital signs, what term describes Ms. Leary's heart rate?

a. hypotensive **b.** febrile **c.** tachycardic **d.** bradypneic

3. Ms. Leary's signs and symptoms are due to:

a. decreased thyroid hormones **b.** increased thyroid hormones **c.** dehydration **d.** overhydration

4. The thyroid storm:

a. came about suddenly

b. has been occurring for a long period of time

c. is diagnosed with a measure of serum electrolytes

d. requires an MRI to confirm Dr. Hilinski's diagnosis

B. Construct *terms related to anatomy and function of the thyroid gland, parathyroid glands, and the thymus gland. Fill in the blanks.* **LO 12.1 and 12.5**

1. Thyroid hormone T4: ______________________/______________________/ine

2. Abnormal thinness: ______________________/______________________

3. Endocrine glands embedded in the back of the thyroid: ______________________/______________________/**oid**

4. Hormone that moves calcium from the blood into the bone: ______________________/______________________/______________________

Lesson 12.2 (cont'd) Disorders of the Thyroid and Parathyroid Glands

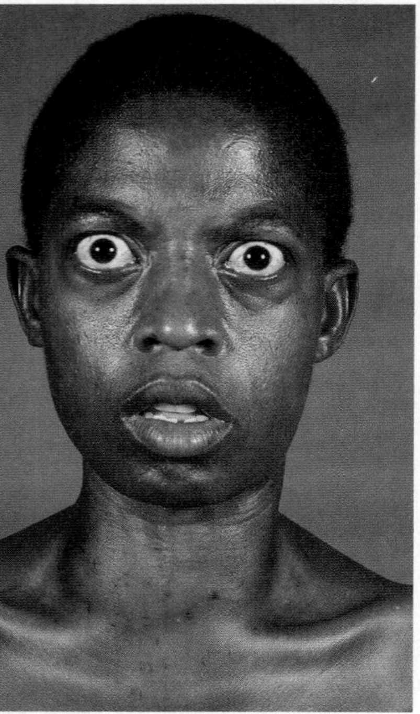

▲ **FIGURE 12.6**
Hyperthyroidism May Cause the Eyes to Protrude (Exophthalmos).
Dr. M.A. Ansary/Science Source

Hyperthyroidism (Thyrotoxicosis) (LO 12.5)

The symptoms of **hyperthyroidism** (excessive thyroid hormone production) are those of an increased body metabolism. These include tachycardia (rapid heart rate), hypertension, sweating, shakiness, anxiety, weight loss despite increased appetite, and diarrhea.

Graves disease is an autoimmune disorder *(see Chapter 7)* in which an antibody stimulates the thyroid to produce and secrete excessive amounts of thyroid hormone into the blood. It presents with **exophthalmos** (bulging of the eyes) *(Figure 12.6),* a **goiter** (an enlarged thyroid gland) *(Figure 12.7),* and a non-pitting, waxy edema of the lower leg.

Hypothyroidism (LO 12.2 and 12.5)

Hypothyroidism is the opposite of hyperthyroidism and results from an inadequate production of thyroid hormone. This decreases the body's metabolism. Primary hypothyroidism affects 10% of older women. Symptoms develop gradually and include hair loss; dry, scaly skin; a puffy face and eyes; slow, hoarse speech; weight gain; constipation; and a high sensitivity to cold temperatures. No specific cause has been found.

Severe hypothyroidism is called **myxedema.** In developing countries, a common cause of this is a lack of **iodine** in the diet. In the United States, iodine is added to table salt to prevent hypothyroidism. Iodine is also found in dairy products and seafood.

Thyroiditis is an inflammation of the thyroid gland. It presents most commonly as **Hashimoto thyroiditis,** an autoimmune disease with lymphocytic infiltration of the gland. Hypothyroidism results, necessitating lifelong thyroid hormone replacement therapy.

Cretinism *(Figure 12.8)* is a congenital form of thyroid deficiency that severely retards mental and physical growth. If diagnosed and treated early with thyroid hormones, the patient can achieve significant improvement.

Thyroid cancer usually presents as a symptomless nodule in the thyroid gland. It can metastasize (spread) to cervical and mediastinal lymph nodes, and to the liver, lungs, and bones. A total **thyroidectomy** with local lymph node dissection is the first step in treating thyroid cancer.

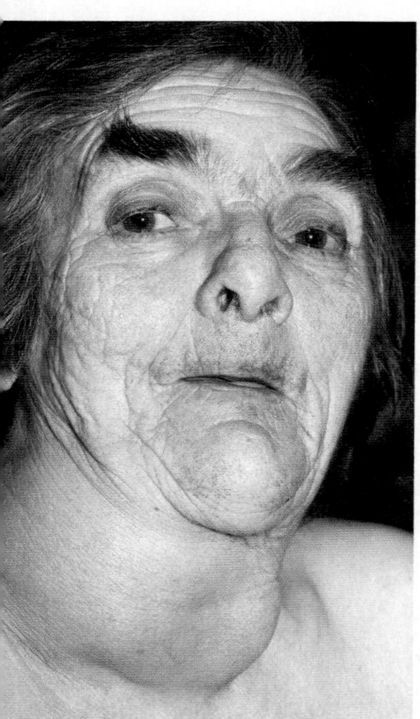

▲ **FIGURE 12.7**
Elderly Woman with Hypothyroidism and Goiter.
Dr P. Marazzi/Science Source

Case Report 12.2 *(continued)*

Thyroid storm is the condition Ms. Norma Leary presented with in the Emergency Department. It is the most extreme state of **hyperthyroidism,** with severely exaggerated effects of the thyroid hormones causing **hyperpyrexia, tachycardia,** agitation, and delirium. The weight loss prior to her illness becoming acute was part of her undiagnosed hyperthyroidism.

Disorders of the Parathyroid Glands (LO 12.5)

Hypoparathyroidism is a deficiency of parathyroid hormone (PTH) that lowers levels of blood calcium. Most symptoms of this are neuromuscular (in nerve and muscle tissue), ranging from tingling in the fingers, to muscle cramps, to the painful muscle spasms of **tetany** (not **tetanus,** which is caused by a toxin acting on the central nervous system).

Hyperparathyroidism is an excess of PTH and is more common than hypoparathyroidism. It is usually caused by one of the four glands enlarging and working out of pituitary control. It leads to calcium depletion in bones (making bones brittle), high blood calcium levels, and kidney stones.

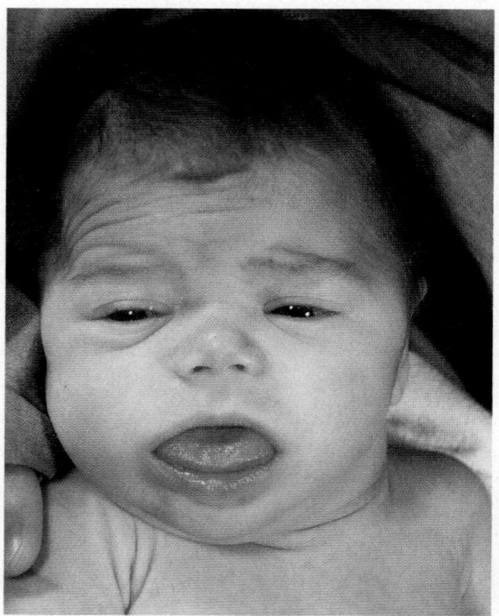

▶ **FIGURE 12.8**
Infant with Cretinism.
Mediscan/Alamy Stock Photo

Word Analysis and Definition

S = Suffix P = Prefix R = Root R/CF = Combining Form

WORD	PRONUNCIATION	ELEMENTS		DEFINITION
cretin cretinism	**KREH**-tin **KREH**-tin-izm	 S/ R/	French *cretin* **-ism** *condition, process* **cretin-** *cretin*	Severe congenital hypothyroidism Condition of severe congenital hypothyroidism
exophthalmos	ek-sof-**THAL**-mos	P/ R/	**ex-** *out* **-ophthalmos** *eye*	Protrusion of the eyeball
goiter	**GOY**-ter		Latin *throat*	Benign enlargement of the thyroid gland
Graves disease	**GRAVZ** diz-**EEZ**		Robert Graves, Irish physician, 1796–1853	Hyperthyroidism with toxic goiter
Hashimoto disease	hah-shee-**MOH**-toe diz-**EEZ**		Hakaru Hashimoto, Japanese surgeon, 1881–1934	Autoimmune disease of the thyroid gland
hyperparathyroidism (**Note:** *Two suffixes and two prefixes*) **hypoparathyroidism**	**HIGH**-per-par-ah-**THIGH**-royd-izm **HIGH**-poh-par-ah-**THIGH**-royd-izm	S/ S/ P/ P/ R/ P/	**-ism** *condition* **-oid-** *resembling* **hyper-** *excessive* **-para-** *adjacent* **-thyr-** *thyroid* **hypo-** *deficient, below*	Excessive levels of parathyroid hormone Deficient levels of parathyroid hormone
hyperpyrexia	**HIGH**-per-pie-**REK**-see-ah	S/ P/ R/	**-ia** *condition* **hyper-** *excessive* **-pyrex-** *fever*	Extremely high body temperature or fever
hyperthyroidism (**Note:** *Two suffixes*) (*Also called* thyrotoxicosis.) **hypothyroidism** (**Note:** *Two suffixes*)	high-per-**THIGH**-royd-izm high-poh-**THIGH**-royd-izm	S/ S/ P/ R/ S/ S/ P/ R/	**-ism** *condition* **-oid-** *resembling* **hyper-** *excessive* **-thyr-** *thyroid* **-ism** *condition* **-oid-** *resembling* **hypo-** *deficient, below* **-thyr-** *thyroid*	Excessive production of thyroid hormones Deficient production of thyroid hormones
iodine	**EYE**-oh-dine *or* **EYE**-oh-deen	S/ R/	**-ine** *pertaining to* **iod-** *violet*	Chemical element, the lack of which causes thyroid disease
myxedema	miks-eh-**DEE**-muh	P/ R/	**myx-** *mucus* **-edema** *swelling*	Nonpitting, waxy edema of the skin in hypothyroidism
tetany	**TET**-ah-nee		Greek *convulsive tension*	Severe muscle twitches, cramps, and spasms
thyroidectomy **thyroiditis**	thigh-roy-**DEK**-toe-me thigh-roy-**DIE**-tis	S/ S/ R/ S/	**-ectomy** *surgical excision* **-oid-** *resembling* **thyr-** *thyroid* **-itis** *inflammation*	Surgical removal of the thyroid gland Inflammation of the thyroid gland
thyrotoxicosis (*also called* **hyperthyroidism**)	**THIGH**-roe-toks-ih-**KOH**-sis	S/ R/CF R/CF	**-sis** *condition* **thyr/o-** *thyroid* **-toxic/o-** *poison*	Disorder produced by excessive thyroid hormone production

EXERCISE

A. Elements: One word or phrase in each of the descriptions in the following questions is in bold. *This is your clue to finding the correct medical term in the word bank. Fill in the blanks with the language of endocrinology. Not all terms will be used.* **LO 12.2 and 12.5**

thyroiditis **tetany** **hyperparathyroidism** **hypoparathyroidism** **thyrotoxicosis** **hyperthyroidism** **myxedema** **thyroidectomy**

1. **Excessive production** of thyroid hormones: ____________________
2. **Swelling** with a waxy substance: ____________________
3. **Deficient** of production of parathyroid hormone: ____________________
4. **Inflammation** of the thyroid gland: ____________________
5. **Removal** of the thyroid gland: ____________________

Lesson 12.2 (cont'd) Diagnostic Procedures for Disorders of the Thyroid Gland (LO 12.5 and 12.8)

Thyroid-stimulating hormone (TSH) levels in the blood are low if the gland is overactive.

Thyroid hormone levels in the blood detail the activity of the gland; the levels are high if the gland is overactive.

Antithyroid antibodies are associated with autoimmune inflammatory diseases of the thyroid.

Isotopic thyroid scans detail the nature of the thyroid enlargement and the function of the gland.

Serum calcitonin level is elevated in medullary carcinoma.

Fine needle aspiration biopsy distinguishes benign from malignant nodules.

Ultrasonography reveals the size of the gland and the presence of nodules.

Therapeutic Procedures for Disorders of the Thyroid Gland (LO 12.5 and 12.8)

Radioactive iodine (I-131) therapy uses the **isotope** of iodine that emits radiation to treat hyperthyroidism and thyroid cancer. When a small dose of the isotope is swallowed, it is absorbed into the bloodstream, taken up from the blood, and concentrated by the cells of the thyroid gland, where it begins destroying the gland's cells.

Hypothyroidism, in most cases, can be treated adequately with a constant daily dose of **levothyroxine (LT4)**. For hypothyroidism due to destruction of thyroid cells, **TSH** levels are monitored. For central (pituitary or hypothalamic) hypothyroidism, $\mathbf{T_4}$ levels are used for monitoring.

Thyroid surgery is indicated for a variety of conditions including **cancerous** and **benign nodules**, **goiters**, and **overactive thyroid glands**. The types of surgery that can be performed include:

- **Excisional biopsy**: removal of a small part of the gland.
- **Lobectomy**: removal of half of the thyroid gland **(hemilobectomy).**
- **Total thyroidectomy**: removal of all thyroid tissue.
- **Near-total thyroidectomy**: removal of all but a very small part of the gland.
- **Endoscopic thyroidectomy**: performed through a single small incision using a flexible lighted tube and video monitor to guide the surgical procedure.
- **Laser ablation**: a minimally invasive procedure used to remove benign thyroid nodules using ultrasound guidance without affecting the surrounding organ.

Thyroid Pharmacology (LO 12.5 and 12.8)

Antithyroid medications prevent formation of thyroid hormones in the gland's cells.

Propylthiouracil and **methimazole** both decrease the amount of thyroid hormone produced by the gland's cells and can be used to treat hyperthyroidism. Unfortunately, they both have the major and frequent side effects of agranulocytosis and aplastic anemia, and are no longer recognized as a front-line medication.

Thyroid replacements are:

- L-thyroxine. This synthetic T_4 is a preferred replacement.
- Liothyronine sodium. This synthetic T_3 has a rapid turnover and has to be monitored frequently.

Word Analysis and Definition

S = Suffix P = Prefix R = Root R/CF = Combining Form

WORD	PRONUNCIATION	ELEMENTS		DEFINITION
ablation	ab-**LAY**-shun	S/ R/	-ion *process* ablat- *take away*	Removal of tissue to destroy its function
aspiration	**AS**-pih-**RAY**-shun	S/ R/	-ion *process* aspirat- *breathe in*	Removal by suction of fluid or gas from a body cavity
isotope **isotopic (adj)**	**EYE**-so-tope	P/ R/ S/ R/	iso- *equal* -tope *part* -ic *pertaining to* -top- *part*	Radioactive element; some of these elements are used in diagnostic procedures Of identical chemical composition
lobectomy	loh-**BEK**-toh-mee	S/ R/	-ectomy *surgical excision* lob- *lobe*	Surgical removal of a lobe of the lungs or the thyroid gland
lymphadenectomy	lim-**FAD**-eh- **NEK**-toh-mee	S/ R/	-ectomy *surgical excision* lymphaden- *lymph node*	Surgical excision of a lymph node
radioactive iodine	**RAY**-dee-oh-**AK**-tiv **EYE**-oh-dine	S/ R/CF R/	-ive *pertaining to* radi/o- *radiation* -act- *performance* iodine *nonmetallic element*	Any of the various tracers that emit alpha, beta, or gamma rays
ultrasonography	**UL**-trah-soh- **NOG**-rah-fee	S/ P/ R/CF	-graphy *recording* ultra- *beyond* son/o- *sound*	Delineation of deep structures using sound waves

EXERCISE

A. Certain kinds of tests are performed for the purpose of arriving at the correct diagnosis for treatment. *Select the correct diagnostic test for each described condition.* **LO 12.5 and 12.8**

1. Is associated with autoimmune inflammatory disease of the thyroid:

a. serum calcitonin levels
b. thyroid-stimulating hormone levels
c. antithyroid antibodies hormone levels
d. fine needle aspiration biopsy

2. Blood test to measure activity of the thyroid gland:

a. serum calcitonin levels
b. thyroid hormone levels
c. antithyroid hormone levels
d. fine needle aspiration biopsy

3. Level becomes elevated in medullary carcinoma:

a. serum calcitonin levels
b. thyroid-stimulating hormone levels
c. antithyroid hormone levels
d. fine needle aspiration biopsy

4. Reveals the size of the gland and the presence of nodules:

a. radioactive iodine therapy
b. fine needle aspiration biopsy
c. ultrasonography
d. serum calcitonin levels

5. Distinguishes benign from malignant nodules:

a. radioactive iodine therapy
b. fine needle aspiration biopsy
c. ultrasonography
d. isotopic thyroid scans

6. Details the nature of the thyroid enlargement and the function of the gland:

a. isotopic thyroid scans
b. fine needle aspiration biopsy
c. ultrasonography
d. serum calcitonin levels

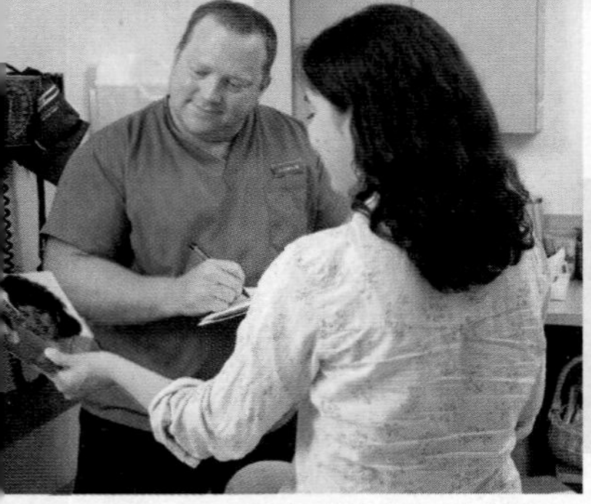

Rick Brady/McGraw-Hill Education

Lesson 12.3

Adrenal Glands and Hormones

Objectives

Your adrenal glands produce several key hormones that help to maintain homeostasis. The information in this lesson will enable you to use correct medical terminology to:

12.3.1 Locate the adrenal glands.

12.3.2 Differentiate between the adrenal cortex and the medulla.

12.3.3 Identify the functions of the hormones produced by the cortex and medulla.

12.3.4 Detail how the body adapts to stress.

12.3.5 Explain common disorders of the adrenal glands.

Adrenal Glands (LO 12.6)

An **adrenal (suprarenal)** gland is anchored like a cap on the upper pole of each kidney *(Figure 12.10 inset)*. The outer layer of the gland—the adrenal cortex *(Figure 12.10)*—synthesizes more than 25 **steroid** hormones known collectively as **adrenocortical** hormones, or corticosteroids. These hormones include:

1. **Glucocorticoids,** mainly **hydrocortisone (cortisol),** which help regulate blood glucose levels, particularly in response to stress. They also have an anti-inflammatory effect, and are often found in dermatologic lotions and ointments;
2. **Mineralocorticoids,** mostly **aldosterone,** which promote sodium retention and potassium excretion by the kidneys; and
3. **Sex steroids,** which include a weak androgen that is converted to testosterone *(see Chapter 14)* and estrogen *(see Chapter 15)*.

The inner layer of the adrenal gland, the adrenal medulla *(Figure 12.10)*, also secretes hormones. These hormones are called **catecholamines,** and principally include **epinephrine (adrenaline)** and **norepinephrine (noradrenaline).** These hormones prepare the body for physical activity and are responsible for the "flight or fight" response.

CASE REPORT 12.3

John Fitzgerald Kennedy (JFK) (1917–1963) was elected president of the United States of America in 1960 at the age of 43 *(Figure 12.9)*. He had health problems from the age of 13, when he was first diagnosed as having **colitis**. At age 27, he had lower back pain that necessitated lower back surgery. He was then diagnosed as having adrenal gland insufficiency (**Addison disease**) with osteoporosis of his lumbar spine. This required lower back surgery on three more occasions. JFK received adrenal hormone replacement therapy for the rest of his life, together with pain medication for his lower back pain, until his assassination in Dallas, Texas, in 1963. In medical retrospect, instead of colitis, JFK probably had **celiac** disease *(see Chapter 9)*, which has strong associations with Addison disease.

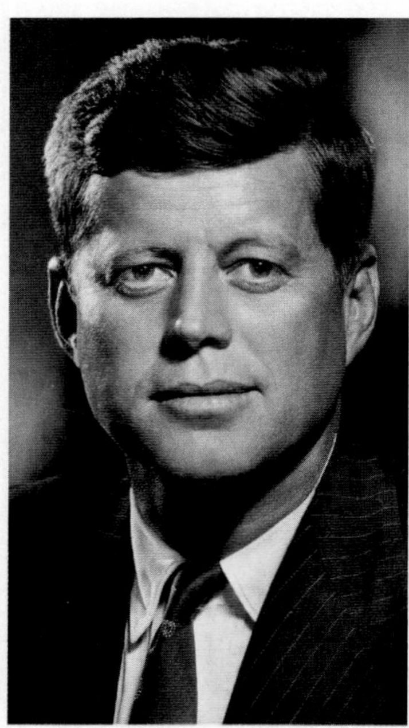

▲ **FIGURE 12.9**
John F. Kennedy.

Bettmann/Getty Images

Disorders of the Adrenal Glands (LO 12.6)

Adrenocortical hypofunction, most commonly seen as **Addison disease,** is caused by the **idiopathic** atrophy (wasting away) of the adrenal cortex. Symptoms are weakness, fatigue, increased susceptibility to infection, and diminished resistance to stress. This disorder is treated with hormone replacement therapy, which John F. Kennedy received until he died.

Adrenocortical hyperfunction most commonly appears as **Cushing syndrome.** Excess production of the steroid hormones produces "moon" **facies** (facial features and expressions), muscle wasting and weakness, kidney stones, and reduced resistance to infection. Most cases are due to a pituitary tumor secreting too much ACTH, causing the adrenal glands to produce an excess of steroids. Sometimes, Cushing syndrome can be produced by the administration of excess steroid medications.

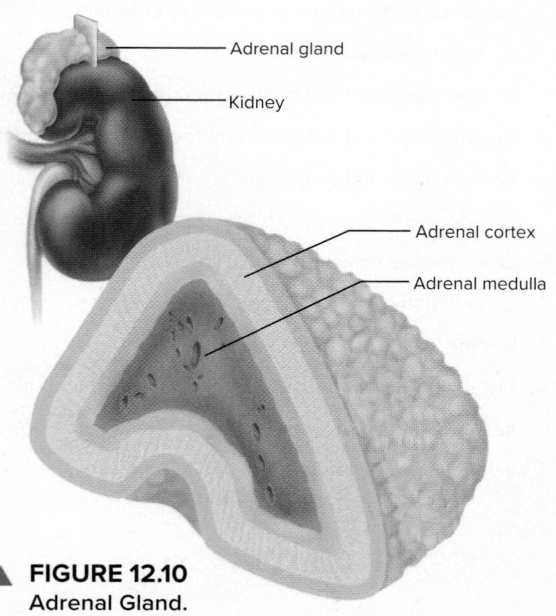

▲ **FIGURE 12.10**
Adrenal Gland.

Word Analysis and Definition

S = Suffix P = Prefix R = Root R/CF = Combining Form

WORD	PRONUNCIATION		ELEMENTS	DEFINITION
Addison disease	**ADD**-ih-son diz-**EEZ**		Thomas Addison, English physician, 1793–1860	An autoimmune disease leading to decreased production of adrenocortical steroids
adrenal (*same as* **suprarenal**)	ah-**DREE**-nal	S/ P/ R/ P/	-al *pertaining to* **ad-** *to, toward* **-ren-** *kidney* **supra-** *above*	Endocrine gland on the upper pole of each kidney
adrenaline (*also called* **epinephrine**)	ah-**DREN**-ah-lin ep-ih-**NEF**-rin	S/ P/ R/	-ine *pertaining to* **epi-** *above* **-nephr-** *kidney*	Main catecholamine produced by the adrenal medulla
adrenocortical	ah-dree-noh-**KOR**-tih-kal	S/ R/CF R/	-al *pertaining to* **adren/o-** *adrenal* **-cortic-** *cortex*	Pertaining to the cortex of the adrenal gland
aldosterone	al-**DOS**-ter-own	S/ R/CF R/	-one *hormone* **ald/o-** *organic compound* **-ster-** *steroid*	Mineralocorticoid hormone of the adrenal cortex
catecholamine	kat-eh-**COAL**-ah-meen	S/ R/	-amine *nitrogen-containing substance* **catechol-** *tyrosine containing*	Major elements produced by the adrenal cortex in the stress response; including epinephrine and norepinephrine
Cushing syndrome	**KUSH**-ing **SIN**-drohm		Harvey Cushing, U.S. neurosurgeon, 1869–1939	Hypersecretion of cortisol (hydrocortisone) by the adrenal gland
facies	**FASH**-eez		Latin *appearance*	Facial features and expressions
glucocorticoid	glu-co-**KOR**-tih-koyd	S/ R/ R/CF	-oid *resembling* **-cortic-** *cortisone* **gluc/o-** *glucose*	Hormone of the adrenal cortex that helps regulate glucose metabolism
hydrocortisone (*also called* **cortisol**)	high-droh-**KOR**-tih-sohn	S/ R/CF R/	-one *hormone* **hydr/o-** *water* **-cortis-** *cortisone*	Potent glucocorticoid with anti-inflammatory properties
idiopathic	id-ih-oh-**PATH**-ik	S/ R/CF R/	-ic *pertaining to* **idi/o-** *unknown* **-path-** *disease*	Pertaining to a disease of unknown etiology
mineralocorticoid	**MIN**-er-al-oh-**KOR**-tih-koyd	S/ R/CF R/	-oid *resemble* **mineral/o-** *inorganic material* **-cortic-** *cortex*	Hormone of the adrenal cortex that influences sodium and potassium metabolism
norepinephrine (**Note:** *Two prefixes: also called* **noradrenaline**)	**NOR**-ep-ih-**NEFF**-rin	S/ P/ P/ R/	-ine *pertaining to* **nor-** *normal* **-epi-** *above* **-nephr-** *kidney*	Catecholamine hormone of the adrenal gland that is a sympathetic neurotransmitter
steroid	**STER**-oyd	S/ R/	-oid *resembling* **ster-** *solid*	Large family of chemical substances found in many drugs, hormones, and body components

EXERCISE

A. Review *Case Report 12.3 before answering the questions. Correctly answer each question. Fill in the blanks.* **LO 12.2, 12.6, 12.8, and 12.9**

1. Did Kennedy's adrenal glands produce too much or too little hormone? ____________________
2. *Adrenal gland insufficiency* is also known as ____________________.
3. What lumbar spine problem did John F. Kennedy also have? ____________________
4. What was used to treat Kennedy's adrenal gland insufficiency? ____________________
5. What other disease has a *strong association* with Addison disease? ____________________

Lesson 12.3 (cont'd) Diagnostic Procedures for Disorders of the Adrenal Glands (LO 12.6 and 12.8)

Congenital adrenal hyperplasia can be diagnosed in the fetus using amniocentesis and chorionic villus sampling and in the newborn through a heel stick to obtain a blood sample. The test detects elevated levels of 17-hydroxyprogesterone (17-HP) and, as with all screening tests, a confirmatory test(s) has to be performed. Treatment can then be started in the womb or immediately after birth.

Cushing syndrome can be confirmed with three tests: elevated cortisol levels in saliva, elevated cortisol levels in 24-hour urine, and suppression of cortisol production by the synthetic steroid dexamethasone.

Addison disease can be diagnosed based on routine blood tests showing hypercalcemia, hypoglycemia, hyponatremia, and hyperkalemia; the diagnosis is confirmed by the ACTH stimulation test, in which the synthetic pituitary ACTH hormone **tetracosactide** fails to stimulate the production of cortisol.

Pheochromocytoma is diagnosed by measuring **catecholamines** and **metanephrines** in plasma or by 24-hour urinary collection. CT scan or MRI can localize the tumor.

Hyperaldosteronism (Conn syndrome) is diagnosed by high levels of aldosterone and low levels of potassium in blood or urine tests. CT scan or MRI can locate the tumor in the adrenal gland.

Therapeutic Procedures for Disorders of the Adrenal Glands (LO 12.6 and 12.8)

Congenital adrenal hyperplasia, when diagnosed in a female fetus, can require the pregnant mother to take a **corticosteroid** drug such as **dexamethasone** during pregnancy. This drug crosses the placenta to reduce the secretion of the fetal male hormones and allow the female genitals to develop normally. When diagnosed in childhood, dexamethasone or hydrocortisone are needed daily, and in some infant girls who have **ambiguous external genitalia**, reconstructive surgery to correct the appearance and function of the **genitals** is performed.

Addison disease requires lifelong replacement of the absent hormones by taking oral corticosteroids such as hydrocortisone and fludrocortisone.

Pheochromocytoma is treated with surgery to remove the adrenal tumor, usually by **laparoscopic** surgery.

Adrenal cortical carcinomas or benign adenomas are usually treated with surgery.

Adrenal Pharmacology (LO 12.6 and 12.8)

The **adrenal medulla** secretes **epinephrine (adrenaline)**. The **adrenal cortex** synthesizes **steroids** from cholesterol. The outer zona glomerulosa secretes **mineralocorticoids**, which regulate salt and water metabolism (aldosterone) by affecting excretory organs such as the kidney, colon, salivary glands, sweat glands, and brain. The middle zona fasciculata synthesizes **glucocorticoids**, which regulate normal metabolism and resistance to stress (cortisol) by affecting every organ in the body including the brain. The inner zona reticularis secretes adrenal **androgens** that control the development and activity of the male sex organs and male secondary sex characteristics. Androgens are the precursor of all **estrogens**. The primary androgen is testosterone, present in males and females.

Word Analysis and Definition

S = Suffix P = Prefix R = Root R/CF = Combining Form

WORD	PRONUNCIATION	ELEMENTS		DEFINITION
ambiguous	am-**BIG**-you-us		Latin *to wander*	Uncertain
androgen	**AN**-droh-jen	S/ R/CF	-gen *to produce* andr/o- *male*	Hormone that produces masculine characteristics
cortex	**KOR**-teks		Latin *outer covering*	Outer portion of an organ
genital	**JEN**-ih-tal	S/ R/	-al *pertaining to* genit- *primary male or female sex organs*	Relating to the primary male or female sex organs
hyperplasia	high-per-**PLAY**-zee-ah	S/ P/ R/	-ia *condition* hyper- *excessive* -plas- *formation*	Increase in the number of cells in a tissue or organ
medulla	meh-**DULL**-ah		Latin *marrow*	Central part of a structure surrounded by cortex
steroid	**STER**-oyd	S/ R/	-oid *resemble* ster- *solid*	Large family of chemical substances found in hormones, body components, and drugs

Exercises

A. Deconstruct medical terms into their component parts. *Using the terms related to the disorders of the adrenal glands, place the correct element on each blank.* **LO 12.1 and 12.6**

1. Increase in the number of cells in a tissue: ____________ / ____________ / ____________
2. Hormone that produces masculine characteristics: ____________ / ____________
3. Large family of chemical substances found in hormones: ____________ / ____________

B. Explain the therapeutic procedures for disorders of the adrenal glands. *Select the correct answer for each statement.* **LO 12.8**

1. Treatment for this condition requires lifelong hormone replacement with hydrocortisone:
   - **a.** pheochromocytoma
   - **b.** Addison disease
   - **c.** Cushing syndrome
   - **d.** adrenal cortex carcinoma
2. In this condition, it is the mother who takes medication to treat the fetal condition:
   - **a.** congenital adrenal hyperplasia
   - **b.** pheochromocytoma
   - **c.** Addison disease
   - **d.** Cushing syndrome
3. A condition that is often treated with laparoscopic surgery and removal of the adrenal tumor:
   - **a.** Cushing syndrome
   - **b.** Addison disease
   - **c.** pheochromocytoma
   - **d.** congenital adrenal hyperplasia

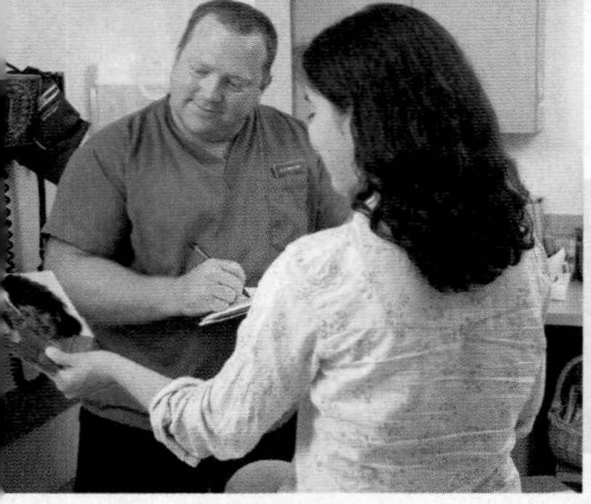
Rick Brady/McGraw-Hill Education

Lesson 12.4

The Pancreas

Objectives

The pancreas measures approximately 6 inches in length, rests across the back of the abdomen, and has many important functions, including the secretion of digestive juices and the production of hormones. The information provided in this lesson will enable the learner to use correct medical terminology to:

12.4.1 Distinguish between the different cells of the pancreas and their secretions.

12.4.2 Identify the functions of the hormones produced by the pancreas.

12.4.3 Explain common disorders of the pancreatic hormones.

CASE REPORT 12.4

You are . . .

. . . a certified medical assistant working with Susan Lee, MD, in her Primary Care Clinic at Fulwood Medical Center.

You are communicating with . . .

. . . Mrs. Martha Jones, who is here for her monthly checkup. She is a 53-year-old type 2 diabetic on insulin. Mrs. Jones has **diabetic retinopathy** and **diabetic neuropathy** of her feet. Bariatric surgery has enabled her to reduce her weight from 275 to 156 pounds. The time is 0930 hrs. She is complaining of having a cold and cough for the past few days. Now, she is feeling drowsy and nauseous and has a dry mouth. As you talk with her, you notice that her speech is slurred. She cannot remember if she gave herself her morning insulin. Examination of her lungs reveals **rales** (wet, crackly lung noises) at her right base.

Her VS: T 97.8, P 120, R 20, BP 100/50. You perform her blood **glucose** measurement. The reading is 600 milligrams per deciliter (mg/dL). A recommended value 2 hours after breakfast is < 145 mg/dL.

Keynotes

- **Glucagon is not the only hormone that raises blood glucose; epinephrine, hydrocortisone, and growth hormone do as well.**
- **Insulin is the only hormone that lowers blood glucose.**

The Pancreas (LO 12.2 and 12.7)

The location and structure of the pancreas are further detailed in *Chapter 9.* Most of your pancreas is an **exocrine** gland (external secretion gland) that secretes digestive juices through a duct *(Figure 12.11a).* Scattered throughout the pancreas are clusters of endocrine cells grouped around blood vessels. These clusters are called **pancreatic islets (islets of Langerhans).** Within the islets are three distinct cell types *(Figure 12.11b):*

1. **Alpha cells:** Secrete the hormone **glucagon** in response to low blood **glucose.** Glucagon's actions are:
   a. In the liver, to stimulate **gluconeogenesis, glycogenolysis,** and the release of glucose into the bloodstream; and
   b. In adipose tissue, to stimulate fat catabolism and the release of free fatty acids.
2. **Beta cells:** Secrete **insulin** in response to a high blood glucose level. Insulin has the opposite effects to those of glucagon, and its actions are:
   a. In muscle and fat cells, to enable them to absorb glucose, and to store glycogen and fat; and
   b. In the liver, to stimulate the conversion of glucose to glycogen.
3. **Delta cells:** Secrete **somatostatin,** which acts within the pancreas to prevent the secretion of glucagon and insulin.

FIGURE 12.11
Pancreas.
(a) Anatomy of the pancreas. (b) Alpha, beta, and delta cells.

Word Analysis and Definition

S = Suffix P = Prefix R = Root R/CF = Combining Form

WORD	PRONUNCIATION		ELEMENTS	DEFINITION
exocrine	**EK**-soh-krin	P/ R/CF	**exo-** *outward* **-crine** *secrete*	A gland that secretes outwardly through excretory ducts
glucagon	**GLU**-kah-gon	S/ R/	**-agon** *to fight* **gluc-** *sugar, glucose*	Pancreatic hormone that supports blood glucose levels
gluconeogenesis	**GLU**-koh-nee-oh-**JEN**-eh-sis	S/ P/ R/CF	**-genesis** *creation* **-neo-** *new* **gluc/o-** *sugar, glucose*	Formation of glucose from noncarbohydrate sources
glucose	**GLU**-kose	S/ R/	**-ose** *full of* **gluc-** *sugar, glucose*	The final product of carbohydrate digestion and the main sugar in the blood
glycogenolysis	**GLYE**-koh-jen-oh-**LYE**-sis	S/ R/CF R/CF	**-lysis** *separate, dissolve* **glyc/o-** *glycogen* **-gen/o-** *create*	Conversion of glycogen to glucose
insulin	**IN**-syu-lin	S/ R/	**-in** *a substance* **insul-** *an island*	Hormone produced by the islet cells of the pancreas
pancreatic islets islets of Langerhans (syn)	pan-kree-**AT**-ik **EYE**-lets **EYE**-lets of **LAHNG**-er-hahnz	S/ R/ S/ R/	**-ic** *pertaining to* **pancreat-** *pancreas* **-et** *little* **isl-** *island* Paul Langerhans, 1847–1888, German anatomist	Areas of pancreatic cells that produce insulin and glucagon
somatostatin	**SOH**-mah-toh-**STAT**-in	S/ R/CF	**-statin** *inhibit* **somat/o-** *body*	Hormone that inhibits release of growth hormone and insulin

Exercises

A. Describe the functions of the pancreas. *Select the correct answer for each of the following statements.* **LO 12.2 and 12.7**

1. The effect of glucagon is:
   a. decrease blood sugar levels **b.** increase blood sugar levels
2. Glucagon is secreted by the _____ cells.
   a. alpha **b.** beta **c.** delta
3. Clusters of alpha, beta, and delta cells in the pancreas are called:
   a. pancreatic clusters **b.** pancreatic islets **c.** pancreatitis **d.** gluconeogenesis
4. The process of gluconeogenesis will cause blood sugar levels to:
   a. increase **b.** decrease **c.** stay the same
5. Storage of glycogen is stimulated by the hormone:
   a. somatostatin **b.** glucagon **c.** insulin

B. Build the correct medical term *that matches the definition. Insert each missing element on the line, and label what type of element it is under the line. Then answer question 5.* **LO 12.1, 12.2, and 12.7**

1. Conversion of glycogen to glucose: ____________ / ____________ /lysis
2. Main sugar in the blood: ____________ /ose
3. Hormone that inhibits release of GH and insulin: ____________ /statin
4. The formation of glucose from noncarbohydrate sources: gluco/____________ /genesis

Lesson 12.4 (cont'd)

Keynotes

- **Type 2 diabetes used to occur over the age of 30, but it is now seen also in obese adolescents and young adults.**
- **The brain is the first organ affected by hypoglycemia.**
- **Hyperglycemia causes damage to vascular endothelial cells at the microvascular and macrovascular levels.**
- **Untreated hyperglycemia can progress to diabetic coma.**

Abbreviations

DM	diabetes mellitus
IDDM	insulin-dependent diabetes mellitus
LADA	latent autoimmune diabetes in adults
MODY	mature-onset diabetes of the young
NIDDM	non-insulin-dependent diabetes mellitus

Diabetes Mellitus (DM) (LO 12.7)

Diabetes mellitus is a condition characterized by hyperglycemia, resulting from an impairment of insulin secretion and/or insulin action. Diabetes affects the body's ability to make use of the energy found in food, disrupting the normal process of carbohydrate, fat, and protein metabolism. It is the world's most prevalent metabolic disease and the leading cause of blindness, renal failure, and gangrene of the lower extremities. There is a spectrum of types of diabetes, the main ones being:

1. **Type 1 diabetes,** also called **insulin-dependent diabetes mellitus (IDDM),** accounts for 10 to 15% of all cases of DM. It is the predominant type of DM found in patients under the age of 30. When symptoms become apparent, 90% of the pancreatic insulin-producing cells have already been destroyed by **autoantibodies** (antibodies that attack the patient's own system).
2. **Type 2 diabetes,** also called **non-insulin-dependent diabetes mellitus (NIDDM),** accounts for 85 to 90% of all DM cases. Nearly 18 million people in the United States have been diagnosed with type 2 DM. Not only is there an impairment of insulin response, but there is also a decreased glucose uptake by tissues due to insulin resistance. In addition to contributing to type 2 DM, insulin resistance leads to other common disorders like hypertension, hyperlipidemia, and coronary artery disease.
3. **Latent autoimmune diabetes in adults (LADA or Type 1.5)** accounts for roughly 10% of people with diabetes. It occurs in adults who have the same autoantibodies as Type 1 diabetics, but there is no need for insulin treatment in the first 6 months after diagnosis. It is a more slowly progressing variation of Type 1 diabetes.
4. **Gestational diabetes** occurs in about 5% of pregnancies. While most cases of gestational diabetes resolve after the pregnancy, a woman who has this complication of pregnancy has a 30% chance of developing type 2 DM within 10 years.
5. **Mature-onset diabetes of the young (MODY)** is a selection of genetically linked forms of diabetes usually found in thin people under 55 years of age. Many forms of MODY will respond to small doses of insulin or to sulfonylurea drugs.

Hypoglycemia (LO 12.7)

Hypoglycemia is present when blood glucose is below 70 mg/dL. Because brain metabolism depends primarily on glucose, the brain is the first organ affected by hypoglycemia. This disorder presents clinically as an impaired mental efficiency, followed by shakiness, anxiety, confusion, tremor, seizures, and, if untreated, loss of consciousness. Symptomatic hypoglycemia is sometimes called **insulin shock.** Low blood glucose can be raised to normal in minutes by taking 10 to 20 g carbohydrate (3 to 4 ounces), such as orange, apple, or grape juice, or a sugar-containing soft drink.

Hyperglycemia (LO 12.7)

In **hyperglycemia,** the classic symptoms are **polyuria** (excessive urination), **polydipsia** (excessive thirst), and **polyphagia** (excessive hunger), with unexplained weight loss.

Symptomatic hyperglycemia is how type 1 DM usually presents. Type 2 DM can be symptomatic or asymptomatic, and is often found during a routine health exam.

Because of high glucose levels, hyperglycemia damages capillary endothelial cells in the retina, renal glomerulus *(see Chapter 13),* and neurons in peripheral nerves *(see Chapter 10).* Of all diabetics, 85% develop some degree of **diabetic retinopathy;** 30% develop diabetic **nephropathy,** which can progress to end-stage renal disease *(see Chapter 13).* Diabetic **neuropathy** causes sensory defects with numbness, tingling, and **paresthesias** (abnormal skin sensations) in the feet and/or hands.

In larger blood vessels, hyperglycemia contributes to endothelial cell-lining damage and atherosclerosis. Coronary artery disease and peripheral vascular disease with claudication *(see Chapter 6)* are complications. Hyperglycemia is the most common cause of foot ulcers and gangrene of the lower extremity, sometimes requiring **amputation.** The risk of infection is increased by the cellular hyperglycemia and the circulatory deficits.

The complications of hyperglycemia can be kept at bay by stringent control of blood glucose levels.

Word Analysis and Definition

S = Suffix P = Prefix R = Root R/CF = Combining Form

WORD	PRONUNCIATION	ELEMENTS		DEFINITION
amputation	am-pyu-**TAY**-shun	S/ R/	**-ation** *a process* **amput-** *to prune, lop off*	Process of removing a limb, part of a limb, a breast, or other projecting part
autoantibody (**Note:** *Two prefixes*)	awe-toe-**AN**-tee-bod-ee	P/ P/ R/	**auto-** *self, same* **-anti-** *against* **-body** *body*	Antibody produced in response to an antigen from the host's own tissue
coma **comatose (adj)**	**KOH**-mah **KOH**-mah-toes	 S/ R/	Greek *deep sleep* **-ose** *full of* **comat-** *coma*	State of deep unconsciousness In a state of coma
diabetes mellitus	dye-ah-**BEE**-teez **MEL**-ih-tus		**diabetes,** Greek *a siphon* **mellitus,** Latin *sweetened with honey*	Metabolic syndrome caused by absolute or relative insulin deficiency and/or ineffectiveness
diabetic (adj)	dye-ah-**BET**-ik	S/ R/	**-ic** *pertaining to* **diabet-** *diabetes*	Pertaining to or suffering from diabetes
hyperglycemia	**HIGH**-per-gly-**SEE**-me-ah	S/ P/ R/	**-emia** *a blood condition* **hyper-** *above* **-glyc-** *glucose*	High level of glucose (sugar) in the blood
hyperglycemic (adj)	**HIGH**-per-gly-**SEE**-mik	S/	**-emic** *pertaining to a blood condition*	Pertaining to or having hyperglycemia
hypoglycemia	**HIGH**-poh-gly-**SEE**-me-ah	S/ P/ R/	**-emia** *a blood condition* **hypo-** *below, deficient* **-glyc-** *glucose*	Low level of glucose (sugar) in the blood
hypoglycemic (adj)	**HIGH**-poh-gly-SEE-mik	S/	**-emic** *pertaining to a blood condition*	Pertaining to or suffering from low blood sugar
nephropathy	neh-**FROP**-ah-thee	S/ R/CF	**-pathy** *disease* **nephr/o-** *kidney*	Any disease of the kidney
neuropathy	nyu-**ROP**-ah-thee	S/ R/	**-pathy** *disease* **neur/o-** *nerve*	Any disease of the nervous system
paresthesia **paresthesias (pl)**	par-es-**THEE**-ze-ah	S/ P/ R/	**-ia** *condition* **par-** *abnormal* **-esthes-** *sensation*	An abnormal sensation; e.g., tingling, burning, pricking
polydipsia	pol-ee-**DIP**-see-ah	S/ P/ R/	**-ia** *condition* **poly-** *many, excessive* **-dips-** *thirst*	Excessive thirst
polyphagia	pol-ee-**FAY**-jee-ah	S/ P/ R/	**-ia** *condition* **poly-** *many, excessive* **-phag-** *eat*	Excessive eating
polyuria	pol-ee-**YOU**-ree-ah	S/ P/ R/	**-ia** *condition* **poly-** *many, excessive* **-ur-** *urine*	Excessive production of urine
retinopathy	ret-ih-**NOP**-ah-thee	S/ R/CF	**-pathy** *disease* **retin/o-** *retina of the eye*	Degenerative disease of the retina

EXERCISE

A. Diabetes *is the world's most prevalent metabolic disease. Many patients have diabetes as a concurrent condition with other health problems, which always makes it a consideration in treatment and the prescribing of medications. Test your knowledge of this disease by answering the following questions. Select the correct answer that completes each statement.* **LO 12.7**

1. Diabetes is the leading cause of:

a. blindness **b.** renal failure **c.** gangrene **d.** all of these

2. The first organ affected by hypoglycemia is the:

a. kidney **b.** heart **c.** pancreas **d.** brain **e.** liver

3. Impairment of insulin response and decreased insulin effectiveness is termed insulin:

a. production **b.** resistance **c.** autoantibodies **d.** control **e.** conversion

4. Most cases of gestational diabetes resolve after:

a. medication **b.** treatment **c.** testing **d.** pregnancy **e.** surgery

Lesson 12.4 (cont'd) Diabetes Mellitus (continued) (LO 12.7)

Keynotes

- **Diabetic ketoacidosis is a medical emergency.**
- **Maintaining normal plasma glucose levels is the basis for good management of DM.**
- **Many insulin-dependent diabetics need multiple subcutaneous insulin injections each day.**

Abbreviations

BUN	blood urea nitrogen
DKA	diabetic ketoacidosis
Hb A1c	glycosylated hemoglobin, hemoglobin A1c

Diabetic ketoacidosis (DKA) is a state of marked hyperglycemia with dehydration, **metabolic acidosis** (abnormal increase in blood acidity), and **ketone** formation. This is seen mostly in type 1 DM and usually results from a lapse in insulin treatment, an acute infection, or a trauma that makes the usual insulin treatment inadequate.

DKA presents with polyuria, vomiting, and lethargy and can progress to coma. The ketone **acetone** can be smelled on the breath. DKA is a medical emergency. There is a 2% to 5% mortality rate from circulatory collapse if the DKA is not promptly controlled.

Diabetic coma is a severe medical emergency, caused by hyperglycemia.

Insulin shock is another severe medical emergency, caused by hypoglycemia.

A blood glucose test will differentiate hypoglycemia from hyperglycemia.

Case Report 12.4 *(continued)*

Mrs. Martha Jones is in the early stages of a diabetic **ketoacidosis** coma, probably initiated by a right lower-lobe pneumonia. A urine specimen was obtained. Dr. Lee was notified. Blood was taken for a full chemistry panel, and arterial blood gases were drawn. Dr. Lee treated Mrs. Jones immediately with an IV infusion of **saline** solution and IV **insulin.** She was admitted to the hospital.

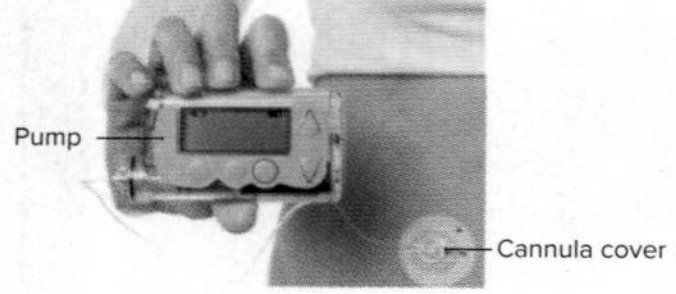

▲ **FIGURE 12.12** Photograph of Insulin Pump—with Cannula Inserted in the Subcutaneous Tissue of the Abdominal Wall.

Oscar Gimeno Baldo/Alamy Images

Treatment of Diabetes Mellitus (LO 12.7)

The basic principle of diabetes treatment is to avoid hyperglycemia and hypoglycemia. The areas of treatment are as follows:

- **Diet and exercise** to achieve weight reduction of 2 pounds per week in overweight type 2 DM patients is essential.
- **Patient education** is necessary so that the patient understands the disease process, can recognize the indications for seeking immediate medical care, and will follow a foot care regimen.
- **Plasma glucose monitoring** is an essential skill that all diabetics must learn. Patients on insulin must learn to adjust their insulin doses. Home glucose analyzers use a drop of blood obtained from the fingertip or forearm by a spring-powered lancet. The frequency of testing varies individually.
- **Assessment of the patient** should be performed on routine physician visits for symptoms or signs of complications.
- **Periodic laboratory evaluation** includes **BUN** and serum creatinine (kidney function), lipid profile, ECG, and an annual complete ophthalmologic evaluation.

Glycosylated hemoglobin (Hb A1c) is used to monitor plasma glucose control during the preceding 1 to 3 months.

Oral antidiabetic drugs are used for type 2 DM but not type 1 DM. There are numerous drugs available, and they produce their effect in four main ways:

- Stimulate the beta cells of the pancreas to produce more insulin. **Sulfonylureas** are an example; the oldest one, chlorpropamide (Diabinese), has been available for 50 years. The second-generation sulfonylureas include glipizide (Glucotrol) and glyburide (Micronase). **Meglitinides**–repaglinide (Prandin)–act in the same way.
- Decrease glucose production by the liver. **Biguanides**–metformin (Glucophage)–act in this way.
- Block the breakdown of starches in the intestine. **Alpha-glucosidase inhibitors**–acarbose (Precose)–act in this way.
- Increase insulin production and decrease glucose production. **DPP-4 inhibitors**–sitagliptin (Januvia)–are an example of this type.

Combinations of these different-acting drugs are often used.

Injectable insulin preparations are used in type 1 DM and sometimes in type 2 DM. They are classified by their speed of action *(see table below.)*

The injectable insulins are supplied in vials, cartridges, and prefilled pens.

For some patients requiring frequent doses of insulin, continuous subcutaneous insulin infusion is given by an implanted battery-powered, programmable pump *(Figure 12.12).* This pump provides continuous insulin through a small needle in the abdominal wall.

PHARMACOLOGY: CLASSES OF INSULIN (LO 12.7)

Insulin Type	Onset of Action*	Peak of Action*	Duration of Action*	Examples
Rapid acting	15 min	30–60 min	3–5 hr	Humalog, NovoLog
Regular acting	30–60 min	100–120 min	5–8 hr	Humulin R, Novolin R
Intermediate acting (NPH)	1–3 hr	7–8 hr	18–24 hr	Humulin N, Novolin N
Long acting	4–8 hr	minimal peak effects	16–24 hr	Lantus, Levemir
Premixed	30 min	2–4 hrs	14–24 hrs	Humulin 70/30, Novolin 70/30

*min = minutes; hr = hours.

Word Analysis and Definition

S = Suffix P = Prefix R = Root R/CF = Combining Form

WORD	PRONUNCIATION	ELEMENTS		DEFINITION
acetone	**ASS**-eh-tone		Latin *vinegar*	Ketone that is found in blood, urine, and breath when diabetes mellitus is out of control
ketoacidosis	**KEY**-toe-ass-ih-**DOE**-sis	S/ R/CF R/	-osis *condition* **ket/o-** *ketone* **-acid-** *acid*	Excessive ketones in the blood, making it acidic
ketone ketosis	**KEY**-tone key-**TOE**-sis	 S/ R/	Greek *acetone* -osis *condition* **ket-** *ketone*	Chemical formed in uncontrolled diabetes or in starvation Excessive production of ketones
lethargy lethargic (adj)	**LETH**-ar-jee le-**THAR**-jik		Greek *drowsiness*	Abnormal drowsiness in depth or length of time
metabolic acidosis	met-ah-**BOL**-ik ass-ih-**DOE**-sis	S/ R/ S/ R/	-ic *pertaining to* **metabol-** *change* -osis *condition* **acid-** *acid*	Decreased pH in blood and body tissues as a result of an upset in metabolism
saline	**SAY**-leen		Latin *salt*	Salt solution, usually sodium chloride

EXERCISES

A. Medications: Diabetics will deal with medications for the rest of their lives. *Select the one drug that is the correct answer for each statement.* **LO 12.7 and 12.8**

1. Act(s) by stimulating the beta cells to secrete insulin:

a. metformin **b.** sulfonylureas **c.** alpha-glucosidase inhibitors

2. Suppress(es) hepatic glucose production:

a. metformin **b.** meglitinides **c.** glipizide

3. Blocks the breakdown of starches in the intestine:

a. acarbose **b.** repaglinide **c.** sitagliptin

B. Test your knowledge of the treatment of patients with diabetes mellitus by identifying statements as T for true and F for false. **LO 12.7 and 12.8**

1. All patients with diabetes mellitus should follow the same plasma glucose monitoring schedule. **T F**

2. An important part of self-monitoring is foot care. **T F**

3. Ketosis can be treated at home. **T F**

4. The HbA1c is a record of blood sugar control over the preceding 6 to 8 months. **T F**

5. Glucophage works by consuming glucose in the blood. **T F**

Additional exercises available in connect

Chapter Review exercises, along with additional practice items, are available in Connect!

The Urinary System

The Essentials of the Language of Urology

CHAPTER 13

Rick Brady/McGraw-Hill Education

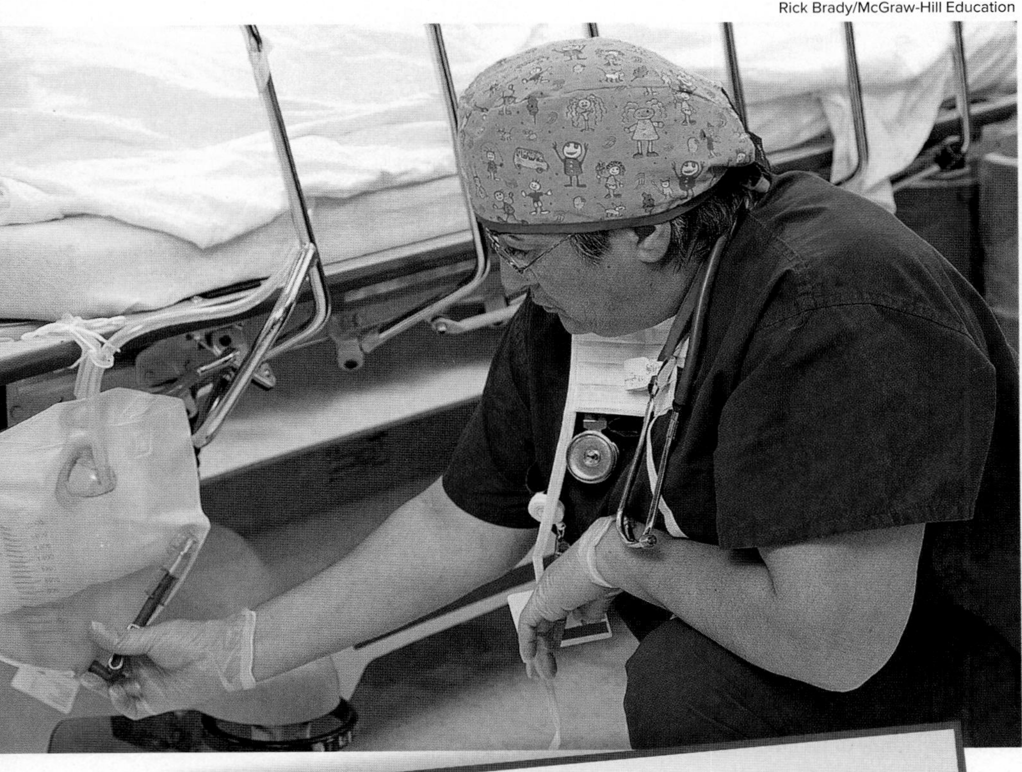

Learning Outcomes

In order to understand and to assess Mr. Hughes' situation, define and recognize the areas of concern, communicate with Dr. Johnson and the patient, and document the patient's progress, you need to be able to:

LO 13.1 **Use roots, combining forms, suffixes, and prefixes to construct and analyze (deconstruct) medical terms related to the urinary system.**

LO 13.2 **Spell and pronounce correctly medical terms related to the urinary system in order to communicate them with accuracy and precision in any health care setting.**

LO 13.3 **Define accepted abbreviations related to the urinary system.**

LO 13.4 **Relate the structure of the kidneys and ureters to their functions and disorders.**

LO 13.5 **Relate the structure of the urinary bladder and urethra and associated organs to their functions and disorders.**

LO 13.6 **Describe the diagnostic and therapeutic procedures and the pharmacologic agents used for disorders of the urinary system.**

LO 13.7 **Apply your knowledge of medical terms relating to the urinary system to documentation, medical records, and medical reports.**

LO 13.8 **Translate the medical terms relating to the urinary system into everyday language in order to communicate clearly with patients and their families.**

CASE REPORT 13.1

You are . . .

. . . a surgical physician assistant working with **urologist** Phillip Johnson, MD, at Fulwood Medical Center.

You are communicating with . . .

. . . Mr. Nelson Hughes, a 58-year-old school principal. You are making your afternoon hospital visits to Dr. Johnson's patients. Earlier today, you assisted at Mr. Hughes' surgery. A **laparoscopic** radical **nephrectomy** (kidney removal) for a **TNM** Stage II **renal** cell carcinoma (cancer) with no evidence of local invasion or lymph node involvement (metastasis) was performed. Your job is to assess Mr. Hughes' postoperative state and determine whether postoperative complications exist.

Abbreviation

TNM tumor, node, metastasis (tumor staging method)

In your future career, being able to communicate comfortably, accurately, and effectively with the health professionals involved in the diagnosis and treatment of problems with the urologic system is key. You may work directly and/or indirectly with one or more of the following:

- **Urologists** are specialists in the diagnosis and treatment of diseases of the urinary system.
- **Nephrologists** are specialists in the diagnosis and treatment of diseases of the kidney.
- **Urologic nurses** and **nurse practitioners** are registered nurses with advanced academic and clinical experience in urology.

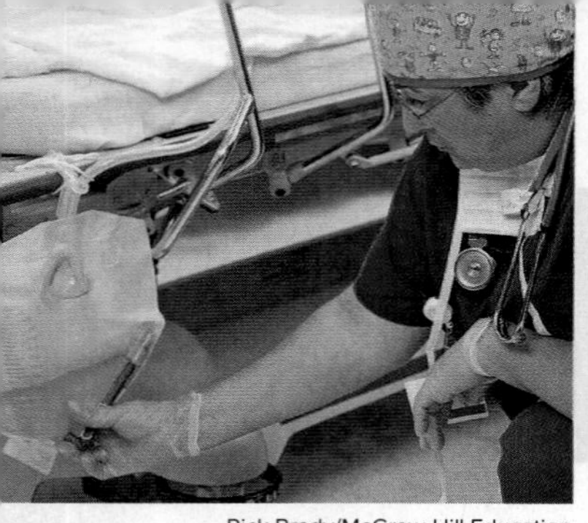
Rick Brady/McGraw-Hill Education

Lesson 13.1

Urinary System, Kidneys, and Ureters

Objectives

Your body's metabolism continually produces metabolic waste products. If these wastes are not eliminated, they will poison your body. Your ***urinary*** *system carries the major burden of excreting these wastes, and within this system, the kidney is the organ that does the actual eliminating. So, the kidney is a vital organ to understand, and it brings with it a whole new set of terminology.*

In this lesson, the information will enable you to use correct medical terminology to:

13.1.1 Name and locate the organs of the urinary system.

13.1.2 Identify the structures and functions of the kidneys and ureters.

13.1.3 Describe disorders of the kidneys and ureters.

Keynotes

- The kidney removes waste products from the blood by a process of filtration.
- Each renal cortex contains about 1 million nephrons, the functional filtration unit of the kidney.
- The filtrate from the kidney's filtration process is urine. It consists of excess water, electrolytes, and urea.

Urinary System (LO 13.4 and 13.5)

Your **urinary system** *(Figure 13.1)* consists of **six organs:**

- Two **kidneys**
- Two **ureters**
- A single **urinary bladder**
- A single **urethra**

The process of removing metabolic wastes is called excretion, and it's essential in maintaining your body's homeostasis *(see Chapter 2).* Metabolic wastes include carbon dioxide, excess water and electrolytes, **nitrogenous** compounds including **ammonia** (from the breakdown of proteins), and **urea.** If these wastes are not eliminated, they will poison the entire body.

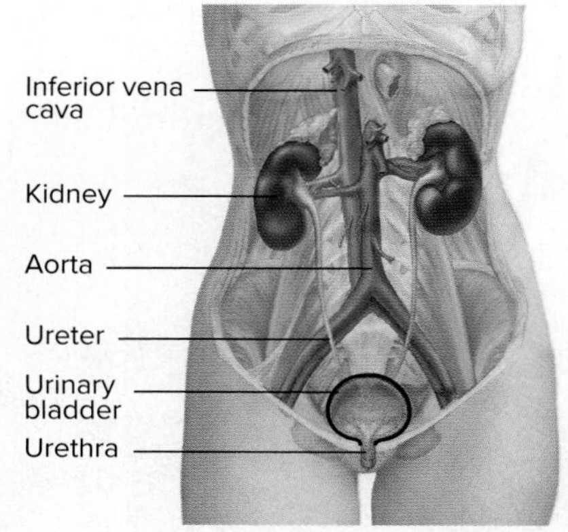

FIGURE 13.1 Urinary System.

The Kidneys (LO 13.4)

Each of your kidneys is a bean-shaped organ about the size of your clenched fist. One kidney is located on each side of the vertebral column and lies against the deep muscles of your back *(Figure 13.1).*

Waste-laden blood enters your kidney at its **hilum** (an opening for nerves and vessels) *(Figure 13.2)* through the **renal** artery. Excess water, urea, and other waste products are **filtered** from the blood by the more than 1 million **nephrons** in each kidney's cortex. The renal artery *(Figure 13.2)* divides into smaller and smaller arterioles, each of which then enters a nephron and divides into a network of capillaries known as a **glomerulus** *(Figure 13.3),* which is encased in **Bowman's capsule.** Because the blood is under pressure and the capillaries are permeable, much of the fluid from the blood filters through the capillary walls into the surrounding renal tubules, including the loop of Henle. The tubules join to form the collecting duct, and collecting ducts join to form **calyces,** which join to form the **ureter** *(Figure 13.2).* The ureters carry the **filtrate,** now called **urine,** from the kidneys to the urinary **bladder.**

The **excretion functions of the kidneys** are to:

- **Filter** blood to eliminate wastes;
- **Regulate** blood volume and pressure by eliminating or conserving water; and
- **Maintain homeostasis** by controlling the amounts of water and electrolytes that are eliminated.

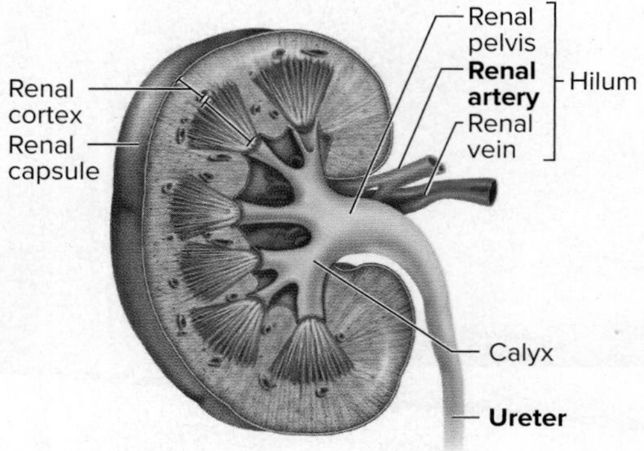

FIGURE 13.2 Section of Kidney.

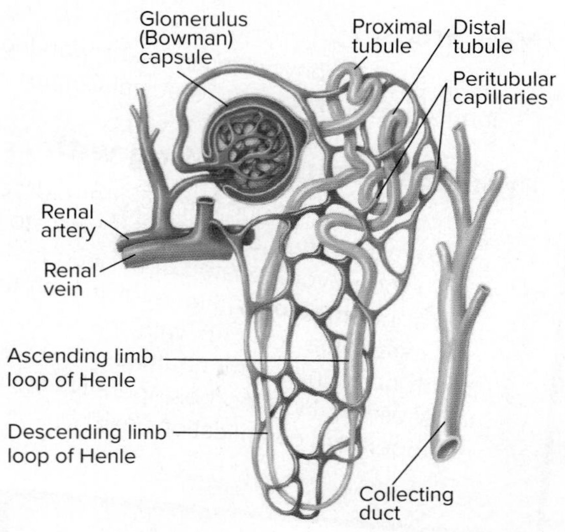

FIGURE 13.3 Nephron.

Word Analysis and Definition

S = Suffix P = Prefix R = Root R/CF = Combining Form

WORD	PRONUNCIATION	ELEMENTS		DEFINITION
ammonia	ah-**MOAN**-ih-ah	S/ R/	-ia *condition* **ammon-** *ammonia*	Toxic breakdown product of amino acids (proteins)
bladder	**BLAD**-er		Old English *bladder*	Hollow sac that holds fluid; e.g., urine or bile
calyx **calyces (pl)** **calices (syn)**	**KAY**-licks **KAY**-lih-seez		Greek *cup of a flower*	Funnel-shaped structure
filter (noun or verb)	**FIL**-ter		Latin *strain through material*	Porous substance used to separate liquids and gases from particulate matter; or to subject a substance to the action of a filter
filtrate	**FIL**-trate	S/ R/	**-ate** *composed of, pertaining to* **filtr-** *strain through*	Liquid that has passed through a filter
filtration	fil-**TRAY**-shun	S/	**-ation** *process*	Process of passing liquid through a filter
glomerulus	glo-**MER**-you-lus		Latin *small ball of yarn*	Network of capillaries in a nephron
hilum **hila (pl)**	**HIGH**-lum **HIGH**-lah		Latin *small bit*	The opening where the nerves and blood vessels enter and leave an organ
kidney	**KID**-nee		Old English *kidney*	Organ of excretion
nephron	**NEF**-ron		Greek *kidney*	Filtration unit of the kidney; composed of glomerulus and renal tubule
nephrology	neh-**FROL**-oh-jee	S/ R/CF	-logy *study of* **nephr/o-** *kidney*	Medical specialty of diseases of the kidney
nephrologist	neh-**FROL**-oh-jist	S/	**-logist** *one who studies, specialist*	Medical specialist in disorders of the kidney
nitrogenous (adj)	ni-**TRO**-jen-us	S/ R/CF R/	**-ous** *pertaining to* **nitr/o-** *nitrogen* **-gen-** *create*	Containing or generating nitrogen
renal (adj)	**REE**-nal	S/ R/	**-al** *pertaining to* **ren-** *kidney*	Pertaining to the kidney
urea	you-**REE**-ah		Greek *urine*	End product of nitrogen metabolism
ureter	you-**REE**-ter		Greek *urinary canal*	Tube that connects each kidney to the urinary bladder
ureteral (adj)	you-ree-**TER**-al	S/ R/	-al *pertaining to* **ureter-** *ureter*	Pertaining to a ureter
urine	**YUR**-in		Latin *urine*	Fluid and dissolved substances excreted by the kidney
urinary (adj)	**YUR**-in-ary	S/ R/	-ary *pertaining to* **urin-** *urine*	Pertaining to urine
urinate (verb) **urination**	**YUR**-in-ate yur-ih-**NAY**-shun	S/ S/	-ate *composed of, pertaining to* -ation *process*	To pass urine Process of passing urine
urology	yur-**ROL**-oh-jee	S/ R/CF	-logy *study of* **ur/o-** *urinary system*	Medical specialty that studies the urinary system
urologist **urological (adj)**	yur-**ROL**-oh-jist yur-roh-**LOJ**-ik-al	S/ S/	-logist *one who studies, specialist* -ical *pertaining to*	Specialist in urology Pertaining to urology

EXERCISE

A. Construct *the following terms related to the urinary system by inserting the correct elements. Fill in the blanks.* **LO 13.1 and 13.4**

1. specialist in the urinary system: ____________ / ____________
2. containing or generating nitrogen: ____________ / ____________ / ____________
3. pertaining to the ureter: ____________ / ____________
4. study of diseases of the kidney: ____________ / ____________
5. pertaining to the kidney: ____________ / ____________
6. liquid that has passed through a filter: ____________ / ____________

Lesson 13.1 (cont'd) Disorders of the Kidneys (LO 13.4)

Keynotes

- 25 to 30% of all renal cancers relate directly to smoking.
- As little as 1 milliliter of blood will turn the urine red.
- The acute form of glomerulonephritis has a 100% recovery rate.

Case Report 13.1 *(continued)*

Mr. Nelson Hughes had been well until a few months before his surgery, when he noticed a vague, aching pain in the left side of his abdomen. One week prior to his surgery, he suddenly passed bright red urine. A urinalysis showed red blood cells **(hematuria)** and a physical examination revealed an enlarged left kidney. **Intravenous pyelogram (IVP)** (Figure 13.4) and other imaging tests showed a tumor 3 inches in diameter in the center of his left kidney. His bone scan was normal, indicating no metastases to the bones.

Renal cell carcinoma, the most common form of kidney cancer, occurs twice as often in men as in women. The cancer develops in the lining cells of the renal tubules, which is why Mr. Hughes had hematuria. Radical **nephrectomy** is the most common treatment for renal cell carcinoma.

Wilms tumor, or **nephroblastoma,** is a malignant childhood kidney tumor, usually occurring between the ages of 3 and 8. It is treated effectively with a combination of surgery and chemotherapy.

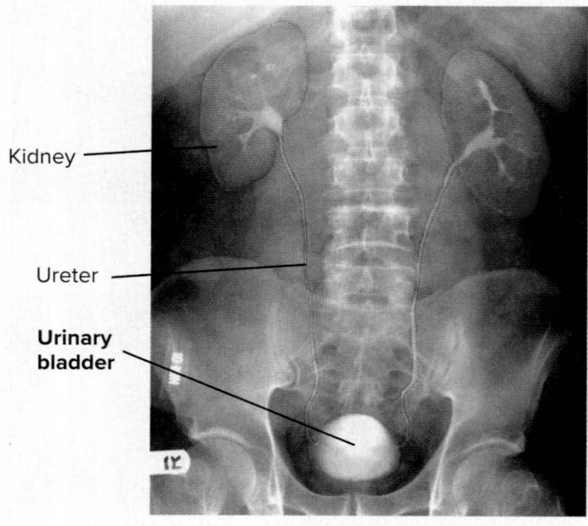

▲ **FIGURE 13.4**
Colored Intravenous Pyelogram (IVP).
Science History Images/Alamy Stock Photo

Renal adenomas (benign kidney tumors) are usually asymptomatic (produce no symptoms), are discovered by chance, and are not life threatening.

Hematuria (blood in the urine) can be caused by lesions or stones anywhere in the urinary system. These lesions may result from trauma, infections, and congenital diseases like sickle cell anemia. In microscopic hematuria, the urine is not red, and red blood cells can be seen only under a microscope or identified by a urine dipstick.

Acute glomerulonephritis is an inflammation of the kidney's filtration unit (the nephron). It damages the glomerular capillaries and allows protein and red blood cells to leak into the urine. It can develop rapidly after a strep throat infection, especially in children.

Chronic glomerulonephritis can occur with no history of kidney disease and present as kidney failure. It also occurs in **diabetic nephropathy** and can be associated with autoimmune diseases like lupus erythematosus (a disease of the connective tissues).

Nephrotic syndrome is caused by different disorders that damage the kidneys, causing large amounts of protein to leak into the urine, so the level of protein in the blood drops. The most obvious symptom is fluid retention, with edema of the ankles and legs. This is treated with **diuretics,** by restricting salt in the diet, and by reducing fluid intake. Minimal change disease *(Table 13.1)* is the most common cause in children. Membranous nephropathy *(Table 13.1)* is the most common cause in adults.

▼ **TABLE 13.1**
TYPES OF NEPHROTIC SYNDROME (LO 13.4)

Disease (as Seen on Biopsy)	Description
Minimal change disease	Most common in children; responds to steroids
Focal segmental glomerulosclerosis (FSGS)	Cause unknown; little response to treatment
Membranous nephropathy	Cause unknown; may respond to immunosuppressive treatment
Diabetes	Occurs if blood sugar has been poorly controlled

Abbreviation

IVP intravenous pyelogram

Word Analysis and Definition

S = Suffix P = Prefix R = Root R/CF = Combining Form

WORD	PRONUNCIATION	ELEMENTS		DEFINITION
diuretic (adj) (**Note:** *The "a" is dropped from dia to enable the word to flow.*) **diuresis (noun)**	die-you-**RET**-ik die-you-**REE**-sis	S/ P/ R/ S/	**-etic** *pertaining to* **di(a)-** *complete* **-ur-** *urine* **-esis** *condition*	Agent that increases urine output Excretion of large volume of urine
glomerulonephritis	glo-**MER**-you-low-nef-**RYE**-tis	S/ R/CF R/	**-itis** *inflammation* **glomerul/o-** *glomerulus* **-nephr-** *kidney*	Infection of the glomeruli of the kidney
hematuria	he-mah-**TYU**-ree-ah	S/ R/	**-uria** *urine* **hemat-** *blood*	Blood in the urine
nephrectomy	neh-**FREK**-toe-me	S/ R/	**-ectomy** *surgical excision* **nephr-** *kidney*	Surgical removal of a kidney
nephroblastoma **Wilms tumor**	**NEF**-roh-blas-**TOE**-mah WILMZ **TOO**-mor	S/ R/CF R/	**-oma** *tumor, mass* **nephr/o-** *kidney* **-blast-** *immature cell* Max Wilms, German surgeon, 1867–1918	Cancerous kidney tumor of childhood
nephropathy	neh-**FROP**-ah-thee	S/ R/CF	**-pathy** *disease* **nephr/o-** *kidney*	Any disease of the kidney
nephrotic syndrome **nephrosis** (*same as* **nephrotic syndrome**)	neh-**FROT**-ik **SIN**-drohm neh-**FROH**-sis	S/ R/CF S/ R/	**-tic** *pertaining to* **nephr/o-** *kidney* **-osis** *condition* **nephr-** *kidney*	Glomerular disease with marked loss of protein
pyelogram	**PIE**-el-oh-gram	S/ R/CF	**-gram** *record, recording* **pyel/o-** *renal pelvis*	X-ray image of renal pelvis and ureters using contrast media

EXERCISES

A. After reading Case Report 13.1 and 13.1 (continued), *answer the following questions. Select the correct answer.* **LO 13.6 and 13.8**

1. "Bright red urine" would indicate the presence of ________ in the urine.
   a. pus **b.** blood **c.** cancer cells **d.** crystals **e.** sugar

2. The diagnostic test that analyzed the contents of the urine:
   a. bone scan **b.** pyelogram **c.** nephrectomy **d.** palpation **e.** urinalysis

3. Which diagnostic test determined that Mr. Hughes did not have bone metastases?
   a. intravenous pyelogram **b.** radical nephrectomy **c.** bone scan **d.** PET scan **e.** urinalysis

4. Has the cancer spread to other parts of the body?
   a. Yes **b.** No

B. Differentiate *the types of kidney disorders. Match the kidney disorder in the first column with its correct description in the second column. Fill in the blanks.* **LO 13.4**

_____ **1.** renal adenoma — **a.** condition diagnosed only in children

_____ **2.** nephroblastoma — **b.** malignant condition of the kidney; develops in the cells of the renal tubules

_____ **3.** nephrotic syndrome — **c.** can develop as a result of strep throat infection

_____ **4.** renal cell carcinoma — **d.** benign and usually asymptomatic

_____ **5.** acute glomerulonephritis — **e.** condition that causes leakage of proteins into the urine; edema of the ankles and legs is a common sign

Lesson 13.1 (cont'd) Disorders of the Kidneys (continued) (LO 13.4)

Interstitial nephritis is an inflammation (often acute and temporary) of the kidney tissue between the renal tubules. It can be an allergic reaction to or a side effect of drugs like penicillin or ampicillin, **NSAIDs,** and diuretics.

Pyelonephritis is an infection of the renal parenchyma, calyces, and pelvis. This usually occurs as part of a total urinary tract infection **(UTI),** beginning in the urinary bladder *(see the next lesson in this chapter).* It has a high mortality rate in the elderly and in people with a compromised immune system.

Polycystic kidney disease (PKD) is an inherited disease. Large fluid-filled cysts grow within the kidneys and press against the kidney tissue. Eventually, the kidneys cannot function effectively.

Acute renal failure (ARF) makes the kidneys suddenly stop filtering waste products from the blood. Initially, **oliguria** and then **anuria** are associated with confusion, seizures, and coma.

The causes of acute renal failure include: severe burns; trauma; septicemia; toxins like mercury and excess alcohol; excessive amounts of drugs like aspirin and ibuprofen; and antibiotics like streptomycin and gentamycin.

When caring for a patient who has ARF, the goal is to treat the underlying disease. **Dialysis** may be necessary while the kidneys are healing.

Chronic renal failure (CRF), or **chronic kidney disease (CKD),** is a gradual loss of renal function. Symptoms and signs may not appear until the kidney's level of functioning is less than 25% of normal. The causes of chronic renal failure are diabetes, hypertension, kidney disease (including chronic glomerulonephritis, nephrotic syndrome), and lead poisoning.

Uremia is the complex of symptoms resulting from excess nitrogenous waste products in the blood, as seen in renal failure.

End-stage renal disease (ESRD) means the kidneys are functioning at less than 10% of their normal capacity. At this point, life cannot be maintained, and either dialysis or a kidney transplant is needed.

Dialysis is an artificial method of removing waste materials and excess fluid from the blood. It is not a cure but can prolong life. There are several types of kidney dialysis:

- **Hemodialysis** *(Figure 13.5)* filters the blood through an artificial kidney machine **(dialyzer).** Most patients require 12 hours of hemodialysis a week, usually in three sessions.
- **Peritoneal dialysis** uses a dialysis solution that is infused into and drained out of your abdominal cavity through a small, flexible, **implanted** catheter. The dialysis solution extracts wastes and excess fluid from the network of capillaries in the peritoneal lining of the abdominal cavity.
- **Continuous ambulatory peritoneal dialysis (CAPD)** is performed by the patient at home through an implanted abdominal catheter *(Figure 13.6),* usually four times a day, 7 days a week.
- **Continuous cycling peritoneal dialysis** uses a machine to automatically infuse dialysis solution into and out of the abdominal cavity during sleep.

Kidney transplant provides a better quality of life than dialysis—if a suitable donor can be found. The donor has to match the recipient's blood type, cell surface proteins, and antibodies. A **sibling** or a blood relative can often qualify as a donor. If not, tissue banks across the country can search for a kidney from an accident victim or a donor who has died.

Keynotes

- Acute interstitial nephritis causes 15% of all cases of acute renal failure.
- Acute renal failure is usually reversible.
- Chronic renal failure has no cure.

Abbreviations

ARF	acute renal failure
CAPD	continuous ambulatory peritoneal dialysis
CKD	chronic kidney disease
CRF	chronic renal failure
ESRD	end-stage renal disease
NSAID	nonsteroidal anti-inflammatory drug
PKD	polycystic kidney disease
UTI	urinary tract infection

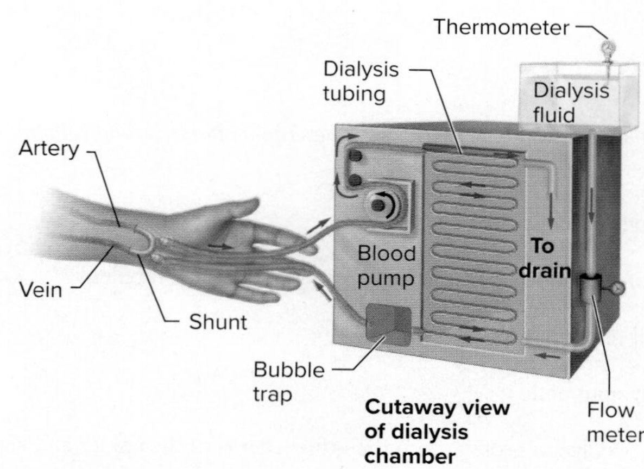

▲ **FIGURE 13.5**
Hemodialysis.

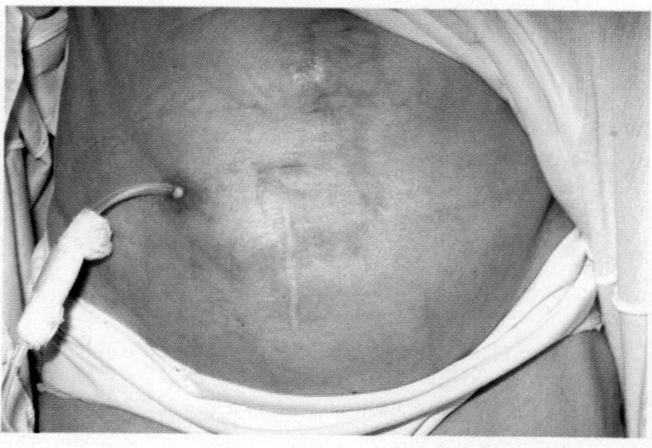

▲ **FIGURE 13.6**
Continuous Ambulatory Peritoneal Dialysis.

Medical-on-line/Alamy

Word Analysis and Definition

S = Suffix P = Prefix R = Root R/CF = Combining Form

WORD	PRONUNCIATION	ELEMENTS		DEFINITION
anuria	an-**YOU**-ree-ah	S/ P/ R/	-ia *condition* an- *a lack of, no* -ur- *urine*	Absence of urine production
dialysis **hemodialysis**	die-**AL**-ih-sis **HE**-moh-die-**AL**-ih-sis	P/ S/ R/CF	dia- *complete* -lysis *destruction* hem/o- *blood*	An artificial method of filtration to remove excess waste materials and water from the body An artificial method of filtration to remove excess waste materials and water directly from the blood
nephritis	neh-**FRY**-tis	S/ R/	-itis *inflammation* nephr- *kidney*	Inflammation of the kidney
oliguria	ol-ih-**GYUR**-ee-ah	S/ P/ R/ R/	-ia *condition* olig *scanty* olig- *scanty* -ur- *urine*	Scanty production of urine
polycystic	pol-ee-**SIS**-tik	S/ P/ R/	-ic *pertaining to* poly- *many* -cyst- *sac, bladder, cyst*	Composed of many cysts
pyelonephritis	**PIE**-eh-loh-neh-**FRY**-tis	S/ R/CF R/	-itis *inflammation* pyel/o- *renal pelvis* -nephr- *kidney*	Inflammation of the kidney and renal pelvis
sibling	**SIB**-ling	S/ R/	-ling *small* sib- *relative*	Brother or sister
transplant	**TRANZ**-plant	P/ R/	trans- *across* -plant *insert, plant*	The act of transferring tissue from one person to another
uremia	you-**REE**-me-ah	S/ R/	-emia *a blood condition* ur- *urine*	The complex of symptoms arising from renal failure

EXERCISES

A. Abbreviations *are commonly used in written and verbal communication. Demonstrate your understanding of kidney disorders by selecting the correct kidney disorder abbreviation that completes each sentence. Not all terms will be used.* **LO 13.3**

CRF **ARF** **PKD** **ESRD**

1. An athlete has sprained her knee. She self-treats it with very large doses of ibuprofen, which can lead to ______.
2. Diabetes that is not well managed can lead to ______ .
3. An inherited disease in which fluid-filled sacs are present within the kidney is known as _______.

B. Identify *the meanings of the word elements in each term. Select the correct answer that completes each statement.* **LO 13.1 and 13.4**

1. The meaning of the prefix in the term *transplant* is:
   a. across **b.** condition **c.** insert **d.** remove
2. The meaning of the prefix in the term *oliguria* is:
   a. urine **b.** scanty **c.** condition **d.** blood
3. The meaning of the suffix in the term *dialysis* is:
   a. urine **b.** condition **c.** destruction **d.** inflammation
4. The prefix *an-* means:
   a. in addition to **b.** move across **c.** surgically remove **d.** lack of
5. The prefix *poly-* means:
   a. sac **b.** fluid **c.** scanty **d.** many

CASE REPORT 13.2

Clinical Note Emergency Department, Fulwood Medical Center 9/12/19

Mr. Justin Leandro, a 37-year-old construction worker, presented at 1520 hrs. He complained of a sudden onset of excruciating pain in his right abdomen and back an hour previously, while at work. The pain is spasmodic and radiates down into his **groin.**

He has vomited once, and keeps having the urge to urinate. He has no previous medical history of significance.

VS: T 99.4°F, P 92, R 20, BP 130/86.

Patient's abdomen is slightly distended, with tenderness in the right upper and lower quadrants and **flank.** A **dipstick** test showed blood in his urine.

Provisional diagnosis by Mark Eagle, MD: stone in the right ureter.

An IV line was started, and 2 mg of morphine sulfate was given by IV push at 1540 hrs. He is going to X-ray STAT for KUB and IVP.

—Andrea Facundo, EMT-P, 1555 hrs.

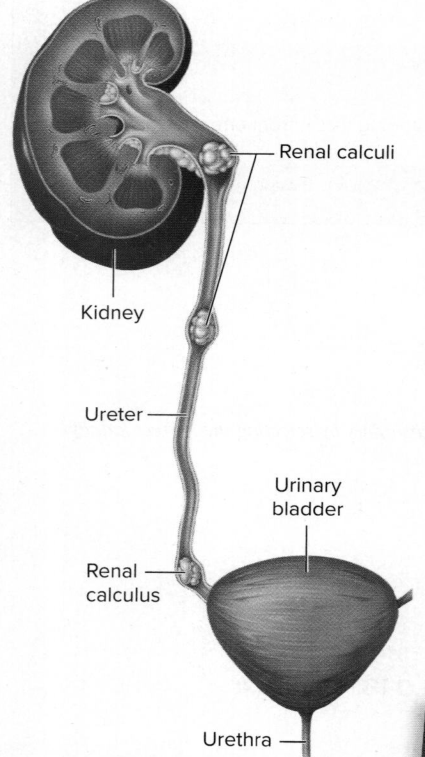

▲ **FIGURE 13.7**
Renal Calculi.
Calculi can become lodged at sites along the urinary tract.

The Ureters (LO 13.4 and 13.7)

Each ureter is a muscular tube, about 10 inches long and ¼ inch wide. The ureters carry urine from the renal pelvis to the urinary bladder. Each ureter lies on the posterior abdominal wall. This is why Mr. Leandro had pain in his back.

The ureters pass obliquely through the bladder's muscle wall. As pressure builds in the filling bladder, the muscle wall compresses the ureters and prevents urine from being forced back up the ureters to the kidneys **(reflux).**

In addition to gravity, muscular **peristaltic** waves, originating in the renal pelvis, squeeze urine down the ureters and squirt it into the bladder. The peristaltic waves are intermittent (come and go), which is why Mr. Leandro's pain was spasmodic.

Kidney and Ureteral Stones (Nephrolithiasis) (LO 13.4 and 13.7)

Stones **(calculi)** begin in the pelvis of the kidney as a tiny grain of undissolved material, usually the minerals uric acid or calcium oxalate *(Figure 13.7)*. When the urine flows out of the kidney, this grain of material is left behind. Over time, more material is deposited and a stone is formed. Most stones enter one of the ureters while they are still small enough to pass down the ureter into the bladder and out of the body in urine.

Case Report 13.2 *(continued)*

Mr. Leandro's KUB (X-ray of **k**idney, **u**reter, and **b**ladder) showed a suspicious lesion halfway down his right ureter. IVP confirmed that this was a stone (renal **calculus**) blocking the ureter and showed the pelvis of the right kidney to be slightly dilated.

Mr. Leandro's stone was large enough to be lodged in the ureter, blocking the flow of urine, with the backflow pressure leading to **hydronephrosis** of the kidney.

Mr. Leandro was kept in the hospital overnight with IV pain medication but did not pass the stone. **Extracorporeal shock wave lithotripsy (ESWL)** was successful in crumbling the stone. He urinated through a strainer so that the stone fragments could be recovered and chemically analyzed.

Abbreviations

ESWL	extracorporeal shock wave lithotripsy
IV	intravenous
KUB	X-ray of abdomen to show Kidneys, Ureters, and Bladder

Word Analysis and Definition

S = Suffix P = Prefix R = Root R/CF = Combining Form

WORD	PRONUNCIATION	ELEMENTS		DEFINITION
calculus **calculi (pl)**	**KAL**-kyu-lus **KAL**-kyu-lie		Latin *pebble*	Small stone
dipstick	**DIP**-stik			A strip of plastic or paper bearing squares of reagent that change color to indicate presence of chemicals
extracorporeal	**EKS**-tra-kor-**POH**-ree-al	S/ P/ R/	-eal *pertaining to* extra- *outside* -corpor- *body*	Outside the body
flank	**FLANK**		Latin *broad*	Side of the body between the pelvis and the ribs
groin	**GROYN**		Old English *groin*	Crease where the thigh joins the abdomen
hydronephrosis **hydronephrotic (adj)**	**HIGH**-droh-neh-**FRO**-sis **HIGH**-droh-neh-**FROT**-ik	S/ R/CF R/CF S/	-osis *condition* hydr/o- *water* -nephr/o- *kidney* -tic *pertaining to*	Dilation of the pelvis and calyces of a kidney Pertaining to or suffering from the dilation of the pelvis and calyces of the kidney
lithotripsy **lithotripter**	**LITH**-oh-trip-see **LITH**-oh-trip-ter	S/ R/CF S/	-tripsy *crushing* lith/o- *stone* -tripter *crusher*	Crushing stones by sound waves Instrument that generates sound waves
nephrolithiasis	**NEF**-roe-lih-**THIGH**-ah-sis	S/ R/CF R/	-iasis *condition, state of* nephr/o- *kidney* -lith- *stone*	Presence of a kidney stone
peristalsis	per-ih-**STAL**-sis	P/ R/	peri- *around* -stalsis *constrict*	Waves of alternate contraction and relaxation of the muscle wall of a tube

EXERCISES

A. After reading Case Report 13.2 and 13.2 (continued), *answer the following questions. Select the correct answer to complete each statement or answer each question.* **LO 13.3, 13.4, 13.6, 13.7, and 13.8**

1. If Mr. Leandro's pain had a "sudden onset," it is termed:

a. acute **b.** chronic

2. Where is the renal calculus located?

a. the organ that filters blood to make urine
b. the organ that breaks down toxins
c. tube that leads from the bladder to the outside of the body
d. tube that leads from the kidney to the bladder

3. Which of the following is the treatment that removed the renal calculus?

a. IVP **b.** ESWL **c.** KUB **d.** EMT-P

B. Match *the element in the first column with the correct meaning in the second column.* **LO 13.1**

_____ **1.** extra **a.** body

_____ **2.** lith **b.** crushing

_____ **3.** corpor **c.** water

_____ **4.** tripsy **d.** stone

_____ **5.** hydro **e.** outside

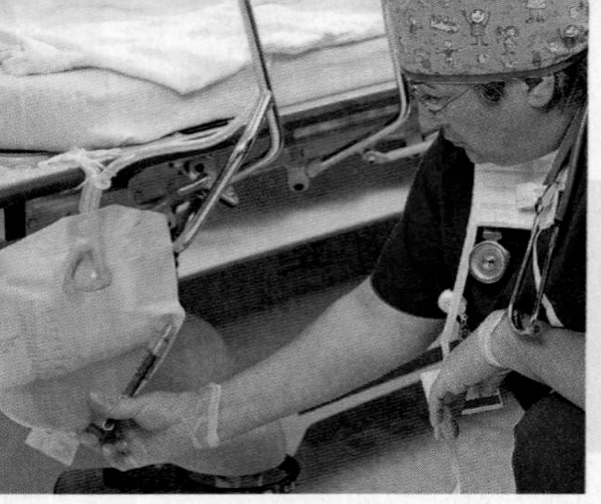

Rick Brady/McGraw-Hill Education

Lesson 13.2

Urinary Bladder and Urethra

Objectives

*The urinary bladder is a temporary storage place for urine before it is **voided** through the **urethra.** A moderately full bladder contains about 500 mL (1 pint) of urine. The maximum capacity of the bladder is around 750 to 800 mL (1½ pints). **Urination,** or emptying of the bladder, is also called **micturition.** The information in this lesson will enable you to use correct medical terminology to:*

13.2.1 Describe the structure and functions of the urinary bladder.

13.2.2 Contrast the differences in structure of the male and female urethras and the incidence of urinary tract infections in the two sexes.

13.2.3 Discuss common disorders of the bladder and urethra.

CASE REPORT 13.3

You are . . .

. . . a medical assistant working in the office of Dr. Susan Lee, a primary care physician, at Fulwood Medical Center.

You are communicating with . . .

. . . Mrs. Caroline Dobson, a 32-year-old housewife. You have asked her the reason for her visit to the office today.

Mrs. Dobson: "Since yesterday afternoon, I've had a lot of pain low down in my belly and in my lower back. I keep having to go to the bathroom every hour or so to pee. It's often difficult to start, and it burns as it comes out. I've had this problem twice before when I was pregnant with my two kids, so I've started drinking cranberry juice. I've been shivering since I woke up this morning, and the last urine I passed was pink. Was that due to the cranberry juice?"

The Urinary Bladder and Urethra (LO 13.5)

Urinary Bladder (LO 13.5)

The urinary bladder is a hollow, muscular organ on the floor of the pelvic cavity, posterior to the pubic symphysis *(Figure 13.8).*

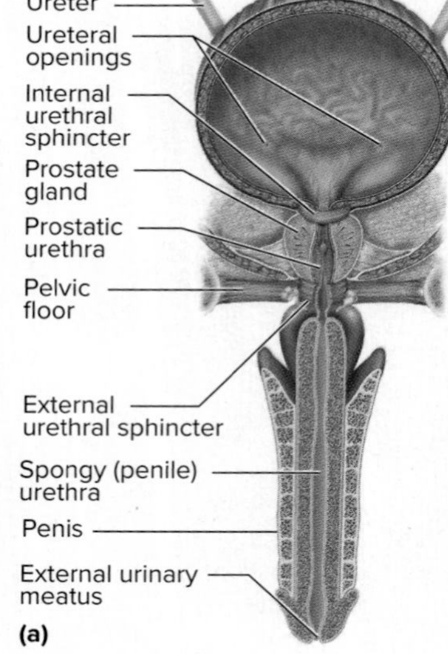

▲ **FIGURE 13.8**
Urinary Bladder.
(a) Male anatomy. (b) Female anatomy.

Urethra (LO 13.5)

The urethra, a thin-walled tube, transports urine from the floor of the bladder to the outside. The base of the bladder's muscular wall is thickened to form the **internal urethral sphincter.** As the urethra passes through the skeletal muscles of the pelvic floor, the **external urethral sphincter** provides voluntary control of urination.

In the male *(Figure 13.8a),* the urethra is 7 to 8 inches long and passes through the penis. In the female *(Figure 13.8b),* the urethra is only about 1½ inches long, and it opens to the outside just above the vagina.

In both the male and female, the opening of the urethra to the outside is called the **external urinary meatus.**

Micturition (LO 13.5)

When the bladder contains about 200 mL or 7 fluid ounces (just less than a cup) of urine, stretch receptors in its wall trigger the **micturition reflex.** Parasympathetic nerves stimulate the bladder's muscle wall to contract and the internal sphincter to relax, and the need to urinate feels urgent. However, voluntary control of the external sphincter can keep that sphincter contracted and can hold urine in the bladder until urination is initiated voluntarily. Involuntary micturition during sleep in older children or adults is called **enuresis.**

Word Analysis and Definition

S = Suffix P = Prefix R = Root R/CF = Combining Form

WORD	PRONUNCIATION	ELEMENTS		DEFINITION
enuresis	en-you-**REE**-sis	S/ R/	-esis *condition* enur- *urinate* in	Involuntary bedwetting
meatus	me-**AY**-tus		Latin *a passage*	The external opening of a passage
micturition (noun)	mik-choo-**RISH**-un	S/ R/	-ition *process* mictur- *pass urine*	Act of passing urine
micturate (verb)	**MIK**-choo-rate	S/	-ate *pertaining to*	Pass urine
reflex	**REE**-fleks		Latin *to bend back*	An involuntary response to a stimulus
sphincter	**SFINK**-ter		Greek *a band*	A band of muscle that encircles an opening; when it contracts, the opening squeezes closed
urethra (**Note:** *One "e" = one tube.*)	you-**REE**-thra		Greek *passage for urine*	Tube that carries urine from bladder to outside
urethral	you-**REE**-thral	R/ S/	urethr- *urethra* -al *pertaining to*	Pertaining to the urethra
void (verb)	**VOYD**		Latin *to empty*	To evacuate urine or feces
voluntary involuntary	**VOL**-un-tare-ee in-**VOL**-un-tare-ee	P/	Latin *voluntary* in- *not*	Acting in obedience to the will Independent of or contrary to the will

EXERCISES

A. Reread *Case Report 13.3 and review all the terms and elements related to the urinary bladder and urethra. Fill in the blanks.*

LO 13.2, 13.5, and 13.7

1. Is Mrs. Dobson suffering from eneuresis? ______________________

2. Has Mrs. Dobson ever had this condition before? ______________________

3. If Dr. Lee feels that Mrs. Dobson might need a referral to a specialist, what kind of specialist would she recommend? ______________________

4. Which two medical terms are used to correctly document Mrs. Dobson's use of the words "to pee"? ______________________

5. What substance may be in Mrs. Dobson's urine, as indicated by the urine's pink color? ______________________

B. Apply your knowledge *of the language of urology to answer the following questions relating to chapter and lesson objectives. Fill in the blanks.*

LO 13.2 and 13.5

1. Describe the location, structure, and function of the urinary bladder:

   Location: ______________________

   Structure: ______________________

   Function: ______________________

2. What is the function of a sphincter? ______________________

3. Which of the two urethral sphincters is voluntary? ______________________

   ____

4. What is the medical term that is used to describe the external opening of the urethra? ______________________

   ____

Lesson 13.2 (cont'd) Disorders of the Urinary Bladder and Urethra

(LO 13.2, 13.5, and 13.8)

Keynotes

- Ten million doctor visits each year are for UTIs.
- Incontinence is not a way of life. It can be helped.
- Cigarette smoking contributes to more than 50% of bladder cancers.

Abbreviation

UTI	urinary tract infection

Urinary Tract Infection (UTI) (LO 13.5)

A urinary tract infection occurs when bacteria invade and multiply in the urinary tract. The bacteria's point of entry is through the urethra. Because the female urethra is shorter than that of the male and opens to the surface near the anus *(Figure 13.9)* bacteria from the GI tract, like *E. coli,* can more easily invade the female urethra. This is why women are more prone to UTIs than men. Once UTIs have occurred, they often recur.

Case Report 13.3 *(continued)*

Mrs. Dobson described many of the symptoms of cystitis. She had **suprapubic** and lower back pain. She had increased frequency of micturition with **dysuria** (difficulty with and pain or burning on urination). Her pink urine is probably **hematuria.**

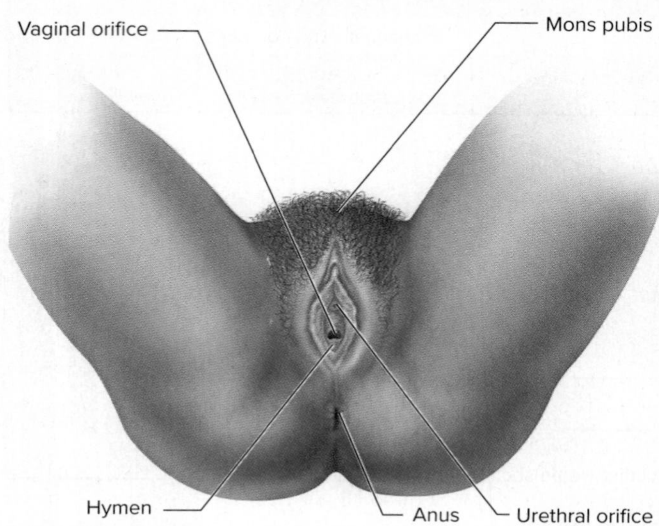

FIGURE 13.9
Female External Genitalia.

An infection of the urethra is called **urethritis; cystitis** is an infection of the urinary bladder. If cystitis is untreated, infection can spread up the ureters to the renal pelvis, causing **pyelitis.** The infection can then travel to the renal cortex and nephrons, causing pyelonephritis.

Pyelonephritis, an inflammation of the renal parenchyma, calyces, and pelvis, is commonly caused by bacterial infection that has spread up the urinary tract, often in association with structural abnormalities in the urinary tract, kidney stones, prostate disease, or **vesicoureteral reflux.** 70 to 80% of the infections are caused by *E. coli* and require aggressive, appropriate antibiotic therapy.

The diagnosis of a UTI can be made through a urinalysis. A culture of the infection-causing organism and testing of its sensitivity to different antibiotics allows the appropriate antibiotic therapy to be prescribed. Cranberry juice can make the urine more acidic and resistant to infection.

Urinary Incontinence (LO 13.5)

Urinary incontinence is a loss of bladder control, which results in wet clothes and bedding. About 12 million adults in America have this condition. Urinary incontinence is most common in women over the age of 50, and it's also seen frequently in elderly men. However, aging alone is not a cause of urinary incontinence.

- **Stress incontinence** is the loss of urine when pressure is exerted on the bladder by coughing, laughing, exercising, or lifting.
- **Urge incontinence** is a sudden, intense urge to urinate followed by an involuntary loss of urine.
- **Overflow incontinence** is the frequent or constant dribbling of urine. It can occur with a damaged bladder; blocked urethra; nerve damage from diabetes, multiple sclerosis, or spinal cord injury; and in men with prostate gland hypertrophy.
- **Functional incontinence** occurs in older adults when a physical or mental impairment prevents them from getting to the toilet in time.
- **Mixed incontinence** is when there are more than one type of incontinence producing symptoms.
- **Total incontinence** is the continuous leakage of urine day and night.

Urinary Retention (LO 13.5)

Urinary retention is the abnormal, involuntary holding of urine in the bladder. **Acute retention** can be caused by an obstruction in the urinary system, like an enlarged prostate in the male. Neurologic problems, like multiple sclerosis, can also be responsible. **Chronic retention** can be caused by an untreated obstruction in the urinary tract, like an enlarged prostate gland.

Bladder Cancer (LO 13.5)

Bladder cancer is more common in men than in women. In fact, it's the fourth most common cancer in men and the eighth most common in women.

Word Analysis and Definition

S = Suffix P = Prefix R = Root R/CF = Combining Form

WORD	PRONUNCIATION	ELEMENTS		DEFINITION
cystitis	sis-**TIE**-tis	S/ R/	-itis *inflammation* cyst- *bladder*	Inflammation of the urinary bladder
dysuria	dis-**YOU**-ree-ah	S/ P/ R/	-ia *condition* dys- *bad, difficult* -ur- *urine*	Difficulty or pain with urination
incontinence **incontinent**	in-**KON**-tin-ence in-**KON**-tin-ent	S/ P/ R/ S/	-ence *state of* in- *not* -contin- *hold together* -ent *pertaining to*	Inability to prevent discharge of urine or feces Denoting incontinence
pyelitis	pie-eh-**LYE**-tis	S/ R/	-itis *inflammation* pyel- *renal pelvis*	Inflammation of the renal pelvis
pyelonephritis	**PIE**-eh-loe-neh-**FRIE**-tis	S/ R/ R/CF	-itis *inflammation* nephr- *kidney* pyel/o *pelvis*	inflammation of the kidney and renal pelvis
retention	ree-**TEN**-shun		Latin *hold back*	Holding back in the body what should normally be discharged (e.g., urine)
suprapubic	**SOO**-prah-**PYU**-bik	S/ P/ R/	-ic *pertaining to* supra- *above* -pub- *pubis*	Above the symphysis pubis
urethritis	you-ree-**THRI**-tis	S/ R/	-itis *inflammation* urethr- *urethra*	Inflammation of the urethra
vesicoureteral reflux	**VEE**-sik-oh-you-**REE**-ter-al **REE**-flucks	S/ R/CF R/ P/ R/	-al *pertaining to* vesic/o- *bladder* -ureter- *ureter* re- *back* -flux *flow*	Backward flow of urine from the bladder into the ureter.

Exercise

A. Define *the different types of disorders related to the urinary bladder and urethra. Choose the correct answer that completes each statement.* **LO 13.5**

1. The portal of entry for bacteria to infect the urinary bladder is the:

a. urethra **b.** ureter **c.** blood **d.** kidney

2. The medical term that defines infection of the bladder is:

a. pyelitis **b.** cystitis **c.** incontinence **d.** retention

3. Diagnosis of a bladder infection is confirmed via:

a. blood test **b.** X-ray of the bladder **c.** ultrasound **d.** urinalysis

4. The medical term incontinence is defined as a(n)

a. inability to empty the bladder
b. loss of the micturition reflex
c. loss of bladder control
d. infection of the bladder and urethra

5. The condition of vesicourethral reflux can be described as:

a. abnormal collection of minerals in the urine
b. inability to empty the bladder
c. backward flow of urine from bladder into the ureter
d. pain with urination

Lesson 13.2 (cont'd) Diagnostic Procedures (LO 13.6)

Methods of Urine Collection

- Random urine collection is taken with no precautions regarding contamination. It is often used for collecting drug testing samples.
- Early morning urine collection is used to determine the ability of the kidneys to concentrate urine following overnight dehydration.
- Clean-catch, midstream urine specimen is collected after the external urethral meatus is cleaned. The first part of the urine is passed, and the sterile collecting vessel is introduced into the urinary stream to collect the last part.
- Twenty-four-hour urine collection is used to determine the amount of protein being excreted and to estimate the kidneys' filtration ability.
- Suprapubic transabdominal needle aspiration of the bladder is used in newborns and small infants to obtain a pure sample of urine.
- Catheterization of the bladder can be used as a last resort to obtain a urine specimen. A soft plastic or rubber tube (catheter) is inserted through the urethra into the bladder to drain and collect urine.

Urinalysis (LO 13.3 and 13.6)

A **dipstick** (a plastic strip bearing paper squares of reagent) is the most cost-effective method of screening urine *(Figure 13.10).* After the stick is dipped into the urine specimen, the color change in each segment of the dipstick is compared to a color chart on the container. Dipsticks can screen for pH, specific gravity, protein, blood, glucose, ketones, bilirubin, **nitrite,** and leukocyte esterase *(see below).*

A **routine urinalysis (UA)** in the lab can include the following tests:

- **Visual observation** examines color and clarity. Normal, healthy urine is pale yellow or amber in color and clear. Cloudiness indicates excess cells or cellular material. Red and cloudy indicates red blood cells.
- **Odor** of normal urine has a slight "nutty" scent. Infected urine has a foul odor. **Ketosis** gives urine a fruity odor.
- **pH** measures how acidic or alkaline urine is.
- **Specific gravity (SG)** measures how dilute or concentrated the urine is.
- **Protein** is not normally detected in urine; its presence **(proteinuria)** indicates infection or urinary tract disease.
- **Glucose** in the urine **(glycosuria)** is a spillover of sugar into the urine when the nephrons are damaged or diseased, or blood sugar is high in uncontrolled diabetes.
- **Ketones** are present in the urine in diabetic **ketoacidosis** *(see Chapter 12)* or in starvation.
- **Leukocyte esterase** indicates the presence of white blood cells in the urine, which can point to a UTI.
- **Urine culture** from a clean-catch specimen *(see box)* is the definitive test for a UTI.

A **microscopic urinalysis** is performed on the solids deposited by centrifuging a specimen of urine. It can reveal:

- **Red blood cells (RBCs), white blood cells (WBCs),** and renal tubular epithelial cells stick together to form **casts,** WBCs stick together to form casts, and bacteria.

Other Diagnostic Procedures (LO 13.3 and 13.6)

Other diagnostic procedures used to test for urinary bladder and urethra infections include:

- **KUB.** An X-ray of the abdomen shows the kidneys, ureters, and bladder.
- **Intravenous pyelogram (IVP).** A contrast material containing iodine is injected intravenously, and its progress through the urinary tract is recorded on a series of X-ray images.
- **Retrograde pyelogram.** Contrast material is injected through a urinary catheter into the ureters and kidneys to locate stones and other obstructions.
- **Voiding cystourethrogram (VCUG).** Contrast material is inserted into the bladder through a catheter and X-rays are taken as the patient voids.
- **CT scan.** X-ray images show cross-sectional views of the kidneys and bladder.
- **MRI.** Magnetic fields are used to generate cross-sectional images of the urinary tract.
- **Ultrasound imaging.** High-frequency sound waves and a computer generate noninvasive images of the kidneys.
- **Renal angiogram.** X-rays with contrast material are used to assess blood flow to the kidneys.
- **Cystoscopy.** A pencil-thin, flexible, tube-like optical instrument is inserted through the urethra into the bladder to examine the bladder's lining and to take a biopsy if needed *(Figure 13.11).*

Abbreviations

IVP	Intravenous pyelogram
RBC	red blood cell
SG	specific gravity
UA	urinalysis
VCUG	voiding cystourethrogram
WBC	white blood cell

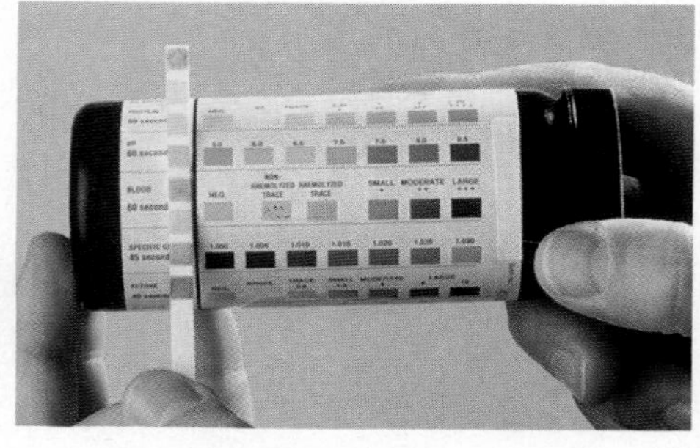

▲ **FIGURE 13.10** Urinalysis Dipstick Being Compared Against Color Chart on Container.

Saturn Stills/Science Source

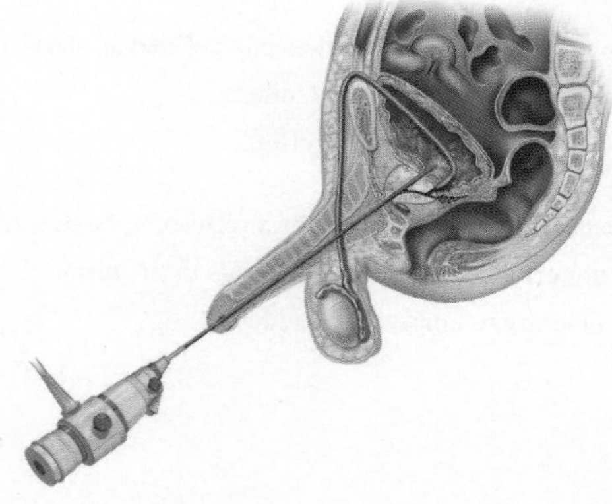

▲ **FIGURE 13.11** Cystoscopy.

Word Analysis and Definition

S = Suffix P = Prefix R = Root R/CF = Combining Form

WORD	PRONUNCIATION	ELEMENTS		DEFINITION
cast	KAST		Latin *pure*	A cylindrical mold formed by materials in kidney tubules
cystoscope cystoscopy	**SIS**-toh-skope sis-**TOS**-koh-pee	S/ R/CF S/	-scope *instrument for viewing* cyst/o- *bladder* -scopy *to examine*	An endoscope inserted to view the inside of the bladder The process of using a cystoscope
cystourethrogram	sis-toh-you-**REETH**-roe-gram	S/ R/CF R/CF	-gram *a record* cyst/o- *bladder* -urethr/o- *urethra*	X-ray image during voiding to show structure and function of bladder and urethra
glycosuria (**Note:** *The "s" is added to make the word flow.*)	**GLYE**-koh-**SYU**-ree-ah	S/ R/CF R/	-ia *condition* glyc/o- *glucose* -ur- *urinary system*	Presence of glucose in urine
ketone ketosis ketoacidosis	**KEY**-tone key-**TOE**-sis **KEY**-toe-as-ih-**DOE**-sis	 S/ R/CF R/CF	Greek *acetone* -sis *abnormal condition* ket/o- *ketones* -acid/o- *acid, low pH*	Chemical formed in uncontrolled diabetes or in starvation Excess production of ketones Excessive production of ketones, making the blood acid
nitrite	**NI**-trite		Greek *niter, saltpeter*	Chemical formed in urine by *E. coli* and other microorganisms
proteinuria	pro-tee-**NYU**-ree-ah	S/ R/ R/	-ia *condition* protein- *protein* -uri- *urine*	Presence of protein in urine
retrograde	**RET**-roh-grade	P/ R/	retro- *backward* -grade *going*	Reversal of a normal flow; for example, back from the bladder into the ureters
urinalysis	you-rih-**NAL**-ih-sis	S/ R/CF	-lysis *to separate* urin/a- *urine*	Examination of urine to separate it into its elements and define their kind and/or quantity

EXERCISES

A. Apply your knowledge *of medical language to this exercise. Select the best answer.* **LO 13.6**

1. An X-ray image taken during voiding: **a.** retrograde pyelogram **b.** angiogram **c.** cystourethrogram
2. Presence of glucose in urine: **a.** hematuria **b.** polyuria **c.** glycosuria
3. Urine collection method to test for proteinuria: **a.** catheterization **b.** 24 hour **c.** clean catch
4. Reversal of normal flow: **a.** reflex **b.** retrograde **c.** regenerate
5. Excessive ketones in the blood, making it acid: **a.** ketosis **b.** ketoacidosis **c.** ketone
6. Separate urine into its elements: **a.** urinalysis **b.** cystourethrogram **c.** retrograde pyelogram

B. Demonstrate your knowledge *of abbreviations and the medical terms they represent. Insert the medical terms that each abbreviation represents. Fill in the blanks.* **LO 13.2, 13.3, and 13.6**

1. KUB ____________________
2. UA ____________________
3. IVP ____________________
4. VCUG ____________________

C. Employ *the language of urology and match the correct diagnostic procedure in the first column with the correct statement in the second column.* **LO 13.3 and 13.6**

_____ **1.** KUB **a.** uses contrast material
_____ **2.** cystoscopy **b.** X-ray
_____ **3.** renal angiogram **c.** invasive procedure to view the inside of the urinary bladder
_____ **4.** CT scan **d.** cross-sectional views
_____ **5.** ultrasound imaging **e.** noninvasive procedure that uses sound waves to view internal structures

Lesson 13.2 (cont'd)

Therapeutic Procedures (LO 13.6)

Abbreviations

BPH	benign prostate hyperplasia
CAPD	continuous ambulatory peritoneal dialysis
CCPD	continuous cycling peritoneal dialysis
ESWL	extracorporeal shock wave lithotripsy
TURP	transurethral resection of the prostate

Renal Stones (LO 13.4)

Renal stones are of four types: calcium oxalate stone are the most common; uric acid stones are more common in men; struvite stones occur mostly in women with UTIs; cystine stones are very rare. For renal stones that do not pass down the ureter into the bladder and out of the body in urine, there are several treatment options:

- **Watchful waiting.** With pain medication to relieve symptoms, the hope is that the stone can be passed.
- **Extracorporeal shock wave lithotripsy (ESWL).** With ESWL, a machine called a **lithotripter** from outside the body generates sound waves that crumble the stone into small pieces that can pass down the ureter into the bladder and be voided.
- **Ureteroscopy.** A small, flexible **ureteroscope** is passed through the urethra and bladder into the ureter. Devices can be passed through the endoscope to remove or fragment the stone.
- **Percutaneous nephrolithotomy.** A **nephroscope** is inserted through the skin and into the kidney to locate and remove the stone.
- **Open surgery.** A surgical incision is made to expose the ureter and remove the stone; this is rarely done.

Kidney Failure (LO 13.4)

Dialysis is an artificial method of removing waste materials and excess fluid from the blood in end-stage renal disease. It is not a cure, but can prolong life. There are several types of kidney dialysis: In treatment of acute renal failure (ARF), the goal is to treat the underlying disease. Dialysis may be necessary while the kidneys are healing.

- **Hemodialysis** (*Figure 13.12*) filters the blood through an artificial kidney machine (**dialyzer**). Most patients require 12 hours of dialysis weekly, usually in three sessions.
- **Peritoneal dialysis** uses a solution that is infused into and drained out of the patient's abdominal cavity through a small flexible catheter implanted into the patient's abdominal cavity. The dialysis solution extracts wastes and excess fluid from the blood through the network of capillaries in the peritoneal lining of the abdominal cavity.
  - **Continuous ambulatory peritoneal dialysis (CAPD)** (*Figure 13.13*) is performed by the patient at home usually four times each day, seven days a week.
  - **Continuous cycling peritoneal dialysis (CCPD)** uses a machine to automatically infuse dialysis solution into and out of the abdominal cavity during sleep.

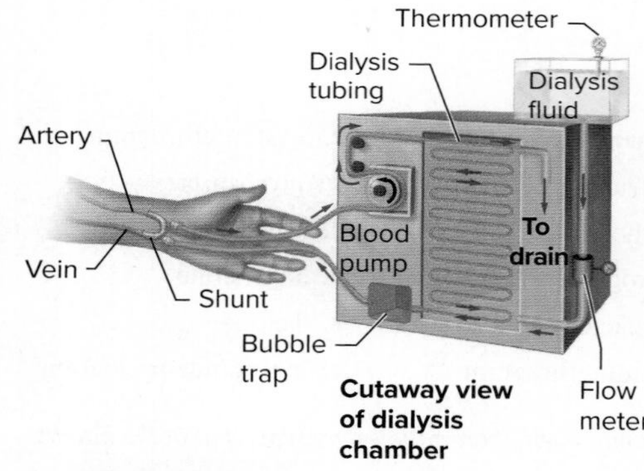

▲ **FIGURE 13.12**
Hemodialysis.

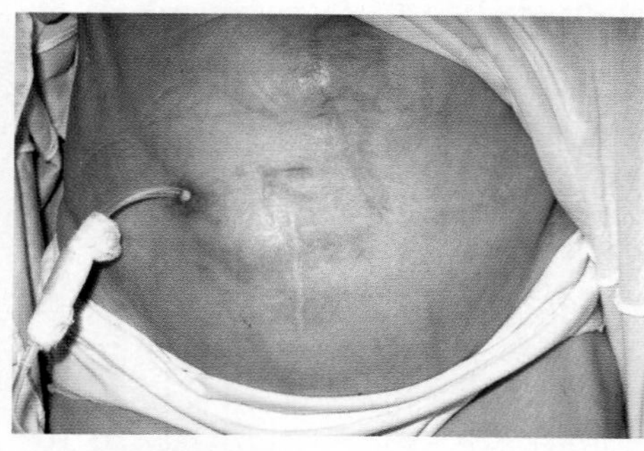

▲ **FIGURE 13.13**
Continuous Ambulatory Peritoneal Dialysis.
Medical-on-line/Alamy

A **kidney transplant** provides a better quality of life than dialysis, provided a suitable donor can be found. A **sibling** or blood relative can often qualify as a donor. If not, tissue banks across the country can search for a kidney from an accident victim or a donor who has died.

Urinary Bladder (LO 13.4)

Cystoscopy can be used therapeutically to remove stones and to perform a transurethral resection of the prostate (**TURP**) to remove tissue from the inner portion of the prostate gland in men with benign prostatic hyperplasia (**BPH**).

For acute or chronic lower urinary tract obstruction in which the urethra is blocked, a flexible urethral catheter (**Foley catheter**) is passed into the bladder. The catheter can be left indwelling, or the patient can perform clean intermittent catheterization. If a Foley catheter cannot be passed, a suprapubic tube can be placed through the lower anterior abdominal wall into the bladder.

Treatment for urinary incontinence depends on the cause. If a medical or surgical problem is present, then the incontinence can go away when the problem is treated. **Bladder training** and **biofeedback** lengthen the time between the urges to go to the toilet. **Kegel exercises** strengthen the muscles of the pelvic floor. Medications, for example oxybutynin, are used for urge incontinence. Surgery can pull up the bladder and secure it if pelvic floor muscles are weak (**cystopexy**). Absorbent underclothing is available.

Word Analysis and Definition

S = Suffix P = Prefix R = Root R/CF = Combining Form

WORD	PRONUNCIATION	ELEMENTS		DEFINITION
ambulatory	**AM**-byu-lah-tor-ee	S/ R/	-ory *relating to* ambulat- *walk*	Relating to walking
catheter	**KATH**-eh-ter		Greek *to send down*	Hollow tube that allows passage of fluid into or out of a body cavity, organ, or vessel.
cystopexy	**SIS**-toh-pek-see	S/ R/CF	-pexy *surgical fixation* cyst/o- *bladder*	Surgical procedure to support the urinary bladder
dialysis dialyzer hemodialysis	die-AL-ih-sis die-**A**-lie-zer **HEE**-moh-die-**AL**-ih-sis	P/ R/ S/ R/CF	dia- *complete* -lysis *to separate* -lyzer *separator* hem/o *blood*	An artificial method of filtration to remove excess waste materials and water from the body. Machine that performs dialysis. An artificial machine-based method to remove wastes from the blood
extracorporeal	**EKS**-trah-kor-**POH**-ree-al	S/ P/ R/	-eal *pertaining to* extra- *outside* -corpor- *body*	Outside the body
Kegel exercises	**KEE**-gal **EKS**-er-size-ez		Arnold Kegel, 1894–1981, American gynecologist	Contraction and relaxation of the pelvic floor muscles to improve urethral and rectal sphincter function
lithotripsy lithotripter	**LITH**-oh-trip-see **LITH**-oh–trip-ter	S/ R/CF S/	-tripsy *to crush* lith/o- *stone* -tripter *crusher*	Crushing stones by sound waves Instrument that generates the sound waves
nephrolithotomy	**NEF**-roh-lih-**THOT**-oh-mee	S/ R/CF R/CF	-tomy *surgical incision* nephr/o- *kidney* lith/o- *stone*	Incision to remove a renal stone
nephroscope nephroscopy	**NEF**-roh-skope neh-**FROS**-koh-pee	S/ R/CF S/	-scope *instrument for viewing* nephr/o- *kidney* -scopy *to examine*	Endoscope to view the inside of the kidney Visual examination of the kidney
percutaneous	**PER**-kyu-**TAY**-nee-us	S/ P/ R/CF	-us *pertaining to* per- *through* cutane/o- *skin*	Pertaining to through the skin
transplant	**TRANZ**-plant	P/ R/	trans- *across* -plant *insert, plant*	The act of transferring tissue from one person to another
ureteroscope ureteroscopy	you-**REE**-ter-oh-skope you-**REE**-ter-**OS**-koh-pee	S/ R/CF S/	-scope *instrument for viewing* ureter/o *ureter* -scopy *to examine*	Endoscope to view the inside of the ureter Endoscopic examination of the inside of the ureter

Exercises

A. Abbreviations are used in written and verbal communication. *Complete each sentence with the correct abbreviations. Use the provided abbreviations to fill in the blanks.* **LO 13.3 and 13.6**

BPH **CAPD** **CCPD** **ESWL** **TURP**

1. The nephrologist recommended that the patient have ______________________ to assist in the passing of his kidney stones.
2. Because of his ______________________, Mr. Plaza suffered from overflow incontinence.
3. Mrs. Doskos prefers to receive her dialysis while she sleeps, and therefore the nephrologist recommended ______________________ to dialyze her blood.
4. ______________________ is used to remove sections of an enlarged prostate.
5. ______________________ allows the patient to walk around while receiving dialysis.

B. Construct terms using word elements. *Given the definition, complete each medical term with the correct missing element. Fill in the blanks. The first one has been done for you.* **LO 13.1 and 13.6**

1. Relating to walking — ambulat/ory
2. Surgical procedure to support the urinary bladder. — cysto/ ______________
3. Visual examination of the kidney. — ______________ /scopy
4. Pertaining to through the skin. — ______________ /cutaneo/us
5. Incision to remove a stone. — nephro/litho/ ______________
6. Artificial method to remove wastes from the blood. — ______________ /dia/lysis

Lesson 13.2 (cont'd) Urinary Tract Pharmacology

(LO 13.2 and 13.6)

The kidneys represent 0.5% of total body weight but receive approximately 25% of the total arterial blood pumped by the heart. When necessary, **diuretics** are prescribed to increase the output of urine in order to maintain homeostasis. There are several types of diuretics:

1. **Thiazides** are medium-potency diuretics used in mild heart failure and moderate hypertension. Examples are chlorothiazide (Diuril) and hydrochlorothiazide (HydroDiuril). A major side effect is loss of potassium.

2. **Loop diuretics** have a strong but brief diuresis and are the most potent diuretics available. The most commonly used is furosemide (Lasix), and it also has a major side effect of potassium loss.

3. **Potassium-sparing diuretics** such as spironolactone (Aldactone), which has been used since 1959 and is gradually being replaced by newer agents such as eplerenone (Inspra), are used for reducing cardiovascular risk following myocardial infarction. **Hyperkalemia** can be a side effect. All of these are not potent diuretics.

4. **Carbonic anhydrase inhibitors** such as acetazolamide (Diamox) are not in use as diuretics anymore, but they are used in open-angle glaucoma (*see Chapter 11*) and to prevent altitude sickness in mountain climbers.

5. An **osmotic diuretic,** such as mannitol (Osmitrol), is given intravenously and used occasionally to prevent renal failure or decrease intracranial pressure.

Alcohol also acts as a diuretic.

Uric acid, in the form of sodium urate crystals, contributes to the formation of kidney stones and produces the pain of gout when deposited in joints. **Uricosuric agents,** such as probenecid (Probalan), increase the excretion of uric acid by the kidneys and are used to prevent recurrences of kidney stones and to treat gout.

Medications used to treat incontinence include:

- **Anticholinergics,** which calm an overactive bladder and include oxybutynin (Ditropan), tolterodine (Detrol), and darifenacin (Enablex).

- **Antidepressants** imipramine (Tofranil) and duloxetine (Cymbalta) may be used to treat stress incontinence.

Word Analysis and Definition

S = Suffix P = Prefix R = Root R/CF = Combining Form

WORD	PRONUNCIATION	ELEMENTS		DEFINITION
anticholinergic	**AN**-tee-koh-lih-**NER**-jik	S/ P/ R/ R/	**-ic** *pertaining to* **anti-** *against* **-cholin-** *choline* **-erg-** *work*	Antagonistic to parasympathetic nerve fibers
antidepressant	**AN**-tee-dee-**PRESS**-ant	S/ P/ P/ R/	**-ant** *pertaining to* **anti-** *against* **de-** *without* **-press-** *press close, press down*	An agent used to counteract depression
hyperkalemia	**HIGH**-per-kah-**LEE**-me-ah	S/ P/ R/	**-emia** *blood condition* **hyper-** *excess* **-kal-** *potassium*	An excessive amount of potassium in the blood
osmosis **osmotic (adj)**	os-**MOH**-sis os-**MOT**-ik	S/ R/ S/	**-sis** *process* **osmo-** *push* **-tic** *pertaining to*	The passage of a solvent across a cell membrane
potent	**POH**-tent		Latin *power*	Possessing strength, power
thiazide	**THIGH**-ah-zide	S/ R/	**-ide** *having a special quality* **thiaz-** *blue dye*	Abbreviated form of benzothiadiazide, a class of diuretic
uric acid	**YUR**-ik **ASS**-id		Latin *relating to urine*	A chemical of white crystals poorly soluble in urine
uricosuric	**YUR**-ih-koh-**SU**-rik	S/ R/CF	**-suric** *excess* **uric/o** *urine*	Pertaining to excessive amounts of uric acid in urine

EXERCISE

A. Deconstruct *the following medical terms into their elements.* **LO 13.1**

1. osmotic ______________ / ______________
R, R/CF S

2. uricosuric ______________ / ______________
R, R/CF S

3. antidepressant ______________ / ______________ / ______________ / ______________
P P R, R/CF S

4. hyperkalemia ______________ / ______________ / ______________
P R, R/CF S

5. thiazide ______________ / ______________
R, R/CF S

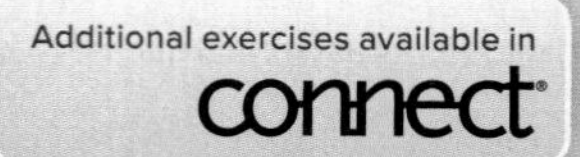

Chapter Review exercises, along with additional practice items, are available in Connect!

The Male Reproductive System

CHAPTER 14

The Essentials of the Language of the Male Reproductive System

Rick Brady/McGraw-Hill Education

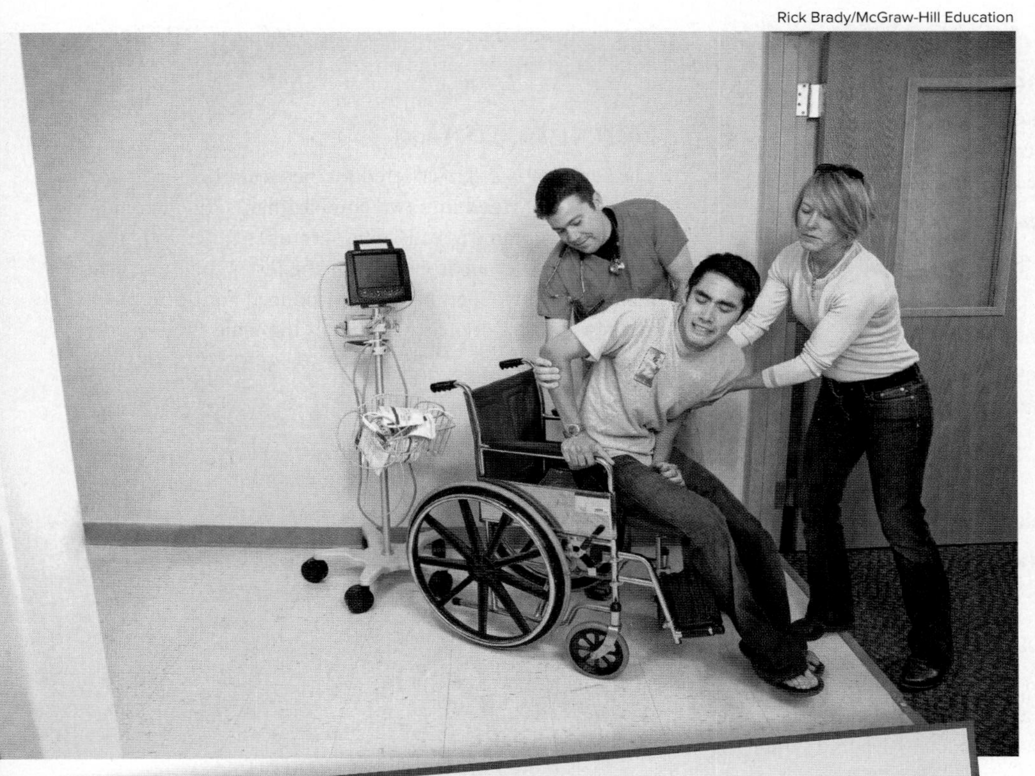

CASE REPORT 14.1

You are . . .

. . . an EMT-P working in the Emergency Department at Fulwood Medical Center.

You are communicating with . . .

. . . Joseph Davis, a 17-year-old high school senior, who has been brought in by his mother at 0400 hrs.

Joseph is complaining of **(c/o)** a sudden onset of pain in his left **testicle,** which began 3 hours earlier and woke him up. The pain is intense and has made him vomit. VS: T 99.2°F, P 88, R 15, BP 130/70. An examination reveals his left testicle to be enlarged, warm, and tender. His abdomen is normal to palpation.

At your request, Dr. Helinski, the emergency physician on duty, examines Joseph immediately. He diagnoses a **torsion** (twisting) of the patient's left testicle.

Learning Outcomes

As you set up the next stage of Joseph's treatment, immediate clinical decisions will need to be made. You will have to communicate clearly with Dr. Helinski, other health professionals, the patient, and the patient's family. You will also need to document the patient's care. In order to participate effectively in this process, you must be able to:

LO 14.1 **Use roots, combining forms, suffixes, and prefixes to construct and analyze (deconstruct) medical terms related to the male reproductive system.**

LO 14.2 **Spell and pronounce correctly medical terms related to the male reproductive system in order to communicate them with accuracy and precision in any health care setting.**

LO 14.3 **Define accepted abbreviations related to the male reproductive system.**

LO 14.4 **Describe the anatomy of the perineum, scrotum, testes, and spermatic cords and their functions, disorders, and treatments.**

LO 14.5 **Relate the anatomy and anatomical positions of the five accessory glands of the male reproductive system to their functions and disorders.**

LO 14.6 **Describe disorders of the prostate gland and their diagnosis and treatment.**

LO 14.7 **Relate the structure of the penis to its functions, disorders, and treatments.**

LO 14.8 **Explain the causes of male infertility and their treatments.**

LO 14.9 **Identify sexually transmitted diseases, their prevention, and treatments.**

LO 14.10 **Describe diagnostic and therapeutic procedures and pharmacology used to treat disorders of the male reproductive system.**

LO 14.11 **Apply your knowledge of medical terms relating to the male reproductive system to documentation, medical records, and medical reports.**

LO 14.12 **Translate the medical terms relating to the male reproductive system into everyday language in order to communicate clearly with patients and their families.**

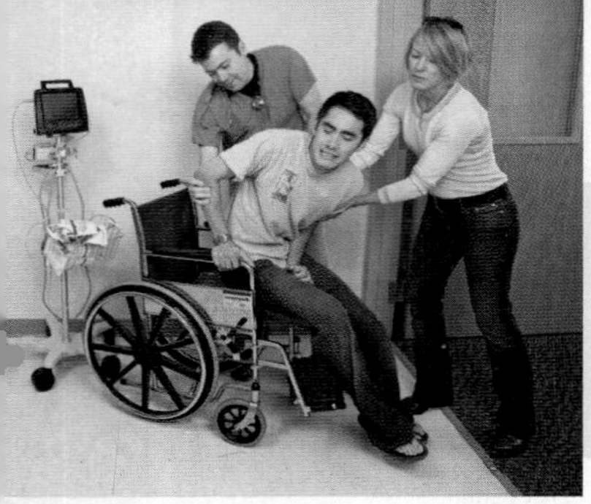

Rick Brady/McGraw-Hill Education

Lesson 14.1

The Male Reproductive System

Objectives

Unlike every other organ system, the reproductive system is not essential for an individual human to survive. However, without the reproductive system, the human species could not survive. The information in this lesson will enable you to use correct medical terminology to:

14.1.1 Identify the components of the male reproductive system.

14.1.2 Describe the male external genitalia.

14.1.3 Explain the structure and functions of the testes.

14.1.4 Outline the process of **spermatogenesis** and the structure of a sperm.

14.1.5 Distinguish common disorders of the testes.

Abbreviation

c/o complaining of

Male Reproductive System (LO 14.4, 14.5, and 14.7)

The **male reproductive organ system** *(Figure 14.1)* consists of the primary and secondary sex organs, and the accessory glands. These are categorized as follows:

1. The **primary sex organs,** or **gonads,** are the two **testes.**
2. The **secondary sex organs** include:
   a. The **penis;**
   b. The **scrotum;** and
   c. A system of ducts, including the **epididymis, ductus (vas) deferens,** and **urethra.**
3. The accessory glands include:
   a. The **prostate;**
   b. The **seminal vesicles;** and
   c. The **bulbourethral glands.**

Perineum (LO 14.4)

The external **genitalia** (the penis, scrotum, and testes) occupy the **perineum,** a diamond-shaped region between the thighs. The perineum borders the pubic symphysis anteriorly and the coccyx posteriorly *(Figure 14.2).* The anus is also in the perineum.

Scrotum (LO 14.4)

The scrotum is a skin-covered sac between the upper thighs. It is divided into two compartments. Each compartment contains a testis. The scrotum's function is to provide a cooler environment for the testes than that inside the body. **Sperm** are best produced and stored at a few degrees cooler than that of the male's internal body temperature.

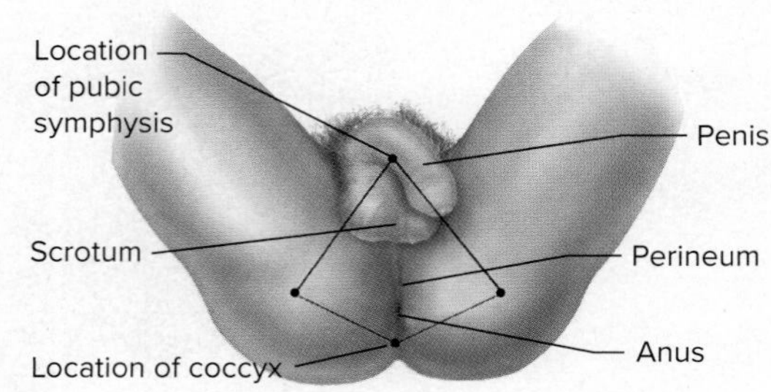

▲ **FIGURE 14.2**
Male Perineum.

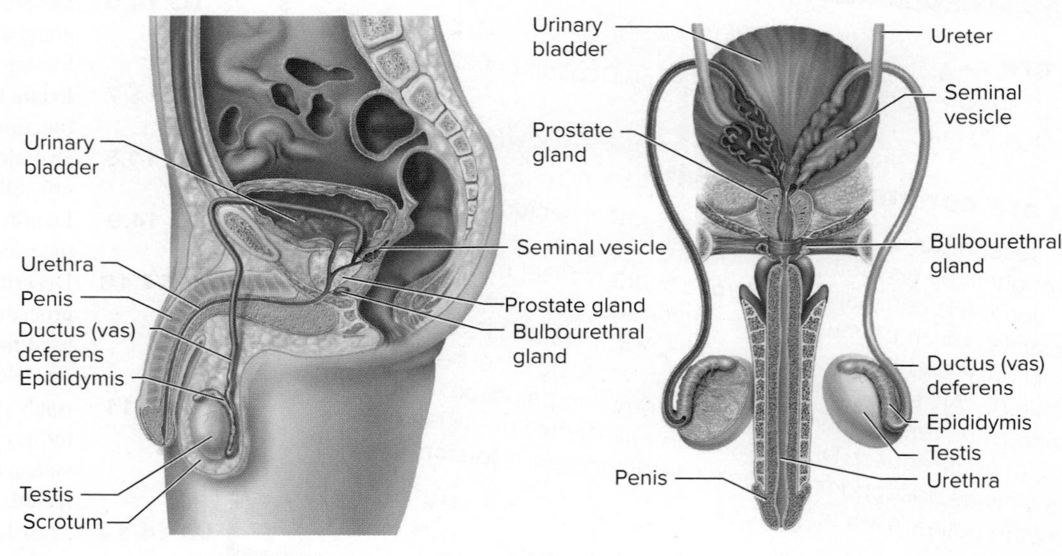

▶ **FIGURE 14.1**
Male Reproductive System.
(a) Male pelvic cavity, midsagittal section.
(b) Male reproductive organs.

Word Analysis and Definition

S = Suffix P = Prefix R = Root R/CF = Combining Form

WORD	PRONUNCIATION	ELEMENTS		DEFINITION
bulbourethral	**BUL**-boh-you-**REE**-thral	S/ R/CF R/	**-al** *pertaining to* **bulb/o-** *bulb* **-urethr-** *urethra*	Pertaining to the bulbous penis and urethra
ductus deferens (*same as* **vas deferens**)	**DUK**-tus **DEH**-fuh-renz VAS		ductus, Latin *to lead* deferens, Latin *carry away* vas, Latin *vessel, canal*	Tube that receives sperm from the epididymis
epididymis	**EP**-ih-**DID**-ih-miss	P/	**epi-** *above* **-didymis** *testis*	Coiled tube attached to testis
genitalia (Note: *Two suffixes*) **genital (adj)**	**JEN**-ih-**TAY**-lee-ah **JEN**-ih-tal	S/ S/ R/	**-ia** *condition* **-al-** *pertaining to* **genit-** *primary male or female sex organs*	External and internal organs of reproduction Pertaining to reproduction or to the male or female sex organs
gonad **gonads (pl)** **gonadal**	**GO**-nad **GO**-nadz go-**NAD**-al	 R/ S/	Greek *seed* **gonad-** **-al** *pertaining to*	Testis or ovary Pertaining to the testis or ovary
penis **penile (adj)**	**PEE**-nis **PEE**-nile	 S/ R/	Latin *tail* **-ile** *pertaining to* **pen-** *penis*	Conveys urine and semen to the outside Pertaining to the penis
perineum **perineal (adj)**	**PER**-ih-**NEE**-um **PER**-ih-**NEE**-al	 S/ R/	Greek *perineum* **-al** *pertaining to* **perine-** *perineum*	Area between the thighs, extending from the coccyx to the pubis Pertaining to the perineum
scrotum **scrotal (adj)**	**SKRO**-tum **SKRO**-tal	 S/ R/	Latin *scrotum* **-al** *pertaining to* **scrot-** *scrotum*	Sac containing the testes Pertaining to the scrotum
seminal vesicle	**SEM**-in-al **VES**-ih-kull	S/ R/ S/ R/	**-al** *pertaining to* **semin-** *semen* **-le** *small* **vesic-** *sac containing fluid*	Sac of the ductus deferens that produces seminal fluid
sperm **spermatozoa (pl)** **spermatic (adj)** **spermatogenesis**	SPERM **SPER**-mat-oh-**ZOH**-ah **SPER**-mat-ik **SPER**-mat-oh-**JEN**-eh-sis	 S/ R/CF S/ S/	Greek *seed* **-zoa** *animal* **spermat/o-** *sperm* **-ic** *pertaining to* **-genesis** *creation, formation*	Mature male sex cell Sperm (plural) Pertaining to sperm The process by which male germ cells differentiate into sperm
testicle **testicular (adj)** **testis** **testes (pl)**	**TES**-tih-kul tes-**TICK**-you-lar **TES**-tis **TES**-teez	 S/ R/	Latin *small testis* **-ar** *pertaining to* **testicul-** *testicle* Latin *testis*	One of the male reproductive glands Pertaining to the testicle Same as testicle
torsion	**TOR**-shun		Latin *to twist*	The act or result of twisting

EXERCISES

A. Use *medical terms related to the anatomy of the male reproductive system. Select the correct answer to complete each statement.* **LO 14.4**

1. The penis, scrotum, and testes collectively are known as:

a. primary sex organs **b.** accessory glands **c.** secondary sex organs **d.** external genitalia **e.** the perineum

2. The male gonads are the:

a. scrotum **b.** penis **c.** prostate **d.** ductus deferens **e.** testes

3. The medical term that refers to the area between the thighs is the:

a. perineum **b.** raphae **c.** spermatic cord **d.** genitalia **e.** varicocele

B. Using *the information presented in Case Report 14.1, document the case in the patient's record. Use the following terms to fill in the blanks. One term will be used twice.* **LO 14.2**

testicular **testes** **testicle**

This patient presented to the ED because of pain in his left (1.) __________. Both (2.) _____________ were examined, but the left (3.) ______________was enlarged, warm, and tender. The emergency physician on duty diagnosed (4.) ______________torsion. Patient will be scheduled for surgery immediately.

Lesson 14.1 (cont'd)

Testes and Spermatic Cord (LO 14.4)

Testes (LO 14.4)

In the adult male, each testis is a small, oval organ that measures about 2 inches long and ¾ of an inch wide *(Figure 14.3)*. Each testis is covered by a serous membrane–the **tunica vaginalis**–which has outer and inner layers that are separated by serous fluid.

Inside the testis are some 250 lobules (small lobes); each contains three or four **seminiferous tubules,** which produce **semen.** Within these tubules are several layers of germ cells that are in the process of developing into sperm. Between the seminiferous tubules are the interstitial (occurring between tissues) cells. These cells produce hormones called **androgens.**

Testosterone is the major androgen produced by the interstitial cells of the testes. Its effects include the stimulation of the following activities:

1. **Spermatogenesis,** *(Figure 14.4)* which is the process of production of spermatozoa (sperm).
2. The development of the male secondary sex characteristics at puberty, which include:
   - **a.** The enlargement of the testes, scrotum, and penis.
   - **b.** The development of the pubic, axillary, body, and facial hair.
   - **c.** The secretion of sebum in skin, which can result in acne *(Chapter 3)*.
3. A burst of growth at puberty, including an increased muscle mass, a higher basal metabolic rate **(BMR),** and a larger larynx (which deepens the voice).
4. Stimulating the brain to increase the male's **libido** (sex drive).

Keynotes

- The sperm count of a 65-year-old man is approximately one-third of the count when he was 20.
- The spermatic cord can be palpated through the skin of the scrotum.

Abbreviation

BMR basal metabolic rate

Spermatic Cord (LO 14.4)

The blood vessels and nerves to the testes–which arise in the abdominal cavity–pass through the inguinal, or groin, canal, where they join with connective tissue. This forms the **spermatic cord** that suspends each testis in the scrotum *(Figure 14.3)*. The left testis is suspended lower than the right. Within the cord exist:

- an artery
- a **plexus** of veins
- nerves
- a thin muscle
- the ductus (vas) deferens into which sperm are deposited when they leave the testis

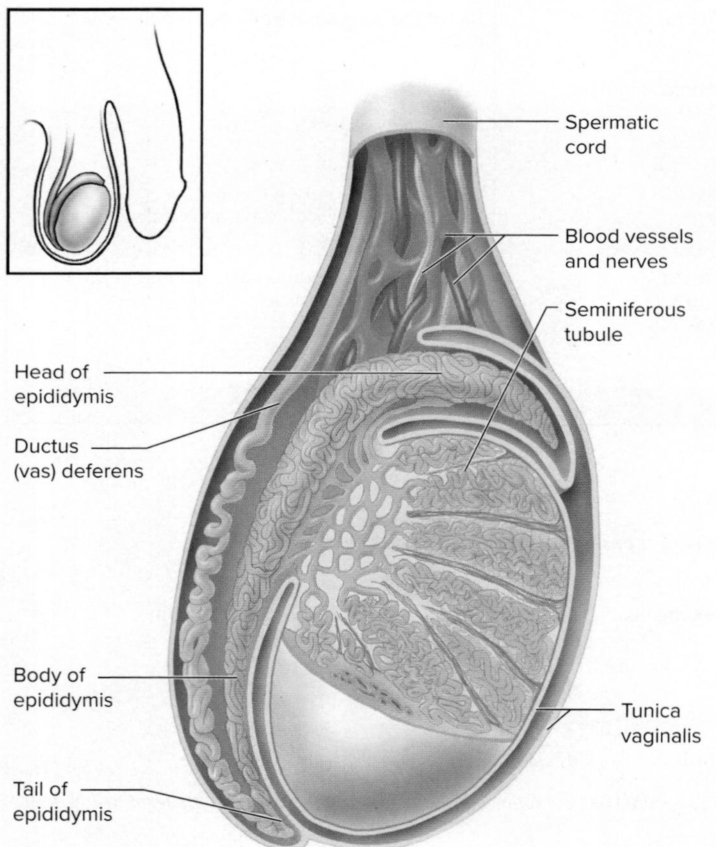

▲ **FIGURE 14.3**
The Testis and Associated Structures.

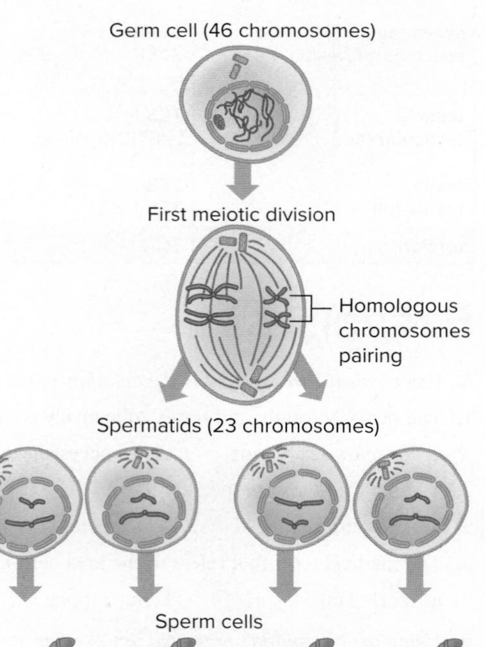

▲ **FIGURE 14.4**
Spermatogenesis.

Word Analysis and Definition

S = Suffix P = Prefix R = Root R/CF = Combining Form

WORD	PRONUNCIATION	ELEMENTS		DEFINITION
androgen	**AN**-droh-jen	S/ R/CF	-gen *create, produce* andr/o- *masculine*	Hormone that promotes masculine characteristics
libido	lih-**BEE**-doh		Latin *lust*	Sexual desire
plexus **plexuses (pl)**	**PLEK**-sus **PLEK**-sus-ez		Latin *braid*	A weblike network of joined nerves
semen **seminiferous (adj)**	**SEE**-men sem-ih-**NIF**-er-us	 S/ R/ R/	Latin *seed* -ous *pertaining to* semin/i- *semen* -fer- *to bear, carry*	Penile ejaculate containing sperm and seminal fluid Pertaining to carrying semen
testosterone	tes-**TOSS**-ter-own	S/ R/CF	-sterone *steroid* test/o- *testis*	Powerful androgen produced by testes
tunica vaginalis	**TYU**-nih-kah vaj-ih-**NAHL**-iss	 S/ R/	tunica, Latin *coat* -alis *pertaining to* vagin- *sheath, vagina*	Covering, particularly of a tubular structure The tunica vaginalis is the sheath of the testis and epididymis

EXERCISES

A. Write *the correct medical term to answer the question.* **LO 14.2, 14.3, and 14.4**

1. What is the name of the serous membrane that covers the testis? ______________________

2. The term *seminiferous* pertains to: ______________________

3. What is another medical term for sex drive? ______________________

4. What does the abbreviation BMR stand for? ______________________

5. What structure supports the testes? ______________________

B. Use *medical terms related to the testes and spermatic cord. Select the correct answer to complete each statement.* **LO 14.4**

1. The major androgen of the male reproductive system:

a. estrogen **b.** testosterone **c.** semen **d.** cortisone **e.** spermatid

2. That which suspends each testis in the scrotum is the:

a. spermatic cord **b.** ductus deferens **c.** dartos muscle **d.** interstitial cells **e.** tunica

3. The ductus deferens is the:

a. plexus of veins in the spermatic cord

b. structure that produces sperm

c. the tube carries sperm through the spermatic cord

d. covering of each testis

Lesson 14.1 (cont'd) Testes and Spermatic Cord (continued)

Keynotes

- The testis in testicular torsion will die in approximately 6 hours unless the blood supply is restored.
- Self-examination of the testes (TSE) for swelling or tenderness should be performed monthly by all men.

Abbreviations

TSE	testicular self-examination
STD	sexually transmitted disease

Sperm (LO 14.4)

A mature sperm has a pear-shaped head and a long tail. The sperm's head contains these three segments *(Figure 14.5)*:

- The **nucleus,** which contains 23 chromosomes;
- The **cap,** which contains enzymes used to penetrate the egg; and
- The **basal body** of the tail.

The tail is further divided into three segments and is responsible for movement as the sperm swims up the female reproductive tract.

Case Report 14.1 *(continued)*

Joseph Davis presented with typical symptoms and signs of testicular torsion. The affected testis rapidly became painful, tender, swollen, and inflamed. Emergency surgery was performed, and the testis and cord were manually untwisted through an incision in the scrotum. The testis was stitched to surrounding tissues to prevent a recurrence of the torsion.

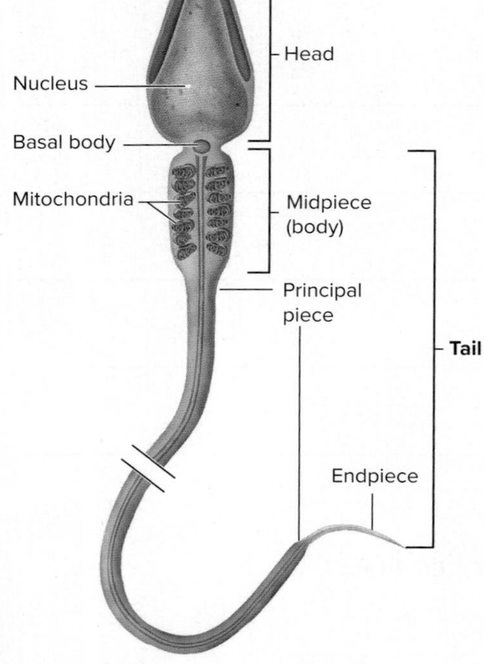

▲ **FIGURE 14.5**
Mature Sperm.

Disorders of the Testes (LO 14.4)

Testicular torsion is the twisting of a testis on its spermatic cord. The testicular artery in the twisted cord becomes blocked, and the blood supply to the testis is cut off. The condition occurs in men between puberty and age 25. In half the cases, it starts in bed at night, as it did for Joseph Davis in Case Report 14.1.

Varicocele is a condition in which the veins in the spermatic cord become dilated and painful as varicose veins. If it is uncomfortable, it can be treated by surgically tying off the affected veins.

Hydrocele is a collection of excess fluid in the space between the visceral and parietal layers of the tunica vaginalis of the testis *(Figure 14.6)*. It is most common after age 40. The diagnosis can be confirmed by transillumination *(Figure 14.6),* shining a bright light on the scrotal swelling to see the shape of the testis through the surrounding translucent excess fluid.

Spermatocele is a collection of sperm in a sac formed in the epididymis, which is the sperm-containing tube attached to a testicle. It occurs in about 30% of men, is benign, and rarely causes symptoms. It does not require treatment unless it becomes uncomfortable.

Cryptorchism occurs when a testis fails to descend from the abdomen into the scrotum before a boy is 12 months old.

Epididymitis is an inflammation of the epididymis; **epididymoorchitis (orchitis)** is an inflammation of the epididymis and testis. Orchitis, an inflammation of the testis, is usually a consequence of epididymitis. In each of these cases, the inflammation is most commonly caused by a bacterial infection spreading from an infection in the urinary tract or prostate. These infections can also be caused by sexually transmitted diseases **(STDs),** like gonorrhea or chlamydia.

A viral cause of orchitis is mumps. In males past puberty who develop mumps, 30% will develop orchitis, and 30% of those will develop resulting testicular atrophy. A bilateral infection can result in infertility. Mumps is avoidable by immunization in childhood.

Testicular cancer is the most common cancer in males aged 20-39 years. One of the first signs is often a lump in the testis, which may be found through self-examination of the testes. Metastasis is uncommon, but it can be seen in the lungs, in the abdominal and cervical lymph nodes, and occasionally in the brain.

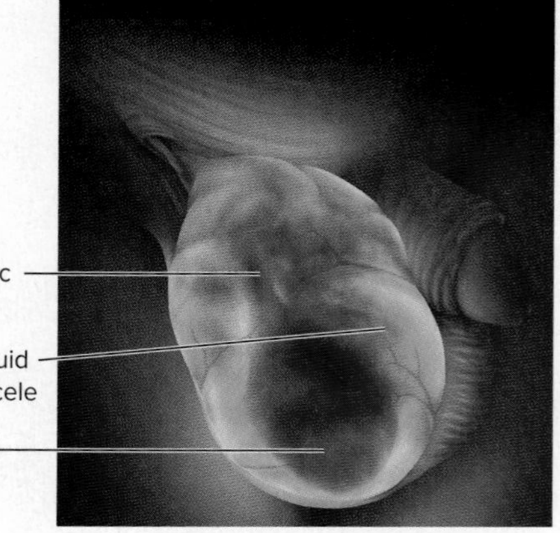

▶ **FIGURE 14.6**
Transillumination of Hydrocele Showing Testis and Spermatic Cord.
Brian Evans/Science Source

Word Analysis and Definition

S = Suffix P = Prefix R = Root R/CF = Combining Form

WORD	PRONUNCIATION	ELEMENTS		DEFINITION
cryptorchism	krip-**TOR**-kizm	S/ P/ R/	**-ism** *condition* **crypt-** *hidden* **-orch-** *testicle*	Failure of one or both testes to descend into the scrotum
epididymitis	**EP**-ih-did-ih-**MY**-tis	S/ R/	**-itis** *inflammation* **epididym-** *epididymis*	Inflammation of the epididymis
epididymoorchitis *(same as* **orchitis***)* (**Note:** *One of the two consecutive "i"s is not used.*)	ep-ih-**DID**-ih-moh-or-**KIE**-tis	S/ R/CF R/	**-itis** *inflammation* **epididym/o-** *epididymis* **-orchi-** *testicle*	Inflammation of the epididymis and testicle
hydrocele	**HIGH**-droh-seal	S/ R/CF	**-cele** *swelling* **hydr/o-** *water*	Collection of fluid in the space of the tunica vaginalis
inguinal	**IN**-gwin-al	S/ R/	**-al** *pertaining to* **inguin-** *groin*	Pertaining to the groin
orchiectomy	or-key-**ECK**-toe-me	S/ R/	**-ectomy** *surgical excision* **orchi-** *testicle*	Removal of one or both testes
orchiopexy	**OR**-key-oh-**PEK**-see	S/ R/CF	**-pexy** *surgical fixation* **orchi/o-** *testicle*	Surgical fixation of a testis in the scrotum
orchitis (**Note:** *One of the two consecutive "i"s is not used.*)	or-**KIE**-tis	S/	**-itis** *inflammation*	Inflammation of the testis
spermatocele	**SPER**-mat-oh-seal	S/ R/CF	**-cele** *swelling* **spermat/o-** *sperm*	Cyst of the epididymis that contains sperm
varicocele	**VAIR**-ih-koh-seal	S/ R/CF	**-cele** *swelling* **varic/o-** *varicosity*	Varicose veins of the spermatic cord

EXERCISES

A. Construct *medical terms related to disorders of the testes. Fill in the blanks.* **LO 14.1 and 14.4**

1. Inflammation of the epididymis: ______________________/itis
2. Failure of a testicle to descend into the scrotum: ______________________/______________________ /ism
3. Swelling containing fluid: ______________________/cele
4. Inflammation of the testis: orch/ ______________________
5. Varicose veins of the spermatic cord: varico/ ______________________

B. Build your knowledge *of the language of the male reproductive system by correctly answering the questions regarding the elements in the following terms. Select the best answer.* **LO 14.1 and 14.4**

1. In the term *hydrocele,* the R/CF means:
 a. testis **b.** water **c.** sperm
2. In the term *cryptorchism,* the element *crypt* means:
 a. outside of **b.** behind **c.** hidden
3. In the term *spermatocele,* the suffix means:
 a. water **b.** swelling **c.** sperm
4. In the term *epididymitis,* which element means inflammation?
 a. epi **b.** epididym **c.** itis
5. In the term *epididymoorchitis,* the element *orchi* means:
 a. threadlike **b.** testicle **c.** hidden

Study Hint

Before you attempt to answer the question, divide each term into its components with a slash. This will help you identify which element is referred to in the question.

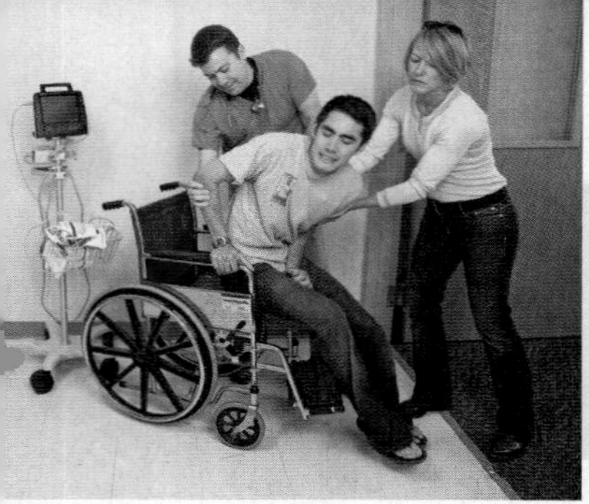

Rick Brady/McGraw-Hill Education

Lesson 14.2

Spermatic Ducts, Accessory Glands, and Penis

CASE REPORT 14.2

You are . . .

. . . a surgical technologist (LCC-ST) working for urologist Phillip Johnson, MD, in the Urology Clinic at Fulwood Medical Center.

You are communicating with . . .

. . . Mr. Ronald Detrick, a 60-year-old man, who has been referred to the Urology Clinic.

Patient Interview

Mr. Detrick complains of having to get out of bed to urinate four or five times at night. He has difficulty starting urination, has a weak stream, and feels he is not emptying his bladder completely. He has lost interest in sex. His physical examination is unremarkable except that a digital rectal examination (DRE) reveals a diffusely enlarged **prostate** with no nodules.

Objectives

*The male prostate and urethra have both **urological** and **reproductive** functions, as the flow of urine and semen goes through both organs. Disorders of the prostate and urethra produce symptoms and signs that arise in both areas. The information provided in this lesson will enable you to use correct medical terminology to:*

14.2.1 Trace the pathway taken by a sperm cell from a testis to the sperm cell's ejaculation.

14.2.2 Identify the structure and functions of the prostate and other male accessory glands.

14.2.3 Describe the origins and functions of semen.

14.2.4 Discuss common disorders of the prostate gland.

14.2.5 Integrate the structures and functions of the penis and its disorders.

Keynotes

- Semen is derived from the secretions of several glands:
  - 5% comes from the testicles and epididymis (sperm).
  - 50% to 80%, from the seminal vesicles.
  - 15% to 33%, from the prostate gland.
  - 2% to 5%, from the bulbourethral glands.
- A normal sperm count is in the range of 75 to 150 million sperm per milliliter (mL) of semen. A normal ejaculation consists of 2 to 5 mL of semen.

Abbreviations

DRE	digital rectal examination
LCC-ST	Liaison Council on Certification for the Surgical Technologist
mL	milliliter

Spermatic Ducts (LO 14.5)

As the sperm cells mature in the testes over a 60-day period, they move down the seminiferous tubules into the epididymis for storage. The epididymis adheres to the posterior side of the testis. It is a single-coiled duct or tube in which the sperm are stored for 12 to 20 days until they mature and become **motile** (capable of movement).

To be ejaculated, the sperm move into the ductus (vas) deferens, the **ejaculatory** duct, and finally the urethra to reach the outside of the body.

The ductus (vas) deferens is a muscular duct that travels up from the epididymis in the scrotum, passes behind the urinary bladder, and joins with the duct of the seminal vesicle to form the ejaculatory duct, which empties sperm and semen into the urethra.

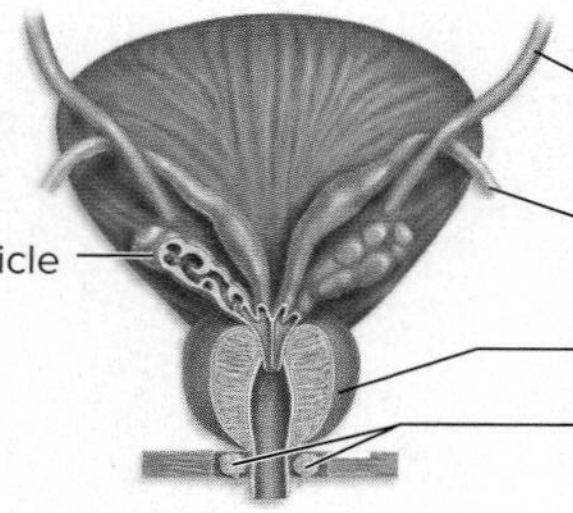

Accessory Glands (LO 14.5)

The five accessory glands *(Figure 14.7)* are:

1. The two **seminal vesicles,** located on the posterior surface of the urinary bladder, hold fluid that mixes with the sperm in the vas deferens. The fluid is rich in sugar to provide nourishment for the sperm and has clotting properties that make the semen sticky.
2. The single **prostate gland** is close in size and shape to the average walnut. The prostate gland is located immediately below the bladder and anterior to the rectum. It surrounds the urethra and the ejaculatory duct. It is composed of 30 to 50 glands that open directly into the urethra; these glands secrete fluid that nourishes and protects sperm. During ejaculation, the prostate squeezes this fluid into the urethra to form part of semen.
3. The two **bulbourethral glands,** are located one on either side of the membranous urethra. Each gland has a short duct leading into the spongy (penile) urethra. When sexually aroused, the glands produce a fluid that neutralizes any acidity in the urethra to make a more hospitable environment in which the sperm can travel.

FIGURE 14.7
The Five Accessory Glands of the Male Reproductive System.

Word Analysis and Definition

S = Suffix P = Prefix R = Root R/CF = Combining Form

WORD	PRONUNCIATION		ELEMENTS	DEFINITION
ejaculate (can be a verb or a noun)	ee-**JACK**-you-late	S/ R/	**-ate** *composed of, pertaining to* **ejacul-** *shoot out*	To expel suddenly; *or* the semen expelled in ejaculation
ejaculation (noun)	ee-**JACK**-you-**LAY**-shun	S/	**-ation** *process*	Process of expelling semen suddenly
ejaculatory (adj)	ee-**JACK**-you-lah-**TOR**-ee	S/	**-atory** *pertaining to*	Pertaining to ejaculation
motile	**MOH**-til	S/ R/	**-ile** *pertaining to* **mot-** *to move*	Capable of spontaneous movement
motility	moh-**TILL**-ih-tee	S/ R/	**-ity** *condition, state* **motil-** *to move*	The ability for spontaneous movement
prostate	**PROS**-tate **(Note:** *not* **PROS**-trate, *which means exhausted)*		Greek *one standing before*	Gland surrounding the beginning of the urethra
prostatic (adj)	pros-**TAT**-ik	S/ R/	**-ic** *pertaining to* **prostat-** *prostate*	Pertaining to the prostate

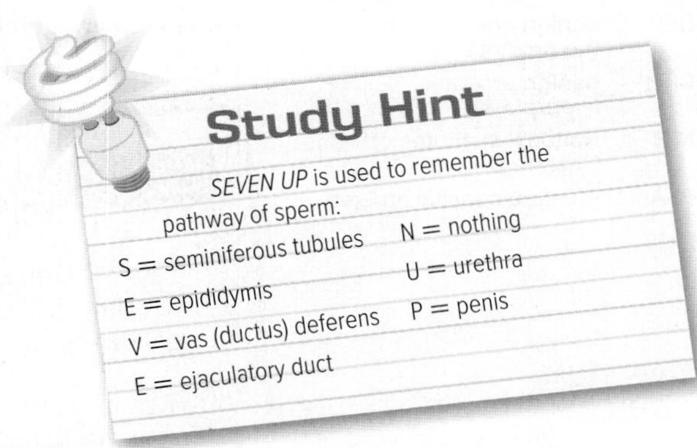

EXERCISES

A. Review *Case Report 14.2 and then answer the following questions. Fill in the blanks.* **LO 14.2, 14.3, 14.5, and 14.11**

1. Does Mr. Detrick have a strong libido? ______________________________

2. What does the abbreviation *DRE* mean? ______________________________

3. Which gland had an abnormality? ______________________________

4. Did Dr. Johnson find any other abnormalities? (yes or no) ______________________________

5. What is responsible for Mr. Detrick's symptoms? ______________________________

B. Recall and review. *Become familiar with the terms pertaining to the spermatic ducts and accessory gland and how they depict clinical conditions related to the male reproductive system. Fill in the blanks.* **LO 14.1 and 14.5**

1. After leaving the testis, sperm are stored in the________.

2. The ____________ glands secrete a fluid that neutralizes the pH in the male urethra.

3. The walnut-sized gland of the male reproductive system is the ________ gland.

4. What is the abbreviation for the procedure in which a finger is inserted into the rectum to evaluate the prostate gland? ______

5. The structure that empties semen into the urethra is the ______ duct.

Keynotes

- Survival from prostate cancer is up to 80% if it is detected before it spreads outside the gland.
- Male infertility is involved in 40% of the 2.6 million infertile married couples in the United States. [Source: National Institutes of Health (NIH)]
- Vasectomy is almost 100% successful in producing male sterility.

Abbreviations

BEP	benign enlargement of the prostate
BPH	benign prostatic hyperplasia
NIH	National Institutes of Health
PSA	prostate-specific antigen

Disorders of the Prostate Gland (LO 14.6)

Benign prostatic hyperplasia (BPH), also known as benign prostatic hypertrophy or **benign enlargement of the prostate (BEP)**—a noncancerous enlargement of the prostate—can cause symptoms starting around age 45; by age 80, some 90% of men have symptoms. This enlargement is one of **hyperplasia** (number of cells) rather than **hypertrophy** (size of cells), and it compresses the prostatic urethra to produce symptoms including:

- Difficulty starting and stopping the urine stream.
- **Nocturia** (excessive nighttime urination), **polyuria** (excessive urine production), and dysuria (difficulty or pain in urination).

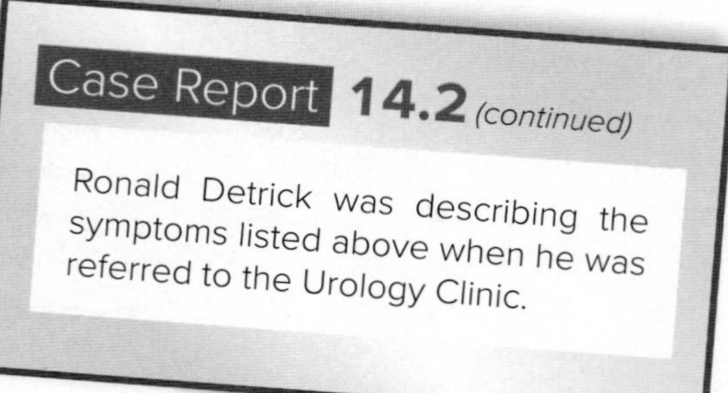

Prostatic cancer affects 10% of men over the age of 50, and its incidence is increasing. It forms hard nodules in the periphery of the gland and is often asymptomatic (produces no symptoms) in its early stages, as it does not compress the urethra.

Prostatitis is an inflammation of the prostate gland that causes groin pain and difficulty and discomfort when urinating.

Male Infertility (LO 14.8)

Infertility is the inability of a couple to conceive after one year of unprotected intercourse. **Male infertility** is the man's inability to produce or deliver fully functioning sperm. The main causes of male infertility are:

- Impaired sperm production, due to cryptorchidism, anorchism (absence of one or both testes), testicular trauma, testicular cancer, or orchitis after puberty.
- Impaired sperm delivery, due to infections and blockage of spermatic ducts.
- **Sperm disorders,** in which sperm are underdeveloped, abnormally shaped, unable to move properly, produced in abnormally low numbers **(oligospermia),** or not produced at all **(azoospermia).**
- **Varicoceles,** in which the dilated scrotal veins impair sperm production by preventing proper drainage of blood within the testes.
- Testosterone deficiency **(hypogonadism).** Phthalates in plastics and dioxins in paper are examples of environmental endocrine disrupters that can contribute to testosterone deficiency.

Word Analysis and Definition

S = Suffix P = Prefix R = Root R/CF = Combining Form

WORD	PRONUNCIATION	ELEMENTS		DEFINITION
azoospermia	a-zoh-oh-**SPER**-me-ah	S/ P/ R/ R/	-ia *condition* a- *without* -zoo- *animal* -sperm- *seed*	Absence of living sperm in the semen
oligospermia	**OL**-ih-go-**SPER**-me-ah	P/	oligo- *too few*	Deficient numbers of sperm in the semen
hyperplasia	**HIGH**-per-**PLAY**-zee-ah	S/ P/ R/	-ia *condition* hyper- *excessive* -plas- *molding, formation*	Increase in the *number* of the cells in a tissue or organ
hypertrophy **(Note:** *See Study Hint below.)*	high-**PER**-troh-fee	S/	-trophy *development*	Increase in the *size* of the cells in a tissue or organ
hypogonadism	**HIGH**-poh-**GOH**-nad-izm	S/ P/ R/	-ism *condition* hypo- *deficient* -gonad- *testis or ovary*	Deficient gonad production of sperm, eggs, or hormones
infertility	in-fer-**TIL**-ih-tee	S/ P/ R/	-ity *condition* in- *not* -fertil- *able to conceive*	Failure to conceive
nocturia	nok-**TYU**-ree-ah	S/ P/ R/	-ia *condition* noct- *night* -ur- *urine*	Excessive urination at night
polyuria	pol-ee-**YOU**-ree-ah	S/ P/ R/	-ia *condition* poly- *excessive* -ur- *urine*	Excessive production of urine
prostatitis	pros-tah-**TIE**-tis	S/ R/	-itis *inflammation* prostat- *prostate*	Inflammation of the prostate
resectoscope	ree-**SEK**-toe-skope	S/ R/CF	-scope *instrument for viewing* resect/o- *cut off*	Endoscope for the transurethral removal of lesions
transurethral	**TRANS**-you-**REE**-thral	S/ P/ R/	-al *pertaining to* trans- *across, through* -urethr- *urethra*	Procedure performed through the urethra

Study Hint

Word association for **hypertrophy:**

Hypertrophy relates to an increase in **size.**

Remember that sports **trophies** come in all **sizes.**

EXERCISES

A. Translate *medical terms into everyday language. Use the terms below to correctly fill in the blanks. Not all terms will be used.* **LO 14.1, 14.2, 14.6, and 14.12**

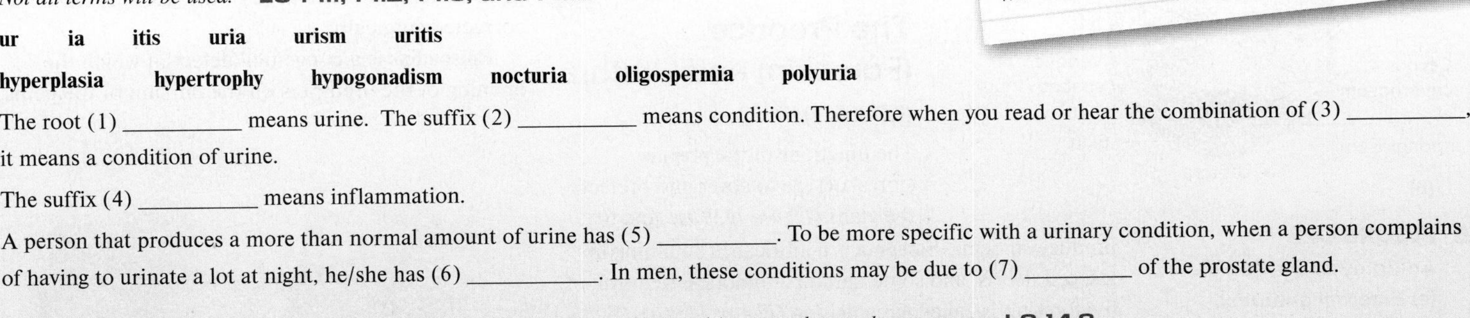

ur ia itis uria urism uritis

hyperplasia hypertrophy hypogonadism nocturia oligospermia polyuria

The root (1) __________ means urine. The suffix (2) __________ means condition. Therefore when you read or hear the combination of (3) __________, it means a condition of urine.

The suffix (4) __________ means inflammation.

A person that produces a more than normal amount of urine has (5) __________. To be more specific with a urinary condition, when a person complains of having to urinate a lot at night, he/she has (6) ___________. In men, these conditions may be due to (7) _________ of the prostate gland.

B. Remember *the definitions related to male infertility. Select the correct answer(s) to complete each statement.* **LO 14.8**

1. Male infertility is defined as the inability to: (choose two answers)

a. produce sperm **c.** secrete adequate amounts of prostatic fluid
b. have unprotected sex **d.** deliver fully functioning sperm

2. The term **hypogonadism** is defined as:

a. undescended testicle(s) **b.** lack of seminal fluid **c.** testosterone deficiency **d.** reduced production of sperm

3. A lack of sperm production can be caused by: (choose all that apply)

a. dioxins in paper **b.** decreased libido **c.** dilated scrotal veins **d.** absence of one or both testicles

Lesson 14.2 (cont'd)

Keynotes

- Erectile dysfunction occurs in some 20 million American men.
- Erectile dysfunction can be associated with diabetes, stroke, multiple sclerosis, hypertension, cigarette smoking, radiation therapy, drugs such as antidepressants and cholesterol-lowering medications, and loss of interest in one's sexual partner.

Penis (LO 14.7)

The **penis** *(Figure 14.8(a))* is an important male external body structure, which is specifically designed to meet its two main functions:

- To enable urine to flow to the outside.
- To deposit semen in the female vagina around the cervix.

The external, visible part of the penis is composed of the **shaft** and the more sensitive **glans.** The external urethral meatus is located at the tip of the glans. The skin of the penis continues over the glans as the **prepuce,** otherwise known as the foreskin. A ventral fold of tissue called the **frenulum** attaches the foreskin to the glans.

The shaft of the penis contains these three **erectile** vascular bodies *(Figure 14.8(b)):*

- The paired **corpora cavernosa** (columns of erectile tissue found in the penis) are located dorsolaterally.
- The single **corpus spongiosum** is located inferiorly. It contains the urethra and goes on to form the glans.

Erection occurs when the corpora cavernosa fill with blood, causing the erectile bodies to distend and become rigid. It is a parasympathetic nervous system response to stimulation.

Ejaculation occurs when the sympathetic nervous system stimulates the smooth muscle of the ductus deferens, ejaculatory ducts, and the glands in the prostate to contract.

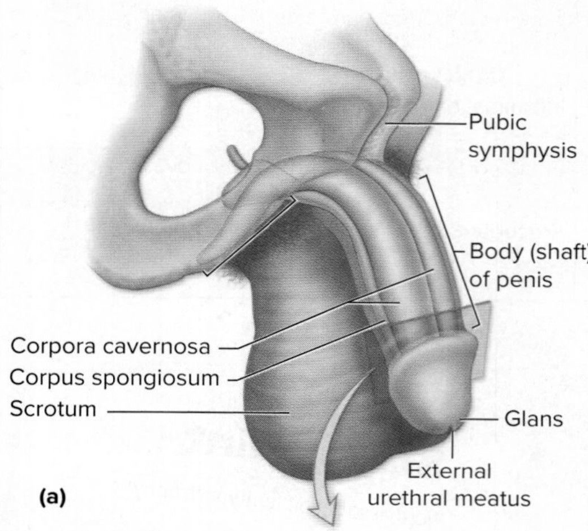

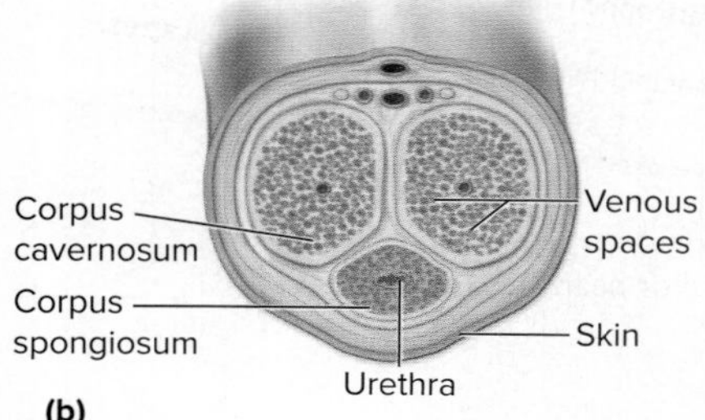

▲ **FIGURE 14.8**
Anatomy of the Penis.
(a) External anatomy.
(b) Cross-sectional view.

The Prepuce (Foreskin) and Urethra (LO 14.7)

The functions of the **prepuce** (foreskin) are to cover and protect the glans *(Figure 14.9(b)),* and to produce smegma. **Smegma** is a lubricant containing lipids, cell debris, and some natural antibiotics. Removal of the foreskin is called **circumcision** *(Figure 14.9(a)).*

Disorders of the Penis (LO 14.7)

Disorders involving the penis range from minor injuries to STDs to cancer. These conditions are outlined below.

Trauma to the penis can vary from being caught in a pants' zipper to being fractured while erect during vigorous sexual intercourse.

Priapism is a persistent, painful erection that occurs when blood cannot escape from the erectile tissue. It can be caused by drugs like epinephrine, by blood clots, or by spinal cord injury.

Cancer of the penis occurs most commonly on the glans and is rare in circumcised men.

Sexually transmitted diseases (STDs) are discussed in detail later in this chapter and in *Chapter 15.*

Erectile dysfunction (ED), or **impotence,** is the inability to have a satisfactory erection. Treatment is aimed at addressing any underlying disease.

Premature ejaculation is more common than erectile dysfunction. It occurs when a man ejaculates so quickly during intercourse that it causes distress or embarrassment to one or both partners.

Disorders of the Prepuce (LO 14.7)

- **Balanitis** is an infection of the glans and foreskin with bacteria or yeast.
- **Phimosis** is a condition in which the foreskin is tight because of a small opening and cannot be retracted over the glans for cleaning. It can lead to balanitis.
- **Paraphimosis** is a condition in which the retracted foreskin cannot be pulled forward to cover the glans.

Disorders of the Penile Urethra (LO 14.7)

Urethritis is an inflammation of the urethra. It can be caused by bacteria, STDs, viruses, and chemical irritants from **spermicides** and contraceptive gels.

Urethral stricture is scarring that narrows the urethra. It results from infection or injury.

Hypospadias is a congenital defect in which the opening of the urethra is on the undersurface of the penis instead of at the head of the glans. It can be corrected surgically.

Epispadias is a congenital defect in which the opening of the urethra is on the dorsum of the penis.

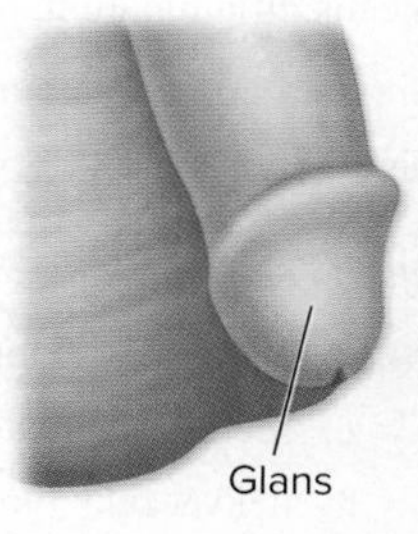

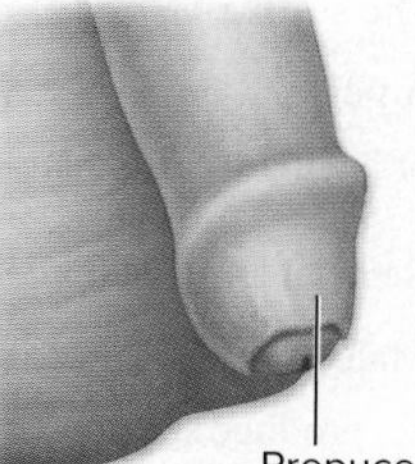

▲ **FIGURE 14.9**
Prepuce.
(a) Circumcised penis. (b) Uncircumcised penis.

Abbreviations

ED	erectile dysfunction
STD	sexually transmitted disease

Word Analysis and Definition

S = Suffix P = Prefix R = Root R/CF = Combining Form

WORD	PRONUNCIATION		ELEMENTS	DEFINITION
balanitis	bal-ah-**NIE**-tis	S/ R/	-itis *inflammation* balan- *glans penis*	Inflammation of the glans and prepuce of the penis
cavernosa	kav-er-**NOH**-sah	S/ R/	-osa *like* cavern- *cave*	Resembling a cave
circumcision	ser-kum-**SIZH**-un	S/ P/ R/	-ion *action, condition* circum- *around* -cis- *to cut*	To remove part or all of the prepuce
corpus **corpora (pl)**	**KOR**-pus kor-**POR**-ah		Latin *body*	Major part of a structure
epispadias	ep-ih-**SPAY**-dee-as	S/ P/ R/	-ias *condition* epi- *above* -spad- *tear or cut*	Condition in which the urethral opening is on the dorsum of the penis
erectile **erection**	ee-**REK**-tile ee-**REK**-shun	S/ R/ S/	-ile *pertaining to* erect- *to set up, straight* -ion *action, condition*	Capable of erection or being distended with blood Distended and rigid state of an organ
frenulum	**FREN**-you-lum		Latin *small bridle*	Fold of mucous membrane between the glans and the prepuce
glans	GLANZ		Latin *acorn*	Head of the penis or clitoris
hypospadias	high-poh-**SPAY**-dee-as	S/ P/ R/	-ias *condition* hypo- *below* -spad- *tear or cut*	Urethral meatus on the underside of the penis
impotence	**IM**-poh-tence		Latin *inability*	Inability to achieve an erection
paraphimosis	**PAR**-ah-fih-**MOH**-sis	S/ P/ R/	-osis *condition* para- *abnormal* -phim- *muzzle*	Condition in which a retracted prepuce cannot be pulled forward to cover the glans
phimosis	fih-**MOH**-sis	S/ R/	-osis *condition* phim- *muzzle*	A condition where the prepuce cannot be retracted
prepuce *(same as* **foreskin**)	**PREE**-puce		Latin *foreskin*	Fold of skin that covers the glans penis
priapism	**PRY**-ah-pizm		Priapus, mythical Roman god of procreation	Persistent erection of the penis
smegma	**SMEG**-mah		Greek *ointment*	Oily material produced by the glans and prepuce
spermicide **spermicidal (adj)**	**SPER**-mih-side sper-mih-**SIGH**-dal	S/ R/CF S/	-cide *destroy* sperm/i- *sperm* -al *pertaining to*	Agent that destroys sperm Pertaining to the killing of sperm; *or* destructive to sperm
spongiosum	spun-jee-**OH**-sum	S/ R/	-um *tissue* spongios- *sponge*	Spongelike tissue

Exercise

A. Language of urology: *Refine your knowledge of urological terminology by selecting the correct term to complete the statement. Select the best choice. Be precise, and watch the spelling!* **LO 14.2 and 14.7**

1. Condition in which a retracted prepuce cannot be pulled forward to cover the glans:

   a. hypospadias **b.** phimosis **c.** spongiosum **d.** paraphimosis

2. To remove all or part of the prepuce:

   a. circumcision **b.** circumscion **c.** circummcision **d.** circumsion

3. Skin that covers the glans penis:

   a. forskin **b.** fourskin **c.** forksin **d.** foreskin

4. Fold of mucous membrane:

   a. frennulum **b.** freeulum **c.** freenulum **d.** frenulum

Sexually Transmitted Diseases (STDs) (LO 14.3 and 14.9)

According to the Centers for Disease Control and Prevention **(CDC),** 15 million new cases of sexually transmitted diseases **(STDs)** are reported annually in the United States. Adolescents and young adults have the greatest risk of contracting STDs.

Chlamydia is known as the "silent" disease because up to 75% of infected women and men have no symptoms. When there are signs, a vaginal or penile discharge and irritation with dysuria (difficult or painful urination) are common. Highly accurate urine tests and DNA probes are available for diagnosis. Treatment is with oral antibiotics. If left untreated, chlamydia can spread higher into the female reproductive tract and cause **pelvic inflammatory disease (PID).** It can also be passed on to a newborn during childbirth and cause eye infections or pneumonia. For this reason, newborns receive antibiotic eyedrops.

Trichomoniasis ("trich") is caused by the parasite ***Trichomonas*** *vaginalis.* In women, it can produce a frothy yellow-green vaginal discharge with irritation and itching of the vulva. Because it is a "ping-pong" infection that goes back and forth between partners, both individuals should be treated.

Gonorrhea is spread by unprotected sex and can be passed on to a baby in childbirth, causing a serious eye infection. As with chlamydia, newborns receive antibiotic eyedrops to prevent eye infections from gonorrhea. Symptoms include a vaginal discharge, bleeding, and dysuria. Laboratory testing on a swab taken from the surface of the infected area can confirm the diagnosis. DNA probes are also available. Gonorrhea can be treated with a single dose of an antibiotic. However, it is developing resistance to antibiotics.

Syphilis is transmitted sexually and can spread through the bloodstream to every organ in the body. **Primary syphilis** begins 10 to 90 days after infection as an ulcer or **chancre** at the infection site. Four to ten weeks later, if the primary syphilis is not treated, **secondary syphilis** appears as a rash on the palms of the hands and the soles of the feet. Swollen glands and muscle and joint pain accompany the rash. **Tertiary syphilis** can occur years after the primary infection and cause permanent damage to the brain, with dementia.

Genital herpes simplex is a disease caused by the virus herpes simplex 2 **(HSV2).** It manifests with painful genital sores *(Figure 14.10),* which can recur throughout life *(Figures 14.10 and 14.11).* There is no cure for genital herpes. Antiviral medications can provide a clinical benefit by limiting the **replication** of the virus. **Herpes of the newborn** *(Figure 14.11)* occurs when a pregnant woman with genital herpes sores delivers her baby vaginally and transmits the virus to the baby.

Human papilloma virus (HPV) causes genital warts in both men and women. HPV can also cause changes to the cells in the cervix. Some strains of the virus can increase a woman's risk for cervical cancer. More than 90% of abnormal **Pap** smears are caused by HPV infections. A vaccine is available that can prevent lasting infections with strains that cause cervical cancers and genital warts. The vaccine can be given to females aged 9 to 26, before they are sexually active. The vaccine can be given to males aged 9 to 26 years to reduce the likelihood of acquiring genital warts.

Molluscum contagiosum is a virus that can be sexually transmitted and produces small, shiny bumps that contain a milky-white fluid. They can disappear and reappear anywhere on the body.

Human immunodeficiency virus (HIV) is a virus that attacks the immune system and usually leads to **acquired immune deficiency syndrome (AIDS).** HIV is carried in body fluids and transmitted during unprotected sex. Sharing needles can spread the virus. The virus can also pass from an infected pregnant woman to her unborn child, so she must take medications to protect the baby.

There is no cure for HIV or AIDS, but combinations of anti-HIV medications can be taken to stop the **replication** of the virus in the cells of the body, and to stop the progression of the disease. However, the development of resistance to the drugs is a problem.

HIV damages the immune system, allowing infections to develop that the body would normally cope with easily. These are **opportunistic infections** and include herpes simplex, candidiasis, syphilis, and tuberculosis **(TB).**

Keynotes

- Three million cases of chlamydia are recognized annually in the United States and can be prevented by abstinence or by using a condom.
- Infection with gonorrhea can be prevented by abstinence or by using a condom.
- Three million cases of trichomoniasis occur annually in the United States and could be prevented by abstinence or by using a condom.

Abbreviations

AIDS	acquired immunodeficiency syndrome
CDC	Centers for Disease Control and Prevention
HIV	human immunodeficiency virus
HPV	human papilloma virus
HSV2	herpes simplex virus 2
Pap	Papanicolaou (test, stain)
PID	pelvic inflammatory disease
STD	sexually transmitted disease
TB	tuberculosis

Vesicles

▲ **FIGURE 14.10**
Genital Herpes Simplex in Male.

Biophoto Associates/Science Source/Getty Images Plus

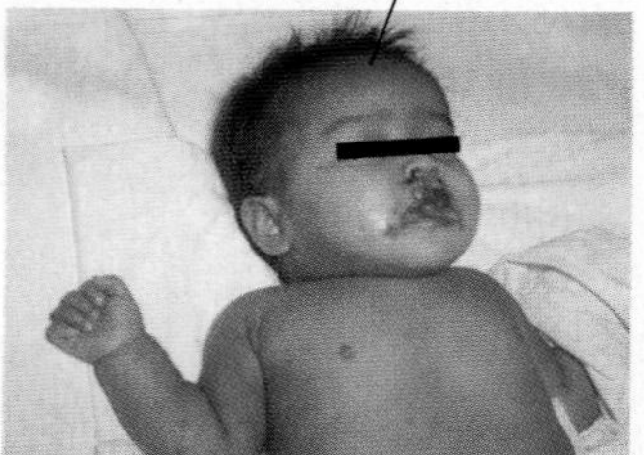

◀ **FIGURE 14.11**
Newborn Infant with Herpes Simplex.

Source: JD Millar/Centers for Disease Control and Prevention

Word Analysis and Definition

S = Suffix P = Prefix R = Root R/CF = Combining Form

WORD	PRONUNCIATION	ELEMENTS		DEFINITION
acquired immunodeficiency syndrome (AIDS)	ah-**KWIRED** **IM**-you-noh-dee-**FISH**-en-see **SIN**-drohm	 S/ R/CF R/ P/ R/	acquired, Latin *obtain* **-ency** *condition* **immun/o-** *immune response* **-defici-** *lacking, inadequate* **syn-** *together* **-drome** *running*	Infection with the HIV virus Combination of signs and symptoms associated with a particular disease process
chancre	**SHAN**-ker		Latin *cancer*	Primary lesion of syphilis
chlamydia	klah-**MID**-ee-ah		Latin *cloak*	An STD caused by infection with *Chlamydia*, a species of bacteria
condom	**KON**-dom		Old English *sheath or cover*	A sheath or cover for the penis or vagina to prevent conception and infection
gonorrhea	gon-oh-**REE**-ah	S/ R/CF	**-rrhea** *flow, discharge* **gon/o-** *seed*	Specific contagious sexually transmitted infection
human immunodeficiency virus (HIV)	**HYU**-man **IM**-you-noh-dee-**FISH**-en-see **VIE**-rus	R/ S/ R/CF R/	**human** *human being* **-ency** *condition* **immun/o-** *immune response* **-defici-** *lacking, inadequate* virus, Latin *poison*	Etiologic agent of acquired immunodeficiency syndrome (AIDS)
human papilloma virus (HPV)	**HYU**-man pap-ih-**LOW**-mah **VIE**-rus	R/ S/ R/	**human** *human being* **-oma** *tumor* **papill-** *pimple* virus, Latin *poison*	Causes warts on the skin and genitalia and can increase the risk for cervical cancer
molluscum contagiosum (**Note:** *"S" in "sum" added to enable word to flow.*) (*modern word contagious*)	moh-**LUS**-kum kon-**TAY**-jee-oh-sum	S/ R/ R/CF	**-um** *structure* **mollusc-** *soft* **contagi/o-** *transmissible by contact*	STD caused by a virus
opportunistic infection (**Note:** *TWO suffixes*)	**OP**-or-tyu-**NIS**-tik in-**FEK**-shun	S/ S/ R/	**-ic** *pertaining to* **-ist-** *agent, specialist* **opportun-** *take advantage of*	An infection that causes disease when the immune system is compromised for other reasons
replication	rep-lih-**KAY**-shun	S/ R/	**-ation** *process of* **replic-** *reply*	Reproduction to produce an exact copy
syphilis	**SIF**-ih-lis		Principal character in a Latin poem	Sexually transmitted disease caused by a spirochete
Trichomonas **trichomoniasis**	trik-oh-**MOH**-nas **TRIK**-oh-moh-**NIE**-ah-sis	R/CF R/ S/ R/	**trich/o-** *hair* **-monas** *single unit* **-iasis** *condition* **-mon-** *single*	A parasite causing an STD Infection with *Trichomonas vaginalis*

Exercise

A. Construct *the correct medical term to match the definition that is given. Insert the appropriate element on the line.* **LO 14.1, 14.2, and 14.9**

1. Infection with *Trichomonas*: _______________ / _______________ / _______________

2. Reproduction to make an exact copy: _______________ / _______________

3. General term that means that an infection occurred due to a compromised immune system:

   _______________ / _______________ / _______________

4. Contagious STD infection that can often be treated with one shot of antibiotics:

   _______________ / _______________

5. Term that means soft *structure*:

   _______________ / _______________

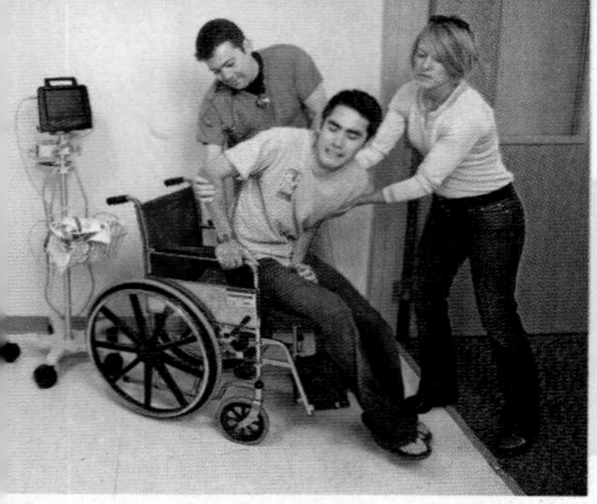

Rick Brady/McGraw-Hill Education

Lesson 14.3

Procedures and Pharmacology

Objectives

The information provided in this lesson will enable you to:

14.3.1 Identify diagnostic procedures used in disorders of the urinary system.

14.3.2 Describe therapeutic procedures used in disorders of the urinary system.

14.3.3 Discuss the pharmacology of drugs used in the treatment of disorders of the urinary system.

Keynote

- **Vasectomy** is almost 100% successful in producing male sterility.
- **Vasovasostomy** is a microsurgical procedure to suture back together **(anastomosis)** the cut ends of the ductus deferens if requested sometime after vasectomy.

Abbreviations

DRE	digital rectal examination
PDE5	phosphodiesterase type 5 inhibitor
PSA	prostate-specific antigen
TUIP	transurethral incision of the prostate
TURP	transurethral resection of the prostate

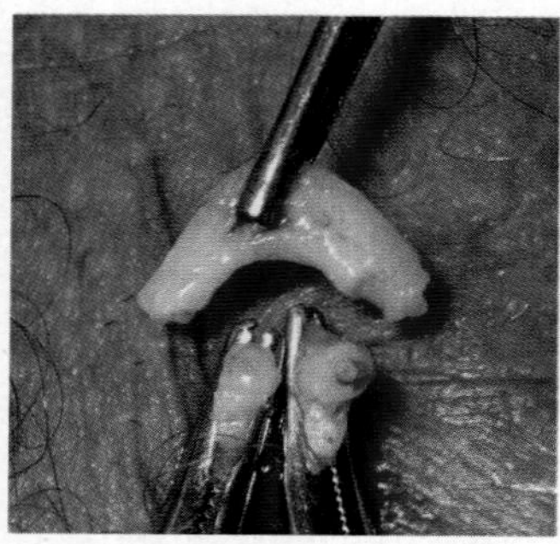

▲ **FIGURE 14.12** Vasectomy being performed.

SPL/Science Source

Diagnostic Procedures (LO 14.10)

A **digital rectal examination (DRE),** in which a lubricated, gloved finger is inserted into the rectum, is part of a routine physical examination in men and women. In men it is used to check for enlargement or other abnormalities of the prostate gland.

Prostate-specific antigen (PSA) is a protein produced by cells of the prostate gland, and the PSA test measures the level of PSA in a man's blood. The level is increased in cancer of the prostate, benign prostatic hyperplasia (BPH), and acute prostatitis.

Prostate biopsy is commonly performed under ultrasound guidance to remove samples of tissue for pathologic analysis. MRI-guided biopsies or a hybrid of MRI images with ultrasound also can be used.

Therapeutic Procedures (LO 14.10)

Circumcision, the removal of the foreskin, can be indicated in an adult for pathological phimosis, **refractory** balanoposthitis, and chronic urinary tract infections. In many religions, circumcision is a ritual in the neonatal period or at varying ages before puberty. In the United States, 85% of all males are circumcised in the neonatal period. In Europe, less than 20% are circumcised.

Orchiopexy is a **surgical** procedure to move an undescended testicle (**cryptorchid**) from the abdomen into the scrotum and permanently fix it there.

Orchiectomy (**orchidectomy)** is the removal of one or both testicles performed for testicular cancer, sex reassignment surgery for transgender men, and advanced prostate cancer to stop the production of testosterone.

Urethrotomy is incision of the urethra to relieve stricture caused by injury or infection.

Benign prostatic hypertrophy (BPH) can be treated surgically by **transurethral resection of the prostate** (**TURP**), in which a **resectoscope** is inserted through the penile urethra to remove prostate tissue obstructing the urethra; transurethral incision of the prostate (**TUIP**), in which the urethra is widened by incision in the neck of the bladder and in the prostate gland; laser surgery, which removes prostate tissue by **ablation** (melting) or **enucleation** (cutting) through insertion of a scope through the penile urethra; or open simple **prostatectomy**, in which the portion of the prostate gland blocking urine flow is removed through incisions or **laparoscopy** in the abdomen.

Cancer of the prostate can be treated with **active surveillance** for early-stage, asymptopmatic, slow-growing lesions; external beam **radiation therapy** or **brachytherapy**, in which many rice-sized radioactive seeds are implanted in the prostate; **cryosurgery**, in which small needles containing a very cold gas are inserted in the cancer using ultrasound images as guidance; **radical prostatectomy**, to remove the prostate gland, surrounding tissue, and lymph nodes surgically; and **chemotherapy.**

In a **vasectomy**, performed under local anesthesia, the ductus deferens is pulled through a small incision in the scrotum and cut in two places, a 1-centimeter segment is removed, and the ends are cauterized and tied *(Figure 14.12)*. The procedure to reverse (repair) a vasectomy is called a **vasovasostomy**.

Pharmacology (LO 14.10)

BPH can be treated medically with **alpha blockers** to relax the bladder neck muscles and muscle fibers in the prostate gland and/or **5-alpha reductase inhibitors,** which block hormones that spur the growth of the gland.

Prostate cancer can be treated with **hormone therapy** using medications that stop the body from producing testosterone, which prostate cancer cells need to grow, or **anti-androgens** that block testosterone from reaching the cancer cells.

Prostatitis is usually a bacterial infection and requires treatment with appropriate **antibiotics**.

Treatment of the underlying cause of **erectile dysfunction** can relieve the difficulty of maintaining an erection, and phosphodiesterase type 5 inhibitors (PDE5) such as *Viagra* and *Cialis* are now in common use. Less common treatments are a penile prosthesis or a penile pump.

Word Analysis and Definition

S = Suffix **P = Prefix** R = Root R/CF = Combining Form

WORD	PRONUNCIATION	ELEMENTS		DEFINITION
ablation	ab-**LAY**-shun	S/ P/ R/	**-ion** *action* **ab-** *away from* **-lat-** *to take*	Removal of tissue to destroy its function
brachytherapy	brah-kee-**THAIR**-ah-pee	P/ R/CF	**brachy-** *short* **-therapy** *treatment*	Radiation therapy in which the source of irradiation is implanted in the tissue to be treated
circumcision	ser-kum-**SIZH**-un	S/ P/ R/	**-ion** *process, action* **circum-** *around* **-cis-** *to cut*	To remove part or all of the prepuce
cryosurgery	cry-oh-**SUR**-jer-ee	S/ R/CF R/	**-ery** *process of* **cry/o-** *icy cold* **-surg-** *operate*	Use of liquid nitrogen or argon gas to freeze and kill abnormal tissue
digital	**DIJ**-ih-tal	S/ R/	**-al** *pertaining to* **digit-** *finger or toe*	Pertaining to a finger or toe
enucleation	ee-nu-klee-**A**-shun	S/ P/ R/	**-ation** *process* **e-** *out of, from* **-nucle-** *kernel*	Removal of an entire structure without rupture
orchiectomy (**orchidectomy**)	or-kee-**ECK**-toh-mee	S/ R/	**-ectomy** *surgical excision* **orchi-** *testicle*	Removal of one testis or both testes
orchiopexy	**OR**-kee-oh-**PEK**-see	S/ R/CF	**-pexy** *surgical fixation* **orchi/o-** *testicle*	Surgical fixation of a testis in the scrotum
prostatectomy	pross-tah-**TEK**-toh-mee	S/ R/	**-ectomy** *surgical excision* **prostat-** *prostate*	Surgical removal of the prostate
radical surgery	**RAD**-ih-kal **SUR**-jeh-ree	 S/ R/	**radical** Latin *root* **-ery** *condition, process of* **surg-** *operate*	Surgical procedure in which the affected organ is removed along with the blood and lymph supply to that organ.
resection	ree-**SEK**-shun	S/ P/ R/	**-ion** *action* **re-** *back* **-sect-** *cut off*	Removal of a specific part of an organ or structure
surgical	**SUR**-jih-kal	S/ R/	**-ical** *pertaining to* **surg-** *operate*	Relating to surgery
urethrotomy	you-ree-**THROT**-oh-mee	S/ R/CF	**-tomy** *surgical incision* **urethr/o-** *urethra*	Incision of a stricture of the urethra
vasectomy	vah-**SEK**-toh-mee	S/ R/	**-ectomy** *surgical excision* **vas-** *duct*	Excision of a segment of the ductus (vas) deferens
vasovasostomy (also called **vasectomy reversal**)	**VAY**-soh-vay-**SOS**-toh-mee	S/ R/CF	**-stomy** *new opening* **vas/o-** *duct*	Reanastomosis of the ductus deferens to restore the flow of sperm

EXERCISE

A. Construct medical terms. *Fill in the blanks.* **LO 14.1 and 14.10**

1. Use of liquid nitrogen to freeze abnormal tissue. ____________/surgery
2. Removal of a specific part of an organ or tissue. re/____________/ion
3. Excision of a section of the ductus deferens. vas/____________
4. Surgical fixation of a testis in the scrotum. ____________/pexy
5. Pertaining to a finger or toe. ____________/al
6. Removal of tissue to destroy its function. ____________/lat/ion
7. Removal of entire structure without rupture. e/____________/ation
8. Radiation therapy for which the source of radiation is implanted into the tissue to be treated. ____________/therapy

Additional exercises available in connect

Chapter Review exercises, along with additional practice items, are available in Connect!

The Female Reproductive System

The Essentials of the Languages of Gynecology and Obstetrics

CHAPTER 15

Rick Brady/McGraw-Hill Education

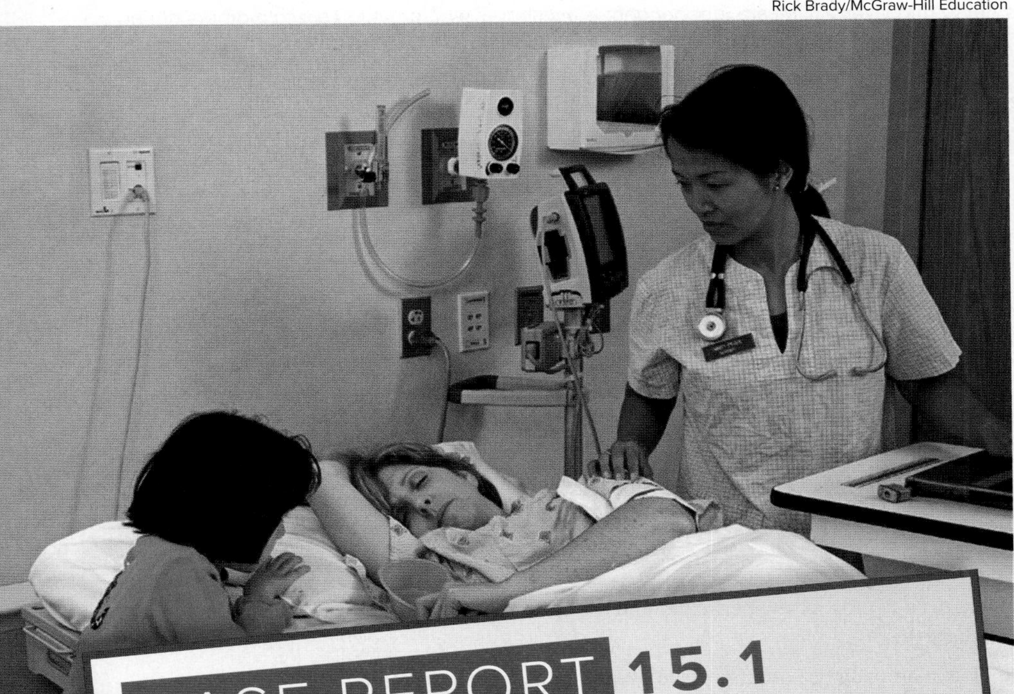

CASE REPORT 15.1

You are . . .

. . . a licensed practical nurse **(LPN)** working in the Emergency Department at Fulwood Medical Center.

You are communicating with . . .

. . . Ms. Lara Baker, a 32-year-old single mother who works in the billing department of the medical center. You have been asked to take her vital signs. For the past couple of days, she has had muscle aches and a feeling of general uneasiness that she thought were due to her heavy menstrual period. In the past 3 hours, she has developed a severe headache with nausea and vomiting. A diffuse rash over her trunk that looks like sunburn is now spreading to her upper arms and thighs. VS: T 104.2°F, P 120 and irregular, R 20, BP 86/50. As you took her VS, you noted that she did not seem to understand where she was. She was unable to pass a urine specimen. For this patient, the treatment she receives in the next few minutes is vital for her survival. You have your supervising nurse and the emergency physician come to see her immediately. As you participate in this patient's care, clear communication among the team members is essential.

Learning Outcomes

As a health care professional in the area of **gynecology** and **obstetrics,** it's essential that you become familiar with not only the functions and structures of the female reproductive system, but also with its associated medical terminology. In order to provide patients with the best possible care, you will need to be able to:

LO 15.1 **Use roots, combining forms, suffixes, and prefixes to construct and analyze (deconstruct) medical terms related to the female reproductive system.**

LO 15.2 **Spell and pronounce correctly medical terms related to the female reproductive system in order to communicate them with accuracy and precision in any health care setting.**

LO 15.3 **Define accepted abbreviations related to the female reproductive system.**

LO 15.4 **Relate the anatomy of the external genitalia and the female reproductive tract to their functions, disorders, and treatments.**

LO 15.5 **Identify the ovarian hormones and their relation to and use in menopause.**

LO 15.6 **Detail the causes of female infertility, their treatments, and the methods of contraception.**

LO 15.7 **Discuss gynecologic diagnostic and therapeutic procedures and pharmacology.**

LO 15.8 **Describe conception, implantation, and development of the embryo, fetus, and placenta during pregnancy, and their disorders.**

LO 15.9 **Explain the stages of delivery and the disorders of childbirth.**

LO 15.10 **Detail obstetric diagnostic and therapeutic procedures and pharmacology.**

LO 15.11 **Relate the structure of the breast to its disorders and to the development of lactation.**

LO 15.12 **Define diagnostic and therapeutic procedures and pharmacology for disorders of the breast.**

LO 15.13 **Apply your knowledge of medical terms relating to the female reproductive system to documentation, medical records, and medical reports.**

LO 15.14 **Translate the medical terms relating to the female reproductive system into everyday language in order to communicate clearly with patients and their families.**

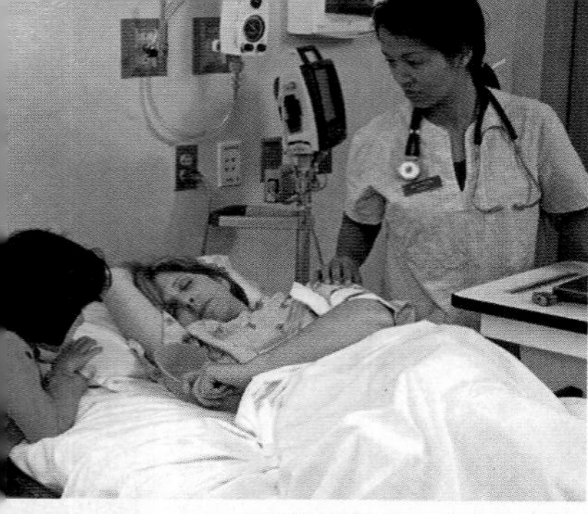

Rick Brady/McGraw-Hill Education

Objectives

The female reproductive system is dormant or undeveloped until puberty, when the ***ovaries*** *begin to secrete significant amounts of the sex hormones* ***estrogen*** *and* ***progesterone****. Then, the external genitalia become more prominent, pubic hair develops, the* ***vagina*** *becomes lubricated, and the breasts begin to enlarge. The information in this lesson will enable you to use correct medical terminology to:*

15.1.1 Describe the essential structures and functions of the external genitalia, vagina, and accessory glands.

15.1.2 Describe common disorders of the external genitalia and vagina.

Abbreviations

LPN	licensed practical nurse
(GYN)	Gynecologists
(OB)	Obstetricians
(OB/GYN)	Obstetrical–gynecological nurse practitioners
(CNM)	Certified midwives/nurse-midwives

The health professionals involved in the diagnosis and treatment of problems with the female reproductive system include:

- **Gynecologists** (GYN) are physicians who are specialists in diseases of the female reproductive tract.
- **Obstetricians** (OB) are physicians who are specialists in the care of women during pregnancy and childbirth.
- **Neonatologists** are physicians who are pediatric subspecialists in disorders of the newborn, particularly ill or premature infants.
- **Perinatologists** are physicians who are obstetric subspecialists in the care of the mother and fetus who are at higher-than-normal risk for complications.
- **Certified midwives/nurse-midwives** (CNM) are independent practitioners who provide care to mothers during pregnancy, delivery, and birth, and to mothers and newborn infants for 6 weeks after birth.
- **Obstetrical–gynecological nurse practitioners** are registered nurses who have acquired skills in the management of health and illness for women throughout their life cycle.

Lesson 15.1

External Genitalia and Vagina

External Genitalia (LO 15.4)

The female external genitalia occupy most of the perineum and are collectively called the **vulva.** The structures of the vulva (Figure 15.1a) include the:

- **Mons pubis,** a mound of skin and adipose or fatty tissue overlying the symphysis pubis.
- **Labia majora,** a pair of thick folds of skin, connective tissue, and adipose tissue.
- **Labia minora,** a pair of thin folds of hairless skin immediately internal to the labia majora. Anteriorly, the labia minora join together to form the prepuce (hood) of the **clitoris.** The clitoris is a small erectile body capped with a glans. Posteriorly, these structures merge with the labia majora.
- **Vestibule,** the area enclosed by the labia minora. It contains the urinary and vaginal openings.

Deep into the labia majora on each side of the vaginal orifice (opening) is a pea-sized greater vestibular **(Bartholin)** gland (Figure 15.1b). These glands secrete mucus to lubricate the vulva and vagina, and this secretion increases during sexual intercourse.

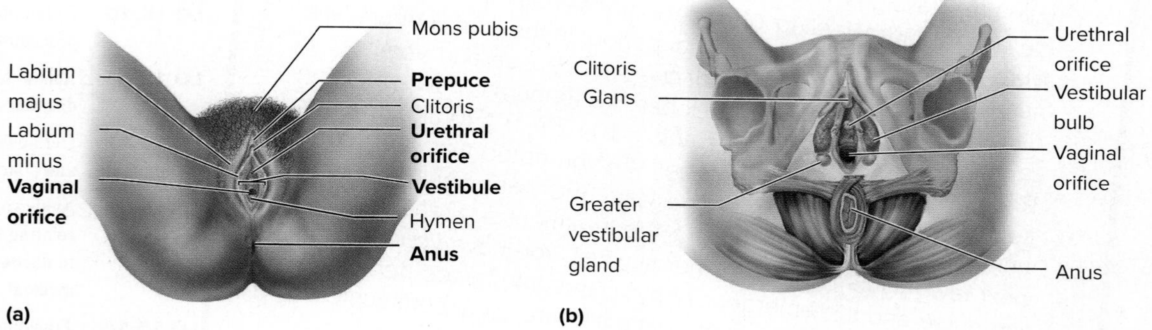

▲ **FIGURE 15.1**
Female Perineum and Vulva.
(a) Surface anatomy. (b) Subcutaneous structures.

Word Analysis and Definition

S = Suffix P = Prefix R = Root R/CF = Combining Form

WORD	PRONUNCIATION		ELEMENTS	DEFINITION
cervix cervical (adj) (**Note:** *This term also means* pertaining to the neck region.)	**SER**-viks **SER**-vih-kal	 S/ R/	Latin *neck* **-al** *pertaining to* **cervic-** *neck*	Lower part of the uterus Pertaining to the cervix
clitoris	**KLIT**-oh-ris		Greek *clitoris*	Erectile organ of the vulva
estrogen	**ES**-troh-jen	S/ R/CF	**-gen** *produce* **estr/o** *woman*	Generic term for hormones that stimulate female secondary sex characteristics
fornix fornices (pl)	**FOR**-niks **FOR**-nih-seez		Latin *a vault*	Arch-shaped, blind-ended part of the vagina behind and around the cervix
gynecology (GYN) gynecologist gynecologic (adj)	guy-nih-**KOL**-oh-jee guy-nih-**KOL**-oh-jist **GUY**-nih-koh-**LOJ**-ik	S/ R/CF S/ S/ R/CF R/	**-logy** *study of* **gynec/o-** *woman, female* **-logist** *one who studies, specialist* **-ic** *pertaining to* **gynec/o-** *woman, female* **-log-** *to study*	Medical specialty of diseases of the female reproductive tract Specialist in gynecology Pertaining to gynecology
hymen	**HIGH**-men		Greek *membrane*	Thin membrane partly occluding the vaginal orifice
labium labia (pl)	**LAY**-bee-um **LAY**-bee-ah		Greek *lip*	Fold of the vulva
majus majora (pl)	**MAY**-jus mah-**JOR**-ah		Latin *greater*	Bigger or greater; e.g., the labia majora
minus minora (pl)	**MY**-nus mih-**NOR**-ah		Latin *smaller*	Smaller or lesser; e.g., the labia minora
mons pubis	MONZ **PYU**-bis		mons, Latin *mountain* pubis, Latin *pubic bone*	Fleshy pad with pubic hair, overlying the pubic bone
obstetrics (OB) obstetrician	ob-**STET**-riks ob-steh-**TRISH**-un	 S/ R/	Latin *a midwife* **-ician** *expert, specialist* **obstetr-** *midwifery*	Medical specialty for the care of women during pregnancy and the postpartum period Medical specialist in obstetrics
ovary ovaries (pl) ovarian (adj)	**OH**-vah-ree **OH**-vah-reez oh-**VAIR**-ee-an	 S/ R/	Latin *egg* **-an** *pertaining to* **ovari-** *ovary*	One of the paired female reproductive glands Pertaining to the ovary(ies)
progesterone (**Note:** *Two suffixes*)	pro-**JESS**-ter-own	S/ S/ P/ R/	**-one** *hormone, chemical substance* **-er-** *agent, one who does* **pro-** *before* **-gest-** *pregnancy*	Hormone that prepares the uterus for pregnancy
vagina vaginal (adj)	vah-**JIE**-nah **VAJ**-ih-nal	 S/ R/	Latin *sheath* **-al** *pertaining to* **vagin-** *vagina*	The female genital canal extending from the uterus to the vulva Pertaining to the vagina
vulva vulvar (adj)	**VUL**-vah **VUL**-var	 S/ R/	Latin *a wrapper or covering* **-ar** *pertaining to* **vulv-** *vulva*	Female external genitalia Pertaining to the vulva

EXERCISE

A. Some Latin and Greek terms cannot be further deconstructed into prefix, root, or suffix. *Match the meaning in the first column with the correct medical term in the second column.* **LO 15.4**

______	**1.** a covering or wrapper	**a.** labia
______	**2.** a vault	**b.** vulva
______	**3.** lesser	**c.** vagina
______	**4.** lip	**d.** fornix
______	**5.** pubic bone	**e.** pubis
______	**6.** sheath	**f.** minora

Lesson 15.1 (cont'd)

Keynotes

- Bacterial vaginosis is associated with increased risk of gonorrhea and HIV infection.
- Of all adult women, 75% have at least one genital yeast infection in their lifetimes.
- Ten million office visits annually are for vulvodynia.

Vagina (LO 15.4)

The **vagina,** or birth canal, is a fibromuscular tube that measures 4 to 5 inches long. It connects the vulva with the uterus *(Figure 15.2)* and has three main functions:

- To discharge menstrual fluid;
- To receive the penis and semen; and
- To deliver a baby.

The vagina is located between the rectum and the urethra. The urethra is embedded in the anterior wall of the vagina.

At its posterior end, the vagina extends beyond the **cervix** of the uterus and forms arch-shaped blind spaces called the anterior and posterior **fornices.** The lower end of the vagina contains numerous crosswise folds. These folds project into the vaginal opening to form the **hymen,** which stretches across the opening. The hymen contains one or two openings to allow menstrual fluid to escape.

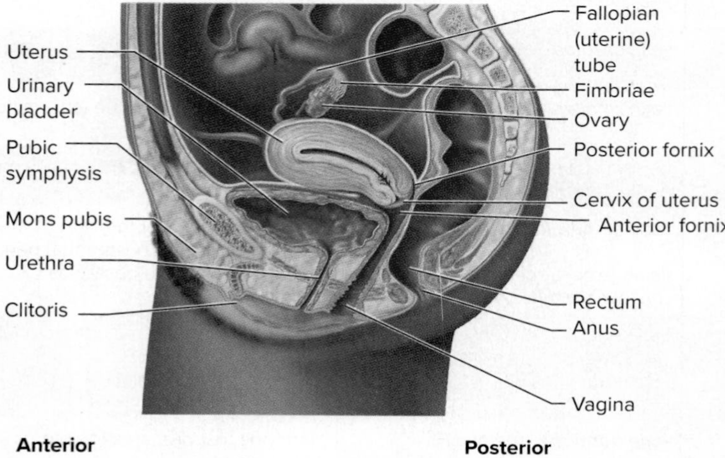

▲ **FIGURE 15.2**
Female Reproductive Organs.

Disorders of the Vulva and Vagina (LO 15.4)

Bacterial vaginosis is the most common cause of **vaginitis** in women of childbearing age. The main symptom is an abnormal vaginal discharge with a fishlike odor. With bacterial vaginosis, different types of invading bacteria outnumber the vagina's normal bacteria. This disorder is diagnosed by a lab exam of a vaginal swab specimen, and it is treated with antibiotics.

Toxic shock syndrome is a life-threatening illness caused by toxins (poisons) circulating in the bloodstream. Bacteria in the vagina are encouraged to grow by the presence of a superabsorbent **tampon** that is not changed frequently *(see Case Report 15.1).* These bacteria produce toxins that are absorbed into the bloodstream. Other risk factors for toxic shock syndrome include skin wounds and surgery.

Vulvovaginal candidiasis is a common cause of genital itching or burning with a "cottage-cheese" vaginal discharge. It is caused by an overgrowth of the yeast fungus ***Candida*** and can occur after taking antibiotics. Treatment is with antifungal drugs.

Vulvovaginitis *(Figure 15.3)* can be caused by allergic and irritative agents found in vaginal hygiene products, spermicides, detergents, and synthetic underwear.

Vulvodynia is a chronic, severe pain around the vaginal orifice, which feels raw. Painful intercourse **(dyspareunia)** is common. The vulva may look normal or be slightly swollen. The etiology (cause) is unknown. Treatment varies from local anesthetics and creams to biofeedback therapy with exercises for the pelvic floor muscles. Surgical removal of the affected area **(vestibulectomy)** has been tried with variable results.

Vaginal cancers are uncommon, comprising only 1% to 2% of gynecologic malignancies. They can be effectively treated with surgery and radiation therapy.

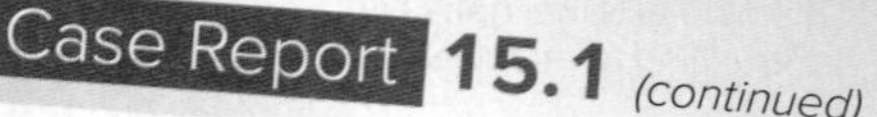

Case Report 15.1 *(continued)*

Ms. Lara Baker presented to the Emergency Department with toxic shock syndrome. Because of her heavy period, she was using a superabsorbent tampon.

She was admitted to intensive care. The tampon was removed and cultured. IV fluids and antibiotics were administered. Her kidney and liver functions were monitored. The causative organism was *Staphylococcus aureus*. She recovered well but had a second episode 6 months later.

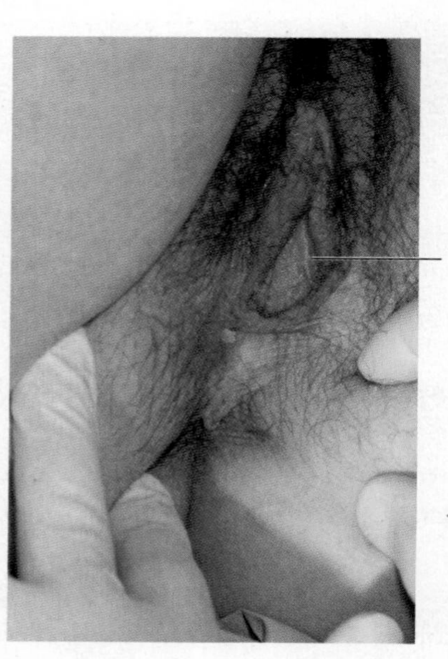

◀ **FIGURE 15.3**
Patient with Vulvovaginitis.

Dr P. Marazzi/Science Source

Word Analysis and Definition

S = Suffix P = Prefix R = Root R/CF = Combining Form

WORD	PRONUNCIATION	ELEMENTS		DEFINITION
dyspareunia	dis-pah-**RUE**-nee-ah	S/ P/ R/	-ia *condition* dys- *painful* -pareun- *lying beside, sexual intercourse*	Pain during sexual intercourse
tampon	**TAM**-pon		French *plug*	Plug or pack in a cavity to absorb or stop bleeding
toxin	**TOK**-sin		Greek *poison*	Poisonous substance formed by a cell or organism
toxic	**TOK**-sick	S/ R/	-ic *pertaining to* tox- *poison*	Pertaining to a toxin
vaginosis vaginitis	vah-jih-**NOH**-sis vah-jih-**NIE**-tis	S/ R/ S/	-osis *condition* vagin- *vagina* -itis *inflammation*	A disease of the vagina Inflammation of the vagina
vestibulectomy	ves-tib-you-**LEK**-toe-me	S/ R/	-ectomy *surgical excision* vestibul- *entrance*	Surgical excision of the vulva
vulvodynia	vul-voh-**DIN**-ee-uh	S/ R/CF	-dynia *pain* vulv/o- *vulva*	Chronic vulvar pain
vulvovaginal vulvovaginitis	**VUL**-voh-**VAJ**-ih-nal **VUL**-voh-vaj-ih-**NIE**-tis	S/ R/CF R/ S/	-al *pertaining to* vulv/o- *vulva* -vagin- *vagina* -itis *inflammation*	Pertaining to the vulva and vagina Inflammation of the vulva and vagina

Exercises

A. After reading *Case Report 15.1 (continued), answer the following questions. Select the correct answer.* **LO 15.4**

1. What is Ms. Baker's diagnosis?

a. vulvodynia **b.** toxic shock syndrome **c.** dyspareunia

2. The causative agent for her condition is:

a. bacterial **b.** viral

3. Antibiotics were given to her via:

a. mouth **b.** vagina **c.** veins **d.** arteries

B. Deconstruct *medical terms related to disorders of the vulva and vagina. Fill in the chart.* **LO 15.1**

Medical Term	Suffix	Meaning of Suffix	Root/Combining Form	Meaning of Root/Combining Form
dyspareunia	**1.**	**2.**	**3.**	**4.**
vaginosis	**5.**	**6.**	**7.**	**8.**
vestibulectomy	**9.**	**10.**	**11.**	**12.**
toxic	**13.**	**14.**	**15.**	**16.**
vaginitis	**17.**	**18.**	**19.**	**20.**

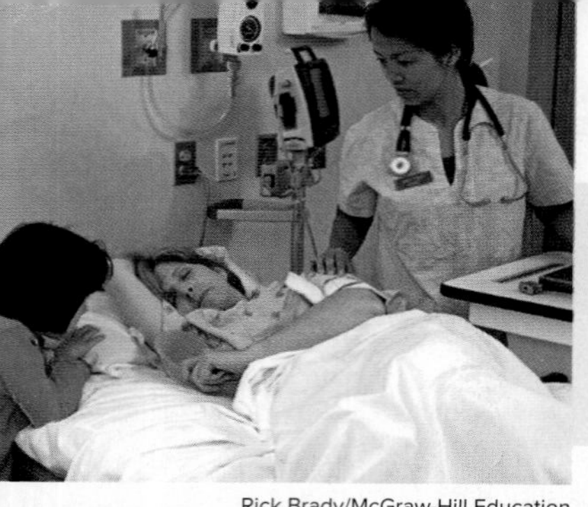

Rick Brady/McGraw-Hill Education

Lesson 15.2

Ovaries, Uterine (Fallopian) Tubes, and Uterus

Objectives

The primary female sex organs are the ***ovaries.*** *The related internal accessory organs include a pair of* ***uterine tubes,*** *a* ***uterus,*** *and a vagina. Women are born with all the eggs* ***(ova)*** *that they will release in their lifetimes, but it is not until puberty that the eggs mature and start to leave the ovary. The ovarian hormones, estrogen and progesterone, are involved in puberty,* ***menstruation,*** *and* ***pregnancy.*** *These complex interactions are the core of the female human reproductive system and an essential part of understanding the human body. The information in this lesson will enable you to use correct medical terminology to:*

15.2.1 Describe the structure and functions of an ovary.

15.2.2 List the functions of estrogen and progesterone.

15.2.3 Explain the structures and functions of the ovaries, uterine (fallopian) tubes, and uterus.

15.2.4 Discuss common disorders of the ovaries, uterine tubes, and uterus.

Abbreviations

CHES	certified health education specialist
GYN	gynecology
PCOS	polycystic ovarian syndrome

CASE REPORT 15.2

You are . . .

. . . a certified health education specialist **(CHES)** employed by Fulwood Medical Center.

You are communicating with . . .

. . . Ms. Claire Marcos, a 21-year-old student referred to you by Anna Rusak, MD, a gynecologist. Ms. Marcos has been diagnosed with polycystic ovarian syndrome **(PCOS),** and your task is to develop a program of self-care as part of her overall plan of therapy. From her medical record, you see that she presented with irregular, often-missed **menstrual** periods since the beginning of puberty; persistent acne; a loss of hair from the front of her scalp; and an inability to control her weight. She is 5 feet 4 inches tall and weighs 150 pounds. You are expected to counsel her about her self-care program involving exercise, diet, and the use of birth control medications.

Anatomy of the Female Reproductive Tract (LO 15.2 and 15.4)

Ovaries (LO 15.4)

Each **ovary** is an almond-shaped organ about 1 inch long and ½ inch in diameter. The ovaries are held in place by ligaments that attach them to the pelvic wall and uterus *(Figure 15.4).* The ovaries' main functions are to:

- produce and release eggs and
- secrete hormones that affect puberty, menstruation, and pregnancy.

FIGURE 15.4
Ovaries.
The ovaries are located on each side against the lateral walls of the pelvic cavity. The right uterine (fallopian) tube is retracted to reveal the ovarian ligament.

Word Analysis and Definition

S = Suffix P = Prefix R = Root R/CF = Combining Form

WORD	PRONUNCIATION	ELEMENTS		DEFINITION
fallopian tubes (also called *uterine tubes*)	fah-**LOW**-pee-an		Gabrielle Fallopio, Italian anatomist, 1523–1562	Uterine tubes connected to the fundus of the uterus
menses (noun) **menstruation (noun)** **menstruate (verb)** **menstrual (adj)**	**MEN**-seez men-stru-**AY**-shun **MEN**-stru-ate **MEN**-stru-al	 S/ R/ S/ S/	Latin *month* -ation *process* menstru- *menses* -ate *composed of, pertaining to* -al *pertaining to*	Monthly uterine bleeding Same as *menses* Act of menstruation Pertaining to menstruation
ovum **ova (pl)**	**OH**-vum **OH**-vah		Latin *egg*	Egg

EXERCISES

A. Review *Case Report 15.2 along with the reading to fill in the blank with the correct answer to complete each statement.* **LO 15.2, 15.3, and 15.13**

1. In her past medical history, which symptom did Ms. Marcos have relating to her menstrual period?
____ menstrual periods

2. What medication was prescribed for Ms. Marcos? _______________________

3. Give the abbreviation for the type of medical doctor that referred Ms. Marco to you: _______________________

4. Ms. Marcos's acne and weight gain are likely due to (use the abbreviation): _______________________

B. Identify *the meanings of the word elements and terms related to the structures of the female reproductive system. Select the correct asnswer.* **LO 15.1 and 15.4**

1. Which term has an element meaning *menses?*
   a. menstruate **b.** fallopian **c.** ova

2. Which term refers to *egg?*
   a. menses **b.** fallopian **c.** ova

3. What other term means the same thing as *menses?*
   a. uterine **b.** fallopian **c.** menstruation

4. The plural of ovum is
   a. oval **b.** oveas **c.** ova

5. What is another name for the fallopian tubes?
   a. urinary tubes **b.** uterine tubes **c.** ureteral tubes

Anatomy of the Female Reproductive Tract (continued)

Keynote

- Menarche cannot occur until a girl has at least 17% body fat.

Uterine (Fallopian) Tubes (LO 15.4)

Each **uterine (fallopian) tube** is a canal about 4 inches long that extends from the uterus and opens to the abdominal cavity near an ovary. At the ovarian end, the outer third of the tube flares out into finger-like folds, each of which is called a **fimbria.** At ovulation, the **fimbriae** enclose the ovary *(Figure 15.5).* The tubes' main functions are to enable sperm and eggs to meet and fertilize.

Uterus (LO 15.4)

The **uterus** is a thick-walled, muscular organ in the pelvic cavity. The main functions of the uterus are to cradle and nourish the fetus from conception to birth and to produce a woman's monthly menstrual flow (period). Anatomically, the uterus is divided into these three regions:

- The **fundus** is the broad, curved upper region between the lateral attachments of the uterine (fallopian) tubes;
- The **body** is the midportion; and
- The **cervix** is the cylindrical inferior portion that projects into the vagina.

The inner lining of the uterus is called the **endometrium;** the muscular layer is called the **myometrium.** The lower end of the uterine cavity communicates with the vagina through the **cervical canal** that has an external **os** (opening) into the vagina.

Ovarian Hormones (LO 15.5)

The ovaries of the sexually mature female secrete the hormones estrogen and progesterone.

Estrogens are produced in the ovarian follicles and their sexual functions are to:

1. Convert girls into sexually mature women through **thelarche, pubarche,** and **menarche;**
2. Regulate the menstrual cycle; and
3. Be involved in pregnancy when it occurs.

Progesterone is produced by the ovary's corpus luteum and also by the adrenal glands *(see Chapter 12).* Its sexual functions are to:

1. Prepare the lining (endometrium) of the uterus for implantation of the egg *(Figure 15.5);*
2. Inhibit lactation during pregnancy; and
3. Produce menstrual bleeding if pregnancy does not occur.

The ovaries also secrete small amounts of androgens, which are male hormones.

Sexual Cycle (LO 15.4 and 15.5)

The sexual cycle averages 28 days in length and includes the **menstrual** cycle. Physiologists recognize the beginning of the sexual cycle as **menstruation,** which occurs for the first 3 to 5 days. After menstruation, developing ovarian follicles mature, and one of them releases an oocyte around day 14. After this ovulation, the lining of the uterus hypertrophies, and the residual ovarian follicle becomes a secretory gland, which then **involutes** around day 26 to form an inactive scar called a **corpus luteum.** At this time, the arteries supplying the lining of the uterus contract. This leads to ischemia, tissue necrosis, and the start of menstruation.

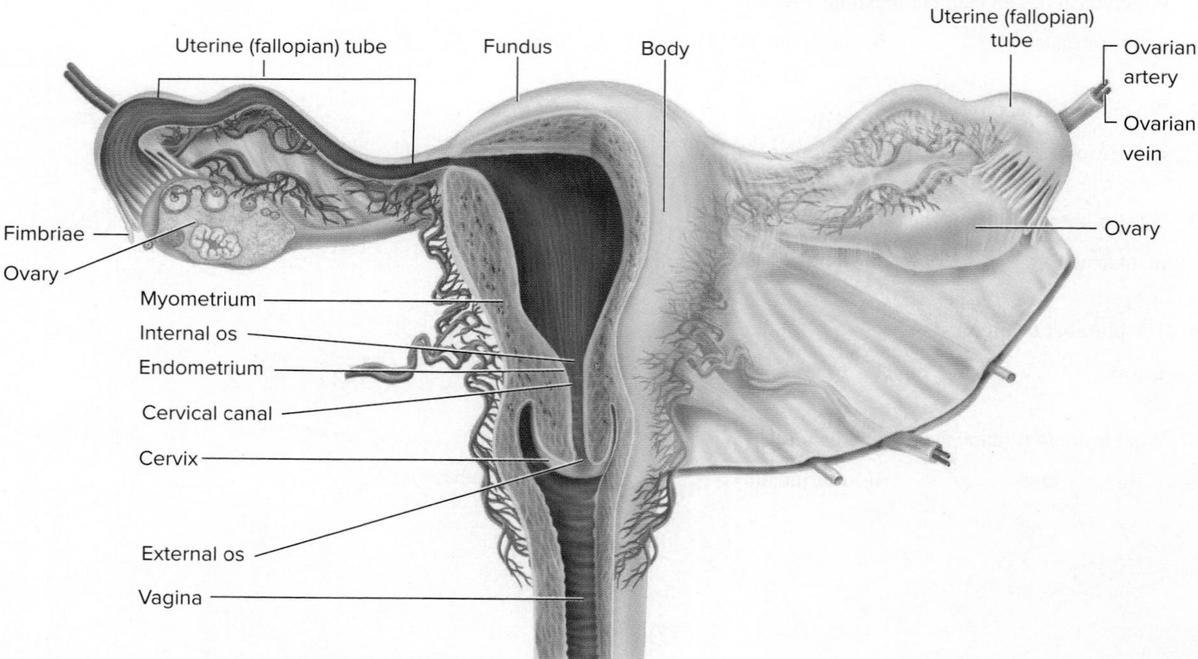

FIGURE 15.5 Female Reproductive Tract.

Word Analysis and Definition

S = Suffix P = Prefix R = Root R/CF = Combining Form

WORD	PRONUNCIATION		ELEMENTS	DEFINITION
corpus luteum	**KOR**-puss **LOO**-tee-um		corpus Latin *body* luteum Latin yellow	Yellow structure formed at the site of a ruptured ovarian follicle
endometrium endometrial (adj)	en-doh-**ME**-tree-um en-doh-**ME**-tree-al	S/ P/ R/CF S/	-um *tissue* **endo-** *within, inside* **-metr/i-** *uterus* -al *pertaining to*	Inner lining of the uterus Pertaining to the inner lining of the uterus
fimbria fimbriae (pl)	**FIM**-bree-ah **FIM**-bree-ee		Latin *fringe*	Fringelike structure
fundus	**FUN**-dus		Latin *bottom*	The upper, rounded top of the uterus above the openings of the fallopian tubes
involution involute (verb)	in-voh-**LOO**-shun in-**VOH**-loot	S/ P/ R/	-ion *process* **in-** *in* **-volut-** *shrink*	A decrease in size.
menarche	meh-**NAR**-key	S/ R/	-arche *beginning* **men-** *month*	First menstrual period
myometrium	my-oh-**MEE**-tree-um	S/ R/CF R/CF	-um *tissue* **my/o-** *muscle* **-metr/i-** *uterus*	Muscle wall of the uterus
os	**OS**		Latin *mouth*	Opening into a canal; e.g., the cervix
pubarche	pyu-**BAR**-key	S/ R/	-arche *beginning* **pub-** *pubis*	Onset of development of pubic and axillary hair
thelarche	thee-**LAR**-key	S/ R/	-arche *beginning* **thel-** *breast, nipple*	Onset of breast development
uterus uterine (adj) uterine tubes (also called **falloplan tubes)**	**YOU**-ter-us **YOU**-ter-in **You**-ter-ine TUBES fah-**LOH**-pee-an TUBES	 S/ R/	Latin *womb* -ine *pertaining to* **uter-** *uterus* Gabrielle Falloppio, Italian anatomist, 1523–1562	Organ in which an egg develops into a fetus Pertaining to the uterus Tubes connected from the uterus to the abdominal cavity. Carry the ovum from the ovary to the uterus.

EXERCISES

A. Meet lesson and chapter objectives *with the language of the female reproductive system. Fill in the blanks.* **LO 15.2, 15.4, and 15.5**

1. Which body cavity contains the uterus? ____________________
2. What is the main function of the uterine tubes? ____________________
3. What two functions does the uterus have? ____________________
____
4. In the female reproductive system, where does the os open into? ____________________
5. What hormone is released by the ovarian follicles? ____________________
6. What is the medical term that means the *first* menstrual period? ____________________

B. Select *the correct pair of terms related to the question.* **LO 15.2, 15.4, and 15.5**

1. Which two terms are structures inside the uterus?
   - **a.** myocardium and pericardium
   - **b.** perineum and periosteum
   - **c.** endocardium and myocardium
   - **d.** myometrium and endometrium
   - **e.** sphincter and meatus
2. Name the regions of the uterus:
   - **a.** fundus and os
   - **b.** fundus, os, and body
   - **c.** fundus, cervix, and body
   - **d.** hypogastric, cervical, and fundus
3. Which pair of terms is associated with the production of progesterone?
   - **a.** pubarche and menarche
   - **b.** fundus and cervix
   - **c.** adrenal glands and corpus luteum
   - **d.** fornix and myometrium
   - **e.** fimbriae and urethra

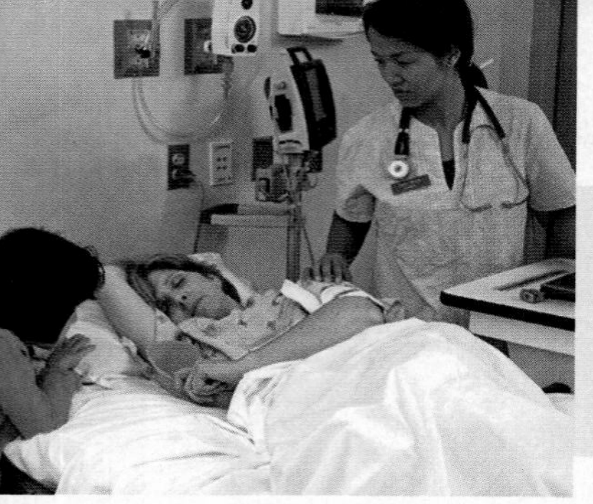
Rick Brady/McGraw-Hill Education

Lesson 15.3

Disorders of the Female Reproductive Tract

Objectives

In order to care for a female patient who is experiencing reproductive tract disorders, you will need to effectively communicate with the patient, and with any of the other health care professionals involved in her case. The information provided in this lesson will enable you to use correct medical terminology to:

15.3.1 Describe common disorders of the ovaries, fallopian tubes, and uterus.

15.3.2 Identify the causes of and treatments for infertility.

15.3.3 Discuss different methods of contraception and their failure rates.

Keynotes

- The peak incidence of ovarian cancer is in the 50- and 60-year age groups.
- Oral contraceptives are 80% to 90% effective in relieving symptoms of PMS.

Abbreviations

GYN	gynecology
PCOS	polycystic ovarian syndrome
PMS	premenstrual syndrome

Case Report 15.2 *(continued)*

When Ms. Claire Marcos first presented in the gynecology clinic, Dr. Rusak examined her abdomen and pelvis. The doctor was able to palpate both enlarged ovaries on vaginal examination. A vaginal ultrasound scan showed multiple small cysts in each ovary. Dr. Rusack diagnosed Ms. Marcos with **polycystic ovarian syndrome,** and prescribed birth control pills because they contain estrogen and progesterone. The pills can correct the hormone imbalance, regulate Ms. Marcos' menses, and lower the level of testosterone to diminish her acne and hair loss problems.

Disorders of the Ovaries (LO 15.4 and 15.5)

Ovarian Cysts (LO 15.4 and 15.5)

Ovarian cysts are fluid-filled sacs that can form, often during ovulation. They are usually benign and symptom-free unless they twist, bleed, or rupture.

Polycystic ovarian syndrome (PCOS), in which multiple follicular cysts form in both ovaries *(Figure 15.6)* is the disorder Ms. Marcos presented with. The repeated cyst formation prevents any eggs from maturing or being released, so ovulation does not occur and progesterone is not produced. Without progesterone, a female's menstrual cycle is irregular or absent.

Ovarian cysts produce androgens, which prevent ovulation and produce acne, the male-pattern hair loss from the front of the scalp, and weight gain. Women with PCOS are also at increased risk for endometrial cancer, type 2 diabetes, high blood cholesterol, hypertension, and heart disease.

Ovarian cancer is the second most common gynecologic cancer after endometrial cancer. However, ovarian cancer accounts for more deaths than any other gynecologic cancer. Symptoms develop late in the disease process and are usually vague. Treatment is to surgically remove the tumor and administer chemotherapy. The 5-year survival rate is below 20%.

Primary amenorrhea occurs when a girl has not menstruated by age 16. This can occur with or without other signs of puberty.

Causes of primary amenorrhea include: drastic weight loss from malnutrition, dieting, bulimia, or anorexia nervosa; extreme exercise, as in some young gymnasts; extreme obesity; and chronic illness. Treatment is directed at the basic cause.

Secondary amenorrhea occurs when a woman who has menstruated normally misses three or more periods in a row and she is not pregnant or in her **menopause.**

The causes of secondary amenorrhea include: ovarian disorders, such as polycystic ovarian syndrome; excessive weight loss, low body fat percentage (e.g., as in gymnasts), or excessive exercise (e.g., as in marathon runners); and certain drugs, including antidepressants.

Primary dysmenorrhea, or **premenstrual syndrome (PMS)** refers to pain or discomfort associated with menstruation. The pain often begins 1 or 2 days before menses, peaks on the first day, and then slowly subsides.

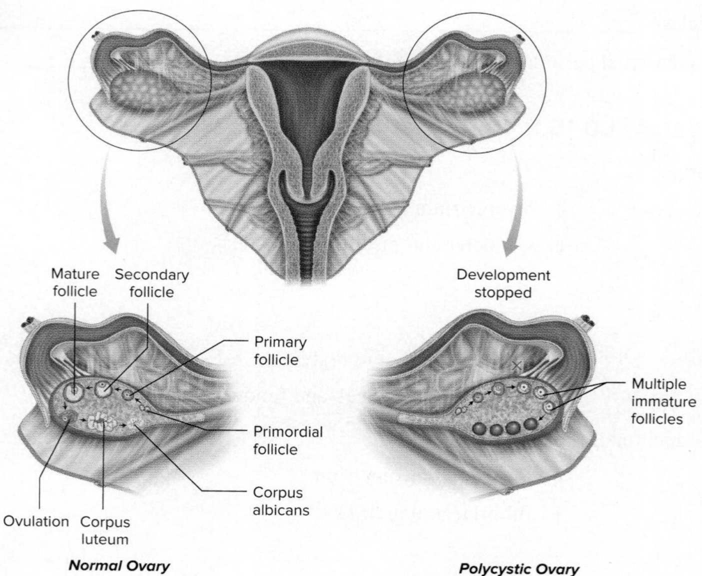

FIGURE 15.6 Polycystic Ovary.

Word Analysis and Definition

S = Suffix P = Prefix R = Root R/CF = Combining Form

WORD	PRONUNCIATION	ELEMENTS		DEFINITION
amenorrhea	a-men-oh-**REE**-ah	S/ P/ R/CF	-rrhea *flow, discharge* a- *without* -men/o- *menses*	Absence or abnormal cessation of menstrual flow
dysmenorrhea	dis-men-oh-**REE**-ah	S/ P/ R/CF	-rrhea *flow, discharge* dys- *painful or difficult* men/o- *menses*	Painful and difficult menstruation
menopause (**Note:** *This term has no suffix, only a combining form and root.)*	**MEN**-oh-paws	R/ R/CF	-pause *cessation* men/o- *menses*	Permanent ending of menstrual periods
menopausal (adj)	**MEN**-oh-paws-al	S/	-al *pertaining to*	Pertaining to the menopause
polycystic	pol-ee-**SIS**-tik	S/ P/ R/	-ic *pertaining to* poly- *many* -cyst- *sac*	Composed of many cysts
premenstrual	pree-**MEN**-stru-al	S/ P/ R/	-al *pertaining to* pre- *before* -menstru- *menses*	Pertaining to the time immediately before the menses
primary	**PRY**-mair-ee		Latin *first*	The first disease or symptom, after which others may occur as complications
secondary	**SEK**-ond-air-ee		Latin *following or second*	Diseases or symptoms following a primary disease or symptom

EXERCISES

A. Critical thinking. *Use Case Report 8.2 (continued) along with the reading to answer the following questions.* **LO 15.3, 15.4, 15.5, and 15.13**

1. Ms. Marcos's ovaries were enlarged due to:

a. cancer **b.** endometriosis **c.** cysts **d.** testosterone

2. The abbreviation for her condition is:

a. PMS **b.** FSH **c.** GnRH **d.** PCOS

3. A consequence of her condition is that she does not:

a. create oocytes **b.** release oocytes **c.** produce testosterone **d.** have an appetite

4. Her condition is associated with what other condition?

a. heart disease **b.** peptic ulcer **c.** decreased fat storage **d.** hematuria

B. Apply your knowledge *of the medical terminology for the female reproductive system by selecting the correct answer to each of the following questions. Select the best answer.* **LO 15.1 and 15.4**

1. The permanent ending of menstrual periods is:

a. menopause **b.** dysmenorrhea **c.** amenorrhea

2. *Premenstrual* happens:

a. before menses **b.** after menses **c.** in the middle of menses

3. The gynecologic malignancy that accounts for the most deaths is:

a. cervical cancer **b.** breast cancer **c.** ovarian cancer

4. Pick the term that contains a prefix, root, and suffix:

a. menopause **b.** secondary **c.** premenstrual

5. In the medical term *dysmenorrhea,* the prefix *dys* means:

a. without **b.** first **c.** painful

Keynote

- Residual scarring of the fallopian tube from salpingitis is a common cause of infertility.

Abbreviation

FUS	focused ultrasound surgery
PID	pelvic inflammatory disease
STD	sexually transmitted disease

CASE REPORT 15.3

You are . . .

. . . a women's health nurse practitioner working with Anna Rusak, MD, a gynecologist at Fulwood Medical Center.

You are communicating with . . .

. . . Mrs. Carol Isbell, a 29-year-old woman c/o severe **dysmenorrhea** since the age of 15. Mrs. Isbell has been unable to conceive after 2 years of unprotected intercourse. She experiences severe, cramping lower abdominal pain for 2 days before, during, and 2 days after her periods, which are very heavy. She also has lower abdominal pain on intercourse. Her physical examination is unremarkable except that her pelvic examination shows several tender masses on each side of a normal-sized uterus. Dr. Rusak has also examined her and agreed with your diagnosis of **endometriosis.** Mrs. Isbell is to have an ultrasound examination.

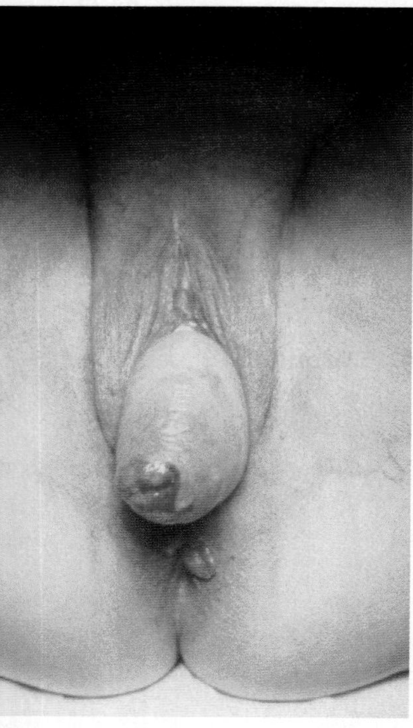

▲ **FIGURE 15.7** Prolapsed Uterus Protruding from the Vagina.

BSIP/UIG/Getty Images

Disorders of the Female Reproductive Tract

Disorders of the Uterus and Uterine (Fallopian) Tubes (LO 15.4)

Endometriosis is said to affect 1 in 10 American women of childbearing age. Here, the endometrium becomes implanted outside the uterus on the uterine tubes, the ovaries, and the pelvic peritoneum. The displaced endometrium continues to go through its monthly cycle. It thickens and bleeds, leads to cysts and scar tissue, and produces pain. The cause of endometriosis is unknown.

Salpingitis is an inflammation of the uterine (fallopian) tubes and is part of pelvic inflammatory disease **(PID).** A bacterial infection, often from a sexually transmitted disease **(STD),** spreads from the vagina through the cervix and uterus. Symptoms are lower abdominal pain, fever, and a vaginal discharge.

Uterine Prolapse (LO 15.4)

The uterus is normally supported by the pelvic floor's muscles, ligaments, and connective tissue. However, a difficult childbirth, aging, obesity, lack of exercise, chronic coughing, and chronic constipation can weaken these tissues, causing the uterus to descend into the vaginal canal *(Figure 15.7).* Uterine prolapse can be accompanied by prolapse of the bladder and anterior vaginal wall **(cystocele),** or by prolapse of the rectum and posterior wall of the vagina **(rectocele).**

Retroversion of the uterus is a normal variation, found in 20% of women. In retroversion, the body of the uterus is tipped backward instead of forward **(anteversion).** It can also be caused by lax pelvic muscles and ligaments, pelvic adhesions (scar tissue in the pelvis following salpingitis), or pelvic inflammatory disease. Retroversion by itself does not cause symptoms, and treatment is not usually necessary.

Uterine Fibroids (LO 15.4)

Uterine **fibroids** are noncancerous growths that appear during childbearing years. Three out of four women have them, but only one out of four women experiences their symptoms, which include **menorrhagia, metrorrhagia, polymenorrhea,** lower back pain, and pelvic pain.

Fibroids are also called **fibromyomas, leiomyomas,** or **myomas** *(Figure 15.8).* They arise in the **myometrium** and produce a pale, firm, rubbery mass separate from the surrounding tissue. They vary in size from seedlings to large masses that distort the uterus. They can protrude into the uterine cavity, causing menorrhagia, or project outside the uterus and press on the bladder or rectum, thereby producing symptoms.

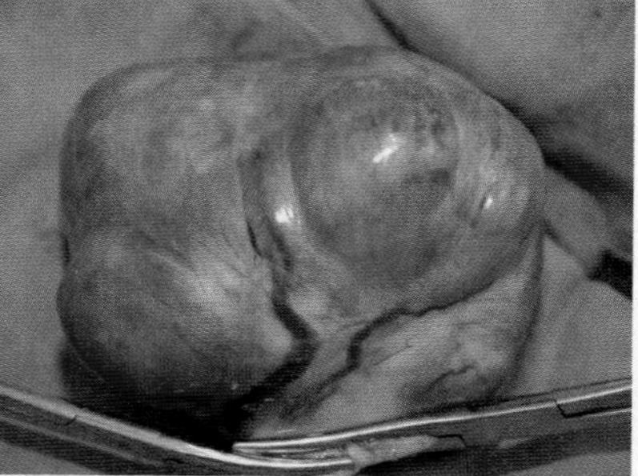

◀ **FIGURE 15.8** Large Tri-fold Fibroid in the Uterus.

Universal Images Group North America LLC / Alamy Stock Photo

Word Analysis and Definition

S = Suffix P = Prefix R = Root R/CF = Combining Form

WORD	PRONUNCIATION	ELEMENTS		DEFINITION
anteversion	an-teh-**VER**-shun	S/ P/ R/	**-ion** *action, condition* **ante-** *forward* **-vers-** *turn*	Forward displacement or tilting of a structure (in this case, the uterus)
cystocele	**SIS**-toh-seal	S/ R/CF	**-cele** *hernia* **cyst/o-** *bladder*	Hernia of the bladder into the anterior wall of the vagina
endometriosis	**EN**-doh-me-tree-**OH**-sis	S/ P/ R/CF	**-osis** *condition* **endo-** *within, inside* **-metr/i-** *uterus*	Endometrial tissue that functions outside the uterus
fibroid	**FIE**-broyd	S/ R/	**-oid** *resembling* **fibr-** *fiber*	Uterine tumor resembling fibrous tissue
fibromyoma	**FIE**-broh-my-**OH**-mah	S/ R/CF R/	**-oma** *tumor, mass* **fibr/o-** *fiber* **-my-** *muscle*	Benign neoplasm derived from smooth muscle and containing fibrous tissue
leiomyoma (also called *fibroid*)	**LIE**-oh-my-**OH**-mah	S/ R/CF R/	**-oma** *tumor, mass* **lei/o-** *smooth* **-my-** *muscle*	Benign neoplasm derived from smooth muscle
menorrhagia	men-oh-**RAY**-jee-ah	S/ R/CF	**-rrhagia** *flow, discharge* **men/o-** *menses*	Excessive menstrual bleeding
metrorrhagia	**MEH**-troh-**RAY**-jee-ah	S/ R/CF	**-rrhagia** *flow, discharge* **metr/o-** *uterus*	Irregular uterine bleeding between menses
myoma	my-**OH**-mah	S/ R/	**-oma** *tumor, mass* **my-** *muscle*	Benign tumor of muscle
polymenorrhea	**POL**-ee-men-oh-**REE**-ah	S/ P/ R/CF	**-rrhea** *flow* **poly-** *many, excessive* **men/o-** *menses*	More than normal frequency of menses
rectocele	**REK**-toe-seal	S/ R/CF	**-cele** *hernia* **rect/o-** *rectum*	Hernia of the rectum into the vagina
retroversion	reh-troh-**VER**-shun	S/ P/ R/	**-ion** *action, condition* **retro-** *backward* **-vers-** *turn*	Tipping backward of the uterus
salpingitis	sal-pin-**JIE**-tis	S/ R/	**-itis** *inflammation* **salping-** *tube*	Inflammation of the uterine (fallopian) tube

Study Hint

The combining form *metr/o* will be used to describe bleeding that is irregular. The combining form *men/o* will be used to describe bleeding that occurs at regular intervals.

Exercise

A. **Build the language of gynecology** *by completing the medical term with the correct element. Fill in the blanks.* **LO 15.1 and 15.4**

1. benign neoplasm derived from smooth muscle: leio/ ________________ / ______________________
2. irregular bleeding between menses: metro/________________
3. permanent ending of menstrual periods: ____________________ /pause
4. uterine tumor resembling fibrous tissue: ____________________ /oid

Note: *Although the suffix* **-oma** *means tumor (or mass), it is not necessarily a malignancy. Fibromyomas, leiomyomas, and myomas are all benign neoplasms or tumors.*

Disorders of the Female Reproductive Tract (continued)

Endometrial Cancer (LO 15.4)

Keynotes

- More than 600,000 hysterectomies are performed each year in the United States.
- In postmenopausal women, the risk of heart disease becomes almost the same as that of men.

Endometrial cancer is the fourth most common cancer in women, after lung, breast, and colon cancer. Each year, 40,000 new cases are diagnosed in the United States, mostly in women between ages 60 and 70. The most frequent symptom is vaginal bleeding after menopause.

Cervical cancer is less common than endometrial cancer, but 50% of cervical cancer cases occur between ages 35 and 55. Some 10,000 new cases are diagnosed in the United States each year. Early cervical cancer produces no symptoms. In the **precancerous** stage, abnormal cells **(dysplasia)** are found only in the outer layer of the cervix. Thirteen types of human papilloma virus (HPV) can convert these **dysplastic** cells to cancer cells.

Other Causes of Abnormal Uterine Bleeding (LO 15.4)

Dysfunctional uterine bleeding is a term that's used when no cause can be found for a patient's menorrhagia.

Endometrial polyps are benign extensions of the endometrium that can cause irregular and heavy bleeding.

Menopause (LO 15.5)

Menopause is diagnosed when a woman has not menstruated for a year and is not pregnant. In this normal, natural, biological process of reproductive aging, levels of estrogen and progesterone start to decline around the age of 40, and most women stop menstruating between the ages of 45 and 55.

Without estrogen and progesterone, the uterus, vagina, and breasts atrophy, and more bone is lost than is replaced. Blood vessels constrict and dilate in response to changing hormone levels and can cause the characteristic menopausal "hot flashes."

Word Analysis and Definition

S = Suffix P = Prefix R = Root R/CF = Combining Form

WORD	PRONUNCIATION	ELEMENTS		DEFINITION
cancer cancerous (adj)	**KAN**-ser **KAN**-ser-us	 S/ R/	Latin *crab* -ous *pertaining to* cancer- *cancer*	General term for a malignant neoplasm Pertaining to a malignant neoplasm
dysfunctional	dis-**FUNK**-shun-al	S/ P/ R/	-al *pertaining to* dys- *painful, difficult* -function- *perform*	Difficulty in performing
dysplasia **dysplastic (adj)**	dis-**PLAY**-zee-ah dis-**PLAS**-tik	S/ P/ R/ S/	-ia *condition* dys- *painful, difficult* -plas- *development, formation* -tic *pertaining to*	Abnormal tissue formation Pertaining to or showing abnormal tissue formation
menopause **(Note:** *This term has no suffix, only a combining form and a root.)*	**MEN**-oh-pawz	R/ R/CF	-pause *cessation* men/o- *menses*	Permanent ending of menstrual periods
menopausal (adj.)	**MEN**-oh-pawz-al	S/	-al *pertaining to*	Pertaining to the menopause

EXERCISES

A. Deconstruct *the following medical terms into their elements with slashes. Then define the terms. Fill in the blanks.* **LO 15.1 and 15.4**

1. *menopause* __________ / __________

   Definition: ____________________

2. *dysfunctional* __________ / __________ / __________

   Definition: ____________________

3. *menopausal* __________ / __________ / __________

   Definition: ____________________

4. *dysplastic* __________ / __________ / __________

   Definition: ____________________

B. You are reviewing a patient chart for a patient at a gynelocologic clinic for a follow-up appointment regarding her lab results. *Select a medical term below to correctly complete each sentence. Each term will be used only once, but not all terms will be used.* **LO 15.2, 15.4, and 15.13**

dysfunction **dysplasia** **dysplastic** **menopause** **menopausal**

Mrs. Volinsky has not menstruated in 11 years and therefore is in (1) __________ This is appropriate for her age of 68 years. The pathology report notes that she has (2) __________ cells obtained from a swab of her cervix. During her last visit, she was prescribed hormones to treat her (3) __________ symptoms. Today, the nurse practioner will discuss further diagnsotic tests to confirm a diagnosis of cervical cell (4) __________.

Lesson 15.3 (cont'd)

Female Infertility and Contraception (LO 15.6)

Female Infertility (LO 15.6)

Infertility is the inability to become pregnant after 1 year of unprotected intercourse. It affects 10% to 15% of all couples. The causes of infertility include:

- The female factor alone in 35% of cases.
- The male factor alone in 30% of cases.
- Male and female factors in 20% of cases.
- Unknown factors in 15% of cases.

Causes of female infertility include scarring of the uterine tubes, structural abnormalities of the uterus, and infrequent ovulation, all of which were addressed earlier in this chapter.

Keynotes

- In women, fertility begins to decrease as early as age 30, and pregnancy rates are very low after age 44.
- Approximately 20% of women now have their first child at age 35 or older.
- In 20% to 30% of female infertility problems, no identifiable cause is found.
- The success rate for IVF is approximately 30% for each egg retrieval.
- Unprotected sex has a failure rate of 85%, with resulting pregnancy.

Abbreviations

IUD	intrauterine device

Contraception (LO 15.5 and 15.6)

Contraception is the prevention of pregnancy. There are several common methods of contraception, including the approaches outlined below.

- **Behavioral methods:** These include **abstinence, coitus interruptus,** and the **rhythm method.** The latter two methods have a 20% failure rate.
- **Barrier methods:**
  - **Condoms** are available for males and females *(Figure 15.9).* They have a 5% to 10% failure rate.
  - **Diaphragms** *(Figure 15.10)* and **cervical caps** consist of a latex or rubber dome that is inserted into the vagina and placed over the cervix. When used with a spermicide, they have a 5% to 10% failure rate.
  - **Spermicidal foams and gels** are inserted into the vagina. Used on their own, they have a 25% failure rate.
- **Intrauterine devices (IUDs):** These are T-shaped flexible plastic or copper devices inserted into the uterus and left in place for 1 to 4 years. The failure rate is less than 3%.
- **Hormonal methods:**
  - **Oral contraceptives** (birth control pills) utilize a mixture of estrogen and progesterone to prevent follicular development and ovulation. They have a 5% failure rate, usually due to inconsistent pill taking.
  - **Estrogen/progestin patches** deliver the hormones transdermally (through the skin). Their failure rate is below 1%.
  - **Injected progestins,** like Depo-Provera, are given by injection every 3 months. Their failure rate is below 1%.
  - **Implanted progestins,** like Norplant, are contained in porous silicone tubes that are inserted under the skin and slowly release the progestin for up to 5 years. Their failure rate is below 1%.
  - **Morning-after pills,** like Plan B, contain large doses of progestins to inhibit or delay ovulation. They are a backup when taken within 72 hours of unprotected intercourse. Their failure rate is around 10%.
  - **Mifepristone (RU486),** when taken with a prostaglandin, induces a miscarriage. It has an 8% failure rate.

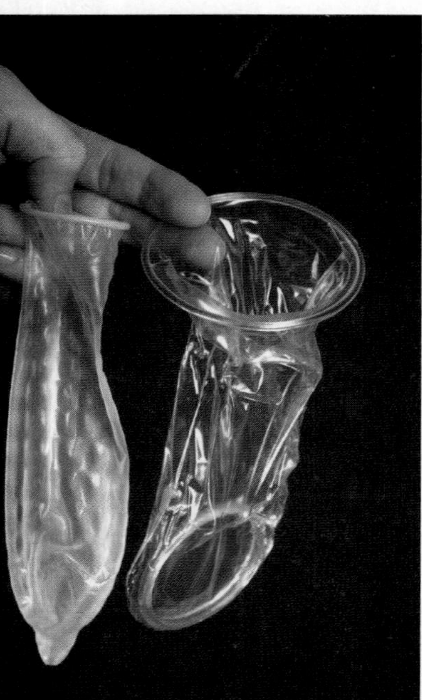

▲ **FIGURE 15.9** Male and Female Condoms.

Jill Braaten/McGraw-Hill Education

Surgical Methods (LO 15.6)

- **Tubal ligation** ("getting your tubes tied") is performed with laparoscopy. Both uterine (fallopian) tubes are cut, a segment is removed, and the ends are tied off and cauterized shut. The contraception failure rate is below 1%.

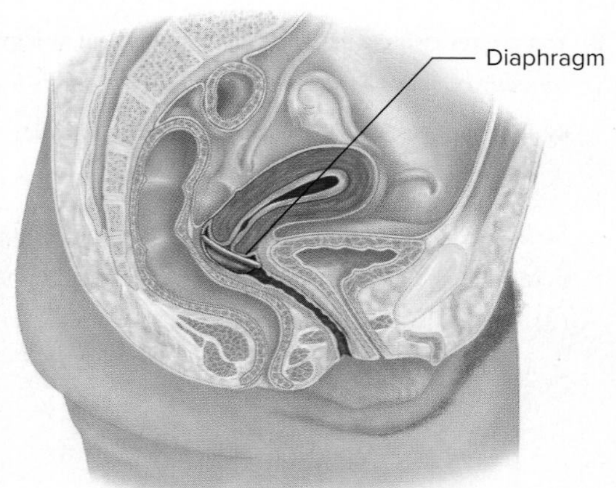

▲ **FIGURE 15.10** Diaphragm in Place.

Word Analysis and Definition

S = Suffix P = Prefix R = Root R/CF = Combining Form

WORD	PRONUNCIATION	ELEMENTS		DEFINITION
coitus **postcoital (adj)**	**KOH**-it-us post-**KOH**-ih-tal	 S/ P/ R/	Latin *come together* **-al** *pertaining to* **post-** *after* **-coit-** *sexual intercourse*	Sexual intercourse After sexual intercourse
contraception	kon-trah-**SEP**-shun	S/ P/ R/	**-ion** *action, condition* **contra-** *against* **-cept-** *receive*	Prevention of pregnancy
contraceptive	kon-trah-**SEP**-tiv	S/	**-ive** *quality of*	An agent that prevents conception
diaphragm (**Note:** *Also the term for the muscle that separates the thoracic and abdominal cavities.*)	**DIE**-ah-fram		Greek *partition or wall*	A ring and dome-shaped material inserted into the vagina to prevent pregnancy
insemination	in-sem-ih-**NAY**-shun	S/ P/ R/	**-ation** *process* **in-** *in* **-semin-** *semen*	Introduction of semen into the vagina
inseminate (verb)	in-**SEM**-ih-nate	S/	**-ate** *pertaining to*	To introduce semen into the vagina
in vitro fertilization (IVF)	**IN VEE**-troh **FER**-til-ih-**ZAY**-shun	P/ S/ R/	**in** *in* **vitro,** Latin *glass* **-ization** *process of creating* **fertil-** *able to conceive*	Process of combining sperm and egg in a laboratory dish and placing resulting embryos inside the uterus
progestin	pro-**JESS**-tin	S/ P/ R/	**-in** *substance* **pro-** *before* **-gest-** *produce, gestation*	A synthetic form of progesterone

EXERCISES

A. Match *the definitions in the first column with the correct medical term in the second column. Fill in the blanks.* **LO 15.3, 15.5, and 15.6**

_____ **1.** synthetic form of progesterone	**a.** diaphragm
_____ **2.** agent that prevents conception	**b.** pregnant
_____ **3.** sexual intercourse	**c.** insemination
_____ **4.** introduction of semen into vagina	**d.** coitus
_____ **5.** having conceived	**e.** progestin
_____ **6.** egg and sperm in a lab dish	**f.** contraceptive
_____ **7.** ring and dome-shaped contraceptive device	**g.** IVF

B. Discuss female infertility. *Select the best answer that completes each statement.* **LO 15.6**

1. Statistically speaking, the most common cause of infertility is attributed to the:

a. unknown factors **b.** male and female factors **c.** male factors only **d.** female factors only

2. In order to be diagnosed with infertility, a female must be unable to conceive for a minimum of:

a. 3 months **b.** 6 months **c.** 1 year **d.** 2 years

3. Fertility begins to decrease in women around the age of:

a. 25 **b.** 30 **c.** 35 **d.** 40

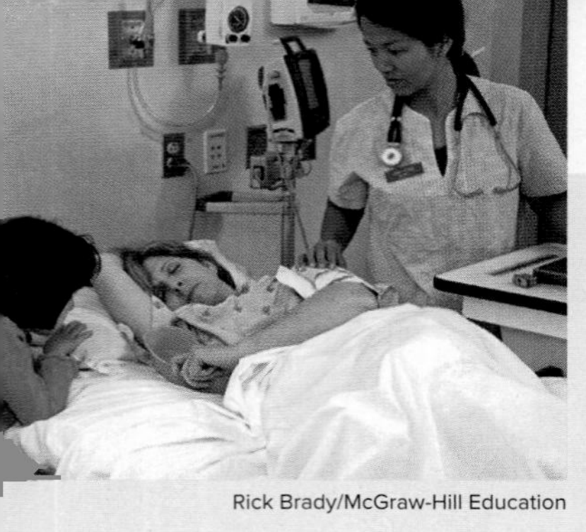

Rick Brady/McGraw-Hill Education

Lesson 15.4

Gynecologic Diagnostic and Therapeutic Procedures and Pharmacology

Objectives

15.4.1 Identify diagnostic procedures used in the treatment of gynecologic disorders.

15.4.2 Describe therapeutic procedures used in the treatment of gynecologic disorders.

15.4.3 Discuss the pharmacology of drugs used in the treatment of gynecologic disorders.

Abbreviations

D and C	dilation and curettage
LEEP	loop electrosurgical excision procedure
Pap	Papanicolaou—a Greek gynecologist

Gynecologic Diagnostic Procedures (LO 15.7)

Palpation is routinely used to feel the structures of the reproductive system.

Laparoscopy directly examines the uterus, fallopian tubes, and ovaries through a **laparoscope** inserted into the abdominal cavity through a small incision in the abdominal wall. Carbon dioxide can be pumped through the laparoscope to inflate the abdominal cavity so that the pelvic organs can be seen more clearly.

Cervical biopsy is a procedure to remove tissue from the cervix for pathological testing for precancerous lesions or cervical cancer.

Colposcopy uses an instrument with a magnifying lens and a light called a **colposcope** to examine the lining of the vagina and cervical canal. Both colposcopy and cervical biopsy are often performed because a Pap test result was abnormal.

Hysteroscopy is the examination of the inside of the uterus using a thin, flexible, lighted tube called a **hysteroscope** to look for abnormalities of the cervical canal and endometrium.

Hysterosalpingography is a procedure in which X-rays (**hysterosalpingograms**) are taken after a radiopaque dye is injected through the cervix into the uterus through a slender catheter to outline the interior of the uterus and fallopian tubes *(see Figure 15.11)*. It can be used to help define the cause of female infertility or to confirm that a sterilization procedure to block the uterine tubes is successful.

Endometrial biopsy—biopsy of the lining of the uterus—is performed to determine the cause of abnormal uterine bleeding and to check the effects of hormones on the endometrium.

Dilation and curettage (D and C) is a surgical procedure in which the cervix is dilated so that the cervical canal and uterine endometrium can be scraped to remove abnormal tissues for pathological examination.

Loop electrosurgical excision procedure (LEEP) uses a wire loop heated by electricity to remove tissue from the vagina and cervix for pathological examination.

After a complete history and physical examination, including vagina and pelvic organs, other diagnostic tools to determine the cause(s) for infertility include:

- **Hormone blood levels** of progesterone, estrogens, and FSH.
- **Ultrasound** of the abdomen, which can show the shape and size of the uterus, and vaginal ultrasound, which can show the shape and size of the ovaries.
- **Laparoscopy**, which allows inspection of the outside of the uterus and ovaries and removal of any scar tissue blocking tubes.
- **Postcoital testing,** in which the cervix is examined soon after unprotected intercourse to see if sperm can travel through into the uterus.

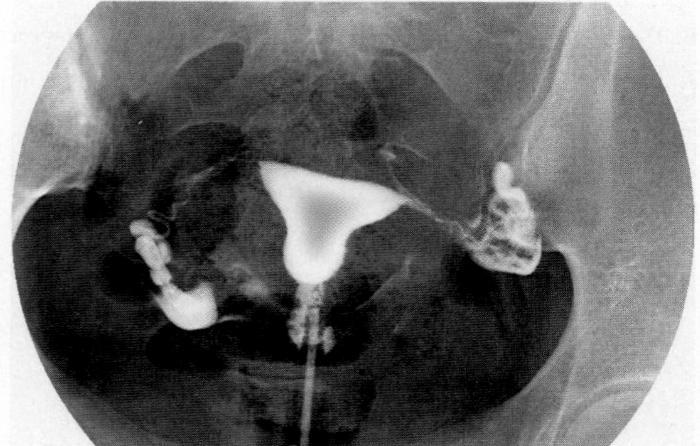

▲ **FIGURE 15.11**
Hysterosalpingogram of a Normal Uterus, Cervix, Uterine Tubes, and Ovaries.

Du Cane Medical Imaging Ltd/Science Source

Word Analysis and Definition

S = Suffix P = Prefix R = Root R/CF = Combining Form

WORD	PRONUNCIATION	ELEMENTS		DEFINITION
biopsy **Note:** The "o" in the root *bio* is dropped from the spelling.	**BIE**-op-see	S/ R/CF	**-opsy** *to view* **bio-** *life*	Removal of living tissue for laboratory examination
colposcopy **colposcope**	kol-**POS**-koh-pee **KOL**-poh-scope	S/ R/CF S/	**-scopy** *to view* **colp/o-** *vagina* **-scope** *instrument for viewing*	Examination of vagina and cervix with an endoscope Endoscope to view the vagina and cervix
conization	koh-nih-**ZAY**-shun	S/ R/	**-ation** *process* **coniz-** *cone*	Surgical excision of a cone-shaped piece of tissue
cryosurgery	cry-oh-**SUR**-jer-ee	S/ R/CF R/	**-ery** *process of* **cry/o-** *icy, cold* **-surg-** *operate*	Use of liquid nitrogen or argon gas to freeze and kill tissue
curette **curettage**	kyu-**RET** kyu-reh-**TAHZH**	 S/ R/	French *cleanse* **-age** *related to* **curett-** *to cleanse*	Instrument with sharpened edges for scraping Scraping of the interior of a cavity
dilation	die-**LAY**-shun		Latin *to spread out*	Artificial enlargement of an opening or hollow structure
excision	eck-**SIZH**-un	S/ R/	**-ion** *action* **excis-** *cut out*	Surgical removal of part or all of a structure
hysterosalpingogram **hysteroscope** **hysteroscopy**	**HIS**-ter-oh-sal-**PING**-oh-gram **HIS**-ter-oh-skope his-ter-**OS**-koh-pee	S/ R/CF R/CF S/ S/	**-gram** *a record* **hyster/o-** *uterus* **-salping/o-** *uterine tube* **-scope** *instrument for viewing* **-scopy** *to view*	Radiograph of uterus and uterine tubes after injection of contrast material Endoscope to visually examine the uterine cavity Visual examination of the uterine cavity
laparoscope **laparoscopy**	**LAP**-ah-roh-skope lap-ah-**ROS**-koh-pee	S/ R/CF S/	**-scope** *instrument for viewing* **lapar/o** *abdomen* **-scopy** *to view*	Endoscope to view the contents of the abdomen Endoscopic examination of the contents of the abdomen
palpate (verb) **palpation (noun)**	**PAL**-pate pal-**PAY**-shun	 S/ R/	Latin *to touch* **-ion** *process, action* **palpat-** *touch, stroke*	To examine with the fingers and hands Examination using the fingers and hands
postcoital	post-**KOH**-ih-tal	S/ P/ R/	**-al** *pertaining to* **post-** *after* **-coit-** *sexual intercourse*	After sexual intercourse

EXERCISES

A. Define gynecologic diagnostic procedures. *Select the correct answer to complete each statement.* **LO 15.7**

1. The term **palpate** means to:

a. smell **b.** touch **c.** excise **d.** incise

2. A diagnostic test for infertility in which the cervix is viewed after unprotected sexual intercourse:

a. hysteroscopy **b.** biopsy **c.** postcoital testing **d.** ultrasound

3. The injection of dye followed by an X-ray of the uterus and uterine tubes is termed:

a. hysterosalpingography **b.** postcoital testing **c.** mammography **d.** endometrial biopsy

4. A **colposcope** is used to:

a. view the vagina and cervical canal **b.** X-ray the uterus **c.** view the internal os of the cervix **d.** remove cells from the uterus

Lesson 15.4 (cont'd) Gynecologic Diagnostic Procedures (continued) (LO 15.7)

Pap Test (LO 15.7)

Pap test screens for cervical cancer. In a Pap test, the doctor brushes cells from the cervix *(Figure 15.12).* The cells are smeared onto a slide or rinsed into a special liquid and sent to the laboratory for examination. This test enables abnormal cells (see *Figure 15.13*), precancerous or cancerous, to be detected. It is the most successful and accurate test for early detection of abnormalities. Current screening guidelines were last updated in March 2012 by the National Cancer Institute, the American Cancer Society, and other national organizations. According to the guidelines, a Pap test should be scheduled as follows:

- **Initial Pap test**–at age 21.
- **Age 21 to 29**–every 3 years.
- **Age 30 to 65**–Pap and HPV cotesting every 5 years or Pap alone every 3 years.
- **Age 65 onward**–continue screening if risk factors are present including HIV infection, **immunosuppression**, previous treatment for precancerous cervical lesion or cervical cancer. Schedule individually with your doctor.
- **Any abnormal result** at any age mandates working out the best schedule for follow-up testing with your doctor.
- A Pap test is best performed 10 to 20 days after the first day of the **last menstrual period (LMP).**

More than 90% of abnormal Papanicolaou **(Pap)** smears are caused by HPV infections. A vaccine is now available that can prevent lasting infections from the two HPV strains that cause 70% of cervical cancers and another two strains that cause 90% of genital warts.

Pelvic ultrasound uses sound waves to scan and picture the pelvic organs.

Swabs are used to determine the causative agents for infections. A sterile cotton swab is rubbed against the infected tissue to obtain a sample of the cells and secretions. The swab is then sent to the laboratory for testing.

DNA probes can be used to test for the presence of gonorrhea and chlamydia.

Diagnostic studies for fibroids include endometrial biopsy, **transabdominal ultrasound**, **transvaginal ultrasound**, **hysteroscopy**, computed tomography (CT), and magnetic resonance imaging (MRI).

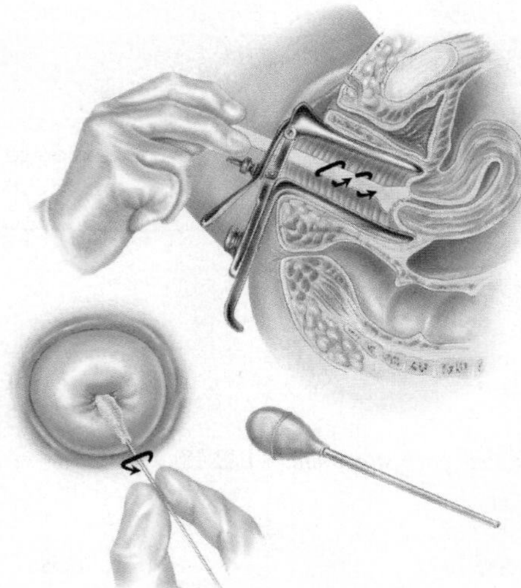

▲ **FIGURE 15.12**
Pap Smear Being Performed.

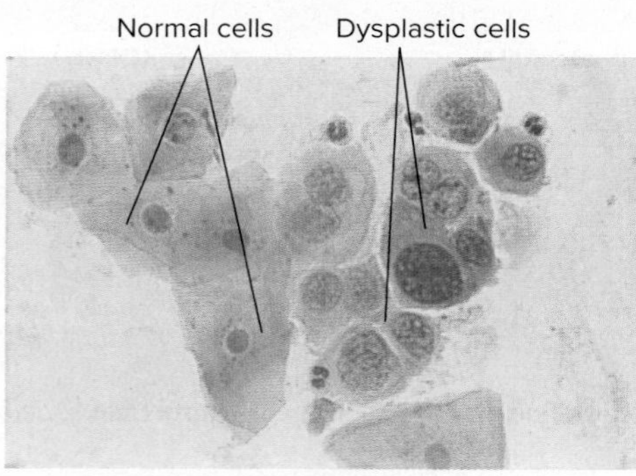

▲ **FIGURE 15.13**
Abnormal Pap Smear with Dysplastic Cells.

Parviz M. Pour/Science Source

Word Analysis and Definition

S = Suffix P = Prefix R = Root R/CF = Combining Form

WORD	PRONUNCIATION		ELEMENTS	DEFINITION
hysteroscopy	his-ter-**OS**-koh-pee	S/ R/CF	-scopy *view* hyster/o *uterus*	Visual inspection of the uterine cavity using an endoscope
cytologist	Sigh-**TOL**-oh-jist	S/ R/CF	-logist *specialist* cyt/o- *cell*	Specialist in the study of the anatomy, physiology and pathology of the cell
immunosuppression	**IM**-you-noh-suh-**PRESH**-un	S/ R/CF R/	-ion *process* immun/o- *immune response* -suppress *press under*	Suppression of the immune response by an outside agent, such as a drug
Pap test	PAP TEST		George Papanicolaou 1883–1962, Greek-U.S. physisician and cytologist	Examination of cells taken from the cervix
swab	SWOB		Old English *to sweep*	Wad of cotton used to remove or apply something from/to a surface
ultrasound	**ULL**-trah-sound	P/ R/	ultra- *higher* -sound *noise*	Very high frequency sound waves

Exercises

A. Test your understanding *of the Pap test by answering these questions. Select the correct answer for each question.* **LO 15.7**

1. How often should a 30- to 40-year-old woman have a Pap test on its own?

a. annually **b.** biannually **c.** every three years **d.** every five years

2. What causes the majority of abnormal Pap smears?

a. improper specimen collection **b.** poor hygiene **c.** infection by the human papilloma virus **d.** overgrowth of yeast in vagina

3. The optimal time to perform a Pap smear is ______________________ days after the last menstrual period.

a. 2–3 **b.** 4–6 **c.** 8–12 **d.** 10–20

B. Construct medical terms. *Complete medical terms related to gynecologic diagnostic procedures. Be precise! Fill in the blanks.* **LO 15.1 and 15.7**

1. Use of very high frequency sound waves ______________ /sound

2. Specialist in the study of the anatomy, physiology and pathology of the cell cyto/ ______________

3. Visual inspection of the uterine cavity using an endoscope hystero/ ______________

Abbreviations

HRT	hormone replacement therapy
IVF	in vitro fertilization
LEEP	loop electrosurgical excision procedure

Gynecologic Therapeutic Procedures (LO 15.7)

Hysterectomy—removal of the uterus—is performed because of uterine fibroids, uterine cancer, and endometriosis. **Subtotal hysterectomy** is removal of the upper uterus, leaving the cervix in place. **Total hysterectomy** is removal of the whole uterus and cervix. **Radical hysterectomy** removes the whole uterus, the cervix, and the top of the vagina; ovaries also may be removed. **Abdominal hysterectomy** is completed through an abdominal incision; **vaginal hysterectomy** through a vaginal incision; **laparoscopic hysterectomy** using a laparoscope and small abdominal incisions; **robot-assisted laparoscopic hysterectomy** using sophisticated robotic surgical tools through a laparoscope.

Oophorectomy is surgical removal of one or both ovaries.

Myomectomy removes fibroids surgically, leaving the uterus in place.

Endometrial ablation removes a thin layer of the uterine endometrium to reduce heavy menstrual bleeding in women who do not plan to have future children.

Tubal ligation prevents future pregnancies.

Sacral colpopexy treats pelvic organ prolapse by suspending the vaginal vault to the sacral promontory using a graft or surgical mesh. Treatment can be an individually fitted vaginal **pessary** inserted into the vagina to support the uterus. Surgical procedures such as **sacral colpopexy,** in which a mesh is inserted into the pelvic floor, or a **vaginal hysterectomy,** in which the uterus is removed through the vagina, achieve good results.

Colporrhaphy is surgical repair of a vaginal wall because of a **cystocele** (protrusion of the urinary bladder into the vagina) or a **rectocele** (protrusion of the rectum into the vagina).

Salpingitis is inflammation of the uterine tube. Treatment is with appropriate antibiotics. If a pelvic abscess has developed, it may be necessary to remove the damaged tube **(salpingectomy).**

Treatment options for fibroids are numerous and include:

- **Expectant management,** or watchful waiting.
- **Myomectomy**, removal of the fibroids surgically, leaving the uterus in place.
- **Hormone therapy,** which uses **GnRH agonists** to cause estrogen and progesterone levels to fall so that menstruation stops and fibroids shrink.
- **Hysterectomy**, major surgery that is performed by many gynecologists as a last resort.

Treatment for dysfunctional uterine bleeding (DUB) is with oral contraceptives. If that fails, **dilation and curettage (D&C)** may be effective. This procedure involves dilating the entrance to the uterus through the cervix so that a thin instrument can be inserted to scrape or suction away the lining of the uterus and take tissue samples. An alternative treatment is **endometrial ablation,** in which a heat-generating tool or a laser removes or destroys the lining of the uterus and prevents or reduces menstruation. Endometrial ablation and hysterectomy are used in women who have finished childbearing.

Endometrial cancer is staged at the time of any surgical procedure into four groups, depending on its localization to the uterus or its spread outside. Surgery is the most common treatment. It can be a total hysterectomy, in which the uterus and cervix are removed, or a radical hysterectomy, in which the uterine tubes and ovaries are removed and a pelvic lymph node dissection is also done. If the cancer has spread to other parts of the body, progesterone therapy, radiation therapy, and chemotherapy are used.

Treatment for cervical cancer depends on the stage of the cancer. In preinvasive cancer, when it is only in the outer layer of the lining of the cervix, treatment can include:

- **Conization.** A cone-shaped piece of tissue from around the abnormality is removed with a scalpel.
- **Loop electrosurgical excision procedure (LEEP).** A wire loop carries an electrical current to slice off cells from the mouth of the cervix.
- **Laser surgery.** A laser beam is used to kill precancerous and cancerous cells.
- **Cryosurgery.** Freezing is used to kill the precancerous and cancerous cells.

In an invasive stage when cancer has invaded the cervix and beyond, treatment can include total or radical hysterectomy, chemotherapy, and radiation therapy.

Infertility treatment is directed at the the underlying cause. If the cause of infertility is infrequent ovulation, the patient can be treated with hormones to stimulate release of the egg. These hormones include clomiphene citrate and injectable forms of FSH, LH, and GnRH.

Surgical procedures to initiate pregnancy include:

- **Intrauterine insemination.** Sperm are inserted directly into the uterus via a special catheter.
- **In vitro fertilization (IVF).** Eggs and sperm are combined in a laboratory dish, and two resulting embryos are placed inside the uterus. This can result in twins.

Word Analysis and Definition

S = Suffix P = Prefix R = Root R/CF = Combining Form

WORD	PRONUNCIATION	ELEMENTS		DEFINITION
ablation	ab-**LAY**-shun	S/ P/ R/	-ion *action* ab- *away from* -lat- *to take*	Removal of tissue to destroy its function
agonist	**AG**-on-ist		Greek *contest*	Agent that combines with receptors on cells to initiate drug actions
colpopexy	**KOL**-poh-pek-see	S/ R/CF	-pexy *surgical fixation* colp/o- *vagina*	Surgical fixation of the vagina
colporrhaphy	col-**POR**-ah-fee	R/CF R/	colp/o- *vagina* -rrhaphy *suture*	Suture of a rupture of the vagina
curettage	kyu-reh-**TAHZH**	S/ R/	-age *related to* curett- *to cleanse*	Scraping of the interior of a cavity
estrogen estriol	**ES**-troh-jen **ESS**-tree-ol	S/ R/CF R/CF S/	-gen *create* estr/o- *woman* estr/i- *woman* -ol *chemical name*	Generic term for hormones that stimulate secondary sex characteristics One of the three main estrogens
hysterectomy	his-ter-**EK**-toh-mee	S/ R/	-ectomy *surgical excision* hyster- *uterus*	Surgical removal of the uterus
insemination inseminate (verb)	in-sem-ih-**NAY**-shun in-**SEM**-ih-nate	S/ P/ R/ R/	-ation *process* in- *in* -semin- *scatter seed* -ate *process*	Introduction of semen into the vagina To introduce semen into the vagina
in vitro fertilization (IVF)	IN **VEE**-troh **FER**-til-eye-**ZAY**-shun	 S/ R/	in vitro Latin *in glass* -ization *process of creating* fertil- *able to conceive*	Process of combining sperm and egg in a laboratory dish and placing the resulting embryos inside the uterus
myomectomy	my-oh-**MEK**-toh-mee	S/ R/ S/	-ectomy *surgical excision* my- *muscle* -om- *tumor*	Surgical removal of a fibroid
oophorectomy	**OH**-oh-for-**EK**-toh-mee	S/ R/	-ectomy *surgical excision* oophor- *ovary*	Surgical removal of the ovary(ies)
salpingectomy	sal-pin-**JEK**-toh-mee	S/ R/	-ectomy *surgical excision* salping- *uterine tube*	Surgical removal of uterine tube(s)

Exercises

A. Apply your knowledge of the language of gynecology. *Match the word element in the first column with its correct meaning in the second column.* **LO 15.1 and 15.7**

	Term	Meaning
______	**1.** *oophor-*	**a.** to cleanse
______	**2.** *-ectomy*	**b.** uterine tube
______	**3.** *hyster/o*	**c.** ovary
______	**4.** *-pexy*	**d.** uterus
______	**5.** *salping/o*	**e.** surgical removal
______	**6.** *semin-*	**f.** surgical fixation
______	**7.** *curette-*	**g.** scatter seed
______	**8.** *colp/o*	**h.** vagina

Lesson 15.4 Gynecologic Pharmacology (LO 15.7)

(cont'd)

Hormone replacement therapy (HRT)–medications to relieve menopausal symptoms by replacement of diminished circulating estrogen and progesterone hormones–have to be given in effective forms. **Estrogen** when taken orally is converted by the liver to estrone, a weaker estrogen. When estrogen, as **synthetic estradiol,** is used **transdermally** as a patch, gel, or vaginal **pessary,** it enters the bloodstream as a more effective **bioidentical** estrogen with fewer side effects. Similarly, **micronized** bioidentical progesterone is more effective and has fewer side effects than synthetic **progestin.** However, long-term **hormone therapy,** as it is now called, is no longer routinely recommended. When taken for more than a few years, it increases the risk of breast cancer.

Oral contraceptives usually contain the synthetic forms of the hormones progesterone (progestin) and estrogen (ethinyl estradiol). They work by (1) preventing ovulation, (2) thickening the cervical mucus to help prevent sperm from entering the uterus, and (3) making implantation in the uterine endometrium more difficult. They are taken for three weeks every month.

The **Minipill** contains only the synthetic progestin, and is taken every day, and functions in the same three ways as the oral contraceptives. It also stops the woman's menstrual period.

Depo-Provera is also a progestin-only drug given by intramuscular injection every three months.

Bacterial vaginosis is treated with antibiotics such as clindamycin. **Vulvovaginal candidiasis** can be treated by applying miconazole (*Monistat*) or clotrimazole (*Desenex*) vaginally, and, if necessary, taking fluconazole (*Diflucan)* orally.

Treatment for STDs

- **Trichomoniasis** infection of the vagina can be treated with a single oral dose of metronidazole (*Flagyl*). Because it is a "ping-pong" infection between partners, both individuals should be treated.
- Treatment for **chlamydia** is with oral antibiotics such as doxycycline, erythromycin, or azithromycin.
- **Gonorrhea** can be treated with a single dose of an antibiotic such as cefixime, but its causative agent, *Neisseria gonorrhoeae,* is developing resistance to antibiotics.
- Antibiotics such as azithromycin and ceftriaxone are effective in the treatment of **chancroid.**
- The lesions of **molluscum contagiosum** are treated with podophyllin ointment, or liquid nitrogen and laser surgery can be used.

Treatment for **vulvodynia** varies from local anesthetics and creams to biofeedback therapy with exercises to the muscles of the pelvic floor. Surgical removal of the affected area **(vestibulectomy)** has been tried with variable results.

There is no cure for genital herpes. Three antiviral medications can provide clinical benefit by limiting the **replication** of the virus. These are acyclovir (*Zovirax*), valacyclovir (*Valtrex*), and famcyclovir (*Famvir*). In people who have recurrent outbreaks, medication taken every day can reduce the recurrences by 70% to 80%.

Clomiphene (*Clomid*) is an oral medication used for stimulating ovulation by causing production of **gonadotrophins** by the pituitary gland (*see Chapter 12*).

The HPV vaccine (*Gardasil*) is offered to girls and women aged 9 to 26 and to boys and men of the same age group.

There is no cure for HIV or AIDS, but combinations of anti-HIV medications are taken to stop the replication of the virus in the cells of the body and stop the progression of the disease. Development of resistance to the drugs is a problem.

Word Analysis and Definition

S = Suffix P = Prefix R = Root R/CF = Combining Form

WORD	PRONUNCIATION	ELEMENTS		DEFINITION
estradiol	ess-trah-**DIE**-ol	S/ R/	-diol *chemical name* estra- *woman*	The most potent natural estrogen
pessary	**PESS**-ah-ree		Greek *an oval stone*	Appliance inserted into the vagina to support the uterus
synthetic	sin-**THET**-ik	S/ P/ R/	-ic *pertaining to* syn- *together* -thet- *arrange*	Built up or put together from simpler compounds
transdermal	trans-**DER**-mal	S/ P/ R/	-al *pertaining to* trans- *across* -derm- *skin*	Going across or through the skin
vestibulectomy	vess-tib-you-**LEK**-toe-me	S/ R/	-ectomy *surgical excision* vestibul- *entrance*	Surgical excision of the vulva

Exercise

A. Demonstrate your knowledge of gynecologic pharmacology. *Select the correct answer that completes the sentence or answers the question.* **LO 15.4 and 15.7**

1. A pharmacologic method to treat vulvodynia is:

a. transdermal estradiol **b.** micronized bioidentical progesterone **c.** topical anesthetic cream **d.** *Gardasil injection*

2. A medication used to promote ovulation:

a. clomiphene **b.** podophyllin ointment **c.** Minipill **d.** acyclovir

3. Miconazole and clotrimazole are used to treat:

a. chlamydia **b.** vulvodynia **c.** infertility **d.** fungal infections

4. An increased risk of breast cancer is seen with which type of long-term pharmacologic therapy?

a. pessary **b.** antibiotic **c.** hormone **d.** antiviral

5. Which type of medication is used to reduce, not cure, herpes outbreaks?

a. metronidazole **b.** liquid nitrogen **c.** valacyclovir **d.** Gardasil

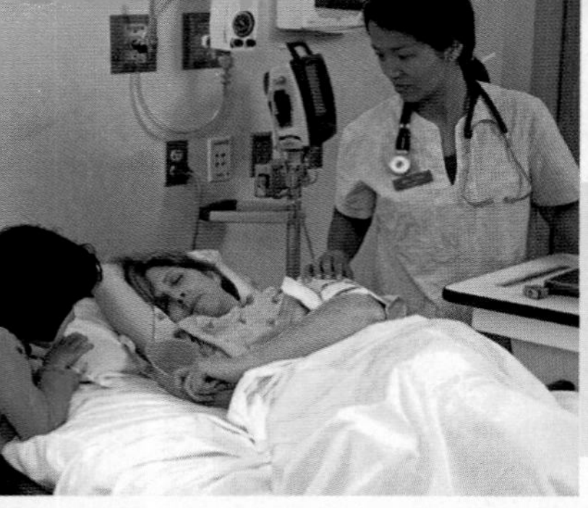

Rick Brady/McGraw-Hill Education

Objectives

For any health care professional involved in the care of a patient who is pregnant, it's necessary to be aware and informed of all aspects concerning pregnancy, childbirth, and their related conditions. The information in this lesson will enable you to use correct medical terminology to:

15.5.1 Describe conception and implantation.

15.5.2 Identify the characteristics of an embryo and **fetus.**

15.5.3 List the functions of the placenta.

15.5.4 Discuss the mechanisms of pregnancy **(PGY)** and childbirth and their common disorders.

Lesson 15.5

Pregnancy

CASE REPORT 15.4

You are . . .

. . . an obstetric assistant **(OA)** employed by Garry Joiner, MD, an obstetrician at Fulwood Medical Center.

You are communicating with . . .

Mrs. Gloria Maggay, a 29-year-old housekeeper. Her last menstrual period was 8 weeks ago, and she has a positive home **pregnancy** test. This is her first pregnancy. She has breast tenderness and mild nausea. For the past 2 days, she has had some cramping, right-sided, lower abdominal pain and this morning had vaginal spotting. Her VS are T 99°F, P 80, R 14, BP 130/70. While you are waiting for Dr. Joiner to come and examine her, Mrs. Maggay complains of feeling faint and has a sharp, severe pain in the right side of her lower abdomen. Her pulse rate has increased to 92. You need to recognize what is happening and to use the correct medical terminology as you talk with Dr. Joiner.

Conception and Development (LO 15.8)

Conception (LO 15.8)

When released from the ovary, an egg takes 72 hours to travel to the uterus–but it must be **fertilized** within 12 to 24 hours to survive. Therefore, **fertilization** must take place in the distal third of the uterine tube.

During unprotected intercourse, with male ejaculation, between 200 and 600 million sperm are deposited in the vagina near the cervix. The journey through the uterus into the uterine tube takes about an hour. Some 2,000 to 3,000 sperm reach the egg. Several of these sperm penetrate the outer layers of the egg to clear the path for the one sperm that will penetrate all the way into the egg to **fertilize** it *(Figure 15.14)*. Once fertilized, the egg becomes a **zygote.**

Implantation (LO 15.8)

While still in the uterine tube, the zygote divides; a fluid-filled cavity develops, and the zygote becomes a **blastocyst** (its first two weeks as a developing **embryo**). A week after fertilization, the blastocyst enters the uterine cavity and burrows into the endometrium, and **implantation** occurs. A group of cells in the blastocyst differentiate into the embryo. Other cells from the blastocyst, together with endometrial cells, form the **placenta.**

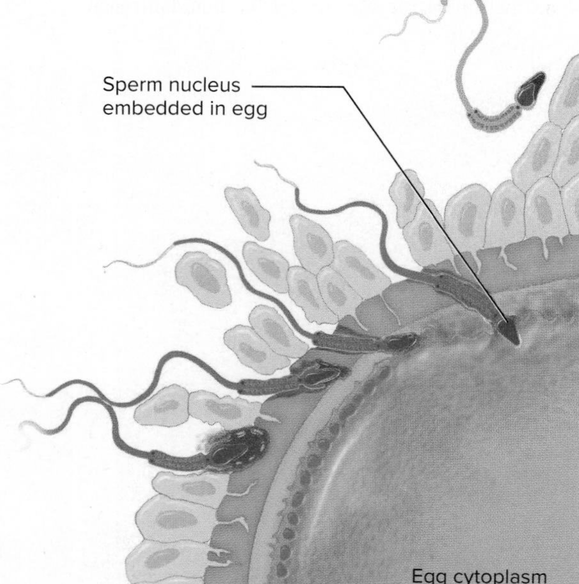

FIGURE 15.14 Fertilization.

Abbreviations

OA	obstetric assistant
PGY	pregnancy

Word Analysis and Definition

S = Suffix P = Prefix R = Root R/CF = Combining Form

WORD	PRONUNCIATION		ELEMENTS	DEFINITION
blastocyst	**BLAS**-toe-sist	S/ R/CF	**-cyst** *cyst, bladder* **blast/o-** *germ or immaturecell*	First 2 weeks of the developing embryo
embryo	**EM**-bree-oh		Greek *a young one*	Developing organism from conception until the end of the second month
embryonic (adj)	em-bree-**ON**-ic	S/ R/	**-ic** *pertaining to* **embryon-** *embryo*	Pertaining to the embryo
fertilize (verb)	**FER**-til-ize		Latin *make fruitful*	Penetration of the oocyte (ovum) by sperm
fertilization (noun)	**FER**-til-ih-**ZAY**-shun	S/ R/	**-ation** *process* **fertiliz-** *make fruitful*	Union of a male sperm and a female egg
fetus	**FEE**-tus		Latin *offspring*	Human organism from the end of the eighth week after conception to birth
fetal (adj)	**FEE**-tal	S/ R/	**-al** *pertaining to* **fet-** *fetus*	Pertaining to the fetus
implantation	im-plan-**TAY**-shun	S/ P/ R/	**-ation** *process* **im-** *in* **-plant-** *to plant, insert*	Attachment of a fertilized egg to the endometrium
placenta	plah-**SEN**-tah		Latin *a cake*	Organ that allows metabolic exchange between the mother and the fetus
zygote	**ZIGH**-goat		Greek *joined together*	Cell resulting from the union of the sperm and egg

EXERCISES

A. Tracing the pathway of embryo implantation. *You are given the terminology –put it in the correct order of the implantation process. Fill in the blanks.* **LO 15.2 and 15.8**

embryo fertilization blastocyst zygote egg

1. ______________________________
2. ______________________________
3. ______________________________
4. ______________________________
5. ______________________________

B. Describe *conception and implantation. Select the correct answer to complete each statement.* **LO 15.8**

1. Fertilization occurs when a(n)
   - **a.** ovum travels down the uterine tube
   - **b.** blastocyst implants into the placenta
   - **c.** sperm penetrates all the way into the egg
   - **d.** blastocyst enters the uterine cavity
2. Implantation occurs when a(n)
   - **a.** ovum travels down the uterine tube
   - **b.** blastocyst burrows into the endometrium
   - **c.** sperm penetrates all the way into the egg
   - **d.** blastocyst enters the uterine cavity

C. Deconstruct *medical terms into their elements. Fill in the blanks.* **LO 15.1 and 15.8**

1. **embryonic:** ______________ / ______________
2. **blastocyst:** ______________ / ______________
3. **implantation:** ______________ / ______________ / ______________

Lesson 15.5 (cont'd) Conception and Development (continued) (LO 15.8)

Abbreviation

CVS chorionic villus sampling

Placenta (LO 15.8)

The placenta is a disc of tissue that increases in size as pregnancy proceeds *(Figure 15.15).* The surface facing the fetus is smooth and gives rise to the **umbilical cord.** The surface attached to the uterine wall consists of treelike structures called **chorionic villi.** The cells of the villi keep the maternal and fetal circulations separate, but they are very thin and allow the exchange of gases, nutrients, and waste products.

The functions of the placenta are to:

- **Transport** nutrients and oxygen from the mother to the fetus;
- **Transport** nitrogenous wastes and carbon dioxide from the fetus to the mother, who can excrete them;
- **Transport** maternal antibodies and hormones to the fetus; and
- **Secrete** hormones like estrogen and progesterone.

Unfortunately, some undesirable matter and many medications can cross the placenta. These include: the HIV and rubella viruses; bacteria that cause syphilis; alcohol; nicotine and carbon monoxide from smoking; and drugs ranging from aspirin to heroin and cocaine. All of these can have detrimental effects on the fetus.

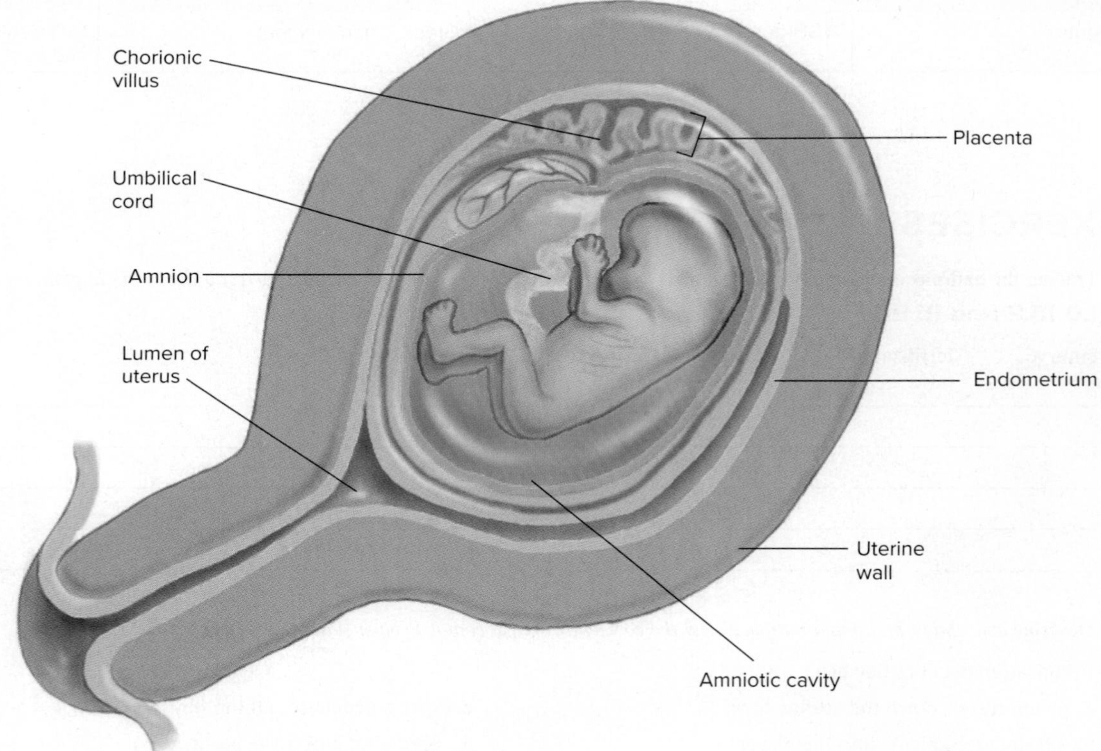

▲ **FIGURE 15.15**
Embryo and Placenta at 13 Weeks.

Word Analysis and Definition

S = Suffix P = Prefix R = Root R/CF = Combining Form

WORD	PRONUNCIATION		ELEMENTS	DEFINITION
chorion chorionic (adj)	**KOH**-ree-on koh-ree-**ON**-ik	S/ R/	Greek *membrane* -ic *pertaining to* **chorion-** *chorion*	The fetal membrane that forms the placenta Pertaining to the chorion
chorionic villus	**VILL**-us		villus, Latin *shaggy hair*	Vascular process of the embryonic chorion to form the placenta
conception	kon-**SEP**-shun		Latin *something received*	Fertilization of the egg by sperm to form a zygote

Exercises

A. Precision in documentation *includes using the correct form (noun, verb, adjective) of the medical term. Practice precision in this written language of obstetrics. Fill in the blanks.* **LO 15.2 and 15.8**

1. embryo embryonic

In the ____________________ stage of gestation, the ____________________ forms in the first 8 weeks of human development.

2. chorionic chorion

The ____________________ villi keep the maternal and fetal circulations separate. The ____________________ is the fetal membrane that forms the placenta.

B. Functions of the placenta. *Fill in each blank with either the term fetus or mother.* **LO 15.2 and 15.8**

1. Transportation of nitrogenous wastes and carbon dioxide moves from the ____________________ (a) to the ____________________ (b).

2. Transportation of maternal antibodies goes from the ____________________ (a) to the ____________________ (b).

3. Transportation of nutrients and oxygen goes from the ____________________ (a) to the ____________________ (b).

C. Challenge your knowledge *of the language of obstetrics by answering the following questions. Fill in the blanks.* **LO 15.2 and 15.8**

1. Where does the umbilical cord originate? ____________________

2. To what structure are the chorionic villi attached in the reproductive system? ____________________

3. The structure that keeps the maternal and fetal circulations separate: ____________________

Lesson 15.5 (cont'd)

Conception and Development (continued) (LO 15.8)

Keynote

- Preeclampsia and eclampsia threaten the life of both mother and fetus.

Abbreviations

OR	operating room
POC	products of conception

Embryo (LO 15.8)

The **embryonic period** occurs from week 2 until week 8. During this time, most of the embryo's external structures and internal organs are formed, together with the placenta, umbilical cord, **amnion** (the amniotic fluid-filled membrane around the fetus), and **chorion.** The amnion grows to envelop the embryo. At the eighth week, all the embryo's organ systems are present. The embryo is just over 1 inch long and is now officially a **fetus.**

Case Report 15.4 *(continued)*

Mrs. Gloria Maggay's symptoms are indicative of an **ectopic** pregnancy. The sudden increase in pain and the rise in pulse rate can signal that the tube has ruptured and is hemorrhaging into the abdominal cavity. The gynecologist should see Mrs. Maggay immediately and take her to the operating room **(OR)** for laparoscopic surgery to stop the bleeding and evacuate the **products of conception (POC).**

Fetus (LO 15.8)

The fetal period lasts from the eighth week until birth. At the eighth week, the heart is beating. By the twelfth week, the bones have begun to calcify, and the external genitalia can be differentiated as male or female. In the fourth month, downy hair called **lanugo** appears on the body. In the fifth month, skeletal muscles become active, and the baby's movements are felt between 16 and 22 weeks of **gestation** *(Figure 15.16).* A protective substance called **vernix caseosa** covers the skin. In the sixth and seventh months, there is an increase in weight gain and body fat is deposited.

At 38 weeks, the baby is at full-term and ready for birth.

Gestation is divided into **trimesters:** The first trimester is up to week 12; the second from weeks 13 to 24; and the third from week 25 to birth.

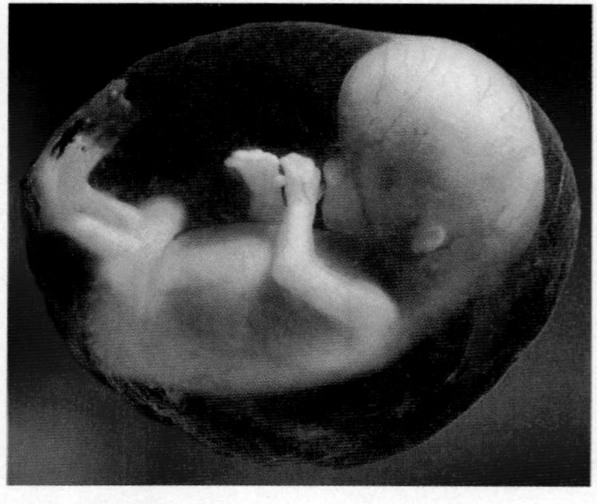

▲ **FIGURE 15.16**
Developing Fetus at 20 Weeks.

Steve Allen/Getty Images

Disorders of Pregnancy (LO 15.8)

The paragraphs below explain the disorders in pregnancy that you will need to be familiar with when caring for a pregnant patient.

Ectopic Pregnancy (LO 15.8)

In an **ectopic pregnancy,** there is an obstruction in the fallopian tube. As a result, the fertilized egg will be prevented from moving into the uterus. Instead, the egg will continue its development in the uterine (fallopian) tube. Tubal disorders that cause ectopic pregnancy include previous salpingitis, pelvic inflammatory disease (PID), and endometriosis.

Preeclampsia and Eclampsia (LO 15.8)

Preeclampsia is a sudden, abnormal increase in maternal blood pressure after the 20th week of pregnancy, with edema (swelling) of the face, hands, and feet. It is also accompanied by proteinuria (protein in the urine). Severe preeclampsia can lead to stroke, bleeding disorders, and death of the mother and fetus.

Eclampsia is a life-threatening condition, characterized by the signs and symptoms of preeclampsia, with the addition of convulsions. Management involves immediate admission to the hospital and control of the mother's blood pressure. The baby is delivered as soon as the mother is stabilized, regardless of its maturity.

Amniotic Fluid Abnormalities (LO 15.8)

Amniotic fluid abnormalities occur in the second trimester, when the fetus breathes in and swallows amniotic fluid. This promotes development of the gastrointestinal tract and lungs. In the third trimester, the total amount of amniotic fluid is about 1 quart and is mostly fetal urine.

Oligohydramnios is a condition involving too little amniotic fluid. It is associated with an increase in the risk of birth defects and poor fetal growth. Its etiology is unknown.

Polyhydramnios is the opposite of oligohydramnios, and involves too much amniotic fluid. It causes abdominal discomfort and breathing difficulties for the mother. It is associated with **preterm delivery,** placental problems, and poor fetal growth.

Word Analysis and Definition

S = Suffix P = Prefix R = Root R/CF = Combining Form

WORD	PRONUNCIATION	ELEMENTS		DEFINITION
amnion	**AM**-nee-on		Greek *membrane around fetus*	Membrane around the fetus that contains amniotic fluid
amniotic (adj)	am-nee-**OT**-ik	S/ R/CF	-tic *pertaining to* amni/o- *amnion, fetal membrane*	Pertaining to the amnion
ectopic	ek-**TOP**-ik	S/ R/	-ic *pertaining to* ectop- *on the outside, displaced*	Out of place, not in a normal position
gestation	jes-**TAY**-shun	S/ R/	-ion *action, condition* gestat- *pregnancy*	From conception to birth
gestational (adj)	jes-**TAY**-shun-al	S/	-al *pertaining to*	Pertaining to gestation
lanugo	la-**NYU**-go		Latin *wool*	Fine, soft hair on the fetal body
oligohydramnios	**OL**-ih-goh-high-**DRAM**-nee-os	P/ R/ R/	oligo- *scanty, too little* -hydr- *water* -amnios *amnion*	Too little amniotic fluid
polyhydramnios	**POL**-ee-high-**DRAM**-nee-os	P/	poly- *many, excessive*	Too much amniotic fluid
preeclampsia	pree-eh-**KLAMP**-see-uh	S/ P/ R/	-ia *condition* pre- *before* -eclamps- *shining forth*	Hypertension, edema, and proteinuria during pregnancy
preterm (*same as* premature)	pree-**TERM**	P/ R/	pre- *before* -term *limit, end*	Baby delivered before 37 weeks of gestation
trimester	**TRY**-mes-ter		Latin *of 3 months' duration*	One-third of the length of a full-term pregnancy
vernix caseosa	**VER**-nicks kay-see-**OH**-sah		vernix, Latin *varnish* caseosa, Latin *cheese*	Cheesy substance covering the skin of the fetus

Exercises

A. After reading Case Report 15.4 and 15.4 *(continued), answer the following questions. Select the best answer.* **LO 15.8, 15.13, and 15.14**

1. Which of the following symptoms did Mrs. Maggay develop while she was in the office?

a. decreased pulse rate **c.** severe right-sided abdominal pain

b. vaginal spotting **d.** mild nausea

2. Mrs. Maggay is most liking suffering from:

a. fertilized egg implanted in a uterine tube **c.** prolapsed uterus

b. endometrial tissue occurring outside of the uterus **d.** rupture of the appendix

3. The event that has elevated Mrs. Maggay's condition to an emergency is:

a. large amount of blood entering the abdomen **c.** labor has begun

b. increased and irregular heart rate **d.** intense nausea and vomiting

B. Define the meaning of the word elements. *Select the correct answer that completes each statement.* **LO 15.1**

1. The word element that means **scanty**:

a. poly- **b.** hyper- **c.** oligo- **d.** ectop- **e.** -amnios

2. The word element **ectop-** means:

a. limit **b.** pertaining to **c.** amnion **d.** on the outside **e.** shining forth

3. The word element **-eclamps** means:

a. cheese **b.** shining forth **c.** tension **d.** bleeding **e.** nausea

Lesson 15.5 (cont'd) Disorders of Pregnancy (continued) (LO 15.8)

Abbreviation

GDM	gestational diabetes mellitus

Gestational Diabetes Mellitus (GDM) (LO 15.8)

In some pregnant women, the amount of insulin they can produce decreases and this leads to hyperglycemia. For the mother, gestational diabetes mellitus **(GDM)** increases the risk of preeclampsia and future type 2 diabetes. For the **neonate** (newborn child), it increases the risk of **perinatal** mortality, birth trauma, and **neonatal** hypoglycemia. Later in life, both mother and child are at increased risk for developing type 2 diabetes and obesity.

Hyperemesis Gravidarum (LO 15.8)

Eighty percent of pregnant women experience some degree of "morning sickness." It is at its worst between 2 and 12 weeks of pregnancy and resolves in the second trimester. For a few women, nausea is persistent, and vomiting is extreme and can lead to dehydration. This condition is called **hyperemesis gravidarum.** Severe cases may have to be admitted to the hospital for IV fluids.

Teratogenesis (LO 15.8)

Teratogenesis is the production of fetal abnormalities–**congenital malformations**–by a chemical agent affecting the mother during the early development of the fetus, while organs and structures are being formed. All medications readily cross the placenta. **Teratogens** include alcohol, isoretinoin (acne medication), valproic acid (an anticonvulsant), and the rubella virus.

Childbirth (LO 15.9)

Labor contractions begin about 30 minutes apart. They have to be intermittent because each contraction shuts down the maternal blood supply to the placenta and to the fetus. Labor pains are due to ischemia of the uterine muscle during contractions.

Labor is divided into three stages *(Figure 15.17)* each of which is usually longer in a **primipara** than in a **multipara.** Another term for pregnant is **gravid,** and a pregnant woman can be called **gravida.** A woman in her first pregnancy is called a **primigravida.**

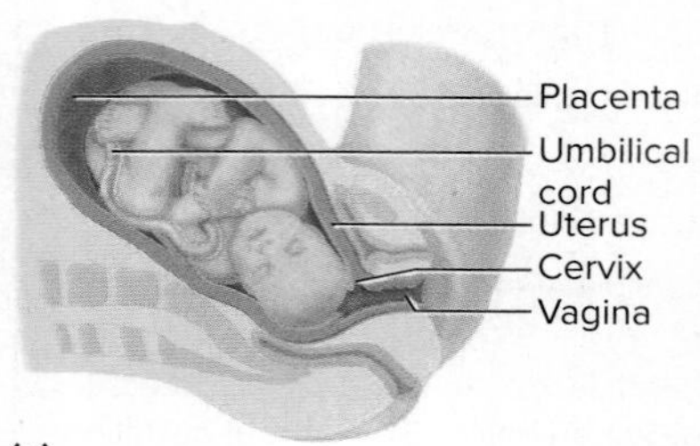

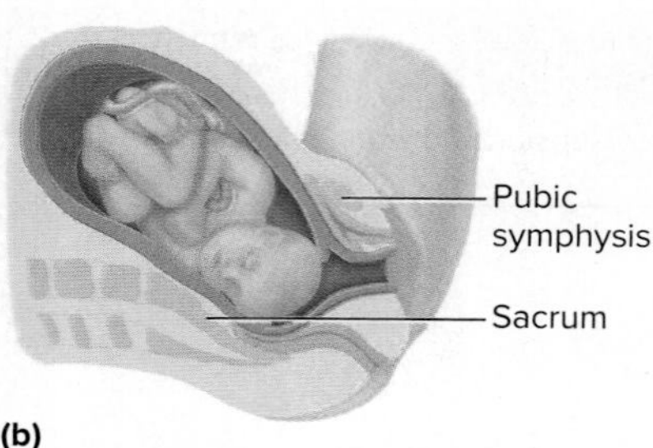

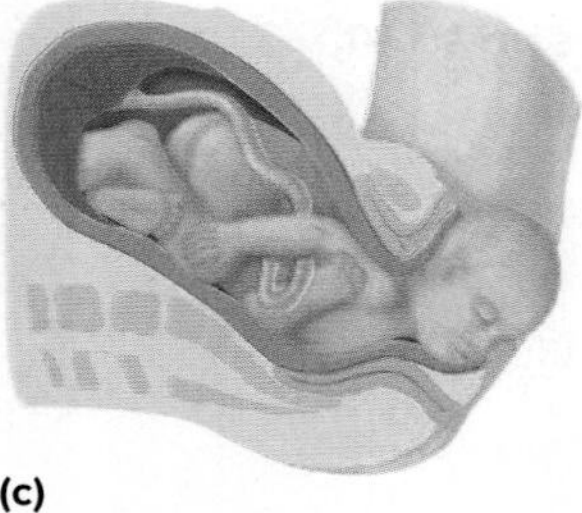

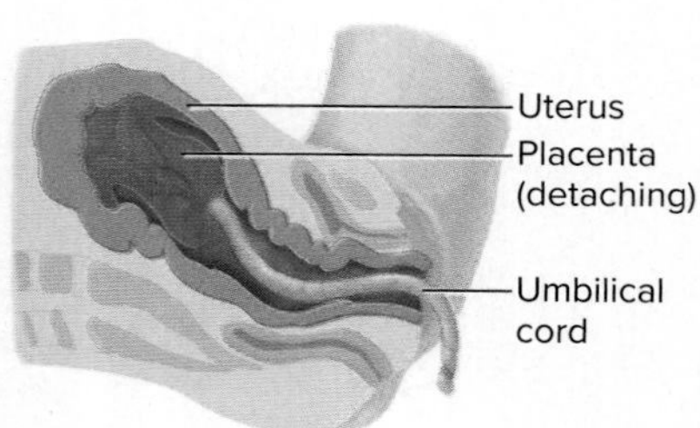

▲ **FIGURE 15.17**
The Stages of Childbirth.
(a) First stage: Early dilation.
(b) First stage: Late dilation.
(c) Second stage: Expulsion of the fetus.
(d) Third stage: Expulsion of the placenta.

First Stage—Dilation of the Cervix (LO 15.9)

This is the longest stage of labor. It can be a few minutes in a multipara to more than 1 day in a primipara. **Dilation** is the widening of the cervical canal to the same diameter as that of the baby's head *(Figure 15.17b).* At the same time that dilation occurs, the wall of the cervix becomes thinner–a process called **effacement.** During dilation, the fetal membranes rupture, and the "waters break" as amniotic fluid is released.

Second Stage—Expulsion of the Fetus (LO 15.9)

While the uterus continues to contract, the baby's head generates additional pain as it stretches the cervix and vagina. When the head reaches the vaginal opening and stretches the vulva, the head is said to be **crowning** and the baby can be delivered *(Figure 15.18).* Sometimes, this process can be helped by performing an **episiotomy** and making an incision in the perineum.

After the baby is delivered, blood in the placental vein is drained into the baby, and the umbilical cord is clamped in two places and cut between the two clamps.

Third Stage—Expulsion of the Placenta (LO 15.9)

After the baby is delivered, the uterus continues to contract. It pushes the placenta off the uterine wall and expels it from the vagina *(Figure 15.17d).*

Puerperium (LO 15.9)

The 6 weeks **postpartum** (after the birth) are called the **puerperium.** The uterus shrinks **(involution)** through self-digestion **(autolysis)** of uterine cells by their own enzymes. This generates a vaginal discharge called **lochia** that lasts about 10 days.

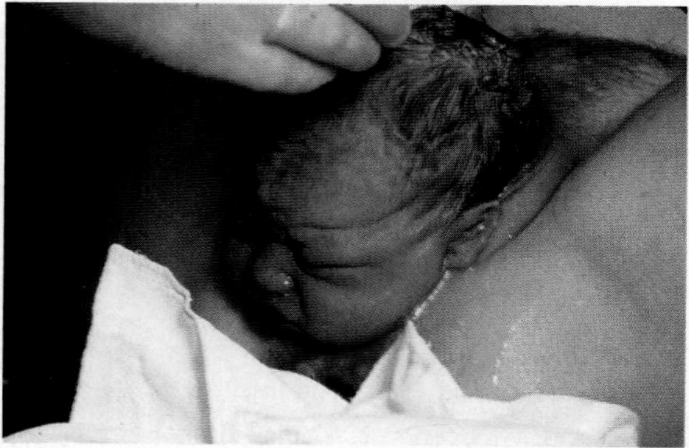

▲ **FIGURE 15.18**
Delivery of the Head.
D. Van Rossum/Science Source

Word Analysis and Definition

S = Suffix P = Prefix R = Root R/CF = Combining Form

WORD	PRONUNCIATION	ELEMENTS		DEFINITION
autolysis	awe-**TOL**-ih-sis	P/ R/	**auto-** *self, same* **-lysis** *destruction*	Destruction of cells by enzymes within the cells
dilation	die-**LAY**-shun	S/ R/	**-ion** *process* **dilat-** *open out*	Stretching or enlarging an opening
effacement	ee-**FACE**-ment	S/ R/	**-ment** *resulting state* **efface-** *wipe out*	Thinning of the cervix in relation to labor
episiotomy	eh-piz-ee-**OT**-oh-me	S/ R/CF	**-tomy** *surgical incision* **episi/o-** *vulva*	Surgical incision of the vulva
gravid **gravida**	**GRAV**-id **GRAV**-ih-dah		Latin *pregnant* Latin *pregnant woman*	Pregnant A pregnant woman
hyperemesis	high-per-**EM**-eh-sis	P/ R/	**hyper-** *excessive* **-emesis** *vomiting*	Excessive vomiting
labor	**LAY**-bore		Latin *toil, suffering*	Process of expulsion of the fetus
lochia	**LOW**-kee-uh		Greek *relating to childbirth*	Vaginal discharge following childbirth
multipara	mul-**TIP**-ah-ruh	P/ R/	**multi-** *many* **-para** *to bring forth*	Woman who has given birth to two or more children
neonate **neonatal (adj)** (**Note:** *The "e" in the root is dropped because of the following vowel.*)	**NEE**-oh-nate **NEE**-oh-**NAY**-tal	R/CF R/ S/	**neo-** *new* **-nate** *born* **-al** *pertaining to*	A newborn infant Pertaining to the newborn infant or the newborn period
perinatal	per-ih-**NAY**-tal	S/ P/ R/	**-al** *pertaining to* **peri-** *around* **-nat-** *birth*	Around the time of birth
postpartum	post-**PAR**-tum	P/ R/	**post-** *after* **-partum** *childbirth, to bring forth*	After childbirth
primigravida	pree-mih-**GRAV**-ih-dah	P/ R/	**primi-** *first* **-gravida** *pregnancy*	A woman in her first pregnancy
primipara	pry-**MIP**-ah-ruh	P/ R/	**primi-** *first* **-para** *to bring forth*	Woman giving birth for the first time
puerperium (**Note:** *This term is composed of roots only.*)	pyu-er-**PER**-ee-um	R/ R/	**puer-** *child* **-perium** *a bringing forth*	Six-week period after birth in which the uterus involutes
teratogen **teratogenic (adj)** **teratogenesis**	**TER**-ah-toe-jen **TER**-ah-toe-**JEN**-ik **TER**-ah-toe-**JEN**-eh-sis	S/ R/CF S/ S/	**-gen** *create, produce* **terat/o-** *monster, malformed fetus* **-ic** *pertaining to* **-esis** *condition*	Agent that produces fetal deformities Capable of producing fetal deformities Process involved in producing fetal deformities

EXERCISE

A. Elements: *Several of these elements you have seen before, and you will certainly see them again in other terms. Learn an element once, and recognize it all the time. Select the best answer to each question.* **LO 15.1 and 15.9**

1. The term that contains the prefix meaning *many* is:

a. primipara **b.** lochia **c.** multipara

2. The term that contains the suffix meaning *incision* is:

a. episiotomy **b.** effacement **c.** dilation

3. The term that contains the root meaning *destruction* is:

a. autolysis **b.** involution **c.** effacement

4. The term that contains the root meaning *child* is:

a. gravid **b.** multipara **c.** puerperium

Lesson 15.5 (cont'd)

Keynotes

Every newborn ***(neonate)*** is either:

- Premature, less than 37 weeks' gestation;
- Full-term, between 37 and 42 weeks' gestation; or
- Post-term, longer than 42 weeks' gestation.

Abbreviations

C-section	cesarean section
OB	obstetrics
PPH	postpartum hemorrhage
RDS	respiratory distress syndrome

Disorders of Childbirth (LO 15.9)

Fetal distress, due to lack of oxygen, is an uncommon complication of labor, but it is detrimental if not recognized. During labor, there is electronic fetal heart monitoring. Treatment is to give the mother oxygen or increase IV fluids. If distress persists, the baby is delivered as quickly as possible by forceps extraction, vacuum extractor, or **cesarean section (C-section).**

An **abnormal position of the fetus** occurs at the beginning of labor if the baby is not a head-first **(vertex)** presentation facing rearward. Abnormal positions include:

- **Breech:** The buttocks present first *(Figure 15.19).*
- **Face:** The face, instead of the top of the head, presents first.
- **Shoulder:** The shoulder and upper back are trying to exit the uterus first.

If the baby cannot be turned into a vertex presentation, a C-section is usually performed.

In addition, other conditions can occur involving an abnormal placement of the baby's umbilical cord. In **prolapsed umbilical cord,** the cord precedes the baby down the birth canal. Pressure on the cord can cut off the baby's blood supply, which is still being provided through the umbilical arteries.

In **nuchal cord,** the cord is wrapped around the baby's neck during delivery. This occurs in 20% of deliveries.

Premature rupture of the membranes occurs in 10% of normal pregnancies and increases the risk of infection of the uterus and fetus.

Gestational Classification (LO 15.9)

Prematurity occurs in about 8% of newborns. The earlier the baby is born, the more life-threatening problems occur.

Because their lungs are underdeveloped, premature babies can develop **respiratory distress syndrome (RDS),** also called **hyaline membrane disease.** Their lungs are not mature enough to produce **surfactant,** a mixture of lipids and proteins that keeps the alveoli from collapsing. As a result, this prevents the respiratory exchange of oxygen and carbon dioxide.

An immature liver can impair the excretion of bilirubin (yellowish bile pigment) *(see Chapter 9),* and premature babies become jaundiced. High levels of bilirubin can produce **kernicterus,** in which deposits of bilirubin in the brain cause brain damage.

Postmaturity is much less common than prematurity. Its etiology is unknown, but the placenta begins to shrink, making it difficult to supply sufficient nutrients to the baby. For the baby, this leads to: hypoglycemia; loss of subcutaneous fat; dry, peeling skin; and, if oxygen is lacking, fetal distress. The baby can pass stools **(meconium)** into the amniotic fluid. In its distress, the baby can take deep gasping breaths and inhale the meconium fluid. This leads to **meconium aspiration syndrome** and respiratory difficulty at birth.

An **abortion** is the expulsion of an embryo or fetus from the uterus before the 20th week of gestation. It can be spontaneous (occurring from natural causes) or induced medically or surgically.

Placental Disorders (LO 15.9)

Placenta abruptio is the separation of the placenta from the uterine wall before delivery of the baby. The baby's oxygen supply is cut off, and fetal distress appears quickly. It is an **obstetric (OB)** emergency, and usually a **C-section** is performed.

Placenta previa is a low-lying placenta between the baby's head and the internal os of the cervix. It can cause severe bleeding during labor, and a C-section may be necessary.

In a **retained placenta,** all or part of the placenta and/or membranes remain behind in the uterus 30 minutes to an hour after the baby has been delivered. The result of a retained placenta is heavy uterine bleeding called **postpartum hemorrhage (PPH).** Manual removal of the retained placenta may be necessary under spinal, epidural, or general anesthesia *(Figure 15.20).*

FIGURE 15.19 Breech Presentation.

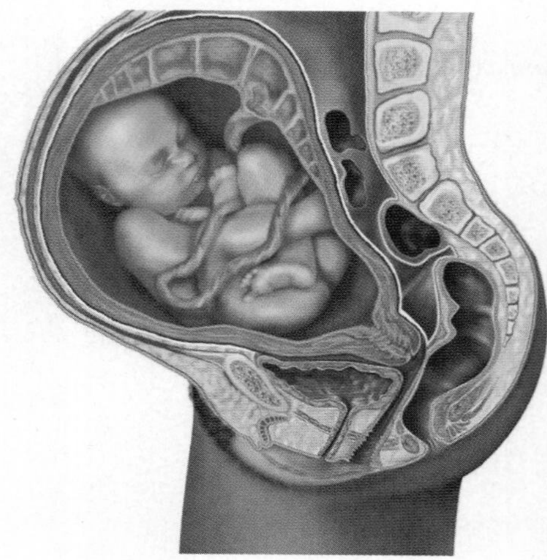

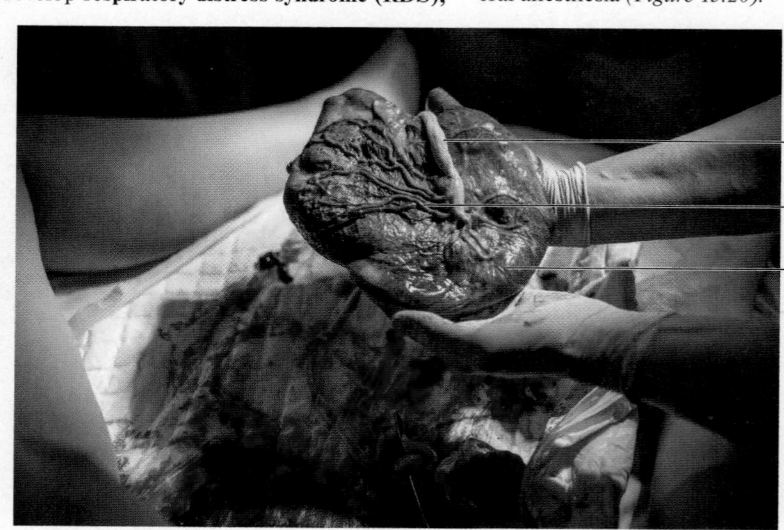

FIGURE 15.20 Placenta (Afterbirth).

AzmanL/Getty Images

Word Analysis and Definition

S = Suffix P = Prefix R = Root R/CF = Combining Form

WORD	PRONUNCIATION	ELEMENTS		DEFINITION
abortion	ah-**BOR**-shun	S/ R/	-ion *action* **abort-** *fail at onset*	Spontaneous or induced expulsion of the embryo or fetus from the uterus at 20 weeks or less
breech	**BREECH**		Old English *trousers*	Buttocks-first presentation of the fetus at delivery
cesarean section (c-section)	seh-**ZAH**-ree-an **SEK**-shun		Roman law under the Caesars required that pregnant women who died be cut open and the fetus be extracted	Extraction of the fetus through an incision in the abdomen and uterine wall
kernicterus	ker-**NICK**-ter-us	R/ R/	**kern-** *nucleus* **-icterus** *jaundice*	Bilirubin staining of the basal nuclei of the brain
meconium	meh-**KOH**-nee-um		Greek *a little poppy*	The first bowel movement of the newborn
nuchal cord	**NYU**-kul KORD		nuchal, French *the back (nape) of the neck*	Loop(s) of umbilical cord around the fetal neck
placenta abruptio	plah-**SEN**-tah ab-**RUP**-she-oh		abruptio, Latin *to break off*	The premature detachment of the placenta
placenta previa	plah-**SEN**-tah **PREE**-vee-ah	P/ R/	**pre-** *before, in front of* **-via** *the way*	Condition in which the placenta is positioned between the fetus and the cervix
postmature	post-mah-**TYUR**	P/ R/	**post-** *after* **-mature** *ripe, ready*	Infant born after 42 weeks of gestation
postmaturity	post-mah-**TYUR**-ih-tee	S/	-ity *condition, state*	Condition of being postmature
premature (slang term "preemie")	pree-mah-**TYUR**	P/ R/	**pre-** *before* **-mature** *ripe, ready*	Occurring before the expected time
prematurity (same as *preterm*)	pree-mah-**TYUR**-ih-tee	S/	-ity *condition, state*	Condition of being premature
surfactant	sir-**FAK**-tant		*surface active agent*	A protein and fat compound that creates surface tension to hold the lung alveolar walls apart
vertex	**VER**-teks		Latin *whorl*	Topmost point of the vault of the skull

EXERCISES

A. Elements. Real familiarity with obstetrical and reproductive terms means you can look at an element and identify it as either a prefix (P), root (R), or suffix (S). *Identify each element by inserting its type and meaning in the appropriate columns. The first one is done for you. Fill in the blanks.* **LO 15.1 and 15.9**

Element	Type	Meaning of the Element
post	**P**	**after**
ity	**1.**	**2.**
kern	**3.**	**4.**
via	**5.**	**6.**
mature	**7.**	**8.**
pre	**9.**	**10.**
abort	**11.**	**12.**

B. Describe the disorders of childbirth. *Match the disorder in the first column with its correct description in the second column. Fill in the blanks.* **LO 15.9**

Term Meaning

______ **1.** prolapsed umbilical cord — **a.** cord is wrapped around the baby's neck during delivery

______ **2.** placenta previa — **b.** cord comes before the baby during delivery

______ **3.** kernicterus — **c.** brain damage due to bilirubin deposits

______ **4.** nuchal cord — **d.** separation of the placenta from the uterine wall before delivery

______ **5.** placenta abruptio — **e.** placenta is positioned over the internal os of the cervix

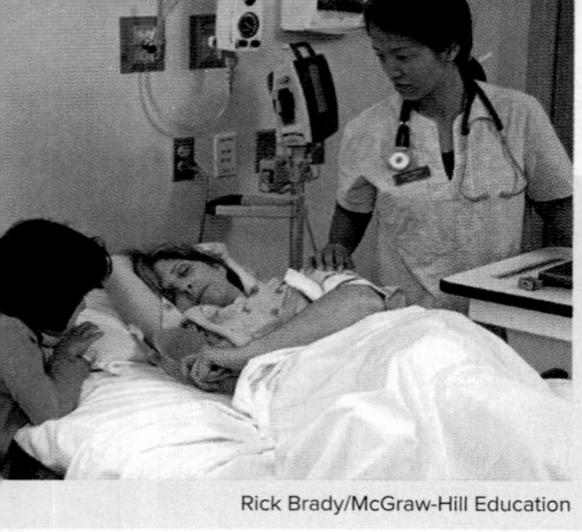
Rick Brady/McGraw-Hill Education

Lesson 15.6

Obstetrical Diagnostic and Therapeutic Procedures and Pharmacology

Lesson Objectives

15.6.1 Identify diagnostic procedures used in the treatment of obstetric problems.

15.6.2 Describe therapeutic procedures used in the treatment of obstetric problems.

15.6.3 Discuss the pharmacology of drugs used in the treatment of obstetric problems.

Obstetrical Diagnostic Procedures (LO 15.10)

Prenatal Screening Tests (LO 15.10)

These tests can help determine if the pregnancy is at a higher risk for the baby to have a specific problem; the test does not diagnose a problem, only whether it is more or less likely. There is no risk of miscarriage from these tests.

First trimester screening is done between the 11th and 13th weeks of pregnancy. It combines **maternal** blood testing for **human chorionic gonadotropin (hCG)** (the pregnancy hormone) and **pregnancy-associated plasma protein A (PAPP-A)** with an ultrasound measurement of the back of the baby's neck (**nuchal translucency–NT).** Women with higher than average NT measurements and/or higher or lower than average hCG or PAPP-A values *might* be at risk for having a baby with Down Syndrome or with another rare chromosomal problem, Trisomy 18.

Chorionic villus sampling (CVS) also uses ultrasound guidance to insert a needle through the abdomen or a catheter through the cervix to obtain a sample of placental tissue that can be tested for fetal chromosomal abnormalities. The main advantage of CVS is that it can be performed between 9 and 13 weeks of pregnancy, earlier than amniocentesis (*see below*).

Second trimester screening is done between the 15th and 18th weeks of gestation. Called the **quad screen,** it measures the levels of four substances in a pregnant woman's blood: **alpha-fetoprotein (AFP), hCG, unconjugated estriol,** and **dimeric inhibin.** These chemicals are made by the placenta and fetus. Women with high or low levels of these substances *may* be at risk for having a baby with Down Syndrome, Trisomy 18, a **neural tube defect** such as **spina bifida**, or an abdominal wall defect in which abdominal contents protrude through the abdominal wall.

Cystic fibrosis screening is a blood test to determine the presence of the gene that causes CF. Both parents have to be carriers of the gene for the baby to be at risk for CF.

Ultrasound can be used to show most of the organs and bones of the baby in utero. In addition to the screenings described above, ultrasound can be used between 18 and 20 weeks of pregnancy to provide a detailed picture of the baby's anatomy, its size, and growth. Ultrasound carries no known risks and is the most frequently used method of prenatal screening.

Diagnostic Tests

Diagnostic tests, as distinct from screening tests, can confirm the presence of the congenital anomaly suggested by the screening test.

Amniocentesis uses ultrasound guidance to insert a thin needle through the abdominal wall into the amniotic sac around the baby to remove a small amount of amniotic fluid. This fluid contains fetal skin fibroblasts that can be tested for abnormalities. Amniocentesis is performed between 15 and 20 weeks to diagnose chromosome abnormalities and neural tube defects.

Therapeutic Procedures

During labor, there is electronic fetal heart monitoring to determine whether the baby is in distress. Treatment is to give the mother oxygen or increase IV fluids. If distress persists, the baby is delivered as quickly as possible by **forceps extraction**, vacuum extractor, or **cesarean section** (**C-section**).

Abbreviations

AFP	alpha-fetoprotein
CVS	chorionic villus sampling
hCG	human chorionic gonadotropin
NT	nuchal translucency
PAPP-A	pregnancy-associated plasma protein A

Word Analysis and Definition

S = Suffix P = Prefix R = Root R/CF = Combining Form

WORD	PRONUNCIATION		ELEMENTS	DEFINITION
amniocentesis	**AM**-nee-oh-sen**TEE**-sis	S/ R/CF	**-centesis** *puncture* **amni/o-** *amnion*	Removal of amniotic fluid for diagnostic purposes
cesarean section (C-section) (syn)	seh-**ZAH**-ree-an **SEK**-shun		Roman law under the Caesars required that pregnant women who died be cut open and the fetus extracted	Extraction of the fetus through an incision in the abdomen and uterine wall
chorion **chorionic** **chorionic villus**	**KOH**-ree-on koh-ree-**ON**-ik koh-ree-**ON**-ik **VILL**-us	 S/ R/	Greek *membrane* **-ic** *pertaining to* **chorion-** *chorion* **villus** Latin *shaggy hair*	Outer fetal membrane that becomes the placenta Pertaining to the chorion Vascular process of the embryonic chorion to form the placenta
diagnostic	die-ag-**NOS**-tik	S/ P/ R/	**-tic** *pertaining to* **dia-** *complete* **-gnos-** *recognize an abnormal condition*	Pertaining to establishing the cause of a disease
forceps extraction	**FOR**-seps ek-**STRAK**-shun		**forceps** Latin *a pair of tongs* **extraction** Latin *to draw out*	Assisted delivery of the baby by an instrument that grasps the head of the baby
gonadotropin	**GO**-nad-oh-**TROH**-pin	S/ R/CF	**-tropin** *nourishing* **gonad/o** *gonad*	Hormone capable of promoting gonad function
maternal	mah-**TER**-nal	S/ R/	**-al** *pertaining to* **matern-** *mother*	Pertaining to, or derived from, the mother
neural **neural tube**	**NYU**-ral **NYU**-ral TYUB	S/ R/	**-al** *pertaining to* **neur-** *nerve*	Pertaining to any structure composed of nerve cells Embryologic tubelike structure that forms the brain and spinal cord
nuchal	**NYU**-kul		French *the back (nape) of the neck*	The back (nape) of the neck
screen **screening**	**SKREEN** **SKREEN**-ing	 S/ R/	Middle English *screne* **-ing** *process* **screen-** *a system for separating*	A test to determine the presence or absence of a disease. A testing process that determines the presence or absence of a disease
translucent	tranz-**LOO**-sent	S/ P/ R/	**-ent** *pertaining to* **trans-** *across, through* **-luc-** *light*	Allowing light to pass through

Exercises

A. Describe the meaning of abbreviations related to obstetrical screening tests. *Given the abbreviation, select its correct description.* **LO 15.3 and 15.10**

1. PAPP-A is used to screen for:

a. spina bifida **b.** fetal alcohol syndrome **c.** Down Syndrome **d.** cystic fibrosis

2. Amniocentesis at 15 and 20 weeks is used to test diagnose:

a. nuchal translucency **b.** neural tube defects **c.** fetal alcohol syndrome **d.** cystic fibrosis

3. How is NT measured?

a. maternal blood testing **b.** fetal blood testing **c.** amniocentesis **d.** ultrasound

B. Construct medical terms related to obstetrics. *Given the definition, complete the described medical terms by inputting the correct word element.* **LO 15.1 and 15.10**

1. Hormone capable of promoting gonad function: gonado/________________

2. To puncture the amniotic sac: amnio/ ________________

3. Pertaining to the mother: ________________ /al

4. Allowing light to pass through: ________________ /luc/ent

5. Pertaining to a nerve: ________________ /al

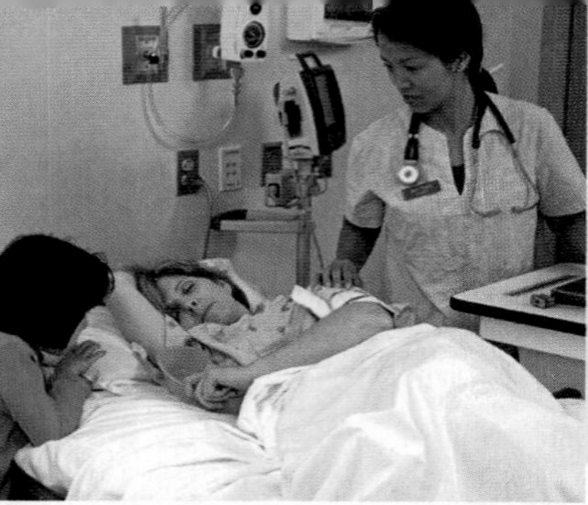

Rick Brady/McGraw-Hill Education

Lesson 15.7

The Female Breast

Objectives

Until the relatively recent introduction of bottles filled with liquid supplied by cows or soybeans, the milk produced by the female breast was essential for the survival of the human species. Nourishment of the infant remains the breast's major function. It is important to complete your understanding of the female reproductive system by being able to use correct medical terminology to:

15.7.1 Describe the anatomy of the breast and the mammary gland.

15.7.2 Explain the physiology and mechanisms of lactation.

15.7.3 Discuss common disorders of the breast.

Keynote

- There is no relation between breast size and the ability to breastfeed.

CASE REPORT 15.5

You are . . .

. . . a surgical technologist working with Charles Walsh, MD, a surgeon at Fulwood Medical Center.

You are communicating with . . .

. . . Mrs. Victoria Post, a 62-year-old woman who has discovered a lump in her right breast. Mrs. Post found the lump in her right breast together with some lumps in her right armpit on self-examination. She had not examined her breasts for about 6 months. She began her menopause at age 52. Her mother and a sister died of breast cancer. Physical examination shows a 2-cm firm, painless lesion in the upper outer quadrant of her right breast, and several small, painless lymph nodes in her right axilla. Dr. Walsh has scheduled her for a biopsy of the breast lesion and for DNA testing.

The Breast (LO 15.11)

Anatomy of the Breast (LO 15.11)

The female breasts can be both beautiful and functional. They help to give a woman her distinctive feminine shape, and, after childbirth, they provide natural nourishment for an infant. Each adult female breast has a **body** located over the pectoralis major muscle and an **axillary tail** extending toward the armpit. The **nipple** projects from the breast and contains multiple openings of the main milk ducts. The reddish-brown **areola** surrounds the nipple. The small bumps on its surface are called **areolar glands.** These are sebaceous glands whose secretions prevent chapping and cracking during breastfeeding.

The **nonlactating breast** consists mostly of adipose and connective tissues. It has a system of ducts that branch through the connective tissue and converge on the nipple.

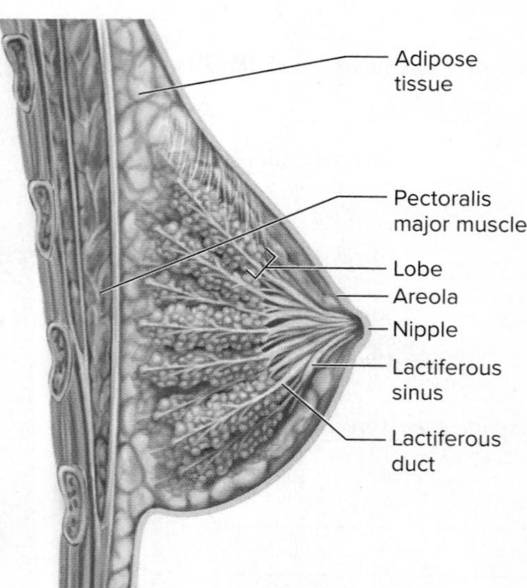

▲ **FIGURE 15.21**
Anatomy of the Lactating Breast.

Mammary Gland (LO 15.11)

When the **mammary** gland develops during pregnancy, it is divided into 15 to 20 lobes that contain the secretory **alveoli** that produce milk. The main milk ducts, called **lactiferous ducts** *(Figure 15.21)* drain each lobe immediately before opening onto the nipple.

Lactation (LO 15.11)

In late pregnancy, the secretory alveoli and lactiferous ducts contain **colostrum.** This is the first secretion from the breasts during pregnancy. Colostrum contains more protein but less fat than human milk. It also contains high levels of **immunoglobulins** *(see Chapter 7)* that give the infant protection from infections. Colostrum begins to be replaced by milk 2 or 3 days after the baby's birth, and this replacement is complete by day 5.

The essential stimulus to milk production is the baby's sucking. This stimulates the pituitary gland to produce **prolactin,** which in turn stimulates milk production, and **oxytocin** *(see Chapter 12),* which causes milk to be ejected from the alveoli into the duct system.

After **lactation** completely stops, **involution** of the mammary gland occurs. The epithelial cells of the alveoli are lost through **apoptosis** (programmed cell death), the ducts shrink in size, and adipose and connective tissues return to be the major breast tissues.

Word Analysis and Definition

S = Suffix P = Prefix R = Root R/CF = Combining Form

WORD	PRONUNCIATION	ELEMENTS		DEFINITION
apoptosis	**AP**-op-**TOE**-sis	P/ R/	apo- *separation from* -ptosis *drooping*	Programmed normal cell death
areola areolar (adj)	ah-**REE**-oh-lah ah-**REE**-oh-lar	S/ R/	Latin *small area* -ar *pertaining to* areol- *areolar*	Circular reddish area surrounding the nipple Pertaining to the areola
colostrum	koh-**LOSS**-trum		Latin *foremilk*	The first breast secretion at the end of pregnancy
involution involute (verb)	in-voh-**LOO**-shun in-voh-**LUTE**	S/ P/ R/	-ion *action, condition* in- *in* -volut- *roll up, shrink*	Decrease in size
lactation (noun) lactate (verb) lactiferous (adj)	lak-**TAY**-shun **LAK**-tate lak-**TIF**-er-us	S/ R/ S/ S/ R/	-ation *action, process of* lact- *milk* -ate *composed of, pertaining to* -ous *pertaining to* -ifer- *to bear, carry*	Production of milk To produce milk Pertaining to or yielding milk
mammary	**MAM**-ah-ree	S/ R/	-ary *pertaining to* mamm- *breast*	Pertaining to the lactating breast
nipple	**NIP**-el		Old English *small nose*	Projection from the breast into which the lactiferous ducts open
oxytocin	**OCK**-see-**TOE**-sin	S/ R/ R/	-in *substance* oxy- *oxygen* -toc- *labor*	Pituitary hormone that stimulates the uterus to contract
prolactin	pro-**LAK**-tin	S/ P/ R/	-in *substance* pro- *before* -lact- *milk*	Pituitary hormone that stimulates the production of milk

Exercises

A. Find the false statements in the following choices. *Choose T if the statement is True. Choose F if the statement is False.* **LO 15.11**

1. The lactiferous ducts produce milk. T F
2. In late pregnancy, the breast secretory alveoli and lactiferous ducts contain colostrum. T F
3. High levels of immunoglobulins are in breast milk. T F
4. The essential stimulus for milk production is suckling of the breast. T F
5. The suckling of the nipple produces estrogen. T F
6. Milk flows from the lactiferous duct to the lactiferous sinus to the nipple. T F

B. Spelling *your documentation correctly is a mark of an educated professional. Read the following statements, and insert the correctly spelled term in the blanks.* **LO 15.2 and 15.11**

1. The circular, reddish area surrounding the nipple is the *(aireola/areola)* ____________.
2. After complete cessation of lactation, involution of the *(mamery/mammary)* ____________ gland occurs.
3. Programmed cell death is known as *(apotosis/apoptosis)* ____________.
4. The first breast secretion at the end of pregnancy is known as *(colestrium/colostrum)* ____________.

C. Construct *medical terms related to the breast. Fill in the blanks with the correct word element.* **LO 15.1 and 15.11**

1. Pituitary hormone that stimulates the uterus to contract: ________ / ________ / ________
2. Programmed natural cell death: ________ / ________
3. Pituitary hormone that stimulates the production of milk: ________ / ________ / ________
4. Pertaining to or yielding milk: ________ / ________ / ________
5. Decrease in size: ________ / ________ / ________

Lesson 15.7
(cont'd)

Keynote

- There is some disagreement whether routine mammograms should begin at age 40 or 50 and whether they should be performed annually or every 2 years.

Abbreviations

BRCA1, BRCA2	breast cancer genes
BSE	breast self-examination
PMS	premenstrual syndrome

Case Report 15.5 *(continued)*

Mrs. Victoria Post's biopsy confirmed that the lump was cancer. DNA testing showed the presence of the **BRCA1 gene,** which explained the occurrence of breast cancer in her mother and sister. Mrs. Post is to attend a consultation with her surgeon, Dr. Walsh, and her **geneticist,** Ingrid Hughes, MD, PhD, to determine what treatment should be undertaken. For example, because of her high risk of cancer, should she have her left breast, currently cancer-free, removed? With BRCA1, there is also a 20% to 40% risk of ovarian cancer. Therefore, should her ovaries also be removed?

Disorders of the Breast (LO 15.11)

Mastitis, an inflammation of the breast, can occur in association with breastfeeding if the nipple or areola is cracked or traumatized. **Mastalgia** (breast pain) is the most common benign breast disorder. This pain may be associated with breast tenderness or **PMS.**

Paget disease of the nipple presents as a scaling, crusting lesion of the nipple, sometimes with a discharge from the nipple *(Figure 15.22).* It is indicative of an underlying cancer that must be the focus of diagnosis and treatment.

Nipple discharge, particularly if it is bloody and only from one breast, is an indication of an underlying disorder like breast cancer and should be investigated.

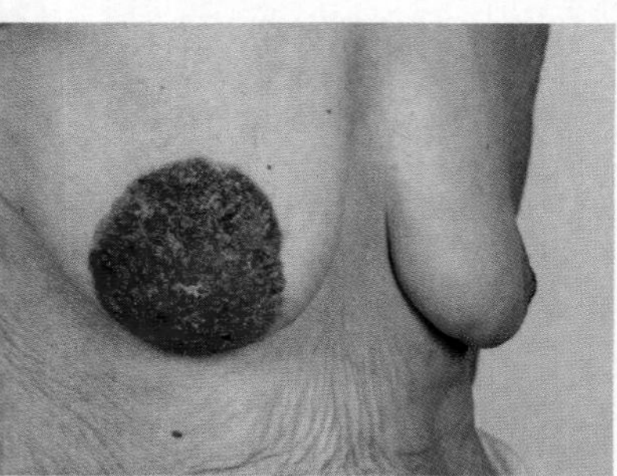

▲ **FIGURE 15.22**
Paget Disease of the Nipple Is Associated with Breast Cancer.

Clinical Photography, Central Manchester University Hospitals NHS Foundation Trust, UK/Science Source

Fibroadenomas are confined, small, benign tumors that can be either cystic or solid, and can be multiple. These tumors can be surgically removed.

Fibrocystic breast disease presents as a dense, irregular, cobblestone consistency of the breast, often with intermittent breast discomfort. It occurs in over 60% of all women and is considered by many doctors as a normal condition.

Breast cancer affects one in eight women in their lifetimes. Risk factors include: a family history, particularly if a woman carries either the **BRCA1** or **BRCA2 gene;** the use of postmenopausal estrogen therapy; and an early menarche and late menopause.

Some breast cancers are discovered as a lump by the patient, which is why **monthly breast self-examinations (BSEs)** are important. Another 40% are discovered on routine **mammograms** *(Figure 15.23).* Routine **mammography** reduces breast cancer mortality by 25% to 30%. Breast cancer rarely occurs in males.

Most breast cancers occur in the upper and outer quadrants of the breast. If cancer is suspected, a biopsy should be planned. Currently, it's common to perform a **stereotactic biopsy,** where a needle biopsy is done during mammography. Breast cancer can metastasize to the lymph nodes, lungs, liver, bones, brain, and skin. The surgical treatments available for breast cancer include:

- **Lumpectomy:** the tumor is removed and the surrounding breast tissue is preserved.
- Simple **mastectomy:** the breast with skin and the nipple is removed.
- Modified radical mastectomy: a simple mastectomy with lymph node dissection.
- Radical mastectomy: a modified mastectomy that includes the removal of lymph nodes and the pectoralis major muscle.

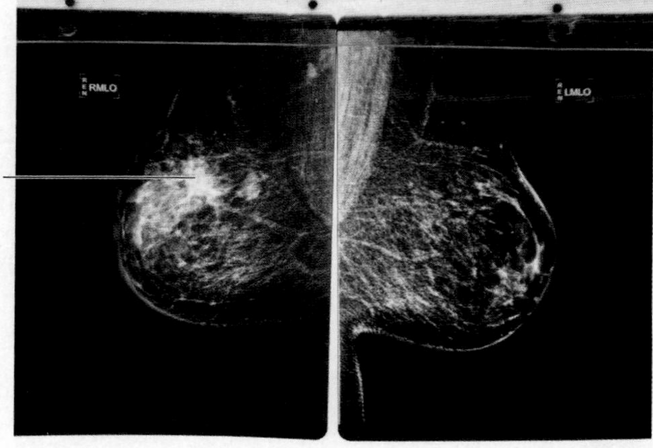

▲ **FIGURE 15.23**
Mammogram Showing Breast Cancer and a Normal Breast.

Alan Nissa/Shutterstock

Additional radiotherapy and chemotherapy are also used.

Galactorrhea occurs when a woman produces milk when she's not breastfeeding. This can occur in association with hormone therapy, antidepressants, a pituitary gland tumor, and the use of street drugs like cocaine, heroin, and marijuana. In most cases, the milk production ceases with time.

Gynecomastia is an enlargement of the breast that can be unilateral or bilateral. It can occur in both sexes. It is usually associated with either liver disease, marijuana use, or drug therapy involving estrogens, calcium channel blockers, and **antineoplastic** drugs. Gynecomastia remits or disappears after the drug is withdrawn. Occasionally, cosmetic surgery is needed.

Word Analysis and Definition

S = Suffix P = Prefix R = Root R/CF = Combining Form

WORD	PRONUNCIATION	ELEMENTS		DEFINITION
antineoplastic	**AN**-tee-nee-oh-**PLAS**-tik	S/ P/ R/CF R/	**-tic** *pertaining to* **anti-** *against* **-ne/o-** *new* **-plas-** *growth*	Pertaining to the prevention of the growth and spread of cancer cells
fibroadenoma	**FIE**-broh-ad-en-**OH**-muh	S/ R/CF R/	**-oma** *tumor* **fibr/o-** *fiber* **-aden-** *gland*	Benign tumor containing much fibrous tissue
fibrocystic disease	fie-broh-SIS-tik diz-**EEZ**	S/ R/CF R/	**-ic** *pertaining to* **fibr/o-** *fiber* **-cyst-** *cyst*	Benign breast disease with multiple tiny lumps and cysts
galactorrhea	gah-**LAK**-toe-**REE**-ah	S/ R/CF	**-rrhea** *flow* **galact/o-** *milk*	Abnormal flow of milk from the breasts
gene genetics geneticist (**Note:** *Two suffixes*)	**JEEN** jeh-**NET**-iks jeh-**NET**-ih-sist	 S/ R/ S/	Greek *origin, birth* **-ics** *knowledge* **genet-** *origin* **-ist** *specialist*	Functional segment of DNA molecule Science of the inheritance of characteristics A specialist in genetics
gynecomastia	**GUY**-nih-koh-**MAS**-tee-ah	S/ R/CF R/	**-ia** *condition* **gynec/o-** *female* **-mast-** *breast*	Enlargement of the breast
lumpectomy	lump-**ECK**-toe-me	S/ R/	**-ectomy** *surgical excision* **lump-** *piece*	Removal of a lesion with preservation of surrounding tissue
mammogram mammography	**MAM**-oh-gram mah-**MOG**-rah-fee	S/ R/CF S/	**-gram** *a record* **mamm/o-** *breast* **-graphy** *process of recording*	The record produced by X-ray imaging of the breast Process of X-ray examination of the breast
mastalgia	mass-**TAL**-jee-uh	S/ R/	**-algia** *pain* **mast-** *breast*	Pain in the breast
mastectomy	mass-**TECK**-toe-me	S/ R/	**-ectomy** *surgical excision* **mast-** *breast*	Surgical excision of the breast
mastitis	mass-**TIE**-tis	S/ R/	**-itis** *inflammation* **mast-** *breast*	Inflammation of the breast
Paget disease	**PAJ**-et diz-**EEZ**		Sir James Paget, 1814–1899, English surgeon	Scaling, crusting lesion of the nipple, often associated with an underlying cancer of the breast
stereotactic	**STER**-ee-oh-**TAK**-tic	S/ R/CF R/	**-ic** *pertaining to* **stere/o-** *three-dimensional* **-tact-** *orderly arrangement*	A precise three-dimensional method to locate a lesion

EXERCISES

A. Review *the terms related to disorders of the breast. Insert the term that is being described. Fill in the blanks.* **LO 15.2 and 15.11**

1. Pain in the breast: ____________________
2. Inflammation of the breast: ____________________
3. A small, benign tumor of the breast: ____________________
4. Enlargement of the breast: ____________________
5. Benign breast disease with multiple tiny bumps and cysts: ____________________

B. Deconstruct medical terms to understand their meanings. *Fill in the blanks with the correct definition.* **LO 15.1 and 15.11**

1. The suffix in the term **galactorrhea** means: ____________________
2. The root in the term **mastalgia** means: ____________________
3. The combining form in the term **galactorrhea** means: ____________________
4. The suffix in the term **mastitis** means: ____________________
5. The suffix in the term **gynecomastia** means: ____________________

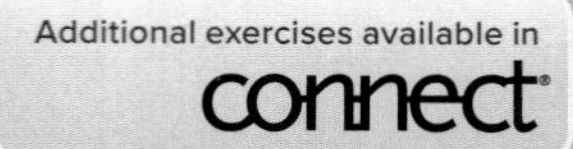

Chapter Review exercises, along with additional practice items, are available in Connect!

Infancy to Old Age

The Languages of Pediatrics and Geriatrics

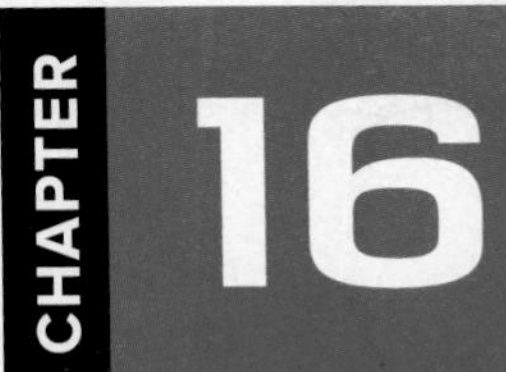

Rick Brady/McGraw-Hill Education

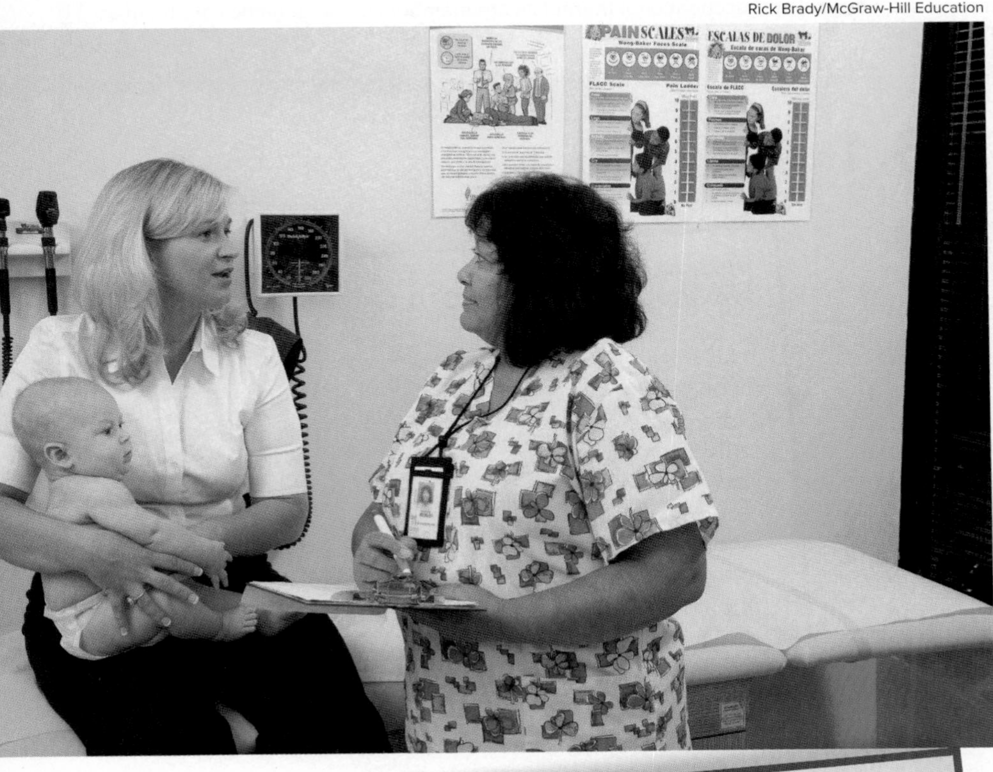

Learning Outcomes

Immediately after birth and in the whole neonatal period dramatic and rapid changes occur in the growth and development of cells, tissues, and body systems. These changes slow down through infancy, childhood, adolescence and young adulthood until **maturity,** which occurs at different ages for different body systems. In general, maturity occurs in the late twenties. Eventually and inevitably, different physiological changes in cells, tissues, and body systems lead to a progressive deterioration and decline in function. This process is called **senescence** and is manifest as the changes that occur in aging and eventually in death. In order to communicate with your colleagues and patients about this process, you will need to:

- **LO 16.1** **Use roots, combining forms, suffixes, and prefixes to construct and analyze (deconstruct) medical terms related to pediatrics and geriatrics.**
- **LO 16.2** **Spell and pronounce correctly medical terms related to pediatrics and geriatrics to communicate them with accuracy and precision in any health care setting.**
- **LO 16.3** **Define accepted abbreviations related to pediatrics and geriatrics.**
- **LO 16.4** **Describe the method of evaluation of a newborn's physical status.**
- **LO 16.5** **Relate the adaptations of each body system that occur in the neonatal period to their functions.**
- **LO 16.6** **Distinguish the different developmental disorders of childhood and adolescence.**
- **LO 16.7** **Identify the significance of the medical terms used in aging and senescence.**
- **LO 16.8** **Compare the changes of senescence in the different body systems.**
- **LO 16.9** **Discuss the medical issues in dying and death.**
- **LO 16.10** **Apply your knowledge of medical terms relating to pediatrics and geriatrics to documentation, medical records, and medical reports.**
- **LO 16.11** **Translate the medical terms relating to pediatrics and geriatrics into everyday language in order to communicate clearly with patients and their families.**

CASE REPORT 16.1

You are . . .

. . . a pediatric medical assistant employed by Sandra Mendes, MD, a **pediatrician** at Fulwood Medical Center. You are working in her Well-Baby Clinic.

You are communicating with . . .

. . . Mrs. Anna Hotteling, a 35-year-old mother, who has brought her 10-week-old daughter, Carol, to the Well-Baby Clinic. Carol, Mrs. Hotteling's first baby, was born via a normal vaginal delivery at term. She weighed 7 pounds 2 ounces. She had normal **Apgar** scores. Carol had persistent jaundice when seen at 2 weeks of age. She is being breastfed. You ask Mrs. Hotteling if she has any concerns.

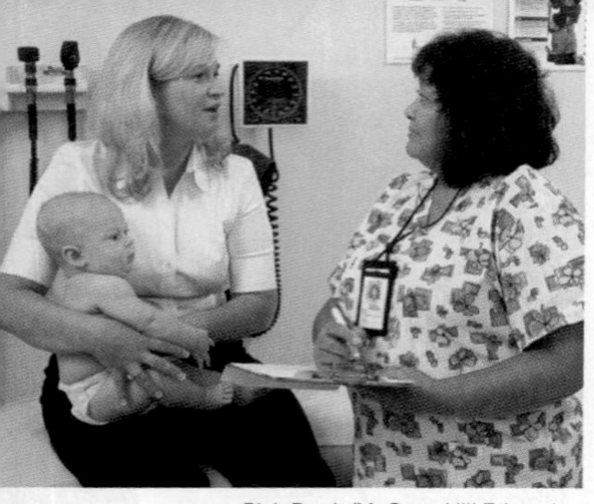

Rick Brady/McGraw-Hill Education

The **health professionals** involved in the treatment of children and the elderly include:

- **Neonatologists** are physicians who are pediatric subspecialists in disorders of the newborn, particularly ill, or premature infants.
- **Pediatricians** are physicians who are specialists in disorders of childhood and adolescence.
- **Geriatricians** are physicians who are specialists in the process of and problems of aging.
- **Gerontologists** are professionals who are specialists in the process of and general problems of aging.
- **Geriatric nurse practitioners** are nurses with special training in the care of the elderly.
- **Social workers, nutritionists, physical and occupational therapists** are members of the geriatric care team as needs for their services arise.

Objectives

In order to comprehend and identify where ***neonates*** *are in their development and to communicate with their mothers, as well as your colleagues, about their growth progress, you must be able to:*

16.1.1 Name the anatomic and physiologic **adaptations** that occur at birth and in the **neonatal** period.

16.1.2 Apply correct medical terminology to common congenital **anomalies** that interfere with normal development.

16.1.3 Describe the medical terminology of disorders in growth and development in the neonatal period.

Abbreviations

APGAR	activity, pulse, grimace, appearance, respiration
SIDS	sudden infant death syndrome

Lesson 16.1

Neonatal Period

Case Report 16.1 *(continued)*

Mrs. Anna Hotteling, the mother, has several areas of concern. A friend's baby recently died of **SIDS** (sudden infant death syndrome). How can Mrs. Hotteling prevent this from happening to her child? Carol wants to feed every 2 to 3 hours day and night, and Mrs. Hotteling is exhausted. How long will this go on, and for how long should she continue breastfeeding? Mrs. Hotteling also wants to know what her baby can see and how she should communicate with her.

Neonatal Adaptations (LO 16.1, 16.3, 16.4, 16.5, and 16.10)

Fetal life is a preparation for birth, and at the end of the first 8 weeks, all the fetus' organ systems are in place *(Figure 16.1)*. From then until birth, the organs grow and acquire the functional capabilities to support life outside the mother. Sometimes a part of this process may fail, causing a developmental abnormality in the **fetus.**

At birth, normal organ development is not yet complete, but the **neonate** *(Figure 16.2)* or newborn infant suddenly has to **adapt** to a totally different environment: life outside the womb. Each of the neonate's organ systems has to adapt to this new environment, and then go on to complete its development during childhood. This developmental process is why children are not just "little adults," and why **pediatricians** are needed to practice the specialty of **pediatrics.**

Immediately after birth, the neonate is evaluated for her **Apgar score** at 1 minute and again at 5 minutes of life. This score gives health care providers an immediate assessment of the baby's condition at birth. The five measurements of **A**ctivity, **P**ulse, **G**rimace, **A**ppearance, and **R**espiration are each scored on a 3-point scale: 0 (poor), 1, or 2 (normal). The total score obtainable is between 0 and 10. A score of 7 or above is normal. A score below 7 indicates the baby needs special immediate care, including oxygen and further airway suctioning. The Apgar score does not predict long-term health, intellectual status, or outcome.

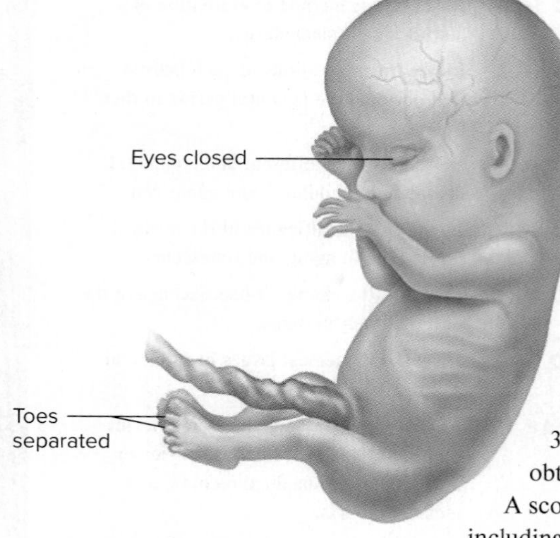

▲ **FIGURE 16.1**
Fetus at 8 Weeks (56 Days).

▲ **FIGURE 16.2**
Full-Term Infant (38 Weeks).

Word Analysis and Definition

S = Suffix P = Prefix R = Root R/CF = Combining Form

WORD	PRONUNCIATION		ELEMENTS	DEFINITION
adaptation **adapt (verb)**	ad-ap-**TAY**-shun a-**DAPT**	S/ R/	-ation *process* adapt- *to adjust*	Change in the function or structure of an organ or organism to meet new conditions
anomaly **anomalies (pl)**	ah-**NOM**-ah-lee		Greek *irregularity*	Structural abnormality present at birth
Apgar score	**AP**-gar SKOR		Virginia Apgar, U.S. anesthesiologist, 1909–1974	Evaluation of a newborn's status
fetus **fetal (adj)**	**FEE**-tus **FEE**-tal	 S/ R/	Latin *offspring* -al *pertaining to* fet- *fetus*	Human organism from the end of the eighth week after conception to birth Pertaining to the fetus
maturity **mature**	mah-**CHUR**-ih-tee mah-**CHUR**	S/ R/	-ity *condition, state* matur- *ripe, ready*	A state of full development or growth Fully developed
neonate **neonatal (adj)** (**Note:** *The "e" is dropped as it is followed by another vowel, "a."*) **neonatologist**	**NEE**-oh-nate **NEE**-oh-NAY-tal **NEE**-oh-nay-**TOL**-oh-jist	R/CF R/CF S/ R/ S/	neo- *new* -nat/e *born* -al *pertaining to* -nat- *born* -logist *one who studies, specialist*	A newborn infant Pertaining to the newborn infant or the newborn period Medical specialist in disorders of the newborn
pediatrics **pediatrician**	pee-dee-**AT**-riks **PEE**-dee-ah-**TRISH**-an	S/ R/ R/ S/	-ics *knowledge* -iatr- *medical treatment* ped- *child* -ician *expert*	Medical specialty of treating children during development from birth through adolescence Medical specialist in disorders of childhood and adolescence

EXERCISES

A. Demonstrate *your understanding of medical professionals. Insert the medical professional being described. Fill in the blanks.* **LO 16.2**

1. Physician that specializes in the process and problems of aging: __________
2. Physician specializing in disorders of the newborn: __________
3. Nurses with special training in the care of the elderly: ________
4. Physician specializing in the care of children and adolescents: __________

B. Match *the meaning in the first column with the correct element in the second column. The elements are ones you will see in terms throughout this chapter. Knowledge of these elements will help to increase your medical vocabulary. Fill in the blanks.* **LO 16.1**

______	**1.** new	**a.** nate
______	**2.** expert	**b.** ics
______	**3.** medical treatment	**c.** ped
______	**4.** knowledge	**d.** ician
______	**5.** to adjust	**e.** neo
______	**6.** child	**f.** al
______	**7.** born	**g.** iatr
______	**8.** pertaining to	**h.** ation
______	**9.** process	**i.** adapt

C. Construct *medical terms that relate to the neonatal period. Fill in the blanks with the correct word element.* **LO 16.1 and 16.2**

1. Pertaining to the fetus: ____________________/____________________
2. Medical specialty of treating children during development from birth through adolescence: ______________/ ______________/______________
3. Change in function of an organ to meet new conditions: ____________________/____________________

Lesson 16.1 (cont'd) Neonatal Adaptations (continued) (LO 16.1, 16.3, 16.4, 16.5, and 16.10)

Keynote

- Meconium is the first stool a baby passes.

Cardiovascular System (CVS) Adaptations (LO 16.1, 16.3, and 16.5)

In utero (when the fetus is still in the uterus), the fetus is dependent on the placenta and umbilical cord to provide oxygen and nutrients, and to remove carbon dioxide and fetal wastes. At birth, the two major divisions of the cardiovascular system **(CVS)**—the pulmonary and systemic circulations *(see Chapter 6)*—become separate and operational.

Congenital (meaning inherited or existing at birth) cardiovascular defects are present in about 1% of births. Before birth, a **patent** (open) vessel called the ductus arteriosus connects the aorta and pulmonary artery. Normally, this closes within a few hours of birth. However, when it doesn't close, the patent ductus arteriosus **(PDA)** allows blood that should normally flow through the aorta and nourish the body to be shunted to the lungs. Children with a PDA grow slowly, tire easily, and develop pneumonia. A small patent ductus can close spontaneously. A ductus can be closed with medication, by surgically tying it, or by inserting a plug.

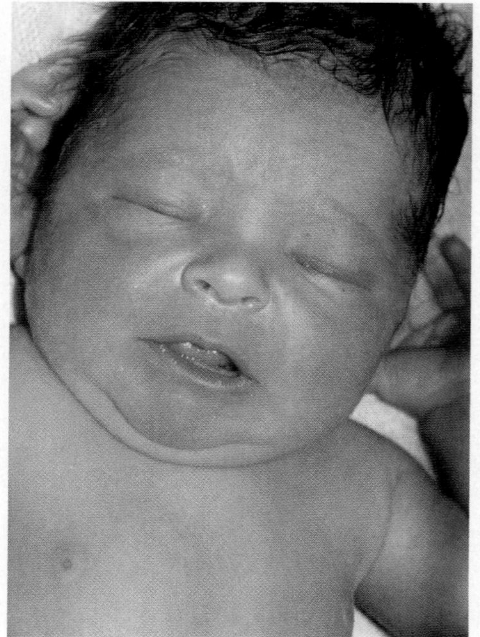

▲ **FIGURE 16.3**
Cyanotic ("Blue") Baby.

St Bartholomew's Hospital, London/ Science Source

Septal defects occur when the baby is born with an opening ("hole in the heart") in the septum (wall) that separates the right and left sides of the heart. An opening between the two upper chambers is called an **atrial septal defect (ASD).** An opening between the two lower chambers is called a **ventricular septal defect (VSD).** Small defects often close on their own during the first year of life; if not, they can be closed surgically.

Cyanosis occurs when the body fails to pump a sufficient amount of blood to the lungs. As a result, the blood being pumped through the body doesn't provide enough oxygen to the tissues. Neonates with cyanosis are called "blue babies" because of their **cyanotic** blue skin *(Figure 16.3).* One type of cyanotic heart disease is the **tetralogy of Fallot (TOF),** in which four heart defects all shunt blood away from the lungs. Children with TOF do not grow, are **dyspneic,** and require open-heart surgery to correct the defects.

Abbreviations

ASD	atrial septal defect
CVS	cardiovascular system
HMD	hyaline membrane disease
PDA	patent ductus arteriosus
RDS	respiratory distress syndrome
SIDS	sudden infant death syndrome
TOF	tetralogy of Fallot
TTN	transient tachypnea of the newborn
VSD	ventricular septal defect

Respiratory Adaptations (LO 16.1, 16.3, and 16.5)

Respiratory adaptations occur immediately at birth when the baby takes its first breath spontaneously, unless the baby's respiratory function is depressed by too much sedation or anesthesia in the mother.

The development of the chemical **surfactant** is necessary for the growth of fully functioning lungs. When surfactant is deficient, the lung alveoli collapse; this prevents a normal exchange of gases. This deficiency occurs in premature infants born before the 37th week of gestation and produces **respiratory distress syndrome (RDS),** previously called **hyaline membrane disease (HMD).** The more premature the baby, the greater its risk of developing RDS. Infants with RDS are at risk for cerebral ischemia, hemorrhage, and neonatal death.

Meconium aspiration syndrome occurs in newborns who are stressed in utero or at the time of delivery. The distress causes the fetus to expel **meconium** into the amniotic fluid. Deep gasping for breath by the distressed fetus causes the aspiration (or inhalation) of meconium into the lungs. This is treated using **intubation** and **suction** to remove the meconium-stained fluid from the lungs.

Transient tachypnea of the newborn (TTN) occurs most often in C-sections and **precipitate** (unduly rapid) vaginal deliveries. With TTN, amniotic fluid remains in the infant's lungs and causes a self-limiting respiratory distress.

Sudden infant death syndrome (SIDS) may be caused by a failure of cardiorespiratory control mechanisms to mature. It is the sudden death of an infant with no identifiable cause found after a thorough investigation and autopsy. It occurs during sleep and peaks between 2 and 3 months, and can be prevented by placing infants on their backs to sleep *(Figure 16.4).*

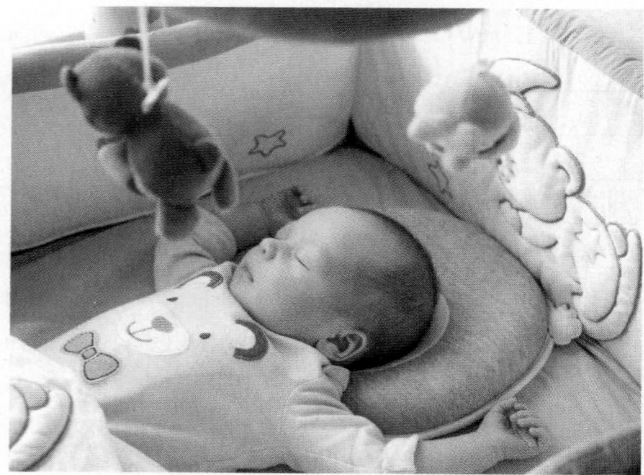

▲ **FIGURE 16.4**
Infant Sleeping on Back.

DigitalMammoth/Shutterstock

Word Analysis and Definition

S = Suffix P = Prefix R = Root R/CF = Combining Form

WORD	PRONUNCIATION	ELEMENTS		DEFINITION
cyanosis **cyanotic (adj)**	sigh-ah-**NO**-sis sigh-ah-**NOT**-ik	S/ R/ S/ R/CF	**-osis** *condition* **cyan-** *blue* **-tic** *pertaining to* **cyan/o-** *blue*	Blue discoloration of skin, lips, and nail beds due to low levels of oxygen in the blood Pertaining to or marked by cyanosis
dyspnea **dyspneic (adj)**	disp-**NEE**-ah disp-**NEE**-ik	P/ R/ S/	**dys-** *bad, difficult* **-pnea** *breathe* **-ic** *pertaining to*	Difficulty breathing Pertaining to or suffering from difficulty in breathing
Fallot	fah-**LOW**		Etienne Louis Arthur Fallot, French physician, 1850–1911	First described the tetralogy of the four heart defects
hyaline membrane disease	**HIGH**-ah-line **MEM**-brain diz-**EEZ**	S/ R/ R/ P/ R/	**-ine** *pertaining to* **hyal-** *glass* **membrane** *cover* **dis-** *apart from* **-ease** *normal function*	Respiratory distress syndrome of the newborn
in utero	IN **YOU**-ter-oh	R/CF	**uter/o** *uterus*	Within the womb; not yet born
meconium	meh-**KOH**-nee-um		Greek *a little poppy*	The first bowel movement of the newborn
patent	**PAY**-tent		Latin *lie open*	Open
precipitate labor	pree-**SIP**-ih-tate **LAY**-bore		precipitate, Latin *to throw down* labor, Latin *toil, suffering*	A very rapid labor and delivery
surfactant	sir-**FAK**-tant		surface, *active agent*	A protein and fat compound that creates surface tension to hold the lung alveolar walls apart
suction	**SUK**-shun		Latin *sucking*	Use of a catheter to clear the upper airway or other tubes
tetralogy	te-**TRAL**-oh-jee	P/ R/	**tetra-** *four* **-logy** *study of*	A set of four congenital heart defects occurring together

EXERCISES

A. Abbreviations: *Incorporate your knowledge of abbreviations from this lesson into the following patient documentation. Fill in the blanks, using the choices below; there are more choices than answers.* **LO 16.3 and 16.10**

RDS ASD SIDS TOF TTN VSD PDA

1. Diagnostic testing confirms ____________________, an opening between the two lower chambers of the infant's heart. Patient will be scheduled for open-heart surgery early next week.
2. Due to a precipitate delivery, and amniotic fluid remaining in the lungs, this infant has ____________________.
3. Because this infant's cardiorespiratory mechanisms have failed to mature, he is at great risk for ____________________.
4. The septal defect in this infant has been confirmed on testing as being between the two upper heart chambers. ____________________
5. One type of cyanotic heart disease is ____________________.

B. These terms *are related to cardiovascular and respiratory adaptations of the newborn. Fill in the blanks with the appropriate explanations.* **LO 16.2 and 16.5**

1. patent ____________________
2. in utero ____________________
3. dyspnea ____________________
4. meconium ____________________
5. precipitate (delivery) ____________________

Lesson 16.1 (cont'd)

Neonatal Adaptations (continued) (LO 16.1, 16.3, 16.4, 16.5, and 16.10)

Keynote

- A baby is born with more than 100 billion brain cells. In the first months and years of life, **connections are made (wiring)** to form complex circuits that allow for thinking, feelings, and behaviors.

Thermoregulation and Adaptations (LO 16.3 and 16.5)

Thermoregulation simply means the body's ability to maintain a steady temperature. This is especially important for newborns. Because an infant has a larger ratio of surface area to body volume than an adult, it loses heat more easily. This is particularly true if the infant's body surface is wet, and it's the reason that a newborn is dried, wrapped, and placed in a warmer soon after birth. **Hypothermia** (very low body temperature) is more likely to occur in premature or small-for-date **(SFD)** neonates.

Brain and Neurologic Adaptations (LO 16.3 and 16.5)

A newborn baby's brain is one-quarter of its adult size. A pediatrician monitors the growth of the baby's brain by charting increases in the baby's head circumference. At birth, only the spinal cord and brainstem are well developed. The cortex is primitive. All of the newborn's kicking, grasping, **rooting** (searching for the nipple), and crying behaviors are functions of the brainstem, which is why they are involuntary and/or not well coordinated.

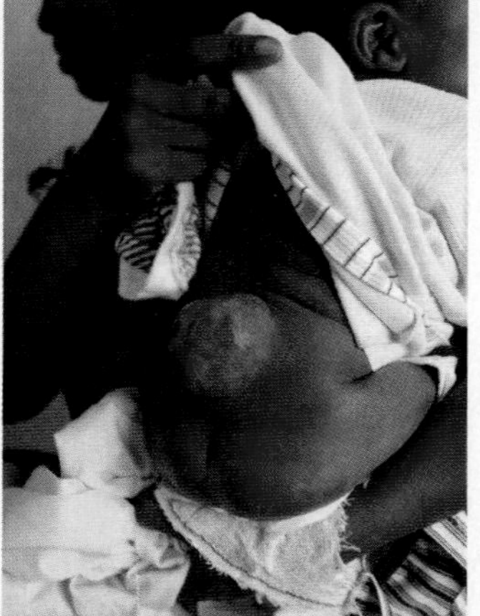

▲ **FIGURE 16.5** Child with Spina Bifida Cystica.

BSIP/UIG/Getty Images

Congenital Neurologic Abnormalities (LO 16.3 and 16.5)

There are some congenital neurologic abnormalities that can severely affect the neonate's quality of life, and its ability to carry on living.

Anencephaly is the absence of the cerebral hemispheres, which is incompatible with life.

Microcephaly is characterized by small cerebral hemispheres, leading to motor and mental retardation.

An **encephalocele** is a protrusion of nervous tissue and meninges through a defect in the skull.

Hydrocephalus is an enlargement of the ventricles with excessive cerebral spinal fluid (CSF), and is the most common cause of a visibly large head in the neonate *(see Chapter 10).*

Spina bifida is a failure of the vertebral column to close over the spinal cord in the lumbar and sacral regions. **Spina bifida occulta** occurs when the vertebral arches fail to unite and there is no neurologic involvement *(see Chapter 10).* When the vertebral defect is more open, nervous tissue can protrude through it in a sac. In **spina bifida cystica** *(Figure 16.5),* the sac can contain **meninges (meningocele),** part of the spinal cord **(myelocele),** or both **(myelomeningocele)** *(see Chapter 10).*

Abbreviation

SFD	small for date

Neonatal seizures are a common and sometimes serious neonatal disorder. These seizures can be primary—caused by an intracranial process like meningitis or a cerebral hemorrhage from a difficult birth—or secondary, caused by a systemic or metabolic problem like hypoxia, hypoglycemia, or hypocalcemia. Treatment is directed to the underlying condition.

Skeletal Adaptations (LO 16.3 and 16.5)

The skeletal system can fail in utero and produce congenital abnormalities in different parts of the newborn's body.

Craniofacial malformations most often present in the form of **cleft lip** and **cleft palate,** which occur once in 800 births *(Figure 16.6).* A cleft palate interferes with feeding and speech development. The end treatment is surgical closure.

Developmental dysplasia of the hip (congenital dislocation of the hip) occurs more commonly in female infants and following a breech delivery. A hip ultrasound can confirm this diagnosis. Treatment is with padded diapers to keep the affected femur abducted. Surgery may be necessary.

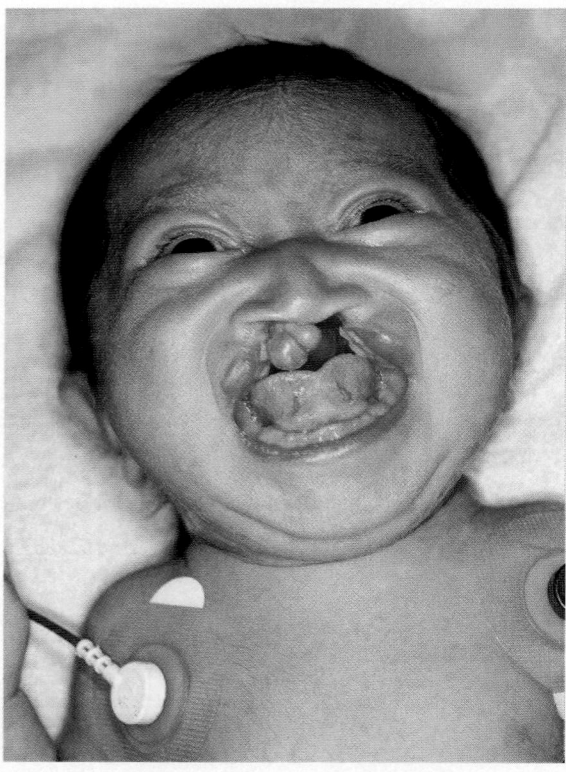

▲ **FIGURE 16.6** Infant with Cleft Lip and Palate.

Scott Camazine/Alamy Images

Word Analysis and Definition

S = Suffix P = Prefix R = Root R/CF = Combining Form

WORD	PRONUNCIATION	ELEMENTS		DEFINITION
anencephaly	**AN**-en-**SEF**-ah-lee	P/ R/	**an-** *without* **-encephaly** *condition of the brain*	Born without cerebral hemispheres
bifid **spina bifida**	**BI**-fid **SPY**-nah **BIH**-fih-dah		bifid, Latin *split into two* spina, Latin *backbone*	Separated into two parts Failure of one or more vertebral arches to close during fetal development
cleft lip **cleft palate**	KLEFT LIP KLEFT PAL-ate		cleft, Latin *fissure, separation of parts*	Congenital defect of the upper lip Congenital defect of the palate
craniofacial	**KRAY**-nee-oh-**FAY**-shal	S/ R/CF R/	**-al** *pertaining to* **crani/o-** *cranium* **-faci-** *face*	Pertaining to both the face and the cranium
dysplasia **dysplastic (adj)**	dis-**PLAY**-zee-ah dis-**PLAS**-tik	S/ P/ R/ S/	**-ia** *condition* **dys-** *bad, difficult* **-plas-** *molding, formation* **-tic** *pertaining to*	Abnormal tissue formation Pertaining to or showing abnormal tissue formation
encephalocele	en-**SEF**-ah-loh-seal	S/ R/CF	**-cele** *swelling, hernia* **encephal/o-** *brain*	Congenital defect of the cranium with herniation of brain tissue
hydrocephalus	high-droh-**SEF**-ah-lus	P/ R/	**hydro-** *water* **-cephalus** *head*	Enlarged head due to excess CSF in the cerebral ventricles
hypothermia	high-poh-**THER**-me-ah	P/ S/ R/	*hypo- below* **-ia** *condition* **-therm-** *heat*	Very low core body temperature
microcephaly **microcephalic (adj)**	**MY**-kroh-SEF-ah-lee **MY**-kroh-SEF-ah-lik	P/ R/ S/	**micro-** *small* **-cephaly** *condition of the head* **-ic** *pertaining to*	Small head Pertaining to or suffering from a small head
myelocele	**MY**-eh-low-seal	S/ R/CF	**-cele** *hernia, swelling* **myel/o-** *spinal cord*	Protrusion of the spinal cord through a defect in the vertebral arch
myelomeningocele	**MY**-eh-low-meh-**NING**-oh-seal	S/ R/CF R/CF	**-cele** *hernia, swelling* **myel/o-** *spinal cord* **-mening/o-** *meninges*	Protrusion of the spinal cord and meninges through a defect in the vertebral arch of one or more vertebrae

EXERCISES

A. Construct *the correct medical term based on the statement given. Insert the element on the line to construct the term.* **LO 16.1 and 16.5**

1. pertaining to both the face and the cranium: ______________ /______________ /______________

2. small head: ______________ /______________ /______________

3. very low core body temperature: ______________ /______________ /______________

4. congenital defect of the cranium with herniation of brain tissue: ______________ /______________

B. Use the language *of pediatrics to answer the following questions. Select the correct answer to complete each statement or answer each question.* **LO 16.5**

1. Which term means "absence of cerebral hemispheres" :

a. microcephaly **b.** anencephaly **c.** myelocele

2. Which element means *spinal cord?*

a. micro **b.** an **c.** cele **d.** myel/o

3. The element *cephaly* means:

a. condition of the brain **b.** condition of the head **c.** spinal cord **d.** cranium

4. Which of these two terms is *incompatible with life?*

a. microcephaly **b.** anencephaly

Lesson 16.1 (cont'd) Neonatal Adaptations (continued) (LO 16.1, 16.3, 16.4, 16.5, and 16.10)

Keynote

- Breast milk provides valuable antibodies, digestive enzymes, and hormones that infants need. It is non-allergenic.

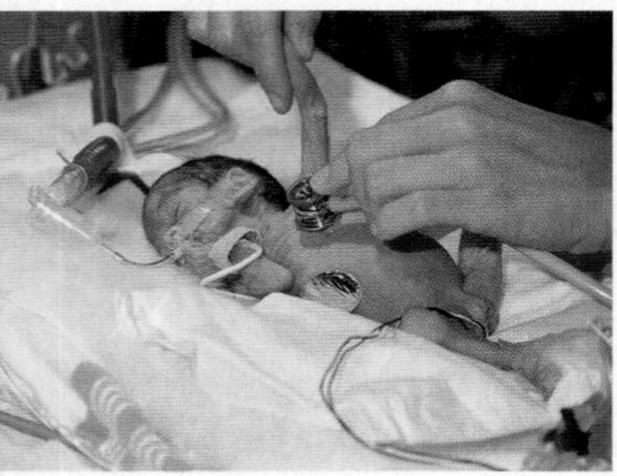

▲ **FIGURE 16.7** Premature Baby.

Susan Leavines/Science Source

Growth Adaptations (LO 16.1, 16.3, and 16.5)

The neonate's failure to grow fully in the uterus has two main causes:

1. **Inadequate nutrition** (caused by poor placental function). Here, the newborn is below the 10th percentile of babies of the same gestational age. This is called **small for gestational age (SGA).** Good nutrition after delivery will enable the neonate's growth to accelerate to normal.
2. **Premature labor** (the infant is born before 37 weeks of gestation). The premature infant *(Figure 16.7)* weighs less than 5½ pounds, has little subcutaneous fat or hair, and has low spontaneous activity. Immature development of the central nervous system (CNS) leads to poor sucking and swallowing. Premature infants may have to be fed by IV or by **gavage** (stomach tube).

Occasionally, labor does not start until after 42 weeks' gestation and produces a **postmature infant** *(Figure 16.8).* Past term, the placenta atrophies and may calcify, so the fetus receives insufficient nutrition in the days after term. As a result, postmature infants have decreased subcutaneous fat and dry, peeling skin *(Figure 16.8).*

Failure to thrive (FTT) is the term used for an infant or young child who is not growing and developing as expected. There are two main reasons for the failure:

1. **Organic disorders,** like chronic illness (e.g., **celiac disease**), genetic (e.g., Down syndrome), metabolic (e.g., fetal alcohol syndrome, or **FAS**), and hormone disorders (e.g., pituitary dwarfism).
2. **Psychosocial disorders,** including poverty, lack of education about feeding, neglect or abuse, and parental mental illness or substance abuse.

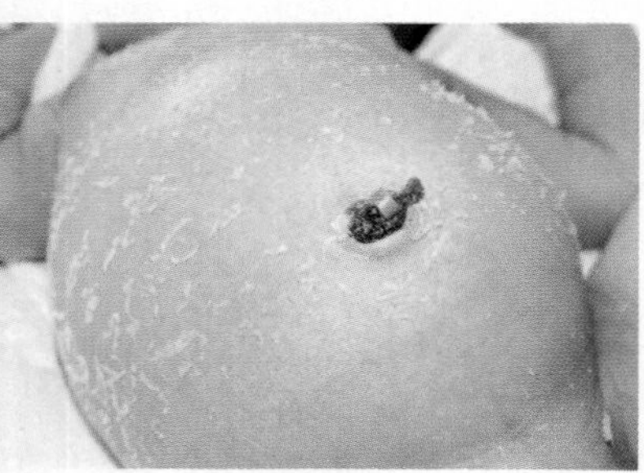

▲ **FIGURE 16.8** Postmature Infant with Skin Changes.

Vipada Kanajod/Shutterstock

Urinary System Adaptations (LO 16.1, 16.3, and 16.5)

Congenital urinary tract disorders include the following conditions:

- Renal **agenesis,** in which one or both kidneys are absent;
- Blockage of urinary flow in utero, causing hydronephrosis of the kidneys;
- **Polycystic kidney disease,** one of the most common genetic disorders; and
- **Hypospadias of the penis,** in which the urethra does not extend to the end of the penis and instead, opens along its underside *(see Chapter 13).*

Abbreviations

FAS	fetal alcohol syndrome
FTT	failure to thrive
SGA	small for gestational age

Digestive System Adaptations (LO 16.1, 16.3, and 16.5)

Until 6 months of age, the baby needs only breast milk or commercially prepared formula. Around 1 month of age, a feeding routine will be established.

Esophageal **atresia**—incomplete formation of the esophagus—is often associated with a **fistula** (abnormal passage) between the esophagus and the trachea. This leads to feeding difficulties and respiratory distress in the neonate's first few days of life.

An immature digestive system may be the cause of **colic,** in which the neonate cries for hours at a time until one or both of its parents feel like joining in. Twenty-five percent of all infants have colic, which begins between the third and sixth weeks, and usually disappears by the twelfth week. There is no known treatment.

Food intolerance, which is totally different from a food allergy *(see the next spread),* is an adverse digestive system reaction to food that does not involve the immune system. It can be a metabolic reaction to a digestive enzyme deficiency like **lactase deficiency** *(see Chapter 9),* causing an intolerance to cows' milk.

Hematologic Adaptations (LO 16.1, 16.3, and 16.5)

The newborn infant has an excess of red blood cells (RBCs). When RBCs are broken down, bilirubin is produced *(see Chapter 7).* Because the neonate's liver is immature and cannot process bilirubin quickly, excess bilirubin is deposited in the tissues, producing jaundice. In the first 3 days after birth, neonatal jaundice affects 60% of full-term and 80% of premature infants. In most infants, no specific treatment is needed. More severe cases respond to **phototherapy,** which employs blue wavelengths of light to convert bilirubin to less toxic chemicals that can be excreted in bile or urine.

Word Analysis and Definition

S = Suffix P = Prefix R = Root R/CF = Combining Form

WORD	PRONUNCIATION	ELEMENTS		DEFINITION
agenesis	a-**JEN**-eh-sis	P/ R/	a- *without* -genesis *creation, production*	Failure to develop any organ or any part
atresia	a-**TREE**-zee-ah	P/ R/	a- *without* -tresia *a hole*	Congenital absence of a normal opening or lumen
colic	**KOL**-ik	S/ R/	-ic *pertaining to* col- *colon*	Spasmodic, crampy pains in the abdomen
fistula	**FIS**-tyu-lah		Latin *pipe, tube*	Abnormal passage
gavage	guh-**VAHZH**		French *to force-feed geese (to make pate de foie gras)*	To feed by a stomach tube
intolerance	in-**TOL**-er-ance		Latin *impatient*	Inability of the small intestine to digest and dispose of a particular dietary substance
lactase	**LAK**-tase	S/ R/	-ase *enzyme* lact- *milk*	Enzyme that breaks down lactose (milk sugar) to glucose and galactose
phototherapy	foh-toe-**THAIR**-ah-pee	S/ R/CF	-therapy *treatment* phot/o- *light*	Treatment using light rays

EXERCISES

A. Documentation: *Use the terminology* and *the abbreviations related to neonatal adaptations to correctly fill in the following patient documentation.* **LO 16.5 and 16.10**

1. This infant's mother has been an alcoholic for the past year and a half. Infant was born suffering from (use the abbreviation)____________.
2. This preemie falls below the 10th percentile and is (use the abbreviation)____________.
3. Because of difficulty in swallowing, this infant is being fed by ____________.
4. Patient was born with only the right kidney present. Diagnosis: renal ____________.
5. Because of jaundice, this infant will receive 8 hours of ____________ each day until discharge.

B. Assess *the information in the following statements. Fill in the blanks with the medical term to correctly complete each sentence.* **LO 16.2 and 16.5**

1. Inadequate nutrition of the fetus can be caused by poor ____________ function.
2. Premature infants may have to be fed by IV or ____________.
3. Renal agenesis occurs when one or more of the ____________ is absent at birth.

C. Match *the element in the first column to its meaning in the second column.* **LO 16.1**

1. _____ *tresia*	**a.** creation
2. _____ *genesis*	**b.** milk
3. _____ *col*	**c.** light
4. _____ *lact*	**d.** a hole
5. _____ *photo*	**e.** colon

Lesson 16.1 (cont'd)

Keynotes

- All newborn babies should receive hearing screening tests before they go home from the hospital.
- By 3 months of age, the baby will smile at the sound of a known voice and turn her head to the direction of the sound.
- In the first 2 years of life, most children have 8 to 10 colds.
- Six percent of children under the age of 3 have food allergies.
- Between 25% and 50% of affected children outgrow their food allergies by age 3.

CASE REPORT 16.2

True Story

A singer in a Master Chorale during her seventh and eighth months of pregnancy was in rehearsal for Handel's ***Messiah*** for a Christmas concert. At home, she frequently practiced her solo, which began, "I know that my redeemer liveth." When her daughter was 6 months old, the mother was changing the baby's diaper and started to sing, "I know that my . . ." The child turned her head and chimed in, "redeemer." Now, at 10 years old, the daughter has absolute pitch—the rare ability to replicate on the piano the note for any sound made in nature.

Neonatal Adaptations (continued) (LO 16.1, 16.3, 16.4, 16.5, and 16.10)

Hearing Adaptations (LO 16.1 and 16.5)

The fetus begins to hear loud noises around the beginning of the third trimester (24 weeks). By the seventh month of pregnancy, the fetus can hear **maternal** speech and, after birth, remember what is heard. **Congenital malformations** of the external auditory canal and middle ear can result in a conductive hearing loss *(see Chapter 11).* Congenital malformations of the inner ear can result in a sensorineural hearing loss *(see Chapter 11).*

Visual Adaptations (LO 16.1 and 16.5)

At birth, a non-anesthetized baby is able to see and focus on an object between 8 and 12 inches away. This distance probably relates to the distance between the mother's and baby's faces during breastfeeding *(Figure 16.9).* For color vision, the baby will see only very brightly colored objects. Full color vision is developed between 3 and 4 months of age.

Immunologic Adaptations (LO 16.1 and 16.5)

The baby is born with immunoglobulin G (IgG) levels *(see Chapter 7)* near those of an adult, having acquired them from the mother through the placenta. These levels of antibody molecules remain high enough in the first 6 months to protect the baby against some infectious diseases, but not against others, like **whooping cough (pertussis)** and **diphtheria.** This is why immunization against these diseases takes place in the first 6 months of life.

In **food allergies,** the body's immune system reacts as though a particular food is harmful (an allergen) and creates immunoglobulin E (IgE) antibodies to it *(see Chapter 7).* This process generates chemicals like histamine that produce the symptoms of a runny nose, itchy skin rash, swelling of the lips, or wheezing. The most common allergens in the neonate are milk, eggs, wheat, soy, and peanuts.

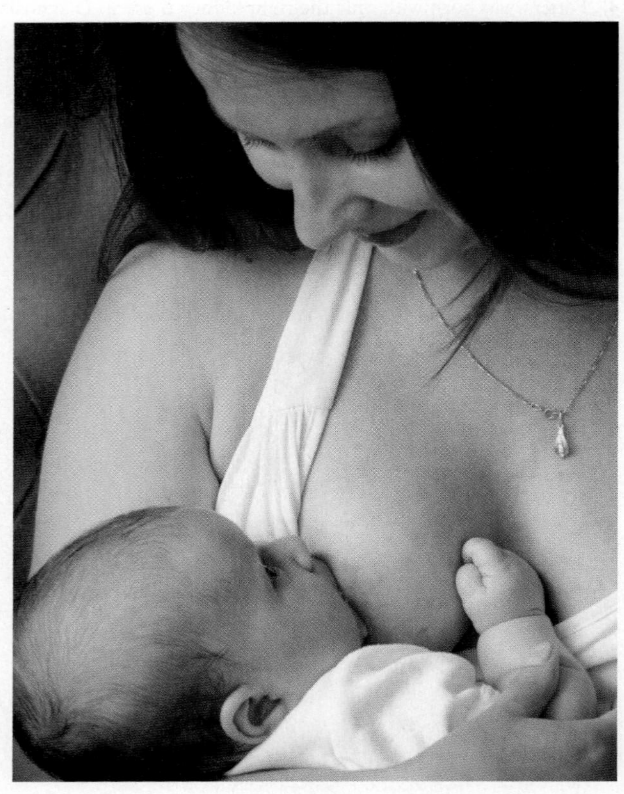

FIGURE 16.9
One-Month-Old Baby Breastfeeds and Interacts with Mother.

Tetiana Mandziuk/Shutterstock

Word Analysis and Definition

S = Suffix P = Prefix R = Root R/CF = Combining Form

WORD	PRONUNCIATION	ELEMENTS		DEFINITION
congenital	kon-**JEN**-ih-tal	S/ P/ R/	-al *pertaining to* con- *together, with* -genit- *birth, bring forth*	Present at birth, either inherited or due to an event during gestation up to the moment of birth
diphtheria	dif-**THEER**-ee-ah		Greek *leather*	Disease with a thick (leathery) coating of the pharynx
malformation	**MAL**-for-**MAY**-shun	S/ P/ R/	-ion *condition* mal- *bad* -format- *to form*	Failure of proper or normal development
maternal	mah-**TER**-nal	S/ R/	-al *pertaining to* matern- *mother*	Pertaining to or derived from the mother
pertussis (also known as whooping cough)	per-**TUSS**-is **WHO**-ping KOFF	P/ R/	per- *intense* -tussis *cough*	Infectious disease with a spasmodic, intense cough ending with a whoop (stridor)

EXERCISES

A. Review *hearing and visual adaptations of the newborn. Fill in the blanks with the correct answer to each question or to complete each statement.* **LO 16.2, 16.5, and 16.10**

1. Newborns are able to see at a distance of ___ to ____ inches.

2. In which trimester can the fetus hear loud noises? ________________

3. What type of hearing loss results from congenital malformations of the external auditory canal and middle ear? ________________

____

4. What type of diagnostic test should all newborns have before they leave the hospital? ________________

5. Congenital malformation of the inner ear can result in ________________ hearing loss.

6. By the 7th month of pregnancy, the fetus can hear maternal ________________.

B. Meet chapter and lesson objectives *by correctly answering the following questions.* **LO 16.2, 16.3, 16.5 and 16.10**

1. The baby's Ig levels are acquired through the ________________.

2. Write a brief definition for *congenital.* ________________

3. In the first six months of life, a child needs immunizations against ________________ and ________________.

4. What immunoglobulin is created in response to a food allergen? ________________

Lesson 16.1 (cont'd) Developmental Disorders of Childhood and Adolescence (LO 16.1 and 16.6)

Certain developmental disorders can occur during childhood and/or **adolescence.** The most common of these conditions are outlined below.

Enuresis occurs in the child who is dry by day, but wets the bed at night without waking up. Fifteen percent of children aged 5 have this condition.

Encopresis is a persistent fecal soiling beyond the age at which toilet training should be complete (i.e., at 3 to 4 years of age).

Eating disorders in early childhood are part of the syndrome **failure to thrive,** and these can include the following:

- **Pica** is the persistent ingestion of nonnutritive substances like dried lead-containing paint, and is associated with iron deficiency anemia and developmental delay.
- **Rumination** disorder occurs between 3 and 12 months and is characterized by the persistent **regurgitation** and re-chewing of food after feeding. It goes away spontaneously.
- Feeding disorder of infancy occurs when a child under 6 years refuses to eat adequately and fails to gain his expected weight. There is no physical explanation found.

Keynote

- Adolescent eating disorders occur 90% of the time in females.

Eating disorders in adolescence include the following:

- **Anorexia nervosa** is a refusal to maintain a normal body weight and occurs more frequently in **adolescent** females. These young women have an inaccurate perception of their body size, weight, and shape.
- **Bulimia (bulimia nervosa)** occurs in females who "binge eat" two or three times per week and then make themselves throw up **(purge).** They tend to fast (not eat) between the binges.
- **Binge-eating disorder** is characterized by binge eating two or three times per week with no compensatory vomiting.

Treatment for adolescent eating disorders requires nutritional support and intense psychiatric care.

Word Analysis and Definition

S = Suffix P = Prefix R = Root R/CF = Combining Form

WORD	PRONUNCIATION	ELEMENTS		DEFINITION
adolescence (state of) **adolescent** (person)	ad-oh-**LESS**-ents ad-oh-**LESS**-ent	S/ R/ S/	-ence *state of, quality of* adolesc- *beginning of adulthood* -ent *end result, pertaining to*	Stage that begins with puberty and ends with physical maturity Pertaining to adolescence or a person in that stage
anorexia	an-oh-**RECK**-see-ah	S/ P/ R/	-ia *condition* an- *without* -orex- *appetite*	Without an appetite; or having an aversion to food
binge eating	BINJ **EE**-ting		binge, Old English *to soak*	Eating with periods of excessive intake
bulimia	buh-**LEEM**-ee-ah		Greek *hunger*	Episodic bouts of excessive eating with compensatory throwing up
encopresis	en-koh-**PREE**-sis		Greek *full of manure*	Repeated soiling with feces
enuresis	en-you-**REE**-sis	S/ R/	-esis *condition* enur- *urinate*	Involuntary bedwetting
pica **purge**	**PIE**-kah PURJ		Latin *magpie* Latin *to cleanse*	Eating substances not considered to be food Consciously throw up or cause bowel evacuation
regurgitation	ree-gur-jih-**TAY**-shun	S/ P/ R/	-ation *process* re- *back, backward* -gurgit- *flood*	Expel contents of the stomach into the mouth, short of vomiting
rumination	**ROO**-min-ay-shun	S/ R/	-ation *process* rumin- *throat*	To bring back food into the mouth to chew over and over

EXERCISES

A. Eating disorders in early childhood. *Select the answer that correctly completes each statement.* **LO 16.6**

1. Eating substances that are considered as nonnutritive:

a. rumination

b. pica

c. regurgitation

d. bulimia

2. Persistent fecal soiling beyond the age of toilet training:

a. rumination

b. enuresis

c. anorexia nervosa

d. encopresis

3. Eating disorders can be a part of the syndrome:

a. failure to thrive

b. encopresis

c. enuresis

B. Match *the element in the first column to its meaning in the second column.* **LO 16.1**

1. _____ *rumin* **a.** appetite

2. _____ *re* **b.** flood

3. _____ *enur* **c.** condition

4. _____ *orex* **d.** back

5. _____ *gurgit* **e.** urinate

6. _____ *esis* **f.** throat

Lesson 16.1 (cont'd) Developmental Disorders of Childhood and Adolescence (continued) (LO 16.1, 16.3, and 16.6)

Keynote

- Autism is a spectrum of disorders.

Attention deficit hyperactivity disorder (ADHD) affects 4% to 8% of school-age children, boys three times as often as girls. ADHD has three major components:

1. **Inattention,** with an inability to pay attention to details, carelessness, distractibility, and problems with organization;
2. **Hyperactivity,** shown by fidgeting, squirming, always being on the go, and talking excessively; and
3. **Impulsiveness,** shown by interrupting, intruding, and acting inappropriately.

The etiology is unknown, but some areas of the brain are known to be smaller in patients with ADHD. There is no evidence that parenting plays any role in the development of ADHD. Treatment is with **stimulants,** like Ritalin, or antidepressants, like Prozac, in combination with special educational interventions, parent training to support the child, and **cognitive behavioral therapy.** This form of therapy identifies the thinking that is causing unwanted feelings and behaviors, and tries to replace this thinking with thoughts that lead to more desirable behaviors.

Learning disability (LD) refers to a group of disorders with difficulties in the acquisition and use of listening, speaking, reading, writing, and reasoning abilities. LD is not associated with obvious problems like bad eyesight and lack of intellectual ability, but instead refers to a discrepancy between a child's capacity to learn and level of achievement. The term **dyslexia** is used for a learning disability characterized primarily by a difficulty with reading and spelling.

Oppositional defiant disorder (ODD) shows a persistent pattern of defiance, disobedience, and hostility to parents and teachers. Children with ODD blame others for their mistakes and frequently lose their tempers.

Conduct disorder (CD) occurs between 9 and 17 years and is expressed by fighting, bullying, cruelty, and early substance abuse. Running away from home is common, and some young women can go into prostitution. Of all children with CD, 25% to 50% become antisocial adults.

Therapy for these disruptive disorders is difficult. Behavioral therapy and psychotherapy can help patients express and control their anger. The only two therapeutic programs shown to be effective both involved parent training to help their children.

Obsessive compulsive disorder (OCD) is an anxiety disorder with recurrent unwanted thoughts **(obsessions)** and repetitive behaviors **(compulsions** or **rituals)** like hand washing, counting, and cleaning. Treatment involves finding the right medication (from the many anti-anxiety and antidepressant options) and using cognitive-behavioral therapy.

An **autism spectrum disorder (ASD)** is characterized by varying degrees of impairment in social interactions and communication skills. These disorders are associated with repetitive and **stereotyped** patterns of behavior. This spectrum varies from a severe form called **autism** to a milder and higher-functioning form called **Asperger syndrome.** If a child has symptoms of these disorders, but does not meet specific criteria for their diagnosis, the term **pervasive developmental disorder, not otherwise specified (PDD-NOS)** is used.

Abbreviations

ADHD	attention deficit hyperactivity disorder
ASD	autism spectrum disorder
CD	conduct disorder
LD	learning disability
OCD	obsessive compulsive disorder
ODD	oppositional defiant disorder
PDD-NOS	pervasive developmental disorder, not otherwise specified

Word Analysis and Definition

S = Suffix P = Prefix R = Root R/CF = Combining Form

WORD	PRONUNCIATION		ELEMENTS	DEFINITION
Asperger syndrome (disorder)	**AHS**-per-ger **SIN**-drohm	 P/ R/	Hans Asperger, Austrian pediatrician, 1906–1980 **syn-** *together* **-drome** *running*	Developmental disorder of children Combination of signs and symptoms associated with a particular disease process
autism	**AWE**-tizm		Greek *self*	Developmental disorder of children
cognitive behavioral therapy	**KOG**-nih-tiv be-**HAYV**-yur-al **THAIR**-ah-pee	S/ R/ S/ S/ R/ R/	**-ive** *quality of* **cognit-** *thinking* *-al pertaining to* **-ior-** *pertaining to* **behav-** *mental or motor activity* **therapy** *treatment*	Psychotherapy that emphasizes thoughts and attitudes in one's behavior
compulsion **compulsive (adj)**	kom-**PUL**-shun kom-**PUL**-siv	S/ R/ S/	**-ion** *action, condition* **compuls-** *to drive, compel* **-ive** *quality of*	Uncontrollable impulses to perform an act repetitively Possessing uncontrollable impulses to perform an act repetitively
dyslexia (noun) **dyslexic (adj)**	dis-**LEK**-see-ah dis-**LEK**-sik	S/ P/ R/ S/	**-ia condition** **dys- difficult, painful** **-lex-** *word* **-ic** *pertaining to*	Impaired reading and writing ability below the person's level of intelligence Pertaining to or suffering from dyslexia
hyperactivity	**HIGH**-per-ac-**TIV**-ih-tee	S/ P/ R/	**-ity** *state, condition* **hyper-** *excessive* **-activ-** *movement*	Excessive restlessness and movement
impulsive	im-**PUL**-siv	S/ P/ R/	**-ive** *quality of* **im-** *not* **-puls-** *to drive*	Unable to resist performing inappropriate actions
inattention	**IN**-ah-**TEN**-shun	S/ P/ R/	**-ion** *condition* **in-** *not* **-attent-** *awareness*	Lack of concentration and direction
obsession (noun) **obsessive (adj)**	ob-**SESH**-un ob-**SES**-iv	 S/ R/	Latin *to besiege* **-ive** *quality of* **obsess-** *besieged by thoughts*	Persistent, recurrent, uncontrollable thoughts or impulses Possessing persistent, recurrent, uncontrollable thoughts or impulses
stereotype	**STER**-ee-oh-tipe	S/ R/CF	**-type** *particular kind, model* **stere/o-** *three-dimensional*	An image held in common by members of a group
stimulus **stimuli (pl)** **stimulant**	**STIM**-you-lus **STIM**-you-lie **STIM**-you-lant	 S/ R/	Latin *goad, incite* **-ant** *forming* **stimul-** *excite, strengthen*	Something that excites or strengthens the functional activity of an organ or part An agent that excites or strengthens

EXERCISES

A. Use *what you have just learned in this chapter and match the description in the first column to the abbreviation in the second column.* **LO 16.3 and 16.6**

1. _________ varying degrees of impairment in social and communication skills — **a.** ODD

2. _________ expressed by fighting, bullying, and cruelty — **b.** OCD

3. _________ persistent pattern of defiance, disobedience, and hostility — **c.** ASD

4. _________ anxiety disorder with recurrent unwanted thoughts and repetitive behaviors — **d.** CD

B. Use medical terms *related to developmental disorders of children and adolescents. Fill in the blanks with the term being described.* **LO 16.2 and 16.6**

1. An agent that excites or strengthens: ______________________

2. Unable to resist performing inappropriate actions: ______________________

3. Uncontrollable impulses to perform an act repetitively: ______________________

4. Excessive restlessness and movement: ______________________

5. Lack of concentration and direction: ______________________

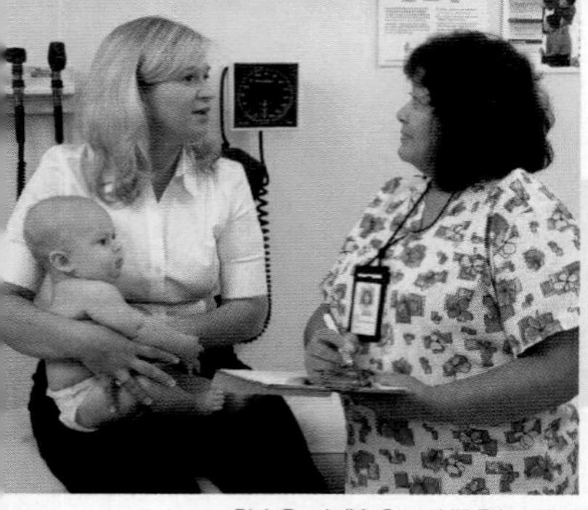
Rick Brady/McGraw-Hill Education

Lesson 16.2

Aging, Senescence, and Death

Objectives

Although most of us don't like to think about death—particularly our own and that of our loved ones—it is a natural, inevitable, and important reality. This is especially true if you're a health care professional who happens to be working with a patient who will soon be facing death. The information in this lesson will enable you to:

16.2.1 Distinguish **aging** from **senescence.**

16.2.2 Use correct medical terminology to describe changes that occur with senescence in major organ systems.

16.2.3 Discuss the medical terminology involved in the preparations for death.

Keynotes

- **Aging** is the decline in function through late adulthood and old age.
- **Senescence** is the inevitable changes in cells and tissues leading to the decline of function in old age and death.
- **Life expectancy** is the average length of life for any given population.
- The documented longest lived persons are **Jeanne Calment,** a French woman who died in 1997 at the age of 122 years and 164 days, and Kane Tanaka, a Japanese man who was 116 years and 211 days old as of August 1, 2019.

CASE REPORT 16.3

You are . . .

. . . a medical assistant working in the **Geriatric** Clinic at Fulwood Medical Center.

You are communicating with . . .

. . . 85-year-old Mr. Mathew Hickman, who has an early **dementia.** Mr. Hickman also has a slow-growing prostate cancer, for which he has opted to have no treatment. With the help of his two daughters and his day care providers, he is struggling to stay at home. His daughter, Sandra Hotteling, is with him.

Mr. Hickman: "I'm still here, you know, somewhere inside this frail old body. I can remember yesteryear, though I'm a bit hazy about today. I can't hear like I used to. But I can still put my own socks on and tie my shoes. I'm not frightened of death, but the process of getting there scares the heck out of me. I've lived my life with dignity. I want to live my death the same way, you know, and leave in peace."

Senescence of Organ Systems (LO 16.7 and 16.8)

Organ systems begin to show signs of **senescence** at very different ages and do not degenerate at the same speed. Most physiologic studies show general peak physical performance in the twenties.

Integumentary system changes in our bodies begin in our forties. The cells that produce melanin called melanocytes *(see Chapter 3)* die, and our hair becomes gray and thinner. Our skin gets paper-thin, loses its elasticity, hangs loose, and wrinkles *(Figure 16.10).* Flat brown-black spots, **senile lentigines (age spots),** appear on the backs of our hands and other areas exposed to sunlight.

Our special senses start to decline in our twenties, including our visual acuity. In our forties, presbyopia *(see Chapter 11)* appears, and many people develop cataracts in old age. Hearing loss occurs as the ossicles become stiffer and the number of cochlear hair cells declines *(see Chapter 11).* (This is the reason for Mr. Hickman's hearing loss.) Our ability to taste and smell are blunted late in life, as taste cells and olfactory buds decline in number.

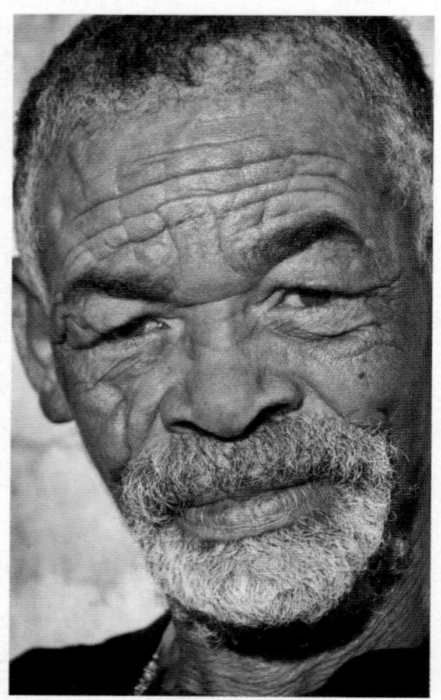
▲ **FIGURE 16.10**
Senescence of the Skin. An old African man.
Tish1/Shutterstock

Skeletal system changes appear in our thirties, when osteoblasts become less active than osteoclasts. This results in osteopenia, which goes on to become osteoporosis, particularly in postmenopausal women. Joints in the older age groups have less synovial fluid and thinner articular cartilage, leading to osteoarthritis *(see Chapter 4).*

Muscular system *(see Chapter 5)* changes occur with age as we lose muscle mass and strength **(sarcopenia).** As muscle atrophies (shrinks and weakens), we have fewer muscle fibers to do the work and the available blood supply to these muscles is decreased.

Word Analysis and Definition

S = Suffix P = Prefix R = Root R/CF = Combining Form

WORD	PRONUNCIATION	ELEMENTS		DEFINITION
aging **aged**	**A**-jing **A**-jid		Latin *aging*	The decline in function through late adulthood and old age. Having lived to advanced age
dementia	da-**MEN**-sha	S/ P/ R/	**-ia** *condition* **de-** *removal, take away* **-ment-** *mind*	Chronic, progressive, irreversible loss of the mind's cognitive and intellectual functions
geriatrics **geriatrician**	jer-ee-**AT**-riks jer-ee-ah-**TRISH**-an	R/ R/ S/	**-iatrics** *medical knowledge* **ger-** *old age* **-ian** *one who does*	Medical specialty that deals with the problems of old age Medical specialist in the process and problems of aging
gerontology **gerontologist**	jer-on-**TOL**-oh-jee jer-on-**TOL**-oh-jist	S/ R/CF S/	**-logy** *study of* **geront/o-** *old age* **-logist** *specialist*	Study of the process and general problems of aging Specialist in the process and general problems of aging
lentigo **lentigines (pl)**	len-**TIE**-go len-**TIHJ**-ih-neez		Greek *lentil*	Age spot; small, flat, brown-black spot in the skin of older people
sarcopenia	sar-koh-**PEE**-nee-ah	S/ R/CF	**-penia** *deficiency* **sarc/o-** *flesh*	Progressive loss of muscle mass and strength in aging
senescence **senescent**	seh-**NES**-ens seh-**NES**-ent	 S/ S/ R/	Latin *to grow old* **-ence** *the quality of* **-ent** *end result, pertaining to* **senesc-** *growing old*	The changes in cells and tissues leading to the decline of function in old age and death. Growing old
senile **senility**	**SEE**-nile seh-**NIL**-ih-tee	S/ R/ S/ R/	**-ile** *pertaining to* **sen-** *old age* **-ity** *condition* **senil-** *senile*	Characteristic of old age Mental disorders occurring in old age

EXERCISES

A. Senescence *of the organ system. Insert the correct answer that completes each statement. Fill in the blanks.* **LO 16.2, 16.7, and 16.8**

1. The plural form of lentigo: ____________________

2. Progressive loss of muscle mass and strength: ____________________

3. Chronic, progressive, irreversible loss of the mind's cognitive and intellectual functions: ____________________

4. Mental disorders occurring in old age: ____________________

B. Review *of elements will make them easier to remember and apply to medical terms. Match the element to its definition.* **LO 16.1**

1. _____ sen — **a.** growing old
2. _____ ile — **b.** deficiency
3. _____ de — **c.** pertaining to
4. _____ senesc — **d.** old age
5. _____ penia — **e.** removal, take away

Lesson 16.2 (cont'd)

Senescence of Organ Systems (continued) (LO 16.7 and 16.8)

Nervous system changes begin around age 30, when our brain weighs twice as much as it does at age 75. Motor coordination, balance, intellectual function, and short-term memory decline more quickly than long-term memory and language skills.

Cardiovascular systems always show coronary artery atherosclerosis from an early age. As a result, when aging myocardial cells die, our heart wall gets thinner and weaker and cardiac output declines. This causes the decline in physical capabilities with aging. The atherosclerotic plaques narrow arteries and trigger thrombosis, leading to strokes and heart attacks *(see Chapter 6).* In veins, valves become weaker and blood flows back and pools in the legs, leading to poor venous return to the heart and heart failure.

Respiratory system changes are noticeable in our thirties, when pulmonary ventilation declines (a factor in the gradual loss of stamina). Our rib cage becomes less flexible; our lungs, less elastic, with fewer alveoli. Our respiratory health declines and hypoxic degenerative changes occur in all the other organ systems.

Urinary system changes begin in our twenties, when the number of nephrons starts to decline. Later in life, many of the remaining glomeruli become atherosclerotic. The **glomerular filtration rate (GFR)** decreases, and our kidneys become less efficient. For example, drug doses in the elderly need to be reduced because drugs cannot be cleared from the blood as rapidly.

Immune system function declines in the elderly as the amounts of lymphatic tissue and red bone marrow decrease with age. This leads to a reduction in both cellular and humoral (antibody) immunity. This means that the elderly have less protection against infectious diseases and cancer.

Keynotes

- Exercise and good nutrition help prevent osteopenia.
- Exercise and good nutrition help prevent muscle degeneration.
- Exercising your brain enhances the quality of life in old age.
- Exercise and good nutrition extend longevity and enhance the quality of life.
- Because of lowered immunity, vaccinations against influenza and other seasonal infections are recommended for the elderly.
- PVS and MCS differ from coma, in which the person is unresponsive and his or her eyes are closed.

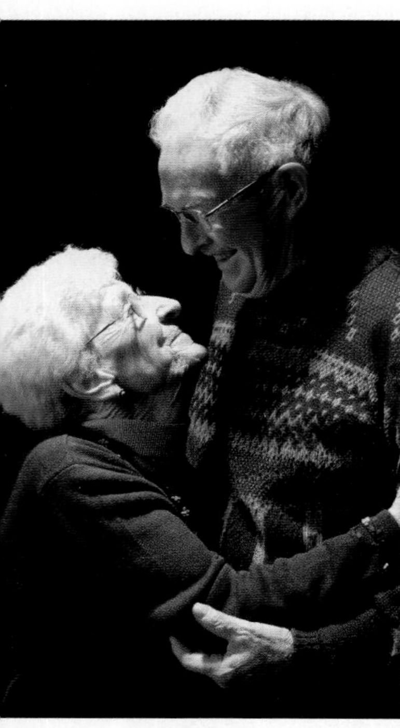

▲ **FIGURE 16.11** Elderly Couple.

Darren Greenwood/Design Pics

Abbreviations

BD	brain death
GFR	glomerular filtration rate
MCS	minimally conscious state
PVS	persistent vegetative state

Dying and Death (LO 16.9)

Death is unavoidable. Just as fetal life in the womb is a preparation for birth, living and aging are a preparation for death. The process of dying, rather than death itself, is of concern to most elderly people. Dying should be dignified and free from physical and emotional pain.

A **hospice** provides **palliative care** and support for the emotional and spiritual needs of terminally ill patients and their loved ones at an in-patient facility or in the patient's home. Palliative care is designed to provide pain and symptom management to maintain the highest quality of life for as long as life remains.

There is no universally accepted moment of biological death. In most states in the United States, death is now defined in terms of **brain death (BD),** in which there is no cerebral or brainstem activity and the EEG is flat for a specific length of time *(Figure 16.12).* The two other conditions involving brain damage and loss of brain function that cause medical difficulty are:

1. **Persistent vegetative state (PVS)** occurs in people who suffer enough brain damage (usually from trauma) that they are unaware of themselves or their surroundings, although their eyes remain open. They still have certain reflexes and can breathe and pump blood because the brainstem still functions. With medical care and artificial feeding, these patients can survive for decades.
2. **Minimally conscious state (MCS)** is a condition of severely altered **consciousness** in which minimal, inconsistent evidence of awareness of self or surroundings is demonstrated. PET scans of MCS patients show cortical function, for example, when the patients' loved ones speak to them. They are more likely to improve than are PVS patients. Trauma is a common cause of MCS.

If the cause of death is uncertain or a crime is suspected, an **autopsy (postmortem)** is performed.

◀ **FIGURE 16.12** Electroencephalogram Shows Brain Death.

argus/Shutterstock

Word Analysis and Definition

S = Suffix P = Prefix R = Root R/CF = Combining Form

WORD	PRONUNCIATION	ELEMENTS		DEFINITION
autopsy (same as **postmortem**) **postmortem**	**AWE**-top-see post-**MOR**-tem	 S/ P/ R/	Greek *see with one's own eyes* -em *condition* **post-** *after* -mort- *death*	Examination of the body and organs of a dead person to determine the cause of death
coma	**KOH**-mah		Greek *deep sleep*	State of deep unconsciousness
consciousness **conscious** **unconscious**	**KON**-shus-ness **KON**-shus un-**KON**-shus	S/ R/ P/	-ness *quality, state* **conscious-** *to be aware* Latin *to be aware* **un-** *not*	The state of being aware of and responsive to the environment Having present knowledge of oneself and one's surroundings Not conscious, lacking awareness
death	DETH		Old English *to die*	Total and permanent cessation of all vital body functions
hospice	**HOS**-pis		Latin *lodging*	Provides supportive and palliative care
influenza	in-flew-**EN**-zah		Latin *caused by the influence of the heavenly bodies*	Acute viral infection of upper and lower respiratory tracts
longevity	lon-**JEV**-ih-tee	S/ R/	-ity *condition* **longev-** *long life*	Duration of life beyond the normal expectation
palliative care	**PAL**-ee-ah-tiv **KAIR**	S/ R/ R/	-ive *quality of* **palliat-** *reduce suffering* **care** *be responsible for*	To relieve symptoms and pain without curing
vegetative	**VEJ**-eh-tay-tiv	S/ R/	-ive *quality of* **vegetat-** *growth*	Functioning unconsciously, as plant life is assumed to do

EXERCISES

A. Differentiate between medical terms associated with death and dying. *Match the term in the first column with its correct definition in the second column.* **LO 16.9**

	Term		Definition
______	**1.** hospice	**a.**	cessation of life
______	**2.** minimally conscious state	**b.**	patient is completely unaware of surroundings
______	**3.** palliative care	**c.**	facility to provide care for dying patients and their families
______	**4.** vegetative state	**d.**	patient that has minimal awareness of self or surroundings
______	**5.** death	**e.**	care that treats but does not cure

B. Abbreviations *for terms related to death and dying. Insert the abbreviation that the statement is describing.* **LO 16.3 and 16.9**

1. Person inconsistently displays evidence of awareness of self or surroundings: ______________________________

2. Person is unaware of themselves or their surroundings: ______________________________

3. Person lacks cerebral and brainstem activity: ______________________________

C. Review *the terms related to death and dying. Insert the correct medical term that answers each question.* **LO 16.7 and 16.9**

1. What is another term for autopsy? ______________________________

2. What condition is described as a state of deep unconsciousness? ______________________________

3. What is the medical term for an acute viral infection of the upper and lower respiratory tracts? ______________________________

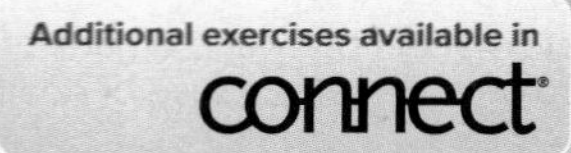

Chapter Review exercises, along with additional practice items, are available in Connect!

Word Parts and Abbreviations

Note: For easy identification, the word parts in this appendix appear in the same colors as in the Word Analysis and Definition boxes: suffix, prefix, root, root/combining form. Any term that is used in the text in both root and combining form is shown only in this appendix as a combining form.

Word Part	Definition
a-	not, without
a-	variant of ad
ab-	away from
abdomin/o	abdomen
ability	competence
ablat	take away
-able	capable
abort	fail at onset, expel nonviable fetus
abras	scrape off
absorpt	to swallow, take in
ac-	toward
-ac	pertaining to
-acea	condition, remedy
acid/o	acid, low pH
acin	grape
acous	hearing
acr/o	peak, topmost, extremity, highest point
acromi/o	acromion
act	to do, perform, performance
activ	movement
acu	needle
acu-	sharp
acumin	to sharpen
ad-	to, toward, into
adapt	to adjust
-ade	process
aden/o	gland
adenoid	adenoid
adip	fat
adjust	alter
adjuv	give help
adolesc	beginning of adulthood
adren/o	adrenal gland

Word Part	Definition
aer/o	air, gas
affer	move toward the center
ag-	to
-age	pertaining to
agglutin	sticking together, clumping
-ago	disease
agon	to fight
-agon	to fight
agor/a	marketplace
-agra	severe pain
-al	pertaining to
alanine	an amino acid, protein synthesized in muscle
albicans	white
albin/o	white
albumin	albumin
ald/o	organic compound
-ale	pertaining to
alges	sensation of pain
-algia	pain, painful condition
aliment	nourishment
-alis	pertaining to
alkal	base
all/o	strange, other
allo-	strange, other
alopec-	baldness, mange
alpha-	first letter in the Greek alphabet
alveol	alveolus, air sac
-aly	condition
ambly-	dull
ambulat	to walk, walking
amin/o	nitrogen containing
-amine	nitrogen-containing substance

S = Suffix P = Prefix R = Root R/CF = Combining Form

WORD PART	DEFINITION
ammon	ammonia
amni/o	amnion, fetal membrane
amnios	amnion
amph-	around
ampull	bottle-shaped
amput	to prune, cut off
amyl	starch
an-	not, lack of, without
-an	pertaining to
an/o	anus
ana-	away from, excessive
anabol	build up
analysis	process to study whole in terms of its parts
analyst	one who separates
anastom	provide a mouth
-ance	condition, state of
-ancy	state of
andr/o	male, masculine
aneurysm	dilation
angi/o	blood vessel, lymph vessel
angina	sore throat, chest pain radiating to throat
ankyl	stiff
-ant	forming, pertaining to
ant-	against
ante-	before, forward, in front of
anter	before, front part
anthrac	coal
anti-	against
aort	aorta
apo-	different from, separation from
appendic	appendix
apse	clasp
aqu-	water
-ar	pertaining to
arachn	cobweb, spider
-arche	beginning
areol	areola, small area
aria	air
-arian	one who is

WORD PART	DEFINITION
-aris	pertaining to
aroma	smell, sweet herb
array	place in order
arter	artery
arteri/o	artery
arteriosus	like an artery
arthr/o	joint
articul	joint
-ary	pertaining to
asbest	asbestos
ascit	fluid in the belly
-ase	enzyme
aspartate	an amino acid
aspergill	aspergillus
aspirat	to breathe on
assay	evaluate
assist	aid, help
asthm	asthma
astr/o	star
-ata	action, place, use
-ate	composed of, pertaining to
-ated	pertaining to a condition
atel	incomplete
ather/o	porridge, gruel, fatty substance
athet	without position, uncontrolled
-atic	pertaining to
-ation	a process
-ative	pertaining to, quality of
-ator	agent, instrument, person or thing that does something
-atory	pertaining to
atri/o	entrance, atrium
-atric	treatment
attent	awareness
attenu	to weaken
audi/o	hearing
audit	hearing
aur-	ear
auscult	listen to

S = Suffix P = Prefix R = Root R/CF = Combining Form

Word Part	Definition
auto-	self, same
avail	useful
axill	armpit, axilla
ayur-	life
azot	nitrogen
-back	back, toward the starting point
bacteri/o	bacteria
balan	glans penis
bar	pressure
bari	weight
bas/o	base, opposite of acid
basal	deepest part
basil	base, support
be	life
behav	mental or motor activity
beta	second letter of Greek alphabet
bi-	two, twice, double
bi/o	life
-bil	able
bil/i	bile
-blast	germ cell, immature cell
blast/o	germ cell, immature cell
blephar/o	eyelid
body	body, mass, substance
bov	cattle
brachi/o	arm
brachii	of the arm
brachy-	short
brady-	slow
bride	rubbish, rubble
bronch/i	bronchus
bronch/o	bronchus
brucell	pathologist David Bruce
buccinat	cheek
bulb/o	bulb
burs	bursa
calc/i	calcium
calcan	calcaneous
calcul	stone, little stone

Word Part	Definition
callos	thickening
calor	heat
canal	duct or channel
cancer	cancer
candid	*Candida*
capill	hairlike, capillary
capit	head
capn	carbon dioxide
caps	box, cover, shell
capsul	box
carb/o	carbon
carboxy	group of organic compounds
carcin/o	cancer
card	heart
cardi/o	heart
care	be responsible for
carotene	yellow-red pigment
carotid	large neck artery
carp/o	bones of the wrist
cartilag	cartilage
cata-	down
catabol	break down
catechol	tyrosine-containing
catheter	insert, catheter
caud	tail
cav	hollow space
cava	cave
cavern	cave
cec	cecum
-cele	cave, hernia, swelling
celi	abdomen
cellul	cell, small cell
cent-	hundred
-centesis	to puncture
centr/o	central
ceph	head
cephal/o	head
-cephalus	head
cephaly	condition of the head

S = Suffix P = Prefix R = Root R/CF = Combining Form

Word Part	Definition
ceps	head
cept	to receive
cerebell	little brain, cerebellum
cerebr/o	brain
cerumin	cerumen
cervic	neck
cess	going forward
chancr	chancre
chem/o	chemical
chemic	chemical
-chete	hair
-chezia	pass a stool
chir/o	hand
chlor	green
chol/e	bile
cholangi	bile duct
cholecyst	gallbladder
choledoch/o	common bile duct
chondr/o	cartilage, rib, granule
chorion	chorion, membrane
chrom/o	color
chromat	color
chron/o	time
chym/o	chyme
-cidal	pertaining to killing
cide	to kill
cili	hairlike structure
circulat	circular route
circum-	around
cirrh	yellow
cis	to cut
cit/i	cell
-clast	break, break down
claudic	limp
claustr/o-	confined space
clav	clavicle
clave	lock
clavicul	clavicle
-cle	small

Word Part	Definition
clitor	clitoris
clon	cutting used for propagation, tumult
-clonus	violent action
co-	with, together
coagul/o	clot, clump
coarct	press together, narrow
cobal	cobalt
cocc	round bacterium
coccus	berry, spherical bacterium
cochle	cochlear
code	information system
cognit	thinking
coit	sexual intercourse
col-	with, together
col	colon
coll	collect, glue
coll/a	glue
colon/o	colon
coloniz	form a colony
colp/o	vagina
com	take care of
com-	with, together
comat	coma
combin	combine
comminut	break into pieces
commodat	adjust
compat	tolerate
compet	strive together
complex	woven together
compli	fulfill
compress	press together
compuls	drive, compel
con-	with, together
concav	arched, hollow
concept	become pregnant
concuss	shake or jar violently
condyl	knuckle
confus	bewildered
congest	accumulation of fluid

S = Suffix P = Prefix R = Root R/CF = Combining Form

Word Part	Definition
coni	dust
coniz	cone
conjunctiv	conjunctiva
connect	join together
conscious	awareness
constip	press together
constrict	to narrow
contagi/o	transmissible by contact
contaminat/o	to corrupt, make unclean
contin	hold together
contra-	against
contract	draw together, pull together
contus	bruise
convalesc	recover
cor	heart
cori	skin
corne/o	cornea
coron	crown, coronary
corpor/e	body
corpus	body
cortic/o	cortex, cortisone
cortis	cortisone
cost	rib
crani/o	cranium, skull
crease	groove
creat	flesh
creatin	creatine
crete	to separate
cretin	cretin
crimin	distinguish
crine	secrete
crista	crest
-crit	to separate
cry/o	cold
crypt-	hidden
cub	cube
cubit	elbow
cubitus	elbow, ulna
cune/i	wedge

Word Part	Definition
cur	cleanse, cure
curat	to care for
curett	to cleanse
cursor	run
cusp	point
cutan/e	skin
cyan/o	dark blue
-cyst	cyst, bladder
cyst/o	bladder, sac, cyst
cysteine	an amino acid
cyt/o	cell
-cyte	cell
cyte	cell
dacry/o	tears, lacrimal duct
dai	day
de-	without, out of, removal, from
defec	clear out waste
defici	failure, lacking, inadequate
degenerat	deteriorate
deglutit	to swallow
del	visible
deliri	confusion, disorientation
delt	triangle
delus	deceive
dem	the people
demi-	half
dendr/o	treelike
dent	tooth
depend	rely on
depress	press down
derm/a	skin
-derma	skin
dermat/o	skin
dermis	skin
-desis	bind together, fixation of bone or joint
di-	two
dia-	complete
diabet	diabetes
diagnost	decision

S = Suffix P = Prefix R = Root R/CF = Combining Form

WORD PART	DEFINITION
dialectic	argument
dialy	separate
diaphor	sweat
diaphragm/a	diaphragm
diastol	diastole, relaxation
dict	consent, surrender
didym/o	testis
didymis	testis
diet	a way of life
different	not identical
digest	to break down food
digit	finger or toe
dilat	open up, expand, widen
dips	thirst
dis-	apart, away from
discipl	understand
disciplin	disciple, instruction
dist	away from the center
-dium	appearance
diuret	increase urine output
diverticul	byroad
dorm	sleep
dors	back
dorsi	of the back
drome	running
drop	liquid globule
duce	to lead
ducer	to lead, leader
duct	to lead, lead
ductus	leading
duoden	twelve, duodenum
dur	dura
dura	hard
dwarf	miniature
dynam/o	power
-dynia	pain
dys-	bad, difficult, painful
e-	out of, from
-eal	pertaining to

WORD PART	DEFINITION
ease	normal function, freedom from pain
ec-	out, outside
ech/o	sound wave
echin	hedgehog
eclamps	shining forth
eco-	environment
-ectasis	dilation
-ectomy	excision, surgical excision
ectop	on the outside, displaced
eczem/a	eczema
-ed	pertaining to
edema	edema, swelling
-ee	person who is the object of an action
efface	wipe out
effer	move out from the center
effus	pour out
ejacul	shoot out
ejaculat	shoot out
elasma	plate
elect	choice
electr/o	electric, electricity
elimin	throw away, expel
-elle	small
-em	condition
em-	in, into
-ema	quality of, quantity of
emac/i	make thin
embol	plug
embryon	embryo, fertilized egg
emesis	vomiting
-emesis	to vomit, vomiting
emet	to vomit
emia	a blood condition
-emia	a blood condition
-emic	pertaining to a blood condition
emmetr-	measure
emuls	suspend in a liquid
en-	in

S = Suffix P = Prefix R = Root R/CF = Combining Form

Word Part	Definition
-ence	forming, quality of, state of
enceph	brain
encephal/o	brain
encephaly	condition of the brain
-ency	condition, state of, quality of
end-	inside, within
endo-	inside, within
-ent	end result, pertaining to
enter/o	intestine
entery	condition of the intestine
enur	urinate
environ	surroundings
-eon	one who does
eosin/o	dawn
ependym	lining membrane
epi-	above, upon, over
epilept	seizure
epiphys/i	growth
episi/o	vulva
equi-	equal
equin	horse
equip	to fit out
-er	agent, one who does
erect	straight, to set up
erg/o	work
-ergy	process of working
-ery	process of
erysi-	red
erythemat	redness
erythr/o	red
-escent	process
-esis	condition
eso-	inward
esophag/e	esophagus
essent	existence
esthes	sensation, perception
esthet	sensation, perception
estr/o	woman
ethm	sieve

Word Part	Definition
eti/o	cause
-etic	pertaining to
-etics	pertaining to
-ette	little
eu-	good, normal
ex-	away from, out, out of
exacerbat	increase, aggravate
examin	test, examine
excis	cut out
excret	separate, discharge
exo-	outside, outward
expect	await
expir	breathe out
extra-	out of, outside
faci	face
factor	maker
farct	area of dead tissue
fasc/i	fascia
febr	fever
fec	feces
feed	to give food, nourish
femor	femur
fer	to bear, to carry
ferrit	iron
fertil	able to conceive
fertiliz	to make fruitful
fet/o	fetus
fibr/o	fiber, fibrous
fibrill	small fiber
fibrin/o	fibrin
fibul	fibula
-fication	remove
fida	split
field	definite area
filar	roundworm
filtr	strain through
fiss	split
fistul	tube, pipe
flammat	flame

S = Suffix P = Prefix R = Root R/CF = Combining Form

Word Part	Definition
flat	flatus
flatul	excessive gas
flavin	yellow
flex	bend
fluid	flowing
fluo-	fluorine
fluor/o	flux, flow
flux	flow
foc	center, focus
follicul	follicle
foramin	opening, foramen
fore-	in front
-form	appearance of, resembling
format	to form
fract	break
fraction	small amount
free	free
frequ	repeated, often
front	front, forehead
fructos	fruit sugar
function	perform
fund/o	fundus
fung/i	fungus
fusion	to pour
galact/o	milk
gall	bile
gastr/o	stomach
gastrin	stomach hormone
gastrocnem	calf of leg
gemin	twin, double
gen/o	produce, create
-gen	create, produce, form
gen-	birth
-gene	production, give birth
gener	create, produce
genesis	origin, creation, production
-genesis	creation, origin, formation, source
genet	origin
-genic	creation, producing

Word Part	Definition
genit	bring forth, birth, primary male or female sex organ
genitor	offspring
ger	old age
geront/o	old age
gest	gestation, pregnancy, produce
gestat	gestation, pregnancy, to bear
gigant	giant
gingiv	gums
gland	gland
glauc	lens opacity, grey
gli/o	glue, supportive tissue of nervous system
-glia	glue, supportive tissue of nervous system
globin/o	protein
globul	globular, protein
glomerul/o	glomerulus
gloss/o	tongue
glott	mouth of windpipe
glottis	mouth of windpipe
gluc/o	glucose, sugar
glut	buttocks
glutin	glue, stick
glyc/o	glycogen, glucose, sugar
glycer	glycerol, sweet
gnath	jaw
gnose	use knowledge
gnosis	knowledge
gomph	bolt, nail
gon/o	seed
gonad/o	gonads, testes, or ovaries
gong	daily practice
-grade	going
graft	splice, transplant
-graft	tissue for transplant
graine	head pain
-gram	a record, recording
grand-	big
grand	big
granul/o	granule, small grain

S = Suffix P = Prefix R = Root R/CF = Combining Form

Word Part	Definition
-graph	to record, write
-grapher	one who records
-graphy	process of recording
gravida	pregnant
gravis	serious
gru	to move
guan	dung
gurgit	flood
gynec/o	woman, female
habilitat	restore
hale	breathe
halit	breath
hallucin	imagination
hallux	big toe
hem/o	blood
hemangi/o	blood vessel
hemat/o	blood
heme	red iron-containing pigment
hemi-	half
-hemia	blood condition
hepar	liver
hepat/o	liver
herb/i	plant
herni/o	hernia, rupture
herp	blister
hetero-	different
hiat	opening
hist	derived from histidine
hist/o	tissue
holist	entire, whole
hom/i	man
home/o	the same
homo-	same, alike
hormon	chemical messenger, hormone
human	human being
humor	fluid
hyal	glass
hydr/o	water
hyp-	below
hyper-	above, beyond, excess, excessive

Word Part	Definition
hypn/o	sleep
hypo-	below, deficient, smaller, low, under
hyster/o	uterus
-ia	condition
-iac	pertaining to
-ial	pertaining to
-ian	one who does, specialist
-ias	condition
-iasis	abnormal condition
iatr	medical treatment, physician
-iatric	relating to medicine, medical knowledge
iatrics	medical knowledge
-iatrist	practitioner, one who treats
-iatry	treatment, field of medicine
-ibility	able to do
-ible	can do, able to
-ic	pertaining to
-ica	pertaining to
-ical	pertaining to
-ician	expert
-ics	knowledge
ict	seizure
icterus	jaundice
-id	having a particular quality, pertaining to
-ide	having a particular quality
idi/o	unknown, personal
ifer	to bear, carry
-ify	to become
-il	a thing
-ile	pertaining to
ile/o	ileum
ili/o	ilium (hip bone)
im-	in, not
imag	likeness
immun/o	immune, immune response, immunity
immune	protected from
immuniz	make immune
impair	worsen
impede	obstruct

S = Suffix P = Prefix R = Root R/CF = Combining Form

Word Part	Definition
-imus	most
-in	substance, chemical compound
in-	not, into, in
incis	cut into
incub	sit on, lie on, hatch
index	to declare
-ine	pertaining to
infant	infant
infect	internal invasion, infection
infer	below, beneath
infest	invade, attack
inflammat	set on fire
inflat	blow up
infra-	below, beneath
-ing	quality of, doing
ingest	carry in
inguin	groin
inhal	breathe in
inhibit	repress
inject	force in
ino	sinew
insect/i	insect
insert	put together
inspir	breathe in
insul	island
integr	whole
integument	covering of the body
inter-	between
interstiti	space between tissues
intestin	gut, intestine
intra-	inside, within
intrins	on the inside
intus-	within
iod	violet, iodine
-ion	action, condition
-ior	pertaining to
-iosum	pertaining to
-ious	pertaining to
irrig	to water

Word Part	Definition
-is	belonging to, pertaining to
isch	to block
ischi	ischium
-ism	condition, process
-ismus	take action
iso-	equal
-ist	agent, specialist
-istic	pertaining to
-isy	inflammation
-ites	associated with
-ition	process
-itis	inflammation, infection
-ity	condition, state
-ium	structure
-ius	pertaining to
-ive	nature of, quality of, pertaining to
-iz	subject to
-ization	process of inserting or creating
-ize	action, affect in a specific way, policy
-ized	affected in a specific way
-izer	affects in a particular way, line of action
jejun	jejunum
jugul	throat
junct	joining together
juxta-	beside, near, close to
kal	potassium
kary/o	nucleus
kel/o	tumor
kerat	keratin, hard protein
kerat/o	cornea
kern	nucleus
ket/o	ketone
keton	ketone
ketone	organic compound
kin	motion
kinase	enzyme
kinesi/o	movement
kinet	motion
-kinin	move in

S = Suffix P = Prefix R = Root R/CF = Combining Form

WORD PART	DEFINITION
klept/o	to steal
kyph/o	bent, humpback
labi	lip
labyrinth	inner ear
lacer	to tear
lacrim	tears, tear duct
lact	milk
lactat	secrete milk
lapar/o	abdomen in general
lapse	clasp, fall together
-lapse	fall together, slide
laryng/o	larynx
lash	end of whip
lat	to take
lateral	at the side
latiss	wide
-le	small
lei/o	smooth
-lemma	covering
-lepsy	seizure
lept	thin, small
-let	small
leuk/o	white
lex	word
librium	balance
ligament	ligament
ligat	tie up, tie off
lign	line
-ling	small
lingu	tongue
lip/o	fat
lipid	fat
lith/o	stone
liv	life, live
load	to carry
lob	lobe
locat	a place
log	to study
-logist	one who studies, specialist

WORD PART	DEFINITION
logous	relation
logy	study of
-logy	study of
longev	long life
lord/o	curve, swayback
lubric	make slippery
lucid	bright, clear
lumb	lower back, loin
lump	piece
lun	moon
lupus	wolf
-lus	small
lute	yellow
luxat	dislocate
ly	break down, separate
-ly	every
lymph/o	lymph, lymphatic system
lymphaden/o	lymph node
lymphangi/o	lymphatic vessels
lys/o	decompose, dissolve
lysis	destruction
-lysis	destruction, dissolve, separation
lyt	dissolve, destroy
-lyte	soluble
-lytic	relating to destruction
lyze	destruct, dissolve
macro-	large
macul	spot
magnet	magnet
mak	makes
-maker	one who makes
mal	bad, difficult, inadequate
mal-	bad, difficult
-malacia	abnormal softness
malign	harmful, bad
malleol	small hammer, malleolus
mamm/o	breast
man	frenzy, madness
man/o	pressure

S = Suffix P = Prefix R = Root R/CF = Combining Form

Word Part	Definition
mandibul	mandible
-mania	frenzy, madness
manic	affected by frenzy
manipul	handful, use of hands
marker	sign
mast	breast
mastic	chew
mastoid	mastoid process
mater	mother
matern	mother
matur(e)	ripe, ready, fully developed
maxilla	maxilla
medi	middle
media	middle
mediastin/o	mediastinum
medic	medicine
medulla	middle
mega-	enormous
-megaly	enlargement
mei	lessening
mela	black
melan/o	melanin, black pigment
mellit	sweetened with honey
membran/o	cover, skin
men/o	menses, monthly, month
mening/o	meninges, membranes
menisc	crescent, meniscus
menstr/u	menses, occurring monthly
ment	mind, chin
-ment	action, state, resulting state
mere	part
mero-	partial
meso-	middle
meta-	after, beyond, subsequent to
metabol	change
-meter	measure, instrument to measure
metr/o	uterus
-metric	pertaining to measurement
-metrist	skilled in measurement

Word Part	Definition
-metry	process of measuring
mi-	derived from *hemi*, half
micr/o	small
micro-	small
mictur	pass urine
mid-	middle
mileusis	lathe
milli	one-thousandth
miner	mines
mineral/o	inorganic material
miss	send
mit	thread
mito-	thread
mitr	having two points
mitt	send
mod	nature, form, method
molec	mass
mollusc	soft
mon	single
monas	single unit
monil	type of fungus
mono-	one, single
morbid	disease
morph/o	shape
mort	death
mot	move
motiv	move
muc/o	mucus, mucous membrane
mucosa	lining of a cavity
multi-	many
mune	in service
muscul/o	muscle
mut	silent
muta	genetic change
mutil	to maim
my/o	muscle
myc/o	fungus
myel/o	spinal cord, bone marrow
myelin	in the spinal cord, myelin

S = Suffix P = Prefix R = Root R/CF = Combining Form

WORD PART	DEFINITION
myo-	to blink
myop	to blink
myos	muscle
myring/o	tympanic membrane, eardrum
myx-	mucus
narc/o	stupor
nas	nose
nat	born, birth
nate	born, birth
natr/i	sodium
natur/o	nature
ne/o	new
nebul	cloud
necr/o	death
neo-	new
nephr/o	kidney
nerv	nerve
-ness	quality, state
neur/o	nerve, nervous tissue
neutr/o	neutral
nici	lethal
nitr/o	nitrogen
noct-	night
noia	to think
nom	law
non-	no, not
nor-	normal
norm-	normal
nos/o	disease
nucle/o	nucleus
nucleol	small nucleus
nutri	nourish
nutrit	nourishment
o/o	egg
oblong	elongated
obsess	besieged by thoughts
obstetr	pregnancy and childbirth
occipit	back of head
occulta	hidden

WORD PART	DEFINITION
ocul/o	eye
-ode	way, road, path
odont	tooth
odyn/o	pain
-oid	resembling
-ol	alcohol, chemical, substance
-ola	small
-ole	small
olfact	smell
oligo-	scanty, too little
om/o	body, tumor
-oma	tumor, mass
onc/o	tumor
-one	chemical substance, hormone
onych/o	nail
ophthalm/o	eye
ophthalmos	eye
-opia	sight
opportun	take advantage of
-opsis	vision
-opsy	to view
opt/o	vision
optic	eye
-or	a doer, one who does, that which does something
or/o	mouth
orbit	orbit
orchi/o	testicle
ordin	arrange
orex	appetite
organ	organ, tool, instrument
orth/o	straight
orthot	correct
-orum	function of
-ory	having the function of
os	mouth
-osa	full of, like
-ose	full of
-osis	abnormal condition

S = Suffix P = Prefix R = Root R/CF = Combining Form

Word Part	Definition
osmo	push
osmol	concentration
oss/e	bone
oste/o	bone
-osus	condition
ot/o	ear
-otomy	incision
-ous	pertaining to
ov/i	egg
ovari	ovary
ovul	ovum, egg
ox	oxygen
-oxia	oxygen condition
oxid	oxidize
oxy	oxygen
pace	step
palat	palate
palliat	reduce suffering
palm	palm
palpat	touch, stroke
palpit	throb
pan-	all
pancreat	pancreas
panto-	entire
papill/o	pimple
par-	abnormal, beside
para	to bring forth
para-	adjacent to, alongside, beside, abnormal
parasit	parasite
paresis	weakness
pareun	lying beside, sexual intercourse
pariet	wall
paroxysm	irritate; sudden, sharp attack
particul	little piece
partum	childbirth, to bring forth
pat	lie open
patell	patella
patent	lie open
-path	disease

Word Part	Definition
path/o	disease
pathet	suffering
-pathic	pertaining to a disease
pathy	disease, emotion
-pathy	disease
paus	cessation
pause	cessation
pector	chest
ped	child, foot
pedicul	louse
pelas	skin
pelv	pelvis
pen	penis
-penia	deficient, deficiency
peps	digestion
pepsin/o	pepsin
pept	digest
per-	through, intense
perforat	bore through
perfus	to pour
peri-	around
perine	perineum
peripher	external boundary, outer part, outer edge
periton/e	stretch over, peritoneum
perium	a bringing forth
perm/e	pass through
pes	foot
pesti	pest
petit	small
petit-	small
-pexy	fixation, surgical fixation
phaco-	lens
phag/o	to eat
phage	to eat
-phage	to eat
phagia	swallowing
-phagia	swallowing, eating
phalang/e	phalanx, finger, toe
pharmac/o	drug

S = Suffix P = Prefix R = Root R/CF = Combining Form

WORD PART	DEFINITION
pharyng/o	pharynx
pharynx	pharynx, throat
phenol	benzene derivative
phenyl	chemical group
pheo-	gray
pher/o	to carry
-pheresis	removal
-phil	attraction
-phile	attraction
-philia	attraction
phim	muzzle
phleb/o	vein
phob	fear
-phobia	fear
phon/o	sound, voice
phor	bear, carry
phosphat	phosphorus
phot/o	light
phren	mind
phylac	protect
phylaxis	protection
-phyll	leaf
physema	blowing
physi/o	body
physis	growth
phyt/o	plant
pia	delicate
pituit	pituitary
pituitar	pituitary
plak	plate, plaque
plant	insert, plant
planus	flat surface
plas	molding, formation, growth
-plasia	formation
-plasm	something formed
plasm/o	to form
-plasty	formation, repair, surgical repair
plate	flat
pleg	paralysis

WORD PART	DEFINITION
plete	filled
pleur	pleura
plexy	stroke
-pnea	breathe
pneum/o	air, lung
pneumat	structure filled with air
pneumon	air, lung
pod	foot
-poiesis	to make
-poiet	the making
-poietin	the maker
poikilo-	irregular
point	to pierce
pol	pole
polio	gray matter
pollut	unclean
poly-	excessive, many, much
polyp	polyp
poplit/e	ham, back of knee
por/o	opening
post-	after
poster	back part
pract	efficient, practical
prand/i	breakfast
pre-	before, in front of
precis	accurate
pregn	with child, pregnant
presby	old person
press	press close, press down, squeeze
prevent	prevent
primi-	first
pro-	before, in front, projecting forward
proct/o	anus and rectum
product	lead forth
prolifer	bear offspring
pronat	bend down
prosta	prostate
prosthet	artificial part
prot/e	first

S = Suffix P = Prefix R = Root R/CF = Combining Form

Word Part	Definition
protein	protein
proto-	first
provision	provide
proxim	nearest to the center
prurit	itch
pseudo-	false
psych/o	mind, soul
psyche	mind, soul
pteryg	wing
ptosis	drooping, falling
-ptosis	drooping
ptysis	spit
pub	pubis
puer	child
pulmon/o	lung
puls	to drive
pump	pump
punct	puncture
pupill-	pupil
pur	pus
purul	pus
py/o	pus
pyel/o	renal pelvis
pylor	gate, pylorus
pyr/o	fire, heat
pyrex	fever
pyrid	heat
quadrant	quadrant
quadri-	four
radi/o	radius, X-ray, radiation
radic	root
re-	again, back, backward
recept	receive
rect/o	rectum
reflex	bend back
refract	bend
regul	to rule, control
remiss	send back, give up
ren	kidney

Word Part	Definition
replic	reply
rescein	resin
resect/o	cut off
resid/u	left over, what is left over
resist	to withstand
respire/a	to breathe
restor	renew
resuscit	revive from apparent death
reticul	fine net, network
retin/o	retina
retinacul	hold back
retro-	backward
rhabd/o	rod shaped, striated
rheumat	a flow, rheumatism
rhin/o	nose
rhythm	rhythm
rib/o	like a rib
ribo	a sugar, pentose
ribo-	from ribose, a sugar
rigid	stiff
rose	rose
rotat	rotate
-rrhagia	excessive flow, discharge
-rrhaphy	suture
rrhea	flow, discharge
-rrhoid	flow
rrhyth	rhythm
rrhythm	rhythm
-rubin	rust colored
rumin	throat
sacchar	sugar
sacr/o	sacrum
sagitt	arrow
saliv	saliva
salping/o	fallopian tube, uterine tube
salpinx	trumpet
san	sound, healthy
sanit	health
sapon	soap

S = Suffix P = Prefix R = Root R/CF = Combining Form

WORD PART	DEFINITION
sarc/o	flesh, muscle, sarcoma
satur	to fill
scapul	scapula
schiz/o	to split, cleave
scintill	spark
scler/o	hardness, white of eye
scoli/o	crooked
scope	instrument for viewing
-scope	instrument for viewing, instrument to examine
-scopy	to examine, to view
scorb	scurvy
scrot	scrotum
seb/o	sebum
sebac/e	wax
sebum	wax
secret	secrete, produce, separate
sect	cut off
sedat	to calm
sedent	sitting
segment	section
seiz	to grab
self	me, own individual
semi-	half
semin/i	semen
seminat	scatter seed
sen	old age
senesc	growing old
senil	senile
sens	feel
sensitiv	feeling
sensor/i	sensation, sensory
separat	move apart
seps	decay, infection
sept/o	septum, partition
ser/o	serum
serum	serum
sib	relative
-side	glycoside

WORD PART	DEFINITION
sigm	Greek letter "S"
silic	silicon, glass
simi	ape, monkey
simul	imitate
sin/o	sinus
sinus	sinus
sipid	flavor
-sis	abnormal condition, process
sit/u	place
skelet	skeleton
smear	spread
soc	partner
soci/o	society, social
soma	body
somat/o	body
-some	body
somn/o	sleep
son/o	sound
sorbit	fruit of a tree
sorpt	swallow
spad	tear or cut
spasm	spasm, sudden involuntary tightening
spast	tight
specif	species
sperm/i	sperm
spermat/o	sperm
sphen	wedge
spher/o	sphere
sphygm/o	pulse
spin/a	spine
spin/o	spine, spinal cord
spir/o	to breathe
spirat	breathe
spirit/u	spirit
spiro-	spiral, coil
splen/o	spleen
spongios	sponge
spor	spore
stable	steady

S = Suffix P = Prefix R = Root R/CF = Combining Form

WORD PART	DEFINITION
stag	standing place
stalsis	constrict, constriction
staphyl/o	bunch of grapes
stasis	stagnate, to stand still
-stasis	stop, stand still, control
stat	stationary
-static	stopped, standing still
-statin	inhibit
stax	fall in drops
steat	fat
stein	stone
sten/o	narrow, contract
ster	solid, steroid
stere/o	three-dimensional
steril	sterile, make sterile
stern	chest, breastbone
-steroid	steroid
-sterol	steroid
-sterone	steroid
steth/o	chest
sthen	strength
stigmat	focus
stimul	excite, strengthen
stin	partition
stip	press
stiti	space
stoma	mouth
-stomy	new opening
stone	stone, pebble
storm	crisis
strab	squint
strat	layer
strept/o	twisted
strict	narrow
study	inquiry
su/i	self
sub-	below, under, underneath
suct	suck
suffic/i	enough

WORD PART	DEFINITION
sulf	sulfur
super	above, excessive
super-	above, excessive
supinat	bend backward
supplement	supply to remedy a deficiency
suppress	pressed under, push under
supra-	above
surfact	surface
surg	operate
suscept	to take up
-sylated	linked
sym-	together
symptomat	collection of symptoms
syn-	together
syndesm	bind together
synov	synovial membrane
syring/o	tube, pipe
system	the body as a whole
systol/e	contraction, systole
tachy-	rapid
tact	orderly arrangement
tag	touch
tain	hold
talip	ankle bone
tamin	touch
tampon	plug
tangent	touch
tars	ankle
tax	coordination
tempor/o	time, temple
ten/o	tendon
tendin	tendon
tens	pressure
-tensin	tense, taut
terat/o	monster, malformed fetus
term	limit, end
test/o	testis, testicle
testicul	testicle, testis
tetra-	four

S = Suffix P = Prefix R = Root R/CF = Combining Form

Word Part	Definition
thalam	thalamus
thalamus	thalamus
thalass	sea
thel	breast, nipple
then	motion
thenar	palm
therap/o	healing, treatment
therapeut	healing, treatment
-therapist	one who treats
therapy	treatment
-therapy	treatment
therm/o	heat
thesis	arrange, place, organize
thet	arrange, place, organize
thi	sulfur
thora	chest
thorac/o	chest
thorax	chest
thromb/o	blood clot, clot
thym	thymus gland
thyr/o	thyroid
tibi	tibia
-tic	pertaining to
-tion	process, being
-tiz	pertaining to
toc	labor, birth
toler	endure
tom/o	cut, slice, layer
-tome	instrument to cut
-tomy	surgical incision
ton/o	pressure, tension
tonsil	tonsil
tonsill/o	tonsil
tope	part, location
topic	local
-tous	pertaining to
tox	poison
-toxic	able to kill
toxic/o	poison

Word Part	Definition
trache/o	trachea, windpipe
tract	draw, pull
tranquil	calm
trans-	across, through
traumat	wound, injury
tresia	a hole
tri-	three
trich/o	hair
-tripsy	crushing
-tripter	crusher
trochle	pulley
trop	turn, turning
troph	development, nourishment
trophy	development, nourishment
-tropic	a turning, change
-tropin	nourishing, stimulation
tryps	friction
tub	tube
tubercul	swelling, nodule, tuberculosis
tubul	small tube
tussis	cough
tympan/o	eardrum, tympanic membrane
-type	model, particular kind
typh	typhus
ulcer	a sore
-ule	little, small
-ulent	abounding in
uln	ulnar
ultra-	higher, beyond
-um	tissue, structure
umbilic	navel, umbilicus
un	one
un-	not
uni-	one
ur/o	urine, urinary system
-ure	process, result of
uresis	to urinate
uret	ureter, urine, urination
ureter/o	ureter

S = Suffix P = Prefix R = Root R/CF = Combining Form

Word Part	Definition
urethr/o	urethra
-uria	urine
urin	urine
-us	pertaining to
uter/o	uterus
uve	uvea
uvul	uvula
vaccin	vaccine, giving a vaccine
vag	vagus nerve
vagin	sheath, vagina
valgus	turn out
valv	valve
varic/o	varicosity; dilated, tortuous vein
vas/o	blood vessel, duct
vascul	blood vessel
ved	knowledge
veget	plants
vegetat	growth
ven/a	vein
ven/o	vein
ventil	wind
ventr	belly
ventricul	ventricle
vers	turn
-version	change
vert	to turn
vertebr	vertebra
vesic	sac containing fluid
vestibul/o	vestibule, entrance
via	the way
violet	bluish purple
viril	masculine
virus	poison
viscer	internal organs
viscos	viscous, sticky
visu	sight
vita	life
voc	voice
vol	volume

Word Part	Definition
volunt	willing
volut	shrink, roll up
-volut	rolled up
vuls	tear, pull
vulv/o	vulva
whip	to swing
xanth	yellow
xeno-	foreign
-xis	condition
-yl	substance
zea-	to live
-zoa	animal
zyg	zygote
zygomat	cheekbone
zyme	fermenting, enzyme, transform

Abbreviations

Abbreviation	Definition
µg	microgram; one-millionth of a gram
^	increase/ above
v	decrease/ below
1°	primary
2°	secondary
Ab	antibody
ABGs	arterial blood gases
ABO	agents of biologic origin
ABO	a blood group system
AC	acromioclavicular
ACE	angiotensin-converting enzyme
ACL	anterior cruciate ligament
ACLS	advanced cardiac life support
ACTH	adrenocorticotropic hormone
AD	right ear
ADD	attention deficit disorder
ADH	antidiuretic hormone
ADHD	attention deficit hyperactivity disorder
ADL	activity of daily living
AED	automatic external defibrillator
Afib	atrial fibrillation
Ag	antigen
AIDS	acquired immunodeficiency syndrome
AKA	above-knee amputation
ALL	acute lymphocytic leukemia
ALS	amyotrophic lateral sclerosis
AMI	acute myocardial infarction
AMS	altered mental state
ANS	autonomic nervous system
AOM	acute otitis media
AP	anteroposterior
ARDS	adult respiratory distress syndrome
ARF	acute renal failure
ARF	acute respiratory failure
AROM	active range of motion

Abbreviation	Definition
AS	left ear
ASD	atrial septal defect
ASD	autism spectrum disorder
ASHD	arteriosclerotic heart disease
AU	both ears
AV	atrioventricular
AVM	arteriovenous malformation
BBB	blood brain barrier
BD	brain death
BEP	benign enlargement of the prostate
BKA	below-knee amputation
BM	bowel movement
BMD	bone mineral density
BMR	basal metabolic rate
BOM	bilateral otitis media
BP	blood pressure
BPD	borderline personality disorder
BPH	benign prostatic hyperplasia
BPPV	benign paroxysmal positional vertigo
BRCA1	genetic mutation responsible for breast and ovarian cancer (**br**east **ca**ncer 1)
BRCA2	genetic mutation responsible for breast cancer (**br**east **ca**ncer 2)
BSE	bovine spongiform encephalopathy
BSE	breast self-examination
C1	first cervical vertebra
C5	fifth cervical vertebra or nerve
C7	seventh cervical vertebra
CA	cancer
CABG	coronary artery bypass graft
CAD	coronary artery disease
CAO	chronic airway obstruction
CAPD	continuous ambulatory peritoneal dialysis
CBC	complete blood count
CBT	cognitive-behavioral therapy

ABBREVIATION	DEFINITION
CD	conduct disorder
CDC	Centers for Disease Control and Prevention
CF	cystic fibrosis
CHD	congenital heart disease
CHES	certified health education specialist
CHF	congestive heart failure
CJD	Creutzfeldt–Jakob disease
CK	creatine kinase
CKD	chronic kidney disease
CMA	certified medical assistant
CMV	cytomegalovirus
CNA	certified nurse assistant
CNS	central nervous system
c/o	complains of
CO_2	carbon dioxide
COPD	chronic obstructive pulmonary disease
COT	certified occupational therapist
COTA	certified occupational therapist assistant
CP	cerebral palsy
CPAP	continuous positive airway pressure
CPR	cardiopulmonary resuscitation
CPT	cognitive processing therapy
CRF	chronic renal failure
CRH	corticoreleasing hormone
CRP	C-reactive protein
C-section	cesarean section
CSF	cerebrospinal fluid
CT	computed tomography
CVA	cerebrovascular accident
CVP	central venous pressure
CVS	cardiovascular system
CVT	cardiovascular technologist
CXR	chest X-ray
D & C	dilation and curettage
DASH	dietary approaches to stop hypertension
DEXA	dual-energy X-ray absorptiometry
DI	diabetes insipidus
DIC	disseminated intravascular coagulation
DID	dissociative identity disorder

ABBREVIATION	DEFINITION
DIFF	differential white blood cell count
DJD	degenerative joint disease
DKA	diabetic ketoacidosis
dL	deciliter; one-tenth of a liter
DM	diabetes mellitus
DMD	Duchenne muscular dystrophy
DNA	deoxyribonucleic acid
DNR	do not resuscitate
DO	Doctor of Osteopathy
DRE	digital rectal examination
DSM-IV	*Diagnostic and Statistical Manual of Mental Disorders,* Fourth Edition
DVT	deep vein thrombosis
EBV	Epstein–Barr virus
ECG	electrocardiogram
ECT	electroconvulsive therapy
ED	emergency department
ED	erectile dysfunction
EEG	electroencephalogram
EKG	electrocardiogram
EMG	electromyography
EMT	emergency medical technician
EMT-P	emergency medical technician-paramedic
EPCA-2	early prostate cancer antigen-2
ER	emergency room
ERT	estrogen replacement therapy
ESR	erythrocyte sedimentation rate
ESRD	end-stage renal disease
ESWL	extracorporeal shock wave lithotripsy
FAS	fetal alcohol syndrome
FDA	U.S. Food and Drug Administration
FEV1	forced expiratory volume in 1 second
FSH	follicle-stimulating hormone
FTD	fronto-temporal dementia
FTT	failure to thrive
FUS	focused ultrasound surgery
FVC	forced vital capacity
Fx	fracture
g	gram

ABBREVIATION	DEFINITION
GAD	generalized anxiety disorder
GDM	gestational diabetes mellitus
GERD	gastroesophageal reflux disease
GFR	glomerular filtration rate
GH	growth hormone, somatotrophin
GHRH	growth hormone-releasing hormone
GI	gastrointestinal
GI	glycemic index
GL	glycemic load
GnRH	gonadotrophin-releasing hormone
GTT	glucose tolerance test
GYN	gynecology
HAV	hepatitis A virus
Hb	hemoglobin
Hb A1c	glycosylated hemoglobin A-one-C
HBOT	hyperbaric oxygen therapy
HBV	hepatitis B virus
HCG	human chorionic gonadotropin
HCl	hydrochloric acid
Hct	hematocrit
HCV	hepatitis C virus
HDL	high-density lipoprotein
HDN	hemolytic disease of the newborn
Hgb	hemoglobin
HIPAA	Health Insurance Portability and Accountability Act
HIV	human immunodeficiency virus
HMD	hyaline membrane disease
HPI	history of present illness
HPV	human papilloma virus
HRT	hormone replacement therapy
HSV	herpes simplex virus
HSV-1	herpes simplex virus, type 1
HTN	hypertension
HUS	hemolytic uremic syndrome
IBS	irritable bowel syndrome
ICD	implantable cardioverter/defibrillator
IDDM	insulin-dependent diabetes mellitus
Ig	immunoglobulin
IgA	immunoglobulin A

ABBREVIATION	DEFINITION
IgD	immunoglobulin D
IgE	immunoglobulin E
IgG	immunoglobulin G
IgM	immunoglobulin M
IM	intramuscular
INR	international normalized ratio
ITP	idiopathic (immunologic) thrombocytopenic purpura
IU	international unit(s)
IUD	intrauterine device
IV	intravenous
IVC	inferior vena cava
IVF	in vitro fertilization
IVP	intravenous pyelogram
JRA	juvenile rheumatoid arthritis
KUB	X-ray of abdomen to show **k**idneys, **u**reters, and **b**ladder
LADA	latent autoimmune diabetes in adults
LASER	**l**ight **a**mplification by **s**timulated **e**mission of **r**adiation
LCC-ST	certified surgical technologist
LD	learning disability
LDL	low-density lipoprotein
LFT	liver function test
LH	luteinizing hormone
LLQ	left lower quadrant
LOC	loss of consciousness
LPN	licensed practical nurse
LUQ	left upper quadrant
LVN	licensed vocational nurse
mcg	microgram; one-millionth of a gram
MCP	metacarpophalangeal
MCS	minimally conscious state
MCV	mean corpuscular volume
MD	Doctor of Medicine
mg	milligram
MI	myocardial infarction
mL	milliliter
mm^3	cubic millimeter
MOAB	monoclonal antibody
MODY	mature onset diabetes of the young

ABBREVIATION	DEFINITION
MONA	morphine, oxygen, nitroglycerine, and aspirin
MPD	multiple personality disorder
MRA	magnetic resonance angiography
MRI	magnetic resonance imaging
mRNA	messenger RNA
MRSA	methicillin-resistant *Staphylococcus aureus*
MS	multiple sclerosis
MSA	myositis specific antibody
NCI	National Cancer Institute
NIDDM	non-insulin-dependent diabetes mellitus
NIH	National Institutes of Health
NKA	no known allergies
NO	nitric oxide
NRDS	neonatal respiratory distress syndrome
NSAID	nonsteroidal anti-inflammatory drug
O_2	oxygen
OA	obstetric assistant
OA	osteoarthritis
OB	obstetrics
OCD	obsessive compulsive disorder
OD	Doctor of Osteopathy
OD	right eye
ODD	oppositional defiant disorder
OGTT	oral glucose tolerance test
OME	otitis media with effusion
OR	operating room
OS	left eye
OSHA	Occupational Safety and Health Administration
OT	occupational therapy
OT	ophthalmic technician
OT	oxytocin
OTC	over the counter
OU	both eyes
P	pulse rate
PA	pernicious anemia
PA	posteroanterior
PaO_2	partial pressure of arterial oxygen
Pap	Papanicolaou (Pap test, Pap smear)

ABBREVIATION	DEFINITION
PAT	paroxysmal atrial tachycardia
PCL	posterior cruciate ligament
PCOS	polycystic ovarian syndrome
PDA	patent ductus arteriosus
PDD-NOS	pervasive developmental disorder, not otherwise specified
PDT	postural drainage therapy
PE tube	pressure equalization tube
PEEP	positive end-expiratory pressure
PEFR	peak expiratory flow rate
PERRLA	pupils equal, round, reactive to light, and accommodation
PET	positron emission tomography
PFTs	pulmonary function tests
PGY	pregnancy
pH	hydrogen ion concentration
PhD	Doctor of Philosophy
PID	pelvic inflammatory disease
PIP	proximal interphalangeal
PKD	polycystic kidney disease
PMDD	premenstrual dysphoric disorder
PMNL	polymorphonuclear leukocyte
PM&R	physical medicine and rehabilitation
PMS	premenstrual syndrome
PNB	pulseless, nonbreather
PNS	peripheral nervous system
PO	by mouth
POC	products of conception
polio	poliomyelitis
PPH	postpartum hemorrhage
PPS	postpolio syndrome
p.r.n, PRN	when necessary
PSA	prostate-specific antigen
PT	physical therapy, physical therapist
PT	physiotherapy
PT	prothrombin time
PTA	physical therapy assistant
PTCA	percutaneous transluminal coronary angioplasty
PTH	parathyroid hormone
PTSD	posttraumatic stress disorder

ABBREVIATION	DEFINITION
PTT	partial thromboplastin time
PVC	premature ventricular contractions
PVD	peripheral vascular disease
PVS	persistent vegetative state
q.4.h.	every 4 hours
q.i.d.	four times each day
R	respiration rate
RA	rheumatoid arthritis
RBC	red blood cell
RDA	recommended dietary allowance
RDS	respiratory distress syndrome
Rh	Rhesus
Rho-GAM	Rhesus immune globulin
RICE	rest, ice, compression, and elevation
RLQ	right lower quadrant
RN	registered nurse
RNA	ribonucleic acid
ROM	range of motion
RU-486	mifepristone
RUQ	right upper quadrant
SA	sinoatrial
SAD	seasonal affective disorder
SARS	severe acute respiratory syndrome
SBS	shaken baby syndrome
SC	subcutaneous
SCI	spinal cord injury
SET	self-examination of the testes
SFD	small for date
SG	specific gravity
SGA	small for gestational age
SI	sacroiliac
SIDS	sudden infant death syndrome
SLE	systemic lupus erythematosus
SOB	short(ness) of breath
SP	standard precautions
SSRI	selective serotonin reuptake inhibitor
STAT	immediately
STD	sexually transmitted disease
SVC	superior vena cava

ABBREVIATION	DEFINITION
T	temperature
T1	first thoracic vertebra or nerve
T3	triiodothyronine
T4	tetraiodothyronine (thyroxine)
TB	tuberculosis
TBI	traumatic brain injury
TENS	transcutaneous electrical nerve stimulation
THR	total hip replacement
TIA	transient ischemic attack
t.i.d.	(Latin *ter in die*) three times a day
TMJ	temporomandibular joint
TN	trigeminal neuralgia
TNM	**t**umor-**n**ode-**m**etastasis staging system for cancer
TOF	tetralogy of Fallot
tPA	tissue plasminogen activator
TRH	thyrotrophin-releasing hormone
TSH	thyroid-stimulating hormone
TTM	trichotillomania
TTN	transient tachypnea of the newborn
TTP	thrombotic thrombocytopenic purpura
TURP	transurethral resection of the prostate
UA	urinalysis
UP	universal precautions
URI	upper respiratory infection
USDA	U.S. Department of Agriculture
UTI	urinary tract infection
UV	ultraviolet
VEP	visual evoked potential
Vfib	ventricular fibrillation
VS	vital signs
VSD	ventricular septal defect
V-tach	ventricular tachycardia
vWD	von Willebrand disease
vWF	von Willebrand factor
WAD	Word Analysis and Definition (box)
WBC	white blood cell; white blood (cell) count
WNL	within normal limits
WNV	West Nile virus

Diagnostic and Therapeutic Procedures

A compilation of the diagnostic and therapeutic procedural terms used in this book.

A

abdominoplasty Esthetic operation on the abdominal wall (tummy tuck).

ablation Removal of tissue to destroy its function.

activated partial thromboplastin time (APTT) Blood test used to monitor the dose of heparin, an anticoagulant.

adenoidectomy Surgical removal of the adenoid tissue.

alignment Process of bringing the ends of a fractured bone at the break back opposite each other so that they fit together as they did in the original bone.

ambulatory Surgery or any other care provided without an overnight stay in a medical facility.

ambulatory blood pressure monitor Device that provides a record of blood pressure readings over a 24-hour period as patients go about their daily activities.

amniocentesis Removal of amniotic fluid for diagnostic purposes.

amputation Process of removing a limb, part of a limb, a breast, or other projecting part.

anastomosis Surgically made union between two tubular structures.

angiogram Radiographic image of arteries or veins after injection of contrast material.

angiography The process of obtaining an angiogram.

angioplasty Reopening of a blood vessel by surgery.

anoscopy Examination of the anus and lower rectum with a rigid instrument.

Apgar score Evaluation of a newborn's status.

appendectomy Surgical removal of the appendix.

arterial blood gases The measurement of the levels of oxygen and carbon dioxide in the blood—a good indicator of respiratory function.

arteriography X-ray visualization of an artery after injection of contrast material.

arthrocentesis Aspiration of fluid from a joint; used to establish a diagnosis by laboratory examination of the fluid, drain off infected fluid, or insert medication such as local corticosteroids.

arthrodesis Fixation or stiffening of a joint by surgery.

arthrography X-ray of a joint after injection of a contrast medium into the joint to make the inside details of the joint visible.

arthroplasty Replacement of a joint with a prosthesis.

arthroscopy Procedure performed using an arthroscope to examine the internal compartments of a joint or perform a surgical procedure such as debridement, removal of damaged tissue, or repair of torn ligaments.

aspiration Removal by suction of fluid or gas from a body cavity.

atherectomy Surgical removal of atheroma from a blood vessel.

audiometer Electronic device that generates sounds in different frequencies and intensities to test for hearing loss.

auscultation Diagnostic method of listening to body sounds with a stethoscope.

autograft Graft removed from the patient's own skin.

automatic external defibrillator (AED) Device that sends an electric shock to the heart to stop the heart and allow a normal contraction rhythm to resume.

B

bariatric surgery Surgical treatment of obesity.

barium meal Ingestion of barium sulfate to study the distal esophagus, stomach, and duodenum on X-ray.

barium swallow Ingestion of barium sulfate, a contrast material, to show details of the pharynx and esophagus on X-ray.

biopsy Removal of tissue from a living person for laboratory examination.

blepharoplasty Correction of defects in the eyelids.

bone marrow aspiration or biopsy Use of a needle to remove bone marrow cells.

bone mineral density (BMD) Screening test for osteoporosis using a dual-energy X-ray absorptiometry (DEXA) scan.

brace Appliance to support a part of the body in its correct position.

brachytherapy Radiation therapy in which the source of irradiation is implanted in the tissue to be treated.

bronchoscopy Examination of the interior of the tracheobronchial tree with an endoscope.

C

cannula Tube inserted into a blood vessel or cavity as a channel for fluid or gas.

cardiac catheterization Procedure that detects patterns of pressures and blood flows in the heart. A thin tube is guided into the heart under X-ray guidance after being inserted into a vein or artery.

cardiac stress testing Exercise tolerance test that raises the heart rate and monitors the effect on cardiac function.

cardiopulmonary resuscitation Attempt to restore cardiac and pulmonary function.

cardioversion Restoration of a normal heart rhythm by electrical shock. Also called *defibrillation.*

catheterization Introduction of a catheter.

cerebral angiography Injection of a radiopaque dye into the blood vessels of the neck and brain to detect blood vessels that are partially or completely blocked, aneurysms, or arteriovenous malformations.

cerebral arteriography Procedure used to determine the site of bleeding in hemorrhagic strokes, enabling surgery to be performed to stop the bleed or to clip off the aneurysm.

chest X-ray Radiograph image of the chest that can be taken in anteroposterior (AP), posteroanterior (PA), lateral, and sometimes oblique and lateral decubitus positions.

cholangiography Use of a contrast medium to radiographically visualize the bile ducts.

cholecystectomy Surgical removal of the gallbladder.

cholelithotomy Surgical removal of a gallstone(s).

circumcision Removal of part or all of the prepuce of the penis.

clean-catch, midstream urine specimen Sample collected after the external urethral meatus is cleaned. The first part of the urine stream is not collected, and the sterile collecting vessel is introduced into the urinary stream to collect the last part.

clot-busting drugs Drugs injected within a few hours of an MI or thrombotic stroke to dissolve the thrombus. Also called *thrombolytic drugs.*

cognitive behavioral therapy (CBT) A form of psychotherapy that emphasizes the role of thoughts and attitudes in one's feelings and behaviors.

cognitive processing therapy (CPT) Uses a variety of techniques in psychotherapy such as self-discovery and self-instruction.

colonoscopy Examination of the inside of the colon by endoscopy.

colostomy Artificial opening from the colon to the outside of the body.

colpopexy Surgical fixation of a relaxed and prolapsed vagina to the anterior abdominal wall.

computed tomography (CT) Scan in which images of sections of the body are generated by a computer synthesis of X-rays obtained in many different directions in a given plane.

conization Surgical excision of a cone-shaped piece of tissue, e.g., from the outer lining of the cervix.

constant positive airway pressure (CPAP) Attempt to keep alveoli open by maintaining a positive pressure in the airways. A mask is fitted over the nose and mouth and attached to a ventilator.

continuous ambulatory peritoneal dialysis (CAPD) Dialysis performed by the patient at home through an implanted peritoneal catheter, usually 4 times a day, 7 days a week.

continuous cycling peritoneal dialysis Use of a machine to automatically infuse dialysis solution into and out of the abdominal cavity through a peritoneal catheter during sleep.

coronary angiogram Injection of a contrast dye during cardiac catheterization to identify coronary artery blockages.

coronary artery bypass graft surgery (CABG) Procedure in which healthy blood vessels harvested as a graft from the leg, chest, or arm are used to bypass (detour) the blood around blocked coronary arteries.

cryosurgery Use of liquid nitrogen or argon gas in a probe to freeze and kill abnormal tissue.

curette Scoop-shaped instrument for scraping or removing new growths (or earwax).

cystoscopy Insertion of a pencil-thin, flexible, tubelike telescope through the urethra into the bladder to examine directly the lining of the bladder and to take a biopsy if needed.

cystourethrogram X-ray image during voiding to show the structure and function of the bladder and urethra.

D

debridement Removal of injured or necrotic tissue.

defibrillation Restoration of uncontrolled twitching of cardiac muscle fibers to a normal rhythm.

dermabrasion Removal of upper layers of the skin using a high-powered rotating brush.

dermascope An instrument that shines a light on the skin and magnifies a lesion for better diagnostic viewing.

dialysis Artificial method of removing waste materials and excess fluid from blood.

digital rectal examination (DRE) Palpation of the rectum and prostate gland with an index finger.

dilation and curettage (D & C) Dilation of the cervix so that a thin instrument can be inserted to scrape away the lining of the uterus and take tissue samples.

dipstick Plastic strip bearing paper squares of reagent—the most cost-effective method of screening urine. After the stick is dipped in the urine specimen, the color change in each segment of the dipstick is compared to a color chart on the container. Dipsticks can screen for pH, specific gravity, protein, blood, glucose, ketones, bilirubin, nitrite, and leukocyte esterase.

Doppler ultrasound Diagnostic instrument that sends an ultrasonic beam into the body.

E

early morning urine collection Process used to determine the ability of the kidneys to concentrate urine following overnight dehydration.

echocardiography Ultrasound recording of heart function.

echoencephalography Use of ultrasound in the diagnosis of intracranial lesions.

electrocardiogram Record of the electrical signals of the heart.

electrocardiography Interpretation of electrocardiograms.

electroconvulsive therapy (ECT) Passage of electric current through the brain to produce convulsions and treat persistent depression.

electroencephalography Recording of the electrical activity of the brain.

electromyography Recording of electrical activity in muscle.

endarterectomy Surgical removal of plaque from an artery.

endometrial ablation Use of a heat-generating tool or a laser to remove or destroy the lining of the uterus and prevent or reduce menstruation.

endoscope An instrument for the examination of the interior of a hollow or tubular organ.

endoscopy Use of an endoscope to examine the interior of a tubular or hollow organ and perform a biopsy, remove polyps (polypectomy), and coagulate bleeding lesions.

enema Injection of fluid into the rectum and lower bowel.

enteroscopy Examination of the lining of the digestive tract.

episiotomy Surgical incision in the perineum to dilate the opening of the vagina.

evoked responses Use of stimuli for vision, sound, and touch to activate specific areas of the brain and measure their responses with EEG. This provides information about how that specific area of the brain is functioning.

excision Surgical removal of part or all of a structure or organ.

excisional biopsy Removal of a tumor with a surrounding margin of normal tissue.

external fixation Method of maintaining the alignment of a fractured bone by immobilizing the bone through the use of plaster casts, splints, traction, and external fixators such as steel rods and pins.

extracorporeal shock wave lithotripsy (ESWL) Process in which a machine called a *lithotripter* produces shock waves that crumble renal or ureteral stones into small pieces that can pass down the ureter.

F

fasciectomy Surgical removal of fascia.

fecal occult blood test Diagnostic procedure that detects the presence of blood not visible to the naked eye. Trade name: *Hemoccult* test.

fistulectomy Surgical excision of a fistula.

fistulotomy Surgical enlargement or opening up of a fistula.

flexible endoscopy Use of a flexible, slim fiber-optic instrument that transmits light and sends back images to the observer.

forceps extraction Assisted delivery of a baby by an instrument that grasps the head of the baby.

fundoscopy Examination of the retina with an ophthalmoscope.

G

gastroscopy Endoscopic examination of the inside of the stomach.

gavage To feed by a stomach tube.

gingivectomy Surgical removal of diseased gum tissue.

H

heart transplant Surgery in which the heart of a recently deceased person (donor) is transplanted to the recipient after the recipient's diseased heart has been removed.

Hemoccult test Trade name for *fecal occult blood test.*

hemodialysis Process that filters blood through an artificial kidney machine (dialyzer).

hemorrhoidectomy Surgical removal of hemorrhoids.

herniorrhaphy Surgical repair of a hernia.

heterograft Graft from a nonhuman species. Also called *xenograft.*

Holter monitor Continuous ECG recorded on a tape cassette for at least 24 hours as a person works, plays, and rests.

homocysteine Amino acid in the blood. Elevated levels are related to a higher risk of CAD, stroke, and peripheral vascular disease.

homograft Skin graft from another person or a cadaver. Also called *allograft.*

hysterectomy Surgical removal of the uterus.

I

ileostomy Artificial opening from the ileum to the outside of the body.

implantable cardioverter/defibrillator (ICD) Implanted device that senses abnormal rhythms and gives the heart a small electrical shock to return the rhythm to normal.

incision Cut or surgical wound.

internal fixation Use of tissue-compatible materials such as stainless steel and titanium to stabilize fractured bony parts, enabling the patient to return to function more quickly and reducing the incidence of nonunion and malunion (improper healing). The types of internal fixation are wires used as sutures to "sew" the bone fragments together; plates that extend along both or all fragments of bone and are held in place by screws; rods inserted through the medullary cavity of both fragments to align the bones; and screws that can be used on their own as well as with plates.

intradermal injection Introduction of a short, thin needle into the epidermis, thus raising a small wheal. This site is used for allergy and tuberculosis (TB) testing.

intramuscular (IM) injection Use of a long needle that penetrates the epidermis, dermis, and hypodermis to reach into the muscles underneath. Some antibiotics and immunizations are given by this route.

intrauterine insemination Insertion of sperm directly into the uterus via a special catheter to initiate pregnancy.

intravenous pyelogram (IVP) Procedure in which a contrast material containing iodine is injected intravenously and its progress through the urinary tract is then recorded on a series of rapid radiological images.

intubation Insertion of a tube into a canal, hollow organ, or cavity, e.g., into the trachea for anesthesia or control of ventilation.

in vitro fertilization (IVF) Process of combining sperm and egg in a laboratory dish and placing the resulting embryos inside the uterus.

Ishihara color system Test for color vision defects.

J

Jaeger reading card Chart containing type in different sizes of print for testing near vision.

K

keratomileusis Procedure that cuts and shapes the cornea.

keratoplasty Corneal graft or transplant.

keratotomy Incision through the cornea.

kidney transplant Surgery in which the kidney of a donor is transplanted to a recipient; provides a better quality of life than kidney dialysis, if a suitable donor can be found.

KUB X-ray of the abdomen to show **k**idneys, **u**reters, and **b**ladder.

L

laparoscopy Examination of the contents of the abdomen using an endoscope, which can also be used to perform surgery and take samples for biopsy.

laryngoscopy Use of a hollow tube with a light and camera to visualize or operate on the larynx.

laser surgery Use of a concentrated, intense narrow beam of electromagnetic radiation for surgery. (*laser:* **l**ight **a**mplification by **s**imulated **e**mission of **r**adiation.)

LASIK Acronym for laser-assisted in situ keratomileusis.

lipectomy Surgical removal of fatty tissue.

lipid profile Group of blood tests that help determine the risk of CAD and comprise total cholesterol; high-density lipoprotein (HDL), or "good cholesterol"; low-density lipoprotein (LDL), or "bad cholesterol"; and triglycerides.

liposuction Surgical removal of fatty tissue using suction.

lobectomy Surgical removal of a lobe of a structure, for example, a lobe of a lung.

lumbar puncture Use of a hollow needle to remove CSF so that it can be examined in the laboratory. Also called *spinal tap.*

lumpectomy Removal of a lesion with preservation of surrounding tissue.

lymphadenectomy Surgical removal of a lymph gland(s).

lymphangiogram Radiographic images of lymph vessels and nodes following injection of contrast material.

M

magnetic resonance angiography (MRA) Method of visualizing vessels that contain flowing structures by producing a contrast between them and stationary structures.

magnetic resonance imaging (MRI) Diagnostic technique that creates detailed images of structures and tissues in various planes without exposing patients to radiation as in conventional radiography or computed tomography.

mammogram Record produced by X-ray imaging of the breast.

mammoplasty Surgical reshaping of the breasts.

mastectomy Surgical excision of the breast.

mechanical ventilation Process by which gases are moved into and out of the lungs via a ventilator that is set to meet the respiratory requirements of the patient.

mediastinoscopy Examination of the mediastinum using an endoscope inserted through an incision in the suprasternal notch.

myomectomy Surgical removal of a uterine myoma (fibroid).

myringotomy Incision through the tympanic membrane; e.g., for the placement of pressure equalization (PE) tubes to allow an effusion to drain.

N

nebulizer Device used to deliver liquid medicine in a fine mist.

nephrectomy Surgical removal of a kidney.

nephrolithotomy Incision into the kidney for removal of a stone.

nephroscopy Examination of the pelvis of the kidney.

nerve conduction studies Studies that measure the speed at which motor or sensory nerves conduct impulses.

nuclear imaging of the heart Use of an injection of a radioactive substance in association with a cardiac stress test to assess cardiac function.

O

ophthalmoscopy Examination of the retina using an ophthalmoscope.

orchiopexy Surgical fixation of a testis in the scrotum.

ostomy Artificial opening into a tubular structure, for example, ileostomy and colostomy.

otoscopy Examination of the ear using an otoscope.

P

pacemaker Device that regulates cardiac electrical activity. The device generates electronic signals carried along thin, insulated wires to the heart muscle.

palpation Examination with the fingers and hands.

panendoscopy Visual examination of the inside of the esophagus, stomach, and upper duodenum using a flexible fiber-optic endoscope.

Pap test Examination of cells taken from the cervix.

parathyroidectomy Surgical removal of the parathyroid glands.

peak flow meter Instrument used to record the greatest flow of air that can be sustained for 10 milliseconds on forced expiration, the peak expiratory flow rate (PEFR). It is of value in following the course of asthma and in postoperative care to monitor the return of lung function after anesthesia.

percutaneous nephrolithotomy Insertion of a nephroscope through the skin to locate and remove a renal pelvic or ureteral stone.

percutaneous transluminal coronary angioplasty (PTCA) Procedure in which a balloon-tipped catheter is guided to the site of the blockage and inflated to expand the artery from the inside by compressing the plaque against the walls of the artery.

percutaneous transthoracic needle aspiration Insertion of a needle with a cutting chamber through an intercostal space to hook a specimen of parietal pleura for laboratory examination.

peritoneal dialysis Procedure in which a dialysis solution is infused into and drained out of the abdominal cavity through a small, flexible, implanted catheter.

phacoemulsification To break down and remove the lens of the eye using an ultrasound needle.

phlebotomy Process of taking blood from a vein.

photocoagulation Use of a laser beam to form a clot or destroy abnormal capillaries. In the eye, this slows the pace of the visual loss in macular degeneration.

phototherapy Treatment using light rays.

pneumonectomy Surgical removal of a lung.

polypectomy Excision or removal of a polyp.

polysomnography Test to monitor brain waves, muscle tension, eye movement, and oxygen levels in the blood as the patient sleeps.

positive end expiratory pressure (PEEP) Technique in ventilation to keep the alveoli from collapsing in adult and neonatal respiratory distress syndromes.

positron emission tomography (PET) Scan that shows the uptake and distribution of substances such as sugar in tissues to locate abnormal, often malignant, structures.

postural drainage therapy (PDT) Treatment that involves positioning and tilting the patient so that gravity promotes drainage of secretions from lung segments. Chest percussion (tapping) on the chest wall can help loosen, mobilize, and drain the retained secretions.

proctoscopy Examination of the inside of the anus and rectum by endoscopy.

prostatectomy Surgical removal of part or all of the prostate.

prosthesis Manufactured substitute for a missing part of the body.

prothrombin time (PT) Test used to monitor the dose of Coumadin, an anticoagulant. It is reported as an *international normalized ratio (INR)* instead of in seconds.

psychotherapy Treatment of psychiatric disorders based on verbal and nonverbal interventions with the patient.

pulmonary rehabilitation Therapeutic restoration of lung function that includes education, breathing exercises and retraining, exercises for the upper and lower extremities, and psychosocial support.

pulse oximeter Sensor placed on the finger to measure the oxygen saturation of the blood.

pyelogram X-ray image of the renal pelvis and ureters.

Q

quadrantectomy Surgical excision of a quadrant of the breast.

R

radical hysterectomy Surgical removal of the fallopian tubes and ovaries as well as the uterus.

radical mastectomy Complete surgical removal of all breast tissue, the pectoralis major muscle, and associated lymph nodes.

radical prostatectomy Complete surgical removal of the prostate and surrounding tissues.

random urine collection Process in which a sample is taken with no precautions regarding contamination. It is often used for collecting samples for drug testing. "Pee into a cup."

reduction Procedure in which the distal segment of a fractured bone is pulled back into alignment with the proximal segment. Anesthesia may be used.

rehabilitation Therapeutic restoration of an ability to function as before after disease, illness, or injury.

renal angiogram X-ray with contrast material used to assess blood flow to the kidneys.

resection Removal of a specific part of an organ or structure.

retrograde pyelogram Injection of contrast material through a urinary catheter into the ureters to locate stones and other obstructions.

rhinoplasty Surgical procedure to alter the size or shape of the nose.

Rinne test Test for a conductive hearing loss.

S

salpingectomy Surgical removal of a fallopian tube.

sclerotherapy Injection of a solution into a vein to thrombose it.

segmentectomy Surgical excision of a segment of a tissue or organ.

sigmoidoscopy Endoscopic examination of the sigmoid colon.

Snellen letter chart Test for acuity of distant vision.

sphygmomanometer Instrument for measuring arterial blood pressure.

spinal tap Placement of a needle through an intervertebral space into the subarachnoid space to withdraw CSF.

spirometer Device used to measure the volume of air that a patient moves in and out of the respiratory system.

splenectomy Surgical removal of the spleen.

staging Process of determining the extent of the distribution of a neoplasm. The TNM (tumor-node-metastasis) staging system can be used.

stent placement Procedure in which a wire mesh tube, or stent, is placed inside the vessel to reduce the likelihood that an occluded artery will close up again. Some stents (drug-eluting stents) are covered with a special medication to help keep the artery open.

sterilization Process of making sterile.

stethoscope Instrument for listening to cardiac, respiratory, and other sounds.

stoma Artificial opening.

subcutaneous (SC) injection Injection in which a needle pierces the epidermis and dermis to reach the hypodermis (subcutaneous) layer. This site is used for insulin injections and for some immunizations.

suprapubic transabdominal needle aspiration of the bladder Procedure used with newborns and small infants to obtain a pure sample of urine.

suture Process or material that brings together the edges of a wound to enhance tissue healing. Also, a form of fibrous joint to unite two bones.

T

thoracentesis Insertion of a needle through an intercostal space to remove fluid from a pleural effusion for laboratory study or to relieve pressure. Also called *pleural tap.*

thoracoscopy Examination of the pleural cavity with an endoscope.

thoracotomy Incision through the chest wall.

thymectomy Surgical removal of the thymus gland.

thyroidectomy Surgical removal of the thyroid gland.

tomography Radiographic image of a selected slice of tissue.

tonometry Measurement of intraocular pressure.

tonsillectomy Surgical removal of the tonsils.

tracheal aspiration Procedure in which a soft catheter is passed into the trachea to allow brushings and washings to remove cells and secretions from the trachea and main bronchi for diagnostic study.

tracheostomy Insertion of a tube into the windpipe to assist breathing.

tracheotomy The process of making an incision into the trachea.

traction Gentle but continuous application of a pulling force that can align a fracture, reduce muscle spasm, and relieve pain.

transdermal application Administration of some medications through the skin by an adhesive transdermal patch that is applied to the skin. The medication diffuses across the epidermis and enters the blood vessels in the dermis. Contraceptive hormones, analgesics, and antinausea/seasickness medications are examples.

transplant The tissue or organ used or the transfer of tissue from one person to another.

transthoracic Going through the chest wall.

tubal ligation Surgery, using laparoscopy, in which both fallopian tubes are cut, a segment is removed, and the ends are tied off and cauterized shut.

24-hour urine collection Process that determines the amount of protein being excreted daily and estimates the kidneys' filtration ability.

tympanostomy Surgically created new opening in the tympanic membrane to allow fluid to drain from the middle ear.

U

ultrasonography Delineation of deep structures using sound waves.

ureteroscopy Examination of the ureter. A small flexible ureteroscope is passed through the urethra and bladder into the ureter. Devices can be passed through the endoscope to remove or fragment stones.

urinalysis (microscopic) Analysis of the solids deposited by centrifuging a specimen of urine. It can reveal RBCs, WBCs, and renal tubular epithelial cells stuck together to form casts (cylindrical molds of cells) in nephrotic syndrome.

urinalysis (U/A) Examination of urine to separate it into its elements and define their kind and/or quantity. A routine urinalysis in the laboratory can include tests for color, clarity, pH, specific gravity, protein, glucose, ketones, and leukocyte esterase (indicator of infection).

urine culture Culture taken from a clean-catch urine specimen. It is the definitive test for a urinary tract infection.

vasectomy Excision of a segment of the ductus deferens to interrupt the flow of sperm.

vasovasostomy Microsurgical procedure to suture back together the cut ends of the ductus deferens to restore the flow of sperm. Also called *vasectomy reversal.*

venogram Radiograph of veins after injection of radiopaque contrast material.

vestibulectomy Surgical excision of the vulva.

voiding cystourethrogram (VCUG) Imaging in which a contrast material is inserted into the bladder through a catheter and X-rays are taken during voiding.

Weber test Test for sensorineural hearing loss.

xenograft Graft from a nonhuman species. Also called *heterograft.*

Pharmacology

A compilation of pharmacologic terms used in this book.

A

acetaminophen Analgesic (reduces response to pain) and antipyretic (reduces fever).

adrenaline (1) Hormone produced by the adrenal medulla that boosts the supply of oxygen and glucose to the brain and increases heart rate and output. (2) Drug used to treat cardiac arrest and dysrhythmias and relieve bronchospasm in asthma. Also called *epinephrine.*

allergen Substance producing a hypersensitivity (allergic) reaction. Examples are animal fur and dander, penicillins, and foods such as eggs, milk, and wheat.

alpha-glucosidase inhibitors Block the breakdown of starches in the intestine.

analgesic Substance that reduces or relieves the response to pain without producing loss of consciousness. Examples are aspirin and other NSAIDs, acetaminophen, and codeine.

androgen Hormone that promotes masculine characteristics. An example is testosterone.

anesthetic Agent that causes absence of feeling or sensation. Examples of local anesthetics are lidocaine and novocaine; examples of general anesthetics are nitrous oxide, thiopental, and ketamine.

antacid Agent that neutralizes the acidity of stomach contents. Examples are aluminum hydroxide, magnesium hydroxide, and calcium carbonate.

antiarrhythmic Agents that restore normal heart rate and rhythm.

antibiotic Substance that has the capacity to inhibit the growth of or destroy bacteria and other microorganisms. Examples are penicillin, erythromycin, cefotaxime, and flucloxacillin.

anticholinergics Agents antagonistic to parasympathetic nerve fibers.

anticoagulant Substance that prevents clotting. Examples are heparin and Coumadin (warfarin).

antidepressants A class of drugs that alleviate the symptoms of depression.

antidiabetic drugs Medications used to treat diabetes. Those given orally include metformin, acarbose, and thiazolidinediones, such as troglitazone. Insulin is given by injection or inhaled.

antidiuretic Agent that decreases urine production. Examples are vasopressin, amiloride, and chlorpropamide.

antiepileptic Agent capable of preventing or arresting epilepsy. Examples are phenobarbitol, phenytoin, and valproate.

antifungal agents Agents used to prevent and arrest fungal infections. Examples are the topical applications 1% clotremazole (Lomotrin, Mycelex) and 1% terbinafine (Lamisol), which are available without prescriptions.

antihistamine Agent used to treat allergic symptoms because of its action antagonistic to histamine. Examples are benadryl, diphenhydramine, and cimetidine.

anti-inflammatory Agent that reduces inflammation by acting on the body's responses, without affecting the causative agent. Examples are corticosteroids and aspirin.

antimicrobial Agent used to destroy or prevent multiplication of organisms. (See *antibiotic*.)

antineoplastic Agent that prevents the growth and spread of cancer cells. Examples are methotrexate, fluorouracil, and cyclophosphamide.

antipruritic Medication against itching. Examples are calamine lotion, hydrocortisone cream applied topically, and diphenhydramine (Benadryl) taken orally.

antipyretic Agent that reduces fever. Examples are aspirin and acetaminophen.

antiseptic Agent that reduces the number of microorganisms in different situations. Examples are alcohol, chlorhexidine, and providone-iodine.

anxiolytics Class of drugs that relieve the symptoms of anxiety.

atropine Agent used to dilate the pupils.

B

benzothiazide Diuretic that increases the excretion of sodium and potassium with an accompanying volume of water.

beta blocker Agent used in the treatment of a variety of cardiovascular diseases. Examples are propanalol and acebutolol.

biguanides Agents that decrease glucose production in the liver.

bronchodilator Agent that relaxes the smooth muscles of the bronchioles. Examples are theophylline; beta-2 agonists, such as salbutamol and terbutaline; and anticholinergics, such as ipratropium bromide.

C

calcium channel blocker Agent that decreases the force of contraction of the myocardium, dilates coronary arteries, and reduces blood pressure. Examples are amlodipine and verapamil.

chemotherapy Treatment using chemical agents, usually in relation to neoplastic disease. Examples are platinum compounds such as cisplatin or paraplatin.

chronotropic Agents that alter the heart rate.

cleansing agents Soaps, shampoos, and detergents that are used to clean wounds and abrasions or to remove crusts and scales.

coagulant Substance that causes clotting. Thrombin and fibrin glue are used surgically to treat bleeding.

contraceptive Agent that prevents conception. Examples are condoms, diaphragms, and birth control pills using a mixture of estrogen and progesterone.

corticosteroids Hormones produced by the adrenal cortex. Examples are cortisol and aldosterone.

cortisol One of the glucocorticoids produced by the adrenal cortex; has anti-inflammatory effects. Also called *hydrocortisone.*

creams Water-based emulsions with a cooling and soothing effect that are cosmetically well tolerated.

D

decongestant An agent that reduces the swelling and fluid in the nose and sinuses. Examples are pseudoephedrine and phenylephrine.

depressant Substance that diminishes activity, sensation, or tone, particularly in relation to the nervous system. Examples are alcohol, barbiturates, and benzodiazepines.

disease-modifying drug Agent that has partial success in slowing down the accumulation of disabilities in a specific disease process. Examples in multiple sclerosis (MS) include interferons and mitoxantrone.

disinfectant Agent used to destroy pathogenic and other microorganisms on nonliving surfaces. Examples are alcohol, hydrogen peroxide, and hypochlorites.

diuretic Agent that increases urine output. Examples are furosemide, hydrochlorthiazide, spironolactone, and mannitol.

dopamine Chemical neurotransmitter in some specific areas of the brain.

E

epinephrine (1) Hormone produced by the adrenal medulla that boosts the supply of oxygen and glucose to the brain and increases heart rate and output. (2) Drug used to treat cardiac arrest and dysrhythmias and relieve bronchospasm in asthma. Also called *adrenaline.*

estrogen Generic term for hormones that stimulate female secondary sex characteristics.

F

fluorescein Dye that produces a vivid green color under a blue light; used to diagnose corneal abrasions and foreign bodies in the eye.

G

gels Jelly-like watery suspension using a chemical gelling agent for insoluble drugs such as corticosteroids and retinoids.

H

histamine Compound liberated in tissues as a result of injury or an immune response.

hydrocortisone Potent glucocorticoid with anti-inflammatory properties. Also called *cortisol.*

I

immunization Treatment with an agent designed to protect susceptible people from a communicable disease, such as agents that protect against the childhood diseases of measles, rubella, and pertussis.

inotropic Agents that change the force of ventricular contraction.

insulin Hormone produced by the islet cells of the pancreas that promotes glucose use. Injectable insulin preparations are classified by their speed of action.

L

lidocaine Ocular local anesthetic.

loop diuretic Promotes evacuation of urine in the kidney.

M

melatonin Hormone formed and secreted by the pineal gland during darkness. Serotonin is a precursor. It assists in the control of daily body rhythms, stimulates the immune system, and is an antioxidant.

morphine Derivative of opium used as an analgesic or sedative.

mucolytic Agent that attempts to break up mucus to allow it to be cleared more effectively from the airways. Examples are guaifenesin (common in over-the-counter cough medications), potassium iodide, and *N*-acetylcysteine (taken through a nebulizer).

mydriatic Agent that dilates the pupils of the eye.

N

narcotic Drug derived from opium. Examples are heroin, morphine, codeine, and demerol.

neurotransmitter Chemical that crosses a synapse to stimulate or inhibit another neuron or the cell of a muscle or gland. Examples are norepinephrine, serotonin, and dopamine.

O

ointments Agents that contain no water and are oil-based to provide an occlusive layer to retain water in the skin; they are used to treat chronic, dry, and scaly conditions.

opiate Drug derived from opium. Examples are morphine, codeine, heroin, and demerol.

osmotic diuretic Promotes evacuation of water and electrolytes in the kidney.

oxygen Gas given by nasal cannula or by mask and intubation to relieve hypoxia. Patients with severe, chronic COPD can be attached to a portable cylinder of oxygen.

P

pharmacist Person licensed by the state to prepare and dispense drugs.

pharmacology Science of the preparation, uses, and effects of drugs.

pharmacy Facility licensed to prepare and dispense drugs.

placebo Inert, medicinally inactive compound with no intrinsic therapeutic value.

progesterone Hormone used to correct abnormalities of menstruation, and as a contraceptive.

prostaglandin Hormone present in many tissues; first isolated from the prostate gland.

psychedlic A class of drugs that enhance sensory experiences and consciousness.

psychoactive Agent able to alter mood, behavior, and/or cognition. Examples include narcotics, stimulants, antidepressants, and hallucinogens.

R

retinoids Keratolytic agents applied for psoriasis, acne, and photo damage.

S

saline Salt solution, usually sodium chloride.

selective serotonin reuptake inhibitors Class of drugs that prevent the reuptake of serotonin and are used in the treatment of depression.

somatotropin Hormone of the anterior pituitary gland that stimulates the growth of body tissues. Also called *growth hormone (GH).*

spermicide Agent that destroys sperm. Examples are nonoxynol-9 and benzalkonium chloride.

sterilization Elimination of all microorganisms by high-pressure steam (autoclave), dry heat (oven), or radiation.

steroid Large family of chemical substances found in many drugs, hormones, and body components.

stimulant Agent that excites or strengthens. Examples include caffeine, nicotine, and cocaine.

sulfonylureas Agents that stimulate the beta cells of the pancreas to produce more insulin.

surfactant Protein and fat compound that creates surface tension to hold the lung alveolar walls apart.

T

teratogen Agent that produces fetal abnormalities–congenital malformations–while organs and structures are being formed. (All medications readily cross the placenta.) Examples include alcohol, isoretinoin (acne medication), valproic acid (anticonvulsant), and the rubella virus.

testosterone The major androgen that promotes development of male sex characteristics.

thrombolytic Agent injected within a few hours of a myocardial infarction (MI) or stroke to dissolve the thrombus causing the arterial blockage. Examples are streptokinase and tissue plasminogen activator (tPA). Also called *clot-busting drug.*

thyroxine Thyroid hormone T4, tetraiodothyronine.

topical Medication applied to the skin to obtain a local effect. Examples are ointments, creams, gels, lotions, patches, and sprays.

toxin Poisonous substance formed by a living cell or organism. Examples are venom from bee stings, snake bites, and jellyfish stings.

triamcinolone Synthetic corticosteroid.

V

vaccine Agent used to generate immunity and composed of the antigenic components of a killed or attenuated microorganism or its inactivated toxins. See *immunization.*

vasopressin Synthetic hormone causing contraction of smooth muscle.

vitamin Essential organic substance necessary in small amounts for normal cell function.

W

warfarin Anticoagulant; also used as rat poison. Trade name: *Coumadin.*

A

abdomen (**AB**-doh-men) Part of the trunk between the thorax and the pelvis.

abdominal (ab-**DOM**-in-al) Pertaining to the abdomen.

abdominopelvic (ab-**DOM**-ih-no-**PEL**-vik) Pertaining to the abdomen and pelvis.

abdominoplasty (ab-**DOM**-ih-noh-plas-tee) Surgical removal of excess subcutaneous fat from the abdominal wall (tummy tuck).

abduction (ab-**DUCK**-shun) Action of moving away from the midline.

abductor (ab-**DUCK**-tor) Muscle that moves a body part away from the midline.

ablation (ab-**LAY**-shun) Removal of tissue to destroy its function.

abortion (ah-**BOR**-shun) Spontaneous or induced expulsion of the fetus from the uterus at 20 weeks or less.

abrasion (ah-**BRAY**-zhun) Area of skin or mucous membrane that has been scraped off.

abruptio (ab-**RUP**-she-oh) Placenta abruptio is the premature detachment of the placenta.

absorb (ab-**SORB**) To take in.

absorption (ab-**SORP**-shun) Uptake of nutrients and water by cells in the GI tract.

accessory (ak-**SESS**-oh-ree) A muscle or nerve that is auxiliary to a more major structure.

accommodate (ah-**KOM**-oh-date) To adapt to meet a need.

accommodation (ah-kom-oh-**DAY**-shun) The act of adjusting something to make it fit the needs; for example, the lens of the eye adjusts itself.

accommodative (ah-kom-oh-**DAY**-tiv) Pertaining to accommodation.

acetabulum (ass-eh-**TAB**-you-lum) The cup-shaped cavity of the hip bone that receives the head of the femur to form the hip joint.

acetaminophen (ah-seat-ah-**MIN**-oh-fen) Medication that is an analgesic and an antipyretic.

acetone (**ASS**-eh-tone) Ketone that is found in blood, urine, and breath when diabetes mellitus is out of control.

Achilles tendon (ah-**KILL**-eeze) A tendon formed from gastrocnemius and soleus muscles and inserted into the calcaneus bone. Also called *calcaneal tendon.*

achondroplasia (a-kon-droh-**PLAY**-zee-ah) Condition with abnormal conversion of cartilage into bone, leading to dwarfism.

acne (**AK**-nee) Inflammatory disease of sebaceous glands and hair follicles.

acoustic (ah-**KYU**-stik) Pertaining to hearing.

acquired immunodeficiency syndrome (AIDS) (ah-**KWIRED IM**-you-noh-dee-**FISH**-en-see **SIN**-drohm) Infection with the HIV.

acromegaly (ak-roe-**MEG**-ah-lee) Enlargement of the head, face, hands, and feet due to excess growth hormone in an adult.

acromioclavicular (AC) (ah-**CROW**-mee-oh-klah-**VICK**-you-lar) The joint between the acromion and the clavicle.

acromion (ah-**CROW**-mee-on) Lateral end of the scapula, extending over the shoulder joint.

active (**AK**-tiv) Causing action or change.

activities of daily living (ADLs) (ak-**TIV**-ih-teez of **DAY**-lee **LIV**-ing) Daily routines for mobility, personal care, bathing, dressing, eating, and moving.

activity (ak-**TIV**-ih-tee) A goal-directed human action.

acute (ah-**KYUT**) Disease of sudden onset.

adapt (a-**DAPT**) To adjust to different conditions.

adaptation (ad-ap-**TAY**-shun) Change in the function or structure of an organ to meet new conditions.

addict (**ADD**-ikt) One who cannot live without a substance or practice.

addiction (ah-**DIK**-shun) Habitual psychologic and physiologic dependence on a substance or practice.

Addison disease (**ADD**-ih-son diz-**EEZ**) An autoimmune disease leading to decreased production of adrenocortical steroids.

adduction (ah-**DUCK**-shun) Action of moving toward the midline.

adductor (ah-**DUCK**-tor) Muscle that moves a body part toward the midline.

adenocarcinoma (**ADD**-eh-noh-kar-sih-**NOH**-mah) A cancer arising from glandular epithelial cells.

adenoid (**ADD**-eh-noyd) Single mass of lymphoid tissue in the midline at the back of the throat.

adenoidectomy (**ADD**-eh-noy-**DEK**-toh-me) Surgical removal of the adenoid tissue.

adipose (**ADD**-ih-pose) Containing fat.

adolescence (ad-oh-**LESS**-ence) Stage that begins with puberty and ends with physical maturity.

adolescent (ad-oh-**LESS**-ent) Pertaining to adolescence or a person in that stage.

adrenal gland (ah-**DREE**-nal GLAND) The suprarenal gland on the upper pole of each kidney.

adrenaline (ah-**DREN**-ah-lin) One of the catecholamines. Also called *epinephrine.*

adrenocortical (ah-**DREE**-noh-**KOR**-tih-kal) Pertaining to the cortex of the adrenal gland.

adrenocorticotropic (ah-**DREE**-noh-**KOR**-tih-koh-**TROH**-pik) Hormone of the anterior pituitary that stimulates the cortex of the adrenal gland to produce its own hormones.

afferent (**AFF**-eh-rent) Moving toward a center; for example, nerve fibers conducting impulses to the spinal cord and brain.

aged (**A**-jid) Having lived to an advanced age.

agenesis (a-**JEN**-eh-sis) Failure to develop any organ or any part.

agglutinate (ah-**GLUE**-tin-ate) Stick together to form clumps.

agglutination (ah-glue-tih-**NAY**-shun) Process by which cells or other particles adhere to each other to form clumps.

aging (**A**-jing) The process of human maturation and decline.

agranulocyte (a-**GRAN**-you-loh-site) A white blood cell without any granules in its cytoplasm.

aldosterone (al-**DOS**-ter-own) Mineralocorticoid hormone of the adrenal cortex.

alignment (a-**LINE**-ment) Having a structure in its correct position relative to other structures.

alimentary (al-ih-**MEN**-tar-ee) Pertaining to the digestive tract.

alimentary canal (al-ih-**MEN**-tar-ee kah-**NAL**) Digestive tract.

allergen (**AL**-er-jen) Substance producing a hypersensitivity (allergic) reaction.

allergenic (al-er-**JEN**-ik) Pertaining to the capacity to produce an allergic reaction.

allergic (ah-**LER**-jik) Pertaining to or suffering from an allergy.

allergy (**AL**-er-jee) Hypersensitivity to an allergen.

allograft **(AL-oh-graft)** Skin graft from another person or a cadaver. Also called *homograft*.

alloimmune (**AL**-oh-im-**YUNE**) Immune reaction directed against foreign tissue.

alopecia (al-oh-**PEE**-shah) Partial or complete loss of hair, naturally or from medication.

alveolus (al-**VEE**-oh-lus) Terminal element of the respiratory tract where gas exchange occurs. Plural *alveoli.*

Alzheimer disease (**AWLZ**-high-mer diz-**EEZ**) Common form of dementia.

amblyopia (am-blee-**OH**-pee-ah) Failure or incomplete development of the pathways of vision to the brain.

ambulatory (**AM**-byu-**LAY**-tor-ee) Surgery or any other care provided without an overnight stay in a medical facility.

amenorrhea (a-men-oh-**REE**-ah) Absence or abnormal cessation of menstrual flow.

amino acid (ah-**ME**-no **ASS**-id) The basic building block for protein.

ammonia (ah-**MOAN**-ih-ah) Toxic breakdown product of amino acids (proteins).

amniocentesis (**AM**-nee-oh-sen-**TEE**-sis) Removal of amniotic fluid for diagnostic purposes.

amnion (**AM**-nee-on) Membrane around the fetus that contains amniotic fluid.

amniotic (am-nee-**OT**-ik) Pertaining to the amnion.

ampulla (am-**PULL**-ah) Dilated portion of a canal or duct.

amputation (am-pyu-**TAY**-shun) Process of removing a limb, a part of a limb, a breast, or some other projecting part. Verb *amputate.*

amputee (**AM**-pyu-tee) A person with an amputation.

amylase (**AM**-il-ase) One of a group of enzymes that breaks down starch.

amyotrophic (a-my-oh-**TROH**-fik) Pertaining to muscular atrophy.

anabolism (an-**AB**-oh-lizm) The buildup of complex substances in the cell from simpler ones as a part of metabolism.

anal (**A**-nal) Pertaining to the anus.

analgesia (an-al-**JEE**-zee-ah) State in which pain is reduced.

analgesic (an-al-**JEE**-zic) Substance that produces analgesia.

anaphylactic (**AN**-ah-fih-**LAK**-tik) Pertaining to anaphylaxis.

anaphylaxis (**AN**-ah-fih-**LAK**-sis) Immediate severe allergic response.

anastomosis (ah-**NAS**-toh-**MOH**-sis) A surgically made union between two tubular structures. Plural *anastomoses.*

androgen (**AN**-droh-jen) Hormone that promotes masculine characteristics.

anemia (ah-**NEE**-me-ah) Decreased number of red blood cells.

anemic (ah-**NEE**-mik) Pertaining to or suffering from anemia.

anencephaly (**AN**-en-**SEF**-ah-lee) Born without cerebral hemispheres.

anesthesia (an-es-**THEE**-zee-ah) Complete loss of sensation.

anesthesiologist (**AN**-es-thee-zee-**OL**-oh-jist) Medical specialist in anesthesia.

anesthesiology (**AN**-es-thee-zee-**OL**-oh-jee) Medical specialty related to anesthesia.

anesthetic (an-es-**THET**-ik) Agent that causes absence of feeling or sensation.

aneurysm (**AN**-yur-izm) Circumscribed dilation of an artery or cardiac chamber.

angiogram (**AN**-jee-oh-gram) Radiograph obtained after injection of radiopaque contrast material into blood vessels.

angiography (an-jee-**OG**-rah-fee) Radiography of vessels after injection of contrast material.

angioplasty (**AN**-jee-oh-**PLAS**-tee) Recanalization of a blood vessel by surgery.

anomaly (ah-**NOM**-ah-lee) Structural abnormality present at birth.

anorectal junction (**A**-no-**RECK**-tal **JUNK**-shun) Junction between the anus and the rectum.

anorexia (an-oh-**RECK**-see-ah) Without an appetite; *or* having an aversion to food.

anoxia (an-**OCK**-see-ah) Without oxygen.

anoxic (an-**OCK**-sik) Pertaining to or suffering from a lack of oxygen.

antacid (ant-**ASS**-id) Agent that neutralizes the acidity of stomach contents.

antagonist (an-**TAG**-oh-nist) An opposing structure, agent, disease, or process.

antagonistic (an-**TAG**-oh-nist-ik) Having an opposite function.

antecubital (an-teh-**KYU**-bit-al) In front of the elbow.

anterior (an-**TEER**-ee-or) Front surface of body; situated in front.

anteversion (an-teh-**VER**-zhun) Forward displacement or tilting of a structure.

anthracosis (an-thra-**KOH**-sis) Lung disease caused by the inhalation of coal dust.

anthrax (**AN**-thraks) A severe, malignant infectious disease.

antibiotic (**AN**-tih-bye-**OT**-ik) A substance that has the capacity to inhibit growth of and destroy bacteria and other microorganisms.

antibody (**AN**-tee-body) Protein produced in response to an antigen. Plural *antibodies.*

anticoagulant (**AN**-tee-koh-**AG**-you-lant) Substance that prevents clotting.

antidiuretic (**AN**-tih-die-you-**RET**-ik) An agent that decreases urine production.

antidiuretic hormone (ADH) (**AN**-tih-die-you-**RET**-ik **HOR**-mohn) Posterior pituitary hormone that decreases urine output by acting on the kidney. Also called *vasopressin.*

antiepileptic (**AN**-tih-epi-**LEP**-tik) A pharmacologic agent capable of preventing or arresting epilepsy.

antigen (**AN**-tee-jen) Substance capable of triggering an immune response.

antihistamine (**AN**-tih-**HISS**-tah-mean) Drug used to treat allergic symptoms because of its action antagonistic to histamine.

antimicrobial (**AN**-tee-my-**KROH**-bee-al) Agent to destroy or prevent multiplication of organisms.

antineoplastic (**AN**-tee-nee-oh-**PLAS**-tik) Pertaining to the prevention of the growth and spread of cancer cells.

antipruritic (AN-tee-pru-**RIT**-ik) Medication against itching.

antipyretic (**AN**-tee-pie-**RET**-ik) Agent that reduces fever.

antisepsis (an-tee-**SEP**-sis) Inhibiting the growth of infectious agents.

antiseptic (an-tee-**SEP**-tik) An agent or substance capable of affecting antisepsis.

antiserum (an-tee-**SEER**-um) Serum taken from another human or animal that has antibodies to a disease. Also called *immune serum.*

antisocial personality disorder (**AN**-tee-**SOH**-shall per-son-**AL**-ih-tee dis-**OR**-der) Chronic violation of the rights of others.

antrum (**AN**-trum) A closed cavity.

anuria (an-**YOU**-ree-ah) Absence of urine production.

anus (**A**-nus) Terminal opening of the digestive tract through which feces are discharged.

anxiety (ang-**ZI**-eh-tee) Distress and dread caused by fear.

aorta (a-**OR**-tuh) Main trunk of the systemic arterial system.

aortic (a-**OR**-tik) Pertaining to the aorta.

apex (**A**-peks) Tip or end; for example, of the cone-shaped heart.

Apgar score (**AP**-gar SKOR) Evaluation of a newborn's status.

aphthous (**AF**-thus) Painful small oral ulcers (canker sores).

apnea (**AP**-nee-ah) Absence of spontaneous respiration.

apoptosis (**AP**-op-**TOE**-sis) Programmed normal cell death.

appendicitis (ah-pen-dih-**SIGH**-tis) Inflammation of the appendix.

appendicular (**AP**-en-**DICK**-you-lar) Relating to the limbs, e.g., the appendicular skeleton.

appendix (ah-**PEN**-dicks) Small blind projection from the pouch of the cecum.

aqueous humor (**AK**-we-us **HEW**-mor) Watery liquid in the anterior and posterior chambers of the eye.

arachnoid mater (ah-**RACK**-noyd **MAY**-ter) Weblike middle layer of the three meninges.

areola (ah-**REE**-oh-luh) Circular reddish area surrounding the nipple.

areolar (ah-**REE**-oh-lar) Pertaining to the areola.

arrhythmia (a-**RITH**-me-ah) Condition when the heart rhythm is abnormal.

arteriography (ar-teer-ee-**OG**-rah-fee) X-ray visualization of an artery after injection of contrast material.

arteriole (ar-**TIER**-ee-ole) Small terminal artery leading into the capillary network.

arteriosclerosis (ar-**TIER**-ee-oh-skler-**OH**-sis) Hardening of the arteries.

arteriosclerotic (ar-**TIER**-ee-oh-skler-**OT**-ik) Pertaining to or suffering from arteriosclerosis.

artery (**AR**-ter-ee) Thick-walled blood vessel carrying blood away from the heart.

arthritis (ar-**THRI**-tis) Inflammation of a joint or joints.

arthrocentesis (**AR**-throw-sen-**TEE**-sis) Withdrawal of fluid from a joint through a needle.

arthrodesis (ar-throw-**DEE**-sis) Fixation or stiffening of a joint by surgery.

arthrography (ar-**THROG**-rah-fee) X-ray of a joint taken after the injection of a contrast medium into the joint.

arthroplasty (**AR**-throw-plas-tee) Surgery to restore, as far as possible, the function of a joint.

arthroscope (**AR**-thro-skope) Endoscope used to examine the interior of a joint.

arthroscopy (ar-**THROS**-koh-pee) Visual examination of the interior of a joint.

articulate (ar-**TIK**-you-late) Two separate bones have formed a joint.

articulation (ar-tik-you-**LAY**-shun) A joint.

asbestosis (as-bes-**TOE**-sis) Lung disease caused by the inhalation of asbestos particles.

ascites (ah-**SIGH**-teez) Accumulation of fluid in the abdominal cavity.

asepsis (a-**SEP**-sis) Absence of living pathogenic organisms.

Asperger syndrome (**AHS**-per-ger **SIN**-drohm) Developmental disorder of children.

aspiration (**AS**-pih-**RAY**-shun) Removal by suction of fluid or gas from a body cavity. Verb *aspirate.*

asthma (**AZ**-mah) Episodes of breathing difficulty due to narrowed or obstructed airways.

asthmatic (az-**MAT**-ik) Suffering from or pertaining to asthma.

astigmatism (ah-**STIG**-maht-izm) Inability to focus light rays that enter the eye in different planes.

asymptomatic (**A**-simp-toe-**MAT**-ik) Without any symptoms experienced by the patient.

asystole (a-**SIS**-toe-lee) Absence of contractions of the heart.

ataxia (a-**TAK**-see-ah) Inability to coordinate muscle activity, leading to jerky movements.

ataxic (a-**TAK**-sik) Pertaining to or suffering from ataxia.

atelectasis (at-el-**ECK**-tah-sis) Collapse of part of a lung.

atherectomy (ath-er-**EK**-toe-me) Surgical removal of atheroma.

atheroma (ath-er-**ROE**-mah) Lipid deposit in the lining of an artery.

atherosclerosis (**ATH**-er-oh-skler-**OH**-sis) Atheroma in arteries.

athetoid (**ATH**-eh-toyd) Resembling or suffering from athetosis.

athetosis (ath-eh-**TOE**-sis) Slow, writhing involuntary movements.

atonic (a-**TOHN**-ik) Without normal muscular tone.

atopic (a-**TOP**-ik) Pertaining to an allergy.

atopy (**AT**-oh-pee) State of hypersensitivity to an allergen—allergic.

atresia (a-**TREE**-zee-ah) Congenital absence of a normal opening or lumen.

atrial (**A**-tree-al) Pertaining to the atrium.

atrioventricular (AV) (**A**-tree-oh-ven-**TRICK**-you-lar) Pertaining to both the atrium and the ventricle.

atrium (**A**-tree-um) Chamber where blood enters the heart on both right and left sides. Plural *atria.*

atrophy (**A**-troh-fee) Wasting or diminished volume of a tissue or organ.

atropine (**AT**-ro-peen) Pharmacologic agent used to dilate pupils.

attenuate (ah-**TEN**-you-ate) Weaken the ability of an organism to produce disease.

audiologist (aw-dee-**OL**-oh-jist) Specialist in evaluation of hearing function.

audiology (aw-dee-**OL**-oh-jee) Study of hearing disorders.

audiometer (aw-dee-**OM**-eh-ter) Instrument to measure hearing.

audiometric (**AW**-dee-oh-**MET**-rik) Pertaining to the measurement of hearing.

auditory (AW-dih-tor-ee) Pertaining to the sense or the organs of hearing.

aura (AWE-rah) Sensory experience preceding an epileptic seizure or a migraine headache.

auricle (AW-ri-kul) The shell-like external ear.

auscultation (aws-kul-TAY-shun) Diagnostic method of listening to body sounds with a stethoscope.

autism (AWE-tizm) Developmental disorder of children.

autistic (awe-TIS-tik) Pertaining to autism.

autoantibody (awe-toe-AN-tee-bod-ee) Antibody produced in response to an antigen from the host's own tissue.

autograft (AWE-toe-graft) A graft using tissue taken from the same individual who is receiving the graft.

autoimmune (awe-toe-im-YUNE) Immune reaction directed against a person's own tissue.

autologous (awe-TOL-oh-gus) Blood transfusion with the same person as donor and recipient.

autolysis (awe-TOL-ih-sis) Destruction of cells by enzymes within the cells.

autonomic (awe-toh-NOM-ik) Self-governing visceral motor division of the peripheral nervous system.

autopsy (AWE-top-see) Examination of the body and organs of a dead person to determine the cause of death.

avascular (a-VAS-cue-lar) Without a blood supply.

avulsion (a-VUL-shun) Forcible separation or tearing away, often of a tendon from bone.

axial (AK-see-al) Relating to the head and trunk, e.g., the axial skeleton.

axilla (AK-sill-ah) Medical name for the armpit. Plural *axillae.*

axillary (AK-sill-air-ee) Pertaining to the armpit.

axon (ACK-son) Single process of a nerve cell carrying nervous impulses away from the cell body.

azoospermia (a-zoh-oh-SPER-me-ah) Absence of living sperm in the semen.

azotemia (a-zo-TEE-me-ah) Excess nitrogenous waste products in the blood.

B

bacterial (bak-TEER-ee-al) Pertaining to bacteria.

bacterium (bak-TEER-ee-um) A unicellular (single-cell), simple, microscopic organism. Plural *bacteria.*

balanitis (bal-ah-NIE-tis) Inflammation of the glans and prepuce of the penis.

bariatric (bar-ee-AT-rik) Treatment of obesity.

basilar (BAS-ih-lar) Pertaining to the base of a structure.

basophil (BAY-so-fill) A basophil's granules attract basic blue stain in the laboratory.

Bell palsy (BELL PAWL-zee) Paresis, or paralysis, of one side of the face.

biceps brachii (BYE-sepz BRAY-key-eye) A muscle of the arm that has two heads or points of origin on the scapula.

bicuspid (by-KUSS-pid) Having two points. A bicuspid heart valve has two flaps; a bicuspid (premolar) tooth has two points.

bifid (BI-fid) Separated into two parts.

bilateral (by-LAT-er-al) On two sides; for example, in both ears.

bile (BILE) Fluid secreted by the liver into the duodenum.

bile acids (BILE AH-sids) Steroids synthesized from cholesterol.

biliary (BILL-ee-air-ree) Pertaining to bile or the biliary tract.

bilirubin (bill-ee-RU-bin) Bile pigment formed in the liver from hemoglobin.

binge eating (BINJ EE-ting) Eating with periods of excessive intake.

biopsy (BI-op-see) Removing tissue from a living person for laboratory examination.

bipolar disorder (bi-POH-lar dis-OR-der) A mood disorder with alternating episodes of depression and mania.

bladder (BLAD-er) Hollow sac that holds fluid, for example, urine or bile.

blastocyst (BLAS-toe-sist) First 2 weeks of the developing embryo.

blepharitis (blef-ah-RYE-tis) Inflammation of the eyelid.

blepharoplasty (BLEF-ah-roh-PLAS-tee) Surgical repair of the eyelid.

blepharoptosis (BLEF-ah-ROP-toe-sis) Drooping of the upper eyelid.

blood-brain barrier (BBB) (BLUD BRAYN BAIR-ee-er) A selective mechanism that protects the brain from toxins and infections.

bolus (BOH-lus) Single mass of a substance.

botulism (BOT-you-lizm) Food poisoning caused by the neurotoxin produced by *Clostridium botulinum.*

bovine spongiform encephalopathy (BO-vine SPON-jee-form en-sef-ah-LOP-ah-thee) Disease of cattle that can be transmitted to humans, causing Creutzfeldt-Jakob disease. Also called *mad cow disease.*

bowel (BOUGH-el) Another name for *intestine.*

brace (BRACE) Appliance to support a part of the body in its correct position.

brachial (BRAY-kee-al) Pertaining to the arm.

brachialis (BRAY-kee-al-is) Muscle that lies underneath the biceps and is the strongest flexor of the forearm.

brachioradialis (BRAY-kee-oh-RAY-dee-al-is) Muscle that helps flex the forearm.

brachytherapy (brah-kee-THAIR-ah pee) Radiation therapy in which the source of radiation is implanted in the tissue to be treated.

bradycardia (brad-ee-KAR-dee-ah) Slow heart rate (below 60 beats per minute).

bradypnea (brad-ip-NEE-ah) Slow breathing.

brainstem (BRAYN-stem) Comprises the thalamus, pineal gland, pons, fourth ventricle, and medulla oblongata.

breech (BREECH) Buttocks-first presentation of the fetus at delivery.

broad-spectrum (broad-SPECK-trum) An antibiotic with a wide range of activity against a variety of organisms.

bronchiectasis (brong-key-ECK-tah-sis) Chronic dilation of the bronchi following inflammatory disease and obstruction.

bronchiole (BRONG-key-ole) Increasingly smaller subdivisions of bronchi.

bronchiolitis (brong-key-oh-LYE-tis) Inflammation of the small bronchioles.

bronchitis (bron-KI-tis) Inflammation of the bronchi.

bronchoconstriction (**BRONG**-koh-kon-**STRIK**-shun) Reduction in the diameter of a bronchus.

bronchodilator (**BRONG**-koh-die-**LAY**-tor) Agent that increases the diameter of a bronchus.

bronchogenic (**BRONG**-koh-**JEN**-ik) Arising from a bronchus.

bronchopneumonia (**BRONG**-koh-new-**MOH**-nee-ah) Acute inflammation of the walls of smaller bronchioles with spread to lung parenchyma.

bronchoscope (**BRONG**-koh-skope) Endoscope used for bronchoscopy.

bronchoscopy (brong-**KOS**-koh-pee) Examination of the interior of the tracheobronchial tree with an endoscope.

bronchus (**BRONG**-kuss) One of two subdivisions of the trachea. Plural *bronchi.*

bulbourethral (**BUL**-boh-you-**REE**-thral) Pertaining to the bulbous penis and urethra.

bulimia (buh-**LEEM**-ee-ah) Episodic bouts of excessive eating with compensatory throwing up.

bulla (**BULL**-ah) Bubble-like dilated structure. Plural *bullae.*

bundle of His (**BUN**-del of HISS) Pathway for electrical signals to be transmitted to the ventricles. Also called *atrioventricular (AV) bundle.*

bunion (**BUN**-yun) A swelling at the base of the big toe.

bursa (**BURR**-sah) A closed sac containing synovial fluid. Plural *bursae.*

bursitis (burr-**SIGH**-tis) Inflammation of a bursa.

C

cadaver (kah-**DAV**-er) A dead body or corpse.

calcaneal (kal-**KAY**-knee-al) Pertaining to the calcaneus.

calcaneus (kal-**KAY**-knee-us) Bone of the tarsus that forms the heel.

calcitonin (kal-sih-**TONE**-in) Thyroid hormone that moves calcium from blood to bones.

calculus (**KAL**-kyu-lus) Small stone. Plural *calculi.*

callus (**KAL**-us) Bony tissue that forms at a fracture site early in healing.

calyx (**KAY**-licks) Funnel-shaped structure. Plural *calyces.*

cancellous (**KAN**-seh-lus) Bone that has a spongy or lattice-like structure.

cancer (**KAN**-ser) General term for a malignant neoplasm.

Candida (**KAN**-did-ah) A yeastlike fungus.

Candida albicans (**KAN**-did-ah **AL**-bih-kanz) The most common form of *Candida.*

candidiasis (can-dih-**DIE**-ah-sis) Infection with the yeastlike fungus *Candida.* Also called *thrush.*

canker (**KANG**-ker) Nonmedical term for an aphthous ulcer. Also called *mouth ulcer.*

cannula (**KAN**-you-lah) Tube inserted into a blood vessel or cavity as a channel for fluid.

capillary (**KAP**-ih-lair-ee) Minute blood vessel between the arterial and venous systems.

capsular (**KAP**-syu-lar) Pertaining to a capsule.

capsule (**KAP**-syul) Fibrous tissue layer surrounding a joint or other structure.

carbohydrate (kar-boh-**HIGH**-drate) Group of organic food compounds that includes sugars, starch, glycogen, and cellulose.

carbuncle (**KAR**-bunk-ul) Infection of many furuncles in a small area, often on the back of the neck.

carcinogen (kar-**SIN**-oh-jen) Cancer-producing agent.

carcinogenesis (kar-**SIN**-oh-**JEN**-eh-sis) Origin and development of cancer.

carcinoma (kar-sih-**NOH**-mah) A malignant and invasive epithelial tumor.

carcinoma in situ (kar-sih-**NOH**-mah in **SIGH**-too) Carcinoma that has not invaded surrounding tissues.

cardiac (**KAR**-dee-ak) Pertaining to the heart.

cardiogenic (**KAR**-dee-oh-**JEN**-ik) Of cardiac origin.

cardiologist (**KAR**-dee-**OL**-oh-jist) A medical specialist in the diagnosis and treatment of disorders of the heart (cardiology).

cardiology (**KAR**-dee-**OL**-oh-jee) Medical specialty of diseases of the heart.

cardiomegaly (**KAR**-dee-oh-**MEG**-ah-lee) Enlargement of the heart.

cardiomyopathy (**KAR**-dee-oh-my-**OP**-ah-thee) Disease of the heart muscle, the myocardium.

cardiopulmonary resuscitation (**KAR**-dee-oh-**PUL**-moh-nary ree-sus-ih-**TAY**-shun) The attempt to restore cardiac and pulmonary function.

cardiovascular (**KAR**-dee-oh-**VAS**-kyu-lar) Pertaining to the heart and blood vessels.

cardioversion (**KAR**-dee-oh-**VER**-zhun) Restoration of a normal heart rhythm by electric shock. Also called *defibrillation.*

caries (**KARE**-eez) Bacterial destruction of teeth.

carotid (kah-**ROT**-id) Main artery of the neck.

carotid endarterectomy (kah-**ROT**-id **END**-ar-ter-**EK**-toe-me) Surgical removal of diseased lining from the carotid artery to leave a smooth lining and restore blood flow.

carpal (**KAR**-pal) Pertaining to the wrist.

carpus (**KAR**-pus) Collective term for the eight carpal bones of the wrist.

cartilage (**KAR**-tih-lage) Nonvascular, firm connective tissue found mostly in joints.

catabolism (kah-**TAB**-oh-lizm) Breakdown of complex substances into simpler ones as a part of metabolism.

cataplexy (**KAT**-ah-plek-see) Sudden loss of muscle tone with brief paralysis.

cataract (**KAT**-ah-ract) Complete or partial opacity of the lens.

catecholamine (kat-eh-**COAL**-ah-meen) Major element in the stress response; includes epinephrine and norepinephrine.

catheter (**KATH**-eh-ter) Hollow tube to allow passage of fluid into or out of a body cavity, organ, or vessel.

catheterization (**KATH**-eh-ter-ih-**ZAY**-shun) Introduction of a catheter.

catheterize (**KATH**-eh-teh-**RIZE**) To introduce a catheter.

caudal (**KAW**-dal) Pertaining to or nearer to the tailbone.

cautery (**KAW**-ter-ee) Agent or device used to burn or scar a tissue.

cavernosa (kav-er-**NOH**-sah) Resembling a cave.

cavity (**KAV**-ih-tee) Hollow space or body compartment. Plural *cavities.*

cecal (**SEE**-kal) Pertaining to the cecum.

cecum (**SEE**-kum) Blind pouch that is the first part of the large intestine.

celiac (**SEE**-lee-ack) Relating to the abdominal cavity.

celiac disease (**SEE**-lee-ak diz-**EEZ**) Disease caused by sensitivity to gluten.

cell (SELL) The smallest unit of the body capable of independent existence.

cellular (SELL-you-lar) Pertaining to a cell.

cellulitis (SELL-you-LIE-tis) Infection of subcutaneous connective tissue.

cephalic (seh-FAL-ik) Pertaining to or nearer to the head.

cerebellum (ser-eh-BELL-um) The most posterior area of the brain, located between the midbrain and the cerebral hemispheres.

cerebral (SER-ee-bral) Pertaining to the cerebral hemispheres or the brain.

cerebrospinal (SER-ee-broh-SPY-nal) Pertaining to the brain and spinal cord.

cerebrospinal fluid (CSF) (SER-ee-broh-SPY-nal FLU-id) Fluid formed in the ventricles of the brain that surrounds the brain and spinal cord.

cerebrum (SER-ee-brum) Cerebral hemispheres.

cerumen (seh-ROO-men) Waxy secretion of the ceruminous glands of the external ear.

ceruminous (seh-ROO-mih-nus) Pertaining to cerumen.

cervical (SER-vih-kal) Pertaining to the cervix or to the neck region.

cervix (SER-viks) The lower part of the uterus.

cesarean section (seh-ZAH-ree-an SEK-shun) Extraction of the fetus through an incision in the abdomen and uterine wall. Also called *C-section.*

chancre (SHAN-ker) Primary lesion of syphilis.

chemotherapy (KEY-moh-THAIR-ah-pee) Treatment using chemical agents.

chiasm (KYE-asm) X-shaped crossing of the two optic nerves at the base of the brain. Alternative term *chiasma.*

chickenpox (CHICK-en-pocks) Acute, contagious viral disease. Also called *varicella.*

chiropractic (kye-roh-PRAK-tik) Diagnosis, treatment, and prevention of mechanical disorders of the musculoskeletal system.

chiropractor (kye-roh-PRAK-tor) Practitioner of chiropractic.

chlamydia (klah-MID-ee-ah) An STD caused by an infection with *Chlamydia,* a species of bacteria.

cholangiography (KOH-lan-jee-OG-rah-fee) Use of a contrast medium to radiographically visualize the bile ducts.

cholecystectomy (KOH-leh-sis-TECK-toe-me) Surgical removal of the gallbladder.

cholecystitis (KOH-leh-sis-TIE-tis) Inflammation of the gallbladder.

choledocholithiasis (KOH-leh-DOH-koh-li-THIGH-ah-sis) Presence of a gallstone in the common bile duct.

cholelithiasis (KOH-leh-lih-THIGH-ah-sis) Condition of having bile stones (gallstones).

cholelithotomy (KOH-leh-lih-THOT-oh-me) Surgical removal of a gallstone(s).

cholesteatoma (KOH-less-tee-ah-TOE-mah) Yellow, waxy tumor arising in the middle ear.

cholesterol (koh-LESS-ter-ol) Formed in liver cells; is the most abundant steroid in tissues and circulates in the plasma attached to proteins of different densities.

chorea (kor-EE-ah) Involuntary, irregular spasms of limb and facial muscles.

choreic (kor-EE-ik) Pertaining to or suffering from chorea.

chorion (KOH-ree-on) The fetal membrane that forms the placenta.

chorionic (koh-ree-ON-ik) Pertaining to the chorion.

chorionic villus (koh-ree-ON-ik VILL-us) Vascular process of the embryonic chorion to form the placenta.

choroid (KOR-oid) Region of the retina and uvea.

chromosome (KROH-moh-sohm) Body in the nucleus that contains DNA and genes.

chronic (KRON-ik) A persistent, long-term disease.

chyle (KYLE) A milky fluid that results from the digestion and absorption of fats in the small intestine.

chyme (KYME) Semifluid, partially digested food passed from the stomach into the duodenum.

cilium (SILL-ee-um) Hairlike motile projection from the surface of a cell. Plural *cilia.*

circulation (SER-kyu-LAY-shun) Continuous movement of blood through the heart and blood vessels.

circumcision (ser-kum-SIZH-un) To remove part or all of the prepuce.

circumduct (ser-kum-DUCKT) To move an extremity in a circular motion.

circumduction (ser-kum-DUCK-shun) Movement of an extremity in a circular motion.

cirrhosis (sir-ROE-sis) Extensive fibrotic liver disease.

claudication (klaw-dih-KAY-shun) Intermittent leg pain and limping.

clavicle (KLAV-ih-kul) Curved bone that forms the anterior part of the pectoral girdle.

clavicular (klah-VICK-you-lar) Pertaining to the clavicle.

cleft lip (KLEFT LIP) Congenital defect of the upper lip.

cleft palate (KLEFT PAL-ate) Congenital defect of the palate.

clitoris (KLIT-oh-ris) Erectile organ of the vulva.

clonic (KLON-ik) State of rapid successions of muscular contractions and relaxations.

closed fracture (KLOSD FRAK-chur) A bone is broken but the skin over it is intact.

Clostridium botulinum (klos-TRID-ee-um bot-you-LIE-num) Bacterium that causes food poisoning.

clot (KLOT) The mass of fibrin and cells that is produced in a wound.

coagulant (koh-AG-you-lant) Substance that causes clotting.

coagulate (koh-AG-you-late) Form a clot.

coagulation (koh-ag-you-LAY-shun) The process of blood clotting.

coagulopathy (koh-ag-you-LOP-ah-thee) Disorder of blood clotting. Plural *coagulopathies.*

coarctation (koh-ark-TAY-shun) Constriction, stenosis, particularly of the aorta.

coccyx (KOK-sicks) Small tailbone at the lower end of the vertebral column.

cochlea (KOK-lee-ah) An intricate combination of passages; used to describe the inner ear.

cochlear (KOK-lee-ar) Pertaining to the cochlea.

cognition (kog-NIH-shun) Process of acquiring knowledge through thinking, learning, and memory.

cognitive-behavioral therapy (CBT) (KOG-nih-tiv be-HAYV-yur-al THAIR-ah-pee) Psychotherapy that emphasizes thoughts and attitudes in one's behavior.

coitus (**KOH**-it-us) Sexual intercourse.

colic (**KOL**-ik) Spasmodic, crampy pains in the abdomen.

colitis (koh-**LIE**-tis) Inflammation of the colon.

collagen (**KOLL**-ah-jen) Major protein of connective tissue, cartilage, and bone.

collateral (koh-**LAT**-er-al) Situated at the side, often to bypass an obstruction.

Colles fracture (**KOL**-ez **FRAK**-chur) Fracture of the distal radius at the wrist.

colloid (**COLL**-oyd) Liquid containing suspended particles.

colon (**KOH**-lon) The large intestine, extending from the cecum to the rectum.

colostomy (koh-**LOSS**-toe-me) Artificial opening from the colon to the outside of the body.

colostrum (koh-**LOSS**-trum) The first breast secretion at the end of pregnancy.

colpopexy (**KOL**-poh-peck-see) Surgical fixation of the vagina.

coma (**KOH**-mah) State of deep unconsciousness.

comatose (**KOH**-mah-toes) In a state of coma.

comedo (**KOM**-ee-doh) A whitehead or blackhead caused by too much sebum and too many keratin cells blocking the hair follicle. Plural *comedones.*

comminuted fracture (**KOM**-ih-nyu-ted **FRAK**-chur) A fracture in which the bone is broken into small pieces.

competent (**KOM**-peh-tent) Capable of performing a task or function.

complement (**KOM**-pleh-ment) Group of proteins in the serum that finish off the work of antibodies to destroy bacteria and other cells.

complete fracture (kom-**PLEET FRAK**-chur) A bone is fractured into two separate pieces.

compliance (kom-**PLY**-ance) Measure of the capacity of a chamber or hollow viscus (e.g., the lungs) to expand; *or* consistency and accuracy with which a patient follows a treatment regimen.

compression (kom-**PRESH**-un) Squeeze together to increase density and/or decrease a dimension of a structure.

compression fracture (kom-**PRESH**-un **FRAK**-chur) Fracture of a vertebra causing loss of height of the vertebra.

compulsion (kom-**PUL**-shun) Uncontrollable impulses to perform an act repetitively.

compulsive (kom-**PUL**-siv) Possessing uncontrollable impulses to perform an act repetitively.

conception (kon-**SEP**-shun) Fertilization of the egg by sperm to form a zygote.

concha (**KON**-kah) Shell-shaped bone on the medial wall of the nasal cavity. Plural *conchae.*

concussion (kon-**KUSH**-un) Mild brain injury.

condom (**KON**-dom) A sheath or cover for the penis or vagina to prevent conception and infection.

conductive hearing loss (kon-**DUK**-tiv) Hearing loss caused by lesions in the outer ear or middle ear.

condyle (**KON**-dile) Large, smooth, rounded expansion of the end of a bone where it forms a joint with another bone.

confusion (kon-**FEW**-zhun) Mental state in which environmental stimuli are not processed appropriately.

congenital (kon-**JEN**-ih-tal) Present at birth, either inherited or due to an event during gestation up to the moment of birth.

conization (koh-ni-**ZAY**-shun) Surgical excision of a cone-shaped piece of tissue.

conjunctiva (kon-junk-**TIE**-vah) Inner lining of the eyelids.

conjunctival (kon-junk-**TIE**-val) Pertaining to the conjunctiva.

conjunctivitis (kon-junk-tih-**VI**-tis) Inflammation of the conjunctiva.

connective tissue (koh-**NECK**-tiv **TISH**-you) The supporting tissue of the body.

consciousness (**KON**-shus-ness) The state of being aware of and responsive to the environment.

constipation (kon-stih-**PAY**-shun) Hard, infrequent bowel movements.

constrict (kon-**STRIKT**) To become or make narrow.

constriction (kon-**STRIK**-shun) A narrowed portion of a structure.

contagious (kon-**TAY**-jus) Infection can be transmitted from person to person or from a person to a surface to a person.

contaminate (kon-**TAM**-in-ate) To cause the presence of an infectious agent to be on any surface or in any substance.

contamination (**KON**-tam-ih-**NAY**-shun) Presence of an infectious agent on a surface or in substances.

contraception (kon-trah-**SEP**-shun) Prevention of pregnancy.

contraceptive (kon-trah-**SEP**-tiv) An agent that prevents conception.

contract (kon-**TRAKT**) Draw together or shorten.

contracture (kon-**TRAK**-chur) Muscle shortening due to spasm or fibrosis.

contrecoup (**KON**-treh-koo) Injury to the brain at a point directly opposite the point of original contact.

contusion (kon-**TOO**-zhun) Hemorrhage into a tissue (bruising), including the brain.

convulsion (kon-**VUL**-shun) Alternative name for seizure.

cor pulmonale (**KOR** pul-moh-**NAH**-lee) Right-sided heart failure arising from chronic lung disease.

cornea (**KOR**-nee-ah) The central, transparent part of the outer coat of the eye covering the iris and pupil.

corneal (**KOR**-nee-al) Pertaining to the cornea.

coronal (**KOR**-oh-nal) Pertaining to the vertical plane dividing the body into anterior and posterior portions.

coronal plane (**KOR**-oh-nal PLAIN) Vertical plane dividing the body into anterior and posterior portions.

coronary circulation (**KOR**-oh-nair-ee **SER**-kyu-**LAY**-shun) Blood vessels supplying the heart.

corpus (**KOR**-pus) Major part of a structure. Plural *corpora.*

corpus albicans (**KOR**-pus **AL**-bih-kanz) An atrophied corpus luteum.

corpus callosum (**KOR**-pus kah-**LOW**-sum) Bridge of nerve fibers connecting the two cerebral hemispheres.

corpus luteum (**KOR**-pus **LOO**-teh-um) Yellow structure formed at the site of a ruptured ovarian follicle.

corpuscle (**KOR**-pus-ul) A blood cell.

cortex (**KOR**-teks) Outer portion of an organ, such as bone; gray covering of cerebral hemispheres. Plural *cortices.*

cortical (**KOR**-tih-cal) Pertaining to a cortex.

corticosteroid (**KOR**-tih-koh-**STAIR**-oyd) A hormone produced by the adrenal cortex.

corticotropin (**KOR**-tih-koh-TROH-pin) Pituitary hormone that stimulates the cortex of the adrenal gland to secrete corticosteroids.

cortisol (**KOR**-tih-sol) One of the glucocorticoids produced by the adrenal cortex; has anti-inflammatory effects. Also called *hydrocortisone.*

coryza (koh-**RYE**-zah) Viral inflammation of the mucous membrane of the nose. Also called *acute rhinitis.*

coup (KOO) Injury to the brain occurring directly under the skull at the point of contact.

coxa (**COCK**-sah) Hipbone. Plural *coxae.*

cranial (**KRAY**-nee-al) Pertaining to the cranium.

craniofacial (**KRAY**-nee-oh-**FAY**-shal) Pertaining to both the face and the cranium.

cranium (**KRAY**-nee-um) The skull.

cretin (**KREH**-tin) A person with severe congenital hypothyroidism.

cretinism (**KREH**-tin-izm) Condition of severe congenital hypothyroidism.

Creutzfeldt-Jakob disease (**KROITS**-felt **YAK**-op diz-**EEZ**) Progressive incurable neurologic disease caused by infectious prions.

cricoid (**CRY**-koyd) Ring-shaped cartilage in the larynx.

crista ampullaris (**KRIS**-tah am-**PULL**-air-is) Mound of hair cells and gelatinous material in the ampulla of a semicircular canal.

Crohn disease (KRONE diz-**EEZ**) Narrowing and thickening of terminal small bowel. Also called *regional enteritis.*

croup (KROOP) Infection of the upper airways in children, characterized by a barking cough. Also called *laryngotracheobronchitis.*

cruciate (**KRU**-she-ate) Shaped like a cross.

cryosurgery (cry-oh-**SUR**-jer-ee) Use of liquid nitrogen or argon gas in a probe to freeze and kill abnormal tissue.

cryptorchism (krip-**TOR**-kizm) Failure of one or both testes to descend into the scrotum.

curettage (kyu-reh-**TAHJ**) Scraping the interior of a cavity.

curette (kyu-**RET**) Scoop-shaped instrument for scraping the interior of a cavity or removing new growths.

Cushing syndrome (**KUSH**-ing **SIN**-drohm) Hypersecretion of cortisol (hydrocortisone) by the adrenal cortex.

cutaneous (kyu-**TAY**-nee-us) Pertaining to the skin.

cuticle (**KEW**-tih-cul) Nonliving epidermis at the base of the fingernails and toenails.

cyanosis (sigh-ah-**NO**-sis) Blue discoloration of the skin, lips, and nail beds due to low levels of oxygen in the blood.

cyanotic (sigh-ah-**NOT**-ik) Pertaining to or marked by cyanosis.

cyst (SIST) An abnormal, fluid-containing sac.

cystic (**SIS**-tik) Relating to a cyst.

cystic fibrosis (CF) (**SIS**-tik fie-**BROH**-sis) Genetic disease in which excessive viscid mucus obstructs passages, including bronchi.

cystitis (sis-**TIE**-tis) Inflammation of the urinary bladder.

cystocele (**SIS**-toh-seal) Hernia of the bladder into the vagina.

cystoscope (**SIS**-toh-skope) An endoscope inserted to view the inside of the bladder.

cystoscopy (sis-**TOS**-koh-pee) Using a cystoscope to examine the inside of the urinary bladder.

cystourethrogram (sis-toh-you-**REETH**-roe-gram) X-ray image during voiding to show the structure and function of the bladder and urethra.

cytologist (**SIGH**-tol-oh-jist) Specialist in the structure, chemistry, and pathology of the cell.

cytology (**SIGH**-tol-oh-jee) Study of the cell.

cytoplasm (**SIGH**-toh-plazm) Clear, gelatinous substance that forms the substance of a cell except for the nucleus.

cytotoxic (sigh-toh-**TOX**-ik) Destructive to cells.

D

dandruff (**DAN**-druff) Scales in hair from shedding of the epidermis.

death (DETH) Total and permanent cessation of all vital functions.

debridement (day-**BREED**-mon) The removal of injured or necrotic tissue.

decongestant (dee-con-**JESS**-tant) Agent that reduces the swelling and fluid in the nose and sinuses.

decubitus ulcer (de-**KYU**-bit-us **UL**-ser) Sore caused by lying down for long periods of time.

defecation (def-eh-**KAY**-shun) Evacuation of feces from the rectum and anus.

defect (**DEE**-fect) An absence, malformation, or imperfection.

defective (dee-**FEK**-tiv) Imperfect.

defibrillation (de-fib-rih-**LAY**-shun) Restoration of uncontrolled twitching of cardiac muscle fibers to normal rhythm.

defibrillator (de-fib-rih-**LAY**-tor) Instrument for defibrillation.

deformity (de-**FOR**-mih-tee) A permanent structural deviation from the normal.

degenerative (dee-**JEN**-er-a-tiv) Relating to the deterioration of a structure.

deglutition (dee-glue-**TISH**-un) The act of swallowing.

dehydration (dee-high-**DRAY**-shun) Process of losing body water.

delirium (de-**LIR**-ee-um) Acute altered state of consciousness with agitation and disorientation; condition is reversible.

deltoid (**DEL**-toyd) Large, fan-shaped muscle connecting the scapula and clavicle to the humerus.

delusion (dee-**LOO**-zhun) Fixed, unyielding false belief held despite strong evidence to the contrary.

dementia (da-**MEN**-sha) Chronic, progressive, irreversible loss of intellectual and mental functions.

demyelination (dee-**MY**-eh-lin-**A**-shun) Process of losing the myelin sheath of a nerve fiber.

dendrite (**DEN**-dright) Branched extension of the nerve cell body that receives nervous stimuli.

dental (**DEN**-tal) Pertaining to the teeth.

dentine (**DEN**-tin) Dense, ivory-like substance located under the enamel in a tooth. (Also spelled *dentin.*)

dentist (**DEN**-tist) Legally qualified specialist in dentistry.

dentistry (**DEN**-tis-tree) Evaluation, diagnosis, prevention, and treatment of conditions of the oral cavity and associated structures.

deoxyribonucleic acid (DNA) (dee-**OCK**-see-rye-boh-nyu-**KLEE**-ik **ASS**-id) Source of hereditary characteristics found in chromosomes.

dependence (dee-**PEN**-dense) The state of needing or relying on someone or something else.

dependent (dee-**PEN**-dent) Having to rely on someone else.

depressant (de-**PRESS**-ant) Substance that diminishes activity, sensation, or tone.

depression (de-**PRESS**-shun) Mental disorder with feelings of deep sadness and despair.

dermabrasion (der-mah-**BRAY**-zhun) Removal of upper layers of skin by rotary brush.

dermal (**DER**-mal) Pertaining to the skin.

dermascope (**DER**-mah-skope) Instrument that shines a light on the skin and magnifies a lesion.

dermatitis (der-mah-**TYE**-tis) Inflammation of the skin.

dermatologic (der-mah-toh-**LOJ**-ik) Pertaining to the skin and dermatology.

dermatologist (der-mah-**TOL**-oh-jist) Medical specialist in diseases of the skin.

dermatology (der-mah-**TOL**-oh-jee) Medical specialty concerned with disorders of the skin.

dermatomyositis (**DER**-mah-toe-my-oh-**SIGH**-**tis**) Inflammation of the skin and muscles.

dermis (**DER**-miss) Connective tissue layer of the skin beneath the epidermis.

detoxification (dee-**TOKS**-ih-fih-**KAY**-shun) Remove poison from a tissue or substance.

diabetes insipidus (dye-ah-**BEE**-teez in-**SIP**-ih-dus) Excretion of large amounts of dilute urine as a result of inadequate ADH production.

diabetes mellitus (dye-ah-**BEE**-teez **MEL**-ih-tus) Metabolic syndrome caused by absolute or relative insulin deficiency and/or insulin ineffectiveness.

diabetic (dye-ah-**BET**-ik) Pertaining to or suffering from diabetes.

diagnose (die-ag-**NOSE**) To make a diagnosis.

diagnosis (die-ag-**NO**-sis) The determination of the cause of a disease. Plural *diagnoses.*

diagnostic (die-ag-**NOS**-tik) Pertaining to or establishing a diagnosis.

dialysis (die-**AL**-ih-sis) An artificial method of filtration to remove excess waste materials and water from the body.

diaphoresis (**DIE**-ah-foh-**REE**-sis) Sweat or perspiration.

diaphoretic (**DIE**-ah-foh-**RET**-ic) Pertaining to sweat or perspiration.

diaphragm (**DIE**-ah-fram) A ring and dome-shaped material inserted into the vagina to prevent pregnancy; *or* the muscular sheet separating the abdominal and thoracic cavities.

diaphragmatic (**DIE**-ah-frag-**MAT**-ik) Pertaining to the diaphragm.

diaphysis (die-**AF**-ih-sis) The shaft of a long bone.

diarrhea (die-ah-**REE**-ah) Abnormally frequent and loose stools.

diastasis (die-**ASS**-tah-sis) Separation of normally joined parts.

diastole (die-**AS**-toe-lee) Dilation of heart cavities, during which they fill with blood.

diastolic (die-as-**TOL**-ik) Pertaining to diastole.

differential (dif-er-**EN**-shal) A differential white blood cell count lists percentages of the different leukocytes in a blood sample.

diffuse (di-**FUSE**) To disseminate or spread out.

diffusion (di-**FYU**-zhun) The means by which small particles move between tissues.

digestion (die-**JESS**-shun) Breakdown of food into elements suitable for cell metabolism.

digestive (die-**JEST**-iv) Pertaining to digestion.

digital (**DIJ**-ih-tal) Pertaining to a finger or toe.

dilate (**DIE**-late) To perform or undergo dilation.

dilation (die-**LAY**-shun) Stretching or enlarging an opening or a structure.

diphtheria (dif-**THEER**-ee-ah) Disease with a thick, membranous (leathery) coating of the pharynx.

diplegia (die-**PLEE**-jee-ah) Paralysis of all four limbs, with the two legs affected most severely.

dipstick (**DIP**-stick) Strip of plastic or paper bearing squares of reagents that change color in the presence of abnormal chemicals in the urine.

disability (dis-ah-**BILL**-ih-tee) Diminished capacity to perform certain activities or functions.

discipline (**DIS**-ih-plin) Training for proper conduct or action.

disease (diz-**EEZ**) A disorder of body functions, systems, or organs.

disinfectant (dis-in-**FEK**-tant) Agent that disinfects.

disinfection (dis-in-**FEK**-shun) Process of destruction of microorganisms by chemical agents.

dislocation (dis-low-**KAY**-shun) Completely out of joint.

displaced fracture (dis-**PLAYSD FRAK**-chur) A fracture in which the fragments are separated and are not in alignment.

disseminate (dih-**SEM**-in-ate) Widely scattered throughout the body or an organ.

dissociative identity disorder (di-**SO**-see-ah-tiv eye-**DEN**-tih-tee dis-**OR**-der) Part of an individual's personality is separated from the rest, leading to multiple personalities.

distal (**DISS**-tal) Situated away from the center of the body.

diuresis (die-you-**REE**-sis) Excretion of large volumes of urine.

diuretic (die-you-**RET**-ik) Agent that increases urine output.

diverticulitis (**DIE**-ver-tick-you-**LIE**-tis) Inflammation of the diverticula.

diverticulosis (**DIE**-ver-tick-you-**LOW**-sis) Presence of a number of small pouches in the wall of the large intestine.

diverticulum (die-ver-**TICK**-you-lum) A pouchlike opening or sac from a tubular structure (e.g., gut). Plural *diverticula.*

dopamine (**DOH**-pah-meen) Neurotransmitter in specific small areas of the brain.

Doppler (**DOP**-ler) Diagnostic instrument that sends an ultrasonic beam into the body.

Doppler ultrasonography (**DOP**-ler **UL**-trah-soh-**NOG**-rah-fee) Detects direction, velocity, and turbulence of blood flow; used in workup of stroke patients.

dormant (**DOOR**-mant) Inactive.

dorsal (**DOOR**-sal) Pertaining to the back or situated behind.

dorsum (**DOOR**-sum) Upper, posterior, or back surface.

Down syndrome (DOWN **SIN**-drome) A syndrome with variable abnormalities associated with three copies of chromosome 21.

Duchenne muscular dystrophy (**DOO**-shen **MUSS**-kyu-lar **DISS**-troh-fee) Symmetrical weakness and wasting of pelvic, shoulder, and proximal limb muscles.

ductus arteriosus (**DUK**-tus ar-**TEER**-ih-**OH**-sus) Fetal vessel that connects the descending aorta with the left pulmonary artery.

ductus deferens (**DUK**-tus **DEH**-fuh-renz) Tube that receives sperm from the epididymis. Also known as *vas deferens.*

duodenal (du-oh-**DEE**-nal) Pertaining to the duodenum.

duodenum (du-oh-**DEE**-num) The first part of the small intestine; approximately 12 finger-breadths (9 to 10 inches) in length.

dura mater (**DYU**-rah **MAY**-ter) Hard, fibrous outer layer of the meninges.

dysentery (**DIS**-en-tare-ee) Disease with diarrhea, bowel spasms, fever, and dehydration.

dysfunctional (dis-**FUNK**-shun-al) Difficulty in functioning.

dyslexia (dis-**LEK**-see-ah) Impaired reading and writing ability below the person's level of intelligence.

dyslexic (dis-**LEK**-sik) Pertaining to or suffering from dyslexia.

dysmenorrhea (dis-men-oh-**REE**-ah) Painful and difficult menstruation.

dyspareunia (dis-pah-**RUE**-nee-ah) Pain during sexual intercourse.

dyspepsia (dis-**PEP**-see-ah) "Upset stomach," epigastric pain, nausea, and gas.

dysphagia (dis-**FAY**-jee-ah) Difficulty in swallowing.

dysphoria (dis-**FOR**-ee-ah) Psychiatric mood disorder.

dysplasia (dis-**PLAY**-zee-ah) Abnormal tissue formation.

dysplastic (dis-**PLAS**-tik) Pertaining to or showing abnormal tissue formation.

dyspnea (disp-**NEE**-ah) Difficulty breathing.

dyspneic (disp-**NEE**-ik) Pertaining to or suffering from difficulty in breathing.

dysrhythmia (dis-**RITH**-me-ah) An abnormal heart rhythm.

dysuria (dis-**YOU**-ree-ah) Difficulty or pain with urination.

E

echocardiography (**EK**-oh-kar-dee-**OG**-rah-fee) Ultrasound recording of heart function.

echoencephalography (**EK**-oh-en-sef-ah-**LOG**-rah-fee) Use of ultrasound in the diagnosis of intracranial lesions.

eclampsia (ek-**LAMP**-see-uh) Convulsions in a patient with preeclampsia.

ectopic (ek-**TOP**-ik) Out of place, not in a normal position.

eczema (**EK**-zeh-mah) Inflammatory skin disease, often with a serous discharge.

eczematous (ek-**ZEM**-ah-tus) Pertaining to or marked by eczema.

edema (ee-**DEE**-mah) Excessive accumulation of fluid in cells and tissues.

edematous (ee-**DEM**-ah-tus) Pertaining to or marked by edema.

effacement (ee-**FACE**-ment) Thinning of the cervix in relation to labor.

efferent (**EFF**-eh-rent) Moving away from a center; for example, conducting nerve impulses away from the brain or spinal cord.

effusion (eh-**FYU**-zhun) Collection of fluid that has escaped from blood vessels into a cavity or tissues.

ejaculate (ee-**JACK**-you-late) To expel suddenly; *or* the semen expelled in ejaculation.

ejaculation (ee-**JACK**-you-**LAY**-shun) Process of expelling semen suddenly.

ejaculatory (ee-**JACK**-you-**LAY**-tor-ee) Pertaining to ejaculation.

elective (e-**LEK**-tiv) Surgery or a procedure that is not urgent or vital.

electrocardiogram (ECG or **EKG)** (ee-**LEK**-troh-**KAR**-dee-oh-gram) Record of the electrical signals of the heart.

electrocardiograph (ee-**LEK**-troh-**KAR**-dee-oh-graf) Machine that makes the electrocardiogram.

electrocardiography (ee-**LEK**-troh-kar-dee-**OG**-rah-fee) Interpretation of electrocardiograms.

electroconvulsive therapy (ECT) (ee-**LEK**-troh-kon-**VUL**-siv **THAIR**-ah-pee) Passage of electric current through the brain to produce convulsions and treat persistent depression.

electrode (ee-**LEK**-trode) A device for conducting electricity.

electroencephalogram (EEG) (ee-**LEK**-troh-en-**SEF**-ah-low-gram) Record of the electrical activity of the brain.

electroencephalograph (ee-**LEK**-troh-en-**SEF**-ah-low-graf) Device used to record the electrical activity of the brain.

electroencephalography (ee-**LEK**-troh-en-**SEF**-ah-**LOG**-rah-fee) The process of recording the electrical activity of the brain.

electrolyte (ee-**LEK**-troh-lite) Substance that, when dissolved in a suitable medium, forms electrically charged particles.

electromyogram (ee-**LEK**-troh-**MY**-oh-gram) Recording of electric currents associated with muscle action.

electromyography (ee-**LEK**-troh-my-**OG**-rah-fee) Recording of electrical activity in muscle.

electroneurodiagnostic (ee-**LEK**-troh-**NYUR**-oh-die-ag-**NOS**-tik) Pertaining to the use of electricity in the diagnosis of a neurologic disorder.

elimination (e-lim-ih-**NAY**-shun) Removal of waste material from the digestive tract.

emaciated (ee-**MAY**-see-**AY**-ted) Pertaining to or suffering from emaciation.

emaciation (ee-may-see-**AY**-shun) Abnormal thinness.

embolus (**EM**-boh-lus) Detached piece of thrombus, a mass of bacteria, quantity of air, or foreign body that blocks a blood vessel.

embryo (**EM**-bree-oh) Developing organism from conception until the end of the second month.

embryology (em-bree-**OL**-oh-jee) Science of the origin and early development of an organism.

embryonic (em-bree-**ON**-ic) Pertaining to the embryo.

emesis (**EM**-eh-sis) Vomit.

emmetropia (emm-eh-**TROH**-pee-ah) Normal refractive condition of the eye.

empathy (**EM**-pah-thee) Ability to place yourself into the feelings, emotions, and reactions of another person.

emphysema (em-fih-**SEE**-mah) Dilation of respiratory bronchioles and alveoli.

empyema (**EM**-pie-**EE**-mah) Pus in a body cavity, particularly in the pleural cavity.

emulsify (ee-**MUL**-sih-fye) Break up into very small droplets to suspend in a solution (emulsion).

emulsion (ee-**MUL**-shun) The system that contains small droplets suspended in a liquid.

enamel (ee-**NAM**-el) Hard substance covering a tooth.

encephalitis (en-**SEF**-ah-**LIE**-tis) Inflammation of brain cells and tissues.

encephalocele (en-**SEF**-ah-loh-seal) Congenital defect of the cranium with herniation of brain tissue.

encephalomyelitis (en-**SEF**-ah-loh-**MY**-eh-**LIE**-tis) Inflammation of the brain and spinal cord.

encephalopathy (en-sef-ah-**LOP**-ah-thee) Any disorder of the brain.

encopresis (en-koh-**PREE**-sis) Repeated soiling with feces.

endarterectomy (**END**-ar-ter-**EK**-toe-me) Surgical removal of plaque from an artery.

endemic (en-**DEM**-ik) Pertaining to a disease always present in a community.

endocardial (en-doh-**KAR**-dee-al) Pertaining to the endocardium.

endocarditis (**EN**-doh-kar-**DIE**-tis) Inflammation of the lining of the heart.

endocardium (en-doh-**KAR**-dee-um) The inside lining of the heart.

endocrine (**EN**-doh-krin) A gland that produces an internal or hormonal substance.

endocrinologist (**EN**-doh-krih-**NOL**-oh-jist) A medical specialist in endocrinology.

endocrinology (**EN**-doh-krih-**NOL**-oh-jee) Medical specialty concerned with the production and effects of hormones.

endometrial (en-doh-**ME**-tree-al) Pertaining to the inner lining of the uterus.

endometriosis (**EN**-doh-me-tree-**OH**-sis) Endometrial tissue outside the uterus.

endometrium (en-doh-**ME**-tree-um) Inner lining of the uterus.

endorphin (en-**DOR**-fin) A natural substance in the brain that simulates opium.

endoscope (**EN**-doh-skope) Instrument to examine the inside of a tubular or hollow organ.

endoscopy (en-**DOS**-koh-pee) The use of an endoscope.

endotracheal (en-doh-**TRAY**-kee-al) Pertaining to being inside the trachea.

enema (**EN**-eh-mah) An injection of fluid into the rectum.

enteric (en-**TEHR**-ik) Pertaining to the intestine.

enteroscope (**EN**-ter-oh-**SKOPE**) Slender, tubular instrument with light source and camera to visualize the digestive tract.

enteroscopy (en-ter-**OSS**-koh-pee) The examination of the lining of the digestive tract.

enuresis (en-you-**REE**-sis) Bedwetting; urinary incontinence.

enzyme (**EN**-zime) Protein that induces changes in other substances.

eosinophil (ee-oh-**SIN**-oh-fill) An eosinophil's granules attract a rosy-red color on staining.

epicardial (ep-ih-**KAR**-dee-al) Pertaining to the epicardium.

epicardium (ep-ih-**KAR**-dee-um) The outer layer of the heart wall.

epicondyle (ep-ih-**KON**-dile) Projection above the condyle for attachment of a ligament or tendon.

epidemic (ep-ih-**DEM**-ik) Pertaining to an outbreak in a community of a disease or a health-related behavior.

epidermal (ep-ih-**DER**-mal) Pertaining to the epidermis.

epidermis (ep-ih-**DER**-miss) Top layer of the skin.

epididymis (ep-ih-**DID**-ih-miss) Coiled tube attached to the testis.

epididymitis (ep-ih-did-ih-**MY**-tis) Inflammation of the epididymis.

epididymoorchitis (ep-ih-**DID**-ih-moh-or-**KIE**-tis) Inflammation of the epididymis and testicle. Also called *orchitis.*

epidural (ep-ih-**DYU**-ral) Above the dura.

epidural space (ep-ih-**DYU**-ral SPASE) Space between the dura mater and the wall of the vertebral canal.

epigastric (ep-ih-**GAS**-trik) Pertaining to the abdominal region above the stomach.

epigastrium (ep-ih-**GAS**-tri-um) The abdominal region above the stomach.

epiglottis (ep-ih-**GLOT**-is) Leaf-shaped plate of cartilage that shuts off the larynx during swallowing.

epiglottitis (ep-ih-glot-**EYE**-tis) Inflammation of the epiglottis.

epilepsy (**EP**-ih-**LEP**-see) Chronic brain disorder due to paroxysmal excessive neuronal discharges.

epileptic (EP-ih-LEP-tik) Pertaining to or suffering from epilepsy.

epinephrine (ep-ih-**NEF**-rin) Main catecholamine produced by the adrenal medulla. Also called *adrenaline.*

epiphysial (ep-ih-**FIZ**-ee-al) Pertaining to an epiphysis.

epiphysial plate (eh-ih-**FIZ**-ee-al PLATE) Layer of cartilage between the epiphysis and the metaphysis where bone growth occurs.

epiphysis (ep-ih-**FI**-sis) Expanded area at the proximal and distal ends of a long bone to provide increased surface area for attachment of ligaments and tendons.

episiotomy (eh-piz-ee-**OT**-oh-me) Surgical incision of the vulva.

epispadias (ep-ih-**SPAY**-dee-as) Condition in which the urethral opening is on the dorsum of the penis.

epistaxis (ep-ih-**STAK**-sis) Nosebleed.

epithelium (ep-ih-**THEE**-lee-um) Tissue that covers surfaces or lines cavities.

equilibrium (ee-kwi-**LIB**-ree-um) Being evenly balanced.

erectile (ee-**REK**-tile) Capable of erection or being distended with blood.

erection (ee-**REK**-shun) Distended and rigid state of an organ.

erosion (ee-**ROE**-zhun) Form a shallow ulcer in the lining of a structure.

erythroblast (eh-**RITH**-ro-blast) Precursor to a red blood cell.

erythroblastosis (eh-**RITH**-roh-blas-**TOH**-sis) Condition of many immature red cells in blood.

erythrocyte (eh-**RITH**-roh-site) A red blood cell.

erythropoiesis (eh-**RITH**-roh-poy-**EE**-sis) The formation of red blood cells.

erythropoietin (eh-**RITH**-roh-**POY**-ee-tin) Protein secreted by the kidney that stimulates red blood cell production.

eschar (**ESS**-kar) The burnt, dead tissue lying on top of third-degree burns.

Escherichia coli (esh-eh-**RIK**-ee-ah **KOH**-lie) Organism in the intestine; releases an exotoxin that can cause diarrhea.

esophageal (ee-**SOF**-ah-**JEE**-al) Pertaining to the esophagus.

esophagitis (ee-**SOF**-ah-**JI**-tis) Inflammation of the lining of the esophagus.

esophagus (ee-**SOF**-ah-gus) Tube linking the pharynx to the stomach.

esotropia (es-oh-**TROH**-pee-ah) Turning the eye inward toward the nose.

estrogen (**ES**-troh-jen) Generic term for hormones that stimulate female secondary sex characteristics.

ethmoid (**ETH**-moyd) Bone that forms the back of the nose and encloses numerous air cells.

etiology (ee-tee-**OL**-oh-jee) The study of the causes of a disease.

eupnea (yoop-**NEE**-ah) Normal breathing.

eustachian tube (you-**STAY**-shun TYUB) Tube that connects the middle ear to the nasopharynx. Also called *auditory tube.*

euthyroid (you-**THIGH**-royd) Normal thyroid function.

eversion (ee-**VER**-zhun) Turning outward.

evert (ee-**VERT**) To turn outward.

evolve (ee-**VOLV**) To develop gradually.

Ewing sarcoma (**YOU**-ing sar-**KOH**-mah) A malignant neoplasm of bone.

exacerbation (ek-zas-er-**BAY**-shun) Period when there is an increase in the severity of a disease.

excision (ek-**SIZH**-un) Surgical removal of part or all of a structure.

excoriate (eks-**KOR**-ee-ate) To scratch.

excoriation (eks-**KOR**-ee-**AY**-shun) Scratch mark.

excrete (eks-**KREET**) To pass waste products of metabolism out of the body.

excretion (eks-**KREE**-shun) Removal of waste products of metabolism out of the body.

exhale (**EKS**-hail) Breathe out.

exocrine (**EK**-soh-krin) A gland that secretes substances outwardly through excretory ducts.

exophthalmos (ek-sof-**THAL**-mos) Protrusion of the eyeball.

exotropia (ek-soh-**TROH**-pee-ah) Turning the eye outward away from the nose.

expectorate (ek-**SPEK**-toh-rate) Cough up and spit out mucus from the respiratory tract.

expiration (**EKS**-pih-**RAY**-shun) Breathe out.

extension (eks-**TEN**-shun) Straighten a joint to increase its angle.

extracorporeal (**EKS**-tra-kor-**POH**-ree-al) Outside the body.

extrinsic (eks-**TRIN**-sik) Any muscle located entirely on the outside of the structure under consideration; for example, the eye.

F

facies (**FASH**-eez) Facial features and expressions.

fallopian tubes (fah-**LOW**-pee-an) Uterine tubes connected to the fundus of the uterus.

Fallot (fah-**LOW**) First described the tetralogy of congenital heart defects.

fascia (**FASH**-ee-ah) Sheet of fibrous connective tissue.

fasciectomy (fash-ee-**EK**-toe-me) Surgical removal of fascia.

fasciitis (fash-ee-**EYE**-tis) Inflammation of fascia.

fasciotomy (fash-ee-**OT**-oh-me) An incision through a band of fascia, usually to relieve pressure on underlying structures.

febrile (**FEB**-ril or **FEB**-rile) Pertaining to or suffering from fever.

fecal (**FEE**-kal) Pertaining to feces.

feces (**FEE**-seez) Undigested, waste material discharged from the bowel.

femoral (**FEM**-oh-ral) Pertaining to the femur.

femur (**FEE**-mur) The thigh bone.

fertilization (**FER**-til-eye-**ZAY**-shun) Union of a male sperm and a female egg.

fertilize (**FER**-til-ize) Penetration of the egg by sperm.

fetal (**FEE**-tal) Pertaining to the fetus.

fetalis (fee-**TAH**-lis) Erythroblastosis fetalis is a hemolytic disease of the newborn.

fetus (**FEE**-tus) Human organism from the end of the eighth week after conception to birth.

fever (**FEE**-ver) Increased body temperature that is a physiologic response to disease.

fibrillation (fi-brih-**LAY**-shun) Uncontrolled quivering or twitching of the heart muscle.

fibrin (**FIE**-brin) Stringy protein fiber that is a component of a blood clot.

fibrinogen (fie-**BRIN**-oh-jen) Precursor of fibrin in blood-clotting process.

fibroadenoma (**FIE**-broh-ad-en-**OH**-muh) Benign tumor containing much fibrous tissue.

fibroblast (**FIE**-broh-blast) Cell that forms collagen fibers.

fibrocystic disease (fie-broh-**SIS**-tik diz-**EEZ**) Benign breast disease with multiple tiny lumps and cysts.

fibroid (**FIE**-broyd) Uterine tumor resembling fibrous tissue.

fibromyalgia (fie-broh-my-**AL**-jee-ah) Pain in the muscle fibers.

fibromyoma (**FIE**-broh-my-**OH**-mah) Benign neoplasm derived from smooth muscle and containing fibrous tissue.

fibrosis (fie-**BROH**-sis) Repair of dead tissue cells by formation of fibrous tissue.

fibrotic (fie-**BROT**-ik) Pertaining to or affected by fibrosis.

fibula (**FIB**-you-lah) The smaller of the two bones of the lower leg.

fibular (**FIB**-you-lar) Pertaining to the fibula.

filter (**FIL**-ter) Porous substance used to separate liquids or gases from particulate matter; *or* to subject a substance to the action of a filter.

filtrate (**FIL**-trate) That which has passed through a filter.

filtration (fil-**TRAY**-shun) Process of passing liquid through a filter.

fimbria (**FIM**-bree-ah) A fringelike structure on the surface of a cell or microorganism. Plural *fimbriae.*

fissure (**FISH**-ur) Deep furrow or cleft. Plural *fissures.*

fistula (**FIS**-tyu-lah) Abnormal passage. Plural *fistulae* or *fistulas.*

flank (FLANK) Side of the body between pelvis and ribs.

flatulence (**FLAT**-you-lence) Excessive amount of gas in the stomach and intestines.

flatus (**FLAY**-tus) Gas or air expelled through the anus.

flex (FLEKS) To bend a joint so that the two parts come together.

flexion (**FLEK**-shun) Bend a joint to decrease its angle.

flexor (**FLEK**-sor) Muscle or tendon that flexes a joint.

flexure (**FLEK**-shur) A bend in a structure.

flora (**FLO**-rah) Microrganisms covering the exterior and interior surfaces of a healthy animal.

fluorescein (flor-**ESS**-ee-in) Dye that produces a vivid green color under a blue light to diagnose corneal abrasions and foreign bodies.

follicle (**FOLL**-ih-kull) Spherical mass of cells containing a cavity; *or* a small cul-de-sac, such as a hair follicle.

follicular (fo-**LIK**-you-lar) Pertaining to a follicle.

foramen (fo-**RAY**-men) An opening through a structure. Plural *foramina.*

forceps extraction (**FOR**-seps ek-**STRAK**-shun) Assisted delivery of the baby by an instrument that grasps the head of the baby.

foreskin (**FOR**-skin) Skin that covers the glans penis.

fornix (**FOR**-niks) Arch-shaped, blind-ended part of the vagina behind and around the cervix. Plural *fornices.*

fovea centralis (**FOH**-vee-ah sen-**TRAH**-lis) Small pit in the center of the macula that has the highest visual acuity.

frenulum (**FREN**-you-lum) Fold of mucous membrane between the glans and the prepuce.

frontal (**FRON**-tal) Vertical plane dividing the body into anterior and posterior portions.

function (**FUNK**-shun) The ability of an organ or tissue to perform its special work.

fundoscopic (fun-doh-**SKOP**-ik) Pertaining to fundoscopy.

fundoscopy (fun-**DOS**-koh-pee) Examination of the fundus (retina) of the eye.

fundus (**FUN**-dus) Part farthest from the opening of a hollow organ.

fungicide (**FUN**-ji-side) Agent to destroy fungi.

fungus (**FUN**-gus) General term used to describe yeasts and molds. Plural *fungi.*

G

galactorrhea (gah-**LAK**-toe-**REE**-ah) Abnormal flow of milk from the breasts.

gallbladder (**GAWL**-blad-er) Receptacle on the inferior surface of the liver for storing bile.

gallstone (**GAWL**-stone) Hard mass of cholesterol, calcium, and bilirubin that can be formed in the gallbladder and bile duct.

ganglion (**GANG**-lee-on) Collection of nerve cells outside the brain and spinal cord; *or* a fluid-filled cyst. Plural *ganglia.*

gastric (**GAS**-trik) Pertaining to the stomach.

gastrin (**GAS**-trin) Hormone secreted in the stomach that stimulates secretion of HCl and increases gastric motility.

gastritis (gas-**TRY**-tis) Inflammation of the lining of the stomach.

gastrocnemius (gas-trok-**NEE**-me-us) Major muscle in back of the lower leg (the calf).

gastroenteritis (**GAS**-troh-en-ter-**I**-tis) Inflammation of the stomach and intestines.

gastroenterologist (**GAS**-troh-en-ter-**OL**-oh-jist) Medical specialist in gastroenterology.

gastroenterology (**GAS**-troh-en-ter-**OL**-oh-gee) Medical specialty of the stomach and intestines.

gastroesophageal (**GAS**-troh-ee-sof-ah-**JEE**-al) Pertaining to the stomach and esophagus.

gastrointestinal (GI) (**GAS**-troh-in-**TESS**-tin-al) Pertaining to the stomach and intestines.

gastroscope (**GAS**-troh-skope) Endoscope for examining the inside of the stomach.

gastroscopy (gas-**TROS**-koh-pee) Endoscopic examination of the stomach.

gavage (guh-**VAHZH**) To feed by a stomach tube.

gene (**JEEN**) Functional segment of DNA molecule.

geneticist (jeh-**NET**-ih-sist) A specialist in genetics.

genetics (jeh-**NET**-iks) Science of the inheritance of characteristics.

genital (**JEN**-ih-tal) Relating to reproduction or to the male or female sex organs.

genitalia (**JEN**-ih-**TAY**-lee-ah) External and internal organs of reproduction.

geriatrician (jer-ee-ah-**TRISH**-an) Medical specialist in the process and problems of aging.

geriatrics (jer-ee-**AT**-riks) Medical specialty that deals with the problems of aging.

gerontologist (jer-on-**TOL**-oh-jist) Medical specialist in the process and general problems of aging.

gerontology (jer-on-**TOL**-oh-jee) Study of the process and problems of aging.

gestation (jes-**TAY**-shun) From conception to birth.

gestational (jes-**TAY**-shun-al) Pertaining to gestation.

gigantism (**JI**-gan-tizm) Abnormal height and size of the entire body.

gingiva (**JIN**-jih-vah) Tissue surrounding the teeth and covering the jaw.

gingival (**JIN**-jih-val) Pertaining to the gingiva.

gingivectomy (jin-jih-**VEC**-toe-me) Surgical removal of diseased gum tissue.

gingivitis (jin-jih-**VI**-tis) Inflammation of the gums.

glans (**GLANZ**) Head of the penis or clitoris.

glaucoma (glau-**KOH**-mah) Increased intraocular pressure.

glia (**GLEE**-ah) Connective tissue that holds a structure together.

glial (**GLEE**-al) Pertaining to glia or neuroglia.

glioma (gli-**OH**-mah) Tumor of a glial cell.

glomerulonephritis (glo-**MER**-you-low-nef-**RYE**-tis) Infection of the glomeruli of the kidney.

glomerulus (glo-**MER**-you-lus) Plexus of capillaries; part of a nephron. Plural *glomeruli.*

glossodynia (gloss-oh-**DIN**-ee-ah) Painful, burning tongue.

glossopharyngeal (**GLOSS**-oh-fah-**RIN**-jee-al) Ninth (IX) cranial nerve, supplying the tongue and pharynx.

glottis (**GLOT**-is) Vocal apparatus of the larynx.

glucagon (**GLU**-kah-gon) Pancreatic hormone that supports blood glucose levels.

glucocorticoid (glu-co-**KOR**-tih-koyd) Hormone of the adrenal cortex that helps regulate glucose metabolism.

gluconeogenesis (**GLU**-koh-nee-oh-**JEN**-eh-sis) Formation of glucose from noncarbohydrate sources.

glucose (GLU-kose) The final product of carbohydrate digestion and the main sugar in the blood.

gluteal (GLU-tee-al) Pertaining to the buttocks.

gluten (GLU-ten) Insoluble protein found in wheat, barley, and oats.

gluteus (GLU-tee-us) Refers to one of three muscles in the buttocks.

glycogen (GLYE-koh-gen) The body's principal carbohydrate reserve, stored in the liver and skeletal muscle.

glycogenolysis (GLYE-koh-jen-oh-LYE-sis) Conversion of glycogen to glucose.

glycosuria (GLYE-koh-SYU-ree-ah) Presence of glucose in urine.

glycosylated hemoglobin (Hb A1c) (GLYE-koh-sih-lay-ted HE-moh-GLOW-bin) Hemoglobin A fraction linked to glucose; used as an index of glucose control.

goiter (GOY-ter) Enlargement of the thyroid gland.

gomphosis (gom-FOE-sis) Joint formed by a peg and socket. Plural *gomphoses.*

gonad (GO-nad) Testis or ovary. Plural *gonads.*

gonadotropin (GO-nad-oh-TROH-pin) Any hormone that stimulates gonad function.

gonorrhea (gon-oh-REE-ah) Specific contagious sexually transmitted infection.

grade (GRAYD) In cancer pathology, a classification of the rate of growth of cancer cells.

graft (GRAFT) Transplantation of living tissue.

grand mal (GRAHN MAL) Old name for generalized tonic-clonic seizure.

granulation (gran-you-LAY-shun) New fibrous tissue formed during wound healing.

granulocyte (GRAN-you-loh-site) A white blood cell that contains multiple small granules in its cytoplasm.

granulosa cell (gran-you-LOW-sah SELL) Cell lining the ovarian follicle.

Graves disease (GRAVZ diz-EEZ) Hyperthyroidism with toxic goiter.

gravid (GRAV-id) Pregnant.

gravida (GRAV-ih-dah) A pregnant woman.

gray matter (GRAY MATT-er) Regions of the brain and spinal cord occupied by cell bodies and dendrites.

greenstick fracture (GREEN-stik FRAK-chur) A fracture in which one side of the bone is partially broken and the other side is bent. Occurs mostly in children.

groin (GROYN) Crease where the thigh joins the abdomen.

Guillain-Barré syndrome (GEE-yan bah-RAY SIN-drom) Disorder in which the body makes antibodies against myelin, disrupting nerve conduction.

gurney (GURR-knee) A stretcher on wheels used to transport hospital patients.

gynecologic (GUY-nih-koh-LOJ-ik) Pertaining to gynecology.

gynecologist (guy-nih-KOL-oh-jist) Specialist in gynecology.

gynecology (guy-nih-KOL-oh-jee) Medical specialty of diseases of the female.

gynecomastia (GUY-nih-koh-MAS-tee-ah) Enlargement of the breast.

gyrus (JI-rus) Rounded elevation on the surface of the cerebral hemispheres. Plural *gyri.*

H

hairline fracture (HAIR-line FRAK-chur) A fracture without separation of the fragments.

halitosis (hal-ih-TOE-sis) Bad odor of the breath.

hallucination (hah-loo-sih-NAY-shun) Perception of an object or event when there is no such thing present.

hallux valgus (HAL-uks VAL-gus) Deviation of the big toe toward the lateral side of the foot.

Hashimoto disease (hah-shee-MOH-toe diz-EEZ) Autoimmune disease of the thyroid gland. Also called *Hashimoto thyroiditis.*

Haversian canals (hah-VER-shan ka-NALS) Vascular canals in bone. Also called *central canals.*

Heberden node (HEH-ber-den NOHD) Bony lump on the terminal phalanx of the fingers in osteoarthritis.

hemangioma (he-MAN-jee-oh-mah) Abnormal mass of proliferating blood vessels.

hematemesis (he-mah-TEM-eh-sis) Vomiting of red blood.

hematocrit (Hct) (HE-mat-oh-krit) Percentage of red blood cells in the blood.

hematologist (he-mah-TOL-oh-jist) Specialist in hematology.

hematology (he-mah-TOL-oh-jee) Medical specialty of disorders of the blood.

hematoma (he-mah-TOE-mah) Collection of blood that has escaped from the blood vessels into surrounding tissues. Also called *bruise.*

hematuria (he-mah-TYU-ree-ah) Blood in the urine.

heme (HEEM) The iron-based component of hemoglobin that carries oxygen.

hemiparesis (HEM-ee-pah-REE-sis) Weakness of one side of the body.

hemiplegia (hem-ee-PLEE-jee-ah) Paralysis of one side of the body.

hemiplegic (hem-ee-PLEE-jik) Pertaining to or suffering from hemiplegia.

Hemoccult test (HEEM-o-kult TEST) Trade name for a fecal occult blood test.

hemodialysis (HE-moh-die-AL-ih-sis) An artificial method of filtration to remove excess waste materials and water directly from the blood.

hemodynamics (HE-moh-die-NAM-iks) The science of the flow of blood through the circulation.

hemoglobin (HE-moh-GLOW-bin) Red-pigmented protein that is the main component of red blood cells.

hemoglobinopathy (HE-moh-GLOW-bin-OP-ah-thee) Disease caused by the presence of an abnormal hemoglobin in the red blood cells.

hemolysis (he-MOL-ih-sis) Destruction of red blood cells so that hemoglobin is liberated.

hemolytic (he-moh-LIT-ik) Pertaining to the process of destruction of red blood cells.

hemophilia (he-moh-FILL-ee-ah) An inherited disease from a deficiency of clotting factor VIII.

hemoptysis (he-MOP-tih-sis) Bloody sputum.

hemorrhage (HEM-oh-raj) To bleed profusely.

hemorrhoid (HEM-oh-royd) Dilated rectal vein producing painful anal swelling. Plural *hemorrhoids.*

hemorrhoidectomy (HEM-oh-royd-EK-toh-me) Surgical removal of hemorrhoids.

hemostasis (he-moh-**STAY**-sis) Control of or stopping bleeding.

hemothorax (he-moh-**THOR**-ax) Blood in the pleural cavity.

heparin (**HEP**-ah-rin) An anticoagulant secreted particularly by liver cells.

hepatic (hep-**AT**-ik) Pertaining to the liver.

hepatitis (hep-ah-**TIE**-tis) Inflammation of the liver.

hernia (**HER**-nee-ah) Protrusion of a structure through the tissue that normally contains it.

herniate (**HER**-nee-ate) To protrude.

herniation (her-nee-**AY**-shun) Protrusion of an anatomical structure from its normal location.

herniorrhaphy (**HER**-nee-**OR**-ah-fee) Repair of a hernia.

herpes simplex virus (HSV) (**HER**-peez **SIM**-pleks **VIE**-rus) Manifests with painful, watery blisters on the skin and mucous membranes.

herpes zoster (**HER**-peez **ZOS**-ter) Painful eruption of vesicles that follows a nerve root on one side of the body. Also called *shingles.*

heterograft (**HET**-er-oh-graft) A graft using tissue taken from another species. Also called *xenograft.*

hiatal (high-**AY**-tal) Pertaining to a hernia.

hiatus (high-**AY**-tus) An opening through a structure.

hilum (**HIGH**-lum) The site where the nerves and blood vessels enter and leave an organ. Plural *hila.*

histamine (**HISS**-tah-mean) Compound liberated in tissues as a result of injury or an allergic response.

histologist (his-**TOL**-oh-jist) Specialist in histology.

histology (his-**TOL**-oh-jee) Study of the structure and function of cells, tissues, and organs.

Hodgkin lymphoma (**HOJ**-kin lim-**FOH**-mah) Marked by chronic enlargement of lymph nodes spreading to other nodes in an orderly way.

holistic (ho-**LIS**-tik) Pertaining to the care of the whole person in physical, mental, emotional, and spiritual dimensions.

homeostasis (hoh-mee-oh-**STAY**-sis) Maintaining the stability of a system or the body's internal environment.

homograft (**HOH**-moh-graft) Skin graft from another person or a cadaver. Also called *allograft.*

hordeolum (hor-**DEE**-oh-lum) Abscess in an eyelash follicle. Also called *stye.*

hormonal (hor-**MOHN**-al) Pertaining to a hormone.

hormone (**HOR**-mohn) Chemical formed in one tissue or organ and carried by the blood to stimulate or inhibit a function of another tissue or organ.

Horner syndrome (**HOR**-ner **SIN**-drome) Disorder of the sympathetic nerves to the face and eye.

hospice (**HOS**-pis) Provides care to the dying and their families.

human immunodeficiency virus (HIV) (**HYU**-man **IM**-you-noh-dee-**FISH**-en-see **VIE**-rus) Etiologic agent of acquired immunodeficiency syndrome (AIDS).

human papilloma virus (HPV) (**HYU**-man pap-ih-**LOW**-mah **VIE**-rus) Causes warts on the skin and genitalia and can increase the risk for cervical cancer.

humerus (**HYU**-mer-us) Single bone of the upper arm.

humoral immunity (**HYU**-mor-al ihm-**YUNE**-ih-tee) Defense mechanism arising from antibodies in the blood.

Huntington disease (**HUN**-ting-ton diz-**EEZ**) Progressive inherited, degenerative, incurable neurologic disease. Also called *Huntington chorea.*

hyaline (**HIGH**-ah-line) Cartilage that looks like frosted glass and contains fine collagen fibers.

hyaline membrane disease (**HIGH**-ah-line **MEM**-brain diz-**EEZ**) Respiratory distress syndrome of the newborn.

hydrocele (**HIGH**-droh-seal) Collection of fluid in the space of the tunica vaginalis.

hydrocephalus (high-droh-**SEF**-ah-lus) Excess CSF in the cerebral ventricles; may cause enlarged head.

hydrochloric acid (HCl) (high-droh-**KLOR**-ik **ASS**-id) The acid of gastric juice.

hydrocortisone (high-droh-**KOR**-tih-sohn) Potent glucocorticoid with anti-inflammatory properties. Also called *cortisol.*

hydronephrosis (**HIGH**-droh-neh-**FROH**-sis) Dilation of the pelvis and calyces of a kidney.

hydronephrotic (**HIGH**-droh-neh-**FROT**-ik) Pertaining to or suffering from hydronephrosis.

hymen (**HIGH**-men) Thin membrane partly occluding the vaginal orifice.

hyperactivity (**HIGH**-per-ac-**TIV**-ih-tee) Excessive restlessness and movement.

hypercalcemia (**HIGH**-per-cal-**SEE**-me-ah) Excessive level of calcium in the blood.

hypercapnia (**HIGH**-per-**KAP**-nee-ah) Abnormal increase of carbon dioxide in the arterial bloodstream.

hyperemesis (high-per-**EM**-eh-sis) Excessive vomiting.

hyperflexion (high-per-**FLEK**-shun) Flexion of a limb or part beyond the normal limits.

hyperglycemia (**HIGH**-per-gly-**SEE**-me-ah) High level of glucose (sugar) in blood.

hyperglycemic (**HIGH**-per-gly-**SEE**-mik) Pertaining to or having hyperglycemia.

hyperimmune globulin (**HIGH**-per-im-**YUNE GLOB**-youlin) Immunoglobulin prepared from serum of people with a high antibody titer to a specific antigen.

hyperkalemia (**HIGH**-per-kah-**LEE**-me-ah) High level of potassium in the blood.

hypernatremia (**HIGH**-per-nah-**TREE**-me-ah) High level of sodium in the blood.

hyperopia (high-per-**OH**-pee-ah) Able to see distant objects but unable to see close objects.

hyperosmolar (**HIGH**-per-os-**MOH**-lar) Marked hyperglycemia without ketoacidosis.

hyperparathyroidism (**HIGH**-per-para-**THIGH**-royd-izm) Excessive production of parathyroid hormone.

hyperplasia (**HIGH**-per-**PLAY**-zee-ah) Increase in the number of cells in a tissue or organ.

hyperpnea (high-perp-**NEE**-ah) Deeper and more rapid breathing than normal.

hyperpyrexia (**HIGH**-per-pie-**REK**-see-ah) Extremely high body temperature or fever.

hypersecretion (**HIGH**-per-seh-**KREE**-shun) Excessive secretion (of mucus or enzymes or waste products).

hypersensitivity (**HIGH**-per-sen-sih-**TIV**-ih-tee) Exaggerated abnormal reaction to an allergen.

hypersplenism (high-per-**SPLEN**-izm) Condition in which the spleen removes blood components at an excessive rate.

hypertension (**HIGH**-per-**TEN**-shun) Persistent high arterial blood pressure.

hypertensive (**HIGH**-per-**TEN**-siv) Pertaining to or suffering from high blood pressure.

hyperthyroidism (high-per-**THIGH**-royd-izm) Excessive production of thyroid hormones.

hypertrophy (high-**PER**-troh-fee) Increase in size, but not in number, of an individual tissue element.

hypochondriac (high-poh-**KON**-dree-ack) A person who exaggerates the significance of symptoms.

hypochromic (high-poh-**CROW**-mik) Pale in color, as in RBCs when hemoglobin is deficient.

hypodermic (high-poh-**DER**-mik) Pertaining to the hypodermis.

hypodermis (high-poh-**DER**-miss) Tissue layer of skin below the dermis.

hypogastric (high-poh-**GAS**-trik) Abdominal region below the stomach.

hypoglossal (high-poh-**GLOSS**-al) Twelfth (XII) cranial nerve, supplying muscles of the tongue.

hypoglycemia (**HIGH**-poh-gly-**SEE**-me-ah) Low level of glucose (sugar) in the blood.

hypoglycemic (**HIGH**-poh-gly-**SEE**-mik) Pertaining to or suffering from low blood sugar.

hypogonadism (**HIGH**-poh-**GOH**-nad-izm) Deficient gonad production of sperm or eggs or hormones.

hypokalemia (**HIGH**-poh-kah-**LEE**-me-ah) Low level of potassium in the blood.

hyponatremia (**HIGH**-poh-nah-**TREE**-me-ah) Low level of sodium in the blood.

hypoparathyroidism (**HIGH**-poh-par-ah-**THIGH**-royd-izm) Deficient production of parathyroid hormone.

hypophysis (high-**POF**-ih-sis) Another name for *pituitary gland.*

hypopituitarism (**HIGH**-poh-pih-**TYU**-ih-tah-rizm) Condition of one or more deficient pituitary hormones.

hypospadias (high-poh-**SPAY**-dee-as) Urethral opening more proximal than normal on the ventral surface of the penis.

hypotension (**HIGH**-poh-**TEN**-shun) Persistent low arterial blood pressure.

hypotensive (**HIGH**-poh-**TEN**-siv) Pertaining to or suffering from low blood pressure.

hypothalamic (high-poh-thal-**AM**-ik) Pertaining to the hypothalamus.

hypothalamus (high-poh-**THAL**-ah-muss) An area of gray matter lying below the thalamus.

hypothenar eminence (high-poh-**THAY**-nar **EM**-in-nens) The fleshy mass at the base of the little finger.

hypothermia (high-poh-**THER**-me-ah) Very low core body temperature.

hypothyroidism (high-poh-**THIGH**-royd-izm) Deficient production of thyroid hormones.

hypovolemic (**HIGH**-poh-vo-**LEE**-mik) Decreased blood volume in the body.

hypoxia (high-**POCK**-see-ah) Below-normal levels of oxygen in tissues, gases, or blood.

hypoxic (high-**POCK**-sik) Deficient in oxygen.

hysterectomy (his-ter-**EK**-toe-me) Surgical removal of the uterus.

hysteroscopy (**his**-ter-**OS**-koh-pee) Visual inspection of the uterine cavity using an endoscope.

I

ictal (**IK**-tal) Pertaining to, or a condition caused by, a stroke or epilepsy.

idiopathic (**ID**-ih-oh-**PATH**-ik) Pertaining to a disease of unknown etiology.

ileocecal (**ILL**-ee-oh-**SEE**-cal) Pertaining to the junction of the ileum and cecum.

ileocecal sphincter (**ILL**-ee-oh-**SEE**-cal **SFINK**-ter) A band of muscle that encircles the junction of the ileum and cecum.

ileoscopy (ill-ee-**OS**-koh-pee) Endoscopic examination of the ileum.

ileostomy (ill-ee-**OS**-toe-me) Artificial opening from the ileum to the outside of the body.

ileum (**ILL**-ee-um) Third portion of the small intestine.

iliac (**ILL**-ee-ack) A structure related to the ilium (pelvic bone).

ilium (**ILL**-ee-um) Large wing-shaped bone at the upper and posterior part of the pelvis. Plural *ilia.*

immune (im-**YUNE**) Protected from an infectious disease.

immune serum (im-**YUNE SEER**-um) Serum taken from another human or animal that has antibodies to a disease. Also called *antiserum.*

immunity (im-**YUNE**-ih-tee) State of being protected.

immunization (**IM**-you-nih-**ZAY**-shun) Administration of an agent to provide immunity.

immunize (**IM**-you-nize) To make resistant to an infectious disease.

immunodeficiency (**IM**-you-noh-dee-**FISH**-en-see) Failure of the immune system.

immunoglobulin (**IM**-you-noh-**GLOB**-you-lin) Specific protein evoked by an antigen. All antibodies are immunoglobulins.

immunologist (im-you-**NOL**-oh-jist) Medical specialist in immunology.

immunology (im-you-**NOL**-oh-jee) The science and practice of immunity and allergy.

immunosuppression (**IM**-you-noh-suh-**PRESH**-un) Failure of the immune system caused by an outside agent.

impacted (im-**PAK**-ted) Immovably wedged, as with earwax blocking the external canal.

impacted fracture (im-**PAK**-ted **FRAK**-chur) A fracture in which one bone fragment is driven into the other.

impairment (im-**PAIR**-ment) The state of being worse, weaker, or damaged.

impetigo (im-peh-**TIE**-go) Infection of the skin producing thick, yellow crusts.

implant (im-**PLANT**) To insert material into tissues; *or* the material inserted into tissues.

implantable (im-**PLAN**-tah-bul) A device that can be inserted into tissues.

implantation (im-plan-**TAY**-shun) Attachment of a fertilized egg to the endometrium.

impotence (**IM**-poh-tence) Inability to achieve an erection.

impulsive (im-**PUL**-siv) Inability to resist performing inappropriate actions.

in situ (IN **SIGH**-tyu) In the correct place.

in utero (IN **YOU**-ter-oh) Within the womb; not yet born.

in vitro fertilization (IVF) (en **VEE**-troh **FER**-til-eye-**ZAY**-shun) Process of combining sperm and egg in a laboratory dish and placing the resulting embryos inside the uterus.

inattention (**IN**-ah-**TEN**-shun) Lack of concentration and direction.

incision (in-**SIZH**-un) A cut or surgical wound.

incompetence (in-**KOM**-peh-tense) Failure of valves to close completely.

incomplete fracture (in-kom-**PLEET FRAK**-chur) A fracture that does not extend across the bone, as in a hairline fracture.

incontinence (in-**KON**-tin-ence) Inability to prevent discharge of urine or feces.

incontinent (in-**KON**-tin-ent) Denoting incontinence.

incubation (in-kyu-**BAY**-shun) Process to develp an infection.

incus (**IN**-cuss) Middle one of the three ossicles in the middle ear; shaped like an anvil.

independence (in-dee-**PEN**-dense) The state of being able to think and act for oneself.

independent (in-dee-**PEN**-dent) Pertaining to the ability to think and act for oneself.

indigestion (in-dee-**JESS**-chun) Symptoms resulting from difficulty in digesting food.

infancy (**IN**-fan-see) The first year of life.

infant (**IN**-fant) Child in the first year of life.

infarct (in-**FARKT**) Area of cell death resulting from blockage of its blood supply.

infarction (in-**FARKT**-shun) Sudden blockage of an artery.

infect (in-**FEKT**) To invade an organism by a microorganism.

infection (in-**FEK**-shun) Invasion of the body by disease-producing microorganisms.

infectious (in-**FEK**-shus) Capable of being transmitted to a person; *or* a disease caused by the action of a microorganism.

inferior (in-**FEER**-ee-or) Situated below.

infertility (in-fer-**TIL**-ih-tee) Failure to conceive.

infestation (in-fes-**TAY**-shun) Act of being invaded on the skin by a troublesome other species, such as a parasite.

inflammation (in-flah-**MAY**-shun) A complex of cell and chemical reactions in response to an injury or a chemical or biologic agent.

inflammatory (in-**FLAM**-ah-tor-ee) Causing or affected by inflammation.

influenza (in-flew-**EN**-zah) An acute, viral infection of upper and lower respiratory tracts.

infusion (in-**FYU**-zhun) Introduction intravenously of a substance other than blood.

ingestion (in-**JES**-chun) Intake of food, either by mouth or through a nasogastric tube.

inguinal (**ING**-gwin-ahl) Pertaining to the groin.

inhale (**IN**-hail) Breathe in.

insanity (in-**SAN**-ih-tee) Nonmedical term for a person unable to be responsible for his or her actions.

insecticide (in-**SEK**-tih-side) Agent to destroy insects.

inseminate (in-**SEM**-ih-nate) To introduce semen into the vagina.

insemination (in-sem-ih-**NAY**-shun) The introduction of semen into the vagina.

insertion (in-**SIR**-shun) The insertion of a muscle is the attachment of a muscle to a more movable part of the skeleton, as distinct from the origin.

inspiration (in-spih-**RAY**-shun) Breathe in.

instability (in-stah-**BIL**-ih-tee) Abnormal tendency of a joint to partially or fully dislocate.

insufficiency (in-suh-**FISH**-en-see) Lack of completeness of function; for example, for a heart valve to fail to close properly.

insulin (**IN**-syu-lin) A hormone produced by the islet cells of the pancreas.

integument (in-**TEG**-you-ment) Organ system that covers the body, the skin being the main organ within the system.

integumentary (in-**TEG**-you-**MENT**-ah-ree) Pertaining to the covering of the body.

interatrial (**IN**-ter-**AY**-tree-al) Between the atria of the heart.

intercostal (**IN**-ter-**KOS**-tal) The space between two ribs.

intermittent (**IN**-ter-**MIT**-ent) Alternately ceasing and beginning again.

internist (in-**TER**-nist) A physician trained in internal medicine.

interosseous (in-ter-**OSS**-ee-us) A structure between bones; for example, muscles.

interphalangeal (**IN**-ter-fay-**LAN**-jee-al) Finger or toe joint between two phalanges.

interstitial (in-ter-**STISH**-al) Pertaining to spaces between cells in a tissue or organ.

interventricular (**IN**-ter-ven-**TRIK**-you-lar) Between the ventricles of the heart.

intervertebral (**IN**-ter-**VER**-teh-bral) The space between two vertebrae.

intestinal (in-**TESS**-tin-al) Pertaining to the intestine.

intestine (in-**TESS**-tin) The digestive tube from stomach to anus.

intolerance (in-**TOL**-er-ance) Inability of the small intestine to digest and dispose of a particular dietary substance.

intracellular (in-trah-**SELL**-you-lar) Within the cell.

intracranial (in-trah-**KRAY**-nee-al) Within the cranium (skull).

intradermal (in-trah-**DER**-mal) Within the epidermis.

intramuscular (in-trah-**MUSS**-kew-lar) Within the muscle.

intraocular (in-trah-**OCK**-you-lar) Pertaining to the inside of the eye.

intrathecal (**IN**-trah-**THEE**-kal) Within the subarachnoid or subdural space.

intrauterine (**IN**-trah-**YOU**-ter-ine) Inside the uterine cavity.

intravenous (**IN**-trah-**VEE**-nus) Through a vein.

intrinsic (in-**TRIN**-sik) Any muscle located entirely within (inside) the structure under consideration; for example, muscles inside the vocal cords or the eye.

intrinsic factor (in-**TRIN**-sik **FAK**-tor) Makes the absorption of vitamin B_{12} happen.

intubation (**IN**-tyu-**BAY**-shun) Insertion of a tube into the trachea.

intussusception (**IN**-tuss-sus-**SEP**-shun) The slipping of one part of the bowel inside another to cause obstruction.

inversion (in-**VER**-zhun) Turning inward.

invert (in-**VERT**) Turn inward.

involuntary (in-**VOL**-un-tay-ree) Not under control of the will.

involute (in-**VOH**-loot) Regressive changes in a tissue.

involution (in-voh-**LOO**-shun) Decrease in size.

iodine (**EYE**-oh-dine or **EYE**-oh-deen) Chemical element, the lack of which causes thyroid disease.

iris (**EYE**-ris) Colored portion of the eye with the pupil in its center.

irrigation (ih-rih-**GAY**-shun) Use of water to remove wax out of the external ear canal.

ischemia (is-**KEY**-me-ah) Lack of blood supply to tissue.

ischemic (is-**KEY**-mik) Pertaining to or affected by the lack of blood supply to tissue.

ischial (**IS**-key-al) Pertaining to the ischium.

ischium (**IS**-key-um) Lower and posterior part of the hip bone. Plural *ischia.*

Ishihara color system (ish-ee-**HAR**-ah) Test for color vision defects.

islet cells (**EYE**-let SELLZ) Hormone-secreting cells of the pancreas.

islets of Langerhans (**EYE**-lets of **LAHNG**-er-hahnz) Areas of pancreatic cells that produce insulin and glucagon. Also called *pancreatic islets.*

isotope (**I**-so-tope) Radioactive element used in diagnostic procedures.

J

Jaeger reading cards (**YA**-ger) Type of different sizes for testing near vision.

jaundice (**JAWN**-dis) Yellow staining of tissues with bile pigments, including bilirubin.

jejunal (je-**JEW**-nal) Pertaining to the jejeunum.

jejunum (je-**JEW**-num) Segment of small intestine between the duodenum and the ileum.

K

Kaposi sarcoma (kah-**POH**-see sar-**KOH**-mah) A skin cancer seen in AIDS patients.

keloid (**KEY**-loyd) Raised, irregular, lumpy scar due to excess collagen fiber production during healing of a wound.

keratin (**KER**-ah-tin) Protein found in the skin, nails, and hair.

keratoconjunctivitis (**KER**-ah-toe-con-**JUNGK**-tih-**VI**-tis) Inflammation of the cornea and conjunctiva.

keratomileusis (**KER**-ah-toe-my-**LOO**-sis) Cuts and shapes the cornea.

keratotomy (**KER**-ah-**TOT**-oh-mee) Incision in the cornea.

kernicterus (ker-**NICK**-ter-us) Bilirubin staining of the basal nuclei of the brain.

ketoacidosis (**KEY**-toe-ass-ih-**DOE**-sis) Excessive production of ketones, making the blood acid.

ketone (**KEY**-tone) Chemical formed in uncontrolled diabetes or in starvation.

ketosis (key-**TOE**-sis) Excess production of ketones.

kidney (**KID**-nee) Organ of excretion.

kyphosis (ki-**FOH**-sis) A normal posterior curve of the thoracic spine that can be exaggerated in disease.

kyphotic (ki-**FOT**-ik) Pertaining to or suffering from kyphosis.

L

labium (**LAY**-bee-um) Fold of the vulva. Plural *labia.*

labor (**LAY**-bore) Process of expulsion of the fetus.

labyrinth (**LAB**-ih-rinth) The inner ear.

labyrinthitis (**LAB**-ih-rin-**THI**-tis) Inflammation of the inner ear.

laceration (lass-eh-**RAY**-shun) A tear of the skin.

lacrimal (**LAK**-rim-al) Pertaining to tears; *or* bone that forms the medial wall of the orbit.

lactase (**LAK**-tase) Enzyme that breaks down lactose (milk sugar) to glucose and galactose.

lactate (**LAK**-tate) To produce milk.

lactation (lak-**TAY**-shun) Production of milk.

lacteal (**LAK**-tee-al) A lymphatic vessel carrying chyle away from the intestine.

lactiferous (lak-**TIF**-er-us) Pertaining to or yielding milk.

lactose (**LAK**-toes) The disaccharide found in cow's milk.

lanugo (la-**NYU**-go) Fine, soft hair on the fetal body.

laparoscope (**LAP**-ah-roh-skope) Instrument (endoscope) used for viewing the abdominal contents.

laparoscopic (**LAP**-ah-roh-**SKOP**-ik) Pertaining to laparoscopy.

laparoscopy (lap-ah-**ROS**-koh-pee) Examination of the contents of the abdomen using an endoscope.

laryngeal (lah-**RIN**-jee-al) Pertaining to the larynx.

laryngitis (lah-rin-**JEYE**-tis) Inflammation of the larynx.

laryngopharynx (lah-**RIN**-go-**FAH**-rinks) Region of the pharynx below the epiglottis that includes the larynx.

laryngoscope (lah-**RING**-oh-skope) Hollow tube with a light and camera used to visualize or operate on the larynx.

laryngotracheobronchitis (lah-**RING**-oh-**TRAY**-kee-oh-brong-**KIE**-tis) Inflammation of the larynx, trachea, and bronchi. Also called *croup.*

larynx (**LAH**-rinks) Organ of voice production.

laser surgery (**LAY**-zer **SUR**-jer-ee) Use of a concentrated, intense narrow beam of electromagnetic radiation for surgery.

lateral (**LAT**-er-al) Situated at the side of a structure.

latissimus dorsi (lah-**TISS**-ih-muss **DOOR**-sigh) The widest (broadest) muscle in the back.

leiomyoma (**LIE**-oh-my-**OH**-mah) Benign tumor derived from smooth muscle.

lens (LENZ) Transparent refractive structure behind the iris.

lentigo (len-**TIH**-go) Age spot; small, flat, brown-black spot in the skin of older people. Plural *lentigines.*

leptin (**LEP**-tin) Hormone secreted by adipose tissue.

lesion (**LEE**-zhun) Pathologic change or injury in a tissue.

lethargy (LETH-ar-jee) Abnormal drowsiness in depth, length, or time. Adj *lethargic.*

leukemia (loo-KEE-mee-ah) Disease when the blood is taken over by white blood cells and their precursors.

leukemic (loo-KEE-mik) Pertaining to or affected by leukemia.

leukocyte (LOO-koh-site) Another term for a white blood cell. Alternative spelling *leucocyte.*

leukocytosis (LOO-koh-sigh-TOE-sis) An excessive number of white blood cells.

leukopenia (loo-koh-PEE-nee-ah) A deficient number of white blood cells.

libido (lih-BEE-doh) Sexual desire.

life expectancy (LIFE eck-SPEK-tan-see) Statistical determination of the number of years an individual is expected to live.

life span (LIFE SPAN) The age that a person reaches.

ligament (LIG-ah-ment) Band of fibrous tissue connecting two structures.

limbic (LIM-bic) Array of nerve fibers surrounding the thalamus.

linear fracture (LIN-ee-ar FRAK-chur) A fracture running parallel to the length of the bone.

lipase (LIE-paze) Enzyme that breaks down fat.

lipectomy (lip-ECK-toe-me) Surgical removal of adipose tissue.

lipid (LIP-id) General term for all types of fatty compounds; for example, cholesterol, triglycerides, and fatty acids.

lipoprotein (LIP-oh-pro-teen) Bonding of molecules of fat and protein.

liposuction (LIP-oh-suck-shun) Surgical removal of adipose tissue using suction.

lithotripsy (LITH-oh-trip-see) Crushing stones by sound waves.

lithotripter (LITH-oh-trip-ter) Machine that generates sound waves.

liver (LIV-er) Body's largest organ, located in the right upper quadrant of the abdomen.

lobar (LOW-bar) Pertaining to a lobe.

lobe (LOBE) Subdivision of an organ or other part.

lobectomy (low-BECK-toe-me) Surgical removal of a lobe.

lochia (LOW-kee-uh) Vaginal discharge following childbirth.

longevity (lon-JEV-ih-tee) Duration of life beyond the normal expectation.

Loop of Henle (LOOP of HEN-lee) Part of the renal tubule where reabsorption occurs.

lordosis (lore-DOH-sis) A normal forward curvature of the lumbar spine that can be exaggerated in disease.

lordotic (lore-DOT-ik) Pertaining to or suffering from lordosis.

louse (LOWSE) Parasitic insect. Plural *lice.*

lumbar (LUM-bar) Region in the back and sides between the ribs and pelvis.

lumen (LOO-men) The interior space of a tubelike structure.

lumpectomy (lump-ECK-toe-me) Removal of a lesion with preservation of surrounding tissue.

luteal (LOO-tee-al) Pertaining to a corpus luteum.

lutein (LOO-tee-in) Yellow pigment.

luteum (LOO-tee-um) Corpus luteum is the yellow (lutein) body formed after an ovarian follicle ruptures.

lymph (LIMF) A clear fluid collected from body tissues and transported by lymph vessels to the venous circulation.

lymphadenectomy (lim-FAD-eh-NECK-toe-me) Surgical excision of a lymph node(s).

lymphadenitis (lim-FAD-eh-neye-tis) Inflammation of a lymph node(s).

lymphadenopathy (lim-FAD-eh-NOP-ah-thee) Any disease process affecting a lymph node.

lymphangiogram (lim-FAN-jee-oh-gram) Radiographic images of lymph vessels and nodes following injection of contrast material.

lymphatic (lim-FAT-ic) Pertaining to lymph or the lymphatic system.

lymphedema (LIMF-eh-DEE-mah) Tissue swelling due to lymphatic obstruction.

lymphocyte (LIM-foh-site) Small white blood cell with a large nucleus.

lymphoid (LIM-foyd) Resembling lymphatic tissue.

lymphoma (lim-FOH-mah) Any neoplasm of lymphatic tissue.

M

macrocyte (MACK-roh-site) Large red blood cell.

macrocytic (mack-roh-SIT-ik) Pertaining to a macrocyte.

macrophage (MACK-roh-fayj) Large white blood cell that removes bacteria, foreign particles, and dead cells.

macula lutea (MACK-you-lah LOO-tee-ah) Yellowish spot on the back of the retina; contains the fovea centralis.

macule (MACK-yul) Small, flat spot or patch on the skin.

majus (MAY-jus) Bigger or greater; for example, labium majus. Plural *majora.*

malabsorption (mal-ab-SORP-shun) Inadequate gastrointestinal absorption of nutrients.

malformation (MAL-for-MAY-shun) Failure of proper or normal development.

malfunction (mal-FUNK-shun) Inadequate or abnormal function.

malignancy (mah-LIG-nan-see) State of being malignant.

malignant (mah-LIG-nant) Tumor that invades surrounding tissues and metastasizes to distant organs.

malleus (MAL-ee-us) Outer (lateral) one of the three ossicles in the middle ear; shaped like a hammer.

malnutrition (mal-nyu-TRISH-un) Inadequate nutrition from poor diet or inadequate absorption of nutrients.

malunion (mal-YOU-nee-un) The two bony ends of a fracture fail to heal together in the correct position.

mammary (MAM-ah-ree) Relating to the lactating breast.

mammogram (MAM-oh-gram) The record produced by X-ray imaging of the breast.

mammography (mah-MOG-rah-fee) The process of X-ray examination of the breast.

mammoplasty (MAM-oh-plas-tee) Surgical reshaping of the breast.

mandible (MAN-di-bel) Lower jawbone.

mandibular (man-DIB-you-lar) Pertaining to the mandible.

mania (MAY-nee-ah) Mood disorder with hyperactivity, irritability, and rapid speech.

manic (MAN-ik) Pertaining to or suffering from mania.

marrow (MAH-roe) Fatty, blood-forming tissue in the cavities of long bones.

mastalgia (mass-TAL-jee-uh) Pain in the breast.

mastectomy (mass-TECK-toe-me) Surgical excision of the breast.

masticate (MASS-tih-kate) To chew.

mastication (mass-tih-KAY-shun) The process of chewing.

mastitis (mass-TIE-tis) Inflammation of the breast.

mastoid (MASS-toyd) Small bony protrusion immediately behind the ear.

maternal (mah-TER-nal) Pertaining to or derived from the mother.

matrix (MAY-triks) Substance that surrounds and protects cells, is manufactured by the cells, and holds them together.

maturation (mat-you-RAY-shun) Process to achieve full development.

mature (mah-TYUR) Fully developed.

maxilla (mak-SILL-ah) Upper jawbone, containing right and left maxillary sinuses.

maxillary (MAK-sih-lair-ee) Pertaining to the maxilla.

maximus (MAKS-ih-mus) The gluteus maximus muscle is the largest muscle in the body, covering a large part of each buttock.

meatal (me-AY-tal) Pertaining to a meatus.

meatus (me-AY-tus) The external opening of a passage.

meconium (meh-KOH-nee-um) The first bowel movement of the newborn.

medial (ME-dee-al) Nearer to the middle of the body.

mediastinal (ME-dee-ass-TIE-nal) Pertaining to the mediastinum.

mediastinoscopy (ME-dee-ass-tih-NOS-koh-pee) Examination of the mediastinum using an endoscope.

mediastinum (ME-dee-ass-TIE-num) Area between the lungs containing the heart, aorta, venae cavae, esophagus, and trachea.

medius (ME-dee-us) The gluteus medius muscle is partly covered by the gluteus maximus.

medulla (meh-DULL-ah) Central portion of a structure surrounded by cortex.

medulla oblongata (meh-DULL-ah ob-lon-GAH-tah) Most posterior subdivision of the brainstem; continuation of the spinal cord.

medullary (MED-ul-ah-ree) Pertaining to a medulla.

meiosis (my-OH-sis) Two rapid cell divisions, resulting in half the number of chromosomes.

melanin (MEL-ah-nin) Black pigment found in the skin, hair, and retina.

melanoma (mel-ah-NO-mah) Malignant neoplasm formed from cells that produce melanin.

melatonin (mel-ah-TONE-in) Hormone formed by the pineal gland.

melena (mel-EN-ah) The passage of black, tarry stools.

membrane (MEM-brain) Thin layer of tissue covering a structure or cavity.

membranous (MEM-brah-nus) Pertaining to a membrane.

menarche (meh-NAR-key) First menstrual period.

Ménière disease (men-YEAR diz-EEZ) Disorder of the inner ear with acute attacks of tinnitus, vertigo, and hearing loss.

meninges (meh-NIN-jeez) Three-layered covering of the brain and spinal cord.

meningitis (men-in-JIE-tis) Inflammation of the meninges.

meningocele (meh-NIN-goh-seal) Protrusion of the meninges from the spinal cord or brain through a defect in the vertebral column or cranium.

meningococcal (meh-NING-goh-KOK-al) Pertaining to the *meningococcus* bacterium.

meningomyelocele (meh-nin-goh-MY-el-oh-seal) Protrusion of the spinal cord and meninges through a defect in the vertebral arch of one or more vertebrae.

meniscectomy (MEN-ih-SEK-toh-me) Excision (cutting out) of all or part of a meniscus.

meniscus (meh-NISS-kuss) Disc of cartilage between the bones of a joint; for example, in the knee joint. Plural *menisci.*

menopausal (MEN-oh-pawz-al) Pertaining to the menopause.

menopause (MEN-oh-pawz) Permanent ending of menstrual periods.

menorrhagia (men-oh-RAY-jee-ah) Excessive menstrual bleeding.

menses (MEN-seez) Monthly uterine bleeding.

menstrual (MEN-stru-al) Pertaining to menstruation.

menstruate (MEN-stru-ate) The act of menstruation.

menstruation (men-stru-AY-shun) Synonym of *menses.*

mesentery (MESS-en-ter-ree) A double layer of peritoneum enclosing the abdominal viscera.

metabolic (met-ah-BOL-ik) Pertaining to metabolism.

metabolic acidosis (met-ah-BOL-ik ass-ih-DOE-sis) Decreased pH in the blood and body tissues as a result of an upset in metabolism.

metabolism (meh-TAB-oh-lizm) The constantly changing physical and chemical processes occurring in the cell that are the sum of anabolism and catabolism.

metacarpal (MET-ah-KAR-pal) The five bones between the carpus and the fingers.

metacarpophalangeal (MET-ah-KAR-poh-fay-LAN-jee-al) The articulations (joints) between the metacarpal bones and the phalanges.

metastasis (meh-TAS-tah-sis) Spread of a disease from one part of the body to another. Plural *metastases.*

metastasize (meh-TAS-tah-size) To spread to distant parts.

metastatic (meh-tah-STAT-ik) Pertaining to the character of cells that can metastasize.

metatarsal (MET-ah-TAR-sal) Pertaining to the metatarsus.

metatarsus (MET-ah-TAR-sus) The five parallel bones of the foot between the tarsus and the phalanges.

metrorrhagia (MEH-troh-RAY-jee-ah) Irregular uterine bleeding between menses.

microbe (MY-krohb) Short for *microorganism.*

microcephalic (MY-kroh-seh-FAL-ik) Pertaining to or suffering from a small head.

microcephaly (MY-kroh-SEF-ah-lee) An abnormally small head.

microcyte (MY-kroh-site) Small red blood cell.

microcytic (my-kroh-SIT-ik) Pertaining to a small cell.

microorganism (MY-kroh-OR-gan-izm) Any organism too small to be seen by the naked eye.

microscope (MY-kroh-skope) Instrument for viewing something small that cannot be seen in detail by the naked eye.

microscopic (MY-kroh-SKOP-ik) Visible only with the aid of a microscope.

micturate (**MIK**-choo-rate) Pass urine.

micturition (mik-choo-**RISH**-un) Act of passing urine.

migraine (**MY**-grain) Paroxysmal severe headache confined to one side of the head.

mineral (**MIN**-er-al) Inorganic compound usually found in the earth's crust.

mineralocorticoid (**MIN**-er-al-oh-**KOR**-tih-koyd) Hormone of the adrenal cortex that influences sodium and potassium metabolism.

minimus (**MIN**-ih-mus) The gluteus minimus is the smallest of the gluteal muscles and lies under the gluteus medius.

minus (**MY**-nus) Smaller or lesser; for example, labium minus. Plural *minora.*

miosis (my-**OH**-sis) Constriction of the pupil.

mitochondrion (my-toe-**KON**-dree-on) Organelle that generates, stores, and releases energy for cell activities. Plural *mitochondria.*

mitosis (my-**TOE**-sis) Cell division that creates two identical cells, each with 46 chromosomes.

mitral (**MY**-tral) Shaped like the headdress of a Catholic bishop.

modify (**MOD**-ih-fie) Change the form or qualities of something.

molar (**MO**-lar) One of six teeth in each jaw that grind food.

mole (MOLE) Benign localized area of melanin-producing cells.

molecule (**MOLL**-eh-kyul) Very small particle.

molluscum contagiosum (moh-**LUS**-kum kon-**TAY**-jee-**OH**-sum) STD caused by a virus.

monocyte (**MON**-oh-site) Large white blood cell with a single nucleus.

mononeuropathy (**MON**-oh-nyu-**ROP**-ah-thee) Disorder affecting a single nerve.

mononucleosis (**MON**-oh-nyu-klee-**OH**-sis) Presence of large numbers of specific, diagnostic mononuclear leukocytes.

monoplegia (**MON**-oh-**PLEE**-jee-ah) Paralysis of one limb.

monoplegic (**MON**-oh-**PLEE**-jik) Pertaining to or suffering from monoplegia.

mons pubis (MONZ **PYU**-bis) Fleshy pad with pubic hair, overlying the pubic bone.

morbidity (mor-**BID**-ih-tee) The frequency of the appearance of a disease.

morphine (**MOR**-feen) Derivative of opium used as an analgesic or sedative.

mortality (mor-**TAL**-ih-tee) Death rate.

motile (**MOH**-til) Capable of spontaneous movement.

motility (moh-**TILL**-ih-tee) The ability for spontaneous movement.

motor (**MOH**-tor) Structures of the nervous system that send impulses out to cause muscles to contract or glands to secrete.

mouth (MOWTH) External opening of a cavity or canal.

mucin (**MYU**-sin) Protein element of mucus.

mucocutaneous (**MYU**-koh-kyu-**TAY**-nee-us) Junction of skin and mucous membrane; for example, the lips.

mucolytic (**MYU**-koh-**LIT**-ik) Agent capable of dissolving or liquefying mucus.

mucosa (myu-**KOH**-sah) Lining of a tubular structure that secretes mucus. Another name for *mucous membrane.*

mucous (**MYU**-kus) Pertaining to mucus or the mucosa.

mucus (**MYU**-kus) Sticky secretion of cells in mucous membranes.

multipara (mul-**TIP**-ah-ruh) Woman who has given birth to two or more children.

murmur (**MUR**-mur) Abnormal heart sound heard with a stethoscope when a valve closes or opens abnormally.

muscle (**MUSS**-el) A tissue consisting of contractile cells.

musculoskeletal (**MUSS**-kyu-loh-**SKEL**-eh-tal) Pertaining to the muscles and the bony skeleton.

mutation (myu-**TAY**-shun) Change in the chemistry of a gene.

mute (MYUT) Unable or unwilling to speak.

mutism (**MYU**-tizm) Absence of speech.

myasthenia gravis (my-as-**THEE**-nee-ah **GRA**-vis) Disorder of fluctuating muscle weakness.

mydriasis (mih-**DRY**-ah-sis) Dilation of the pupil.

myelin (**MY**-eh-lin) Material of the sheath around the axon of a nerve.

myelitis (**MY**-eh-**LIE**-tis) Inflammation of the spinal cord.

myelocele (**MY**-eh-low-seal) Protrusion of the spinal cord through a defect in the vertebral arch.

myelomeningocele (**MY**-eh-low-meh-**NING**-oh-seal) Protrusion of the spinal cord and meninges through a defect in the vertebral arch of one or more vertebrae.

myocardial (my-oh-**KAR**-dee-al) Pertaining to heart muscle.

myocarditis (**MY**-oh-kar-**DIE**-tis) Inflammation of the heart muscle.

myocardium (my-oh-**KAR**-dee-um) All the heart muscle.

myoma (my-**OH**-mah) Benign tumor of muscle.

myomectomy (my-oh-**MEK**-toe-me) Surgical removal of a myoma (fibroid).

myometrium (my-oh-**MEE**-tree-um) Muscle wall of the uterus.

myopathy (my-**OP**-ah-thee) Any disease of muscle.

myopia (my-**OH**-pee-ah) Able to see close objects but unable to see distant objects.

myositis (my-oh-**SIGH**-tis) Inflammation of muscle tissue.

myringotomy (mir-in-**GOT**-oh-me) Incision in the tympanic membrane.

myxedema (miks-eh-**DEE**-muh) Nonpitting, waxy edema of the skin in hypothyroidism.

N

narcissism (**NAR**-sih-sizm) A state of relating everything to oneself.

narcissistic (**NAR**-sih-**SIS**-tik) Relating everything to oneself.

narcolepsy (**NAR**-koh-lep-see) Involuntary falling asleep.

narcotic (nar-**KOT**-ik) Drug derived from opium or any drug with effects similar to those of opium derivatives.

nares (**NAH**-rees) Nostril. Plural *nares.*

nasal (**NAY**-zal) Pertaining to the nose.

nasogastric (**NAY**-zoh-**GAS**-trik) Pertaining to the nose and stomach.

nasolacrimal duct (**NAY**-zoh-**LAK**-rim-al DUKT) Passage from the lacrimal sac to the nose.

nasopharyngeal (**NAY**-zoh-fah-**RIN**-jee-al) Pertaining to the nasopharynx.

nasopharynx (NAY-zoh-**FAH**-rinks) Region of the pharynx at the back of the nose and above the soft palate.

natal (NAY-tal) Pertaining to birth.

nebulizer (**NEB**-you-liz-er) Device used to deliver liquid medicine in a fine mist.

necrosis (neh-**KROH**-sis) Pathologic death of cells or tissue.

necrotic (neh-**KROT**-ik) Pertaining to or affected by necrosis.

necrotizing fasciitis (neh-kroh-**TIZE**-ing fash-ee-**EYE**-tis) Inflammation of fascia producing death of the tissue.

neonatal (NEE-oh-**NAY**-tal) Pertaining to the newborn infant or the newborn period.

neonate (NEE-oh-nate) A newborn infant.

neonatologist (NEE-oh-nay-**TOL**-oh-jist) Medical specialist in disorders of the newborn.

nephrectomy (nef-**REK**-toe-me) Surgical removal of a kidney.

nephritis (nef-**RY**-tis) Inflammation of the kidney.

nephroblastoma (NEF-roh-blas-**TOE**-mah) Cancerous kidney tumor of childhood. Also known as *Wilms tumor.*

nephrolithiasis (NEF-roe-lih-**THIGH**-ah-sis) Presence of a kidney stone.

nephrolithotomy (NEF-roe-lih-**THOT**-oh-me) Incision for removal of a kidney stone.

nephrologist (nef-**ROL**-oh-jist) Medical specialist in disorders of the kidney.

nephrology (nef-**ROL**-oh-jee) Medical specialty of diseases of the kidney.

nephron (NEF-ron) Filtration unit of the kidney; glomerulus + renal tubule.

nephropathy (nef-**ROP**-ah-thee) Any disease of the kidney.

nephroscope (NEF-roe-skope) Endoscope to view the inside of the kidney.

nephroscopy (nef-**ROS**-koh-pee) To examine the kidney.

nephrosis (nef-**ROH**-sis) Same as *nephrotic syndrome.*

nephrotic syndrome (nef-**ROT**-ik **SIN**-drome) Glomerular disease with marked loss of protein. Also called *nephrosis.*

nerve (NERV) A cord of nerve fibers bound together by connective tissue.

nervous (**NER**-vus) Pertaining to a nerve or the nervous system; *or* easily excited or agitated.

nervous system (**NER**-vus **SIS**-tem) The whole, integrated nerve apparatus.

neural (**NYU**-ral) Pertaining to nervous tissue.

neuralgia (nyu-**RAL**-jee-ah) Pain in the distribution of a nerve.

neuroglia (nyu-**ROG**-lee-ah) Connective tissue holding nervous tissue together.

neurohypophysis (NYU-roh-high-**POF**-ih-sis) Posterior lobe of the pituitary gland.

neurologic (NYU-roh-**LOJ**-ik) Pertaining to the nervous sytem.

neurologist (nyu-**ROL**-oh-jist) Medical specialist in disorders of the nervous system.

neurology (nyu-**ROL**-oh-jee) Medical specialty of disorders of the nervous system.

neuroma (nyu-**ROH**-mah) Any tumor arising from cells in the nervous system.

neuromuscular (NYU-roh-**MUSS**-kyu-lar) A junction where a nerve supplies muscle tissue.

neuron (**NYU**-ron) Technical term for a nerve cell; consists of the cell body with its dendrites and axons.

neuropathy (nyu-**ROP**-ah-thee) Any disorder affecting the nervous system.

neurosurgeon (NYU-roh-**SUR**-jun) One who operates on the nervous system.

neurosurgery (NYU-roh-**SUR**-jer-ee) Operating on the nervous system.

neurotoxin (NYU-roh-tock-sin) Agent that poisons the nervous system.

neurotransmitter (NYU-roh-trans-**MIT**-er) Chemical agent that relays messages from one nerve cell to the next.

neutropenia (NEW-troh-**PEE**-nee-ah) A deficiency of neutrophils.

neutrophil (**NEW**-troh-fill) A neutrophil's granules take up (purple) stain equally, whether the stain is acid or alkaline.

neutrophilia (NEW-troh-**FILL**-ee-ah) An increase in neutrophils.

nevus (**NEE**-vus) Congenital lesion of the skin. Plural *nevi.*

nipple (**NIP**-el) Projection from the breast into which the lactiferous ducts open.

nitrite (**NI**-trite) Chemical formed in urine by *E. coli* and other microorganisms.

nitrogenous (ni-**TRO**-jen-us) Containing or generating nitrogen.

nocturia (nok-**TYU**-ree-ah) Excessive urination at night.

node (NOHD) A circumscribed mass of tissue.

norepinephrine (**NOR**-ep-ih-**NEFF**-rin) Catecholamine hormone of the adrenal gland that is a parasympathetic neurotransmitter. Also called *noradrenaline.*

nosocomial (noh-soh-**KOH**-mee-al) Acquired while in the hospital.

nuchal cord (**NYU**-kul KORD) Loop(s) of umbilical cord around the fetal neck.

nuclear (**NYU**-klee-ar) Pertaining to a nucleus.

nucleolus (nyu-**KLEE**-oh-lus) Small mass within the nucleus.

nucleus (**NYU**-klee-us) Functional center of a cell or structure.

nutrient (**NYU**-tree-ent) A substance in food required for normal physiologic function.

nutrition (nyu-**TRISH**-un) The study of food and liquid requirements for normal function of the human body.

nystagmus (nis-**TAG**-mus) Fast uncontrollable movements of the eye in any direction.

O

obesity (oh-**BEE**-sih-tee) Excessive amount of fat in the body.

oblique fracture (ob-**LEEK FRAK**-chur) A diagonal fracture across the long axis of the bone.

obsession (ob-**SESH**-un) Persistent, recurrent, uncontrollable thoughts or impulses.

obsessive (ob-**SES**-iv) Possessing persistent, recurrent, uncontrollable thoughts or impulses.

obstetrician (ob-steh-**TRISH**-un) Medical specialist in obstetrics.

obstetrics (OB) (ob-**STET**-ricks) Medical specialty for the care of women during pregnancy and the postpartum period.

occipital (ock-**SIP**-it-al) The back of the skull.

occipital lobe (ock-**SIP**-it-al LOBE) Posterior area of the cerebral hemispheres.

occlude (oh-**KLUDE**) To close, plug, or completely obstruct.

occlusion (oh-**KLU**-zhun) A complete obstruction.

occult (oh-**KULT**) Not visible on the surface, hidden.

occult blood (oh-**KULT** BLUD) Blood that cannot be seen in the stool but is positive on a fecal occult blood test.

occupational (**OCK**-you-**PAY**-shun-al) A disorder resulting from exposure to an agent during performance of one's work.

ocular (**OCK**-you-lar) Pertaining to the eye.

olfaction (ol-**FAK**-shun) Sense of smell.

olfactory (ol-**FAK**-toh-ree) Related to the sense of smell.

oligohydramnios (**OL**-ih-goh-high-**DRAM**-nee-os) Too little amniotic fluid.

oligospermia (**OL**-ih-go-**SPER**-me-ah) Too few sperm in the semen.

oliguria (ol-ih-**GYUR**-ee-ah) Scanty production of urine.

omentum (oh-**MEN**-tum) Membrane that encloses the bowels.

onychomycosis (oh-nih-koh-my-**KOH**-sis) Condition of a fungus infection in a nail.

oocyte (**OH**-oh-site) Female egg cell.

oogenesis (oh-oh-**JEN**-eh-sis) Development of a female egg cell.

open fracture (**OH**-pen **FRAK**-chur) The skin over the fracture is broken.

ophthalmia neonatorum (off-**THAL**-me-ah ne-oh-nay-**TOR**-um) Conjunctivitis of the newborn.

ophthalmic (off-**THAL**-mik) Pertaining to the eye.

ophthalmologist (off-thal-**MALL**-oh-jist) Medical specialist in ophthalmology.

ophthalmology (off-thal-**MALL**-oh-jee) Diagnosis and treatment of diseases of the eye.

ophthalmoscope (off-**THAL**-moh-skope) Instrument for viewing the retina.

ophthalmoscopic (**OFF**-thal-moh-**SKOP**-ik) Pertaining to the use of an ophthalmoscope.

ophthalmoscopy (**OFF**-thal-**MOS**-koh-pee) The process of viewing the retina.

opiate (**OH**-pee-ate) A drug derived from opium.

opportunistic (**OP**-or-tyu-**NIS**-tik) An organism or a disease in a host with lowered resistance.

opportunistic infection (**OP**-or-tyu-**NIS**-tik in-**FEK**-shun) An infection that causes disease when the immune system is compromised for other reasons.

optic (**OP**-tik) The eye or vision; *or* second (II) cranial nerve, which carries visual information.

optical (**OP**-tih-kal) Pertaining to the eye or vision.

optometrist (op-**TOM**-eh-trist) Someone skilled in the measurement of vision but who cannot treat eye diseases or prescribe medication.

optometry (op-**TOM**-eh-tree) The profession of the measurement of vision.

oral (**OR**-al) Pertaining to the mouth.

orbit (**OR**-bit) The bony socket that holds the eyeball.

orbital (**OR**-bit-al) Pertaining to the orbit.

orchiectomy (or-key-**ECK**-toe-me) Removal of one or both testes.

orchiopexy (**OR**-key-oh-**PEK**-see) Surgical fixation of a testis in the scrotum.

orchitis (or-**KIE**-tis) Inflammation of the testis. Also called *epididymoorchitis.*

organ (**OR**-gan) Structure with specific functions in a body system.

organelle (**OR**-gah-nell) Part of a cell having specialized function(s).

organism (**OR**-gan-izm) Any whole, living individual animal or plant.

orifice (**OR**-ih-fis) Any opening or aperture.

origin (**OR**-ih-gin) Fixed source of a muscle at its attachment to bone.

oropharyngeal (**OR**-oh-fah-**RIN**-jee-al) Pertaining to the oropharynx.

oropharynx (**OR**-oh-**FAH**-rinks) Region at the back of the mouth between the soft palate and the tip of the epiglottis.

orthopedic (or-tho-**PEE**-dik) Pertaining to the correction and cure of deformities and diseases of the musculoskeletal system; originally, most of the deformities treated were in children. Also spelled *orthopaedic.*

orthopedist (or-tho-**PEE**-dist) Specialist in orthopedics.

orthopnea (or-**THOP**-nee-ah) Difficulty in breathing when lying flat.

orthopneic (or-**THOP**-nee-ik) Pertaining to or affected by orthopnea.

orthotic (or-**THOT**-ik) Orthopedic appliance to correct an abnormality.

orthotist (or-**THOT**-ist) Maker and fitter of orthopedic appliances.

os (OSS) Opening into a canal; for example, the cervix.

ossicle (**OSS**-ih-kel) A small bone, particularly relating to the three bones in the middle ear.

osteoarthritis (**OSS**-tee-oh-ar-**THRI**-tis) Chronic inflammatory disease of the joints, with pain and loss of function.

osteoblast (**OSS**-tee-oh-blast) Bone-forming cell.

osteocalcin (**OSS**-tee-oh-**KAL**-sin) A hormone produced by bone cells.

osteocyte (**OSS**-tee-oh-site) A bone-maintaining cell.

osteogenesis imperfecta (**OSS**-tee-oh-**JEN**-eh-sis im-per-**FEK**-tah) Inherited condition when bone formation is incomplete, leading to fragile, easily broken bones.

osteogenic sarcoma (**OSS**-tee-oh-**JEN**-ik sar-**KOH**-mah) Malignant tumor originating in bone-producing cells.

osteomalacia (**OSS**-tee-oh-mah-**LAY**-she-ah) Soft, flexible bones lacking in calcium (rickets).

osteomyelitis (**OSS**-tee-oh-my-eh-**LIE**-tis) Inflammation of bone tissue.

osteopath (**OSS**-tee-oh-path) Practitioner of osteopathy.

osteopathy (**OSS**-tee-**OP**-ah-thee) Medical practice based on maintaining the balance of the body.

osteopenia (**OSS**-tee-oh-**PEE**-nee-ah) Decreased calcification of bone.

osteoporosis (**OSS**-tee-oh-poh-**ROE**-sis) Condition in which the bones become more porous, brittle, and fragile and more likely to fracture.

ostomy (**OSS**-toe-me) Artificial opening into a tubular structure.

otitis media (oh-**TIE**-tis **ME**-dee-ah) Inflammation of the middle ear.

otolith (**OH**-toe-lith) A calcium particle in the vestibule of the inner ear.

otologist (oh-**TOL**-oh-jist) Medical specialist in diseases of the ear.

otology (oh-**TOL**-oh-jee) Study of the function and diseases of the ear.

otorhinolaryngologist (oh-toe-rye-no-lah-rin-**GOL**-oh-jist) Ear, nose, and throat medical specialist.

otosclerosis (**OH**-toe-sklair-**OH**-sis) Hardening at the junction of the stapes and oval window that causes loss of hearing.

otoscope (**OH**-toe-skope) Instrument for examining the ear.

otoscopic (**OH**-toe-**SKOP**-ik) Pertaining to examination with an otoscope.

otoscopy (oh-**TOS**-koh-pee) Examination of the ear.

ovarian (oh-**VAIR**-ee-an) Pertaining to the ovary(ies).

ovary (**OH**-vah-ree) One of the paired female egg-producing glands. Plural *ovaries.*

ovulate (**OV**-you-late) Release the oocyte from a follicle.

ovulation (**OV**-you-**LAY**-shun) Release of an oocyte from a follicle.

ovum (**OH**-vum) Egg. Also called *oocyte.* Plural *ova.*

oxygen (**OCK**-see-jen) The gas essential for life.

oxyhemoglobin (**OCK**-see-he-moh-**GLOW**-bin) Hemoglobin in combination with oxygen.

oxytocin (**OCK**-see-**TOE**-sin) Pituitary hormone that stimulates the uterus to contract.

P

pacemaker (**PACE**-may-ker) Device that regulates cardiac electrical activity.

palate (**PAL**-ate) Roof of the mouth.

palatine (**PAL**-ah-tine) Bone that forms the hard palate and parts of the nose and orbits.

palliative care (**PAL**-ee-ah-tiv KAIR) To relieve symptoms and pain without curing.

pallor (**PAL**-or) Paleness of the skin.

palm (PAHLM) Flat or anterior surface of the hand.

palmar (**PAHL**-mar) Pertaining to the palm.

palpate (**PAL**-pate) To examine with the fingers and hands.

palpation (pal-**PAY**-shun) Examination with the fingers and hands.

palpitation (pal-pih-**TAY**-shun) Forcible, rapid beat of the heart felt by the patient.

palsy (**PAWL**-zee) Paralysis or paresis from brain damage.

pancreas (**PAN**-kree-as) Lobulated gland, the head of which is tucked into the curve of the duodenum.

pancreatic (**PAN**-kree-**AT**-ik) Pertaining to the pancreas.

pancreatic islets (pan-kree-**AT**-ik **EYE**-lets) Areas of pancreatic cells that produce insulin and glucagon. Also called *islets of Langerhans.*

pancreatitis (**PAN**-kree-ah-**TIE**-tis) Inflammation of the pancreas.

pancytopenia (**PAN**-site-oh-**PEE**-nee-ah) Deficiency of all types of blood cells.

pandemic (pan-**DEM**-ik) Pertaining to a disease attacking the population of a very large area.

panendoscopy (pan-en-**DOS**-koh-pee) A visual examination of the inside of the esophagus, stomach, and upper duodenum using a flexible fiber-optic endoscope.

panhypopituitarism (pan-**HIGH**-poh-pih-**TYU**-ih-tah-rizm) Deficiency of all the pituitary hormones.

Pap test (PAP) Examination of cells taken from the cervix.

papilla (pah-**PILL**-ah) Any small projection. Plural *papillae.*

papilledema (pah-pill-eh-**DEE**-mah) Swelling of the optic disc in the retina.

papillomavirus (pap-ih-**LOH**-mah-vi-rus) Virus that causes warts and is associated with cancer.

papule (**PAP**-yul) Small, circumscribed elevation on the skin.

para (**PAH**-rah) Abbreviation for number of deliveries.

paralysis (pah-**RAL**-ih-sis) Loss of voluntary movement.

paralytic (par-ah-**LYT**-ik) Suffering from paralysis.

paralyze (**PAR**-ah-lyze) To make incapable of movement.

paranasal (**PAR**-ah-**NAY**-zal) Adjacent to the nose.

paranoia (par-ah-**NOY**-ah) Presence of persecutory delusions.

paranoid (**PAR**-ah-noyd) Having delusions of persecution.

paraphimosis (**PAR**-ah-fih-**MOH**-sis) Condition in which a retracted prepuce cannot be pulled forward to cover the glans.

paraplegia (par-ah-**PLEE**-jee-ah) Paralysis of both lower extremities.

paraplegic (par-ah-**PLEE**-jik) Pertaining to or suffering from paraplegia.

parasite (**PAR**-ah-site) An organism that attaches itself to, lives on or in, and derives its nutrition from another species.

parasitic (par-ah-**SIT**-ik) Pertaining to a parasite.

parasympathetic (par-ah-sim-pah-**THET**-ik) Division of the autonomic nervous system; has opposite effects of the sympathetic division.

parathyroid (par-ah-**THIGH**-royd) Endocrine glands embedded in the back of the thyroid gland.

paraurethral (**PAR**-ah-you-**REE**-thral) Situated around the urethra.

parenchyma (pah-**RENG**-kih-mah) Characteristic functional cells of a gland or organ that are supported by the connective tissue framework.

parenteral (pah-**REN**-ter-al) Giving medication by any means other than the gastrointestinal tract.

paresis (par-**EE**-sis) Partial paralysis (weakness).

paresthesia (par-es-**THEE**-ze-ah) An abnormal sensation; for example, tingling, burning, prickling. Plural *parasthesias.*

parietal (pah-**RYE**-eh-tal) Pertaining to the outer layer of the pericardium and the wall of any body cavity; *or* the two bones forming the sidewalls and roof of the cranium.

parietal lobe (pah-**RYE**-eh-tal LOBE) Area of the brain under the parietal bone.

Parkinson disease (**PAR**-kin-son diz-**EEZ**) Disease of muscular rigidity, tremors, and a masklike facial expression.

paronychia (par-oh-**NICK**-ee-ah) Infection alongside the nail.

parotid (pah-**ROT**-id) Parotid gland is the salivary gland beside the ear.

paroxysmal (par-ock-**SIZ**-mal) Occurring in sharp, spasmodic episodes.

particle (**PAR**-tih-kul) A small piece of matter.

particulate (par-**TIK**-you-late) Relating to a fine particle.

passive (**PASS**-iv) Not active.

patella (pah-**TELL**-ah) Thin, circular bone in front of the knee joint and embedded in the patellar tendon. Also called *kneecap.* Plural *patellae.*

patellar (pah-**TELL**-ar) Pertaining to the patella.

patent (**PAY**-tent) Open.

patent ductus arteriosus (**PAY**-tent **DUK**-tus ar-ter-ee-**OH**-sus) An open, direct channel between the aorta and the pulmonary artery.

pathogen (**PATH**-oh-jen) A disease-causing microorganism.

pathogenic (path-oh-**JEN**-ik) Causing disease.

pathologic fracture (path-oh-**LOJ**-ik **FRAK**-chur) Fracture occurring at a site already weakened by a disease process, such as cancer.

pathologist (pa-**THOL**-oh-jist) A specialist in pathology.

pathology (pa-**THOL**-oh-jee) Medical specialty dealing with the structural and functional changes of a disease process or the cause, development, and structural changes in disease.

pectoral (**PEK**-tor-al) Pertaining to the chest.

pectoral girdle (**PEK**-tor-al **GIR**-del) Incomplete bony ring that attaches the upper limb to the axial skeleton.

pectoralis (**PEK**-tor-ah-lis) Pertaining to the chest.

pedal (**PEED**-al) Pertaining to the foot.

pediatrician (**PEE**-dee-ah-**TRISH**-an) Medical specialist in pediatrics.

pediatrics (pee-dee-**AT**-riks) Medical specialty of treating children during development from birth through adolescence.

pediculosis (peh-dick-you-**LOH**-sis) An infestation with lice.

peer (PEER) A person at the same level or standing.

pelvic (**PEL**-vik) Pertaining to the pelvis.

pelvis (**PEL**-viss) A basin-shaped ring of bones, ligaments, and muscles at the base of the spine; *or* a basin-shaped cavity, as in the pelvis of the kidney.

penile (**PEE**-nile) Pertaining to the penis.

penis (**PEE**-nis) Conveys urine and semen to the outside.

pepsin (**PEP**-sin) Enzyme produced by the stomach that breaks down protein.

pepsinogen (pep-**SIN**-oh-jen) Converted by HCl in stomach to pepsin.

peptic (**PEP**-tik) Relating to the stomach and duodenum.

percutaneous (**PER**-kyu-**TAY**-nee-us) Passage through the skin.

perforated (**PER**-foh-ray-ted) Punctured with one or more holes.

perforation (per-foh-**RAY**-shun) A hole through the wall of a structure.

perfuse (per-**FYUSE**) To force blood to flow through a lumen or a vascular bed.

perfusion (per-**FYU**-zhun) The act of perfusing.

pericardial (per-ih-**KAR**-dee-al) Pertaining to the pericardium.

pericarditis (**PER**-ih-kar-**DIE**-tis) Inflammation of the pericardium, the covering of the heart.

pericardium (per-ih-**KAR**-dee-um) A double layer of membranes surrounding the heart.

perimetrium (per-ih-**ME**-tree-um) The covering of the uterus; part of the peritoneum.

perinatal (per-ih-**NAY**-tal) Around the time of birth.

perineal (**PER**-ih-**NEE**-al) Pertaining to the perineum.

perineum (**PER**-ih-**NEE**-um) Area between the thighs, extending from the coccyx to the pubis.

periodontal (**PER**-ee-oh-**DON**-tal) Around a tooth.

periodontics (**PER**-ee-oh-**DON**-tiks) Branch of dentistry specializing in disorders of tissues around the teeth.

periodontist (**PER**-ee-oh-**DON**-tist) Specialist in periodontics.

periodontitis (**PER**-ee-oh-don-**TIE**-tis) Inflammation of tissues around a tooth.

periorbital (per-ee-**OR**-bit-al) Pertaining to tissues around the orbit.

periosteal (**PER**-ee-**OSS**-tee-al) Pertaining to the periosteum.

periosteum (**PER**-ee-**OSS**-tee-um) Fibrous membrane covering a bone.

peripheral (peh-**RIF**-er-al) Pertaining to the periphery or external boundary.

peripheral vision (peh-**RIF**-er-al **VIZH**-un) Ability to see objects as they come into the outer edges of the visual field.

peristalsis (per-ih-**STAL**-sis) Waves of alternate contraction and relaxation of the muscle wall of a tube; for example, of the intestinal wall to move food along the digestive tract.

peritoneal (**PER**-ih-toe-**NEE**-al) Pertaining to the peritoneum.

peritoneum (**PER**-ih-toe-**NEE**-um) Membrane that lines the abdominal cavity.

peritonitis (**PER**-ih-toe-**NIE**-tis) Inflammation of the peritoneum.

pernicious anemia (per-**NISH**-us ah-**NEE**-me-ah) Chronic anemia due to lack of vitamin B_{12}.

pertussis (per-**TUSS**-is) Infectious disease with a spasmodic, intense cough ending on a whoop (stridor). Also called *whooping cough.*

pes planus (PES **PLAY**-nuss) A flat foot with no plantar arch.

pessary (**PES**-ah-ree) Appliance inserted into the vagina to support the uterus.

petechia (peh-**TEE**-kee-ah) Pinpoint capillary hemorrhagic spot in the skin. Plural *petechiae.*

petit mal (peh-**TEE** MAL) Old name for absence seizures.

phacoemulsification (**FAKE**-oh-ee-**MUL**-sih-fih-**KAY**-shun) Breaking down and sucking out a cataract with an ultrasonic needle.

phagocyte (**FAG**-oh-site) Blood cell that ingests and destroys foreign particles and cells.

phagocytic (fag-oh-**SIT**-ik) Pertaining to a phagocyte.

phagocytosis (**FAG**-oh-sigh-**TOE**-sis) Process of ingestion and destruction.

phalanx (**FAY**-lanks) A bone of a finger or toe. Plural *phalanges.*

pharmacist (**FAR**-mah-sist) Person licensed by the state to prepare and dispense drugs.

pharmacology (far-mah-**KOLL**-oh-jee) Science of the preparation, uses, and effects of drugs.

pharmacy (**FAR**-mah-see) Facility licensed to prepare and dispense drugs.

pharyngeal (fah-**RIN**-jee-al) Pertaining to the pharynx.

pharyngitis (fah-rin-**JIE**-tis) Inflammation of the pharynx.

pharynx (**FAH**-rinks) Tube from the back of the nose to the larynx.

phimosis (fih-**MOH**-sis) Prepuce cannot be retracted.

phlebitis (fleh-**BIE**-tis) Inflammation of a vein.

phlebotomist (fleh-**BOT**-oh-mist) Person skilled in taking blood from veins.

phlebotomy (fleh-**BOT**-oh-me) Taking blood from a vein.

phlegm (FLEM) Abnormal amounts of mucus expectorated from the respiratory tract.

phobia (**FOH**-bee-ah) Pathologic fear or dread.

photocoagulation (**FOH**-toe-koh-**AG**-you-**LAY**-shun) Using light (laser beam) to form a clot.

photophobia (foh-toe-**FOH**-bee-ah) Fear of the light because it hurts the eyes.

photophobic (foh-toe-**FOH**-bik) Pertaining to or suffering from photophobia.

photoreceptor (**FOH**-toe-ree-**SEP**-tor) A photoreceptor cell receives light and converts it into electrical impulses.

photosensitive (**FOH**-toe-**SEN**-sih-tiv) Abnormally sensitive to light.

photosensitivity (**FOH**-toe-sen-sih-**TIV**-ih-tee) Light produces pain in the eye.

phototherapy (foh-toe-**THAIR**-ah-pee) Treatment using light rays.

physiatrist (fizz-**I**-ah-trist) A physician who specilizes in physical medicine and rehabilitation.

physiatry (fizz-**I**-ah-tree) Physical medicine.

physical (**FIZZ**-ih-kal) Relating to the body.

pia mater (**PEE**-ah **MAY**-ter) Delicate inner layer of the meninges.

pica (**PIE**-kah) Eating substances not considered to be food.

pineal (**PIN**-ee-al) Pertaining to the pineal gland.

pink eye Conjunctivitis.

pinna (**PIN**-ah) Another name for *auricle.* Plural *pinnae.*

pitting edema (ee-**DEE**-mah) An indentation made by a finger in an edematous area persists for a long time.

pituitary (pih-**TYU**-ih-tar-ee) Pertaining to the pituitary gland.

placenta (plah-**SEN**-tah) Organ that allows metabolic interchange between the mother and the fetus.

placenta abruptio (plah-**SEN**-tah ab-**RUP**-she-oh) Premature detachment of the placenta.

placenta previa (plah-**SEN**-tah **PREE**-vee-ah) Placenta obstructing the fetus during delivery.

plaque (PLAK) Patch of abnormal tissue.

plasma (**PLAZ**-mah) Fluid, noncellular component of blood.

platelet (**PLAYT**-let) Cell fragment involved in the clotting process. Also called *thrombocyte.*

pleura (**PLUR**-ah) Membrane covering the lungs and lining the ribs in the thoracic cavity. Plural *pleurae.*

pleural (**PLUR**-al) Pertaining to the pleura.

pleurisy (**PLUR**-ih-see) Inflammation of the pleura.

plexus (**PLEK**-sus) A weblike network of joined nerves. Plural *plexuses.*

pneumoconiosis (**NEW**-moh-koh-nee-**OH**-sis) Fibrotic lung disease caused by the inhalation of different dusts.

pneumonectomy (**NEW**-moh-**NECK**-toe-me) Surgical removal of a lung.

pneumonia (new-**MOH**-nee-ah) Inflammation of the lung parenchyma (tissue).

pneumonitis (new-moh-**NI**-tis) Synonym for *pneumonia.*

pneumothorax (new-moh-**THOR**-ax) Air in the pleural cavity of the chest.

podiatrist (poh-**DIE**-ah-trist) Practitioner of podiatry.

podiatry (poh-**DIE**-ah-tree) The diagnosis and treatment of disorders and injuries of the foot.

poliomyelitis (**POE**-lee-oh-**MY**-eh-lie-tis) Inflammation of the gray matter of the spinal cord, leading to paralysis of the limbs and muscles of respiration. Abbreviation *polio.*

pollutant (poh-**LOO**-tant) Substance that makes an environment unclean or impure.

pollution (poh-**LOO**-shun) Condition that is unclean, impure, and a danger to health.

polycystic (pol-ee-**SIS**-tik) Composed of many cysts.

polycythemia vera (**POL**-ee-sigh-**THEE**-me-ah **VEH**-rah) Chronic disease with bone marrow hyperplasia, increase in number of RBCs, and increase in blood volume.

polydipsia (pol-ee-**DIP**-see-ah) Excessive thirst.

polyhydramnios (**POL**-ee-high-**DRAM**-nee-os) Too much amniotic fluid.

polymenorrhea (**POL**-ee-men-oh-**REE**-ah) More than normal frequency of menses.

polymorphonuclear (**POL**-ee-more-foh-**NEW**-klee-ahr) White blood cell with a multilobed nucleus.

polymyositis (**POL**-ee-my-oh-**SIGH**-tis) Inflammation of a number of voluntary muscles simultaneously.

polyneuropathy (**POL**-ee-nyu-**ROP**-ah-thee) Disorder affecting many nerves.

polyp (**POL**-ip) Any mass of tissue that projects outward.

polypectomy (pol-ip-**ECK**-toh-mee) Excision or removal of a polyp.

polyphagia (pol-ee-**FAY**-jee-ah) Excessive eating.

polyposis (pol-ee-**POH**-sis) Presence of several polyps.

polysomnography (**POL**-ee-som-**NOG**-rah-fee) Test to monitor brain waves, muscle tension, eye movement, and oxygen levels in the blood as the patient sleeps.

polyuria (pol-ee-**YOU**-ree-ah) Excessive production of urine.

pons (PONZ) Part of the brainstem.

popliteal (pop-**LIT**-ee-al) Pertaining to the back of the knee.

popliteal fossa (pop-**LIT**-ee-al **FOSS**-ah) The hollow at the back of the knee.

portal vein (**POR**-tal) The vein that carries blood from the intestines to the liver.

postcoital (post-**KOH**-ih-tal) After sexual intercourse.

posterior (pos-**TEER**-ee-or) Pertaining to the back surface of the body; situated behind.

postictal (post-**IK**-tal) Transient neurologic deficit after a seizure.

postmature (post-mah-**TYUR**) Infant born after 42 weeks of gestation.

postmaturity (post-mah-**TYUR**-ih-tee) Condition of being postmature.

postmortem (post-**MOR**-tem) Examination of the body and organs of a dead person to determine the cause of death.

postnatal (post-**NAY**-tal) After the birth.

postpartum (post-**PAR**-tum) After childbirth.

postpolio syndrome (PPS) (post-**POE**-lee-oh **SIN**-drome) Progressive muscle weakness in a person previously affected by polio.

postprandial (post-**PRAN**-dee-al) Following a meal.

posttraumatic (post-traw-**MAT**-ik) Occurring after and caused by trauma.

Pott fracture (POT **FRAK**-shur) Fracture of the lower end of the fibula, often with fracture of the tibial malleolus.

precancerous (pree-**KAN**-ser-us) Lesion from which cancer can develop.

precipitate labor (pree-**SIP**-ih-tate **LAY**-bore) A very rapid labor and delivery.

precursor (pree-**KUR**-sir) Cell or substance formed earlier in the development of the cell or substance.

preeclampsia (pree-eh-**KLAMP**-see-uh) Hypertension, edema, and proteinuria during pregnancy.

preemie (**PREE**-me) Slang for *premature baby.*

pregnancy (**PREG**-nan-see) State of being pregnant.

pregnant (**PREG**-nant) Having conceived.

prehypertension (pree-**HIGH**-per-**TEN**-shun) Precursor to hypertension.

premature (pree-mah-**TYUR**) Occurring before the expected time; for example, an infant born before 37 weeks of gestation.

prematurity (pree-mah-**TYUR**-ih-tee) Condition of being premature.

premenstrual (pree-**MEN**-stru-al) Pertaining to the time immediately before the menses.

prenatal (pree-**NAY**-tal) Before birth.

prepatellar (pree-pah-**TELL**-ar) In front of the patella.

prepuce (**PREE**-puce) Fold of skin that covers the glans penis. Same as *foreskin.*

presbyopia (prez-bee-**OH**-pee-ah) Difficulty in nearsighted vision occurring in middle and old age.

preterm (**PREE**-term) Baby delivered before 37 weeks of gestation. Also called *premature.*

previa (**PREE**-vee-ah) Anything blocking the fetus during its birth; for example, an abnomally situated placenta, *placenta previa.*

priapism (**PRY**-ah-pizm) Persistent erection of the penis.

primary (**PRY**-mah-ree) The first of a disease or symptom, after which others may occur as complications arise.

primigravida (pry-mih-**GRAV**-ih-dah) First pregnancy.

primipara (pry-**MIP**-ah-ruh) Woman giving birth for the first time.

prion (**PREE**-on) Small infectious protein particle.

proctitis (prok-**TIE**-tis) Inflammation of the lining of the rectum.

proctoscopy (prok-**TOSS**-koh-pee) Examination of the inside of the anus by endoscopy.

progesterone (pro-**JESS**-ter-own) Hormone that prepares the uterus for pregnancy.

progestin (pro-**JESS**-tin) A synthetic form of progesterone.

prognathism (**PROG**-nah-thizm) Condition of a forward-projecting jaw.

prognosis (prog-**NO**-sis) Forecast of the probable future course and outcome of a disease.

prolactin (pro-**LAK**-tin) Pituitary hormone that stimulates the production of milk.

prolapse (pro-**LAPS**) A sinking down of an organ or tissue.

proliferate (pro-**LIF**-eh-rate) To increase in number through reproduction.

pronate (**PRO**-nate) Rotate the forearm so that the surface of the palm faces posteriorly in the anatomical position.

pronation (pro-**NAY**-shun) Process of lying face down or of turning a hand or foot with the volar (palm or sole) surface down.

prone (PRONE) Lying face down, flat on your belly.

prophylactic (pro-fih-**LAK**-tik) The act or the agent that prevents a disease.

prophylaxis (pro-fih-**LAK**-sis) Prevention of disease.

prostaglandin (**PROS**-tah-**GLAN**-din) Hormone present in many tissues but first isolated from the prostate gland.

prostate (**PROS**-tate) Organ surrounding the urethra at the base of the male urinary bladder.

prostatectomy (pros-tah-**TEK**-toe-me) Surgical removal of the prostate.

prostatic (pros-**TAT**-ik) Pertaining to the prostate.

prostatitis (pros-tah-**TIE**-tis) Inflammation of the prostate.

prosthesis (**PROS**-thee-sis) Manufactured substitute for a missing part of the body.

prosthetic (pros-**THET**-ik) Pertaining to a prosthesis.

prostrate (pros-**TRAYT**) To lay flat or to be overcome by physical weakness and exhaustion.

prostration (pros-**TRAY**-shun) To be lying flat or to be overcome by physical weakness and exhaustion.

protease (**PRO**-tee-ase) Group of enzymes that break down protein.

protein (**PRO**-teen) Class of food substances based on amino acids.

proteinuria (pro-tee-**NYU**-ree-ah) Presence of protein in urine.

prothrombin (pro-**THROM**-bin) Protein formed by the liver and converted to thrombin in the blood-clotting mechanism.

proton pump inhibitor (**PRO**-ton PUMP in-**HIB**-ih-tor) Agent that blocks the enzyme system in the lining of the stomach that produces gastric acid.

provisional diagnosis (pro-**VIZH**-un-al die-ag-**NO**-sis) A temporary diagnosis pending further examination or testing.

proximal (**PROK**-sih-mal) Situated nearest the center of the body.

pruritic (proo-**RIT**-ik) Itchy.

pruritus (proo-**RYE**-tus) Itching.

psoriasis (so-**RYE**-ah-sis) Rash characterized by reddish, silver-scaled patches.

psychedelic (sigh-keh-**DEL**-ik) An agent that intensifies sensory perception.

psychiatric (sigh-kee-**AH**-trik) Pertaining to psychiatry.

psychiatrist (sigh-**KIGH**-ah-trist) Licensed medical specialist in psychiatry.

psychiatry (sigh-**KIGH**-ah-tree) Diagnosis and treatment of mental disorders.

psychologic (sigh-koh-**LOJ**-ik) Pertaining to psychology.

psychological (sigh-koh-**LOJ**-ik-al) Pertaining to psychology.

psychologist (sigh-**KOL**-oh-jist) One who studies and becomes a specialist in psychology.

psychology (sigh-**KOL**-oh-jee) Study of the behavior of the human mind.

psychopath (**SIGH**-koh-path) Person with antisocial personality disorder.

psychosis (sigh-**KOH**-sis) Disorder causing mental disruption and loss of contact with reality.

psychosocial (**SIGH**-koh-**SOH**-shal) Involving both the mind and various social and community aspects of life.

psychosomatic (**SIGH**-koh-soh-**MAT**-ik) Disorders of the body influenced by the mind.

psychotic (sigh-**KOT**-ik) Pertaining to or affected by psychosis.

ptosis (**TOE**-sis) Sinking down of the upper eyelid or an organ.

pubarche (pyu-**BAR**-key) Development of pubic and axillary hair.

puberty (**PYU**-ber-tee) Process of maturing from child to young adult.

pubic (**PYU**-bik) Pertaining to the pubis.

pubis (**PYU**-bis) Alternative name for *pubic bone.*

puerperium (pyu-er-**PER**-ee-um) Six-week period after birth in which the uterus involutes.

pulmonary (**PULL**-moh-**NAR**-ee) Pertaining to the lungs.

pulmonologist (**PULL**-moh-**NOL**-oh-jist) Specialist in treating disorders of the lungs.

pulmonology (**PULL**-moh-**NOL**-oh-jee) Study of the lungs, or the medical specialty of disorders of the lungs.

pulp (PULP) Dental pulp is the connective tissue in the cavity in the center of the tooth.

pupil (**PYU**-pill) The opening in the center of the iris that allows light to reach the lens. Plural *pupillae.*

pupillary (**PYU**-pill-ah-ree) Pertaining to the pupil.

purge (PURJ) Consciously throw up or cause bowel evacuation.

Purkinje fibers (per-**KIN**-jee **FI-berz**) Network of nerve fibers in the myocardium.

purpura (**PUR**-pyu-rah) Skin hemorrhages that are red initially and then turn purple.

purulent (**PURE**-you-lent) Showing or containing a lot of pus.

pustule (**PUS**-tyul) Small protuberance on the skin that contains pus.

pyelitis (pie-eh-**LYE**-tis) Inflammation of the renal pelvis.

pyelogram (**PIE**-el-oh-gram) X-ray image of renal pelvis and ureters.

pyelonephritis (**PIE**-eh-loh-neh-**FRY**-tis) Inflammation of the kidney and renal pelvis.

pyloric (pie-**LOR**-ik) Pertaining to the pylorus.

pylorus (pie-**LOR**-us) Exit area of the stomach.

pyorrhea (pie-oh-**REE**-ah) Purulent discharge.

pyrexia (pie-**REK**-see-ah) An abnormally high body temperature or fever.

pyromania (pie-roh-**MAY**-nee-ah) Morbid impulse to set fires.

Q

quadrant (**KWAD**-rant) One-quarter of a circle; *or* one of four regions of the surface of the abdomen.

quadrantectomy (kwad-ran-**TEK**-toe-me) Surgical excision of a quadrant of the breast.

quadriceps femoris (**KWAD**-rih-seps **FEM**-or-is) An anterior thigh muscle with four heads.

quadriplegia (kwad-rih-**PLEE**-jee-ah) Paralysis of all four limbs.

quadriplegic (kwad-rih-**PLEE**-jik) Pertaining to or suffering from quadriplegia.

R

radial (**RAY**-dee-al) Pertaining to the forearm or to any of the structures (artery, vein, nerve) named after it; *or* diverging in all directions from any given center.

radiation (ray-dee-**AY**-shun) To spread out.

radiologic (**RAY**-dee-oh-**LOJ**-ik) Pertaining to radiology.

radiologist (ray-dee-**OL**-oh-jist) Medical specialist in the use of X-rays and other imaging techniques.

radiology (ray-dee-**OL**-oh-jee) Study of medical imaging.

radius (**RAY**-dee-us) The forearm bone on the thumb side.

rale (RAHL) Crackle heard through a stethoscope when air bubbles through liquid in the lungs. Plural *rales.*

rash (RASH) Skin eruption.

rectocele (**RECK**-toe-seal) Hernia of the rectum into the vagina.

rectum (**RECK**-tum) Terminal part of the colon from the sigmoid to the anal canal.

reflex (**REE**-fleks) An involuntary response to a stimulus.

reflux (**REE**-fluks) Backward flow.

refract (ree-**FRAKT**) Make a change in the direction of, or bend, a ray of light.

refraction (ree-**FRAKT**-shun) The bending of light.

regenerate (ree-**JEN**-eh-rate) Reconstitution of a lost part.

regeneration (ree-**JEN**-eh-**RAY**-shun) The process of reconstitution.

regulate (**REG**-you-late) To control the way in which a process progresses.

regulation (**REG**-you-**LAY**-shun) Control of the way in which a process progresses.

regurgitate (ree-**GUR**-jih-tate) To flow backward; for example, blood through a heart valve.

regurgitation (ree-gur-jih-**TAY**-shun) Expel contents of the stomach into the mouth, short of vomiting.

rehabilitation (**REE**-hah-bill-ih-**TAY**-shun) Therapeutic restoration of an ability to function as before.

remission (ree-**MISH**-un) Period when there is a lessening or absence of the symptoms of a disease.

renal (**REE**-nal) Pertaining to the kidney.

replication (rep-lih-**KAY**-shun) Reproduction to produce an exact copy.

reproduction (ree-pro-**DUK**-shun) The process by which organisms produce offspring.

reproductive (ree-pro-**DUK**-tiv) Pertaining to reproduction.

resection (ree-**SEK**-shun) Removal of a specific part of an organ or structure.

resectoscope (ree-**SEK**-toe-skope) Endoscope for transurethral removal of lesions of the prostate.

residual (reh-**ZID**-you-al) Pertaining to anything left over.

resistance (reh-**ZIS**-tants) Ability of an organism to withstand the effects of an antagonistic agent.

resistant (reh-**ZIS**-tant) Able to resist.

respiration (**RES**-pih-**RAY**-shun) Process of breathing; fundamental process of life used to exchange oxygen and carbon dioxide.

respirator (**RES**-pih-**RAY**-tor) Another name for *ventilator.*

respiratory (**RES**-pih-rah-tor-ee) Pertaining to respiration.

retention (ree-**TEN**-shun) Holding back in the body what should normally be discharged (e.g., urine).

retina (**RET**-ih-nah) Light-sensitive innermost layer of the eyeball.

retinal (**RET**-ih-nal) Pertaining to the retina.

retinoblastoma (**RET**-in-oh-blas-**TOE**-mah) Malignant neoplasm of primitive retinal cells.

retinoids (**RET**-ih-noydz) Keratolytic agents applied for psoriasis, acne, and photodamage.

retinopathy (ret-ih-**NOP**-ah-thee) Any disease of the retina.

retrograde (**RET**-roh-grade) Reversal of a normal flow; for example, back from the bladder into the ureters.

retroversion (reh-troh-**VER**-zhun) Tipping backward of the uterus.

retroverted (**REH**-troh-vert-ed) Tilted backward.

retrovirus (**REH**-troh-vie-rus) Virus with an RNA core.

rhesus factor (**REE**-sus **FAK**-tor) An antigen on the surface of red blood cells of Rh positive individuals. First discovered in Rhesus monkeys.

rheumatic (ru-**MA**-tik) Pertaining to or affected by rheumatism.

rheumatism (**RU**-ma-tizm) Pain in various parts of the musculoskeletal system.

rheumatoid arthritis (RA) (**RU**-mah-toyd ar-**THRI**-tis) Disease of connective tissue, with arthritis as a major manifestation.

rhinitis (rye-**NIE**-tis) Inflammation of the nasal mucosa. Also called *coryza.*

rhinoplasty (**RYE**-no-plas-tee) Surgical procedure to change size or shape of the nose.

rhonchus (**RONG**-kuss) Wheezing sound heard on auscultation of the lungs; made by air passing through a constricted lumen. Plural *rhonchi.*

ribonucleic acid (RNA) (**RYE**-boh-nyu-**KLEE**-ik **ASS**-id) Information carrier from DNA in the nucleus to an organelle to produce protein molecules.

ribosome (**RYE**-boh-sohm) Structure in the cell that assembles amino acids into protein.

rickets (**RICK**-ets) Disease due to vitamin D deficiency, producing soft, flexible bones.

rigidity (ri-**JID**-ih-tee) Increased muscle tone at rest.

Rinne test (**RIN**-eh **TEST**) Test for conductive hearing loss.

root (ROOT) Fundamental or beginning part of a structure.

rooting (**RUE**-ting) A neonatal reflex to turn toward the nipple and open the mouth when a nipple is placed on the cheek.

rosacea (roh-**ZAY**-she-ah) Persistent erythematous rash of the central face.

rotator cuff (roh-**TAY**-tor CUFF) Part of the capsule of the shoulder joint.

rumination (roo-min-**NAY**-shun) To bring back food into the mouth to chew over and over.

rupture (**RUP**-tyur) Break or tear of any organ or body part.

S

sacral (**SAY**-kral) Pertaining to or in the neighborhood of the sacrum.

sacroiliac joint (say-kroh-**ILL**-ih-ak JOINT) The joint between the sacrum and the ilium.

sacrum (**SAY**-crum) Segment of the vertebral column that forms part of the pelvis.

sagittal (**SAJ**-ih-tal) Vertical plane through the body dividing it into right and left portions.

saline (**SAY**-leen) Salt solution, usually sodium chloride.

saliva (sa-**LIE**-vah) Secretion in the mouth from salivary glands.

salivary (**SAL**-ih-var-ee) Pertaining to saliva.

salpingectomy (sal-pin-**JEK**-toe-me) Surgical excision of a fallopian tube.

salpingitis (sal-pin-**JIE**-tis) Inflammation of the uterine tube.

saphenous (**SAPH**-ih-nus) Relating to the saphenous vein in the thigh.

sarcoidosis (sar-koy-**DOH**-sis) Granulomatous lesions of the lungs and other organs; cause is unknown.

sarcoma (sar-**KOH**-mah) A malignant tumor originating in connective tissue.

sarcopenia (sar-koh-**PEE**-nee-ah) Progressive loss of muscle mass and strength with aging.

saturated fatty acid (**SATCH**-you-ray-ted **FAT**-ee **ASS**-id) Lipid that is incapable of absorbing any more hydrogen.

scab (SKAB) Crust that forms over a wound or sore during healing.

scabies (**SKAY**-beez) Skin disease produced by mites.

scald (SKAWLD) Burn from contact with hot liquid or steam.

scapula (**SKAP**-you-lah) Shoulder blade. Plural *scapulae.*

scapular (**SKAP**-you-lar) Pertaining to the scapula.

scar (SKAR) Fibrotic seam that forms when a wound heals.

schizophrenia (skitz-oh-**FREE**-nee-ah) Disorder of perception, thought, emotion, and behavior.

sclera (**SKLAIR**-ah) Fibrous outer covering of the eyeball and the white of the eye.

scleral (**SKLAIR**-al) Pertaining to the sclera.

scleritis (sklair-**RI**-tis) Inflammation of the sclera.

scleroderma (sklair-oh-**DERM**-ah) Thickening and hardening of the skin due to new collagen formation.

sclerose (skleh-**ROSE**) To harden or thicken.

sclerosis (skleh-**ROH**-sis) Thickening or hardening of a tissue; in the nervous system, hardening of nervous tissue by fibrous and glial connective tissue.

sclerotherapy (**SKLAIR**-oh-**THAIR**-ah-pee) Injection of a solution into a vein to thrombose it.

scoliosis (skoh-lee-**OH**-sis) An abnormal lateral curvature of the vertebral column.

scoliotic (**SKOH**-lee-**OT**-ik) Pertaining to or suffering from scoliosis.

scrotal (**SKRO**-tal) Pertaining to the scrotum.

scrotum (**SKRO**-tum) Sac containing testes.

seasonal affective disorder (see-**ZON**-al af-**FEK**-tiv dis-**OR**-der) Depression that occurs at the same time every year, often in winter.

sebaceous glands (seh-**BAY**-shus GLANZ) Glands in the dermis that open into hair follicles and secrete an oily fluid called *sebum.*

seborrhea (seb-oh-**REE**-ah) Excessive amount of sebum.

seborrheic (seb-oh-**REE**-ik) Pertaining to seborrhea.

sebum (**SEE**-bum) Waxy secretion of the sebaceous glands.

secondary (**SEK**-ond-ah-ree) Diseases or symptoms following a primary disease or symptom.

secrete (seh-**KREET**) To produce a chemical substance in a cell and release it from the cell.

secretion (seh-**KREE**-shun) The production of a chemical substance in a cell and its release from the cell.

sedation (seh-**DAY**-shun) State of being calmed.

sedative (**SED**-ah-tiv) Agent that calms nervous excitement.

segment (SEG-ment) A section of an organ or structure.

seizure (SEE-zhur) Event due to excessive electrical activity in the brain.

self-examination (SELF-ek-zam-ih-NAY-shun) Conduct an examination of one's own body.

self-mutilation (self-myu-tih-LAY-shun) Injury or disfigurement made to one's own body.

semen (SEE-men) Penile ejaculate containing sperm and seminal fluid.

semilunar (sem-ee-LOO-nar) Appears like a half moon.

seminal vesicle (SEM-in-al VES-ih-kull) Sac of the ductus deferens that produces seminal fluid.

seminiferous (sem-ih-NIF-er-us) Pertaining to carrying semen.

seminiferous tubule (sem-ih-NIF-er-us TU-byul) Coiled tubes in the testes that produce sperm.

seminoma (sem-ih-NO-mah) Neoplasm of germ cells of a testis.

senescence (seh-NES-ens) The state of being old.

senescent (seh-NES-ent) Growing old.

senile (SEE-nile) Characteristic of old age.

senility (seh-NIL-ih-tee) Mental disorders occurring in old age.

sensation (sen-SAY-shun) The conscious feeling of the effects of a stimulation.

sensorineural hearing loss (SEN-sor-ih-NYUR-al) Hearing loss caused by lesions of the inner ear or the auditory nerve.

sensory (SEN-soh-ree) Having the function of sensation; structures of the nervous system that carry impulses to the brain.

sepsis (SEP-sis) Presence of pathogenic organisms or their toxins in blood or tissues.

septicemia (sep-tih-SEE-mee-ah) Microorganisms circulating in, and infecting, the blood (blood poisoning).

septum (SEP-tum) A thin wall separating two cavities or tissue masses. Plural *septa.*

serotonin (ser-oh-TOE-nin) A neurotransmitter in the central and peripheral nervous systems.

serum (SEER-um) Fluid remaining after removal of cells and fibrin clot from blood.

shock (SHOCK) Sudden physical or mental collapse or circulatory collapse.

shunt (SHUNT) A bypass or diversion of fluid; for example, blood.

sigmoid (SIG-moyd) Sigmoid colon is shaped like an "S."

sigmoidoscopy (sig-moi-DOS-koh-pee) Endoscopic examination of the sigmoid colon.

sign (SINE) Physical evidence of a disease process.

silicosis (sil-ih-KOH-sis) Fibrotic lung disease from inhaling silica particles.

sinoatrial (SA) node (sigh-noh-AY-tree-al NODE) The center of modified cardiac muscle fibers in the wall of the right atrium that acts as the pacemaker for the heart rhythm.

sinus (SIGH-nus) Cavity or hollow space in a bone or other tissue.

sinus rhythm (SIGH-nus RITH-um) The normal (optimal) heart rhythm arising from the sinoatrial node.

sinusitis (sigh-nyu-SIGH-tis) Inflammation of the lining of a sinus.

Sjogren syndrome (SHER-gren SIN-drome) Dryness of the mucous membranes of the eye and mouth.

skeletal (SKEL-eh-tal) Pertaining to the skeleton.

skeleton (SKEL-eh-ton) The bony framework of the body.

Skene glands (SKEEN GLANZ) Paraurethral glands in the anterior wall of the vagina. Also called *paraurethral glands.*

smegma (SMEG-mah) Oily material produced by the glans and prepuce.

Snellen letter chart (SNEL-en) Test for acuity of distance vision.

snore (SNOR) Noise produced by vibrations in the structures of the nasopharynx.

sociopath (SOH-see-oh-path) Person with antisocial personality disorder.

somatic (soh-MAT-ik) Relating to the body in general; *or* a division of the periperal nervous system serving the skeletal muscles.

somatostatin (SOH-mah-toh-STAT-in) Hormone that inhibits release of growth hormone and insulin.

somatotrophin (SOH-mah-toh-TROH-phin) Hormone of the anterior pituitary that stimulates the growth of body tissues. Also called *growth hormone.*

spasm (SPASM) Sudden involuntary contraction of a muscle group.

spasmodic (spaz-MOD-ik) Intermittent contractions.

spastic (SPAS-tik) Increased muscle tone on movement.

specific (speh-SIF-ik) Relating to a particular entity.

specificity (spes-ih-FIS-ih-tee) State of having a fixed relation to a particular entity.

sperm (SPERM) Mature male sex cell. Also called *spermatozoon.*

spermatic (SPER-mat-ik) Pertaining to sperm.

spermatid (SPER-mat-id) A cell late in the development process of sperm.

spermatocele (SPER-mat-oh-seal) Cyst of the epididymis that contains sperm.

spermatogenesis (SPER-mat-oh-JEN-eh-sis) The process by which male germ cells differentiate into sperm.

spermatozoa (SPER-mat-oh-ZOH-ah) Sperm (plural of *spermatozoon*).

spermicidal (sper-mih-SIGH-dal) Pertaining to the killing of sperm; *or* destructive to sperm.

spermicide (SPER-mih-side) Agent that destroys sperm.

sphenoid (SFEE-noyd) Wedge-shaped bone at the base of the skull.

sphincter (SFINK-ter) Band of muscle that encircles an opening; when it contracts, the opening squeezes closed.

sphygmomanometer (SFIG-moh-mah-NOM-ih-ter) Instrument for measuring arterial blood pressure.

spina bifida (SPY-nah BIH-fih-dah) Failure of one or more vertebral arches to close during fetal development.

spina bifida cystica (SIS-tik-ah) Meninges and spinal cord protruding through the absent vertebral arch and having the appearance of a cyst.

spina bifida occulta (OH-kul-tah) The deformity of the vertebral arch is not apparent from the surface.

spinal (SPY-nal) Pertaining to the spine.

spinal tap (SPY-nal TAP) Placement of a needle through an intervertebral space into the subarachnoid space to withdraw CSF.

spine (SPINE) The vertebral column; *or* a short bony projection.

spiral fracture (SPY-ral FRAK-chur) A fracture in the shape of a coil.

spirochete (**SPY**-roh-keet) Spiral-shaped bacterium causing a sexually transmitted disease (syphilis).

spirometer (spy-**ROM**-eh-ter) An instrument used to measure respiratory volumes.

spirometry (spy-**ROM**-eh-tree) Use of a spirometer.

spleen (SPLEEN) Vascular, lymphatic organ in the left upper quadrant of the abdomen.

splenectomy (sple-**NECK**-toe-me) Surgical removal of the spleen.

splenomegaly (sple-noh-**MEG**-ah-lee) Enlarged spleen.

spondylosis (spon-dih-**LOH**-sis) Degenerative osteoarthritis of the spine.

spongiosum (spun-jee-**OH**-sum) Spongelike tissue.

sprain (SPRAIN) A wrench or tear in a ligament.

sputum (**SPYU**-tum) Matter coughed up and spat out by individuals with respiratory disorders.

squamous cell (**SKWAY**-mus SELL) Flat, scalelike epithelial cell.

stabilize (**STAY**-bill-ize) To make or hold firm or steady.

stable (**STAY**-bel) Steady, not varying.

stage (STAYJ) Definition of the extent and dissemination of a malignant neoplasm.

staging (**STAY**-jing) Process of determination of the extent of the distribution of a neoplasm.

stapes (**STAY**-peez) Inner (medial) one of the three ossicles of the middle ear; shaped like a stirrup.

Staphylococcus (**STAF**-ih-loh-**KOK**-us) Genus of gram-positive bacteria that divide in more than one plane to form clusters. Plural *staphylococci.*

starch (STARCH) Complex carbohydrate made of multiple units of glucose attached together.

stasis (**STAY**-sis) Stagnation in the flow of any body fluid.

statin (**STAH**-tin) A class of drugs used to lower blood cholesterol levels.

status (**STAT**-us) A state or condition.

status epilepticus (**STAT**-us ep-ih-**LEP**-tik-us) Latin phrase for being in a prolonged or recurrent seizure for longer than a specific time frame.

stem cell (STEM SELL) Undifferentiated cell found in a differentiated tissue that can divide to yield the specialized cells in that tissue.

stenosis (steh-**NOH**-sis) Narrowing of a canal or passage.

stent (STENT) Wire-mesh tube used to keep arteries open.

stereopsis (ster-ee-**OP**-sis) Three-dimensional vision.

stereotactic (**STER**-ee-oh-**TAK**-tic) A precise three-dimensional method to locate a lesion.

stereotype (**STER**-ee-oh-tipe) An image held in common by members of a group.

sterile (**STER**-il) Free from all living organisms and their spores; *or* unable to fertilize or reproduce.

sterility (ster-**RIL**-ih-tee) Inability to reproduce.

sterilization (**STER**-ih-lih-**ZAY**-shun) Process of making sterile.

sterilize (**STER**-ih-lize) To make sterile.

sternum (**STIR**-num) Long, flat bone forming the center of the anterior wall of the chest.

steroid (**STAIR**-oyd) Large family of chemical substances found in many drugs, hormones, and body components.

stethoscope (**STETH**-oh-skope) Instrument for listening to cardiac and respiratory sounds.

stimulant (**STIM**-you-lant) Agent that excites or strengthens.

stimulation (stim-you-**LAY**-shun) Arousal to increased functional activity.

stimulus (**STIM**-you-lus) Something that excites or strengthens the functional activity of an organ or part. Plural *stimuli.*

stoma (**STOW**-mah) Artificial opening.

strabismus (strah-**BIZ**-mus) Turning of an eye away from its normal position.

strain (STRAIN) Overstretch or tear in a muscle or tendon.

stratum basale (**STRAH**-tum bay-**SAL**-eh) Deepest layer of the epidermis, from which the other cells originate and migrate.

Streptococcus (strep-toe-**KOK**-us) Genus of gram-positive bacteria that grow in chains. Plural *streptococci.*

striated muscle (**STRI**-ay-ted **MUSS**-el) Another term for *skeletal muscle.*

stricture (**STRICK**-shur) Narrowing of a tube.

stridor (**STRY**-door) High-pitched noise made when there is a respiratory obstruction in the larynx or trachea.

stroke (STROHK) Acute clinical event caused by impaired cerebral circulation.

stye (STEYE) Infection of an eyelash follicle.

subarachnoid space (sub-ah-**RACK**-noyd SPACE) Space between the pia mater and the arachnoid membrane.

subclavian (sub-**CLAY**-vee-an) Underneath the clavicle.

subcutaneous (sub-kew-**TAY**-nee-us) Below the skin. Also called *hypodermic.*

subdural space (sub-**DYU**-ral SPASE) Space between the arachnoid and dura mater layers of the meninges.

sublingual (sub-**LING**-wal) Underneath the tongue.

subluxation (sub-luck-**SAY**-shun) An incomplete dislocation when some contact between the joint surfaces remains.

submandibular (sub-man-**DIB**-you-lar) Underneath the mandible.

submucosa (sub-mew-**KOH**-sa) Tissue layer underneath the mucosa.

substernal (sub-**STER**-nal) Under (behind) the sternum or breastbone.

suction (**SUK**-shun) Use of a catheter to clear the upper airway or other tubes.

sulcus (**SUL**-cuss) Groove on the surface of the cerebral hemispheres that separates gyri. Plural *sulci.*

superficial (soo-per-**FISH**-al) Situated near the surface.

superior (soo-**PEER**-ee-or) Situated above.

supinate (**SOO**-pih-nate) Rotate the forearm so that the surface of the palm faces anteriorly in the anatomical position.

supination (soo-pih-**NAY**-shun) Process of lying face upward or of turning a hand or foot so that the palm or sole is facing up.

supine (soo-**PINE**) Lying face up, flat on your spine.

suprapubic (**SOO**-prah-pyu-bik) Above the symphysis pubis.

surfactant (sir-**FAK**-tant) A protein and fat compound that creates surface tension to hold the lung alveolar walls apart.

suture (**SOO**-chur) Two bones are joined together by a fibrous band continuous with their periosteum, as in the skull; *or* a stitch to hold the edges of a wound together; *or* to stitch the edges of a wound together. Plural *sutures.*

swab (SWOB) Wad of cotton used to remove or apply something from/to a surface.

sympathetic (sim-pah-**THET**-ik) Division of the autonomic nervous system operating at an unconscious level.

sympathy (**SIM**-pah-thee) Appreciation and concern for another person's mental and emotional state.

symphysis (**SIM**-feh-sis) Two bones joined by fibrocartilage. Plural *symphyses.*

symptom (**SIMP**-tum) Departure from the normal experienced by a patient.

symptomatic (simp-toe-**MAT**-ik) Pertaining to the symptoms of a disease.

synapse (**SIN**-aps) Junction between two nerve cells or a nerve fiber and its target cell, where electrical impulses are transmitted between the cells.

syncope (**SIN**-koh-pee) Temporary loss of consciousness and posture due to diminished cerebral blood flow.

syndesmosis (sin-dez-**MOH**-sis) Binding together of two bones with ligaments. Plural *syndesmoses.*

syndrome (**SIN**-drohm) Combination of signs and symptoms associated with a particular disease process.

synovial (si-**NOH**-vee-al) Pertaining to synovial fluid and the synovial membrane.

synthesis (**SIN**-the-sis) The process of building a compound from different elements.

synthetic (sin-**THET**-ik) Built up or put together from simpler compounds.

syphilis (**SIF**-ih-lis) Sexually transmitted disease caused by a spirochete.

syringomyelia (sih-**RING**-oh-my-**EE**-lee-ah) Abnormal longitudinal cavities in the spinal cord that cause paresthesias and muscle weakness.

systemic (sis-**TEM**-ik) Relating to the entire organism.

systemic lupus erythematosus (sis-**TEM**-ik **LOO**-pus er-ih-**THEE**-mah-toe-sus) Inflammatory connective tissue disease affecting the whole body.

systole (**SIS**-toe-lee) Contraction of the heart muscle.

systolic (sis-**TOL**-ik) Pertaining to systole.

T

tachycardia (tack-ih-**KAR**-dee-ah) Rapid heart rate (above 100 beats per minute).

tachypnea (tack-ip-**NEE**-ah) Rapid breathing.

talipes (**TAL**-ip-eze) Deformity of the foot involving the talus.

talus (**TAY**-luss) The tarsal bone that articulates with the tibia to form the ankle joint.

tampon (**TAM**-pon) Plug or pack in a cavity to absorb or stop bleeding.

tamponade (tam-poh-**NAID**) Pathologic compression of an organ, such as the heart.

tapeworm (**TAPE**-worm) Intestinal parasitic worm.

tarsal (**TAR**-sal) Pertaining to the tarsus.

tarsus (**TAR**-sus) The collection of seven bones in the foot that form the ankle and instep; *or* the flat fibrous plate that gives shape to the outer edges of the eyelids.

tartar (**TAR**-tar) Calcified deposit at the gingival margin of the teeth.

Tay-Sachs disease (TAY SAKS diz-**EEZ**) Congenital fatal disorder of fat metabolism.

temperament (**TEM**-per-ah-ment) Predisposition to character or personality.

temporal (**TEM**-pore-al) Bone that forms part of the base and sides of the skull.

temporal lobe (**TEM**-pore-al LOBE) Posterior two-thirds of the cerebral hemispheres.

temporomandibular joint (TMJ) (**TEM**-pore-oh-man-**DIB**-you-lar JOYNT) The joint between the temporal bone and the mandible.

tendinitis (ten-dih-**NYE**-tis) Inflammation of a tendon. Also spelled *tendonitis.*

tendon (**TEN**-dun) Fibrous band that connects muscle to bone.

tenosynovitis (**TEN**-oh-sin-oh-**VIE**-tis) Inflammation of a tendon and its surrounding synovial sheath.

teratogen (**TER**-ah-toe-jen) Agent that produces fetal deformities.

teratogenesis (**TER**-ah-toe-**JEN**-eh-sis) Process involved in producing fetal deformities.

teratogenic (**TER**-ah-toe-**JEN**-ik) Pertaining to or capable of producing fetal deformities.

teratoma (ter-ah-**TOE**-mah) Neoplasm of a testis or ovary containing multiple tissues from other sites in the body.

testicle (**TES**-tih-kul) One of the male reproductive glands. Also called *testis.*

testicular (tes-**TICK**-you-lar) Pertaining to the testicle.

testis (**TES**-tis) A synonym for *testicle.* Plural *testes.*

testosterone (tes-**TOSS**-ter-own) Powerful androgen produced by the testes.

tetany (**TET**-ah-nee) Severe muscle twitches, cramps, and spasms.

tetralogy of Fallot (TOF) (te-**TRA**-loh-jee ov fah-**LOW**) Set of four congenital heart defects occurring together.

thalamus (**THAL**-ah-mus) Mass of gray matter underneath the ventricle in each cerebral hemisphere.

thalassemia (thal-ah-**SEE**-mee-ah) Group of inherited blood disorders that produce a hemolytic anemia.

thelarche (thee-**LAR**-key) Onset of breast development.

thenar (**THAY**-nar) The thenar eminence is the fleshy mass at the base of the thumb.

therapeutic (**THAIR**-ah-**PYU**-tik) Pertaining to the treatment of a disease or disorder.

therapy (**THAIR**-ah-pee) Systematic treatment of a disease, dysfunction, or disorder.

thoracentesis (**THOR**-ah-sen-**TEE**-sis) Insertion of a needle into the pleural cavity to withdraw fluid or air. Also called *pleural tap.*

thoracic (**THOR**-ass-ik) Pertaining to the chest (thorax).

thoracic cavity (**THOR**-ass-ik **KAV**-ih-tee) Space within the chest containing the lungs, heart, aorta, venae cavae, esophagus, trachea, and pulmonary vessels.

thoracoscopy (thor-ah-**KOS**-koh-pee) Examination of the pleural cavity with an endoscope.

thoracotomy (thor-ah-**KOT**-oh-me) Incision through the chest wall.

thorax (**THOR**-acks) The part of the trunk between the abdomen and the neck.

thrombin (**THROM**-bin) Enzyme that forms fibrin.

thrombocyte (**THROM**-boh-site) Another name for *platelet.*

thrombocytic (**THROM**-bo-**SIT**-ik) Pertaining to a thrombocyte (platelet).

thrombocytopenia (**THROM**-boh-site-oh-**PEE**-nee-uh) Deficiency of platelets in circulating blood.

thromboembolism (**THROM**-boh-**EM**-boh-lizm) A piece of detached blood clot (embolus) blocking a distant blood vessel.

thrombolysis (throm-**BOH**-lih-sis) Dissolving of a thrombus (clot).

thrombolytic (throm-boh-**LIT**-ik) Able to dissolve a thrombus.

thrombophlebitis (**THROM**-boh-fleh-**BY**-tis) Inflammation of a vein with clot formation.

thrombosis (throm-**BOH**-sis) Formation of a thrombus.

thrombus (**THROM**-bus) A clot attached to a diseased blood vessel or heart lining. Plural *thrombi.*

thrush (THRUSH) Infection with *Candida albicans.*

thymectomy (thigh-**MEK**-toe-me) Surgical removal of the thymus gland.

thymoma (thigh-**MOH**-mah) Benign tumor of the thymus.

thymus (**THIGH**-mus) Lymphoid and endocrine gland located in the mediastinum.

thyroid (**THIGH**-royd) Endocrine gland in the neck; *or* a cartilage of the larynx.

thyroid hormone (**THIGH**-royd **HOR**-mohn) Collective term for the two thyroid hormones, T3 and T4.

thyroid storm (**THIGH**-royd STORM) Medical crisis and emergency due to excess thyroid hormones.

thyroidectomy (thigh-royd-**ECK**-toe-me) Surgical removal of the thyroid gland.

thyroiditis (thigh-royd-**EYE**-tis) Inflammation of the thyroid gland.

thyrotoxicosis (**THIGH**-roe-toks-ih-**KOH**-sis) Disorder produced by excessive thyroid hormone production.

thyrotropin (thigh-roe-**TROH**-pin) Hormone from the anterior pituitary gland that stimulates function of the thyroid gland.

thyroxine (thigh-**ROCK**-sin) Thyroid hormone T4, tetraiodothyronine.

tibia (**TIB**-ee-ah) The larger bone of the lower leg.

tibial (**TIB**-ee-al) Pertaining to the tibia.

tic (TIK) Sudden, involuntary, repeated contraction of muscles.

tic douloureux (tik duh-luh-**RUE**) Painful, sudden, spasmodic involuntary contractions of the facial muscles supplied by the trigeminal nerve. Also called *trigeminal neuralgia.*

tinea (**TIN**-ee-ah) General term for a group of related skin infections caused by different species of fungi.

tinnitus (**TIN**-ih-tus) Persistent ringing, whistling, clicking, or booming noise in the ears.

tissue (**TISH**-you) Collection of similar cells.

tolerance (**TOL**-er-ans) The capacity to become accustomed to a stimulus or drug.

tomography (toe-**MOG**-rah-fee) Radiographic image of a selected slice of tissue.

tone (TONE) Tension present in resting muscles.

tongue (TUNG) Mobile muscle mass in the mouth; bears the taste buds.

tonic (**TON**-ik) State of muscular contraction.

tonic-clonic (**TON**-ik-**KLON**-ik) The body alternates between excessive muscular rigidity (tonic) and jerking muscular contractions (clonic).

tonic-clonic seizure (**TON**-ik-**KLON**-ik **SEE**-zhur) Generalized seizure due to epileptic activity in all or most of the brain.

tonometer (toe-**NOM**-eh-ter) Instrument for determining intraocular pressure.

tonometry (toe-**NOM**-eh-tree) The measurement of intraocular pressure.

tonsil (**TON**-sill) Mass of lymphoid tissue on either side of the throat at the back of the tongue.

tonsillectomy (ton-sih-**LEK**-toh-me) Surgical removal of the tonsils.

tonsillitis (ton-sih-**LIE**-tis) Inflammation of the tonsils.

topical (**TOP**-ih-kal) Medication applied to the skin to obtain a local effect.

torsion (**TOR**-shun) The act or result of twisting.

Tourette syndrome (tur-**ET SIN**-drome) Disorder of multiple motor and vocal tics.

toxic (**TOK**-sick) Pertaining to a toxin.

toxicity (tok-**SIS**-ih-tee) The state of being poisonous.

toxin (**TOK**-sin) Poisonous substance formed by a cell or organism.

trachea (**TRAY**-kee-ah) Air tube from the larynx to the bronchi.

tracheal (**TRAY**-kee-al) Pertaining to the trachea.

tracheostomy (tray-kee-**OST**-oh-me) Incision into the windpipe into which a tube can be inserted to assist breathing.

tracheotomy (tray-kee-**OT**-oh-me) Incision made into the trachea to create a tracheostomy.

tract (TRACKT) Bundle of nerve fibers with a common origin and destination.

traction (**TRAK**-shun) Pulling or dragging force.

trait (TRAYT) A discrete characteristic that has a known quality.

tranquilizer (**TRANG**-kwih-lie-zer) Agent that calms without sedating or depressing.

transdermal (tranz-**DER**-mal) Going across or through the skin.

transfusion (tranz-**FYU**-zhun) Transfer of blood or a blood component from donor to recipient.

transplant (**TRANZ**-plant) The tissue or organ used; *or* the act of transferring tissue from one person to another.

transplantation (**TRANZ**-plan-**TAY**-shun) The moving of tissue or an organ from one person or place to another.

transthoracic (tranz-thor-**ASS**-ik) Going through the chest wall.

transurethral (**TRANZ**-you-**REE**-thral) Procedure performed through the urethra.

transverse (tranz-**VERS**) Horizontal plane dividing the body into upper and lower portions.

transverse fracture (tranz-**VERS FRAK**-chur) A fracture perpendicular to the long axis of the bone.

tremor (**TREM**-or) Small, shaking, involuntary, repetitive movements of hands, extremities, neck, or jaw.

triceps brachii (**TRY**-sepz **BRAY**-key-eye) Muscle of the arm that has three heads or points of origin.

Trichomonas (trik-oh-**MOH**-nas) A parasite causing an STD.

trichomoniasis (**TRIK**-oh-moh-**NIE**-ah-sis) Infection with *Trichomonas vaginalis.*

tricuspid (try-**KUSS**-pid) Having three points; a tricuspid heart valve has three flaps.

trigeminal (try-**GEM**-in-al) The fifth (V) cranial nerve, which has three branches supplying the face.

triglyceride (try-**GLISS**-eh-ride) Lipid containing three fatty acids.

trimester (**TRY**-mes-ter) One-third of the length of a full-term pregnancy.

triplegia (try-**PLEE**-jee-ah) Paralysis of three limbs.

triplegic (try-**PLEE**-jik) Pertaining to or suffering from triplegia.

trochanter (troh-**KAN**-ter) One of two bony prominences near the head of the femur.

tropic (**TROH**-pik) Tropic hormones stimulate other endocrine glands to produce hormones.

tuberculosis (too-**BER**-kyu-**LOW**-sis) Infectious disease that can infect any organ or tissue.

tumor (**TOO**-mor) Any abnormal swelling.

tunica (**TYU**-nih-kah) A covering layer in the wall of a blood vessel or other tubular structure.

tunica vaginalis (**TYU**-nih-kah vaj-ih-**NAHL**-iss) The sheath of the testis and epididymis.

tympanic (tim-**PAN**-ik) Pertaining to the tympanic membrane (eardrum) or tympanic cavity.

tympanostomy (tim-pan-**OS**-toe-me) Surgically created new opening in the tympanic membrane to allow fluid to drain from the middle ear.

U

ulna (**UL**-nah) The medial and larger of the bones of the forearm.

ulnar (**UL**-nar) Pertaining to the ulna or to any of the structures (artery, vein, nerve) named after it.

ultrasonography (**UL**-trah-soh-**NOG**-rah-fee) Delineation of deep structures using sound waves.

ultraviolet (ul-trah-**VIE**-oh-let) Light rays at a higher frequency than the violet end of the spectrum.

umbilical (um-**BILL**-ih-kal) Pertaining to the umbilicus or the center of the abdomen.

umbilicus (um-**BILL**-ih-kuss) Pit in the abdomen where the umbilical cord entered the fetus.

unilateral (you-nih-**LAT**-er-al) Pertaining to one side.

urea (you-**REE**-ah) End product of nitrogen metabolism.

uremia (you-**REE**-me-ah) The complex of symptoms arising from renal failure.

ureter (you-**REE**-ter) Tube that connects a kidney to the urinary bladder.

ureteral (you-**REE**-ter-al) Pertaining to the ureter.

ureteroscope (you-**REE**-ter-oh-scope) Endoscope to view the inside of the ureter.

ureteroscopy (you-**REE**-ter-**OS**-koh-pee) To examine the ureter.

urethra (you-**REE**-thra) Canal leading from the bladder to the outside.

urethritis (you-ree-**THRI**-tis) Inflammation of the urethra.

urinalysis (yur-ih-**NAL**-ih-sis) Examination of urine to separate it into its elements and define their kind and/or quantity.

urinary (**YUR**-in-ary) Pertaining to urine.

urinate (**YUR**-in-ate) To pass urine.

urination (yur-ih-**NAY**-shun) The act of passing urine.

urine (**YUR**-in) Fluid and dissolved substances excreted by the kidney.

urological (yur-oh-**LOJ**-ih-kal) Pertaining to urology.

urologist (you-**ROL**-oh-jist) Medical specialist in disorders of the urinary system.

urology (you-**ROL**-oh-jee) Medical specialty of disorders of the urinary system.

urticaria (ur-tee-**KARE**-ee-ah) Rash of itchy wheals (hives).

uterine (**YOU**-ter-in) Pertaining to the uterus.

uterus (**YOU**-ter-us) Organ in which a fertilized egg develops into a fetus.

uvea (**YOU**-vee-ah) Middle coat of the eyeball–includes the iris, ciliary body, and choroid.

uveitis (you-vee-**EYE**-tis) Inflammation of the uvea.

uvula (**YOU**-vyu-lah) Fleshy projection of the soft palate.

V

vaccinate (**VAK**-sin-ate) To administer a vaccine.

vaccination (vak-sih-**NAY**-shun) Administration of a vaccine.

vaccine (**VAK**-seen) Preparation to generate active immunity.

vagina (vah-**JIE**-nah) Female genital canal extending from the uterus to the vulva.

vaginal (**VAJ**-ih-nal) Pertaining to the vagina.

vaginitis (vah-jih-**NIE**-tis) Inflammation of the vagina.

vaginosis (vah-jih-**NOH**-sis) A disease of the vagina.

vagus (**VAY**-gus) Tenth (X) cranial nerve; supplies many different organs throughout the body.

varicocele (**VAIR**-ih-koh-seal) Varicose veins of the spermatic cord.

varicose (**VAIR**-ih-kos) Characterized by or affected with varices.

varicosities (vair-ih-**KOS**-ih-teez) Collection of varicose veins.

varix (**VAIR**-iks) Dilated, tortuous vein. Plural *varices.*

vasectomy (vah-**SEK**-toe-me) Excision of a segment of the ductus deferens.

vasoconstriction (**VAY**-soh-con-**STRIK**-shun) Reduction in the diameter of a blood vessel.

vasodilation (**VAY**-soh-die-**LAY**-shun) Increase in the diameter of a blood vessel.

vasovasostomy (**VAY**-soh-vay-**SOS**-toe-me) Reanastomosis of the ductus deferens to restore the flow of sperm. Also called *vasectomy reversal.*

vegetative (**VEJ**-eh-tay-tiv) Functioning unconsciously, as plant life is assumed to do.

vein (**VANE**) Blood vessel carrying blood toward the heart.

vena cava (**VEE**-nah **KAY**-vah) One of the two largest veins in the body. Plural *venae cavae.*

venogram (**VEE**-noh-gram) Radiograph of veins after injection of radiopaque contrast material.

venous (**VEE**-nuss) Pertaining to a vein.

ventilation (ven-tih-**LAY**-shun) Movement of gases into and out of the lungs.

ventilator (**VEN**-tih-lay-tor) Device that breathes for the patient.

ventral (**VEN**-tral) Pertaining to the belly or situated nearer to the surface of the belly.

ventricle (**VEN**-trih-kel) Chamber of the heart (pumps blood) or brain (produces cerebrospinal fluid).

venule (**VEN**-yule or **VEEN**-yule) Small vein leading from the capillary network.

vernix caseosa (**VER**-nicks kay-see-**OH**-sah) Cheesy substance covering the skin of the fetus.

verruca (ver-**ROO**-cah) Wart caused by a virus.

vertebra (**VER**-teh-brah) One of the bones of the spinal column. Plural *vertebrae.*

vertebral (**VER**-teh-bral) Pertaining to a vertebra.

vertex (**VER**-teks) Topmost point of the vault of the skull.

vertigo (**VER**-tih-go) Sensation of spinning or whirling.

vesicle (**VES**-ih-kull) Small sac containing liquid; for example, a blister.

vestibular (ves-**TIB**-you-lar) Pertaining to the vestibule.

vestibule (**VES**-tih-byul) Space at the entrance to a canal.

vestibulectomy (ves-tib-you-**LEK**-toe-me) Surgical excision of the vulva.

villus (**VILL**-us) Thin, hairlike projection, particularly of a mucous membrane lining a cavity. Plural *villi.*

virus (**VIE**-rus) Group of infectious agents that require living cells for growth and reproduction.

viscera (**VISS**-er-ah) Internal organs, particularly in the abdomen.

visceral (**VISS**-er-al) Pertaining to the internal organs.

viscosity (viss-**KOS**-ih-tee) The resistance of a fluid to flow.

viscous (**VISS**-kus) Sticky fluid that is resistant to flow.

viscus (**VISS**-kus) Any single internal organ.

visual acuity (**VIH**-zhoo-al ah-**KYU**-ih-tee) Sharpness and clearness of vision.

vitamin (**VYE**-tah-min) Essential organic substance necessary in small amounts for normal cell function.

vitreous (**VIT**-ree-us) Vitreous humor is a gelatinous liquid in the posterior cavity of the eyeball with the appearance of glass.

vocal (**VOH**-kal) Pertaining to the voice.

void (VOYD) To evacuate urine or feces.

voluntary muscle (**VOL**-un-tare-ee **MUSS**-el) Muscle that is under the control of the will.

vomer (**VOH**-mer) Lower nasal septum.

vulva (**VUL**-vah) Female external genitalia.

vulvar (**VUL**-var) Pertaining to the vulva.

vulvodynia (vul-voh-**DIN**-ee-uh) Chronic vulvar pain.

vulvovaginal (**VUL**-voh-**VAJ**-ih-nal) Pertaining to the vulva and vagina.

vulvovaginitis (**VUL**-voh-vaj-ih-**NIE**-tis) Inflammation of the vulva and vagina.

W

warfarin (**WAR**-fuh-rin) Anticoagulant; also used as rat poison; trade name *Coumadin.*

Weber test (**VAY**-ber, **WEB**-er TEST) Test for sensorineural hearing loss.

wheal (WHEEL) Small, itchy swelling of the skin. Wheals raised by an injection do not itch. Also called *hives.*

whiplash (**WHIP**-lash) Symptoms caused by sudden, uncontrolled extension and flexion of the neck, often in an automobile accident.

white matter (WIGHT **MAT**-er) Regions of the brain and spinal cord occupied by bundles of axons.

whooping cough (**HOO**-ping KAWF) Infectious disease with spasmodic, intense cough ending on a whoop (stridor). Also called *pertussis.*

Wilms tumor (WILMZ **TOO**-mor) Cancerous kidney tumor of childhood. Also known as *nephroblastoma.*

wound (WOOND) Any injury that interrupts the continuity of skin or a mucous membrane.

xenograft (**ZEN**-oh-graft) A graft from another species. Also called *heterograft.*

yeast (YEEST) Microscopic fungus.

Z

zygoma (zye-**GO**-mah) Bone that forms the prominence of the cheek.

zygomatic (zye-go-**MAT**-ik) Pertaining to the zygoma.

zygote (**ZYE**-goat) Cell resulting from the union of the sperm and egg.

A

B

E

F

H

I

J

K

L

M

O

P

Q

R

S

T

U

V

W

X

Y

Z